Testosterone

Action, Deficiency, Substitution

Fourth Edition

Testosterone

Action, Deficiency, Substitution

Fourth Edition

Edited by

Eberhard Nieschlag
Emeritus Professor and former Director, Center for Reproductive Medicine and Andrology, University of Münster, Germany

Hermann M. Behre
Director, Center for Reproductive Medicine and Andrology of the University, Halle, Germany

Associate Editor

Susan Nieschlag
Center for Reproductive Medicine and Andrology, University of Münster, Germany

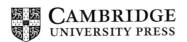

CAMBRIDGE
UNIVERSITY PRESS

CAMBRIDGE UNIVERSITY PRESS
Cambridge, New York, Melbourne, Madrid, Cape Town,
Singapore, São Paulo, Delhi, Mexico City

Cambridge University Press
The Edinburgh Building, Cambridge CB2 8RU, UK

Published in the United States of America
by Cambridge University Press, New York

www.cambridge.org
Information on this title: www.cambridge.org/9781107012905

© Cambridge University Press 2004, 2012

Third edition published 2004
Fourth edition published 2012

Printed and Bound in the United Kingdom by the MPG Books Group

A catalog record for this publication is available from the British Library

Library of Congress Cataloging-in-Publication Data

Testosterone : action, deficiency, substitution / edited by
Eberhard Nieschlag, Hermann M. Behre ; associate editor,
Susan Nieschlag. – 4th ed.
   p. ; cm.
  Includes bibliographical references and index.
  ISBN 978-1-107-01290-5 (Hardback)
  I. Nieschlag, E.   II. Behre, H. M. (Hermann M.), 1961–
III. Nieschlag, S. (Susan)
  [DNLM: 1. Testosterone–therapeutic use.   2. Testosterone–physi-
ology. WJ 875]
615.3′66–dc23

                                                        2011049739

ISBN 978-1-107-01290-5 Hardback

Contents

Contributors

Bruno Allolio
Department of Medicine I, University of Würzburg, Würzburg, Germany

Wiebke Arlt
Division of Medical Sciences, Endocrinology and Metabolism, University of Birmingham, Birmingham, UK

John Bancroft
Kinsey Institute for Research in Sex, Gender, and Reproduction, Indiana University, Bloomington, IN, USA

Shezad Basaria
Boston University School of Medicine, Section of Endocrinology, Diabetes and Nutrition, Boston Medical Center, Boston, MA, USA

Hermann M. Behre
Center for Reproductive Medicine and Andrology of the University, Halle, Germany

Shalender Bhasin
Boston University School of Medicine, Section of Endocrinology, Diabetes and Nutrition, Boston Medical Center, Boston, MA, USA

Steven Boonen
Gerontology and Geriatrics Section, Department of Clinical and Experimental Medicine, KU Leuven, Leuven, Belgium

Cesare Carani
Department of Biomedical, Metabolic and Neural Sciences, University of Modena and Reggio Emilia, Modena, Italy

Kevin S. Channer
Sheffield Hallam University and Royal Hallamshire Hospital, Sheffield, UK

Frank Claessens
Laboratory of Molecular Endocrinology, Department of Cellular and Molecular Medicine, KU Leuven, Leuven, Belgium

Susan R. Davis
Women's Health Research Program, School of Public Health and Preventive Medicine, Department of Epidemiology and Preventive Medicine, Monash University, Melbourne, Victoria, Australia

Samuel R. Denmeade
Johns Hopkins University, Department of Oncology, Baltimore, MD, USA

Flaminia Fanelli
Endocrinology Unit, S. Orsola-Malpighi Hospital, Alma Mater University of Bologna, Bologna, Italy

Evelien Gielen
Laboratory of Molecular Endocrinology, Department of Cellular and Molecular Medicine, KU Leuven, Leuven, Belgium

Wen Guo
Boston University School of Medicine, Section of Endocrinology, Diabetes and Nutrition, Boston Medical Center, Boston, MA, USA

Stefanie Hahner
Department of Medicine I, University of Würzburg, Würzburg, Germany

David J. Handelsman
ANZAC Research Institute and Department of Andrology, Concord Hospital, University of Sydney, Sydney, NSW, Australia

Olaf Hiort
Department of Pediatric Endocrinology and Diabetology, Pediatric and Adolescent Medicine, University of Lübeck, Lübeck, Germany

John T. Isaacs

The Johns Hopkins University, Oncology Center, Baltimore, MD, USA

Ravi Jasuja

Boston University School of Medicine, Section of Endocrinology, Diabetes and Nutrition, Boston Medical Center, Boston, MA, USA

T. Hugh Jones

Robert Hague Centre for Diabetes and Endocrinology, Barnsley Hospital NHS Foundation Trust, Barnsley, and Department of Human Metabolism, University of Sheffield, Sheffield, UK

Jean-Marc Kaufman

Department of Endocrinology, Ghent University Hospital, Ghent, Belgium

C. Marc Luetjens

Division of Research and Safety Assessment, Covance Laboratories GmbH, Münster, Germany

Mario Maggi

Unità di Andrologia, Dipartimento di Fisiopatologia Clinica, Florence, Italy

Robert I. McLachlan

Prince Henry's Institute of Medical Research, Clayton, Victoria, Australia

Eberhard Nieschlag

Center for Reproductive Medicine and Andrology, University of Münster, Münster, Germany

Susan Nieschlag

Center for Reproductive Medicine and Andrology, University of Münster, Münster, Germany

Liza O'Donnell

Prince Henry's Institute of Medical Research, Clayton, Victoria, Australia

Uberto Pagotto

Endocrinology Unit, S. Orsola-Malpighi Hospital, Alma Mater University of Bologna, Bologna, Italy

Valerie Anne Randall

Department of Biomedical Sciences, University of Bradford, Bradford, UK

Vincenzo Rochira

Department of Biomedical, Metabolic and Neural Sciences, University of Modena and Reggio Emilia, Modena, Italy

Laura Roli

Department of Clinical Pathology, Azienda USL of Modena, Modena, Italy

Daniele Santi

Department of Biomedical, Metabolic and Neural Sciences, University of Modena and Reggio Emilia, Modena, Italy

Wilhelm Schänzer

Institute of Biochemistry, Center for Preventive Doping Research, German Sports University Cologne, Cologne, Germany

Carlo Serra

Boston University School of Medicine, Section of Endocrinology, Diabetes and Nutrition, Boston Medical Center, Boston, MA, USA

Manuela Simoni

Department of Biomedical, Metabolic and Neural Sciences, University of Modena and Reggio Emilia, Modena, Italy

Rajan Singh

Boston University School of Medicine, Section of Endocrinology, Diabetes and Nutrition, Boston Medical Center, Boston, MA, USA

Mieke Sinnesael

Clinical and Experimental Endocrinology Section, Department of Clinical and Experimental Medicine, KU Leuven, Leuven, Belgium

Thomas W. Storer

Boston University School of Medicine, Section of Endocrinology, Diabetes and Nutrition, Boston Medical Center, Boston, MA, USA

Ronald S. Swerdloff

Department of Medicine/Endocrinology, Harbor-UCLA Medical Center, Torrance, CA, USA

Mario Thevis
Institute of Biochemistry,
Center for Preventive Doping Research,
German Sports University Cologne, Cologne,
Germany

Thomas G. Travison
Boston University School of Medicine,
Section of Endocrinology, Diabetes and
Nutrition, Boston Medical Center,
Boston, MA, USA

Guy T'Sjoen
Department of Endocrinology, Ghent University
Hospital, Ghent, Belgium

Dirk Vanderschueren
Clinical and Experimental Endocrinology Section,
Department of Clinical and Experimental Medicine,
KU Leuven, Leuven, Belgium

Alex Vermeulen
Department of Endocrinology, Ghent University
Hospital, Ghent, Belgium

Elena Vorona
University Clinics of Münster, Clinic for
Transplantation Medicine, Münster, Germany

Christina C. L. Wang
UCLA Clinical and Translational Science Institute,
Harbor-UCLA Medical Center and Los Angeles
Biomedical Research Institute, Torrance, CA, USA

Gerhard F. Weinbauer
Covance Laboratories GmbH, Münster, Germany

Ralf Werner
Division of Paediatric Endocrinology and Diabetes,
Department of Paediatrics, University of Lübeck,
Lübeck, Germany

Mikhail N. Zacharov
Boston University School of Medicine,
Section of Endocrinology, Diabetes and Nutrition,
Boston Medical Center, Boston, MA, USA

Michael Zitzmann
Center for Reproductive Medicine and Andrology,
University of Münster, Münster, Germany

Preface

Testosterone is the focal point of male reproductive health. Testosterone is responsible for all male characteristics, and testosterone deficiency results in hypogonadism which has an impact on the entire male organism. Testosterone plays an important role in male aging. Many diseases, especially mood disorders, cardiovascular diseases and the metabolic syndrome can be caused by testosterone deficiency, but can also result in hypogonadism. Consequently, testosterone is a key factor in the treatment of male disorders; benefits and risks of such treatment need to be balanced. The potent effects of testosterone also give rise to their misuse, prompting the establishment of sensitive detection systems, but also bearing adverse side-effects. Measuring testosterone in body fluids based on immunoassays was the basis for research in male pathophysiology over decades; however, methodology is currently shifting to gas or liquid chromatography tandem mass spectrometry. The hopes for a male hormonal contraceptive rest on testosterone as its major constituent. As estrogens derived from testosterone play a role in male physiology, testosterone also is of importance for general and sexual health in women. Finally, new therapeutic applications are expected from selective androgen receptor modulators (SARMs).

A tremendous amount of new knowledge has accumulated over the eight years since the third edition of this book on testosterone appeared. The 25 chapters of the current volume, written by worldwide leading experts in their field, encapsulate this progress. The book appeals to the clinician as well as to the basic scientist wishing for an authoritative overview of this central area of male reproductive health.

In order to synchronize the writing of the various chapters, the authors assembled at Castle Hohenkammer in Bavaria in October 2011 for three days, and finalized their writings during that time. This served to unify the work as a whole, and ensures that it represents the most up-to-date reference source on testosterone and its many facets. This coordinated effort of all contributors guarantees a long half-life of this book as an up-to-date reference source.

The editors wish to thank the authors of the various chapters for their excellent compliance and timely submission of manuscripts. We could not have concluded this task without the tireless reading capacity and help from Susan Nieschlag, who as a professional edited all manuscripts; nor would the volume have come to fruition without the skilful assistance of our secretaries Maria Schalkowski and Ina Nelles, who processed the manuscripts expediently. Finally, the project and the meeting would not have been possible without the generous support from Bayer Health Care (formerly Bayer Schering Pharma), the International Society of Andrology (ISA), the European Academy of Andrology (EAA), the German Association for Reproductive Health, the Clinical Research Group for Reproductive Medicine, Galen Pharma, Merck Serono, Ferring Pharmaceuticals and our home institutions, the Centers for Reproductive Medicine and Andrology at the Universities of Münster and Halle.

Chapter

1

The medical and cultural history of testosterone and the testes

Eberhard Nieschlag and Susan Nieschlag

1.1 Introduction

Although the term "hormone" was coined only as late as 1905 (Starling 1905; Henderson 2005), the biological effects of hormones were known for much longer and probably from the early beginnings of humankind. The over- or underproduction of hormones as the fundamental pathophysiological principle in endocrine disorders often produces phenotypical alterations that can be easily recognized. Similarly, elimination of hormones by removing the respective gland or replacing the hormones in a deficient organism is a basic tool of experimental endocrinology. In their exposed scrotal position, the testes are easily accessible for manipulation, be it by accidental or by inflicted trauma. The causal relationship between absence of the glands and the resulting biological effects – before or after puberty – is easily recognizable, and that is why effects of testosterone, or rather its absence, have been known from early on. Victor C. Medvei (1993), the master of the history of endocrinology, summarized this phenomenon by saying "The oldest key to the endocrine treasure trove: the testicles."

Indeed the lack of functional effects of the testes has been noted since antiquity and, in the light of modern science, these observations are often entertaining for today's reader, but at the same time they are also educational for the medical scholar. In addition, they reflect the socio-cultural environment of the time when they were observed or exploited, so that the history of testosterone and the testes is not only of medical interest, but also of interest to the general public.

The authors of this chapter are not trained historians, but the first author has a keen interest in the history of medicine, as documented early by his first medical publication dealing with the biography of Otto Deiters (1834–1863), the describer of the Deiters' cells and nucleus (Nieschlag 1965). While specializing in endocrinology and andrology, historical events surrounding testosterone were collected along with the scientific studies, culminating in the request by the Royal College of Physicians (London) in 2005 to commemorate the hundredth anniversary of the term "hormone" by a talk on "The history of testosterone," thus precipitating more systematic research on the subject. Since then a more complete but still patchy picture has been developed, which is presented here. As it is impossible to give a full history of

---

Testosterone: Action, Deficiency, Substitution, ed. Eberhard Nieschlag and Hermann M. Behre, Assoc. ed. Susan Nieschlag.
Published by Cambridge University Press. © Cambridge University Press 2012.

testosterone and the testes here, and many developments occurred simultaneously in various epochs, the material is summarized under three more or less systematic subheadings as follows (1.2–1.4). Nevertheless, this is not a systematic review, but rather a collection of historical highlights.

1.2 From antiquity to the age of enlightenment

1.2.1 Ancient Egypt

One of the oldest hypogonadal patients whose image has been preserved appears to be Vizier Hemiunu, the architect of the pyramid of Giza. The statue in his mausoleum dating from 2531 BC (Roemer-Pelizaeus Museum, Hildesheim) shows a seated man with straight hairline, no beard, bilateral gynecomastia and myxedematous lower legs. In contrast, other statues from that period show well-built athletic men; for instance the statue of Amenemhat II (1919–1884 BC) (which travelled in 2011 from the Egyptian Museum in Berlin to be exhibited in the Metropolitan Museum in New York). The plaque on Hemiunu's statue describes his achievements as an architect, but does not mention a wife or children as was customary at the time, indicating that he may have been infertile. He could have suffered from hypopituitarism including hypogonadism, perhaps caused by a prolactinoma, but Klinefelter syndrome would also be a possible diagnosis.

1.2.2 Greco-Roman period

Aristotle (384–322 BC), the universal genius and philosopher of the Hellenistic era, observed and wrote on *The Generation of Animals*, in which he described the generation of visible organs in fertilized chicken eggs. He knew the effects of castration in men as well as in animals, and described its consequences for animal husbandry. For humans, he developed the fascinating hypothesis that the right testis produces boys and the left testis girls. This could be based on case reports of men with unilateral anorchia or traumatic loss of one testis. To date no study could be traced verifying or falsifying this hypothesis, and a proposed controlled clinical study to be performed today would most likely not be met by agreement of an ethics committee. This also demonstrates how misleading case reports may be.

Aristotle also developed a theory of fertilization: semen is the activating agonist of the "soul" fertilizing the passive female soil. Like his other work, this theory had a long-lasting effect on science and was only superseded by Leeuwenhoek and Spallanzani about 2000 years later (see below).

Also dating from the Hellenistic time (about 300 BC) until the first century AD, the fertility cult around Diana/Artemis Ephesina was popular in the entire Greco-Roman world, and was especially promoted by the emperors Trajan (53–117) and Hadrian (76–138). This cult had its origin in the temple of Artemis in Ephesos, the Artemision, where the "magna mater" was worshipped. The statues, of which an excellent example can be seen in the National Archaeological Museum in Naples, are characterized by multiple oval objects fixed to the goddess's frontal thorax. Until quite recently these were interpreted as breasts, but were in reality bull or ram testes whose bearers were sacrificed to the goddess, following which their testes were fixed to the originally wooden statue, then emanating fertility and potency to the worshipper. This cult is thus based on knowledge of the powers of generation connected with the testes.

1.2.3 Castration through the times

In Greek mythology castration already occurred among the first generation of gods. Gaea, mother earth, grew out of the chaos and produced Uranos by parthenogenesis, with whom she then generated the titan Chronos. When Uranos prevented Gaea from creating children with their son Chronos, she induced Chronos to castrate his father. This episode has been depicted beautifully in a fresco by Giorgio Vasari (1511–1574) in the Palazzo Vecchio in Florence. Uranos' testes, thrown into the sea, caused the water to foam, and out of these bubbles the foam-born goddess of love Aphrodite (= Venus) was born. Quite extraordinary events in terms of reproductive physiology!

In the real world, castration has been practiced for socio-cultural purposes since antiquity. Its major purpose was to generate obedient slaves who were loyal to their masters or rulers and who, being infertile, could not create competing offspring. Set to guarding harems, they also, and in larger numbers, obtained influential administrative and political positions as in China, and formed elite troops (Mitamura 1992; Flaig 2009).

Although most likely already practiced earlier, the earliest documentation of creating eunuchs in China dates back to about 1300 BC. The Chinese eunuch system, with several thousands at a time, continued until the end of the imperial system in 1912. In the nineteenth century there were still about 2000 eunuchs at the imperial court in Beijing. The last Chinese eunuch died at the age of 93 in 1996. Only the fact that imperial eunuchs could obtain high-ranking positions and considerable power as well as wealth makes it plausible that adult men underwent this gruesome operation. It was performed by "licensed surgeons" just outside the imperial court in Beijing, by cutting off testes *and* penis. About 25% of the volunteers did not survive this bloody operation. The severed genitals were kept in a box, as shown in the film "The Last Emperor" (1987), and were eventually buried with their owner.

Eunuchs probably already existed in ancient Egypt. From the times of the legendary Queen Semiramis (about 800 BC) eunuchs were reported from Assyria, and the system developed and continued into the Islamic world in the Middle East and North Africa. Over centuries, slaves were deported from Sub-Saharan Africa to the Islamic cities and courts, and many of the slaves who survived the exhausting march through the desert were then castrated to serve as laborers, guards, administrators and even soldiers (Barth 1857). It is astonishing that these tasks could be fulfilled without the anabolic effects of testosterone.

It has been estimated that the transatlantic deportation of Africans to the Americas between 1450 and 1870 comprised about 11.5 million people, while the entire Islamic deportation of slaves from Africa between 650 and 1920 amounted to 17 million people, and several million of these African slaves were castrated. This constant drain of manpower effectively prevented economic and cultural development of Sub-Saharan Africa. In medieval times slaves were also exported from Europe to the Islamic countries. These slaves were mainly from Eastern European (Slavic) and Central Asian countries. There were well-established slave routes through Europe, and Verdun has the questionable historical fame of having been the European center for castration of slaves on their way from the East to the South at those times (Flaig 2009).

Castration has also been practiced as lawful punishment. In medieval Scandinavia, castration combined with blinding was administered for high treason, especially when the insurgent was a close relative whom one did not want to kill directly. As told in the Islendinga Saga, Sturla of the Sturlungar Clan in Iceland castrated and blinded his rebelling relative Oraekja Snorrason in 1236 (personal communication from U. Ebel, Chair of Scandinavian Sciences, University of Münster, 2007). When the Normans migrated south they also introduced this penal practice in the areas they invaded. When he established his reign in Britain after 1066, William the Conqueror abolished the Anglo-Saxon death penalty and replaced it by castration and blinding: "I also forbid that anyone shall be slain or hanged for any fault, but let his eyes be put out and let him be castrated" (Van Eickels 2004). As a further example, in Sicily in 1194 King William III was castrated and blinded after a rebellion against Emperor Henry VI. This episode forms the historical background for Klingsor's castration in the *Parsifal* epos (Tuchel 1998). The Toulouse Law Codex of 1296 described (and depicted) castration for high treason.

Throughout the centuries, castration was applied to beaten enemies by victorious soldiers for revenge and as a measure to eliminate the enemies without outright killing. When Italian troops invaded Ethiopia and lost the battle of Aduwa in 1896, supposedly 7000 Italian soldiers were castrated (Melicow 1977). As reported by Babtschenko (2007), this still happened on both sides during the Chechen War in the Caucasus in 1996.

Castration has also been reported as self-mutilation for religious reasons since ancient times in order to make a life of chastity easier. The early church father Origines (186–254) is one of the most prominent examples. In the eleventh to fourteenth centuries the sect of the Catharers, with their strongholds in Southern France, promulgated self-castration as part of a "pure" life. More recently, castration was practiced in Southern Russia among members of the Scoptic sect founded in the eighteenth century, and the medical consequences were documented (Wilson and Roehrborn 1999). The largest contemporary group of castrates are the hijras in India. They function as professional well-wishers at birth rites, and receive considerable financial rewards. Several thousand of them exist.

Castration has also been used as revenge for seduction and adultery through the centuries. For example, Paris has been reported to have castrated

Peritanos after he had seduced his famous wife Helena (Lehrs 1832). The case of the great medieval theologian and philosopher Peter Abaelard (1079–1142) has been celebrated in history and literature. As master of the cathedral school in Paris he seduced one of his disciples, Heloise (1100–1164), whose uncle then had Abaelard castrated by paid criminals. Despite the lack of testosterone, one of the most romantic love stories documented by literature developed (Podlech 1990). This type of revenge continues into most recent times as demonstrated by an incident in Germany in 2011 when the father of a 17-year-old girl castrated her 57-year-old lover (Holzhaider 2011). These people had migrated to Germany from Kazakhstan and might have brought rules of self-justice with them.

Castration before puberty maintains the high voice of boys, so that soprano and alto voices with the acoustic volume of an adult male result. Such high-pitched voices were considered desirable among music lovers, especially at times when women were not allowed to sing in church or in operatic performances. Prepubertal castrates belonged to casts of operas in the seventeenth and eighteenth centuries; in the Vatican choirs these voices could be heard until the early twentieth century. Some of these castrates became famous soloists, such as Carlo Farinelli (1705–1782) or Domenico Annibaldi (1705–1779) (Melicow 1983; Ortkemper 1993; Jenkins 1998). The middle Italian city of Nurcia was a center for the operation on young boys. However, most of the thousands of prepubertal castrates lost their virility in vain as they did not achieve the promised career as a singer, developed only mediocre voices and were ridiculed by their contemporaries. An impression of the castrato voice, although of very low recording quality, is preserved from the last Vatican castrato, Alessandro Moreschi (1858–1922), in one of the earliest gramophone recordings, made in 1902 (available today on CD). Today countertenors applying a trained falsetto sing the castrato roles in, for example, Händel operas, but their head voices probably only approximate those of seventeenth-century castrati. Another impression of the enormous artistic talents of the castrati is provided by the recordings of the mezzo-soprano Cecilia Bartoli, who trained her voice to sing the extremely demanding arias by Nicola Porpora (1686–1768), Georg Friedrich Händel (1685–1759) and others (Bartoli 2009).

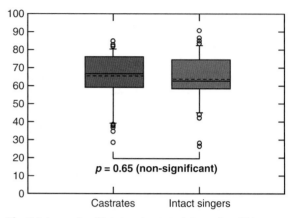

Fig. 1.1 Longevity of intact and castrated singers ($n = 50$ in each group) born between 1580 and 1859 (matched pairs of intact and castrated singers with similar birth dates were formed). (Box and whisker plots: solid line = median; broken line = mean value) (Nieschlag *et al.* 1993).

Prepubertal castration provides an involuntary experiment on the influence of testosterone on longevity. A retrospective comparison of the life expectancy of singers born between 1580 and 1859 and castrated before puberty, in order to preserve their high voices, against intact singers born at the same time, did not reveal a significant difference between the lifespan of intact and castrated singers (Fig.1.1; Nieschlag *et al.* 1993). This would imply that the presence or absence of normal male testosterone levels has no influence on life expectancy.

1.2.4 Power through polyorchidism

While removal of the testes was used to punish or to weaken the enemy or to obtain specific effects as a consequence of the lack of testosterone, a supernumerary testis was always considered a sign of extraordinary virility and sexual vigor. Several such cases have been reported anecdotally. The Venetian Condottiero Bartolomeo Colleoni (1400–1475), whose success on the battlefield as well as in the bedroom was legion (Frigeni–Careddu 1996), advertised his physical abnormality by showing three testes in his coat of arms ("*Colleoni*" in Italian means "testes"; nowadays spelled "*coglioni*").

Allegedly, in 1539 Philipp Magnanimus, Count of Hesse (1504–1567), a protagonist of the Protestant reformation, was granted permission by Martin Luther to have two wives simultaneously: Christine von Sachsen (1505–1549) and Margarethe von der Saale (1522–1566), because of his three testes.

Because at that time bigamy was forbidden upon penalty of death, Philipp got in even more trouble with the Holy Roman Emperor than his ambitions as a religious reformer had caused. A third testis had already been diagnosed in the boy, but without ultrasound, biopsy or post-mortem examination it remains unclear what these third structures in his and other famous people's scrotums were – possibly real testes or large spermatoceles? Whatever it was, this diagnosis had a tremendous impact on the person and on historical events.

1.2.5 First description of testicular morphology and sperm

The declaration of the Netherlands as an independent state during the Thirty Years War (1618–1648), and legalized at the Westphalian Peace Treaty in Münster in 1648, resulted in an enormous upswing in economy, culture and science in this country. The medical sciences also boomed, based on proper research, especially in anatomy, as shown in Rembrandt's painting "Anatomy of Dr. Tulp" (1632).

The reproductive sciences benefited from this boom as well. It was Regnier de Graaf (1641–1673) who not only described the Graafian follicle (1672), but also published a book about the anatomy of the male reproductive tract as well as the treatment of its disorders (de Graaf 1668). He produced very detailed drawings and descriptions of the male genital organs, and was the first to discover that the testes were composed of a "collection of minute vessels or tubules which confect semen; if these tubules were disentangled without being broken and tied to one another, they would far exceed 20 Dutch ells in length." Having first described this in the edible dormouse, he then went on to the human: a classical case of translational medicine. Unfortunately, de Graaf became involved in a quarrel with his contemporary, Jan Swammerdam (1637–1680), about the question of who had first described the follicles, and during that phase he died under nebulous circumstances at the young age of 32 (Setchell 1974).

A few years after Regnier de Graaf's early and mysterious death, his friend Antoni A. Leeuwenhoek (1632–1723), together with the student Johan Hamm, used his newly invented prototype of a microscope and described the "little animals of the sperm" in a letter to the Royal Society in London in 1677 (van Leeuwenhoek 1948). Considering the primitive appearance of his microscope, the details of his morphological descriptions of sperm are amazing, and it is even more amazing that 300 years later we are still quarreling about normal and abnormal sperm morphology (Kremer 1979).

But it took another century until Lazzaro Spallanzani (1729–1799), a priest and scientist in Modena, artificially inseminated frogs and dogs and demonstrated the real function of sperm (Spallanzani 1779). By using sperm that he had preserved on ice he also became the father of cryopreservation, without which modern reproductive medicine and medicine in general would be unthinkable.

He was a very systemic investigator and insisted – quite in contrast to others at the time – that experiments needed to be repeated before results could be accepted (Gaeto 1999), a principle that prevails until today.

The anatomist Franz Leydig (1821–1908) in Würzburg described the interstitial cells of the testes in 1850 (Leydig 1850). Although he did not know their function, they still carry his name (Christensen 1996). Finally in Milan, in 1865 Enrico Sertoli (1842–1910) discovered the supporting cells in the seminiferous tubules (Sertoli 1865), also carrying his name to date (Virdis 2005).

Thus, over roughly two centuries the basic morphological elements of the testes had been described, as well as the one major product of the testes, the sperm. Even the function of sperm and fertilization had been elucidated, so that the time had come to explore the basis of testicular endocrine function.

1.2.6 Proof of endocrine function

Although the endocrine function of the testes was known through their physiological and clinical effects, their nature remained completely obscure. While William Harvey (1578–1657) had discovered the role of the heart and blood circulation in 1628, in some medical schools Galen's (AD 129–216) concept of the four bodily humors prevailed well into the nineteenth century. Against this background, it is not surprising that the idea of a hormone working as a signal transduced by circulating blood took so long to be born.

John Hunter (1728–1793) is considered by some to be the father of endocrinology, as he transplanted testes in chickens. However, his outstanding achievement as a scientist notwithstanding, he transplanted testes in order to demonstrate the "vital principle" of living organs. As a surgeon in the Seven Years' War (1756–1763), he saw the need for transplantation of organs and limbs, and this is what stimulated his research. He never described his testis transplantations himself, but we learn about them through a scholar, Dr. W. Irvine, in a letter to Professor Th. Hamilton in Glasgow in 1771: "…Nay more, he has many hens just now into whose abdomen when young, he has put the testes of a cock just separated from his body and his testis has got blood vessels and nerves from the part of the abdomen or viscera to which it is applied…" Far from any endocrine thought, the goal was to demonstrate the survival of the transplant (Barker Jorgensen 1971).

Such thoughts were precipitated by Arnold Adolph Berthold's (1803–1861) experiments, which also concerned transplanting chicken testes. As published in 1849, he castrated four cocks: two received an ectopic transplantation of one testis, the two others remained untreated, and he observed "They crowed quite considerably, often fought among themselves and with other young roosters and showed a normal inclination to hens… Since the testes can no longer remain in connection with their original nerves after being transplanted to a strange place… it follows that the consensus in question must be affected through the productive relationship of the testes, that is to say, through their action on the blood, and then through the suitable ensuing action of the blood on the organism as a whole." (Berthold 1849). The paper describes only four animals and comprises only four pages – in contrast to the extensive style of the time – but was epochal. However, Berthold's rival at the University of Göttingen, Rudolf Wagner (1805–1864) was jealous, tried to repeat the experiments, but failed and declared them as rubbish (Wagner 1852). And as he became the full professor of physiology, his opinion prevailed. Berthold's personality did not allow him to fight for recognition of his findings (Simmer and Simmer 1961; Simmer 1980).

As blood circulation, the essential morphological elements of the testes and the biological and clinical effects of their endocrine action were known, history could have continued straight from here to the discovery of testosterone, but due to these interpersonal quarrels and other unhappy events, further developments took an oblique route.

1.3 Detours on the way to modern medicine

1.3.1 Organotherapy

As it was known that removal of the testes caused the clinically evidenced symptoms of hypogonadism, including impotence, prescribing ingestion of testes to remedy the symptoms was a medical reflex inherent in organotherapy, practiced since antiquity. Thus the Roman Gaius Plinius Secundus (AD 23–79) recommended the consumption of animal testes to treat symptoms of testosterone deficiency. Slightly more refined was the prescription of testicular extracts for the same purpose in Arabic medicine, for example by Mensue the Elder (777–837) in Baghdad. Also, in China, raw and desiccated testes were prescribed, documented at least in the twelfth century by Hsue Shu-Wei. Around the same time, Albertus Magnus (1193–1280) in Cologne, better known as a philosopher, recommended powdered hog testes, but refined his recipe by offering the powder in wine (Medvei 1993).

Since early documentation, these potions continued to be prescribed and consumed up into the twentieth century. In the 1920s Testifortan® became a financially successful drug for treatment of impotence (Hirschfeld 1927). Its main constituent was testis extracts and yohimbine, and after the war 17α-methyltestosterone was added without changing the name. Another famous preparation from the 1920s and still marketed today is Okasa® which, among other components, also contains *testis sicca* and thereby small amounts of testosterone, as we could determine in the 1970s (unpublished data). However, as the testes synthesize testosterone but do not store it, the daily production of an adult man of about 6–8 mg is contained in roughly 1 kg of (bull) testes, and even if this amount of testosterone were to be consumed, the testosterone taken orally would be inactivated by the first-pass effect in the liver (Nieschlag *et al.* 1977). Therefore, all testicular organ therapy administered orally can only be considered as a placebo medication, which, however, may not be without its own effects (Bundesärztekammer 2011). Ultimately this type of testicular organotherapy was terminated by the advent of phosphodiesterase inhibitors.

Organotherapy literally exploded at the end of the nineteenth century when Charles E. Brown-Séquard (1847–1894), who until then was a well-reputed scientist and member of several scientific academies, published the results of his famous self-experimentation in the Lancet (Brown-Séquard 1889). He gave himself 1-ml injections of a mixture of one part testicular vein blood, one part semen and one part juice extracted from dog or guinea-pig testes daily, and after 20 days made astonishing observations on himself: "A radical change took place in me... I had regained at least all the strength I possessed a good many years ago. I was able to make experiments for several hours. After dinner I was able to write a paper on a difficult subject. My limbs, tested with a dynamometer, gained 6 to 7 kg in strength. The jet of urine and the power of defecation became stronger."

Certainly all these were placebo effects, but the world had obviously waited for such quackery, because in no time the "extracts of animal organs by the Brown-Séquard method" were sold all over the (western) world, and factories sprung forth in Europe as well as in America, for example next to Central Park in New York (Borell 1976). There must have been a real craze for these products, and physicians concerned about the image of the young field of endocrinology started worrying. The famous neurosurgeon Harvey W. Cushing (1869–1939), and the president of the Association of the Study of Internal Secretions, E. H. Rynearson even talked about "endocriminology" in the context of this organotherapy (Hamblen 1950). This assessment of the medical scene at the time is also reflected in contemporary cartoons and comic songs from the early twentieth century. Eventually, this type of quackery stimulated science and decent pharmaceutical companies to search for real hormones.

1.3.2 Testis transplantations

However, before science succeeded in that attempt there was another sad approach to treat hypogonadism and bring about rejuvenation and treatment for all sorts of disorders: the transplantation of testes. G. Frank Lydston (1858–1923) in Chicago was one of the first to perform human testicular transplantation from donors after experimentation in animals (Lydston 1915; Schultheiss and Engel 2003). V. D. Lespinase (1913) published his experience with transplanting human testes to patients for rejuvenation, and Leo Stanley (1920) reported 20 cases of transplantation of testes from executed prisoners to other inmates who reported signs of revitalization.

Later on he turned to animals as sources for his testicular grafts and reported satisfaction on the part of the patients including 13 physicians (Stanley 1923).

These surgeons had followers in many parts of the world, for example even in Iceland where, in 1929, the surgeon Jonas Sveinsson transplanted testis slices from a poor farmer in need of money to a rich Norwegian businessman who, he then claimed, satisfied his 23-year-old wife so that he even had three children with her (Sveinsson 1969). In the Soviet Union, experimentation with human testicular transplantation continued at least into the 1980s (Shumankov and Gotsiridze 1978). The only testicular transplantation resulting in fertility of the recipient was performed by Sherman J. Silber (Silber and Rodriguez-Rigau 1980) between twin brothers.

In Vienna, Eugen Steinach (1861–1944) performed vasoligation for rejuvenation (Steinach 1920), and one of his followers, Serge Voronoff (1866–1951) turned to xenotransplantation and used monkey testes to be transplanted for rejuvenation (Voronoff 1920; 1923). He first offered his surgery in Paris, but after some scandals continued his questionable operations in Algiers, where he was obviously visited by patients from all over the world. Voronoff had followers in many countries who xenotransplanted animal testes or pieces thereof to patients in need of rejuvenation, also in the USA, where this type of treatment caused great interest among the laymen and the media (e.g. Gayton 1922). As unrest among the medical profession continued to grow, in 1927 the Royal Society of Medicine (London) sent an international committee to Voronoff in Algiers, which concluded that Voronoff's claims were all poppycock (Parkes 1965). This, and the success of upcoming steroid biochemistry finally terminated this malpractice.

However, in a transformed fashion it continued as cellular therapy by injecting suspensions of fresh cells of sheep embryos including testis cells, also for rejuvenation and revitalization, well into the second half of the twentieth century (Niehans 1952; 1960).

Meanwhile, science has progressed and, in the age of cell biology, testicular transplantation continues with the aim of inducing fertility, but now uses isolated germ cells (Brinster and Zimmermann 1994; Schlatt et al. 2002), and fertility has indeed been restored by this method in gamma-irradiated cocks (Trefil et al. 2006). Whether this may become a method to treat male infertility, for example in

Klinefelter patients (Wistuba 2010), remains to be seen, but at least it is pursued on a rational scientific basis – as far as our present knowledge goes.

1.4 Twentieth-century science and medicine

1.4.1 The rise of steroid biochemistry

Berthold's unique discovery was superseded by organotherapy, but it was not permanently forgotten: Moritz Nussbaum (1850–1915), professor of anatomy in Bonn, repeated Berthold's experiments and confirmed the results in frogs (Nussbaum 1909), as did Eugen Steinach in rats (Steinach 1910). Finally, A. Pézard confirmed Berthold's original results in cocks (Pézard 1911), and the search for the active androgenic substance in the testes began.

From observation of the cock's comb growing under the influence of transplanted testes, Moore *et al.* (1929) established the standardized capon comb's test, measuring androgenic activity in square centimeters of comb surface. This first bioassay facilitated determination of androgenic activity in body products as well as in chemical solutions. S. Loewe and H. E. Voss (1930) used the biological effects of androgens on the accessory sex organs and developed the "cytological regeneration test," which was based on regrowth of the seminal vesicle epithelium under androgenic substances (Loewe–Voss test). The then still hypothetical male hormone was called "androkinin."

Simultaneously, steroid biochemistry emerged and the great breakthroughs were the discovery of the ring structure of steroids and bile acids at the National Institute of Medical Research in London (Rosenheim and King 1932) and at the Bavarian Academy of Sciences in Munich (Wieland and Dane 1932). A heated discussion started about whether there were three or four rings in the steroid structure and, if four rings, whether the fourth had five or six carbon atoms. Under the sponsorship of the Health Organization of the League of Nations (the predecessor of the World Health Organization, WHO), famous chemists including Edmund A. Doisy, Adolf Butenandt and Guy Marrian assembled at University College London and reached the consensus that steroids had four rings, and the fourth ring had five carbon atoms (Butenandt 1980). Shortly before, these eminent researchers, including Ernest Laqueur, had isolated pregnanediol and estrone from pregnant mare urine provided by

various drug companies cooperating with scientists in order to replace the miscredited organotherapy and to bring proper hormone substitution to patients (see Table 1.1) (Simmer 1982).

1.4.2 Testosterone is born

In 1931 Butenandt isolated the androgenic steroid, androsterone (androstan-3α-ol-17-one), from urine, for which he required 15 000 liters provided by young

Table 1.1 Early isolation of reproductive steroids (for references see the text)

1928 Pregnanediol	Guy Frederick Marrian Dept. Physiology and Biochemistry, University College London	Crystalline material from pregnant mare urine provided by BRITISH DRUG HOUSES
1929 Estrone	Edward Albert Doisy Dept. Biological Chemistry, St. Louis	
1929 Estrone	Adolf Butenandt Chemistry Laboratory, University of Gottingen	Raw extracts and crystals from pregnant mare urine provided by SCHERING
1929 Estrone	Ernst Laqueur Pharmacotherapeutic Laboratory, Amsterdam	Benzene extracts from pregnant mare urine provided by ORGANON
1931 Androsterone	Adolf Butenandt Chemistry Laboratory, University of Gottingen	Extracted from 15 000 liters of urine provided by the Prussian Police Academy in Berlin and processed by SCHERING
1935 Testosterone	Ernst Laqueur Pharmacotherapeutic Laboratory, Amsterdam	Isolated from bull testes Provided by ORGANON

policemen from Berlin, which was then processed by Schering to obtain 15 mg of this first androgen (Butenandt 1931). In 1935 Ernst Laqueur (1866–1947) and his group in Amsterdam extracted and isolated 10 mg testosterone (androsten-17α-ol-3-one) from 100 kg of bull testes, which they found more active than androsterone, and named it "testosterone" (David *et al.* 1935). In the same year Butenandt and Hanisch (1935) as well as Ruzicka and Wettstein (1935) published the chemical synthesis of testosterone. This marked the beginning of modern clinical pharmacology and endocrinology of testosterone, and male reproductive physiology.

Soon after its synthesis testosterone became clinically available, first in the form of pellets (Deansley and Parkes 1937; Parkes 1965) and then as injectable esters, that is, testosterone propionate, with a short half-life. And, from the mid-1950s on, the longer-acting testosterone enanthate (Junkmann 1952; 1957) appeared, which remained the major testosterone preparation for half a century. Also in 1935, 17α-methyltestosterone was synthesized and its oral effectiveness was demonstrated (Ruzicka *et al.* 1935). However, due to its 17α-structure it turned out to be liver toxic (Werner *et al.*1950; Nieschlag 1981), a fact which gave testosterone in general a bad name among physicians, as this toxicity was also suspected for testosterone without reason; eventually in the 1980s this androgen became obsolete for clinical use in Europe. In the late 1970s the orally effective testosterone undecanoate, absorbed from the gut via the lymph to avoid the first-pass effect in the liver, was added to the spectrum of testosterone preparations used clinically (Coert *et al.* 1975; Nieschlag *et al.* 1975) (see also Chapter 15).

In the 1950s and 1960s the pharmaceutical industry became more interested in new androgens than in testosterone itself, and concentrated its androgen research on the chemical modification of steroid molecules in order to disentangle the various effects of testosterone and produce predominantly erythropoietic or anabolic steroids (Kopera 1985). In 1956 contemporary textbooks on androgens had already described 256 androgenic steroids (Dorfman and Shipley 1956), and by 1976 the number had increased to more than 1000 (Kochakian 1976).

However, it proved impossible to produce androgens with only *one* effect out of the spectrum of testosterone activities; at best, one of these effects could be emphasized, but the other effects remained. The steroid with pure anabolic effects on muscles or bones to treat cachexia, osteoporosis or small stature, or pure erythropoietic effect for the treatment of anemia without androgenization could not be found. Nevertheless, anabolic and similar steroids were clinically used, but disappeared again in the wake of evidence-based medicine (Kopera 1985). However, they continued their existence for illegal use and abuse for doping in sports and bodybuilding (see Chapters 24 and 25). Regrettably, at that time the pharmaceutical industry neglected the chance to develop testosterone preparations better suited for the substitution of hypogonadal patients than the existing testosterone esters. It remains to be seen whether the current search for selective androgen receptor modulators (SARMs) will take a more rewarding course than did anabolic steroids (see Chapter 21).

From the 1970s the newly developed testosterone immunoassays (see Chapter 4) made serial testosterone determinations in blood possible and, when applied to pharmacokinetic studies, it turned out that all available testosterone preparations resulted in unphysiologically high or low serum levels which were undesirable in substitution therapy. Clinicians assembled at a workshop on androgen therapy sponsored by the WHO, and US National Institutes of health (NIH) and Food and Drug Administration (FDA) in 1990 came to the conclusion: "The consensus view was that the major goal of therapy is to replace testosterone levels at as close to physiologic concentrations as is possible" (World Health Organization 1992), and demanded that new testosterone preparations better suited for clinical use be manufactured.

In the mid-1990s, transdermal testosterone patches applied to the scrotal skin became the first transdermal testosterone preparation in clinical use (Bals-Pratsch *et al.* 1986). They had been invented by Virgil Place at ALZA in Palo Alto, a company specializing in new forms of delivery of known drugs (Atkinson *et al.* 1998). However, although clinical results with this preparation were excellent, and for the first time physiological serum levels could be achieved under testosterone substitution, physicians were reluctant to prescribe a medication to be applied to the scrotum and preferred a subsequently developed non-scrotal system (Meikle *et al.* 1992). This, however, caused unpleasant skin reactions as it required an enhancer to drive testosterone through the skin. For this reason the advent of the first transdermal testosterone gel was welcome. This gel became available in 2000 for the treatment of male hypogonadism, first in the USA and later also in other countries (Wang *et al.* 2000). Finally in 2004 the intramuscular testosterone undecanoate preparation entered the market and soon achieved great popularity as a real testosterone depot preparation (see Chapter 15).

Testosterone undecanoate had originally been used in oral capsules (see above), but had been turned into an injectable preparation by Chinese investigators using tea seed oil as a vehicle (Wang *et al.* 1991). When the author came across it at an exhibition accompanying an andrology symposium in Beijing in 1993, samples were brought to Germany, injected into monkeys and showed a surprisingly long half-life. A long half-life was confirmed in volunteering hypogonadal men who all showed serum levels in the normal range (Behre *et al.* 1999). When finally a company was interested in this fascinating preparation, it was "Europeanized" by using castor oil as vehicle and was developed as Nebido® for clinical use (Nieschlag 2006).

1.4.3 Early descriptions of syndromes of hypogonadism

It may not have been a coincidence, but rather a sign of heightened interest in the hypogonadism clinics, that at the same time as testosterone became available for clinical use (i.e. when rational treatment became possible), the major syndromes of primary and secondary hypogonadism were first described: that is, the Klinefelter syndrome (Klinefelter *et al.* 1942) and the Kallmann syndrome (Kallmann *et al.* 1944). Pasqualini and Bur (1950) described the first case of the fertile-eunuch syndrome, characterized by all symptoms of lack of testosterone, but active spermatogenesis; Del Castillo *et al.* (1947) published the first five cases suffering from Sertoli-cell-only syndrome. Also at that time the symptoms of the aging male were first described systematically, but unfortunately wrongly termed as "male climacteric" (Werner 1945), starting a controversial discussion that continues until today (see Chapter 16). E. C. Reifenstein (1947) first described a syndrome with partial androgen insensitivity (PAIS) that carries his name to date, and J. M. Morris (1953) published the first cases of complete androgen insensitivity (CAIS) as "testicular feminization in male pseudo-hermaphroditism" – of course without

knowing anything about the androgen receptor or androgen receptor mutations (see Chapter 3).

At the same time, Huggins also posted his warning about testosterone influencing prostate carcinoma (Huggins and Hodges 1941), which led to castration (euphemistically called "orchidectomy") as the major treatment of prostate carcinoma, and prevailed until quite recently when androgen deprivation therapy (ADT) by gonadotropin-releasing hormone (GnRH) analogs or antiandrogens was introduced instead or in addition to castration (maximal androgen blockade = MAB). Huggins' statement, "Cancer of the prostate is activated by androgen injections" induced a general fear of testosterone, especially among urologists, that prevented testosterone treatment in many patients who might have needed it. Only recently it became clear that neither endogenous serum testosterone levels (Endogenous Hormones and Prostate Cancer Collaborative Group 2008) nor testosterone treatment (Raynaud 2006) have an impact on prostate carcinogenesis, and now testosterone treatment under careful supervision is even considered for patients after radical prostatectomy suffering from testosterone deficiency (Morgenthaler 2007). However, orchidectomy will continue in the foreseeable future to remain the major option for treatment of prostate carcinoma (Damber and Aus 2008). Thus, castration continues to be recommended for therapeutic purposes as it had already been promulgated during Greco-Roman times and the Middle Ages for the treatment of leprosy, epilepsy, gout, priapism, excessive masturbation and insanity (Melicow 1977), reflecting the knowledge or rather the lack of knowledge of the respective period. There remains the hope that research will eventually result in more humane and patient-friendly methods of treatment as we have witnessed the transition from castration to ADT for treating sexual offenders (Gooren 2011).

1.5 Key messages

- The importance of the testes for normal male function and reproduction has been known since antiquity.
- Correspondingly, castration has also been practiced since antiquity to produce obedient slaves, harem custodians, civil servants and soldiers, as well as for punishment and revenge.

- Prepubertal castration was exercised between the sixteenth and nineteenth century to obtain voluminous high-pitched voices for singing in operas and churches.
- Following the description of the morphological structure of the testes, their endocrine function was established by A. A. Berthold in 1849.
- Organotherapy with testes extracts and (xeno-) transplantation of testes were big business in the first half of the twentieth century, based on placebo effects.

- In 1935 testosterone was chemically identified and synthesized and since then has been available for clinical use – and also for abuse.
- In order to avoid inactivation in the liver and to prolong action, testosterone has been esterified, and the clinically most widely used esters became testosterone propionate, enanthate, cypionate and finally undecanoate.
- Transdermal testosterone patches and gels represent the most recent developments in testosterone preparations.

1.6   References

Atkinson LE, Chang YL, Snyder PJ (1998) Long-term experience with testosterone replacement through scrotal skin. In: Nieschlag E, Behre HM (eds) *Testosterone: Action, Deficiency, Substitution*, 2nd edn. Springer, Heidelberg, pp 365–388

Babtschenko A (2007) *Die Farbe des Krieges*. Rowohlt, Hamburg

Bals-Pratsch M, Knuth UA, Yoon YD, Nieschlag E (1986) Transdermal testosterone substitution therapy for male hypogonadism. *Lancet* ii:943–946

Barker Jorgensen CB (1971) John Hunter, A. A. Berthold and the origins of endocrinology. *Acta Hist Scient Natural Medicinal* 24:1–54

Barth H (1857) *Reisen und Entdeckungen in Nord-und Central-Afrika in den Jahren 1849 bis 1855*. Justus Perthes, Gotha

Bartoli C (2009) *Sacrificium: the School for Castratos*, CD and booklet. Decca Music Group, London

Behre HM, Abshagen K, Oettel M, Hubler D, Nieschlag E (1999) Intramuscular injection of testosterone undecanoate for the treatment of male hypogonadism: phase I studies. *Europ J Endocrinol* 140:414–419

Berthold AA (1849) Über die Transplantation der Hoden. *Arch Anat Physiol Wiss Med*:42–46

Borell M (1976) Brown-Séquard's organotherapy and its appearance in America at the end of the nineteenth century. *Bull Hist Med* 50:309–320

Brinster RL, Zimmermann JW (1994) Spermatogenesis following male germ-cell transplantation. *Proc Natl Acad Sci USA* 91:1289–1302

Brown-Séquard E (1889) The effects produced on man by subcutaneous injections of a liquid obtained from the testicles of animals. *Lancet* 20:105–107

Bundesärztekammer (ed) (2011) *Placebo in der Medizin*. Deutscher Ärzteverlag, Cologne

Butenandt A (1931) Über die chemische Untersuchung des Sexualhormons. *Z Angew Chem* 44:905–908

Butenandt A (1980) Die Entdeckungsgeschichte des Oestrons. *Endokrinol Inform* 4:160–163

Butenandt A, Hanisch G (1935) Über Testosteron. Umwandlung des Dehydroandrosterons in Androstendiol und Testosteron; ein Weg zur Darstellung des Testosterons aus Cholesterin. *Hoppe-Seyler's Z Physiol Chem* 237:89–98

Christensen AK (1996) A history of studies on testicular Leydig cells: the first century. In: Payne AH, Hardy M, Russel LD (eds) *The Leydig Cell*. Cache River Press, Vienna, IL

Coert A, Geelen J, de Visser J, van der Vies J (1975) The pharmacology and metabolism of testosterone undecanoate (TU), a new orally active androgen. *Acta Endocrinol* 79:789–800

Damber JE, Aus G (2008) Prostate cancer. *Lancet* 371: 1710–1721

David K, Dingemanse E, Freud J, Laquer E (1935) Über krystallinisches männliches Hormon aus Hoden (Testosteron), wirksamer als aus Harn oder aus Cholesterin bereitetes Androsteron. *Hoppe-Seyler's Z Physiol Chem* 233:281–282

Deansley R, Parkes AS (1937) Factors influencing effectiveness of administered hormones. *Proc R Soc London* 124:279–298

de Graaf R (1668) *Virorum Organis Generationi Inservientibus, de Clysteribus et de Usa Siphonis in Anatomia*. Ex officina Hackiana, Leyden and Rotterdam

Del Castillo EB, Trabucco A, de la Balze FA (1947) Syndrome produced by absence of the germinal epithelium without impairment of the Sertoli or Leydig cells. *J Clin Endocrinol Metab* 7:493–502

Dorfman RL, Shipley RA (1956) *Androgens: Biochemistry, Physiology and Clinical Significance*. John Wiley & Sons,Inc., New York

Endogenous Hormones and Prostate Cancer Collaborative Group (2008) Endogenous sex hormones and prostate cancer: a collaborative analysis of 18 prospective studies. *J Ntl Cancer Inst* 100:170–183

Flaig E (2009) *Weltgeschichte der Sklaverei.* Verlag CH Beck, Munich

Frigeni-Careddu M (1996) *Il Condottiero: Vita, Avventure e Bataglie di Bartolomeo Colleoni.* Sperling and Kupfer Editori, Milan

Gaeto, M (1999) The bicentennial of a forgotten giant: Lazzaro Spallanzani (1729–1799). *Internatl Microbiol* **2**:273–274

Gayton B (1922) *The Gland Stealers.* Lippincott, Philadelphia

Gooren LJ (2011) Ethical and medical considerations of androgen deprivation treatment of male sex offenders. *J Clin Endocrinol Metab* **96**:3628–3637

Hamblen EC (1950) Endocrinology or "endocriminology." Some abuses of endocrine therapy. *Southern Med J* **43**:506–509

Henderson J (2005) Ernest Starling and "hormones": an historical commentary. *J Endocrinol* **184**:5–10

Hirschfeld M (1927) *Die Behandlung der Impotenz in der ärztlichen Praxis.* Institut für Sexualwissenschaft, Berlin

Holzhaider H (2011) Verbotene Liebe. *Süddeutsche Zeitung* March 31, p 10

Huggins C, Hodges CV (1941) Studies on prostatic cancer: I. The effect of castration, of estrogen and of androgen injection on serum phosphatases in metastatic carcinoma of the prostate. *Cancer Res* 293–297

Jenkins JS (1998) The voice of the castrato. *Lancet* **351**:1877–1881

Junkmann K (1952) Über protrahiert wirksame Androgene. *Arch Path Pharmacol* **215**:85–92

Junkmann K (1957) Long-acting steroids in reproduction. *Rec Progr Horm Res* **13**:389–419

Kallmann FJ, Schoenfeld WA, Barrera SE (1944) The genetic aspects of primary eunuchoidism. *Am J Ment Def* **158**:203–236

Klinefelter HF, Reifenstein EC, Albright F (1942) Syndrome characterized by gynecomastia, aspermatogenesis, without A-Leydigism, and increased excretion of follicle-stimulating hormone. *J Clin Endocrinol* **2**:615–627

Kochakian CD (ed) (1976) *Anabolic-Androgenic Steroids.* Springer, Heidelberg

Kopera H (1985) The history of anabolic steroids and a review of clinical experience with anabolic steroids. *Acta Endocrinol Suppl* **271**:11–18

Kremer J (1979) The significance of Antoni van Leeuwenhoek for the early development of andrology. *Andrologia* **II**:243–249

Lehrs (1832) Über die Darstellungen der Helena in der Sage und den Schriftwerken der Griechen. In: *Historische und literarische Abhandlungen der Königlichen Deutschen Gesellschaft zu Königsberg*, Second Collection. Bornträger, Königsberg, p 108

Lespinase VD (1913) Transplantation of the testicle. *J Am Med Assoc* **18**:251–253

Leydig F (1850) Zur Anatomie der männlichen Geschlechtsorgane und Analdrüsen der Säugethiere. *Ztschr Wiss Zool* **2**:1–57

Loewe S, Voss HE (1930) Der Stand der Erfassung des männlichen Sexualhormons (Androkinins). *Klin Wschr* **9**:481–487

Lydston GF (1915) Sex gland implantation. *NY Med J* **51**:601–608

Medvei VC (1993) *The History of Clinical Endocrinology.* Parthenon Publishing Group, New York

Meikle AW, Mazer NA, Moellmer JF, Stringham JD, Tolman KG, Sanders SW, Odell WD (1992) Enhanced transdermal delivery of testosterone across nonscrotal skin produces physiological concentrations of testosterone and its metabolites in hypogonadal men. *J Clin Endocrinol Metab* **74**:623–628

Melicow MM (1977) Castration down the ages. *NY State J Med*:804–808

Melicow MM (1983) Castrati singers and the lost "cords". *Bull NY Acad Med* **59**:744–764

Mitamura T (1992) *Chinese Eunuchs: The Structure of Intimate Politics.* Charles E. Tuttle, Rutland, VT

Moore CR, Gallagher TF, Koch FC (1929) The effects of extracts of testis in correcting the castrated condition in the fowl and in the mammal. *Endocrinology* **13**:367–374

Morgenthaler A (2007) Testosterone deficiency and prostate cancer: emerging recognition of an important and troubling relationship. *Eur Urol* **52**:623–625

Morris JM (1953) The syndrome of testicular feminization in male pseudohermaphrodites. *Am J Obstet Gynecol* **65**:1192–1211

Niehans P (1952) 20 years of cellular therapy. *Med Klin* **47**:2–16

Niehans P (1960) *Introduction to Cellular Therapy.* Pageant, New York

Nieschlag E (1965) Otto Deiters (1834–1863). *Med Welt* **23**:222–226

Nieschlag E (1981) Ist die Anwendung von Methyltestosteron obsolet? *Dtsch Med Wschr* **106**:1123–1125

Nieschlag E (2006) Testosterone treatment comes of age: new options for hypogonadal men. *Clin Endocrinol* **65**:275–281

Nieschlag E, Mauss J, Coert A, Kicovic P (1975) Plasma androgen levels in men after oral administration of testosterone or testosterone undecanoate. *Acta Endocrinol* **79**:366–374

Nieschlag E, Cüppers EJ, Wickings EJ (1977) Influence of sex, testicular development and liver function on the bioavailability of oral testosterone. *Europ J Clin Invest* **7**:145–147

Nieschlag E, Nieschlag S, Behre HM (1993) Life expectancy and testosterone. *Nature* **366**:215

Nussbaum M (1909) Hoden und Brunstorgane des braunen Landfrosches (Rana fusca). *Pflügers Arch Eur J Physiol* **126**:519–577

Ortkemper H (1993) *Engel wider Willen: die Welt der Kastraten.* Henschel-Verlag, Berlin

Parkes AS (1965) The rise of reproductive endocrinology, 1926–1940. *J Endocrinol* 34:XX–XXXii

Pasqualini RQ, Bur GE (1950) Sindrome hipoandrogenico con gametogenesis conservada. Classificacion de la insuficiencia testicular. *Rev Asoc Med Argent* 64:6–10

Pézard A (1911) Sur la détermination des caractères sexuels secondaires chez les gallinacés. *Cpt Rend Scienc* 153:1027

Podlech A (1990) *Abaelard und Heloise. Die Theologie der Liebe.* Piper, Munich

Raynaud JP (2006) Prostate cancer risk in testosterone-treated men. *J Steroid Biochem Mol Biol* 102:261–266

Reifenstein EC Jr (1947) Hereditary familial hypogonadism. *Proc Am Fed Clin Res* 3:86

Rosenheim SO, King H (1932) The ring-system of steroids and bile acids. *Nature* 130:315

Ruzicka L, Wettstein A (1935) Synthetische Darstellung des Testishormons, Testosteron (Androsten 3-on-17-ol). *Helv Chim Acta* 18:1264–1275

Ruzicka L, Goldberg MW, Rosenberg HR (1935) Herstellung des 17alpha-Methyl-testosterons und anderer Androsten – und Androstanderivate. Zusammenhänge zwischen chemischer Konstitution und männlicher Hormonwirkung. *Helv Chim Acta* 18:1487–1498

Schlatt S, Foppiani L, Rolf C, Weinbauer GF, Nieschlag E (2002) Germ cell transplantation into x-irradiated monkey testes. *Hum Reprod* 17:55–62

Schultheiss D, Engel RM (2003) G. Frank Lydston (1858–1923) revisited: therapy by testicular implantation in the early twentieth century. *World J Urol* 21:356–363

Sertoli E (1865) Dell' esistenza di particolori cellule ramificate nei canaliculi seminiferi del testicolo umano. *Il Morgani* 7:31–40

Setchell BP (1974) The contributions of Reinier de Graaf to reproductive biology. *Europ J Obstet Gynec Reprod Biol* 4:1–13

Shumankov VI, Gotsiridze OA (1978) Chirurgische Technik der Hodentransplantation. *Vestn Khir Im II Grek* 121:77–81

Silber SJ, Rodriguez-Rigau LJ (1980) Pregnancy after testicular transplant: importance of treating the couple. *Fertil Steril* 33:454–455

Simmer HH (1980) Arnold Adolph Berthold (1803–1861) – Vorläufer oder Begründer der experimentellen Endokrinologie? *Endokrinol Inform* 3:101–111

Simmer H (1982) Biosynthese der Steroidhormone. *Endokrinol Inform* 2:80–92

Simmer H, Simmer I (1961) Arnold Adolph Berthold (1803–1861). Zur Erinnerung an den hundertsten Todestag des Begründers der experimentellen Endokrinologie. *Dtsch Med Wschr* 86:2186–2192

Spallanzani L (1779) Fecundazione artefiziale. In: *Prodomo Della Nuova Encyclopedia Italiana*, Siena

Stanley LL (1920) Experiences in testicle transplantation. *Cal State J Med* 18:251–253

Stanley LL (1923) An analysis of one thousand testicular substance implantations. *Endocrinol* 7:787–794

Starling EH (1905) The chemical correlation of the functions of the body I. *Lancet* 2:339–341

Steinach E (1910) Geschlechtstrieb und echt sekundäre Geschlechtsmerkmale als Folge der innersekretorischen Funktion der Keimdrüsen. *Zbl Physiol* 24:551–566

Steinach E (1920) *Verjüngung durch experimentelle Neubelebung der alternden Pubertätsdrüse.* Springer-Verlag, Berlin

Sveinsson H (1969) *Lifid er dásamlegt (autobiography).* Helgafell, Iceland

The Last Emperor (1987) Film directed by Bernardo Bertolucci. Columbia Pictures

Trefil P, Micakova A, Mucksova J, Hejnar J, Poplstein M, Bakst MR, Kalina J, Brillard J-P (2006) Restoration of spermatogenesis and male fertility by transplantation of dispersed testicular cells in the chicken. *Biol Reprod* 75:575–581

Tuchel S (1998) *Kastration im Mittelalter.* Droste-Verlag, Düsseldorf

Van Eickels K (2004) Gendered violence: castration and blinding as punishment for treason in Normandy and Anglo-Norman England. *Gender & History* 16:588–602

van Leeuwenhoek A (1948) *Collected Letters of Antoni van Leeuwenhoek* Vol III. Swets and Zeitlinger, Amsterdam

Virdis R (2005) Historical milestones in endocrinology. *J Endocrinol Invest* 28:944–948

Voronoff S (1920) *Testicular Grafting from Ape to Man.* Brentanos Ltd, London

Voronoff S (1923) *Innesti Testicolori.* Quintieri Editore, Milan

Wagner R (1852) Mitteilung einer einfachen Methode zu Versuchen über die Veränderungen thierischer Gewebe in morphologischer und chemischer Beziehung. *Nachr Königl Ges Wiss Göttingen*:97–109

Wang C, Berman N, Longstreth JA, Chuapoco B, Hull L, Steiner B, Faulkner S, Dudley RE, Swerdloff RS (2000) Pharmacokinetics of transdermal testosterone gel in hypogonadal men: application of gel at one site versus four sites: a general clinical research center study. *J Clin Endocrinol Metab* 85:964–969

Wang L, Shi DC, Lu SY, Fang RY (1991) The therapeutic effect of domestically produced testosterone undecanoate in Klinefelter syndrome. *New Drug Mark* **8**:28–32

Werner AA (1945) The male climacteric. *J Am Med Assoc* **127**:705–710

Werner SC, Hamger FM, Kritzler RA (1950) Jaundice during methyltestosterone therapy. *Am J Med* **8**:325–331

Wieland HO, Dane E (1932) Untersuchungen über die Konstitution der Gallensäuren. *Hoppe-Syler's Ztschr Physiol Chem* **210**:268–281

Wilson JD, Roehrborn C (1999) Long-term consequences of castration in men: lessons from the Skoptzy and the eunuchs of the Chinese and Ottoman courts. *J Clin Endocrinol Metab* **84**:4324–4331

Wistuba J (2010) Animal models for Klinefelter's syndrome and their relevance for the clinic. *Mol Hum Reprod* **16**:375–385

World Health Organization, Nieschlag E, Wang C, Handelsman DJ, Swerdloff RS, Wu F, Einer-Jensen N, Waites G (1992) *Guidelines for the Use of Androgens.* WHO, Geneva

Chapter

2

Testosterone: biosynthesis, transport, metabolism and (non-genomic) actions

C. Marc Luetjens and Gerhard F. Weinbauer

2.1 Introduction

Androgens are essential for the development and function of male reproductive organs, for example maturation of secondary sexual characteristics, libido and stimulation of spermatogenesis. Beyond that, androgens influence many somatic organ functions, which are covered in various chapters in this volume. In fact, a large number of organs express androgen receptors (Dankbar *et al.* 1995). Physiological effects of androgens depend on different factors such as number of androgen molecules, distribution of androgens and their metabolites inside the cell, interaction with the receptors, polyglutamine number of the amino-acid sequence in the androgen receptor and receptor activation (Palazzolo *et al.* 2008). In order to achieve sufficient exposure to androgens in target tissues, their peripheral and local levels must be well balanced and the transport mechanisms must be in place. Obviously, production and clearance/excretion rates must be in balance as well. The action of androgens in target cells depends on the amount of steroid which can penetrate into the cells, the extent of metabolic conversions within the cells, the interactions with the receptor proteins and, finally, upon the action of the androgen receptors at the genomic level. Unless mentioned specifically, this chapter refers to human data. It provides a timely overview of this topic and focuses on Leydig cells, regulation of Leydig cell function, steroidogenesis, transport and metabolism of testosterone and genomic/non-genomic androgen actions. For more detailed and extensive descriptions on the various topics, the reader may also find the book *The Leydig Cell in Health and Disease* edited by Payne and Hardy (2007) useful.

2.2 Leydig cells

The Leydig cells are located in the testicular interstitium. These cells are the main source of testosterone, and produce approximately 95% of circulating testosterone in men. Approximately 10–20% of the interstitial area is occupied by Leydig cells, and the human testes contain approximately 200×10^6 Leydig cells. Daily testosterone production from the testis is estimated to be around 6–7 mg. Since most of the peripheral testosterone is derived locally from the testicular Leydig cells, it is not surprising that testicular testosterone concentrations exceed those of sex hormone-binding globulin (SHBG)/androgen binding protein (ABP) by about 200-fold (Jarow *et al.* 2001), indicating a substantial surplus of (free) testosterone in the testis. Relative to

Testosterone: Action, Deficiency, Substitution, ed. Eberhard Nieschlag and Hermann M. Behre, Assoc. ed. Susan Nieschlag. Published by Cambridge University Press. © Cambridge University Press 2012.

concentrations in peripheral blood, testicular testosterone concentrations are indeed approximately 80-fold higher (Coviello *et al.* 2005). The Leydig cell is the only cell expressing all enzymes essential for converting cholesterol into testosterone (Payne 2007). In the Leydig cell, testosterone can also be further metabolized into dihydrotestosterone (DHT) or estradiol.

From the developmental, morphological and functional viewpoint, different types of Leydig cells can be distinguished: stem Leydig cells as founder cells, progenitor Leydig cells as committed stem cells, fetal Leydig cells as terminally differentiated cells in the fetus, and adult Leydig cells as the terminally differentiated Leydig cell (Ge and Hardy 2007). Fetal Leydig cells become neonatal Leydig cells at birth and degenerate thereafter or regress into immature Leydig cells (Prince 2007). Fetal Leydig cells produce testosterone. Immature Leydig cells that mainly produce androstane-3α,17β-diol instead of testosterone have also been described. The proliferation rate of the Leydig cells in the adult testis is rather low and is influenced by luteinizing hormone (LH). The ontogeny of Leydig cells is not entirely clear, and mesonephros, neural crest and celomic sources have been discussed. In the adult testis, Leydig cells develop from perivascular and peritubular, mesenchymal-like cells, and the differentiation of these cells into Leydig cells is induced by LH but also by growth factors and differentiation factors derived from Sertoli cells. Both synthesis and secretion are under regulation of pituitary LH and local factors (Lei *et al.* 2001; Sriraman *et al.* 2005). In general terms, in most mammalian species, the testis goes through a period of independent function before the fetal hypothalamic-pituitary-gonadal axis develops at around mid-gestation (see O'Shaughnessy and Fowler 2011 for review). Later, the fetal testes appear to become pituitary hormone dependent, concurrent with declining Leydig cell function, but increasing Sertoli cell numbers. Rodents and primates appear to represent special cases insofar as rodents are born well before the pituitary-dependent phase of fetal development; whilst in primates the testis is dependent upon placental gonadotropin released during the pituitary-independent phase of development.

Aside from Leydig cells, the remaining testosterone/androgen production with biological significance is derived from adrenal steroidogenesis. The production of steroids is not necessarily limited to endocrine glands, but very small amounts, mainly pregnane derivatives, can also be produced in brain cells, and although the contribution of cells in the nervous system to circulating hormones is very small, local production of steroids can be physiologically very important, especially when transport and clearance are low (Rommerts 2004).

2.3 Testosterone biosynthesis

2.3.1 General aspects

Since Leydig cells cannot store androgens, de novo biosynthesis takes place continuously. The starting point for androgen synthesis is cholesterol, a fundamental metabolic substance, with the typical steroid ring conformation energetically compatible with the transformation into androgens (Fig. 2.1). Unlike most cells that use cholesterol primarily for membrane synthesis, Leydig cells have additional requirements for cholesterol, because it is the essential precursor for all steroid hormones. Luteinizing hormone, as the central regulatory factor, controls both steroidogenesis and Leydig cell cholesterol homeostasis in vivo. Cholesterol can either be incorporated by the cell through receptor-mediated endocytosis from low-density lipoproteins (LDLs), or can be synthesized de novo within the Leydig cell starting from acetyl-coenzyme A. In addition, testosterone signaling regulates lipid homeostasis in Leydig cells, and also affects the synthesis of steroids and modulates the expression of genes involved in de novo cholesterol synthesis (Eacker *et al.* 2008). Cholesterol is stored in cytoplasmic lipid droplets. The number of lipid droplets is inversely related to the rate of androgen synthesis, meaning that a high synthesis rate is accompanied by a low content of lipid droplets and vice versa.

Androgen synthesis requires the conversion of cholesterol to testosterone. This transformation is achieved via five different enzymatic steps, at the end of which the side chain of cholesterol is shortened through oxidation from 27C to 19C. The steroidal A-ring assumes a keto configuration at position 3. The starting point for the transformation of cholesterol into testosterone is the shortening of the side chain through C22 and C20 hydroxylases, followed by cleavage of the bond between C20 and C22, leading to production of pregnenolone (Fig. 2.2). The steps following pregnenolone formation occur in the endoplasmic reticulum, either through the Δ4 or through the Δ5 pathway. The designation Δ4 or Δ5 refers to the localization of the

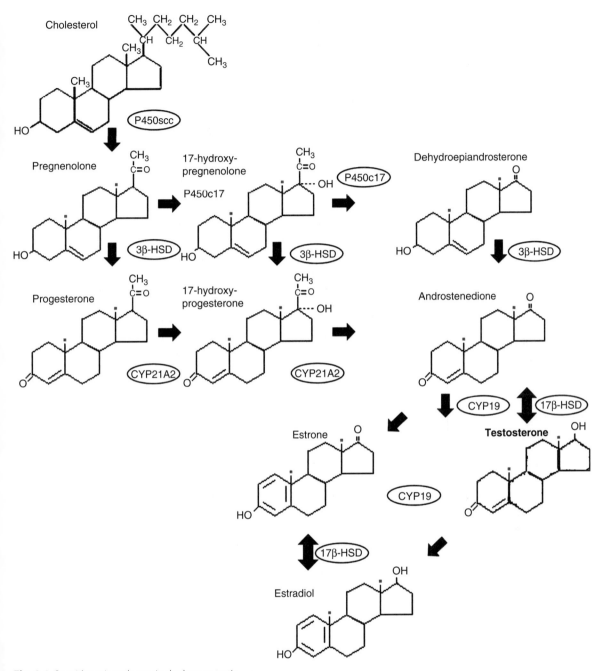

Fig. 2.1 Steroidogenic pathways in the human testis.

double bond in the steroid. The Δ5 pathway is predominant over the Δ4 in human steroid synthesis. Along the Δ4 pathway, pregnenolone is dehydrated to progesterone, a key biological substance. The Δ4 pathway proceeds to the intermediate 17α-hydroxyprogesterone. If the side chain is removed at this stage, the intermediate androstene-3,17-dione is produced, which, through further reduction at position C17, is then transformed into testosterone. In the Δ5 synthesis pathway, testosterone synthesis occurs through the intermediates 17-hydroxypregnenolone and dehydroepiandrosterone (DHEA).

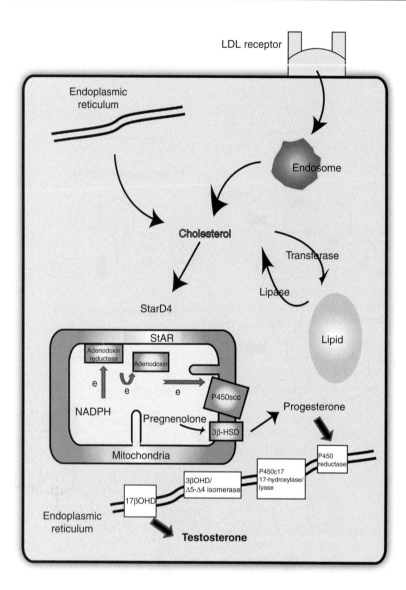

Fig. 2.2 Cholesterol uptake, transport to the inner mitochondrial membrane and mitochondrial side-chain cleavage system yielding pregnenolone in mitochondria, and subsequent metabolism of pregnenolone in endoplasmic reticulum. Normally human steroidic cells take up circulating low-density lipoproteins (LDL) through receptor-mediated endocytosis, directing the cholesterol to endosomes. Cholesterol may also be stored in the endoplasmic reticulum or it may be esterified by acyl-CoA cholesterol transferase and stored in lipid droplets as cholesterol esters. Steroidogenic acute regulatory protein (StAR) plays a key role during steroidogenesis. StAR is localized to the inner mitochondrial membrane and governs cholesterol transport. StAR is responsible for the rapid movement of cholesterol from the outer mitochondrial membrane to the inner mitochondrial membrane, side chain-cleaved and converted by P450scc to pregnenolone. Pregnenolone is biologically inactive and is processed further in the endoplasmic reticulum. Depending on activity and availability of other enzyme systems, other steroids can then be produced further, or different pathways can be employed for synthesis of the same steroid hormone.

Cholesterol is the starting point for biosynthesis of steroids, oxysterols and bile acids. After cholesterol, an insoluble molecule is synthesized de novo or taken up via the LDL receptor or into the cell. Cholesterol available for steroidogenesis is stored in an ester form in lipid droplets, which are hydrolyzed by LH activation of cholesterol ester hydrolase. Cholesterol needs to be transported intracellularly to mitochondria for incorporation into the mitochondrial cristae. The discovery of the steroidogenic acute regulatory protein (StAR) and associated proteins containing StAR-related lipid transfer domains have helped substantially to unravel and understand this limiting step of testosterone synthesis. Steroidogenic acute regulatory protein mRNA expression is triggered by endocrine stimuli and is rapidly and widely distributed among steroidogenic tissues including adrenals and corpora lutea. Steroidogenic acute regulatory protein moves cholesterol from the outer to the inner mitochondrial membrane, but acts exclusively on the outer membrane. The precise mechanism by which StAR's action stimulates the influx of cholesterol remains unclear, but when StAR connects to cholesterol it performs a conformational change that opens a cholesterol-binding pocket (Miller 2007). Following phosphorylation, StAR interacts with voltage-dependent anion channel 1 (VDAC1) on the outer membrane, which processes the phospho-StAR into a smaller intermediate. If VDAC1 is lacking, phospho-StAR is degraded by cysteine proteases, preventing the mitochondrial membrane transport (Bose *et al.* 2008). A number of StAR homologs have also been identified with suspected roles in lipid binding and transfer activities. The physiological importance of StAR is highlighted by the phenotype of patients with an inactivating mutation of the StAR gene. Being unable to produce the necessary amounts of steroids, these patients suffer from life-threatening congenital adrenal hyperplasia (CAH) (King *et al.* 2011).

At the inner mitochondrial membrane site, cytochrome P450ssc (ssc = side-chain cleavage) catalyzes the conversion of cholesterol into pregnenolone. The enzyme cytochrome P450ssc is responsible for the different enzymatic reactions leading to the production of pregnenolone. Like other steroid synthetic enzymes, pregnenolone belongs to the group of mono-oxygenases, containing a prosthetic hemogroup in hemoglobin, and localized on the internal membrane of mitochondria. This reaction consists of three consecutive mono-oxygenations requiring two electrons to activate molecular oxygen: a 22-hydroxylation, 20-hydroxylation and the cleavage of the C20–C22 bond, yielding pregnenolone and isocaproic aldehyde. Pregnenolone diffuses across the mitochondrial membranes and is transformed into testosterone through the enzyme cytochrome P450c17, also belonging to the group of mono-oxygenases and located in the endoplasmic reticulum. Overall, however, the enzymatic system is not capable of transforming every molecule of pregnenolone into testosterone, thus rendering several metabolic intermediates.

2.3.2 Regulation of testosterone synthesis by luteinizing hormone

Luteinizing hormone (LH) is a dimeric glycoprotein containing a glycosylated polypeptide α-subunit and β-subunit that are covalently linked. Luteinizing hormone binds to specific receptors in the testis which are located on Leydig cells, and has a molecular weight of 93 kDa. The LH receptor – like the follicle-stimulating hormone (FSH) and GnRH receptor – belongs to the family of G-coupled receptors. Common to these receptors are seven transmembrane domains that are crucial for the normal functioning of the gonadotropin receptors. The main action of LH is to bind to its receptor in the Leydig cells and to induce the synthesis and release

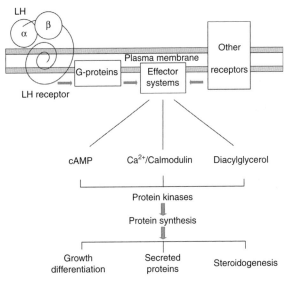

Fig. 2.3 Luteinizing hormone signaling in Leydig cells. Luteinizing hormone binds to the LH receptor, a G-coupled membrane receptor. A great deal of information about the LH/LH receptor interactions has been learned from studies dealing with receptor mutations. Since various effector systems are in place, it has been assumed that factors other than LH can influence Leydig cell steroidogenesis. Based upon Rommerts (2004).

of testosterone (Figs. 2.3 and 2.4). Luteinizing hormone is the most important hormone for regulation of Leydig cell number and functions (Rommerts 2004).

Luteinizing hormone is also *the* key hormone stimulating Leydig cell testosterone synthesis and release via specific receptors. This concept received compelling support from recent clinical and molecular observations. Single mismatch mutations in the transmembrane region were associated with a constitutive activation of the LH receptor in the absence of its ligand, and patients bearing this LH receptor defect showed familial precocious puberty, that is, the premature maturation of the gonad (Kremer *et al.* 1993; Canto *et al.* 2002). There seems to be no functional necessity for LH in the male until the onset of puberty. The first wave of spermatogenesis in fetal mice occurs without LH or relies on maternal human chorionic gonadotropin (hCG) in male fetuses (Huhtaniemi 2000). Luteinizing hormone receptor knock-out (LHRKO) mice have normal testes at birth, and the number of Leydig cells is identical to that of control animals (Zhang *et al.* 2001; Rao and Lei 2002; Lei *et al.* 2004). Human chorionic gonadotropin is also a very potent stimulator of Leydig cell testosterone production. Testosterone is already produced by

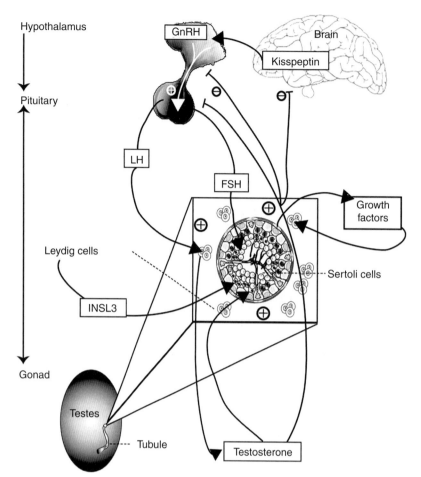

Fig. 2.4 Endocrine and local regulation of Leydig cell steroidogenesis by LH and locally produced factors. Luteinizing hormone is the key regulator of Leydig cell function, and testosterone is the key product of the Leydig cell. A sensitive and rapid negative-feedback loop exists between the Leydig cells and the brain that is mediated via testosterone (and its metabolites DHT and estradiol). Another key product of the Leydig cells is insulin-like factor 3 (INSL3), playing an important role in testicular development and descent. A variety of factors, for instance a plethora of growth factors, is derived from the seminiferous tubules and modulates Leydig cell steroidogenesis – these effects can either be stimulatory or inhibitory.

the fetal testis during the 10th week of gestation, under the stimulation of fetal LH and maternal hCG. The role of maternal hCG in this crucial phase of gonadal development is suggested by the fact that a mutation of the LH β chain leading to a biologically inactive gonadotropin is associated with normal sexual differentiation. Conversely, inactivating mutations of the LH receptor produce a clinical syndrome resembling complete androgen insensitivity, with a phenotype of female external genitalia (Themmen *et al.* 1998).

It has been shown that LH receptors are not only confined to the Leydig cells within the male gonad. The presence of LH/hCG receptors has been demonstrated in endothelial cells of the testicular microvasculature (Ghinea and Milgrom 2001). The relevance of vascular LH/hCG receptors for testicular physiology is currently unknown (Haider 2004). Luteinizing hormone may not be the only factor

stimulating testosterone production, because in studies administering exogenous LH, pulsatile testosterone production seems to increase before LH reaches the Leydig cells through the interstitial space (Setchell *et al.* 2002; Setchell 2004). Also, although LH receptors were believed to be expressed in the gonads only, a number of reports have documented the presence of LH receptors in a variety of organs and tissues. The rat prostate expresses a functional gonadal-sized receptor capable of binding iodinated hCG and stimulating a cAMP response in a LH dose-dependent manner. The main expression was seen in the ventral lobe, which is highly dependent on androgens. Tao *et al.* (1997) have also demonstrated that the human prostate expresses luteinizing hormone receptors. These findings raise the possibility that, in the male, LH exerts extragonadal actions and influences prostatic functions which still remain undefined.

2.3.3 Regulation of Leydig cell function by factors other than luteinizing hormone

Insulin-like factor 3 (INSL3) is a relaxin-like proteohormone produced by Leydig cells (Foresta *et al.* 2004) and signals through a G-coupled receptor (LGR8) that is expressed in Leydig cells and meiotic/postmeiotic testicular human germ cells but not in peritubular and Sertoli cells (Anand-Ivell *et al.* 2006). Compelling evidence is available to indicate that INSL3 is a marker of Leydig cell differentiation and of entry into male puberty (Ferlin *et al.* 2006; Wikström *et al.* 2006). Levels of INSL3 are influenced by hCG/LH, but this effect appears uncoupled from the steroidogenic effects of LH on testosterone synthesis (Bay *et al.* 2006). Since receptors for INSL3 are present on advanced germ cells, it is tempting to assume a local role for INSL3 during spermatogenesis. While the role for spermatogenesis may be unclear, it appears that INSL3 provides a marker for Leydig cell capacity (Ivell and Anand-Ivell 2011).

Growth factors, at least by inference from in-vitro studies, appear to influence Leydig cell function (Chandrashekar and Bartke 2007). Thus, studies have suggested that the local function of inhibin and activin could be a modulation of steroidogenic activity in Leydig cells. Activins inhibit or stimulate Leydig cell steroidogenesis in a species-dependent manner. Generally, insulin-like growth factor 1 (IGF-1) and transforming growth factor alpha (TGF-α) exert a stimulatory activity in the testis, while TGF-β acts as an inhibitor. In the rat, the development of Leydig cells is sustained by an interplay between TGF-α and TGF-β, and LH activity is modulated by IGF-1. In the human Leydig cell the steroidogenic activity is also stimulated by epidermal growth factor (EGF). Thyroid hormone accelerates the differentiation of Leydig cells (Ariyaratne *et al.* 2000) and also stimulates the StAR expression and steroid production in fully developed cells (Manna *et al.* 1999). Glucocorticoids inhibit steroidogenic enzymes and induce apoptosis in rat Leydig cells (Gao *et al.* 2002). The ultimate effects of glucocorticoids in vivo depend very much on local metabolism within the target cells. In this connection, the activity of 11β-hydroxysteroid dehydrogenase as a local amplifier of glucocorticoid action is also of importance (Seckl and Walker 2001). Interestingly, recombinant FSH stimulates testosterone production in men (Levalle *et al.* 1998) and in patients with selective FSH deficiency (Lofrano-Porto *et al.* 2008),

lending further support to the importance of local interactions between Sertoli cells, Leydig cells and peritubular cells in connection with the actions of androgens and gonadotropins.

2.4 Testosterone transport

During transport in plasma, testosterone is mainly bound to albumin or to SHBG which is produced by hepatocytes. Androgen-binding protein, with similar steroid-binding characteristics when compared to SHBG, is produced by Sertoli cells in the testis, and is a β-globulin consisting of different protein subunits. In rats, SHBG is expressed in Sertoli cells, secreted preferentially into the seminiferous tubules, and migrates into the caput epididymidis where it is internalized by epithelial cells and modulates androgen-dependent sperm maturation. Testicular SHBG isoforms are found in sperm and released from sperm during the capacitation reaction. Plasma SHBG has about 95 kDa molecular weight, 30% of which is represented by carbohydrates, and possesses one androgen binding site per molecule. Human testicular SHBG transcripts are expressed in germ cells and contain an alternative exon 1 sequence, appearing to encode an SHBG isoform that is 4–5 kDa smaller than plasma SHBG. The testosterone binding capacity is also much lower compared to the plasma SHBG (Selva *et al.* 2005). In normal men, only 2% of total testosterone circulates freely in blood, while 44% is bound to SHBG and 54% to albumin. The binding affinity of testosterone to albumin is about 100 times lower compared to SHBG. However, since albumin concentration is far higher than that of SHBG, the binding capacity of both proteins for testosterone is approximately the same. The ratio of testosterone bound to SHBG over free SHBG is proportional to SHBG concentration. A direct measurement of free testosterone is impractical in routine practice, so that several equations are used to estimate the free testosterone concentration in serum (see Chapter 4).

Apparently, dissociation of testosterone from binding proteins takes place predominantly in capillaries. The interaction of binding proteins with the endothelial glycocalyx leads to a structural modification of the hormonal binding site and thereby to a change in affinity. As a result testosterone is set free and can diffuse freely into the target cell, or binds together with SHBG to megalin (Fig. 2.5), a cell importer protein (Hammes *et al.* 2005). Megalin is

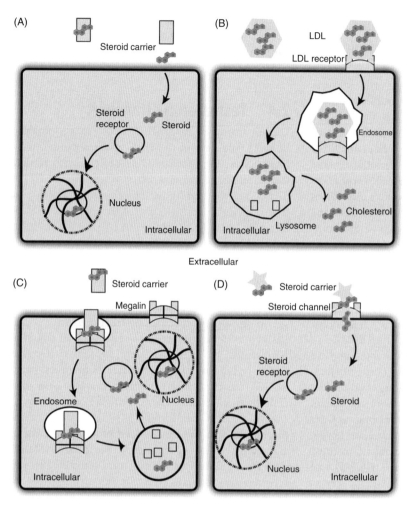

Fig. 2.5 Mechanisms by which steroidal hormones can enter cells. (A) The steroid hormone diffuses freely across the cell membrane, binds to an intracellular receptor and enters the nucleus to regulate gene expression. (B) Receptor-mediated endocytosis of steroid containing lipophilic molecules. The LDL binds its receptor and is taken up, degraded in lysosomes and the steroid cholesterol can enter different metabolic pathways. (C) Receptor-mediated endocytosis of steroids. The entire hormone carrier is endocytotically bound after binding to a carrier protein. Following the intracellular degradation of the carrier, the ligand hormone is released into the free cytoplasm. (D) Transport-mediated uptake of molecules through the membrane. The steroid carrier is recognized by a membrane receptor and the ligand is transported into the cell. See plate section for color version.

expressed in sex-steroid target tissues and is a member of the LDL receptor superfamily of endocytotic proteins. In the serum, 98–99.5% of the sex steroids are protein bound, and endocytosis is quantitatively more relevant for tissue delivery of biologically active steroid hormones than free diffusion. To date several different ways have been described by which steroids can enter the target cells, and which of these are the most relevant pathways to take up the various steroid hormones is still being debated.

Sex hormone-binding globulin binds not only testosterone but also estradiol. The type of binding is influenced by the different SHBG isoforms, but generally testosterone binds threefold higher than estradiol to SHBG. For example, it could be demonstrated that post-translational changes in the carbohydrate structure of SHBG can lead to different binding affinity of the protein to testosterone or estradiol. Sex hormone-binding globulin concentration in serum is under hormonal regulation and primarily regulated through opposing actions of sex steroids on hepatocytes: estrogen stimulates and androgen inhibits SHBG production. Other hormones such as thyroid hormones are also potent stimulators of SHBG production. Sex hormone-binding globulin concentration in men is about one-third to one-half of the concentration found in women. In normal, healthy men with an intact hypothalamic-pituitary-testicular axis, an increase in plasma concentrations of SHBG leads to an acute decrease of free testosterone and simultaneous stimulation of testosterone synthesis, persisting until achievement of normal concentrations.

Testosterone concentrations in the testicular lymphatic circulation and in the venous blood are very similar, but there are essential differences in the flow rate and velocity of both systems. Therefore, transport of testosterone in the general blood circulation occurs mainly through the spermatic vein. Androgens diffuse into interstitial fluid and then enter testicular capillaries or enter capillaries directly from Leydig cells that are in direct contact with the testicular microvasculature. The mechanism for testosterone transport from the Leydig cell into the blood or lymph is not completely known. Probably lipophilic steroids distributed within cells or small cell groups are released through passive diffusion. On the other hand, mouse studies have raised the possibility of an active testosterone transport being important for spermatogenesis (Takamiya *et al.* 1998), showing that gangliosides-associated testosterone transport appeared necessary for complete spermatogenesis.

Steroids such as pregnenolone, progesterone and testosterone not only rapidly pass the Leydig cell membranes, but they can also equilibrate rapidly between different testicular compartments, and the testicular secretion pattern is most likely determined by amounts that are produced inside the tissue, the permeability characteristics of the membranes and the binding proteins in various testicular fluids (Rommerts 2004). As the blood flow is much higher than the flow of interstitial fluid, most of the unconjugated steroids diffuse from the interstitial space to the blood and leave the testis via venous blood. Estradiol is produced by Leydig cells, but the amount is small, with about 20% of peripheral aromatization (Rommerts 2004).

2.5 Testosterone metabolism

Testosterone is the main secretory product of the testis, along with 5α-dihydrotestosterone (DHT), androsterone, androstenedione, 17-hydroxyprogesterone, progesterone and pregnenolone (Fig. 2.6). The transformation of testosterone into DHT takes place principally in the target organs, for example prostate. Androstenedione is important as a precursor for the production of extratesticular estrogens. Biologically active estradiol can be produced as a result of extratesticular aromatization of androstenedione to estrone that is subsequently reduced to estradiol in peripheral tissues. Only a very small portion of the testosterone produced is stored in the testis, and the androgen is mainly secreted in blood. The role of androsterone, progesterone and 17-hydroxyprogesterone in the testis is unknown, but progesterone receptors have been found in some peritubular cells and on spermatozoa

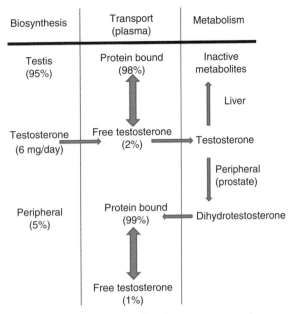

Fig. 2.6 Quantitative aspects of production, transport and metabolism of biologically active androgens. The majority of testosterone is derived from the testis. During peripheral transport, most of the testosterone is bound to transport proteins. In peripheral tissues, testosterone is either metabolized or converted into other active steroids such as DHT or estradiol. Based upon Rommerts (2004).

(Luetjens *et al.* 2006; Modi *et al.* 2007). Using a derivative of progesterone, norethisterone enanthate, no direct effects on testicular/epididymidal function were found (Junaidi *et al.* 2005). Through 5α-reduction, testosterone gives rise to DHT which is three- to sixfold more potent than testosterone. The half-life of testosterone in plasma is only about 12 minutes. Estrogens influence testosterone effects by acting either synergistically or antagonistically. Moreover, estrogens have other specific effects which were originally described to be typical of testosterone. For example, it has been found that inactivating mutations of the estrogen receptor or aromatase activity, preventing estrogen action on the bones, results in continuous linear growth and lack of epiphyseal closure.

Low levels of bioavailable estrogen and testosterone are strongly associated with high bone turnover, low bone mineral density and high risk of osteoporotic fractures. In aromatase-knock-out and estrogen receptor-knock-out male mice, an association between impaired glucose tolerance with insulin resistance and lack of estrogens with elevated testosterone concentrations has been found (Takeda *et al.* 2003). It also seems that aromatase deficiency in men is associated with the occurrence of insulin resistance and diabetes mellitus type 2 during high-dose testosterone treatment (Maffei *et al.* 2004) (see also Chapter 11). The impairment of the estrogen-to-testosterone ratio is thought to be responsible for the development of impaired glucose tolerance and insulin resistance in aromatase-deficiency patients receiving a testosterone replacement therapy (TRT). An imbalance in the ratio of estrogen to androgen tissue levels is also postulated as a major cause in the development of gynecomastia. Furthermore, recent investigations have shown a local neuroprotective effect of newly aromatized estradiol on the brain.

Reduction of testosterone to DHT occurs in the endoplasmic reticulum via the enzyme 5α-reductase located in the microsomes. Testosterone and DHT both bind to the same intracellular androgen receptor to regulate gene expression in the target tissue. Although both hormones interact with the same androgen receptor, testosterone and DHT produce distinct biological responses, and the molecular mechanisms that convey this differential activity are still under debate. Two isoforms of 5α-reductase have been identified in humans. Being nicotinamide adenine dinucleotide phosphate (NADPH)-dependent enzymes, reduction of the double bond at the four to five position in C19 steroids as well as C21 steroids occurs. The gene for 5α-reductase type 1 is located on chromosome 5, encoding for a protein with 259 amino acids, while the gene for the 5α-reductase type 2 is on chromosome 2, encoding for a slightly shorter protein with 254 amino acids. The two isoforms are very similar but show different biochemical properties. Type 1 enzyme works optimally at an alkaline pH, while the optimal pH for type 2 is acidic. Also, the tissue distribution of the two forms is different. Type 1 5α-reductase has been localized in the non-genital skin, liver, brain prostate, ovary and testis; while type 2 is mainly active in classical androgen-dependent tissues, such as the epididymis, genital skin, seminal vesicle, testis and prostate, but also in liver, uterus, breast, hair follicles and placenta. At a cellular level, DHT sustains differentiation and growth and is particularly important for normal sexual development and virilization in men. It also affects muscle mass and the deepening of the voice. Dihydrotestosterone transactivates the androgen receptor, leading to prostate gene transcription and growth.

Overall, testosterone effects result from influences of the hormone itself and of its metabolites estradiol and DHT. Changes in the property of type 2 5α-reductase due to mutation can result in complete androgen insensitivity syndrome (CAIS) or partial androgen insensitivity syndrome (PAIS) (see also Chapter 3). Dihydrotestosterone is eliminated by type 3α-HSD (hydroxysteroid dehydrogenase; aldo-keto reductase (AKR)1C2), which reduces 5α-DHT to 3α-androstanediol. Studies in men have demonstrated that 3α-androstanediol can be converted back to 5α-DHT by AKR1C2 activity only, to stimulate growth of the prostate (Penning *et al.* 2000). In human tissues, five aldo-keto reductase isoforms exist with varying reductase activity on the 3-, 17- and 20-ketosteroid position, with isoform AKR1C2 predominately converting 5α-DHT to 3α-diol. The inactivated metabolites are excreted in the urine. Some androgen metabolites are excreted in their free form; others are glucuronated by the liver before excretion. Recently excreted metabolites have been used in screening assays to uncover doping with exogenous testosterone esters in high-performance athletics (Saudan *et al.* 2006). The 17-glucuronidation of the DHT metabolite androstane-3α,17β-diol is correlated with several metabolic risk factors in men. The ratio of 17G to DHT is associated with total fat mass, its distribution, intrahepatic fat, disturbed lipid profile, insulin resistance and diabetes (Vandenput *et al.* 2007).

2.6 Mechanism of androgen action

2.6.1 Genomic effects of androgens

Testosterone dissociates from SHBG at the target organ and diffuses into the cells. The conversion of testosterone into DHT is organ dependent. This occurs, for example, in the prostate, where DHT is the main biologically active androgen. Hydroxysteroid dehydrogenases regulate ligand access to the androgen receptor in the human prostate. The first step in androgen action is binding to the androgen receptor which belongs to the family of steroid hormone receptors. Along with RoDH, HSDs are involved in the pre-receptor regulation of androgen action. The androgen receptor and other nuclear receptors act as transcriptional factors via a general mechanism in which they bind to their cytosolic ligand, inducing conformational changes, loss of chaperones, dimerization and nuclear translocation.

In the nucleus both (ligand and nuclear receptor) bind to specific sequences of genomic DNA and induce stimulation of RNA synthesis. Chromatin remodeling such as modification of histones plays a role in gene transcription, and many nuclear receptor interacting coregulators perform significant roles in gene transcription. Histone demethylases are key players in the regulation of androgen-mediated transcription. In the absence of androgens, target genes are turned off due to the presence of H3K9 methylation of a lysine residue on histones H3 and H4. In the presence of androgens, H3K9 methylation is removed, which leads to the derepression of androgen target genes (Klose and Zhang 2007). For further detailed information please see the review by Wu and Zhang (2009). Mineralocorticoid, glucocorticoid, thyroid hormone, retinol, fatty acid metabolite, estrogen and progesterone receptors also belong to this family. At least 48 nuclear receptors have been identified in humans (Kishimoto *et al.* 2006). These receptors share substantial functions and are thought to have evolved from a single ancestral gene (Bertrand *et al.* 2004). Orphan nuclear receptors have also been found for which no ligand has yet been identified. Members of this receptor family possess an N-terminal domain, a DNA-binding domain (DBD), a hinge region and a hormone-binding domain.

Nuclear receptors have several functional domains, a constitutionally activating function domain, a highly conserved DNA-binding domain, a nuclear localization signal domain and a ligand-binding domain (LBD). Steroid receptors show high homology with the corresponding DNA-binding and ligand-binding domains in the mineralocorticoid, glucocorticoid and progesterone receptors. In contrast, at the N-terminal domain little similarity with these receptors remains. The nuclear receptors are subdivided into two subfamilies depending on their ligand partners forming homodimers, such as the androgen receptor and other steroid receptors; another subfamily forms heterodimers with only one ligand, such as the thyroid hormone receptor. In most nuclear receptors the binding in a pouch to their ligand at the C-terminal end, made of 12 α-helices, leads to a shift of the most C-terminal α-helix and to an alteration of its activity. Inside the 12 helices, a hydrophobic cave is induced to change its formation and angle which the helix number 12 folds into. This angle is associated with transactivation status of the receptor.

An important characteristic of the N-terminal domain of the androgen receptor is the presence of three short tandem repeats (STRs) CAG, coding for polymorphic polyglutamine, TGG repeats coding for polyproline and GGC repeats for polyglycine. In normal men, about 17–29 glutamine repeats and 13–17 glycine repeats are present. Alleles of small GGC size have been associated with esophageal cancer; while in patients with Kennedy disease, a disease with degenerating motoneurons, up to 72 such glutamine repeats are present. Furthermore, in the androgen receptor, long CAG and GGC alleles are associated with decreased transactivation function and have been associated with cancers in women. In the androgen receptor, low-size CAG (<19 repeats) and GGC (<15 repeats) alleles result in higher receptor activity, and have been associated with earlier age of onset, and a higher grade and more advanced stage of prostate cancer at the time of diagnosis. The number of glutamine repeats of the androgen receptor has been associated with azoospermia or oligozoospermia, but no clear association was found (Asatiani *et al.* 2003; see also Chapter 3).

The androgen receptor gene encoding for two isoforms is located on the X chromosome and spans about 90 kb and codes for a 2 757-base pair open reading frame within a 10.6-kb mRNA. The location of the androgen receptor gene on the X chromosome is preserved in evolutionarily distant animals, such as marsupials and monotremes, and may reflect a developmentally significant association of the androgen receptor gene with other systemic genes. The coding sequence, containing the sequence of nucleotides translated into amino acids, consists of eight exons. The N-terminal domain, the transcriptional regulatory region of the protein, is fully encoded by exon 1, while DNA-binding domain is encoded by exon 2 and 3, and steroid-binding domain by exons 4–8.

Similar to all the other steroid receptors, the DNA-binding domain of the androgen receptor contains two zinc fingers. This domain is about 70 amino acids long and is localized between the N-terminal and the androgen-binding domain. In this part of the sequence, eight cysteines are spatially arranged such that four sulfur atoms keep one zinc atom in place, giving rise to the typical structure of two overlapping helices. Exon 2 and 3 of the androgen receptor encode for the DNA-binding domain. The first zinc finger, encoded by exon 2, is important for the specific binding of the androgen receptor to the second and fifth nucleotide pairs in the first androgen-response element repeat GGTACA of the DNA.

The second zinc finger, encoded by exon 3, stabilizes DNA receptor binding by hydrophobic interactions with the first finger, and contributes to specificity of receptor DNA binding, leading to dimerization of two receptor molecules. In immediate proximity to the DNA-binding domain, a short amino-acid sequence is responsible for the transport of the receptor into the nucleus.

The androgen-binding domain of the androgen receptor encompasses about 30% of the overall receptor (the DNA-binding domain about 10%) and is responsible for the specific binding of androgens. This domain forms a lipophilic pocket based upon 24 amino acids that enables the binding of testosterone or other androgens. Experimental deletion of this domain results in increased gene transcription in vitro. This part of the receptor is necessary for inducible and regulated gene transcription. Regulation of steroid hormone receptor action occurs, in part, by post-translational modifications, such as phosphorylation. The androgen receptor is phosphorylated at a number of sites in response to agonist binding that results in nuclear localization, but usually not in response to antagonists. It has also been shown that phosphorylation is regulated by steroid hormones or forskolin and phorbol esters at different sites. Dihydrotestosterone binds to the androgen receptor with higher affinity than testosterone, mainly because testosterone more quickly dissociates from the receptor. Other steroids such as androstenedione, estradiol and progesterone bind to the androgen receptor with much lower affinity than testosterone. Phosphorylation in the hinge region required for full transcriptional activity is involved in the signal transduction mediated by cyclic AMP and protein kinase C.

Chaperones such as heat shock protein 90 (HSP 90) are responsible for the maintenance of the receptor in the inactive state and are released from the complex. Without its hormone ligand the androgen receptor can bind to homologous or heterologous ligands in the cytoplasm and exert inhibitory effects on cell death processes. The loss of this protein has uncovered functional domains of the receptor and is necessary for nuclear transport. Nuclear transport is mediated by import receptors through a pathway that employs two proteins, importin-α and importin-β. In this nuclear-protein-import pathway, the positively charged nuclear localization signal of the androgen receptor is recognized in the cytoplasm by importin-α that serves as an adaptor to the nuclear transport factor importin-β. The importin-α–importin-β androgen receptor complex then moves through nuclear-pore complexes and dissociates, mediated by a guanosine triphosphatase (GTPase) protein, thus releasing the androgen receptor inside the nucleus.

The actual interaction with DNA occurs through the two zinc fingers in the DNA-binding domain of the androgen receptor. The androgen receptor interacts with DNA in a homodimeric form consisting of two identical hormone receptor complexes. These homodimers bind to DNA sequences known as androgen-responsive elements, which contain typical palindromic sequences, that is, DNA tracts with a nucleotide sequence independent of the reading direction. Before it can bind to the DNA, covalent modifications of the DNA trapping proteins, the histones, have to occur first. At the N-terminal ends of histones various covalent modifications can be carried out, such as acetylation, phosphorylation, ubiquitination and methylation. Depending on the histone modifications, genes will either be expressed or silenced, and the methylation of lysines or arginines has been linked to either transcriptional activation or repression. Lysine residues of the histone tails can be monomethylated, dimethylated or trimethylated. The differentially methylated lysine residues serve as binding sites for various effector proteins which may be co-repressor or coactivators.

Lysine-specific demethylase 1 (LSD1) has the function to silence genes if no nuclear receptor is present but, in the opposite case, to demethylate histones if such a ligand-activated receptor is docking onto the site. During this step, LSD1 forms a chromatin-associated complex with the ligand-activated androgen receptor. Another coactivator is needed to start actual gene expression of the LSD1 chromatin-associated, ligand-activated androgen receptor complex. This again is a demethylase (JHDM2A) which is only associated with DNA in combination with the above-mentioned complex. Two different mechanisms involving demethylases in the transcriptional regulation of the androgen receptor are needed to express androgen target genes (Metzger et al. 2006). The time sequence of events is not known. Up to now many methylation/demethylation enzymes have been found which all may be needed for fine tuning of gene expression. The transcription complex induces mRNA synthesis of androgen-dependent genes and, after mRNA translation, synthesis of new androgen-dependent proteins such as prostate-specific antigen (PSA).

The regulation of androgen receptor expression at the transcriptional and translational level is complex and depends on factors such as age, cell type and tissue. Generally, androgens have a positive effect on stabilization of the receptor protein, so that androgen administration leads to inhibition of receptor degradation and thereby to an increase in androgen receptor protein levels. The effects of androgens on the androgen receptor mRNA are the opposite. In this case, androgen administration leads to downregulation of the androgen receptor mRNA by shortening of the mRNA half-life. Current and future research activities concentrate on selective androgen receptor modulators (SARMs), analogous to the SERMs for the estrogen receptor. This work leads to a general understanding of structure-activity relationships of new pharmacophors of non-steroidal SARMs by structural modification of non-steroidal antiandrogens (see Chapter 21).

Selective androgen receptor modulator pharmacophores can be classified into four categories so far: aryl-propionamide, bicyclic hydantoin, quinoline and tetrahydroquinoline analogs. A characteristic of these molecules is that they are not substrates for aromatase or 5α-reductase. These androgen receptor ligands are intended to act as agonists in anabolic organs (e.g. muscle and bone) but be neutral in androgenic tissues (e.g. prostate and seminal vesicles). Other possible molecular mechanisms related to the tissue selectivity of SARMs include ligand-dependent changes in androgen receptor conformation, differential interaction with the promoter context of target tissue genes, and the differential recruitment of co-regulators in these tissues. These new compounds are now in preclinical animal trials or already in phase I clinical trials. The hope is that SARMs may be of benefit for the treatment of primary or secondary hypogonadism, anemias, osteopenia or osteoporosis, frailty, benign hyperplasia of the prostate (BPH), and may also be of help in designing a hormonal male contraception method.

Androgen receptor defects such as deletions or inactivating mutations can profoundly alter receptor function. The resulting phenotype is highly variable, ranging from under virilization to testicular feminization. Inactivating mutations of the androgen receptor gene in a 46,XY male with testes resulted in a female phenotype, owing to the complete lack of all androgen activity. However, there is no uterus and only a partially formed vagina, and during puberty pubic and axillary hair is scant or absent. Earlier, this syndrome of complete androgen insensitivity (CAIS) was called testicular feminization (see Chapter 3).

2.6.2 Non-genomic effects of androgens

Androgens also exert rapid non-genomic effects, contributing to the physiological actions (Lösel et al. 2003). Most androgenic hormone action is thought to work through direct activation of DNA transcription via high affinity interactions with the androgen receptor. Whereas genomic effects take hours or days to produce their actions, rapid steroid effects are activated within seconds or minutes. These non-genomic actions are not removed by inhibition of transcription or translation and are often activated by membrane-impermeant steroid conjugates. However, rapid pathways of androgen action can modulate transcriptional activity of androgen receptors or other transcription factors (Rahman and Christian 2007).

In recent years, a variety of rapid "non-genomic" effects of sex steroids has been documented for these "nuclear-oriented" ligands (reviewed by Simoncini and Genazzani 2003). Androgens can also activate transcription-independent signaling pathways (Heinlein and Chang 2002). Rapid effects of androgens have been shown on calcium fluxes (Guo et al. 2002) and on intracellular phosphorylation cascades such as the MAP-kinase pathway (Castoria et al. 2003). Membrane effects of androgens have also been implicated in functional responses such as rapid secretion of PSA by prostatic cells (Papakonstanti et al. 2003) and the secretion of GnRH by pituitary cells (Shakil et al. 2002). In NIH 3T3 cells, DNA synthesis is triggered after association between the androgen receptor and the membrane components has occurred under the influence of nanomolar concentrations of androgens. It appears that in these cells the very low density of androgen receptors is not sufficient to stimulate gene transcription (Castoria et al. 2003). Androgen-stimulated gene transcription only occurs when the intracellular receptor concentration is elevated. The membranous effects of low concentrations of "nuclear oriented" receptors could represent a more general mode for steroid action in general.

Not all the membrane effects of androgens (and other sex steroids) are mediated by the classical receptor. There are several good indications that other steroid-binding proteins localized in the plasma membrane are essential for signal transduction, but for many years the structure of these proteins could not be elucidated and therefore this was not a popular subject for study. Recently an alternative receptor for membrane effects of progestins has been cloned (Zhu *et al.* 2003a). The protein has seven transmembrane domains and has similarities with G-protein-coupled receptors. Hybridization analyses have revealed that many mRNAs are present in a variety of human tissues (Zhu *et al.* 2003b). Although a similar protein has not been identified for androgens, it is known that humans can smell very small amounts of androstenone (16 ene-5α-androsten-3-one) as a volatile compound. Since only a very few isomers (but not testosterone) can be detected by the olfactory system, it is very likely that the smell is triggered by specific membrane receptors for androstenone in the olfactory sensory neurons (Snyder *et al.* 1988). It is known that all olfactory receptors are classical G-protein-coupled proteins, and since the alternative membrane receptor for progestins is homologous with G-coupled-receptors, it is not unlikely that alternative androgen receptors in the olfactory system have a similar structure.

The dependency of spermatogenesis on high levels of testosterone cannot be explained by properties of the classical nuclear receptor, and since the levels of testosterone required for maintaining normal spermatogenesis are much higher than the saturation level of the high-affinity androgen receptor, an alternative sensing system with a lower affinity has been postulated (Rommerts 2004). It is interesting to note that the alternative membrane receptor for progestins also has a 10-fold lower affinity than the classical progesterone receptor.

Thus, testosterone can modify the susceptibility of T-cells to infectious diseases. Effects of testosterone on calcium mobility through cell membranes of T-cells have been reported (Benten *et al.* 1997). Since T-cells do not possess the classical androgen receptors, this biological response also indicates the involvement of unconventional plasma membrane receptors for the expression of these androgen effects. Another example of the involvement of

alternative androgen receptors can be found in eels. In eels, nanomolar concentrations of 11-ketotestosterone, for which no nuclear receptor has been found, are essential for maintaining spermatogenesis in vitro. Under these conditions high concentrations of testosterone or DHT were inactive (Miura *et al.* 1991). A number of further examples related to non-genomic androgen actions were reported more recently. Androgens acutely (e.g. within approximately 30 minutes) altered the frequency of the peristaltic activity of small intestine muscle and augmented the amplitude of agonist-induced contractile activity (Gonzalez-Montelongo *et al.* 2011). Further studies linked androgen activities to calcium mobilization and potentially the activation of the Rho pathway. Evidence has also been presented that the orphan G-coupled protein receptor GPRC6A, a widely expressed calcium- and amino-acid-sensing G-coupled receptor, transduces the non-genomic effects of testosterone and also those of other steroids (Pi *et al.* 2011). Interestingly, and conversely, the testosterone-induced rapid signaling was reduced in prostate cancer cells with GPRC6A deficiency. Of similar interest, testosterone suppressed LH secretion in wild-type mice but stimulated LH in GPRC6A−/− null mice.

There is also considerable evidence that the non-genomic effects of steroids are mediated via the nuclear receptors that stimulate signaling pathways in the cytoplasm of target cells (Migliacco *et al.* 2011). Overall, though, albeit there is no longer any doubt about the reality of non-genomic actions of androgens (Bennett *et al.* 2010; Grosse *et al.* 2011), much still needs to be learned about the role of the androgen receptor in non-gonadal tissues; for example why certain tissues develop androgen insensitivity.

2.7 Key messages

- Leydig cells are the main source of testosterone and undergo various developmental and functional stages throughout ontogeny.
- Steroidogenesis is the conversion of cholesterol within mitochondria into pregnenolone. Transformation of pregnenolone into testosterone occurs enzymatically in the endoplasmic reticulum of Leydig cells.

- Luteinizing hormone is the key regulator of Leydig cell steroidogenesis. Involvement of other factors is likely but less well established.
- Steroid hormones diffuse through tissues without apparent specific transport systems.

- In addition to genomic effects of androgens mediated via their nuclear receptor, androgens can also exert non-genomic effects by interacting with cellular membrane receptors.

2.8   References

Anand-Ivell RJ, Relan V, Balvers M, Coiffec-Dorval I, Fritsch M, Bathgate RA, Ivell R (2006) Expression of the insulin-like peptide 3 (INSL3) hormone-receptor (LGR8) system in the testis. *Biol Reprod* 74:945–953

Ariyaratne HB, Mills N, Mason JI, Mendis-Handagama SM (2000) Effects of thyroid hormone on Leydig cell regeneration in the adult rat following ethane dimethane sulphonate treatment. *Biol Reprod* 63:1115–1123

Asatiani K, von Eckardstein S, Simoni M, Gromoll J, Nieschlag E (2003) CAG repeat length in the androgen receptor gene affects the risk of male infertility. *Int J Androl* 26:255–261

Bay K, Matthiesson KL, McLachlan RI, Andersson AM (2006) The effects of gonadotropin suppression and selective replacement on insulin-like factor 3 secretion in normal adult men. *J Clin Endocrinol Metab* 91:1108–1111

Bennett NC, Gardiner RA, Hooper JD, Johnson DW, Gobe GC (2010) Molecular cell biology of androgen receptor signalling. *Int J Biochem Cell Biol* 42:813–827

Benten WP, Lieberherr M, Sekeris CE, Wunderlich F (1997) Testosterone induces Ca2+ influx via non-genomic surface receptors in activated T cells. *FEBS Lett* 407:211–214

Bertrand S, Brunet FG, Escriva H, Parmentier G, Laudet V, Robinson-Rechavi M (2004) Evolutionary genomics of nuclear receptors: from twenty-five ancestral genes to derived endocrine systems. *Mol Biol Evol* 21:1923–1937

Bose M, Whittal RM, Miller WL, Bose HS (2008) Steroidogenic activity of StAR requires contact with mitochondrial VDAC1 and phosphate carrier protein. *J Biol Chem* 283:8837–8845

Canto P, Soderlund D, Ramon G, Nishimura E, Mendez JP (2002) Mutational analysis of the luteinizing hormone receptor gene in two individuals with Leydig cell tumors. *Am J Med Genet* 108:148–152

Castoria G, Lombardi M, Barone MV, Bilancio A, Di Domenico M, Bottero D, Vitale F, Migliaccio A, Auricchio F (2003) Androgen-stimulated DNA synthesis and cytoskeletal changes in fibroblasts by a nontranscriptional receptor action. *J Cell Biol* 161:547–556

Chandrashekar V, Bartke A (2007) Growth factor in Leydig cell function. In: Payne A, Hardy MP (eds) *The Leydig Cell in Health and Disease*. Humana Press, Totowa, NJ, pp 263–277

Coviello AD, Matsumoto AM, Bremner WJ, Herbst KL, Amory JK, Anawalt BD, Sutton PR, Wright WW, Brown TR, Yan X, Zirkin BR, Jarow JP (2005) Low-dose human chorionic gonadotropin maintains intratesticular testosterone in normal men with testosterone-induced gonadotropin suppression. *J Clin Endocrinol Metab* 90:2595–2602

Dankbar B, Brinkworth MH, Schlatt S, Weinbauer GF, Nieschlag E, Gromoll J (1995) Ubiquitous expression of the androgen receptor and testis-specific expression of the FSH receptor in the cynomolgus monkey (Macaca fascicularis) revealed by a ribonuclease

protection assay. *J Steroid Biochem Mol Biol* 55:35–41

Eacker SM, Agrawal N, Qian K, Dichek HL, Gong EY, Lee K, Braun RE (2008) Hormonal regulation of testicular steroid and cholesterol homeostasis. *Mol Endocrinol* 22:623–635

Ferlin A, Arredi B, Zuccarello D, Garolla A, Selice R, Foresta C (2006) Paracrine and endocrine roles of insulin-like factor 3. *J Endocrinol Invest* 29:657–664

Foresta C, Bettella A, Vinanzi C, Dabrilli P, Meriggiola MC, Garolla A, Ferlin A (2004) A novel circulating hormone of testis origin in humans. *J Clin Endocrinol Metab* 89:5952–5958

Gao HB, Tong MH, Hu YQ, Guo QS, Ge R, Hardy MP (2002) Glucocorticoid induces apoptosis in rat leydig cells. *Endocrinology* 143:130–138

Ge R, Hardy MP (2007) Regulation of Leydig cells during pubertal development. Payne A, Hardy MP (eds) *The Leydig Cell in Health and Disease*. Humana Press, Totowa, NJ, pp 55–70

Ghinea N, Milgrom E (2001) A new function for the LH/CG receptor: transcytosis of hormone across the endothelial barrier in target organs. *Semin Reprod Med* 19:97–101

Gonzalez-Montelongo MC, Marin R, Gomez T, Diaz M (2011) Androgens are powerful non-genomic inducers of calcium sensitization in visceral smooth muscle. *Steroids* 75:533–538

Grosse A, Bartsch S, Baniahmad A (2011) Androgen receptor-mediated gene repression. *Mol Cell Endocrinol* Jul 19 [Epub ahead of print]

Guo Z, Benten WP, Krucken J, Wunderlich F (2002) Nongenomic testosterone calcium signaling. Genotropic actions in androgen receptor-free macrophages. *J Biol Chem* **277**:29600–29607

Haider SG (2004) Cell biology of Leydig cells in the testis. *Int Rev Cytol* **233**:181–241

Hammes A, Andreassen TK, Spoelgen R, Raila J, Hubner N, Schulz H, Metzger J, Schweigert FJ, Luppa PB, Nykjaer A, Willnow TE (2005) Role of endocytosis in cellular uptake of sex steroids. *Cell* **122**:751–762

Heinlein CA, Chang C (2002) The roles of androgen receptors and androgen-binding proteins in nongenomic androgen actions. *Mol Endocrinol* **16**:2181–2187

Huhtaniemi I (2000) The Parkes lecture. Mutations of gonadotrophin and gonadotrophin receptor genes: what do they teach us about reproductive physiology? *J Reprod Fertil* **119**:173–186

Ivell R, Anand-Ivell R (2011) Biological role and clinical significance of insulin-like peptide 3. *Curr Opin Endocrinol Diabetes Obes* **18**:210–216

Jarow JP, Chen H, Rosner TW, Trentacoste S, Zirkin BR (2001) Assessment of the androgen environment within the human testis: minimally invasive method to obtain intratesticular fluid. *J Androl* **22**:640–645

Junaidi A, Luetjens CM, Wistuba J, Kamischke A, Yeung CH, Simoni M, Nieschlag E (2005) Norethisterone enanthate has neither a direct effect on the testis nor on the epididymis: a study in adult male cynomolgus monkeys (Macaca fascicularis). *Eur J Endocrinol* **152**:655–661

King SR, Bhangoo A, Stocco DM (2011) Functional and physiological consequences of StAR deficiency: role in lipoid congenital adrenal hyperplasia. *Endocr Dev* **20**:47–53

Kishimoto M, Fujiki R, Takezawa S, Sasaki Y, Nakamura T, Yamaoka K, Kitagawa H, Kato S (2006) Nuclear receptor mediated gene regulation through chromatin remodeling and histone modifications. *Endocr J* **53**:157–172

Klose RJ, Zhang Y (2007) Regulation of histone methylation by demethylimination and demethylation. *Nat Rev Mol Cell Biol* **8**:307–318

Kremer H, Mariman E, Otten BJ, Moll GW Jr, Stoelinga GB, Wit JM, Jansen M, Drop SL, Faas B, Ropers HH, Brunner HG (1993) Cosegregation of missense mutations of the luteinizing hormone receptor gene with familial male-limited precocious puberty. *Hum Mol Genet* **2**:1779–1783

Lei ZM, Mishra S, Zou W, Xu B, Foltz M, Li X, Rao CV (2001) Targeted disruption of luteinizing hormone/human chorionic gonadotropin receptor gene. *Mol Endocrinol* **15**:184–200

Lei ZM, Mishra S, Ponnuru P, Li X, Yang ZW, Rao ChV (2004) Testicular phenotype in luteinizing hormone receptor knockout animals and the effect of testosterone replacement therapy. *Biol Reprod* **71**:1605–1613

Levalle O, Zylbersztein C, Aszpis S, Aquilano D, Terradas C, Colombani M, Aranda C, Scaglia H (1998) Recombinant human follicle-stimulating hormone administration increases testosterone production in men, possibly by a Sertoli cell-secreted nonsteroid factor. *J Clin Endocrinol Metab* **83**:3973–3976

Lofrano-Porto A, Casulari LA, Nascimento PP, Giacomini L, Naves LA, da Motta LD, Layman LC (2008) Effects of follicle-stimulating hormone and human chorionic gonadotropin on gonadal steroidogenesis in two siblings with a follicle-stimulating hormone beta subunit mutation. *Fertil Steril* **90**:1169–1174

Lösel RM, Falkenstein E, Feuring M, Schultz A, Tillmann HC, Rossol-Haseroth K, Wehling M (2003) Nongenomic steroid action: controversies, questions, and answers. *Physiol Rev* **83**:965–1016

Luetjens CM, Didolkar A, Kliesch S, Paulus W, Jeibmann A, Bocker W, Nieschlag E, Simoni M (2006) Tissue expression of the nuclear progesterone receptor in male non-human primates and men. *J Endocrinol* **189**:529–539

Maffei L, Murata Y, Rochira V, Tubert G, Aranda C, Vazquez M, Clyne CD, Davis S, Simpson ER, Carani C (2004) Dysmetabolic syndrome in a man with a novel mutation of the aromatase gene: effects of testosterone, alendronate, and estradiol treatment. *J Clin Endocrinol Metab* **89**:61–70

Manna PR, Tena-Sempere M, Huhtaniemi IT (1999) Molecular mechanisms of thyroid hormone-stimulated steroidogenesis in mouse Leydig tumor cells. Involvement of the steroidogenic acute regulatory (StAR) protein. *J Biol Chem* **274**:5909–5918

Metzger E, Wissmann M, Schule R (2006) Histone demethylation and androgen-dependent transcription. *Curr Opin Genet Dev* **16**:513–517

Migliaccio A, Castoria G, Auricchio F (2011) Analysis of androgen receptor rapid actions in cellular signaling pathways: receptor/src association. *Methods Mol Biol* **776**:361–370

Miller WL (2007) StAR search – what we know about how the steroidogenic acute regulatory protein mediates mitochondrial cholesterol import. *Mol Endocrinol* **21**:589–601

Miura T, Yamauchi K, Takahashi H, Nagahama Y (1991) Hormonal induction of all stages of spermatogenesis in vitro in the male Japanese eel (Anguilla japonica).

Proc Natl Acad Sci USA **88**:5774–5778

Modi DN, Shah C, Puri CP (2007) Non-genomic membrane progesterone receptors on human spermatozoa. *Soc Reprod Fertil Suppl* **63**:515–529

O'Shaughnessy PJ, Fowler PA (2011) Endocrinology of the mammalian fetal testis. *Reproduction* **141**:37–46

Palazzolo I, Gliozzi A, Rusmini P, Sau D, Crippa V, Simonini F, Onesto E, Bolzoni E, Poletti A (2008) The role of the polyglutamine tract in androgen receptor. *J Steroid Biochem Mol Biol* **108**:245–253

Papakonstanti EA, Kampa M, Castanas E, Stournaras C (2003) A rapid, nongenomic, signaling pathway regulates the actin reorganization induced by activation of membrane testosterone receptors. *Mol Endocrinol* **17**:870–881

Payne AH (2007) Steroidogenic enzymes in Leydig cells. In: Payne A, Hardy MP (eds) *The Leydig Cell in Health and Disease.* Humana Press, Totowa, NJ, pp 157–172

Payne AH, Hardy MP (eds) (2007) *The Leydig Cell in Health and Disease.* Humana Press, Totowa, NJ

Penning TM, Burczynski ME, Jez JM, Hung CF, Lin HK, Ma H, Moore M, Palackal N, Ratnam K (2000) Human 3alpha-hydroxysteroid dehydrogenase isoforms (AKR1C1-AKR1C4) of the aldo-keto reductase superfamily: functional plasticity and tissue distribution reveals roles in the inactivation and formation of male and female sex hormones. *Biochem J* **351**:67–77

Pi M, Parrill AL, Quarles LD (2011) GPRC6A mediates the non-genomic effects of steroids. *J Biol Chem* **285**:39953–39964

Prince F (2007) The human Leydig cell: functional morphology and developmental history. In: Payne A, Hardy MP (eds) *The Leydig Cell in Health and Disease.* Humana Press, Totowa, NJ, pp 71–90

Rahman F, Christian HC (2007) Non-classical actions of testosterone: an update. *Trends Endocrinol Metab* **18**:371–378

Rao CV, Lei ZM (2002) Consequences of targeted inactivation of LH receptors. *Mol Cell Endocrinol* **187**:57–67

Rommerts FFG (2004) Testosterone: an overview of biosynthesis, transport, metabolism and non-genomic actions. In: Nieschlag E, Behre HM (eds) *Testosterone: Action, Deficiency, Substitution*, 3rd edn. Cambridge University Press, Cambridge, pp 1–38

Saudan C, Baume N, Robinson N, Avois L, Mangin P, Saugy M (2006) Testosterone and doping control. *Br J Sports Med* **40** (Suppl 1): i21–i24

Seckl JR, Walker BR (2001) Minireview: 11beta-hydroxysteroid dehydrogenase type 1 – a tissue-specific amplifier of glucocorticoid action. *Endocrinology* **142**:1371–1376

Selva DM, Bassas L, Munell F, Mata A, Tekpetey F, Lewis JG, Hammond GL (2005) Human sperm sex hormone-binding globulin isoform: characterization and measurement by time-resolved fluorescence immunoassay. *J Clin Endocrinol Metab* **90**:6275–6282

Setchell BP (2004) Hormones: what the testis really sees. *Reprod Fertil Dev* **16**:535–545

Setchell BP, Pakarinen P, Huhtaniemi I (2002) How much LH do the Leydig cells see? *J Endocrinol* **175**:375–382

Shakil T, Hoque AN, Husain M, Belsham DD (2002) Differential regulation of gonadotropin-releasing hormone secretion and gene expression by androgen: membrane versus nuclear receptor activation. *Mol Endocrinol* **16**:2592–2602

Simoncini T, Genazzani AR (2003) Non-genomic actions of sex steroid hormones. *Eur J Endocrinol* **148**:281–292

Snyder SH, Sklar PB, Pevsner J (1988) Molecular mechanisms of olfaction. *J Biol Chem* **263**:13971–13974

Sriraman V, Anbalagan M, Rao AJ (2005) Hormonal regulation of Leydig cell proliferation and differentiation in rodent testis: a dynamic interplay between gonadotrophins and testicular factors. *Reprod Biomed Online* **11**:507–518

Takamiya K, Yamamoto A, Furukawa K, Zhao J, Fukumoto S, Yamashiro S, Okada M, Haraguchi M, Shin M, Kishikawa M, Shiku H, Aizawa S (1998) Complex gangliosides are essential in spermatogenesis of mice: possible roles in the transport of testosterone. *Proc Natl Acad Sci USA* **95**:12147–12152

Takeda K, Toda K, Saibara T, Nakagawa M, Saika K, Onishi T, Sugiura T, Shizuta Y (2003) Progressive development of insulin resistance phenotype in male mice with complete aromatase (CYP19) deficiency. *J Endocrinol* **176**:237–246

Tao YX, Bao S, Ackermann DM, Lei ZM, Rao CV (1997) Expression of luteinizing hormone/human chorionic gonadotropin receptor gene in benign prostatic hyperplasia and in prostate carcinoma in humans. *Biol Reprod* **56**:67–72

Themmen AP, Martens JW, Brunner HG (1998) Activating and inactivating mutations in LH receptors. *Mol Cell Endocrinol* **145**:137–142

Vandenput L, Mellstrom D, Lorentzon M, Swanson C, Karlsson MK, Brandberg J, Lonn L, Orwoll E, Smith U, Labrie F, Ljunggren O, Tivesten A, Ohlsson C (2007) Androgens and glucuronidated androgen metabolites are associated with metabolic risk factors in men. *J Clin Endocrinol Metab* **92**:4130–4137

Wikström AM, Bay K, Hero M, Andersson AM, Dunkel L (2006) Serum insulin-like factor 3 levels during puberty in healthy boys and boys with Klinefelter syndrome. *J Clin Endocrinol Metab* **91**:4705–4708

Wu SC, Zhang Y (2009) Minireview: role of protein methylation and demethylation in nuclear hormone signaling. *Mol Endocrinol* **23**:1323–1334

Zhang FP, Poutanen M, Wilbertz J, Huhtaniemi I (2001) Normal prenatal but arrested postnatal sexual development of luteinizing hormone receptor knockout (LuRKO) mice. *Mol Endocrinol* **15**:172–183

Zhu Y, Rice CD, Pang Y, Pace M, Thomas P (2003a) Cloning, expression, and characterization of a membrane progestin receptor and evidence it is an intermediary in meiotic maturation of fish oocytes. *Proc Natl Acad Sci USA* **100**:2231–2236

Zhu Y, Bond J, Thomas P (2003b) Identification, classification, and partial characterization of genes in humans and other vertebrates homologous to a fish membrane progestin receptor. *Proc Natl Acad Sci USA* **100**:2237–2242

Chapter 3

Pathophysiology of the androgen receptor

Olaf Hiort, Ralf Werner, and Michael Zitzmann

3.1   Introduction

The final biological steps in the cellular cascade of normal male sexual differentiation are initiated by the molecular action of androgens in androgen-responsive target tissues. Lack of androgenic steroids leads to defective sexual differentiation in embryos with 46,XY karyotype; while their excess is associated with virilization in 46,XX children. Furthermore, androgens lead to specific changes during male puberty and are required for male fertility.

A key player in the translation of androgen action is the androgen receptor (AR), a nuclear transcription factor which can bind various androgenic steroids as ligands and then act via differential DNA targeting and genetic control. With the elucidation of the X-chromosomal localization and the genetic structure of the AR more than 20 years ago (Fig. 3.1), it was thought that most 46,XY patients with presumed defects of androgen action would carry mutations in the coding regions of the *AR* gene. While this holds true for the majority of patients with complete androgen insensitivity syndrome (CAIS), to an increasing proportion patients clinically assigned as partial (PAIS) or minimal androgen insensitivity syndrome (MAIS) do not carry relevant mutations in the AR. Therefore the clarification of the time- and cell-specific mechanisms of androgen action and the factors acting in concert with the AR is of utmost importance. They lead to the cell-specific modulation of androgen-dependent transcription of several hundred target genes (Holterhus *et al.* 2003; 2007).

One example is the subtle modulations of the transcriptional activity induced by the AR that have been assigned to a polyglutamine stretch of variable

Testosterone: Action, Deficiency, Substitution, ed. Eberhard Nieschlag and Hermann M. Behre, Assoc. ed. Susan Nieschlag.
Published by Cambridge University Press. © Cambridge University Press 2012.

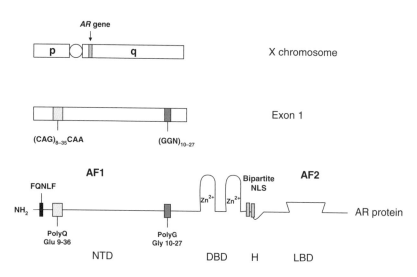

Fig. 3.1 Display of the X chromosome with the androgen receptor (*AR*) gene. Exon 1 contains a variable number of CAG repeats encoding a polyglutamine stretch of variable length in the receptor protein. The number of CAG repeats or length of polyglutamine residues is inversely associated with the transcriptional activity of androgen-dependent genes, and hence androgen effects in target tissues.

length within the N-terminal domain of the receptor. This stretch is encoded by a variable number of CAG triplets in exon 1 of the *AR* gene. First observations of pathologically elongated *AR* CAG repeats in patients with X-linked spinal and bulbar muscular atrophy (XSBMA) showing marked hypoandrogenic traits (La Spada *et al.* 1991) were supplemented by partially conflicting findings of clinical significance also within the normal range of CAG repeat length. The modulatory effect on androgen-dependent gene transcription is linear, and probably mediated by a differential affinity of coactivator proteins to the encoded polyglutamine stretch, such as ARA24 and p160 (Hsiao *et al.* 1999; Irvine *et al.* 2000). As these proteins are ubiquitously but nevertheless non-uniformly expressed, the modulatory effect of the CAG repeat polymorphism on AR target genes is most likely not only dependent on androgenic saturation and AR expression, but also varies from tissue to tissue. To date, an involvement of prostate cancer risk, spermatogenesis, bone density, hair growth, cardiovascular risk factors and psychological implications has been demonstrated.

3.2 Gonadal development and endocrine function

Normal male sexual development is dependent on genetic events of gonadal development as well as on endocrine pathways initiated by hormones secreted from the testes. The gonad is an organ with a bipotential nature that can develop from a single primordium, the genital ridges, either into a testis or an ovary. After formation of the genital ridges, low expression of both male and female pathway genes is initiated, independent of the genetic sex of the embryo. In eutherian mammals, the presence or absence of *SRY* (sex-determining region of the Y chromosome) is the genetic master switch that initiates changes in the ratio of male and female factors to enhance one of the two sex-determining pathways, leading to the differentiation of the gonad into testis or ovary (for a review see Kashimada and Koopman 2010; Piprek 2009; Sekido and Lovell-Badge 2009). In mice *Sry* is expressed in XY gonads only in a short time-window between 10.5 and 12.5 days post-coitum, with a peak at 11.5 days post-coitum in precursors of Sertoli cells, and upregulates Sry-box containing gene 9 (*Sox9*) expression (Hacker *et al.* 1995; Bullejos and Koopman 2001; Sekido and Lovell-Badge 2008). Then *Sry* is downregulated and *Sox9* is maintained by autoregulatory direct and indirect feed-forward loops. Proper and sufficient *Sox9* expression is necessary for recruitment of supporting cell precursors (Sertoli and follicle cell precursors) into the Sertoli cell lineage. *SOX9* can bind to its own testis-specific enhancer (*TES*, testis-specific enhancer of SOX9) via the same DNA-binding motif as *SRY*, and can be recruited by protein–protein interaction with SF1 (Sekido and Lovell-Badge 2008). *SOX9* also upregulates SF1 in early testis development, providing a positive feed-forward loop (Shen and Ingraham 2002). Another positive feed-forward loop necessary for *SOX9* maintenance is upregulation of fibroblast growth factor 9 (*FGF9*) by *SOX9*, which transduces its signals mainly by fibroblast growth factor receptor 2 (FGFR2) and helps to maintain SOX9 expression (Kim *et al.* 2006; 2007). Although early SOX9 expression is not affected in Fgf9 knock-out mice, maintenance of SOX9 expression is abolished, leading to a complete XY, female sex reversal (Kim *et al.* 2006).

Prostaglandin D synthase (PTGDS) is another target of SOX9 and is required to synthesize prostaglandin D_2 (PGD$_2$). Prostaglandin D_2 enhances SOX9 nuclear transport and upregulates SOX9 expression (Malki *et al.* 2005; Wilhelm *et al.* 2005); while SOX9 binds to and activates the promoter of PTGDS, providing another feed-forward loop of SOX9 maintenance (Wilhelm *et al.* 2007). In contrast to Fgf9, knock-out of Ptgds does not disrupt gonadal development (Moniot *et al.* 2009). Fibroblast growth factor 9 and PGD$_2$ may also act as paracrine factors that stimulate proliferation and differentiation of Sertoli progenitor cells. The differentiating Sertoli cells enclose clusters of germ cells and form, together with the peritubular myoid cells, the testis cords, a structure that separates the germ cells and Sertoli cells from the interstitial cells. The Sertoli cells are thought to also coordinate the differentiation of the interstitial steroidogenic Leydig cells and the peritubular myoid cells (Wilhelm *et al.* 2007). Steroid-producing fetal Leydig cells appear 24 hours after Sertoli cell differentiation (Habert *et al.* 2001; Yao *et al.* 2002). Desert hedgehog (DHH), a Sertoli-derived signaling molecule, has been shown to play an important role in fetal Leydig cell differentiation (Yao *et al.* 2002). Ectopic activation of the Hedgehog signaling pathway in fetal ovaries leads to a transformation of SF1-positive somatic cells into functional fetal Leydig cells producing androgens and INSL3 (Barsoum *et al.* 2009; Barsoum and Yao 2010). In mammals, two distinct populations of Leydig cells appear sequentially during testis development: fetal Leydig cells and adult Leydig cells. Fetal Leydig cells start to produce androgens around 13 days post coitum in mice, leading to the masculinization of the male urogenital system (O'Shaughnessy *et al.* 2006). In mice, in contrast to adult Leydig cells, fetal Leydig cells do not express 17β-HSD, and secrete androstenedione, which is converted within the seminiferous tubules, most likely by Sertoli cells, into testosterone (O'Shaughnessy *et al.* 2000). The development of fetal Leydig cells is independent of androgens up to postnatal day five, as evidenced by AR knock-out mice (O'Shaughnessy *et al.* 2002).

In early gestation, two pairs of unipotential ducts, the Wolffian (WD or mesonephric) and Mullerian (MD or paramesonephric) ducts develop in the fetus regardless of the karyotype. Wolffian and Mullerian ducts represent anlagen of the male and female reproductive tracts. If testicular formation is unhindered, the Leydig cells will produce testosterone (in humans at eight weeks of gestation) and the Sertoli cells will produce anti-Mullerian hormone/Mullerian-inhibiting substance (AMH/MIS). High local concentrations of testosterone lead to the stabilization of the Wolffian duct and its development into the separate but connected organs, the epididymis, the vas deferens and the seminal vesicles. The action of testosterone on Wolffian duct stabilization is mediated by the androgen receptor, as shown by AR knock-out mice, and patients with complete androgen sensitivity syndrome (CAIS) that lack Wolffian duct derivates (Yeh *et al.* 2002; Hannema *et al.* 2006; Hannema and Hughes 2007).

Expression of AMH induces regression of the Mullerian ducts in a short period between 8 and 10 weeks of gestation (Taguchi *et al.* 1984). In contrast, absence of AMH action leads to development of Fallopian tubes, the uterus and the upper third of the vagina. To exert the action of AMH, also high concentrations of this hormone and active binding to a membrane receptor in the mesenchymal cells surrounding the Mullerian ducts are necessary. Therefore, reduced excretion of AMH due to lowered numbers of Sertoli cells is responsible for partial uterus formation seen clinically in sex determination disorders (Ostrer 2008).

3.3 Androgens in sexual development

3.3.1 In sexual differentiation of the embryo and fetus

The prostate develops from the urogenital sinus (UGS), a ventral urinary compartment formed after separation of the digestive and urinary tract by the urorectal septum. The sexually dimorphic development of the UGS is dependent on androgens secreted by the Leydig cells of the developing testis (for a review see Marker *et al.* 2003; Meeks and Schaeffer 2011). Androgen-dependent development of the prostate was demonstrated by de novo induction of prostatic buds from male and female urogenital sinuses of rats using organ culture methods (Lasnitzki and Mizuno 1977; 1979; Takeda *et al.* 1986). Although prostate development begins with the development of epithelial buds, the AR is expressed at these stages only in the surrounding mesenchyme (Takeda *et al.* 1986), indicating that paracrine androgen-dependent signals may mediate bud formation. Androgen dependency of prostate development is also shown by the lack of a prostate in AR knock-out mice and in humans with CAIS (Zhou 2010). In addition, some 46,XX DSD (disorders of sexual development) patients suffering from CAH with intrauterine exposure to high androgen levels have developed prostatic tissue (Klessen *et al.* 2005; da Costa Rose Paulino *et al.* 2009). Since the concentration of testosterone in the fetal circulation is relatively low, target cells in the prostate and the external genitalia express 5α-reductase type 2, an enzyme that converts testosterone into the 10-fold more potent androgen DHT (Deslypere *et al.* 1992). Urogenital sinus organ culture experiments with testosterone or DHT led to the conclusion that the effect of testosterone is mediated by conversion to DHT (Lasnitzki and Mizuno 1977). On the other hand, inhibition of 5α-reductase by in-utero application of the 5α-reductase inhibitor finasteride led to a significant decrease in prostate size in rats (Imperato-McGinley *et al.* 1992). In humans with 5α-reductase type 2 deficiency and in mice with targeted disruption of 5α-red 2, the UGS is specified as a prostate but prostate growth and development are greatly reduced (Andersson *et al.* 1991; Mahendroo *et al.* 2001).

Several AR-dependent target genes have been described in fetal prostate development. Nkx3.1 is a homeobox transcription factor expressed early in the developing prostate buds and its expression is androgen dependent. Castration of mice leads to immediate ablation of Nkx3.1 expression (Bieberich *et al.* 1996). Nkx3.1 is a direct target of the AR, and its androgen-dependent transcription is mediated by androgen response elements (AREs) in the 3' UTR of the gene (Thomas *et al.* 2010). Targeted disruption of Nkx3.1 in mice leads to defects in ductal morphology and secretory protein production (Bhatia-Gaur *et al.* 1999). The homeobox genes *Hoxa13*, *Hoxb13* and *Hoxd13* are expressed during UGS development and in the developing prostate (Zeltser *et al.* 1996; Warot *et al.* 1997). A slight testosterone-dependent upregulation of these *Hox* genes was observed in organ cultures of the ventral prostate of newborn rats, but not in the lateral prostate (Huang *et al.* 2007). Sonic hedgehog (SHH; see below) is expressed in the urogenital epithelium (UGE) of prostatic buds and is upregulated by testosterone. Dependency on androgens was confirmed by a five-fold decreased expression of SHH in the absence of DHT in in-vitro organ culture of UGS (Podlasek *et al.* 1999). Although the DHT-dependent development of the prostate is established downstream, effectors of androgen signaling mediating the fetal differentiation of the prostate have been poorly defined.

Up to the seventh week of gestation in humans and day of embryogenesis (E) 16.5 in mice, the external genitalia of male and female embryos are morphologically identical and consist of bipotential anlagen, the genital tubercle (GT), the urogenital folds and the bilateral genital swellings. Under influence of DHT, the GT develops into a penis and the genital swellings fuse and grow into a scrotum. With the growing penis, a ventral urethral groove appears, with lateral urethral folds which fuse, and, together with a distal canalizing urethral plate, forms the urethra. In females the GT develops into a clitoris, and the genital swellings and urogenital folds remain separate and form the labia majora and labia minora (for a review see Yamada *et al.* 2003; 2006). Like the prostate, the GT also develops through epithelial–mesenchymal interactions (Murakami and Mizuno 1986; Kurzrock *et al.* 1999), but the factors mediating the masculinization are not yet known. Recently, the critical time-window for androgen action on genital masculinization has been defined to embryonic stage E15.5 in mice. At this time point the AR is expressed in the mesenchyme as well as in the urethral plate epithelium (UPE) (Miyagawa *et al.* 2009). Targeted disruption of mesenchymal versus epithelial AR showed a demasculinization in male mesenchymal AR knock-out mice, indicating that proper mesenchymal AR signaling is necessary for GT development. In epithelial AR knock-out mice no effect on GT development could be detected (Miyagawa *et al.* 2009). Gene expression analysis of GT from E15.5 mice revealed increased expression of the Wnt inhibitory genes Dickkopf (*DKK*) and secreted frizzled related protein 1 (*SFRP1*) in females, demonstrating a sexually dimorphic expression of Wnt signaling genes in the GT (Nishida *et al.* 2008; Miyagawa *et al.* 2009). A sexually dimorphic Wnt/β-catenin signaling enhanced in the male GT was observed in a BatGAL Wnt/β-catenin indicator mouse line. Forty percent of conditional β-catenin loss of function mutants failed to develop a proper prepuce and midline formation; while female β-catenin gain of function mutants showed enlarged external genitalia with a well-developed prepuce similar to androgen-treated females, but no enlarged anogenital distance (Miyagawa *et al.* 2009). These results made β-catenin a good candidate as a potentially downstream effector of androgen signaling involved in external genitalia masculinization that may act by the canonical β-catenin/Tcf/Lef pathway or as an AR coactivator (Song *et al.* 2003).

Sonic hedgehog is a secreted growth factor expressed in the urethral plate epithelium; whereas its receptor patched1 (PTC1), or its target the transcription factor glioblastoma 1 (GLI1), is expressed in adjacent mesenchyme (Miyagawa *et al.* 2011). The role of Shh in epithelial–mesenchymal interactions and androgen-independent outgrowth of the GT has been acknowledged, and Shh knock-out mice display complete GT agenesis (Haraguchi *et al.* 2001; Perriton *et al.* 2002; Seifert *et al.* 2010). Recently, Miyagawa *et al.* (2011) showed by conditional Gli and Shh knock-out mice that Hedgehog signaling also affects sexually dimorphic mesenchymal differentiation of the GT. Conditional Gli2−/− mice showed a complete loss of Hedgehog responsiveness within the mesenchyme adjacent to the urethral plate epithelium in a lacZ reporter line associated with GT hypoplasia and defects in the ventral midline that are even more prominent in the male than in the female. Demasculinization of the male GT was also associated with decreased sexually dimorphic gene expression in the GT. Interestingly, female Gli2−/− mice do not masculinize with androgen treatment, indicating a requirement of Gli2 for GT masculinization. On the other hand, other androgen effects like enlargement of the anogenital distance are not affected. Conditional gain of function mutants for Shh signaling lead to a partial masculinization of the female GT by prepuce hypertrophy, but no fusion of the urethral folds was observed. In contrast to β-catenin signaling, Shh signaling appears not to be a downstream target, but may act cooperatively with androgen signaling (Miyagawa *et al.* 2011). To date, androgen-dependent effectors of masculinization of the external genitalia other than the androgen receptor have been poorly defined. Participation of Wnt and Hedgehog signaling pathways in sexually dimorphic development of the GT has been demonstrated. Neither targeted deletion nor gain of function mutations in these pathways could mimic complete sex reversal as could the absence of androgens or the AR. Thus other downstream effectors of androgen action must exist, whose identity and role in genital development still remain elusive.

The morphogenetic result of these specific actions of androgens is the irreversible virilization of the external male genitalia. In humans, this process is terminated in the 12th week of gestation. Hence, incomplete masculinization, for example incomplete closure of the midline (hypospadias) during the sensitive window between the 7th and the 12th week cannot be overcome even by high doses of androgens at later stages of development. This fact may seem trivial, but it clearly indicates that the genomic programs provided by the androgen target tissues must have undergone comprehensive and definitive alterations in parallel to the ontogenetic process of external virilization.

3.3.2 In male puberty and adulthood

Puberty is a period of development with two main processes: namely adrenarche and gonadarche. Adrenarche describes the increasing androgenic steroid secretion from the adrenals, which is usually observed between 8 and 10 years in both girls and boys, and is limited to primates (Plant and Witchel 2006). Gonadarche describes the enlargement of the gonads with formation of sex steroids and the induction of fertility. Thus, only gonadarche is fundamental to the process of puberty and reproduction. Gonadarche is triggered by increasing pulsatility of GnRH secretion leading to a release of the pituitary hormones LH and FSH. Luteinizing hormone in turn is responsible for increasing testosterone synthesis in the testes via direct stimulation of the Leydig cells (Plant 2006).

In males, puberty is clinically evident with the enlargement of testes and penis. Testicular volume increases from 1 to 2 cm^3 prepubertally to reach 20–30 cm^3 in adulthood. In addition to changes in secondary hair, and genital changes, increasing testosterone concentrations produce other changes in most tissues of the body (Welsh *et al.* 2009). The larynx increases in size and the voice deepens. Also bone mass and muscle strength increase, a growth spurt occurs, the erythrocyte cell mass increases, the skin thickens, and hair growth on the trunk is enhanced; androgenic hair recession may be induced as well. Furthermore, the internal sex organs such as prostate and seminal vesicles enlarge. Sex steroids, and specifically testosterone, may alter behavior, and central nervous effects include stimulation of sexual libido and aggressiveness.

In conjunction with FSH, testosterone is an essential endocrine factor for spermatogenesis in male

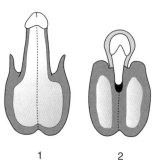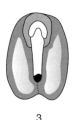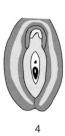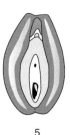

1   2   3   4   5

Fig. 3.2 Clinical grades of ambiguous genitalia. Virilization is diminished from grade 1 towards grade 5. According to Sinnecker *et al.* 1997.

mammals which acts directly on the germinal epithelium via the AR. During hormonal quiescence in prepuberty, germ-cell proliferation is arrested until the juvenile phase. Testosterone alone can induce spermatogenesis if administered during this period (Marshall *et al.* 1984). However, quantitative maintenance of the spermatogenic process cannot be achieved by testosterone alone, but needs the supportive action of FSH (see Chapter 6).

Current concepts state that mammary gland development is mainly dependent on estrogens; numerous studies primarily using mouse models have revealed that estrogen is a critical requirement for ductal elongation during puberty, whereas progesterone and prolactin signaling are crucial during pregnancy and lactation (LaMarca and Rosen 2008). The role of the AR in breast development is unclear.

3.4 Androgen insensitivity in humans

3.4.1 Clinical findings

Defective androgen action caused by cellular resistance to androgens causes the androgen insensitivity syndrome (AIS) (Quigley *et al.* 1995; Hiort *et al.* 1996). The end-organ resistance to androgens results in a wide clinical spectrum of defective virilization of the external genitalia in 46,XY individuals (Fig. 3.2). In AIS, testicular function is apparently normal. However, affected individuals will have a clinical phenotype that is consistent with a varying degree of presumable androgen deficiency, but testis may be of low-normal size and histology in childhood, and Muller structures (oviducts, uterus and upper third of the vagina) are absent due to normal AMH synthesis and action. In this regard, at clinical investigation AIS in childhood is a phenocopy from disorders of androgen synthesis not affecting adrenal function, such as 5α-reductase deficiency or 17β-hydroxysteroid dehydrogenase deficiency.

However, at the time of puberty, the specific clinical appearance of AIS is much more striking. The timing of puberty apparently follows a female pattern (Papadimitriou *et al.* 2006). A main feature of pubertal development is the feminization that occurs in almost all patients with CAIS and PAIS with gonads in situ. Patients with CAIS show a female puberty with normal onset of breast development. This is different in all other forms of 46,XY disorders of sex development, where only virilization might be seen at the time of puberty (Werner *et al.* 2010).

Most strikingly, patients with 5α-reductase deficiency or with 17β-hydroxysteroid dehydrogenase deficiency mostly demonstrate a strong surge in testosterone and DHT, leading to marked virilization and sometimes to gender change if the individual had been raised as a female (Hiort *et al.* 2003).

In AIS, the testes enlarge and histologically show Leydig cell hyperplasia as well as a Sertoli-cell-only pattern without evidence for spermatogenesis. An important feature of CAIS is the insufficiency of sexual hair growth. In some patients with CAIS, pubic hair is reported, but this may appear thinner than normal and may not reach Tanner stage 5 (Sinnecker *et al.* 1997).

In PAIS, a mixture of virilization and feminization may occur. This leads to phallic and testicular enlargement with sexual hair growth on one side, but breast development on the other side. Puberty may not fully develop, although laboratory values for testosterone are measured in the adult reference range (Ahmed *et al.* 2011). The voice may not deepen appropriately and acne is scarce. Body proportions tend to be female or intermediate. Gynecomastia is present in almost all patients with PAIS, as we reported in a recent survey of 15 individuals assigned to male sex (Steltenkamp and Hiort 2007). These features make clinical assessment of androgen insensitivity much easier during puberty and thereafter than during infancy and childhood.

However, within families, the phenotype may vary considerably between MAIS and PAIS, even with the same underlying molecular abnormality (Rodien *et al.* 1996; Holterhus *et al.* 2000).

The fate of the gonads in CAIS is a point of current debate. While the gonads in patients with PAIS and female sex assignment are removed to avoid possible virilization at the time of puberty, this point is not valid in CAIS patients. In the past, their gonads were often removed at the time of diagnosis, at latest at puberty, due to a possible increased risk for malignancy. This has to be weighed against the invasive and psychologically stressing nature of this procedure, which inevitably leads to the need for hormone replacement therapy to induce puberty and maintain adult health in these patients. Mostly, tumors of the gonads occur as type II germ cell tumors, namely classic seminoma in the testis or dysgerminomas in the dysgenetic gonads of disorders of sex determination. Apparently, those disorders that are associated with normal testicular development and histology often depict a maturation delay rather than a preneoplastic change. Therefore, the tumor risk in CAIS is seemingly lower than in other forms of DSD (Cools *et al.* 2011).

This leads to a novel view of leaving the gonads in situ with the possibility that individuals with CAIS synthesize their own sex steroids with the very special CAIS hormonal profile. If the gonads are maintained after puberty, however, the patients should be aware of the lack of long-term outcome data and they should be involved in a regular screening program with imaging of the gonads as well as regular laboratory assessment.

3.4.2 Laboratory assessment of androgen insensitivity

The determination of laboratory values relies on age-dependent reference values during infancy and childhood and is difficult to assess in androgen insensitivity. Bouvattier et al. (2002) reported that in children with CAIS, LH levels were comparably low during mini-puberty (measurement at day 30); while, in PAIS, they rose to a normal level, which corresponds to a reference range of Tanner 4–5. Also, the testosterone levels were low in CAIS infants, but stimulated properly in PAIS. The authors concluded that, due to the impaired pituitary feedback mechanism in androgen insensitivity syndrome, the postnatal surge of gonadotropins and testosterone is missing in CAIS, but may be normal in PAIS. Anti-Mullerian hormone and inhibin B measurements were reported as normal or even elevated, because the inhibited AR expression accounts for the absence of AMH repression during testis development (Boukari *et al.* 2009). Rey *et al.* (1999) reported AMH as a valuable marker of testicular differentiation. While AMH was low in testicular dysgenesis, values were within the normal range in disorders of androgen biosynthesis or action. Inhibin B as a Sertoli cell marker showed a similar response. It was measured low in anorchia or gonadal dysgenesis and normal or elevated in disorders of androgen biosynthesis or AIS compared to normal 46,XY boys (Kubini *et al.* 2000).

At the time of puberty, gonadotropins rise normally. In due course of puberty, FSH might become elevated above the normal range because of secondary testicular atrophy. Luteinizing hormone is in the upper normal male reference range or even elevated. Subsequently, a surge of testosterone is seen that does not correspond to external masculinization, thus giving rise to the diagnosis of androgen insensitivity. Usually, testosterone levels are in the upper male reference range. An androgen sensitivity index has been postulated as the mathematical product of LH and testosterone serum values (Aiman *et al.* 1979) and is helpful in the discrimination of adult patients with MAIS as a cause of male infertility, although it does not differentiate AIS from other causes of hormonal imbalance such as estrogen insufficiency in MAIS (Hiort *et al.* 2000). Thus, the higher the androgen sensitivity index, the more likely is an abnormality of the *AR* gene.

The patients have strong features of feminization, although estradiol levels are not elevated above the male reference range. It can be postulated that either a high degree of intracellular aromatization of testosterone to estradiol or the loss of repression of feminizing genes is responsible for this finding (Doehnert *et al.* 2011).

Before the time of molecular characterization of the *AR* gene, analysis of specific androgen binding in genital skin fibroblasts of patients had been a major diagnostic procedure. In the age of molecular genetics, this type of analysis has been abandoned because it requires the invasive method of a genital skin biopsy to gain the cells to be investigated. As fewer and fewer patients are operated on, biopsies are often not available. Furthermore, androgen binding studies were able to detect only mutations of the AR located in the ligand-binding part of the receptor, while mutations affecting the DNA-binding region of the AR usually have normal androgen binding capacities, but lack transactivational function.

An androgen sensitivity test was described on the basis of the response of serum levels of SHBG after intake of stanozolol, a synthetic anabolic steroid. In normal probands, serum levels of SHBG decline to about 50% of the initial value five to eight days after the start of stanozolol treatment (Sinnecker et al. 1997). In AIS, this response is diminished, correlating somewhat with the phenotypic degree of under-masculinization. While the SHBG test can be valuable as the only available in-vivo test of androgen insensitivity, it has several pitfalls. Namely, stanozolol has been taken off the regular market due to its high potential for misuse as a doping agent and its liver toxicity. Second, due to the endogenous testosterone surge during the first months of life, this test is not sensitive during this important period for diagnosis and management of the child with presumed AIS. And third, the test might fail in patients with somatic mosaicism of a mutation in the AR gene (Sinnecker et al. 1997; Holterhus et al. 1999).Therefore at present it should be proposed only for patients with unclear disorders of androgen action over the age of one year.

3.4.3   Genetics

The AR belongs to the intracellular family of structurally related steroid hormone receptors. Transcriptional regulation through the AR is a complex multistep process involving androgen binding, conformational changes of the AR protein, receptor phosphorylation, nuclear trafficking, DNA binding, cofactor interaction and finally transcription activation. It is now more than 20 years ago that the human AR gene was cloned by several groups and mapped to Xq11–12 (Chang et al. 1988; Trapman et al. 1988; Lubahn et al. 1988; 1989; Tilley et al. 1989). It spans approximately 90 kb and comprises 8 exons, named 1–8 or A–H. Transcription of the AR gene and subsequent splicing usually results in distinct AR-mRNA populations in genital fibroblasts. Translation of the mRNA into the AR protein usually leads to a product migrating at about 110 kDa in Western immunoblots comprising between 910 and 919 amino acids.

The AR shares its particular modular composition of three major functional domains with the other steroid hormone receptors. A large N-terminal domain precedes the DNA-binding domain (DBD) that is connected by a short hinge region to the C-terminal LBD (Fig. 3.1). The N-terminal domain (NTD) is encoded by the first exon and contains the strong ligand-independent transactivation domain named "activation function 1" (AF1) (Simental et al. 1991; Jenster et al. 1995; Chamberlain et al. 1996). The N-terminal domain is proposed to be a highly flexible and disordered domain that adopts a higher structure by induced folding when in contact with transcriptional regulators such as the basal transcription factor TFIIF (RAP74) (Lavery and McEwan 2006; 2008a; 2008b). The N-terminal domain harbors two polymorphic repeats, a polyglutamine repeat of 9–36 residues and a polyglycine repeat of 10–27 glycine residues, and its repeat length affects AR transactivation (Chamberlain et al. 1994; Kazemi-Esfarjani et al. 1995; Wang et al. 2004; Werner et al. 2006a). In contrast to the N-terminal domain, the DNA-binding domain and LBD are highly structured domains, and their crystal structure has been resolved (Matias et al. 2000; Sack et al. 2001; He et al. 2004; Shaffer et al. 2004). The DNA-binding domain is encoded by exon 2 and 3 and consists of two zinc fingers followed by a C-terminal extension. The first zinc finger contains the so-called P-box, an α-helix that makes the base-specific contact with the major groove of the DNA, while the second zinc finger containing the so-called D-box is involved in DNA-dependent dimerization (Claessens et al. 2008). All classical steroid receptors (AR, progesterone receptor (PR), mineralocorticoid receptor and glucocorticoid receptor) can bind to the same hormone-responsive element (Mangelsdorf et al. 1995), but, in addition, AR can bind to selective AREs not bound by the glucocorticoid receptor (Claessens et al. 2001; 2008). The hinge region, encoded in part by exon 3 and 4, is defined as a flexible linker between the DNA-binding domain and the LBD, and contains the bipartite nuclear localization signal (NLS) (Jenster et al. 1992; 1993; Zhou et al. 1994; Cutress et al. 2008). The C-terminal extension of the second zinc finger is also part of the hinge and involved in specificity of selective AREs (Haelens et al. 2003; Schauwaers et al. 2007). The LBD is encoded by exon 4–8 and contains 12 α helices and 4 small β-strands that assemble into a three-layer, sandwich-like structure with a central ligand binding pocket (He *et al.* 2004). Agonist binding leads to a repositioning of helix 12 and seals the ligand binding pocket like a mouse trap (Moras and Gronemeyer 1998). Thereby a hydrophobic cleft is formed called activation function 2 (AF2) that interacts with LxxLL- and FxxLF-like motifs of co-regulators as well as with the 23FQNLF27 motif in the N-terminal domain of the AR. Additional functional subdomains could be identified by in-vitro investigation of artificially truncated, deleted or point-mutated ARs (see http://androgendb.mcgill.ca/). Upon entering target cells, androgens interact very specifically with the ligand-binding pocket of the AR. This initiates an activation cascade with conformational changes and nuclear translocation of the AR. Prior to receptor binding to target DNA, homodimerization of two AR proteins occurs in a ligand-dependent manner. This is mediated by distinct sequences within the second zinc finger of the DNA-binding domain as well as through specific structural N–C-terminal interactions. The AR-homodimer binds to hormone responsive elements which usually consist of two palindromic (half-site) sequences within the promoter of androgen-regulated genes. Through chromatin remodeling, direct interaction with other transcription factors and specific coactivators and co-repressors, a steroid-receptor-specific modulation of the assembly of the preinitiation complex is achieved, resulting in specific activation or repression of target gene transcription.

More than 800 different mutations have been identified in AIS to date (http://androgendb.mcgill.ca/). Extensive structural alterations of the AR can result from complete or partial deletions of the *AR* gene. Smaller deletions may introduce a frame shift into the open reading frame, leading to a premature stop codon downstream of the mutation. Similar molecular consequences arise from the direct introduction of a premature stop codon due to point mutations. Such alterations usually lead to severe functional defects of the AR and are associated with CAIS. Extensive disruption of the AR protein structure can also be due to mutations leading to aberrant splicing of the AR mRNA (Hellwinkel *et al.* 1999; 2001). However, as aberrant splicing can be partial and thus enable expression of the wild-type AR, the AIS phenotype is not necessarily CAIS but may also present with PAIS (Hellwinkel *et al.* 2001). The most common molecular defects of the *AR* gene are missense mutations. They may either result in CAIS or in PAIS because of complete or partial loss of AR

function (Hiort *et al.* 1996). Mutations within the LBD may alter androgen binding but may in addition influence dimerization due to disruption of N–C-terminal structural interactions. Mutations within the DNA-binding domain can affect receptor binding to target DNA. To date, only one patient with complete AIS without an *AR* gene mutation but with clear experimental evidence for an AR-coactivator deficiency as the only underlying molecular mechanism of defective androgen action has been reported (Adachi *et al.* 2000). Cofactors of the AR will presumably play a pivotal role in the understanding of phenotypic variability in AIS. So far, only a few mechanisms contributing to the phenotypic diversity in AIS have been identified in affected individuals. A striking phenotypic variability in a family with partial AIS has been attributed to differential expression of the 5α-reductase type 2 enzyme in genital fibroblasts (Boehmer *et al.* 2001). Another mechanism may be the combination of varying androgen levels during early embryogenesis and partially inactivating mutations of the LBD (Holterhus *et al.* 2000).

Moreover, post-zygotic mutations of the *AR* gene resulting in a somatic mosaicism of mutant and wild-type *AR* genes can contribute to modulation of the phenotype. This can result in a higher degree of virilization than expected from the *AR* mutation alone because of the expression of the wild-type *AR* in a subset of somatic cells. Due to the fact that at least one-third of all de-novo mutations of the *AR* gene occur at the post-zygotic stage, this mechanism is not only important for phenotypic variability in AIS but also crucial for genetic counseling. All kinds of mutations, from missense to nonsense as well as frame shift and splice-site mutations have been identified in AIS patients with somatic mosaicism, and are associated with both PAIS and CAIS (Hiort *et al.* 1998; Holterhus *et al.* 1999; 2001; Kohler *et al.* 2005). Nevertheless, a substantial fraction of mosaic mutations may escape detection because of an unequal distribution of mutant vs. wild-type *AR* in various tissues of an individual. This may result in a low percentage of leukocytes with mutant *AR* that is undetectable by conventional Sanger sequencing.

3.4.4 Functional characterization of mutants in androgen insensitivity syndrome

Diagnosis of AIS is confirmed in most cases by molecular genetic analysis and the detection of aberrations in the *AR* gene. The impact of many mutations on AR function has already been proven (http://androgendb.mcgill.ca/), but the effect of new mutations on protein activity has to be established. Androgen receptor mutations are often recreated in mammalian expression vectors and cotransfected into an AR-negative mammalian cell line together with an androgen-responsive reporter gene. These assays are sensitive for many functions of the AR including hormone binding, protein stability, nuclear transport, DNA binding, or transcriptional activation. Impaired AR function results in reduced reporter gene expression when compared to a wild-type *AR* construct. Mutations associated with complete or severe forms of AIS often demonstrate a good genotype–phenotype correlation in these functional studies. This holds especially true for mutations that disrupt the highly structured LBD or DNA-binding domain, leading to severely impaired ligand or DNA-binding. However, for mutations associated with MAIS or less severe forms of PAIS, experimental evidence is often lacking or scarce.

This is due to the fact that, through different mutations within the AR, the reduced activation of androgen-dependent reporter genes can be highly variable. It depends on the type of mutation and its localization within the gene, but also on the promoter of the experimental target gene (Werner *et al.* 2006b). Furthermore, the conformational changes that will be induced by ligand-binding or chaperone interaction, the post-translational modifications, as well as the trafficking within the cell, and further molecular interaction may influence target gene activation. In particular the cell-dependent expression of coactivators and co-repressors of the AR might modulate the cellular androgen response in a very distinct and highly specific manner (Bebermeier *et al.* 2006). Therefore, the use of different reporter genes and cell lines may be necessary to prove the pathogenicity of a new variation. Detailed functional analysis of distinct features of the mutant AR, such as ligand-binding assays, N–C-terminal interaction assays, EMSA (electrophoretic mobility shift assay) or nuclear localization assays may provide a more pronounced effect on AR function, and support the pathogenic role of a mutation.

The elucidation of androgen-regulated genes is of utmost importance to understand the androgen-dependent cell regulation and, hence, the physiology and pathophysiology of sexual differentiation.

Employing genome-wide analysis in genital skin fibroblasts from patients with complete AIS compared to 46,XY male reference cells, distinct androgen-regulated gene profiles could be assessed which correlated to the genital phenotype (Holterhus *et al.* 2003). In peripheral blood monocytes a different, but also distinct androgen-dependent expression, was verified (Holterhus *et al.* 2009). These patterns were independent of the current endocrine status, but rather reflected an embryonal androgen influence on cell development. This proves that androgens lead to a "fingerprint" of gene expression patterns, which are distinct for cell-type, possibly mirroring genital phenotype in all individuals. Detection of apolipoprotein D as a highly specific androgen-regulated gene in genital skin fibroblasts in response to incubation with DHT (Appari *et al.* 2009) is promising. Its use as a possible biomarker of androgen insensitivity, especially in those patients where a mutation in the *AR* gene cannot be detected, remains to be proved.

3.5 The role of CAG repeat polymorphisms of the androgen receptor in various target organs

3.5.1 Kennedy syndrome: a pathological expansion of the *AR* gene CAG repeats

Kennedy syndrome or X-linked spinal and bulbar muscular atrophy (XSBMA) is a rare inherited neurodegenerative disease characterized by progressive neuromuscular weakness caused by a loss of motor neurons in the brain stem and spinal cord. Disease onset, developing in the third to fifth decade of life, is likely to be preceded by muscular cramps on exertion, tremor of the hands and elevated muscle creatine kinase (Kennedy *et al.* 1968). The initial description of one of the individuals affected with Kennedy syndrome also contains information about gynecomastia, a hypoandrogenic symptom (Kennedy *et al.* 1968). Subsequent reports emphasized the presence of symptoms indicating the development of androgen insensitivity in men with XSBMA, exhibiting varying degrees of gynecomastia, testicular atrophy, disorders of spermatogenesis, elevated serum gonadotropins and also diabetes mellitus (e.g. Arbizu *et al.* 1983). Thus, the *AR* was regarded as a candidate gene for XSBMA, and the expansion of the polyglutamine repeat within the N-terminal region was further recognized as the cause (La Spada *et al.* 1991). The longer the CAG repeat in the *AR* gene, the earlier the onset of the disease is observed and the more severe are the symptoms of hypoandrogenicity (Doyu *et al.* 1992; Choong and Wilson 1998; Mariotti *et al.* 2000; Dejager *et al.* 2002). The absence of any neuromuscular deficit or degeneration in patients with complete androgen insensitivity (CAIS) (Quigley *et al.* 1995) suggests that neurological deficits in XBSMA are not caused by a lack of androgen influence but rather by a neurotoxic effect associated with the pathologically elongated number of CAG repeats, which causes irregular processing of the AR protein and accumulation of end-products (Abdullah *et al.* 1998).

3.5.2 An animal model of the human CAG repeat polymorphism

A "humanized" mouse model of the *AR* gene (CAG)n directly assessed the functional significance of the *AR* gene (CAG)n: the mouse AR was converted to the human sequence by germline gene targeting, introducing alleles with 12, 21 or 48 (CAG)n. The three "humanized" AR mouse lines revealed markedly different seminal vesicle weights indicating androgen effects, despite similar serum testosterone concentrations. Molecular analysis of AR-dependent target gene expression demonstrated Nkx3.1 and clusterin mRNAs to be modulated by the number of (CAG)n in the prostate probasin. Crossed with transgenic-adenocarcinoma-of-mouse-prostate mice, genotype-dependent differences in prostate cancer prevalence were observed (Albertelli *et al.* 2006). This confirms findings of *AR* gene (CAG)n expression in human prostate cancer cells (Coutinho-Camillo *et al.* 2006).

3.5.3 Ethnic differences

The normal range of CAG repeats is 9 to 37, and follows a normal, slightly skewed distribution towards the higher number of triplets (Edwards *et al.* 1992; Platz *et al.* 2000; Hsing *et al.* 2000a; Kuhlenbäumer *et al.* 2001), and symptoms related to XBSMA seem to start at 38 to 40 CAG repeats (Pioro *et al.* 1994). Within the normal range of the AR polyglutamine stretch, significant differences between ethnic groups have been observed. For healthy men of African descent the mean number of CAG repeats ranges between 18 and 20 (Edwards *et al.* 1992; Platz *et al.* 2000) and seems to be even shorter in certain African

subpopulations (Kittles *et al.* 2001). In healthy Caucasians the mean number of CAG repeats is 21 to 22 (Edwards *et al.* 1992; Platz *et al.* 2000), while in East Asians a mean of 22–23 triplets is found (Hsing *et al.* 2000a; Platz *et al.* 2000; van Houten and Gooren 2000; Wang *et al.* 2001). These differences can possibly be held responsible for some variations in androgen-dependent diseases and features which are observed among different ethnicities; for example beard growth or rate of prostate cancer.

3.5.4 Prostate development and malignancy

The prostate is an androgen-regulated organ (see Chapter 13). A substantial difference exists in the incidence of prostate cancer between ethnic groups, with African Americans having a 20- to 30-fold higher incidence than East Asians (Hsing *et al.* 2000b). Such disparity cannot be explained entirely by screening bias in different populations. Also after multiple adjustments for ethnic and screening differences, a significant contrast in incidence rates between African Americans, Caucasians and Asians is found (Ross *et al.* 1998; Platz *et al.* 2000).

It can be assumed that a polymorphism of the *AR* with the capacity to modulate androgen effects has an influence on the fate of malignant cells in the prostate. Thus, with shorter CAG repeats, an earlier onset of the disease would be observed, as well as an association with aggressiveness of the tumor. Investigation of a younger study group would then lead to the supposition of an increased risk of developing prostate cancer. While this would hold true for a specific younger age group, it is likely that the effect cannot be observed when older men are also involved since the overall incidence of prostate cancer is high. Stratification for lifestyle factors and multidimensional matching of controls in a sufficient number of subjects is a prerequisite for relevant investigations: this is best met by eight studies (Giovannucci *et al.* 1997; Stanford *et al.* 1997; Platz *et al.* 1998; Correa-Cerro *et al.* 1999; Hsing *et al.* 2000a; Beilin *et al.* 2001; Latil *et al.* 2001; Balic *et al.* 2002). Seven of these described an independent contribution of the CAG repeat polymorphism to prostate cancer: either to the age of onset or to the general risk of development. The age of the study group, time point and intensity of diagnostic performance varying with the location of the study most likely influence the result as to whether it is seen as earlier onset or higher risk. The putative association with disease stage is also likely to be influenced by such factors. Each triplet may hence account for a 3 to 14% risk for prostate cancer (Stanford *et al.* 1997). In conclusion, it is likely that the genesis of prostate cancer cells is not induced by androgens, but that stronger androgenicity induced by ARs with shorter polyglutamine stretches contributes to a faster development of these cells, and this might be seen either as earlier onset of or as higher risk for prostate cancer, depending on the age of the study group.

Epidemiological findings in research on the incidence of prostate cancer in humans confirm an influence of the *AR* gene (CAG)n polymorphism: a meta-analysis described an odds ratio of 1.19 for prostate cancer with decreasing (CAG)n (Zeegers *et al.* 2004). The modulatory effect on androgen-dependent gene transcription is described to be linear and obviously mediated by a differential affinity of coactivator proteins to the polyglutamine stretch (e.g. ARA24 and p160) (Hsiao *et al.* 1999; Irvine *et al.* 2000).

Another aspect is the putative relation between BPH and the CAG repeat polymorphism of the *AR* gene. BPH consists of the overgrowth of tissue within the transition zone and periurethral area of the prostate. This is histologically defined as epithelial and fibromuscular hyperplasia (Price *et al.* 1990). One factor modulating androgenic exposure is the cellular level of androgens, particularly DHT. The influence of the CAG repeat polymorphism causes variations in such effects as demonstrated by several studies. The two largest studies comparing matched healthy controls ($n = 1041$ and $n = 499$) and BPH patients ($n = 310$ and $n = 449$) described the odds ratio for BPH surgery or an enlarged prostate gland to be 1.92 ($p = 0.0002$) when comparing CAG repeat length of 19 or less to 25 or more. For a six-repeat decrement in CAG repeat length, the odds ratio for moderate or severe urinary obstructive symptoms from an enlarged prostate gland was 3.62 ($p = 0.004$) (Giovannucci *et al.* 1999a;1999b). Similarly, adenoma size was found to be inversely associated with the number of CAG repeats in 176 patients vs. 41 controls (Mitsumori *et al.* 1999). Prostate growth during androgen substitution is also significantly modified by the CAG repeat polymorphism (see below).

3.5.5 Reproductive functions

Stimulation of Sertoli cells by FSH is a prerequisite in primate spermatogenesis, and intratesticular androgen

activity represents an important cofactor that takes positive effect on the supporting function of Sertoli cells. Thus, it can be speculated that the CAG repeat polymorphism within the *AR* gene could have a limited influence on spermatogenesis. Such an effect can be observed as severely impaired spermatogenesis in XSBMA patients (Arbizu *et al.* 1983). The investigation of the possible influence of a polyglutamine stretch of within the normal length on sperm production requires a sample of carefully selected patients in which significant confounders (obstructive symptoms due to infections, congenital aplasia of the vas deferens (CBAVD), impaired spermatogenesis due to hormone disorders, deletions in one of the azoospermia-associated regions of the Y chromosome) have been ruled out.

Control groups consisting of healthy fertile males should be homogenous in terms of ethnic origin (see above). It should be considered that within the cohort of fertile controls, sperm densities below 20 million/ml might occur (Rajpert-De Meyts *et al.* 2002). Unfortunately, a fraction of studies on this subject did not exclude the above-described patients strictly enough. Therefore, it is not surprising that conflicting results emerged when infertile and fertile men were compared in regard to their number of CAG repeats. Some studies reported higher numbers of CAG triplets in infertile men (Tut *et al.* 1997; Legius *et al.* 1999; Dowsing *et al.* 1999; Yoshida *et al.* 1999; Yong *et al.* 2000; Mifsud *et al.* 2001; Patrizio *et al.* 2001; Wallerand *et al.* 2001; Mengual *et al.* 2003), but some did not (Lundberg-Giwercman *et al.* 1998; Dadze *et al.* 2000; Sasagawa *et al.* 2001; van Golde *et al.* 2002; Rajpert-De Meyts *et al.* 2002). A more recent meta-analysis involving 33 reports provides support for an association between increased *AR* gene CAG length and idiopathic male infertility; suggesting that even subtle disruptions in the androgen axis may compromise male fertility (Davis-Dao *et al.* 2007).

When only fertile men covering the whole range of normal sperm concentrations were involved in evaluations, a shorter CAG repeat tract was associated with higher sperm numbers (von Eckardstein *et al.* 2001; Rajpert-De Meyts *et al.* 2002). Nevertheless, a marked variation of sperm density in relation to the *AR* polymorphism was observed. Hence, spermatogenesis is likely to be influenced by the number of CAG repeats within the normal range, but whether this reaches relevance for individuals remains doubtful. The range of sperm concentrations leading to infertility is most likely reached at CAG repeat numbers that are associated with XSBMA. Furthermore, it can be assumed that the proportion of men with longer CAG repeats among infertile patients may, in the case of strict selection criteria excluding all known causes of infertility, appear higher than in a control population. Genetic counseling concerning inheritability of this modulator of spermatogenesis is of very restricted value, since the CAG polymorphism is located on the X chromosome and the specific tract length will affect spermatogenesis of the offspring only as early as in one half of the grandsons.

3.5.6   Bone tissue

Polymorphisms of the estrogen receptor (ER) have repeatedly been demonstrated to modulate quantity and quality of bone tissue in healthy men (e.g. Sapir-Koren *et al.* 2001). As androgen activity influences bone metabolism (see Chapter 8), these observations apply to the CAG repeat polymorphism in the *AR* gene as well: in 110 healthy younger males, a high number of CAG repeats was significantly associated with lower bone density (Zitzmann *et al.* 2001a). This result is corroborated by a negative association between *AR* CAG repeat length and bone density at the femoral neck in a group of 508 Caucasian men aged over 65 years (Zmuda *et al.* 2000a). The same workgroup also observed a more pronounced bone loss at the hip and increased vertebral fracture risk among older men with longer *AR* CAG repeat length (Zmuda *et al.* 2000b). In a group of 140 Finnish men aged 50–60 years, lumbar and femoral bone mineral density values were higher in those men with shorter CAG repeats in comparison to those with longer CAG repeats (Remes *et al.* 2003). The differences reach statistical significance when the groups with CAG repeat length of 15–17 and 22–26 are compared directly. In contrast, in a group of 273 healthy Belgian men aged 71 and 86 years, no influence of the androgen receptor gene polymorphism was seen (Van Pottelbergh *et al.* 2001).

Higher androgenization will lead to higher peak bone mass (Khosla 2002); thus, the *AR* polymorphism effects on bone density are likely to be visible among healthy younger males, while the difference could be mitigated by the overall age-dependent bone loss and may be no longer visible in old men, in whom confounders have exerted influence on bone tissue. Thus, the longer the CAG repeat in the *AR* gene, the lower

peak bone density in males will be, while it is inconclusive whether this effect reaches clinical significance in terms of higher fracture risk.

It has been demonstrated in a larger cohort of soldiers that, even in healthy younger men, shorter *AR* gene CAG repeats may be preventive of stress fractures: Smaller-sized (< 16) *AR* CAG repeats were more prevalent among control subjects (23%) than among patients (13%); the risk for having stress fracture was almost halved if the size of the repeat was shorter than 16 repeats (Yanovich *et al.* 2011).

In women, low androgen levels and, hence, low activation of the AR are present. In addition, two alleles of the *AR* gene will cause an effect less clear in terms of influence exerted by the CAG repeat polymorphism. Nevertheless, reports concerning such impact on bone density in women exist (Sowers *et al.* 1999; Chen *et al.* 2003). As can be expected from physiology, the *AR* polymorphism does not influence the effects of hormone replacement therapy by estrogens on bone tissue in postmenopausal women (Salmen *et al.* 2003).

In addition, the CAG repeat polymorphism affects body composition in young men: absolute muscle (thigh) and (lower) trunk increase as CAG(n) decreases. Expressed relatively, muscle areas and lean body mass increase, while fat mass decreases as CAG (n) decreases. The polymorphism does not affect deep adipose tissues or circulating androgen levels in young men (Nielsen *et al.* 2010).

3.5.7   Cardiovascular risk factors

Testosterone plays an ambiguous role in relation to cardiovascular risk factors, and its respective role has not been fully resolved (see Chapter 10). The interactions between the CAG repeat polymorphism, serum levels of sex hormones, lifestyle factors and endothelium-dependent and independent vessel relaxation of the brachial artery, as well as lipoprotein levels, leptin and insulin concentrations and body composition were described in over 100 eugonadal men of a homogenous population. In agreement with previously demonstrated androgen effects on these parameters, it was demonstrated that androgenic effects were attenuated in persons with longer CAG repeats, while testosterone levels themselves played only a minor role within the eugonadal range. A marked increased prevalence of the metabolic syndrome in older men was seen in those patients with longer CAG repeats than average (Stanworth *et al.* 2008).

Significant positive correlations with the length of CAG repeats were seen for endothelial-dependent vasodilatation, HDL-cholesterol concentrations, body fat content, insulin and leptin levels. These results remained stable in multiple regression analyses correcting for age and lifestyle factors. It was demonstrated by a five-factor model that adverse and beneficial components are mutually dependent (Zitzmann et al. 2001b; 2003a). Within the investigated range of androgen-related cardiovascular risk factors and eugonadal testosterone levels, the CAG repeat polymorphism could play a more dominant role than testosterone itself. Concerning lipid concentrations, corresponding results are reported in men with XSBMA (Dejager et al. 2002). Also in agreement, an inclination to develop diabetes mellitus has been described for these patients (Arbizu et al. 1983). Hence, adverse or beneficial effects of a longer or shorter CAG repeat chain in regard to cardiovascular risk will most likely strongly depend on cofactors. The implications in terms of modulation of cardiovascular risk by androgens apply especially to hypogonadal men receiving testosterone substitution. The pharmacogenetic role in this respect of the CAG repeat polymorphism has yet to be elucidated.

3.5.8   Psychological implications

Testosterone substitution in hypogonadal men improves lethargic or depressive aspects of mood significantly (Burris et al. 1992). Studies exploring the relationship between gonadal function and depressive episodes demonstrated testosterone levels to be markedly decreased in these patients (Unden et al. 1988; Schweiger et al. 1999; Barrett-Connor et al. 1999). Accordingly, treatment with testosterone gel may improve symptoms in men with refractory depression (Pope et al. 2003). The age-dependent decline of testosterone levels is sometimes associated with symptoms of depression. It has been recently demonstrated in 1000 older men that this mood dependency on androgen levels is modified by the CAG repeat polymorphism of the AR gene. Depression scores were significantly and inversely associated with testosterone levels in subjects with shorter CAG repeats, while this was not observed in men with moderate and longer polyglutamine stretches in the AR protein. Low versus high testosterone in such men was associated with a fivefold increased likelihood of depressive mood (Seidman et al. 2001). It can

be speculated that the higher activation rate of the AR in this subgroup revealed effects of declining androgen levels more readily than in subgroups with longer CAG repeats.

In a sample of 172 Finnish men aged 41 to 70 years, the length of CAG repeats was significantly, and independently of testosterone levels, positively associated with symptom scores concerning depression, as expressed by the wish to be dead ($r = 0.45$; $p < 0.0001$), depressed mood ($r = 0.23$; $p = 0.003$), anxiety ($r = 0.15$; $p < 0.05$), deterioration of general well-being ($r = 0.22$; $p = 0.004$) and also decreased beard growth ($r = 0.49$; $p < 0.0001$) (Harkonen et al. 2003). This was later confirmed by a large epidemiological trial involving patients from both psychological and andrological care units in comparison to healthy controls: scores of the Aging Male Symptom Score as well as Depression Scales were markedly elevated in subjects with both lower testosterone concentrations and longer CAG repeats (Schneider et al. 2011a; 2011b).

Another aspect of psychological parameters is represented by the group of externalizing behaviors; these are predominantly found in males and have been associated with androgens (Zitzmann and Nieschlag 2001). The personality traits are attention deficit hyperactivity disorder (ADHD); conduct disorder (CD) and oppositional defiant disorder (ODD). A controlled study in 302 younger men concerning these disorders in relation to the CAG repeat of the AR gene demonstrated a significantly higher prevalence in genotypes with shorter repeat chains. The group also reported an association of short CAG repeats in the AR gene with novelty-seeking behavior (drug abuse, pathological gambling) (Comings et al. 1999).

Confirmingly, in a sample of 183 healthy Swedish men aged 20–75 years, associations of CAG repeat length and scores in the Karolinska Scales of Personality were described. Tendencies indicated positive relationships between shorter CAG trinucleotide repeats and personality scales connected to dominance and aggression (low "Lack of Assertiveness"; high "Verbal Aggression"; high "Monotony Avoidance"). Longer polyglutamine tracts were associated with some neuroticism-related personality scales: high "Muscular Tension," high "Lack of Assertiveness" and high "Psychasthenia" (Jönsson et al. 2001).

In addition, there exists a case report of three Caucasian brothers with mental retardation especially demonstrating a delay in speech development, shy but sometimes aggressive behavior, marfanoid habitus and relatively large testes in combination with abnormally short CAG repeats (eight triplets) (Kooy *et al.* 1999).

3.5.9   Hair growth

Male pattern baldness is described by a loss of scalp hair and affects up to 80% of males by the age of 80 years. A balding scalp is caused by androgens and expression of the AR in the respective hair follicle, and is thus known as androgenetic alopecia (see Chapter 7). One can assume that the influence of the CAG repeat polymorphism on androgenicity causes a variation of androgenetic alopecia. In men with such a clinical condition, significantly shorter CAG repeats were described in comparison to controls by two studies (Sawaya and Shalita 1998; Ellis *et al.* 2001). Thus, the CAG repeat polymorphism is likely to play a role in modulation of androgen influence on male hair pattern, but since statistical significance is weak in a reasonable number of patients due to high interindividual variability, the cosmetic consequence for the individual is questionable.

3.5.10   Pharmacogenetics and hypotheses

Considering the observations in eugonadal men, one can assume that testosterone therapy in hypogonadal men should have a differential impact on androgen target tissue, depending on the number of CAG repeats. In a longitudinal pharmacogenetic study in 131 hypogonadal men, prostate volume was assessed before and under androgen substitution. The length of CAG repeats, sex hormone levels and anthropometric measures were considered. Initial prostate size of hypogonadal men was dependent on age and baseline testosterone levels, but not the CAG repeat polymorphism. However, when prostate size increased significantly during therapy, prostate growth per year and absolute prostate size under substituted testosterone levels were strongly dependent on the *AR* polymorphism, with lower treatment effects in patients with longer repeats. Other modulators of prostate growth were age and testosterone level under treatment. The odds ratio for men with repeats < 20, compared to those with $\geq$ 20, to develop a prostate size of at least 30 ml under testosterone substitution was 8.7 (95% confidence interval (CI) 3.1–24.3; $p <$ 0.001). This first pharmacogenetic study on androgen substitution in hypogonadal men demonstrates a marked influence of the CAG repeat polymorphism on prostate growth (Zitzmann *et al.* 2003b).

Another retrospective approach concerning pharmacogenetic influences in hormonal male contraception demonstrated, as spermatogenesis is partially dependent on intratesticular androgen activity, sperm counts to be more easily suppressed by various pharmacological regimens in men with longer CAG repeats in the subgroup with remnant gonadotropin activity (von Eckardstein *et al.* 2002).

Testosterone levels within the normal range will more or less saturate the androgen receptors present, and it has been demonstrated that androgenic effects will reach a plateau at certain levels, which are probably tissue specific (Zitzmann *et al.* 2002a; 2002b). In agreement with this, a study applying exponentially increasing doses of testosterone to hypogonadal men shows corresponding results (Bhasin *et al.* 2001): androgen effects on various parameters increased linearly with the logarithm of testosterone levels and linearly with the logarithm of the testosterone dose. In practice, this means more or less a plateau effect. Significant increments of androgenic effects caused by rising testosterone levels within the eugonadal range are seen only when the normal range is left and clearly supraphysiological levels are reached. Therefore, it can be assumed that within the range of such a plateau of saturation, genetically determined functional differences in androgen receptor activity can be best observed; while in a condition of hypogonadism, androgenicity will be strongly dependent on androgen levels themselves, as binding to and, hence, activation of androgen receptors will increase until saturation is reached (Fig. 3.3). This model explains why androgen effects are found between hypo- and eugonadal men but can often not be confirmed for various testosterone levels within the eugonadal range. During substitution therapy of hypogonadal men, both effects on androgenicity – increment of testosterone levels from the hypo-into the eugonadal range and modulation of androgen effects within the eugonadal range by the androgen receptor polymorphism – have to be taken into account.

Studies examining the effects of the *AR* gene (CAG)n polymorphism have to consider androgen levels for a proper description of clinical relevance, because involving hypogonadal men will distort results owing to lack of sufficient ligand binding, hence, activation of the AR. Similarly, not considering testosterone levels, possibly compensating for the

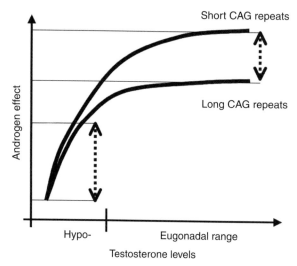

Fig. 3.3 Hypothetical model of androgen effects: within the hypogonadal range, and in comparison to the eugonadal range, differences in androgen effects are determined by testosterone levels. Within the eugonadal range, androgen effects depend rather on the AR polymorphism. As this effect depends on the presence of AR coactivators, the concentrations of which are tissue specific, the shapes of the curves are putatively variable from organ to organ.

effects of the (CAG)n polymorphism, takes an incomplete approach. When examining the effects of androgens, regression models are required to include both testosterone concentrations and the length of the *AR* gene CAG repeat polymorphism. In this light, a recent study in a large cohort of aging men did not demonstrate a relationship of the *AR* gene CAG repeat polymorphism to the risk of heart disease, possibly due to the fact that serum testosterone concentrations were not considered (Page *et al.* 2006).

The weaker androgen action induced by longer (CAG)n will also affect the feedback mechanism of the hypothalamic-pituitary-gonadal (HPG) axis. In healthy men, longer (CAG)n will usually provoke higher LH secretion (Zitzmann *et al.* 2001b; Stanworth *et al.* 2008; Huhtaniemi *et al.* 2009). This can, in persons with intact and fully responsive Leydig cell capacity, result in higher concentrations of testosterone and, hence, compensation of weaker androgen action. As a result of higher testosterone concentrations, its aromatization product estradiol will also be present in higher amounts (Huhtaniemi *et al.* 2009). Such higher estradiol concentrations in these men with intact HPG regulation or feedback mechanisms can even

lead to enhanced effects in estrogen-dependent tissues, such as bones (Limer *et al.* 2009).

However, investigation of men with an intact HPG axis does not focus on the clinically relevant clientele: those men with symptoms of androgen deficiency, those men with disturbances of the HPG axis. Such disorders can be of a milder nature, as seen in late-onset hypogonadism (LOH) (Wang *et al.* 2008) or subjects with the metabolic syndrome (Shabsigh *et al.* 2008), conditions in which both pituitary function and Leydig cell capacity are impaired. In case of longer (CAG)n, these men will present with inadequately low-normal LH concentrations and/or low-normal testosterone levels, but, nevertheless, will require higher concentrations of testosterone to compensate for their attenuated androgen action. Thus, they are likely to present with features of hypogonadism in the presence of normal testosterone levels (Canale *et al.* 2005). Exactly this is the patient group most likely missed for investigation, diagnostics and putative treatment up to this day.

In the case of "classical" hypogonadism (i.e. the (almost) complete breakdown of the HPG axis due to causes of primary or secondary origin), testosterone levels are low and patients require substitution. The findings in men with intact HPG axes demonstrate that men with longer (CAG)n require higher testosterone concentrations for normal androgen action in comparison to men with shorter (CAG)n (Huhtaniemi *et al.* 2009). Thus, hypogonadal persons with longer (CAG)n will then, as do their healthy counterparts, need higher testosterone levels (and, hence, higher testosterone doses) to compensate for mitigated androgen action. Correspondingly, persons with rather short (CAG)n will need lower doses of testosterone substitution in the case of hypogonadism.

3.6 Outlook

Further decoding of the molecular and biochemical pathways is necessary for a comprehensive understanding of normal and abnormal sexual determination and differentiation. Based on the known molecular defects of impaired human sexual development, recent achievements in the field of functional genomics and proteomics offer unique opportunities to identify the genetic programs downstream of these pathways, which are ultimately responsible for structure and function of a normal or abnormal genital phenotype. Hopefully this knowledge will lead to better

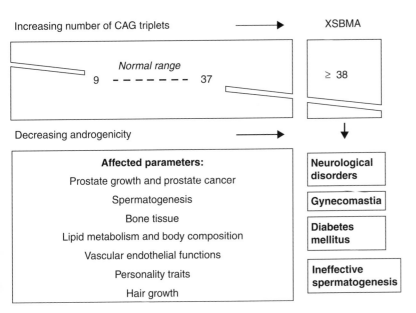

Increasing number of CAG triplets ⟶ XSBMA

Normal range
9 – – – – – – 37   ≥ 38

Decreasing androgenicity ⟶

Affected parameters:
Prostate growth and prostate cancer
Spermatogenesis
Bone tissue
Lipid metabolism and body composition
Vascular endothelial functions
Personality traits
Hair growth

Neurological disorders

Gynecomastia

Diabetes mellitus

Ineffective spermatogenesis

Fig. 3.4 The inverse association between the number of CAG repeats in the *AR* gene and functionality of the AR protein. Longer CAG tracts result in lower transcription of target genes and, thus, lower androgenicity. Expansion of the encoded polyglutamine stretch to beyond probably 38 leads to the neuromuscular disorder X-linked spinal and bulbar muscular atrophy (XSBMA); a condition in which defective spermatogenesis and undervirilization are observed. Conversely, low numbers of CAG repeats are associated with increased androgenicity of susceptible tissues.

medical decisions in patients with androgen insensitivity due to AR defects, and will open pathways for the development of individual therapeutic options.

The highly polymorphic nature of glutamine residues within the AR protein, which is encoded by the CAG repeat polymorphism within the *AR* gene, causes a subtle gradation of androgenicity among individuals. This modulation of androgen effects may be small but continuously present during a man's lifetime, thus exerting effects that are measurable in many tissues as various degrees of androgenicity (Fig. 3.4). It remains to be seen whether these insights are important enough to become part of individually useful laboratory assessments. The pharmacogenetic implication of this polymorphism seems to play an important role as modulator of treatment effects in hypogonadal men. Further studies are required to decide whether these insights should sublimate into individualized aspects of testosterone therapy; for example adaptation of dosage or surveillance intervals.

3.7 Key messages

- Androgen insensitivity has a very variable phenotypic appearance and may be clinically undistinguishable from defects of androgen biosynthesis during childhood.

- During childhood, laboratory analysis is often difficult and lacks specificity and sensitivity.
- In adolescence and adulthood, diagnosis of androgen insensitivity can be made on the grounds of undermasculinization and/or feminization despite high measurable androgen levels.
- Molecular genetic analysis of the androgen receptor gene can detect a relevant mutation only in a subset of patients. The less severe the phenotype, the less likely is the chance of demonstrating a mutation.
- Highly specific tools for early and specific detection of androgen receptor abnormalities must be developed.
- High-throughput analysis is needed to elucidate genetic alterations in factors leading to androgen insensitivity without mutation of the androgen receptor.
- Future research should evolve model systems to better elucidate individualized genotype–phenotype correlations.
- The characterization of other factors of androgen-controlled genital development is mandatory for further insight into the cellular and time-dependent events of androgen action and to define further mechanisms of androgen insensitivity.

- The CAG repeat polymorphism in exon 1 of the AR gene modulates androgen effects: longer triplets attenuate testosterone effects.

- The pharmacogenetic implications of this polymorphism are likely to play a significant role in future testosterone treatment of hypogonadal men.

3.8 References

Abdullah A, Trifiro MA, Panet-Raymond V, Alvarado C, de Tourreil S, Frankel D, Schipper HM, Pinsky L (1998) Spinobulbar muscular atrophy: polyglutamine-expanded androgen receptor is proteolytically resistant in vitro and processed abnormally in transfected cells. *Hum Mol Genet* 7:379–384

Adachi M, Takayanagi R, Tomura A, Imasaki K, Kato S, Goto K, Yanase T, Ikuyama S, Nawata H (2000) Androgen-insensitivity syndrome as a possible coactivator disease. *N Engl J Med* 343:856–862

Ahmed SF, Achermann JC, Arlt W, Balen A, Conway G, Edwards Z, Elford S, Hughes IA, Izatt L, Krone N, Miles H, O'Toole S, Perry L, Sanders C, Simmonds M, Michael Wallace A, Watt A, Willis D (2011) UK guidance on the initial evaluation of an infant or an adolescent with a suspected disorder of sex development. *Clin Endocrinol (Oxf)* 75:12–26

Aiman J, Griffin JE, Gazak JM, Wilson JD, MacDonald PC (1979) Androgen insensitivity as a cause of infertility in otherwise normal men. *N Engl J Med* 300:223–227

Albertelli MA, Scheller A, Brogley M, Robins DM (2006) Replacing the mouse androgen receptor with human alleles demonstrates glutamine tract length-dependent effects on physiology and tumorigenesis in mice. *Mol Endocrinol* 20:1248–1260

Andersson S, Berman DM, Jenkins EP, Russell DW (1991) Deletion of steroid 5 alpha-reductase 2 gene in male pseudohermaphroditism. *Nature* 354:159–161

Appari M, Werner R, Wunsch L, Cario G, Demeter J, Hiort O, Riepe FJ, Holterhus PM (2009) Apolipoprotein D (APOD) is a putative biomarker of androgen receptor function in androgen insensitivity syndrome. *J Mol Med* 87:623–632

Arbizu T, Santamaria J, Gomez JM, Quilez A, Serra JP (1983) A family with adult onset spinal and bulbar muscular atrophy X-linked inheritance and associated testicular failure. *J Neurol Sci* 59:371–382

Balic I, Graham ST, Troyer DA, Higgins BA, Pollock BH, Johnson-Pais TL, Thompson IM, Leach RJ (2002) Androgen receptor length polymorphism associated with prostate cancer risk in Hispanic men. *J Urol* 168:2245–2248

Barrett-Connor E, von Mühlen DG, Kritz-Silverstein D (1999) Bioavailable testosterone and depressed mood in older men: the Rancho Bernardo Study. *J Clin Endocr Metab* 84:573–577

Barsoum IB, Yao HH (2010) Fetal Leydig cells: progenitor cell maintenance and differentiation. *J Androl* 31:11–15

Barsoum IB, Bingham NC, Parker KL, Jorgensen JS, Yao HH (2009) Activation of the Hedgehog pathway in the mouse fetal ovary leads to ectopic appearance of fetal Leydig cells and female pseudohermaphroditism. *Dev Biol* 329:96–103

Bebermeier JH, Brooks JD, Deprimo SE, Werner R, Deppe U, Demeter J, Hiort O, Holterhus PM (2006) Cell-line and tissue-specific signatures of androgen receptor-coregulator transcription. *J Mol Med* 84:919–931

Beilin J, Harewood L, Frydenberg M, Mameghan H, Martyres RF, Farish SJ, Yue C, Deam DR, Byron KA, Zajac JD (2001) A case-control study of the androgen receptor gene CAG repeat polymorphism in Australian prostate carcinoma subjects. *Cancer* 92:941–949

Bhasin S, Woodhouse L, Casaburi R, Singh AB, Bhasin D, Berman N, Chen X, Yarasheski KE, Magliano L, Dzekov C, Dzekov J, Bross R, Phillips J, Sinha-Hikim I, Shen R, Storer TW (2001) Testosterone dose-response relationships in healthy young men. *Am J Physiol Endocrinol Metab* 281:1172–1181

Bhatia-Gaur R, Donjacour AA, Sciavolino PJ, Kim M, Desai N, Young P, Norton CR, Gridley T, Cardiff RD, Cunha GR, Abate-Shen C, Shen MM (1999) Roles for Nkx3.1 in prostate development and cancer. *Genes Dev* 13:966–977

Bieberich CJ, Fujita K, He WW, Jay G (1996) Prostate-specific and androgen-dependent expression of a novel homeobox gene. *J Biol Chem* 271:31779–31782

Boehmer AL, Brinkmann O, Bruggenwirth H, van Assendelft C, Otten BJ, Verleun-Mooijman MC, Niermeijer MF, Brunner HG, Rouwe CW, Waelkens JJ, Oostdijk W, Kleijer WJ, van der Kwast TH, de Vroede MA, Drop SL (2001) Genotype versus phenotype in families with androgen insensitivity syndrome. *J Clin Endocrinol Metab* 86:4151–4160

Boukari K, Meduri G, Brailly-Tabard S, Guibourdenche J, Ciampi ML, Massin N, Martinerie L, Picard JY, Rey R, Lombes M, Young J (2009) Lack of androgen receptor expression in Sertoli cells accounts for the absence of anti-Mullerian hormone repression during early human testis development. *J Clin Endocrinol Metab* 94:1818–1825

Bouvattier C, Carel JC, Lecointre C, David A, Sultan C, Bertrand AM, Morel Y, Chaussain JL (2002) Postnatal changes of T, LH, and FSH in 46,XY infants with mutations in the AR gene. *J Clin Endocrinol Metab* **87**:29–32

Bullejos M, Koopman P (2001) Spatially dynamic expression of Sry in mouse genital ridges. *Dev Dyn* **221**:201–205

Burris AS, Banks SM, Carter CS, Davidson JM, Sherins RJ (1992) A long-term prospective study of the physiologic and behavioural effects of hormone replacement in untreated hypogonadal men. *J Androl* **13**:297–304

Canale D, Caglieresi C, Moschini C, Liberati CD, Macchia E, Pinchera A, Martino E (2005) Androgen receptor polymorphism (CAG repeats) and androgenicity. *Clin Endocrinol (Oxf)* **63**:356–361

Chamberlain NL, Driver ED, Miesfeld RL (1994) The length and location of CAG trinucleotide repeats in the androgen receptor N-terminal domain affect transactivation function. *Nucleic Acids Res* **22**:3181–3186

Chamberlain NL, Whitacre DC, Miesfeld RL (1996) Delineation of two distinct type 1 activation functions in the androgen receptor amino-terminal domain. *J Biol Chem* **271**:26772–26778

Chang CS, Kokontis J, Liao ST (1988) Molecular cloning of human and rat complementary DNA encoding androgen receptors. *Science* **240**:324–326

Chen HY, Chen WC, Wu MC, Tsai FJ, Tsai CH (2003) Androgen receptor (AR) gene microsatellite polymorphism in postmenopausal women: correlation to bone mineral density and susceptibility to osteoporosis. *Eur J Obstet Gynecol Reprod Biol* **107**:52–56

Choong CS, Wilson EM (1998) Trinucleotide repeats in the human androgen receptor: a molecular basis for disease. *J Mol Endocrinol* **21**:235–257

Claessens F, Verrijdt G, Schoenmakers E, Haelens A, Peeters B, Verhoeven G, Rombauts W (2001) Selective DNA binding by the androgen receptor as a mechanism for hormone-specific gene regulation. *J Steroid Biochem Mol Biol* **76**:23–30

Claessens F, Denayer S, Van Tilborgh N, Kerkhofs S, Helsen C, Haelens A (2008) Diverse roles of androgen receptor (AR) domains in AR-mediated signaling. *Nucl Recept Signal* **6**:e008

Comings DE, Chen C, Wu S, Muhleman D (1999) Association of the androgen receptor gene (AR) with ADHD and conduct disorder. *Neuroreport* **10**:1589–1592

Cools M, Wolffenbuttel KP, Drop SL, Oosterhuis JW, Looijenga LH (2011) Gonadal development and tumor formation at the crossroads of male and female sex determination. *Sex Dev* **5**:167–180

Correa-Cerro L, Wohr G, Haussler J, Berthon P, Drelon E, Mangin P, Fournier G, Cussenot O, Kraus P, Just W, Paiss T, Cantu JM, Vogel W (1999) (CAG)nCAA and GGN repeats in the human androgen receptor gene are not associated with prostate cancer in a French-German population. *Eur J Hum Gen* **7**:357–362

Coutinho-Camillo CM, Miracca EC, dos Santos ML, Salaorni S, Sarkis AS, Nagai MA (2006) Identification of differentially expressed genes in prostatic epithelium in relation to androgen receptor CAG repeat length. *Int J Biol Markers* **21**:96–105

Cutress ML, Whitaker HC, Mills IG, Stewart M, Neal DE (2008) Structural basis for the nuclear import of the human androgen receptor. *J Cell Sci* **121**:957–968

da Costa Rose Paulino M, Steinmetz L, Menezes Filho HC, Kuperman H, Della Manna T, Vieira JG, Blasbalg R, Baroni R, Setian N, Damiani D (2009) Search of prostatic tissue in 46,XX congenital adrenal hyperplasia. *Arq Bras Endocrinol Metabol* **53**:716–720

Dadze S, Wieland C, Jakubiczka S, Funke K, Schröder E, Royer-Pokora B, Willers R, Wieacker PF (2000) The size of the CAG repeat in exon 1 of the androgen receptor gene shows no significant relationship to impaired spermatogenesis in an infertile Caucasoid sample of German origin. *Mol Hum Reprod* **6**:207–214

Davis-Dao CA, Tuazon ED, Sokol RZ, Cortessis VK (2007) Male infertility and variation in CAG repeat length in the androgen receptor gene: a meta-analysis. *J Clin Endocrinol Metab* **92**:4319–4326

Dejager S, Bry-Gaillard H, Bruckert E, Eymard B, Salachas F, LeGuern E, Tardieu S, Chadarevian R, Giral P, Turpin G (2002) A comprehensive endocrine description of Kennedy's disease revealing androgen insensitivity linked to CAG repeat length. *J Clin Endocr Metab* **87**:3893–3901

Deslypere JP, Young M, Wilson JD, McPhaul MJ (1992) Testosterone and 5 alpha-dihydrotestosterone interact differently with the androgen receptor to enhance transcription of the MMTV-CAT reporter gene. *Mol Cell Endocrinol* **88**:15–22

Doehnert U, Bertelloni S, Richter-Unruh A, Werner R, Hiort O (2011) Hormone profiles in adolescents and adults with complete androgen insensitivity syndrome. In: Hiort O (ed) *3rd International Symposium on Disorders of Sex Development, Lübeck*. Book of abstracts, Universität zu Lübeck, Lübeck, Germany, p 57

Dowsing AT, Yong EL, Clark M, McLachlan RI, de Kretser DM, Trounson AO (1999) Linkage between male infertility and trinucleotide repeat expansion in the androgen-receptor gene. *Lancet* **354**:640–643

Doyu M, Sobue G, Mukai E, Kachi T, Yasuda T, Mitsuma T, Takahashi A (1992) Severity of X-linked recessive bulbospinal neuronopathy correlates with size of the tandem CAG repeat in androgen receptor gene. *Annals Neurol* **32**:707–710

Edwards A, Hammond HA, Jin L, Caskey CT, Chakraborty R (1992)

Genetic variation at five trimeric and tetrameric tandem repeat loci in four human population groups. *Genomics* 12:241–253

Ellis JA, Stebbing M, Harrap SB (2001) Polymorphism of the androgen receptor gene is associated with male pattern baldness. *J Invest Dermatol* 116:452–455

Giovannucci E, Stampfer MJ, Krithivas K, Brown M, Dahl D, Brufsky A, Talcott J, Hennekens CH, Kantoff PW (1997) The CAG repeat within the androgen receptor gene and its relationship to prostate cancer. *Proc Natl Acad Sci* 94:3320–3323

Giovannucci E, Stampfer MJ, Chan A, Krithivas K, Gann PH, Hennekens CH, Kantoff PW (1999a) CAG repeat within the androgen receptor gene and incidence of surgery for benign prostatic hyperplasia in U.S. physicians. *Prostate* 39:130–134

Giovannucci E, Platz EA, Stampfer MJ, Chan A, Krithivas K, Kawachi I, Willett WC, Kantoff PW (1999b) The CAG repeat within the androgen receptor gene and benign prostatic hyperplasia. *Urology* 53:121–125

Habert R, Lejeune H, Saez JM (2001) Origin, differentiation and regulation of fetal and adult Leydig cells. *Mol Cell Endocrinol* 179:47–74

Hacker A, Capel B, Goodfellow P, Lovell-Badge R (1995) Expression of Sry, the mouse sex determining gene. *Development* 121:1603–1614

Haelens A, Verrijdt G, Callewaert L, Christiaens V, Schauwaers K, Peeters B, Rombauts W, Claessens F (2003) DNA recognition by the androgen receptor: evidence for an alternative DNA-dependent dimerization, and an active role of sequences flanking the response element on transactivation. *Biochem J* 369:141–151

Hannema SE, Hughes IA (2007) Regulation of Wolffian duct development. *Horm Res* 67:142–151

Hannema SE, Scott IS, Rajpert-De Meyts E, Skakkebaek NE,

Coleman N, Hughes IA (2006) Testicular development in the complete androgen insensitivity syndrome. *J Pathol* 208:518–527

Haraguchi R, Mo R, Hui C, Motoyama J, Makino S, Shiroishi T, Gaffield W, Yamada G (2001) Unique functions of Sonic hedgehog signaling during external genitalia development. *Development* 128:4241–4250

Harkonen K, Huhtaniemi I, Makinen J, Hübler D, Irjala K, Koskenvuo M, Oettel M, Raitakari O, Saad F, Pollanen P (2003) The polymorphic androgen receptor gene CAG repeat pituitary-testicular function and andropausal symptoms in ageing men. *Int J Androl* 26:187–194

He B, Gampe RT Jr, Kole AJ, Hnat AT, Stanley TB, An G, Stewart EL, Kalman RI, Minges JT, Wilson EM (2004) Structural basis for androgen receptor interdomain and coactivator interactions suggests a transition in nuclear receptor activation function dominance. *Mol Cell* 16:425–438

Hellwinkel OJ, Bull K, Holterhus PM, Homburg N, Struve D, Hiort O (1999) Complete androgen insensitivity caused by a splice donor site mutation in intron 2 of the human androgen receptor gene resulting in an exon 2-lacking transcript with premature stop-codon and reduced expression. *J Steroid Biochem Mol Biol* 68:1–9

Hellwinkel OJ, Holterhus PM, Struve D, Marschke C, Homburg N, Hiort O (2001) A unique exonic splicing mutation in the human androgen receptor gene indicates a physiologic relevance of regular androgen receptor transcript variants. *J Clin Endocrinol Metab* 86:2569–2575

Hiort O, Sinnecker GH, Holterhus PM, Nitsche EM, Kruse K (1996) The clinical and molecular spectrum of androgen insensitivity syndromes. *Am J Med Genet* 63:218–222

Hiort O, Sinnecker GH, Holterhus PM, Nitsche EM, Kruse K (1998)

Inherited and de novo androgen receptor gene mutations: investigation of single-case families. *J Pediatr* 132:939–943

Hiort O, Holterhus PM, Horter T, Schulze W, Kremke B, Bals-Pratsch M, Sinnecker GH, Kruse K (2000) Significance of mutations in the androgen receptor gene in males with idiopathic infertility. *J Clin Endocrinol Metab* 85:2810–2815

Hiort O, Reinecke S, Thyen U, Jurgensen M, Holterhus PM, Schon D, Richter-Appelt H (2003) Puberty in disorders of somatosexual differentiation. *J Pediatr Endocrinol Metab* 16 (Suppl 2):297–306

Holterhus PM, Wiebel J, Sinnecker GH, Bruggenwirth HT, Sippell WG, Brinkmann AO, Kruse K, Hiort O (1999) Clinical and molecular spectrum of somatic mosaicism in androgen insensitivity syndrome. *Pediatr Res* 46:684–690

Holterhus PM, Sinnecker GH, Hiort O (2000) Phenotypic diversity and testosterone-induced normalization of mutant L712F androgen receptor function in a kindred with androgen insensitivity. *J Clin Endocrinol Metab* 85:3245–3250

Holterhus PM, Bruggenwirth HT, Brinkmann AO, Hiort O (2001) Post-zygotic mutations and somatic mosaicism in androgen insensitivity syndrome. *Trends Genet* 17:627–628

Holterhus PM, Hiort O, Demeter J, Brown PO, Brooks JD (2003) Differential gene-expression patterns in genital fibroblasts of normal males and 46,XY females with androgen insensitivity syndrome: evidence for early programming involving the androgen receptor. *Genome Biol* 4:R37

Holterhus PM, Deppe U, Werner R, Richter-Unruh A, Bebermeier JH, Wunsch L, Krege S, Schweikert HU, Demeter J, Riepe F, Hiort O, Brooks JD (2007) Intrinsic androgen-dependent gene expression patterns revealed by comparison of genital fibroblasts from normal males and individuals with complete and partial androgen insensitivity syndrome. *BMC Genomics* 8:376

Holterhus PM, Bebermeier JH, Werner R, Demeter J, Richter-Unruh A, Cario G, Appari M, Siebert R, Riepe F, Brooks JD, Hiort O (2009) Disorders of sex development expose transcriptional autonomy of genetic sex and androgen-programmed hormonal sex in human blood leukocytes. *BMC Genomics* 10:292

Hsiao PW, Lin DL, Nakao R, Chang C (1999) The linkage of Kennedy's neuron disease to ARA24, the first identified androgen receptor polyglutamine region-associated coactivator. *J Biol Chem* 274:20229–20234

Hsing AW, Gao YT, Wu G, Wang X, Deng J, Chen YL, Sesterhenn IA, Mostofi FK, Benichou J, Chang C (2000a) Polymorphic CAG and GGN repeat lengths in the androgen receptor gene and prostate cancer risk: a population-based case-control study in China. *Cancer Res* 60:5111–5116

Hsing AW, Tsao L, Devesa SS (2000b) International trends and patterns of prostate cancer incidence and mortality. *Int J Cancer* 85:60–67

Huang L, Pu Y, Hepps D, Danielpour D, Prins GS (2007) Posterior Hox gene expression and differential androgen regulation in the developing and adult rat prostate lobes. *Endocrinology* 148:1235–1245

Huhtaniemi IT, Pye SR, Limer KL, Thomson W, O'Neill TW, Platt H, Payne D, John SL, Jiang M, Boonen S, Borghs H, Vanderschueren D, Adams JE, Ward KA, Bartfai G, Casanueva F, Finn JD, Forti G, Giwercman A, Han TS, Kula K, Lean ME, Pendleton N, Punab M, Silman AJ, Wu FC; European Male Ageing Study Group (2009) Increased estrogen rather than decreased androgen action is associated with longer androgen receptor CAG repeats. *J Clin Endocrinol Metab* 94:277–284

Imperato-McGinley J, Sanchez RS, Spencer JR, Yee B, Vaughan ED (1992) Comparison of the effects of the 5 alpha-reductase inhibitor finasteride and the antiandrogen flutamide on prostate and genital differentiation: dose-response studies. *Endocrinology* 131:1149–1156

Irvine RA, Ma H, Yu MC, Ross RK, Stallcup MR, Coetzee GA (2000) Inhibition of p160-mediated coactivation with increasing androgen receptor polyglutamine length. *Hum Mol Genet* 9:267–274

Jenster G, van der Korput JA, Trapman J, Brinkmann AO (1992) Functional domains of the human androgen receptor. *J Steroid Biochem Mol Biol* 41:671–675

Jenster G, Trapman J, Brinkmann AO (1993) Nuclear import of the human androgen receptor. *Biochem J* 293:761–768

Jenster G, van der Korput HA, Trapman J, Brinkmann AO (1995) Identification of two transcription activation units in the N-terminal domain of the human androgen receptor. *J Biol Chem* 270:7341–7346

Jönsson EG, von Gertten C, Gustavsson JP, Yuan QP, Lindblad-Toh K, Forslund K, Rylander G, Mattila-Evenden M, Asberg M, Schalling M (2001) Androgen receptor trinucleotide repeat polymorphism and personality traits. *Psychiatr Genet* 11:19–23

Kashimada K, Koopman P (2010) Sry: the master switch in mammalian sex determination. *Development* 137:3921–3930

Kazemi-Esfarjani P, Trifiro MA, Pinsky L (1995) Evidence for a repressive function of the long polyglutamine tract in the human androgen receptor: possible pathogenetic relevance for the (CAG)n-expanded neuronopathies. *Hum Mol Genet* 4:523–527

Kennedy WR, Alter M, Sung JH (1968) Progressive proximal spinal and bulbar muscular atrophy of late onset. *Neurology* 18:671–680

Khosla S (2002) Oestrogen bones and men: when testosterone just isn't enough. *Clin Endocrinol* 56:291–293

Kim Y, Kobayashi A, Sekido R, DiNapoli L, Brennan J, Chaboissier MC, Poulat F, Behringer RR, Lovell-Badge R, Capel B (2006) Fgf9 and Wnt4 act as antagonistic signals to regulate mammalian sex determination. *PLoS Biol* 4:e187

Kim Y, Bingham N, Sekido R, Parker KL, Lovell-Badge R, Capel B (2007) Fibroblast growth factor receptor 2 regulates proliferation and Sertoli differentiation during male sex determination. *Proc Natl Acad Sci USA* 104:16558–16563

Kittles RA, Young D, Weinrich S, Hudson J, Argyropoulos G, Ukoli F, Adams-Campbell L, Dunston GM (2001) Extent of linkage disequilibrium between the androgen receptor gene CAG and GGC repeats in human populations: implications for prostate cancer risk. *Hum Gen* 109:253–261

Klessen C, Asbach P, Hein PA, Beyersdorff D, Hamm B, Taupitz M (2005) Complex genital malformation in a female with congenital adrenal hyperplasia: evaluation with magnetic resonance imaging. *Acta Radiol* 46:891–894

Kohler B, Lumbroso S, Leger J, Audran F, Grau ES, Kurtz F, Pinto G, Salerno M, Semitcheva T, Czernichow P, Sultan C (2005) Androgen insensitivity syndrome: somatic mosaicism of the androgen receptor in seven families and consequences for sex assignment and genetic counseling. *J Clin Endocrinol Metab* 90:106–111

Kooy RF, Reyniers E, Storm K, Vits L, van Velzen D, de Ruiter PE, Brinkmann AO, de Paepe A, Willems PJ (1999) CAG repeat contraction in the androgen receptor gene in three brothers with mental retardation. *Am J Med Gen* 85:209–213

Kubini K, Zachmann M, Albers N, Hiort O, Bettendorf M, Wolfle J, Bidlingmaier F, Klingmuller D (2000) Basal inhibin B and the testosterone response to human chorionic gonadotropin correlate in prepubertal boys. *J Clin Endocrinol Metab* **85**:134–138

Kuhlenbäumer G, Kress W, Ringelstein EB, Stögbauer F (2001) Thirty-seven CAG repeats in the androgen receptor gene in two healthy individuals. *J Neurol* **248**:23–26

Kurzrock EA, Baskin LS, Li Y, Cunha GR (1999) Epithelial-mesenchymal interactions in development of the mouse fetal genital tubercle. *Cells Tissues Organs* **164**:125–130

LaMarca HL, Rosen JM (2008) Minireview: hormones and mammary cell fate – what will I become when I grow up? *Endocrinology* **149**:4317–4321

Lasnitzki I, Mizuno T (1977) Induction of the rat prostate gland by androgens in organ culture. *J Endocrinol* **74**:47–55

Lasnitzki I, Mizuno T (1979) Role of the mesenchyme in the induction of the rat prostate gland by androgens in organ culture. *J Endocrinol* **82**:171–178

La Spada AR, Wilson EM, Lubahn DB, Harding AE, Fischbeck KH (1991) Androgen receptor gene mutations in X-linked spinal and bulbar muscular atrophy. *Nature* **352**:77–79

Latil AG, Azzouzi R, Cancel GS, Guillaume EC, Cochan-Priollet B, Berthon PL, Cussenot O (2001) Prostate carcinoma risk and allelic variants of genes involved in androgen biosynthesis and metabolism pathways. *Cancer* **92**:1130–1137

Lavery DN, McEwan IJ (2006) The human androgen receptor AF1 transactivation domain: interactions with transcription factor IIF and molten-globule-like structural characteristics. *Biochem Soc Trans* **34**:1054–1057

Lavery DN, McEwan IJ (2008a) Functional characterization of the native NH2-terminal transactivation domain of the human androgen receptor: binding kinetics for interactions with TFIIF and SRC-1a. *Biochemistry* **47**:3352–3359

Lavery DN, McEwan IJ (2008b) Structural characterization of the native NH2-terminal transactivation domain of the human androgen receptor: a collapsed disordered conformation underlies structural plasticity and protein-induced folding. *Biochemistry* **47**:3360–3369

Legius E, Vanderschueren D, Spiessens C, D'Hooghe T, Matthijs G (1999) Association between CAG repeat number in the androgen receptor and male infertility in a Belgian study. *Clin Genet* **56**:166–167

Limer KL, Pye SR, Thomson W, Boonen S, Borghs H, Vanderschueren D, Huhtaniemi IT, Adams JE, Ward KA, Platt H, Payne D, John SL, Bartfai G, Casanueva F, Finn JD, Forti G, Giwercman A, Han TS, Kula K, Lean ME, Pendleton N, Punab M, Silman AJ, Wu FC, O'Neill TW; EMAS Study Group (2009) Genetic variation in sex hormone genes influences heel ultrasound parameters in middle-aged and elderly men: results from the European Male Aging Study (EMAS). *J Bone Miner Res* **24**:314–323

Lubahn DB, Joseph DR, Sullivan PM, Willard HF, French FS, Wilson EM (1988) Cloning of human androgen receptor complementary DNA and localization to the X chromosome. *Science* **240**:327–330

Lubahn DB, Brown TR, Simental JA, Higgs HN, Migeon CJ, Wilson EM, French FS (1989) Sequence of the intron/exon junctions of the coding region of the human androgen receptor gene and identification of a point mutation in a family with complete androgen insensitivity. *Proc Natl Acad Sci USA* **86**:9534–9538

Lundberg-Giwercman Y, Xu C, Arver S, Pousette A, Reneland R (1998) No association between the androgen receptor gene CAG repeat and impaired sperm production in Swedish men. *Clin Genet* **54**:435–436

Mahendroo MS, Cala KM, Hess DL, Russell DW (2001) Unexpected virilization in male mice lacking steroid 5 alpha-reductase enzymes. *Endocrinology* **142**:4652–4662

Malki S, Nef S, Notarnicola C, Thevenet L, Gasca S, Mejean C, Berta P, Poulat F, Boizet-Bonhoure B (2005) Prostaglandin D2 induces nuclear import of the sex-determining factor SOX9 via its cAMP-PKA phosphorylation. *EMBO J* **24**:1798–1809

Mangelsdorf DJ, Thummel C, Beato M, Herrlich P, Schutz G, Umesono K, Blumberg B, Kastner P, Mark M, Chambon P, Evans RM (1995) The nuclear receptor superfamily: the second decade. *Cell* **83**:835–839

Mariotti C, Castellotti B, Pareyson D, Testa D, Eoli M, Antozzi C, Silani V, Marconi R, Tezzon F, Siciliano G, Marchini C, Gellera C, Donato SD (2000) Phenotypic manifestations associated with CAG-repeat expansion in the androgen receptor gene in male patients and heterozygous females: a clinical and molecular study of 30 families. *Neuromusc Dis* **10**:391–397

Marker PC, Donjacour AA, Dahiya R, Cunha GR (2003) Hormonal, cellular, and molecular control of prostatic development. *Dev Biol* **253**:165–174

Marshall GR, Wickings EJ, Nieschlag E (1984) Testosterone can initiate spermatogenesis in an immature nonhuman primate, Macaca fascicularis. *Endocrinology* **114**:2228–2233

Matias PM, Donner P, Coelho R, Thomaz M, Peixoto C, Macedo S, Otto N, Joschko S, Scholz P, Wegg A, Basler S, Schafer M, Egner U, Carrondo MA (2000) Structural evidence for ligand specificity in the binding domain of the human androgen receptor. Implications for pathogenic gene mutations. *J Biol Chem* **275**:26164–26171

Meeks JJ, Schaeffer EM (2011) Genetic regulation of prostate development. *J Androl* **32**:210–217

Mengual L, Oriola J, Ascaso C, Ballesca JL, Oliva R (2003) An increased CAG repeat length in the androgen receptor gene in azoospermic ICSI candidates. *J Androl* **24**:279–284

Mifsud A, Sim CK, Boettger-Tong H, Moreira S, Lamb DJ, Lipshultz LI, Yong EL (2001) Trinucleotide (CAG) repeat polymorphisms in the androgen receptor gene: molecular markers of risk for male infertility. *Fertil Steril* **75**:275–281

Mitsumori K, Terai A, Oka H, Segawa T, Ogura K, Yoshida O, Ogawa O (1999) Androgen receptor CAG repeat length polymorphism in benign prostatic hyperplasia (BPH): correlation with adenoma growth. *Prostate* **41**:253–257

Miyagawa S, Satoh Y, Haraguchi R, Suzuki K, Iguchi T, Taketo MM, Nakagata N, Matsumoto T, Takeyama K, Kato S, Yamada G (2009) Genetic interactions of the androgen and Wnt/beta-catenin pathways for the masculinization of external genitalia. *Mol Endocrinol* **23**:871–880

Miyagawa S, Matsumaru D, Murashima A, Omori A, Satoh Y, Haraguchi R, Motoyama J, Iguchi T, Nakagata N, Hui CC, Yamada G (2011) The role of sonic hedgehog-gli2 pathway in the masculinization of external genitalia. *Endocrinology* **152**:2894–2903

Moniot B, Declosmenil F, Barrionuevo F, Scherer G, Aritake K, Malki S, Marzi L, Cohen-Solal A, Georg I, Klattig J, Englert C, Kim Y, Capel B, Eguchi N, Urade Y, Boizet-Bonhoure B, Poulat F (2009) The PGD2 pathway, independently of FGF9, amplifies SOX9 activity in Sertoli cells during male sexual differentiation. *Development* **136**:1813–1821

Moras D, Gronemeyer H (1998) The nuclear receptor ligand-binding domain: structure and function. *Curr Opin Cell Biol* **10**:384–391

Murakami R, Mizuno T (1986) Proximal-distal sequence of development of the skeletal tissues in the penis of rat and the inductive effect of epithelium. *J Embryol Exp Morphol* **92**:133–143

Nielsen TL, Hagen C, Wraae K, Bathum L, Larsen R, Brixen K, Andersen M (2010) The impact of the CAG repeat polymorphism of the androgen receptor gene on muscle and adipose tissues in 20–29-year-old Danish men: Odense Androgen Study. *Eur J Endocrinol* **162**:795–804

Nishida H, Miyagawa S, Matsumaru D, Wada Y, Satoh Y, Ogino Y, Fukuda S, Iguchi T, Yamada G (2008) Gene expression analyses on embryonic external genitalia: identification of regulatory genes possibly involved in masculinization processes. *Congenit Anom (Kyoto)* **48**:63–67

O'Shaughnessy PJ, Baker PJ, Heikkila M, Vainio S, McMahon AP (2000) Localization of 17beta-hydroxysteroid dehydrogenase/17-ketosteroid reductase isoform expression in the developing mouse testis – androstenedione is the major androgen secreted by fetal/neonatal Leydig cells. *Endocrinology* **141**:2631–2637

O'Shaughnessy PJ, Johnston H, Willerton L, Baker PJ (2002) Failure of normal adult Leydig cell development in androgen-receptor-deficient mice. *J Cell Sci* **115**:3491–3496

O'Shaughnessy PJ, Baker PJ, Johnston H (2006) The foetal Leydig cell – differentiation, function and regulation. *Int J Androl* **29**:90–95; discussion:105–108

Ostrer H (2008) 46,XY disorder of sex development and 46,XY complete gonadal dysgenesis. In: Pagon RA, Bird TD, Dolan CR, Stephens K (eds) *GeneReviews* [Internet].

University of Washington, Seattle [updated Sep 15, 2009]

Page ST, Kupelian V, Bremner WJ, McKinlay JB (2006) The androgen receptor gene CAG repeat polymorphism does not predict increased risk of heart disease: longitudinal results from the Massachusetts Male Ageing Study. *Clin Endocrinol (Oxf)* **65**:333–339

Papadimitriou DT, Linglart A, Morel Y, Chaussain JL (2006) Puberty in subjects with complete androgen insensitivity syndrome. *Horm Res* **65**:126–131

Patrizio P, Leonard DG, Chen KL, Hernandez-Ayup S, Trounson AO (2001) Larger trinucleotide repeat size in the androgen receptor gene of infertile men with extremely severe oligozoospermia. *J Androl* **22**:444–448

Perriton CL, Powles N, Chiang C, Maconochie MK, Cohn MJ (2002) Sonic hedgehog signaling from the urethral epithelium controls external genital development. *Dev Biol* **247**:26–46

Pioro EP, Kant A, Mitsumoto H (1994) Disease expression in a Kennedy's disease kindred is unrelated to CAG tandem repeat size in the androgen receptor gene: characterization in a symptomatic female. *Ann Neurol* **36**:318

Piprek RP (2009) Genetic mechanisms underlying male sex determination in mammals. *J Appl Genet* **50**:347–360

Plant TM (2006) The role of KiSS-1 in the regulation of puberty in higher primates. *Eur J Endocrinol* **155** (Suppl 1):S11–S16

Plant TM, Witchel SF (2006) Puberty in non-human primates and humans. In: Neill JD, Plant TM, Pfaff DW, Challis JRG, de Kretser DM, Richards JS, Wassarman PM (eds) *Knobil and Neill's Physiology of Reproduction*. Academic Press, St Louis, pp 2177–2230

Platz EA, Giovannucci E, Dahl DM, Krithivas K, Hennekens CH, Brown

M, Stampfer MJ, Kantoff PW (1998) The androgen receptor gene GGN microsatellite and prostate cancer risk. *Cancer Epidemiol Biomarkers Prev* 7:379–384.

Platz EA, Rimm EB, Willett WC, Kantoff PW, Giovannucci E (2000) Racial variation in prostate cancer incidence and in hormonal system markers among male health professionals. *J Natl Cancer Inst* 92:2009–2017

Podlasek CA, Barnett DH, Clemens JQ, Bak PM, Bushman W (1999) Prostate development requires Sonic hedgehog expressed by the urogenital sinus epithelium. *Dev Biol* 209:28–39

Pope HG, Cohane GH, Kanayama G, Siegel AJ, Hudson JI (2003) Testosterone gel supplementation for men with refractory depression: a randomized placebo-controlled trial. *Am J Psychiatry* 160:105–111

Price H, McNeal JE, Stamey TA (1990) Evolving patterns of tissue composition in benign prostatic hyperplasia as a function of specimen size. *Hum Pathol* 21:578–585

Quigley CA, De Bellis A, Marschke KB, el-Awady MK, Wilson EM, French FS (1995) Androgen receptor defects: historical, clinical, and molecular perspectives. *Endocr Rev* 16:271–321

Rajpert-De Meyts E, Leffers H, Petersen JH, Andersen AG, Carlsen E, Jorgensen N, Skakkebaek NE (2002) CAG repeat length in androgen-receptor gene and reproductive variables in fertile and infertile men. *Lancet* 359:44–46

Remes T, Vaisanen SB, Mahonen A, Huuskonen J, Kroger H, Jurvelin JS, Penttila IM, Rauramaa R (2003) Aerobic exercise and bone mineral density in middle-aged Finnish men: a controlled randomized trial with reference to androgen receptor aromatase and estrogen receptor alpha gene polymorphisms. *Bone* 32:412–420

Rey RA, Belville C, Nihoul-Fekete C, Michel-Calemard L, Forest MG, Lahlou N, Jaubert F, Mowszowicz I, David M, Saka N, Bouvattier C, Bertrand AM, Lecointre C, Soskin S, Cabrol S, Crosnier H, Leger J, Lortat-Jacob S, Nicolino M, Rabl W, Toledo SP, Bas F, Gompel A, Czernichow P, Chatelain P, Rappaport R, Morel Y, Josso N (1999) Evaluation of gonadal function in 107 intersex patients by means of serum antimullerian hormone measurement. *J Clin Endocrinol Metab* 84:627–631

Rodien P, Mebarki F, Mowszowicz I, Chaussain JL, Young J, Morel Y, Schaison G (1996) Different phenotypes in a family with androgen insensitivity caused by the same M780I point mutation in the androgen receptor gene. *J Clin Endocrinol Metab* 81:2994–2998

Ross RK, Pike MC, Coetzee GA, Reichardt JK, Yu MC, Feigelson H, Stanczyk FZ, Kolonel LN, Henderson BE (1998) Androgen metabolism and Prostate Cancer: establishing a model of genetic susceptibility. *Cancer Res* 58:4497–4504

Sack JS, Kish KF, Wang C, Attar RM, Kiefer SE, An Y, Wu GY, Scheffler JE, Salvati ME, Krystek SR Jr, Weinmann R, Einspahr HM (2001) Crystallographic structures of the ligand-binding domains of the androgen receptor and its T877A mutant complexed with the natural agonist dihydrotestosterone. *Proc Natl Acad Sci USA* 98:4904–4909

Salmen T, Heikkinen AM, Mahonen A, Kroger H, Komulainen M, Pallonen H, Saarikoski S, Honkanen R, Maenpaa PH (2003) Relation of androgen receptor gene polymorphism to bone mineral density and fracture risk in early postmenopausal women during a 5-year randomized hormone replacement therapy trial. *J Bone Miner Res* 18:319–324

Sapir-Koren R, Livshits G, Landsman T, Kobyliansky E (2001) Bone mineral density is associated with

estrogen receptor gene polymorphism in men. *Anthropol Anzeiger* 59:343–353

Sasagawa I, Suzuki Y, Ashida J, Nakada T, Muroya K, Ogata T (2001) CAG repeat length analysis and mutation screening of the androgen receptor gene in Japanese men with idiopathic azoospermia. *J Androl* 22:804–808

Sawaya ME, Shalita AR (1998) Androgen receptor polymorphisms (CAG repeat lengths) in androgenetic alopecia hirsutism and acne. *J Cutan Med Surg* 3:9–15

Schauwaers K, De Gendt K, Saunders PT, Atanassova N, Haelens A, Callewaert L, Moehren U, Swinnen JV, Verhoeven G, Verrijdt G, Claessens F (2007) Loss of androgen receptor binding to selective androgen response elements causes a reproductive phenotype in a knockin mouse model. *Proc Natl Acad Sci USA* 104:4961–4966

Schneider G, Nienhaus K, Gromoll J, Heuft G, Nieschlag E, Zitzmann M (2011a) Depressive symptoms in men aged 50 years and older and their relationship to genetic androgen receptor polymorphism and sex hormone levels in three different samples. *Am J Geriatr Psychiatry* 19:274–283

Schneider G, Nienhaus K, Gromoll J, Heuft G, Nieschlag E, Zitzmann M (2011b) Sex hormone levels, genetic androgen receptor polymorphism, and anxiety in ≥50-year-old males. *J Sex Med* 8:3452–3464

Schweiger U, Deuschle M, Weber B, Korner A, Lammers CH, Schmider J (1999) Testosterone gonadotropin and cortisol secretion in male patients with major depression. *Psychosom Med* 61:292–296

Seidman SN, Araujo AB, Roose SP, McKinlay JB (2001) Testosterone level androgen receptor polymorphism and depressive symptoms in middle-aged men. *Biol Psych* 50:371–376

Seifert AW, Zheng Z, Ormerod BK, Cohn MJ (2010) Sonic hedgehog controls growth of external genitalia by regulating cell cycle kinetics. *Nat Commun* **1**:23

Sekido R, Lovell-Badge R (2008) Sex determination involves synergistic action of SRY and SF1 on a specific Sox9 enhancer. *Nature* **453**:930–934

Sekido R, Lovell-Badge R (2009) Sex determination and SRY: down to a wink and a nudge? *Trends Genet* **25**:19–29

Shabsigh R, Arver S, Channer KS, Eardley I, Fabbri A, Gooren L, Heufelder A, Jones H, Meryn S, Zitzmann M (2008) The triad of erectile dysfunction, hypogonadism and the metabolic syndrome. *Int J Clin Pract* **62**:791–798

Shaffer PL, Jivan A, Dollins DE, Claessens F, Gewirth DT (2004) Structural basis of androgen receptor binding to selective androgen response elements. *Proc Natl Acad Sci USA* **101**:4758–4763

Shen JH, Ingraham HA (2002) Regulation of the orphan nuclear receptor steroidogenic factor 1 by Sox proteins. *Mol Endocrinol* **16**:529–540

Simental JA, Sar M, Lane MV, French FS, Wilson EM (1991) Transcriptional activation and nuclear targeting signals of the human androgen receptor. *J Biol Chem* **266**:510–518

Sinnecker GH, Hiort O, Nitsche EM, Holterhus PM, Kruse K (1997) Functional assessment and clinical classification of androgen sensitivity in patients with mutations of the androgen receptor gene. German Collaborative Intersex Study Group. *Eur J Pediatr* **156**:7–14

Song LN, Herrell R, Byers S, Shah S, Wilson EM, Gelmann EP (2003) Beta-catenin binds to the activation function 2 region of the androgen receptor and modulates the effects of the N-terminal domain and TIF2 on ligand-dependent transcription. *Mol Cell Biol* **23**:1674–1687

Sowers M, Willing M, Burns T, Deschenes S, Hollis B, Crutchfield M, Jannausch M (1999) Genetic markers, bone mineral density, and serum osteocalcin levels. *J Bone Min Res* **14**:1411–1419

Stanford JL, Just JJ, Gibbs M, Wicklund KG, Neal CL, Blumenstein BA, Ostrander EA (1997) Polymorphic repeats in the androgen receptor gene: molecular markers of prostate cancer risk. *Cancer Res* **57**:1194–1198

Stanworth RD, Kapoor D, Channer KS, Jones TH (2008) Androgen receptor CAG repeat polymorphism is associated with serum testosterone levels, obesity and serum leptin in men with type 2 diabetes. *Eur J Endocrinol* **159**:739–746

Steltenkamp S, Hiort O (2007) Pubertal development of 46,XY DSD patients with partial androgen insensitivity due to mutation of the androgen receptor assigned to male sex. *Horm Res* **68**:205

Taguchi O, Cunha GR, Lawrence WD, Robboy SJ (1984) Timing and irreversibility of Mullerian duct inhibition in the embryonic reproductive tract of the human male. *Dev Biol* **106**:394–398

Takeda H, Lasnitzki I, Mizuno T (1986) Analysis of prostatic bud induction by brief androgen treatment in the fetal rat urogenital sinus. *J Endocrinol* **110**:467–470

Thomas MA, Preece DM, Bentel JM (2010) Androgen regulation of the prostatic tumour suppressor NKX3.1 is mediated by its 3′ untranslated region. *Biochem J* **425**:575–583

Tilley WD, Marcelli M, Wilson JD, McPhaul MJ (1989) Characterization and expression of a cDNA encoding the human androgen receptor. *Proc Natl Acad Sci USA* **86**:327–331

Trapman J, Klaassen P, Kuiper GG, van der Korput JA, Faber PW, van Rooij HC, Geurts van Kessel A, Voorhorst MM, Mulder E, Brinkmann AO (1988) Cloning, structure and expression of a cDNA encoding the human androgen receptor. *Biochem Biophys Res Commun* **153**:241–248

Tut TG, Ghadessy FJ, Trifiro MA, Pinsky L, Yong EL (1997) Long polyglutamine tracts in the androgen receptor are associated with reduced trans-activation impaired sperm production and male infertility. *J Clin Endocr Metab* **82**:3777–3782

Unden F, Ljunggren JG, Beck-Friis J, Kjellman F, Wetterberg L (1988) Hypothalamic-pituitary-gonadal axis in major depressive disorders. *Acta Psychiatri Scand* **78**:138–146

van Golde R, Van Houwelingen K, Kiemeney L, Kremer J, Tuerlings J, Schalken J, Meuleman E (2002) Is increased CAG repeat length in the androgen receptor gene a risk factor for male subfertility? *J Urol* **167**:621–623

van Houten ME, Gooren LJ (2000) Differences in reproductive endocrinology between Asian men and Caucasian men—a literature review. *Asian J Androl* **2**:13–20

Van Pottelbergh I, Lumbroso S, Goemaere S, Sultan C, Kaufman JM (2001) Lack of influence of the androgen receptor gene CAG-repeat polymorphism on sex steroid status and bone metabolism in elderly men. *Clin Endocrinol* **55**:659–666

von Eckardstein S, Syska A, Gromoll J, Kamischke A, Simoni M, Nieschlag E (2001) Inverse correlation between sperm concentration and number of androgen receptor CAG repeats in normal men. *J Clin Endocr Metab* **86**:2585–2590

von Eckardstein S, Schmidt A, Kamischke A, Simoni M, Gromoll J, Nieschlag E (2002) CAG repeat length in the androgen receptor gene and gonadotrophin suppression influence the effectiveness of hormonal male contraception. *Clin Endocrinol* **57**:647–655

Wallerand H, Remy-Martin A, Chabannes E, Bermont L, Adessi GL, Bittard H (2001) Relationship between expansion of the CAG repeat in exon 1 of the androgen receptor gene and idiopathic male infertility. *Fertil Steril* **76**:769–774

Wang C, Nieschlag E, Swerdloff R, Behre HM, Hellstrom WJ, Gooren LJ, Kaufman JM, Legros JJ, Lunenfeld B, Morales A, Morley JE, Schulman C, Thompson IM, Weidner W, Wu FC (2008) Investigation, treatment and monitoring of late-onset hypogonadism in males: ISA, ISSAM, EAU, EAA and ASA recommendations. *Eur J Endocrinol* **159**:507–514

Wang G, Chen G, Wang X, Zhong J, Lu J (2001) The polymorphism of (CAG)n repeats within androgen receptor gene among Chinese male population [article in Chinese]. *Zhonghua Yi Xue Yi Chuan Xue Za Zhi [Chinese Journal of Medical Genetics]* **18**:456–458

Wang Q, Udayakumar TS, Vasaitis TS, Brodie AM, Fondell JD (2004) Mechanistic relationship between androgen receptor polyglutamine tract truncation and androgen-dependent transcriptional hyperactivity in prostate cancer cells. *J Biol Chem* **279**:17319–17328

Warot X, Fromental-Ramain C, Fraulob V, Chambon P, Dolle P (1997) Gene dosage-dependent effects of the Hoxa-13 and Hoxd-13 mutations on morphogenesis of the terminal parts of the digestive and urogenital tracts. *Development* **124**:4781–4791

Welsh M, MacLeod DJ, Walker M, Smith LB, Sharpe RM (2009) Critical androgen-sensitive periods of rat penis and clitoris development. *Int J Androl* **33**: e144–e152

Werner R, Holterhus PM, Binder G, Schwarz HP, Morlot M, Struve D, Marschke C, Hiort O (2006a) The A645D mutation in the hinge region of the human androgen receptor (AR) gene modulates AR activity, depending on the context of the polymorphic glutamine and glycine repeats. *J Clin Endocrinol Metab* **91**:3515–3520

Werner R, Schutt J, Hannema S, Ropke A, Wieacker P, Hiort O, Holterhus PM (2006b) Androgen receptor gene mutations in androgen insensitivity syndrome cause distinct patterns of reduced activation of androgen-responsive promoter constructs. *J Steroid Biochem Mol Biol* **101**:1–10

Werner R, Grotsch H, Hiort O (2010) 46, XY disorders of sex development – the undermasculinised male with disorders of androgen action. *Best Pract Res Clin Endocrinol Metab* **24**:263–277

Wilhelm D, Martinson F, Bradford S, Wilson MJ, Combes AN, Beverdam A, Bowles J, Mizusaki H, Koopman P (2005) Sertoli cell differentiation is induced both cell-autonomously and through prostaglandin signaling during mammalian sex determination. *Dev Biol* **287**:111–124

Wilhelm D, Hiramatsu R, Mizusaki H, Widjaja L, Combes AN, Kanai Y, Koopman P (2007) SOX9 regulates prostaglandin D synthase gene transcription in vivo to ensure testis development. *J Biol Chem* **282**:10553–10560

Yamada G, Satoh Y, Baskin LS, Cunha GR (2003) Cellular and molecular mechanisms of development of the external genitalia. *Differentiation* **71**:445–460

Yamada G, Suzuki K, Haraguchi R, Miyagawa S, Satoh Y, Kamimura M, Nakagata N, Kataoka H, Kuroiwa A, Chen Y (2006) Molecular genetic cascades for external genitalia formation: an emerging organogenesis program. *Dev Dyn* **235**:1738–1752

Yanovich R, Milgrom R, Friedman E, Moran DS (2011) Androgen receptor CAG repeat size is associated with stress fracture risk: a pilot study. *Clin Orthop Relat Res* **469**:2925–2931

Yao HH, Whoriskey W, Capel B (2002) Desert Hedgehog/Patched 1 signaling specifies fetal Leydig cell fate in testis organogenesis. *Genes Dev* **16**:1433–1440

Yeh S, Tsai MY, Xu Q, Mu XM, Lardy H, Huang KE, Lin H, Yeh SD, Altuwaijri S, Zhou X, Xing L, Boyce BF, Hung MC, Zhang S, Gan L, Chang C (2002) Generation and characterization of androgen receptor knockout (ARKO) mice: an in vivo model for the study of androgen functions in selective tissues. *Proc Natl Acad Sci USA* **99**:13498–13503

Yong EL, Lim LS, Wang Q, Mifsud A, Lim J, Ong YC, Sim KS (2000) Androgen receptor polymorphisms and mutations in male infertility. *J Endocrinol Invest* **23**:573–577

Yoshida KI, Yano M, Chiba K, Honda M, Kitahara S (1999) CAG repeat length in the androgen receptor gene is enhanced in patients with idiopathic azoospermia. *Urology* **54**:1078–1081

Zeegers MP, Kiemeney LA, Nieder AM, Ostrer H (2004) How strong is the association between CAG and GGN repeat length polymorphisms in the androgen receptor gene and prostate cancer risk? *Cancer Epidemiol Biomarkers Prev* **13**:1765–1771

Zeltser L, Desplan C, Heintz N (1996) Hoxb-13: a new Hox gene in a distant region of the HOXB cluster maintains colinearity. *Development* **122**:2475–2484

Zhou X (2010) Roles of androgen receptor in male and female reproduction: lessons from global and cell-specific androgen receptor knockout (ARKO) mice. *J Androl* **31**:235–243

Zhou ZX, Sar M, Simental JA, Lane MV, Wilson EM (1994) A ligand-dependent bipartite nuclear targeting signal in the human androgen receptor. Requirement for the DNA-binding domain and modulation by NH2-terminal and carboxyl-terminal sequences. *J Biol Chem* **269**:13115–13123

Zitzmann M, Nieschlag E (2001) Testosterone levels in healthy men and the relation to behavioural and physical characteristics: facts and constructs. *Euro J Endocrinol* **144**:183–197

Zitzmann M, Brune M, Kornmann B, Gromoll J, Junker R, Nieschlag E (2001a) The CAG repeat polymorphism in the androgen receptor gene affects bone density and bone metabolism in healthy males. *Clin Endocrinol* **55**:649–657

Zitzmann M, Brune M, Kornmann B, Gromoll J, von Eckardstein S, von Eckardstein A, Nieschlag E (2001b) The CAG repeat polymorphism in the AR gene affects high density lipoprotein cholesterol and arterial vasoreactivity. *J Clin Endocr Metab* **86**:4867–4873

Zitzmann M, Brune M, Nieschlag E (2002a) Vascular reactivity in hypogonadal men is reduced by androgen substitution. *J Clin Endocr Metab* **87**:5030–5037

Zitzmann M, Brune M, Vieth V, Nieschlag E (2002b) Monitoring bone density in hypogonadal men by quantitative phalangeal ultrasound. *Bone* **31**:422–429

Zitzmann M, Gromoll J, von Eckardstein A, Nieschlag E (2003a) The CAG repeat polymorphism in the androgen receptor gene modulates body fat mass and serum levels of leptin and insulin in men. *Diabetologia* **46**:31–39

Zitzmann M, Depenbusch M, Gromoll J, Nieschlag E (2003b) Prostate volume and growth in testosterone-substituted hypogonadal men are dependent on the CAG repeat polymorphism of the androgen receptor gene: a longitudinal pharmacogenetic study. *J Clin Endocrinol Metab* **88**:2049–2054

Zmuda JM, Cauley JA, Kuller LH, Newman AB, Robbins J, Harris T, Ferrell RE (2000a) Androgen receptor CAG repeat polymorphism: a novel marker of osteoporotic risk in men. *Osteoporosis Int* **11** S151: 355

Zmuda JM, Cauley JA, Kuller LH, Zhang X, Palermo L, Nevitt MC, Ferrell RE (2000b) Androgen receptor CAG repeat length is associated with increased hip bone loss and vertebral fracture risk among older men. *J Bone Min Res* **15** S491: M141

Chapter 4

Methodology for measuring testosterone, dihydrotestosterone and sex hormone-binding globulin in a clinical setting

Manuela Simoni, Flaminia Fanelli, Laura Roli, and Uberto Pagotto

4.1 Introduction

Testosterone is a hormone difficult to measure accurately. Yet, its accurate determination is the prerequisite for the correct diagnosis and clinical management of hypogonadism in males and hyperandrogenism in females. In the last decade a number of studies increased awareness of the poor performance of most of the current assays and identified some strategies to improve the accuracy of testosterone testing (Rosner *et al.* 2007; 2010). In the previous edition of this book a chapter was dedicated to the description of the principles, analytical performance and limitations of the existing methodologies for measuring testosterone, DHT and SHBG (Simoni 2004). Here, we will provide an update on the state of the art to help the reader choose the testosterone detection system most suitable for his/her needs in view of the current recommendations.

4.2 Testosterone, dihydrotestosterone and sex hormone-binding globulin in blood

Testosterone and DHT circulate in serum largely bound to transport proteins: that is albumin, which displays low affinity but very high binding capacity, and SHBG, with high affinity and low capacity. A systematic analysis of serum transport of steroid hormones and their interaction with binding proteins revealed an association constant of SHBG of 1.6×10^9 M^{-1} for testosterone and of 5.5×10^9 M^{-1} for DHT at 37 °C (Dunn *et al.* 1981). By comparison the association constant of albumin for testosterone is five orders of magnitude lower (6×10^4 M^{-1}) (Anderson 1974). The relative amounts of protein binding of circulating testosterone in men and women are shown in Table 4.1.

Testosterone: Action, Deficiency, Substitution, ed. Eberhard Nieschlag and Hermann M. Behre, Assoc. ed. Susan Nieschlag. Published by Cambridge University Press. © Cambridge University Press 2012.

Table 4.1 Transport of endogenous testosterone and DHT in male and female serum

	Serum concentration (nM)	Unbound (%)	SHBG (%)	CBG (%)	Albumin (%)
Testosterone					
Adult men	23.0	2.23	44.3	3.56	49.9
Adult women					
Follicular phase	1.3	1.36	66.0	2.26	30.4
Luteal phase	1.3	1.37	65.7	2.20	30.7
Pregnancy	4.7	0.23	95.4	0.82	3.6
DHT					
Adult men	1.70	0.88	49.7	0.22	39.2
Adult women					
Follicular phase	0.65	0.47	78.4	0.12	21.0
Luteal phase	0.65	0.48	78.1	0.12	21.3
Pregnancy	0.93	0.07	97.8	0.04	21.2

Source: Dunn *et al.* (1981).
Abbreviations: CBG, cortisol-binding globulin; SHBG, sex hormone-binding globulin; DHT, dihydrotestosterone.

About 1.5–2% of serum testosterone is free and is believed to represent bioactive testosterone. Free and protein-bound testosterone and DHT are in equilibrium, so that when free hormone is subtracted from circulation because of entry into tissue, new testosterone dissociates from albumin and SHBG, a new equilibrium is promptly reached, and the free-hormone concentration in serum remains constant. Conversely, pathophysiological conditions causing changes in binding protein concentration (e.g. pregnancy, hypo- or hyperthyroidism, growth hormone (GH) excess, treatment with antiepileptic drugs) or displacement of testosterone from SHBG by drugs (e.g. danazol) results in changes in total testosterone concentration in order to maintain constant free testosterone levels.

The measurement of SHBG is valuable for assessment of androgenization and of free testosterone. In earlier times SHBG was measured indirectly, by estimating its binding capacity. The classic method used tritiated DHT as ligand because of its higher affinity to SHBG and lack of binding to cortisol-binding globulin (CBG). Saturating amounts of labeled DHT were added to the samples and SHBG was then precipitated by ammonium sulfate. The amount of labeled DHT precipitated provided a direct measurement of SHBG binding capacity. This method did not allow absolute changes in SHBG protein concentrations to be measured, which can now be assessed by modern immunoradiometric assays. Modern assays have demonstrated that, in general, SHBG binding capacity (expressed in terms of DHT binding) corresponds acceptably to the molar SHBG concentration.

The "free-hormone hypothesis" has been repeatedly challenged in the scientific literature, mainly due to the difficulty of reconciling the existing experimental evidence with appropriate mathematical models of hormone transport (Ekins 1990; Mendel 1992). For instance, the low affinity of testosterone for albumin binding and some experimental data led to the idea that albumin-bound testosterone is readily available for delivery to the tissues (i.e. bioavailable); while only SHBG-bound testosterone is not biologically active (Manni *et al.* 1985). In contrast, SHBG itself has been proposed to interact with cell surface receptors, thereby contributing to the biological activity of androgens (Rosner *et al.* 1999). This novel, putative function of SHBG is of particular interest in the light of the essential lack of any physiological explanation of why primates, unlike all other species, possess such a protein. Sex hormone-binding globulin seems to "buffer" serum testosterone levels, which, beside the physiological circadian rhythm, show only minor circhoral variations despite highly pulsatile LH secretion (Simoni *et al.* 1988; 1992). In contrast, serum testosterone levels oscillate widely in rodents, which do not have SHBG. In addition SHBG reduces the rate of hepatic testosterone degradation. There are no known cases of congenital absence of SHBG in humans, but an analbuminemic strain of rats, a species which does not have circulating SHBG, is normally fertile and shows normal free testosterone levels, arguing for a dispensable role of serum-testosterone-binding proteins (Mendel *et al.* 1989). Similarly, the congenital absence of thyroxin-binding globulin (TBG) in humans is compatible with normal thyroid function (Dussault *et al.* 1977).

Several factors influence SHBG production and, thereby, free testosterone levels. Estrogens stimulate and androgens inhibit SHBG secretion. Administration of 20 µg daily of ethinyl estradiol to men for five weeks resulted in a 150% increase in SHBG and, as a consequence of the reduced free testosterone levels, in a 50% increase in total serum testosterone (Anderson 1974). The estrogen effect is responsible for the higher SHBG serum levels in women compared to men. In pregnancy, SHBG rises to levels 5–10 times higher than in non-pregnant women. In addition, SHBG levels are stimulated by thyroid hormones, resulting in high levels in thyrotoxycosis and low levels in hypothyroidism, and are reduced by GH and cortisol, resulting in low levels in acromegaly and in Cushing syndrome. Finally, SHBG levels are higher in children than in adults and increase in men after the age of 50, contributing to the possible decline of free testosterone levels observed in aging men.

The most important bioactive metabolite of testosterone is DHT. The reduction of testosterone to DHT occurs in those tissues expressing 5α-reductase, and DHT is well measurable in circulation. In eugonadal, adult men, serum DHT concentrations are about 10–12 times lower than testosterone, and DHT is mainly bound to SHBG (Table 4.1). Given the role of DHT in prostate growth, the measurement of serum DHT is of relevance during testosterone treatment, especially when testosterone is administered via the transdermal route (e.g. testosterone gel or patches), since the skin is the primary organ for 5α-reduction.

4.3 Measurement of testosterone

Testosterone measurement is useful in the assessment of a number of clinical conditions such as hypogonadism, hyperandrogenism, diabetes, cardiovascular disease, bone diseases, neurovegetative disorders, aging etc. (see Simoni and Nieschlag 2010), but, despite the importance of testosterone determination for clinical decisions, the different methods in current use are frequently inaccurate and their results inconsistent, especially at low concentrations. This problem is mainly due to the lack of recognized reference standards and is common to all types of assays currently available, from immunoassays to mass spectrometry (MS) methods, with the automated immunoassays

showing the greatest inaccuracy, as demonstrated by proficiency tests results (Wang *et al.* 2004; Rosner *et al.* 2007). Testosterone detection in pediatric and female samples is affected by the physiologically low concentrations of the hormone, the high concentrations of other, interfering, cross-reacting steroids and the age-related variability of matrix and steroid composition (Rauh 2010). As a consequence, no trustworthy age- and sex-specific reference ranges are presently available for this important biomarker. Even in adult males the current reference ranges contain a remarkable "gray zone" at about 8–12 nmol/l, leaving the lowest level of "normality" basically undefined.

Facing these problems, The Endocrine Society, in partnership with the Centers for Disease Control and Prevention and other endorsing organizations, published a consensus statement in October 2010 with the aim of stimulating the cooperation of clinical laboratories, instrument makers, assay manufacturers, medical communities and other stakeholders in thoroughly reviewing the process, from guidelines for patient preparation and specimen handling to a workable standard for the testosterone assay, the true core target. This consensus statement contains seven recommendations to follow to achieve the goal of highly accurate testosterone testing, and a timeline suggesting that standardization of testosterone assay could be achieved by 2012 (Rosner *et al.* 2010). In summary these recommendations include: (1) all stakeholders should work at testosterone assay standardization and production of accurate and reliable tests; (2) experts should work at defining performance criteria ensuring coverage of the full range of expected values; (3) reference intervals in adults and children of both sexes should be established; (4) guidelines for preanalytical steps (patient preparation, specimen collection, etc.) should be prepared; (5) third-party payers and healthcare organizations should promote and reimburse only standardized, accuracy-based tests; (6) research funding agencies and journals should support and publish, respectively, only research work based on standardized testosterone tests; (7) manufacturers and laboratories should further develop new methods for accurate, specific, sensitive and cost-effective testosterone testing. Meanwhile everyone concerned should be aware of the methods available and make an educated choice of the system that better suits his/her needs. A detailed list of the pros and cons of the current methods has been summarized in this consensus statement (Rosner *et al.* 2010).

4.3.1 Mass spectrometry methods

While testosterone immunoassays still dominate in routine laboratories due to their indispensable high-throughput capabilities, their shortcomings, especially inaccuracy and poor reproducibility at low levels, prompted the advancement of a new generation of MS technologies.

The application of gas chromatography combined with mass spectrometry (GC-MS) to the discovery and structural elucidation of steroid hormones and metabolites goes back to the 1960s, and this technique still represents not only the pre-eminent tool for steroid disorder and metabolomic studies (Krone *et al.* 2010), but also the gold standard and reference method used for the validation of other assays. However, this technique did not overcome the need for an extensive sample pretreatment, thus preventing its introduction to routine settings, and GC-MS survives as a prerogative of only a few specialized laboratories. In contrast, the latest advances in the development of quantitative methods by liquid chromatography–tandem mass spectrometry (LC-MS/MS), as witnessed by the exponential number of publications on this topic since the late 1990s, render LC-MS/MS potentially suitable for routine testosterone measurement, as it offers a promising fusion of good accuracy and specificity, high-throughput capabilities, and abatement of both direct and indirect costs of the present immunoassays.

In principle MS acts as a detector for the chromatographic technique to which it is combined, performing, in addition, a further analysis based on the recognition of intrinsic features of the molecules: molecular weight and structure. In quantitative applications, the measurement coincides with the identification of the analyte, providing high specificity.

Chromatographic methods are based on the separation of the molecules in a complex mixture through the interaction between the analyte and the stationary phase contained in the chromatographic column, in the presence of a mobile phase flowing in the system: a liquid solvent or a mixture of solvents in liquid chromatography, and a gas in gas chromatography. The relative affinity between the analyte and the mobile and stationary phase will determine the time needed by the former to reach the detector: retention time is a specific feature of the analyte and is constant in stable chromatographic conditions; the higher the affinity for the stationary phase compared to the mobile phase, the longer the retention time.

4.3.1.1 Gas chromatography–mass spectrometry

In gas chromatography systems the analytes are injected into a capillary column filled with a silica polymer. The analytes interact with the stationary phase until the temperature, regulated by a heating program, reaches the specific boiling point of the analytes that hence become volatile and are carried to the detector by the gas flow. Since a very small number of molecules exhibit the thermo-stability and volatility features required by gas chromatography, strategies of chemical modification of the analytes prior to injection were developed: the so called derivatization. The most common derivatives of testosterone are pentafluoro-benzyloxime-trimethylsilyl-, t-butyldimethylsylil- and pentafluoropropionic anhydride (Fitzgerald *et al.* 2010). The chemical modification is performed on the purified extract: after a liquid-liquid extraction (LLE) involving solvents such as ethylacetate (Fitzgerald *et al.* 2010), diethylether (Taieb *et al.* 2003), dichloromethane or hexane (Wolthers and Kraan 1999), a further clean-up is needed, and is usually accomplished by a gel chromatography on Sephadex LH-20 or water extraction (Shackleton 2010). Before entering the mass spectrometer, usually a single quadrupole, the analyte is ionized by electronic impact, so that Gaussian-shaped peaks of the whole molecule and of its specific fragments, the fragmentography, appear at a specific retention time, and are revealed for their mass-to-charge ratio (m/z). Usually one or two fragments, detected in selected-ion monitoring mode, are used for the quantification.

The abundance of steps in the sample processing and analysis would inevitably result in high imprecision of the assay. This is overcome by the use of stable, isotopically labeled internal standards, in which at least two atoms of hydrogen (H) or ^{12}C are replaced with deuterium (^{2}H) or ^{13}C, reducing the imprecision to the negligible levels required for reference methods. The testosterone internal standard, usually $^{13}C_2$-testosterone or d3-testosterone, is added at the very beginning of sample processing, and, since the stable, isotopically labeled internal standard displays the same physical and chemical properties of the analyte, it will display the same recovery of the analyte in each step and the same efficiency of derivatization, so that the ratio between the analyte and the internal standard remains constant throughout preparation and analysis. The internal standard differs from the analyte in the m/z of the precursor ion and of the fragments, so that it can be specifically identified and quantified by the MS detector. In the quantification by isotopic dilution, the calibration curve is built with the ratio between the signal of the analyte and the signal of the internal standard for each calibration point (y-axis) against the nominal concentration (x-axis). Each sample is quantified through back calculation of the analyte/internal standard ratio found on the calibration curve.

4.3.1.2 Liquid chromatography–tandem mass spectrometry

In liquid chromatography the molecules are resolved for their specific partition coefficient between a flowing mobile phase and the stationary phase. Since large amounts of liquids are continuously eluted at high pressure, the combination with the high *vacuum* system of the MS was hindered until the generation of the atmospheric pressure ionization (API) source in the 1980s. This procedure is able to completely evaporate the liquid solvent and to transfer the charge to the molecules without, or only minimally, altering their structure: this "soft" ionization allows the generation of the ionized molecule, or precursor ion. Liquid chromatography is a versatile technique: the liquid environment allows, theoretically, the analysis of all kinds of molecules, and, when combined with MS, generally requires a reduced volume of sample and less demanding purification than gas chromatography.

The volume of serum required for testosterone measurement largely depends on the ion source and on sensitivity of the mass spectrometer detector, and may usually vary from 0.05 to 0.5 ml (Cawood *et al.* 2005; Kushnir *et al.* 2011). The extraction approach mostly used is LLE, and several examples were reported using methyl tertiary butyl ether (MTBE) (Kushnir *et al.* 2006; Moal *et al.* 2007), diethylether (Cawood *et al.* 2005; Yamashita *et al.* 2009) or ethyl acetate–hexane mixtures (Harwood and Handelsman 2009; Fitzgerald *et al.* 2010). In order to achieve satisfying sensitivity using minimal sample volume, some groups used derivatization strategies generating the testosterone oxime derivative, by incubating the extracted sample either with hydroxylamine solution (Kushnir *et al.* 2006; 2010), or the picolinic acid ester derivative (Yamashita *et al.* 2009). Derivatization requires further purification to remove excess salts, and on-line (Kushnir *et al.* 2010) or off-line (Kushnir *et al.* 2006; Yamashita *et al.* 2009) solid-phase extraction (SPE) approaches have been used. Some groups

treated samples by protein precipitation with acetonitrile (Harwood and Handelsman 2009) or mixtures of methanol/zinc-sulfate (Rauh *et al.* 2006; Ceglarek *et al.* 2009; Kushnir *et al.* 2011) followed by on-line purification on preparative columns mimicking the function of a SPE cartridge (Rauh *et al.* 2006; Guo *et al.* 2006): while steroids are retained on the cartridge, salts and protein residuals are sent to the waste. After clean-up, the sample is directed to the chromatographic column for analysis.

Reverse-phase C18 and C8 columns have been used for testosterone analysis, usually working with water as polar phase and methanol or acetonitrile as organic phases. The pH of the mobile phases can be buffered by addition of formic acid, ammonium acetate or ammonium formate. Compared to the other steroid hormones, testosterone displays a very good revelation efficiency in positive ion mode. All soft ionization approaches have been tested: electrospray ionization (ESI), atmospheric pressure chemical ionization (APCI) and the latest generation of atmospheric pressure photo-ionization (APPI) sources. Ceglarek *et al.* (2009) compared the signal-to-noise ratio (S/N) for several steroids with the three sources, and ESI was reported to give the highest S/N for testosterone, while Kushnir and colleagues (2006) reported higher S/N by APPI for the natural molecule but higher S/N by ESI for the oxime derivative. Since the performance of each source may vary between instruments of the same type, it is difficult to establish a general rule. It has proved wise to validate the best S/N on all the sources available on one's own MS detector.

The appellative "tandem" refers to triple quadrupole mass spectrometry in which the selection of the precursor ion is physically separated from the molecule fragmentation. While in GC-MS the fingerprint of the molecule is generated at the same time as ionization and simultaneous fragmentation of the molecule, the API-MS/MS instruments allow the separation of the ionization and fragmentation steps. In multiple reaction monitoring (MRM) mode, the precursor ion is filtered for its specific m/z by the first quadrupole and fragmented in the second quadrupole, which acts as a collision cell. The third quadrupole filters the specific fragments generated by the analyte further by their m/z. The process is called transition, and for each analyte two transitions, each targeting a different fragment, are monitored: one for the quantification and one for the qualitative confirmation. Similarly to GC-MS, quantification by isotopic dilution is recommended in LC-MS/MS, but, in order to avoid reciprocal isotopic interference, internal standards with the addition of 3 or more amu (M+3) should be chosen. Deuterated isotopes are cheaper and easily available, but ^{13}C isotopes are more stable during sample extraction and ionization, and should be preferred.

One of the great advantages of LC-MS/MS is the possibility of measuring multiple analytes in the same run. In multianalytical methods the choice of sample volume, extraction, chromatographic separation and source should consider the requirements of each analyte. In our own method (Fanelli et al. 2011), testosterone is measured together with eight other steroids starting from 0.9 ml of serum, allowing good sensitivity for the whole panel. We adopted an SPE approach followed by on-line purification in order to lower the noise level, to extend the column life (after 5000 measurements the column performance is not changed) and the source cleanness during the measurement of a large number of samples, preventing the decrease in sensitivity caused by the accumulation of contaminants. Due to the frequently occurring isobaric pairs, a chromatographic gradient of 12.5 min was used, followed by a washing step and a re-equilibration step to ensure specificity of detection. In the case of testosterone, particular attention should be paid to its resolution from the epimer epitestosterone, especially when short chromatography is used. Moreover, in our hands the APCI source provided good sensitivity for all analytes included in the panel. The most relevant publications reporting the currently validated methods to measure serum testosterone by LC-MS/MS are summarized in Table 4.2.

Methods for the direct measurement of free testosterone were also proposed with both LC-MS/MS (Chen et al. 2010) and GC-MS (Van Uytfanghe et al. 2004). Both techniques can achieve satisfying sensitivity to measure free-fraction levels, but the main problem is obtaining the free fraction without altering the equilibrium with the bound fraction. The free fraction was obtained by ultrafiltration, SPE purification, HPLC separation, derivatization and final injection in the GC-MS system, with a sensitivity of 15–20 pmol/l (Van Uytfanghe et al. 2004). In another approach, after ultrafiltration, the procedure is eased by LLE purification and subsequent injection in the LC-MS/MS system, reaching a limit of quantification

of 16 pmol/l (Chen et al. 2010). However, routine measurement of free testosterone will not become feasible until faster and more simple procedures for free-fraction separation are developed.

Interestingly, some groups reported the development of a method for the simultaneous detection of both testosterone and DHT; the latter being a more challenging analyte for which satisfying sensitivities were achieved through derivatization (Yamashita et al. 2009) or with the latest generation of MS detectors (Shiraishi et al. 2008; Harwood and Handelsman 2009; Kulle et al. 2010).

In addition to high specificity and reliability, another important aspect of LC-MS/MS technology is the low cost per sample, which should boost its introduction to routine laboratories. If testosterone is included in the multianalyte LC-MS/MS method, approximately 50–80% of the total costs can be saved by using one LC-MS/MS run instead of individual immunoassays for each analyte. Further resources can be saved considering the consequences of testosterone immunoassay inefficiency, resulting in expenses due to repeated measurements, re-examination of the patients, wrong therapy and unsatisfactory quality of patient care. A present drawback of LC-MS/MS is the requirement of highly experienced, ad-hoc personnel to deal with the analytical difficulties, the complexity of the instruments and the possible pitfalls.

4.3.1.3 Comparative analytical performance and standardization

A number of comparative studies on the accuracy of testosterone measurement by different methods were reported in the last decade. For no other hormone have the analytical methods ever been assessed, questioned and compared to such an extent as for testosterone. The poor reliability of immunoassays was systematically described in comparison to both GC-MS and LC-MS/MS (Table 4.3)

In an early work in 1996, a direct chemiluminescence competitive immunoassay was compared to the GC-MS method developed by the authors, reporting excellent accuracy and precision for male samples but high discrepancies, in terms of correlation and systematic bias, for female samples (Fitzgerald and Herold 1996). In 2003 Taieb et al. extended the comparison to eight automated immunoassays and two direct radioimmunoassays (RIAs) among the most commonly used in worldwide laboratories. The authors reported high inter-assay

Table 4.2 Main features of published LC-MS/MS methods for the measurement of circulating testosterone

Reference	Sample volume (µl); type[a]	Extraction[b]	Derivatization	Chromatography	Total run time (min)	API source	MRM transition Quantifying	MRM transition Qualifying	Internal standard[c]	Calibrator matrix	No. analytes	LLOQ[d]
Guo et al. 2004	760; S	PP + on-line SPE	No	RP-C18	18	APPI	289\97		d2-T	BSA	9	≤100 pg/ml
Cawood et al. 2005	50; S or P	LLE (diethyl ether)	No	RP-C18	4.75	ESI	289\97		d2-T	Stripped S	1	0.3 nmol/l
Guo et al. 2006	200; S	PP + on-line SPE	No	RP-C8	11	APPI	289\109		d2-T	BSA	12	n.d.
Kushnir et al. 2006	100; S	LLE (MTBE) + SPE	Hydroxylamine	RP-C18	3	ESI	e304\112	e304\124	d3-T	BSA	1	0.0345nmol/l
Rauh et al. 2006	100; S or P	PP + on-line SPE	No	RP-C18	6	APCI	289\109	289\97	d5-T	Saline solution	3	0.35 nmol/l
Borrey et al. 2007	200; S	LLE (MTBE) + on-line SPE	Hydroxylamine	RP-C18	3	ESI	e304\124	e304\112	d3-T	BSA	1	0.01 µg/l
Kalhorn et al. 2007	100; S	LLE (ethylacetate: hexane = 1:4)	Hydroxylamine	RP-C18	7	ESI	304\124		d3-T	H₂O	2	500 amol/o.c.
Moal et al. 2007	500; S	LLE (MTBE)	No	RP-C8	20	ESI	289\97		d5-T	BSA	1	<0.17 nmol/l
Tai et al. 2007	1–3 grams; S	SPE + LLE (hexane)	No	RP-C18	62	ESI	289\97		d3-T	MeOH	1	n.d.
Janzen et al. 2008	15; S	PP	No	RP-C18	6	ESI	289\109		d8-17OHP	Steroid free S	10	2.07 nM
Licea-Perez et al. 2008	300; S	LLE (MTBE)	2,3-pyridine-dicarboxylic anhydride	RP-C18	5	ESI	437\286		d3-T	Stripped S	2	0.2 ng/ml
Shiraishi et al. 2008	100; S	LLE (ethylacetate: hexane = 3:2)	No	Hypersil	16	ESI	289\109		d2-T	Steroid free S	2	0.069 nmol/l
Singh 2008	100; S or P	PP + on-line SPE	No	RP-C18	7.5	APCI	289\97	289\109	d3-T	n.d.	1	7 ng/dl
Turpeinen et al. 2008	250–500; S	LLE (diethylether: ethylacetate = 7:3)	No	RP-C18	10	ESI	289\97		d2-T	MeOH	1	0.15 nmol/l

Table 4.2 (cont.)

Ceglarek et al. 2009	100; S	PP + on-line SPE	No	RP-C18	4	APCI	289\97	289\97	d3-T	Saline solution	9	0.05 µg/l
Chen et al. 2009	250; S	LLE (MTBE + 80% MeOH : heptane)	No	RP-C8	6.5	APCI	289\109	289\109	d5-T	MeOH	1	0.056 nmol/l
Harwood and Handelsman 2009	200; S	LLE (ethylacetate : hexane) + on-line SPE	No	RP-C8	>8.5	APPI	289\109		d3-T	BSA	6	10 pg/ml
Yamashita et al. 2009	200; S	LLE (diethyl ether) + SPE	Picolinic acid	RP-C18	12	ESI	394\253	289\97	d3-T	Stripped S	2	1 pg/0.2 ml
Fitzgerald et al. 2010	1000; S or P	LLE (ethylacetate : hexane = 3 : 2)	No	RP-C18	7	ESI	289\109	289\97	d3-T	H_2O	1	5 ng/dl
Kulle et al. 2010	100; P	SPE	No	RP-C18	3.2	ESI	289\97		d8-17OHP	Steroid free P	3	3 ng/dl
Kushnir et al. 2010	200; S	LLE (MTBE) + on-line SPE	Hydroxylamine	RP-C18	3.5	ESI	304\112	304\124	d3-T	BSA	3	10 ng/l
Salameh et al. 2010	150; S or P	On-line SPE	No	RP-C12	4.5	APCI	[e]289\109	[e]289\97	d5-T	n.d.	1	0.3 ng/dl
Fanelli et al. 2011	900; S	PP + off-line SPE + No on-line SPE	No	RP-C8	21	APCI	289\97	289\109	$^{13}C_2$-T	BSA	9	0.019 ng/ml

Abbreviations: n.d., not determined; API, atmospheric pressure ionization; APCI, atmospheric pressure chemical ionization; APPI, atmospheric pressure photo-ionization; ESI, electrospray ionization; RP, reversed phase; APCI, atmospheric pressure chemical ionization; MRM, multiple reaction monitoring; LLOQ, lower limit of quantification; BSA, bovine serum albumin; MTBE, methyl tertiary butyl ether; serum (S), plasma (P).

[a] serum (S), plasma (P).
[b] liquid-liquid extraction (LLE); protein precipitation (PP); solid-phase extraction (SPE).
[c] testosterone (T), 17-hydroxyprogesterone (17OHP).
[d] on column (o.c.).
[e] quantitative or qualitative function not specified.

Table 4.3 Summary of the results of the main comparison studies between immunoassays and GC-MS (a) and LC-MS/MS (b) on samples from men (M), women (W) and children (C)

(a)

Reference	Immunoassay	Producer	Sample	n	Regression	Slope	Intercept	Correlation coefficient	Mean difference (RIA − LC-MS/MS or %RIA/LC-MS/MS)
Fitzgerald and Herold 1996	ACS kit	Ciba Corning Diagnostic Corp	W	44	Linear	$0.72 \times$ GC-MS	1.21 nmol/l	r^2 0.31	0.89 nmol/l
			M	57	Linear	$1.07 \times$ GC-MS	0.19 nmol/l	r^2 0.98	1.2 nmol/l
Taieb et al. 2003	Architect i2000	Abbott Laboratories	W	54	Deming	$1.64 \times$ GC-MS	−0.20 nmol/l	r 0.80	1.26 nmol/l
	ACS-180	Bayer Diagnostic	M	45	Deming	$1.07 \times$ GC-MS	−1.48 nmol/l	r 0.95	−0.21 nmol/l
			W	55	Deming	$1.63 \times$ GC-MS	0.53 nmol/l	r 0.84	2.04 nmol/l
	Immuno-1	Bayer Diagnostic	M	50	Deming	$1.07 \times$ GC-MS	1.19 nmol/l	r 0.95	2.53 nmol/l
			W	55	Deming	$1.47 \times$ GC-MS	−0.48 nmol/l	r 0.68	0.56 nmol/l
	Vidas	Bio-Mérieux	M	50	Deming	$1.10 \times$ GC-MS	−1.48 nmol/l	r 0.96	0.54 nmol/l
			W	51	Deming	$1.16 \times$ GC-MS	−0.58 nmol/l	r 0.75	−0.07 nmol/l
	Immulite 2000	Diagnostic Products Corporation	M	50	Deming	$0.94 \times$ GC-MS	−2.92 nmol/l	r 0.92	−4.67 nmol/l
			W	53	Deming	$2.57 \times$ GC-MS	−0.82 nmol/l	r 0.57	3.23 nmol/l
			M	50	Deming	$0.79 \times$ GC-MS	1.80 nmol/l	r 0.97	−2.46 nmol/l
	Vitros ECi	Ortho-Clinical Diagnostics	W	55	Deming	$1.15 \times$ GC-MS	−0.40 nmol/l	r 0.76	−0.05 nmol/l
	AutoDelfia	Perkin-Elmer	M	50	Deming	$0.94 \times$ GC-MS	−2.03 nmol/l	r 0.97	−3.36 nmol/l
			W	55	Deming	$3.28 \times$ GC-MS	−2.01 nmol/l	r 0.78	2.68 nmol/l
	Elecsys 2010	Roche Diagnostic	M	50	Deming	$0.95 \times$ GC-MS	1.98 nmol/l	r 0.86	0.69 nmol/l
			W	53	Deming	$0.85 \times$ GC-MS	−0.48 nmol/l	r 0.72	−0.74 nmol/l
	RIA Immunotech	Beckman-Coulter	M	50	Deming	$0.93 \times$ GC-MS	−3.02 nmol/l	r 0.96	−4.79 nmol/l
			W	54	Deming	$1.43 \times$ GC-MS	−0.46 nmol/l	r 0.78	0.46 nmol/l
	Coat-A-Count DPC	Dade Behring	M	50	Deming	$0.96 \times$ GC-MS	−2.95 nmol/l	r 0.95	−4.19 nmol/l
			W	51	Deming	$1.45 \times$ GC-MS	−0.56 nmol/l	r 0.89	0.49 nmol/l
			M	50	Deming	$1.06 \times$ GC-MS	−1.36 nmol/l	r 0.92	−0.55 nmol/l

(b)

Reference	Immunoassay	Producer	Sample	n	Regression	Slope	Intercept	Correlation coefficient	Mean difference (RIA − LC-MS/MS or %RIA/LC-MS/MS)
Wang et al. 2004	DPC coat-a-tube RIA	Diagnostic Products Corporation	M	101	Deming	$1.098 \times$ LC-MS/MS	−2.9 ng/dl	ICC 0.968	9.70%
	HUMC-RIA	In house; tracer and antibody by ICN	M	101	Deming	$1.141 \times$ LC-MS/MS	−39.2 ng/dl	ICC 0.948	9.70%

Study	Assay	Manufacturer	Group	N	Method	Equation	Intercept		Corr.	Bias
	Elecsys 2010	Roche Diagnostics	M	101	Deming	$1.167 \times$ LC-MS/MS	−75.5 ng/dl	ICC	0.965	−3.40%
	Vitros ECi	Ortho-Clinical Diagnostics	M	101	Deming	$1.233 \times$ LC-MS/MS	−118.4 ng/dl	ICC	0.954	−11.20%
	Immulite 2000	Diagnostic Products Corporation	M	101	Deming	$0.881 \times$ LC-MS/MS	−28.6 ng/dl	ICC	0.925	−18.70%
	ACS Centaur	Bayer Diagnostic	M	101	Deming	$1.195 \times$ LC-MS/MS	−1.4 ng/dl	ICC	0.919	15.90%
Guo et al. 2004	RIA	ICN Pharmaceuticals	M and W	50	Linear[a]	0.919	−0.064 nmol/l	r	0.971	
Cawood et al. 2005	Extraction RIA	In house	W ≤3 nmol/l	67	n.d.	$0.69 \times$ RIA	−0.15 nmol/l	r^2	0.66	
			M ≤3 nmol/l	29	n.d.	$0.74 \times$ RIA	−0.26 nmol/l	r^2	0.35	
			W >8 nmol/l	13	n.d.	$1.12 \times$ RIA	−1.7 nmol/l	r^2	0.77	
			M >8 nmol/l	n.d.	n.d.	$1.02 \times$ RIA	−0.2 nmol/l	r^2	0.97	
Kushnir et al. 2006	Vitros ECi	Ortho-Clinical Diagnostics	M and W	216	Deming	$1.15 \times$ LC-MS/MS	11.2 ng/dl	r	0.976	
			<50 ng/dl	150						4.1 ng/dl
Rauh et al. 2006	Roche Elecsys	Roche Diagnostics	C (<5 nmol/l)	70	Passing-Bablok	$1.485 \times$ LC-MS/MS	−0.149 nmol/l	r	0.623	
			C (>5 nmol/l)	37		$0.954 \times$ LC-MS/MS	−0.142 nmol/l	r	0.864	
Borrey et al. 2007	RIA Spectria	Orion Diagnostica	W	43	Passing-Bablok	$0.887 \times$ RIA	0.014 µg/l	r^2	0.92	0.031 µg/l
Moal et al. 2007	CIS bio	Shering SA	W and C	59	Deming	$0.972 \times$ LC-MS/MS	0.3 nmol/l	r	0.870	0.23 nmol/l
	Immunotech	Beckman-Coulter	W and C	59	Deming	$1.365 \times$ LC-MS/MS	0.8 nmol/l	r	0.868	1.24 nmol/l

Study	Assay	Manufacturer	Sample	N	Regression	Slope	Intercept		Correlation	
	Spectria-Orion	Orion Diagnostica	W and C	59	Deming	1.177 × LC-MS/MS	0.2 nmol/l	r	0.803	0.38 nmol/l
	Liaison	DiaSorin	W and C	59	Deming	1.114 × LC-MS/MS	0.7 nmol/l	r	0.772	0.81 nmol/l
	Roche Modular E	Roche Diagnostics	W and C	59	Deming	1.153 × LC-MS/MS	0.1 nmol/l	r	0.792	0.32 nmol/l
Ceglarek et al. 2009	Elecsys 2010	Roche Diagnostics	n.d.	57	Passing-Bablok	1.083 × LC-MS/MS	0.089 µg/l	Pearson's r	0.967	9.70%
Shiraishi et al. 2008	Coat-A-Count DPC	Diagnostic Products Corporation	M and W	145	Deming	1.06 × RIA	−20.6 nmol/l	r^2	0.9785	0.15 nmol/l
Singh 2008	Direct ACS:180	Bayer	M	37	n.d.	1.0497 × RIA	8.95 ng/dl	r^2	0.9809	
	Extraction ACS:180	Bayer	W	73	n.d.	0.7231 × RIA	0.2109 ng/dl	r^2	0.8561	
Turpeinen et al. 2008	Spectria coated tube RIA	Orion Diagnostica	>3 nmol/l	121	Linear	0.57 × LC-MS/MS	2.3 nmol/l	r	0.92	−43%
	Extraction RIA	In house	>3 nmol/l	109	Linear	0.85 × LC-MS/MS	0.18 nmol/l	r	0.984	−15%
Chen et al. 2009	Abbott Architect i2000	Abbott Laboratories	>3 nmol/l	<62	n.d.	0.8710 × LC-MS/MS	1.4450 nmol/l	r^2	0.9406	
			<3 nmol/l	<62	n.d.	0.9434 × LC-MS/MS	1.0093 nmol/l	r^2	0.3408	
	Roche Modular E170	Roche Diagnostics	>3 nmol/l	<62	n.d.	0.8898 × LC-MS/MS	0.4237 nmol/l	r^2	0.9483	
			<3 nmol/l	<62	n.d.	0.9657 × LC-MS/MS	0.551 nmol/l	r^2	0.3836	
	DPC Immulite 2500	Diagnostic Products Corporation	>3 nmol/l	<62	n.d.	0.7602 × LC-MS/MS	1.6192 nmol/l	r^2	0.8124	
			<3 nmol/l	<62	n.d.	0.8623 × LC-MS/MS	0.5480 nmol/l	r^2	0.2925	
Harwood and Handelsman 2009	RIA Delfia	Perkin Elmer	M	172	Passing-Bablok	1.333 × LC-MS/MS	0.35 ng/ml	r	0.9631	42%

Study	Assay	Manufacturer	Range/Sex	n	Regression	Equation	Intercept		Correlation	
Salameh et al. 2010	Extraction + LC RIA	In house	<40 ng/dl	n.d.	n.d.	1.0064 × RIA	0.0618 ng/dl	r^2	0.995	
			Entire range	n.d.	n.d.	1.0210 × RIA	1.4997 ng/dl	r^2	0.994	
Brandhorst et al. 2011	Elecsys Testosterone	Roche Diagnostics	M	117	Passing-Bablok	1.06 × LC-MS/MS	0.02 µg/l	Pearson's r	0.974	
			W	119	Passing-Bablok	1.32 × LC-MS/MS	−0.03 µg/l	Pearson's r	0.893	
	Elecsys Testosterone II	Roche Diagnostics	M	117	Passing-Bablok	1.05 × LC-MS/MS	0.03 µg/l	Pearson's r	0.986	
			W	113	Passing-Bablok	1.06 × LC-MS/MS	−0.02 µg/l	Pearson's r	0.956	
Fanelli et al. 2011	Elecsys Modular E170	Roche Diagnostics	M	51	Deming	1.004 × LC-MS/MS	−0.097 ng/ml	r	0.938	−2.50%
			W	111	Deming	1.724 × LC-MS/MS	−0.181 ng/ml	r	0.773	16.80%

Abbreviations: n.d., not determined; RIA, radioimmunoassay; ICC, interclass correlation coefficient; n, number of tested samples.
[a] x-axis and y-axis method not specified.

variability among the 10 immunoassays, and, through the comparison with a GC-MS method, concluded that none of them showed acceptable reliability for the measurement of female or pediatric testosterone levels. Furthermore, two methods were reported to have questionable reliability even in the male range (Taieb *et al.* 2003). In 2004 Wang *et al.* published a similar comparative study between four automated immunoassays, two RIAs and LC-MS/MS on male serum. The authors found that only four methods gave results within ±20% of those obtained by LC-MS/MS in more than 60% of samples. In addition, when samples with testosterone concentrations below 100 ng/dl were considered, all six immunoassays failed to give results with acceptable variability in 55.5 to 90.9% of the samples. The authors concluded that none of the automated immunoassays displayed adequate precision, accuracy and sensitivity to be applied to samples from females and children (Wang *et al.* 2004).

Moal *et al.* (2007) reported another multi-assay comparison where one extractive RIA, two direct RIAs and two automated immunometric platforms were compared to a validated LC-MS/MS method on female and pediatric sera. Confirming previous findings, they reported poor agreement between the immunoassays and LC-MS/MS, in terms of both poor correlation coefficient and variable slope and intercept coefficient by regression analysis. In general, all methods overestimated the results. The authors attributed this problem not only to the poor specificity of the immunoassays, but also to non-linearity of the calibration curves, especially at low doses, where the low-concentration samples appear and high variance is expected (Moal *et al.* 2007).

The poor performance of immunoassays at low concentrations was confirmed by Cawood *et al.* (2005), who verified the accuracy of their LC-MS/MS method with two GC-MS methods. Compared to the LC-MS/MS method, an *in-house* extractive RIA showed good correlation and regression for levels above 8 nmol/l, but poor correlation and regression at levels below 3 nmol/l.

Many other papers reported similar results on the comparison of LC-MS/MS technique and one or more immunoassays of different kinds (Table 4.3). All these efforts provided strong and unambiguous evidence for the need to shift toward a more specific, sensitive and reliable method such as LC-MS/MS. As a consequence many laboratories all over the world

apply their own LC-MS/MS technique, raising the problem of harmonization, validation, calibration, quality control material and, finally, reference intervals using all these different LC-MS/MS methods (Rosner *et al.* 2010).

In the last few years, papers have reported the comparison to GC-MS reference methods of several LC-MS/MS methods, using different preparative methodologies, chromatography and detection strategies (Thienpont *et al.* 2008; Vesper *et al.* 2009). Thienpont *et al.* (2008) reported the comparison of four routinely used LC-MS/MS methods with a reference GC-MS method listed by the Joint Committee for Traceability in Laboratory Medicine (JCTLM). The LC-MS/MS methods reported good intra-laboratory precision in the entire range of clinically relevant values: the median coefficient of variation (CV) was below 6.6% at concentrations > 5 nmol/l, and below 8.5% at concentrations < 5 nmol/l. The regression analysis, in terms of slope and intercept coefficients, the correlation coefficients and the percentage of the difference plot, revealed good agreement of the four LC-MS/MS methods compared to the reference GC-MS method: far better than that obtained by similar studies in which immunoassays were compared to GC-MS (Taieb *et al.* 2003). The authors stated that this improvement in performance should be ascribed to the use of isotope dilution and to the specificity provided by the precursor-to-fragment transitions performed by tandem MS. The authors concluded that the tested LC-MS/MS procedures displayed sufficient levels of sensitivity in defining normogonadal, hypogonadal and female testosterone levels, proper specificity and good accuracy. However, small to medium biases (<9.6%) were reported for three out of four assays (Thienpont *et al.* 2008).

Vesper *et al.* reported the results of the comparison of seven LC-MS/MS methods and one GC-MS/MS method to an LC-MS/MS reference method performed at the National Institute of Standard and Technology (NIST) included in the JCTLM list (Vesper *et al.* 2009). The reported intra-laboratory CV ranged between 2.52 and 25.58% at low levels of testosterone (8.47 ng/dl) and between 1.40 and 11.36% at high levels of testosterone (297 ng/dl). The reported inter-laboratory CV is < 15% at concentrations above 44 ng/dl, but it increased up to 33% at lower levels. The percentage difference between each tested procedure and the reference method is on average 7.5% for concentrations > 100 ng/dl and

15.5% for concentrations < 100 ng/dl. By performing a regression analysis, proportional bias was observed in six assays, while constant bias was observed in four assays. The authors stated that the variability observed among the tested tandem-MS procedures is surprisingly small for testosterone levels above 100 ng/dl; better than what was previously reported for immunoassays. However, the situation worsens at female concentrations, where the increased variability observed could be attributed to several factors: the sensitivity limit of the different assays, intra-laboratory variability, interference in the detection (ion suppression) caused, probably, by phospholipids, and the rounding to different decimal points. When compared directly to the NIST method, the single assays reported a mean difference below or equal to 10%, which is smaller than that reported for immunoassays (Vesper *et al.* 2009).

Both papers concluded by emphasizing the importance of careful validation and standardization of the procedure and of monitoring performance in each laboratory, together with the importance of proper assay calibration and quality control. Finally, they promote the sharing of common calibration materials and participation in external quality assurance programs and/or the comparison with internationally accepted reference methods (Thienpont *et al.* 2008; Vesper *et al.* 2009).

4.3.2 Radioimmunoassay

The first radioimmunoassay for plasma testosterone was developed at the end of the sixties (Furuyama *et al.* 1970). It was based on an antiserum raised against testosterone coupled to bovine serum albumin at position 3 (T-3-BSA), ^{3}H-labelled testosterone as the tracer and bound/free separation by ammonium sulfate precipitation. Plasma testosterone was extracted and chromatographed on alumina columns prior to immunoassay. Radio- and other immunoassays for plasma and serum testosterone were developed by several investigators, for instance Nieschlag and Loriaux (1972). These authors produced their own antiserum by a novel immunization technique (Vaitukaitis *et al.* 1971) and distributed the antiserum freely to other laboratories so that their method became widely used and their papers were ranked as Citation Classics in 1981. Slowly, kit manufacturers took over the development of assays, but while the practicability of the assays consistently

improved, the overall performance of current immunoassays is not much different from that of 40 years ago. For instance, the early assays already showed a lower detection limit of 3–10 pg, as do current assays. Since RIAs are most sensitive at low antibody concentrations, when competition between tracer and unknown is high, high-affinity antibodies are crucial for sensitive assays. However, usually high affinity is better obtained with polyclonal antisera which display elevated cross-reactivity with DHT. A substantial improvement in the sensitivity of testosterone RIAs (and other immunoassays as well) could be achieved by using highly specific monoclonal antibodies with high affinity: a goal very difficult to reach.

In general the current in-house methods for testosterone RIA are the same as the early assays of the seventies and are still in use mainly for research purposes because they are cheap and accurate. An extraction step is necessary to eliminate serum proteins which do not allow the correct interaction of albumin and SHBG-bound testosterone with the antiserum.

The long experience with the traditional RIAs produced well-documented reference intervals in different age and sex groups, and this methodology has several advantages such as high sensitivity, due to the large volume of samples which can be employed, and the possibility of measuring different steroids in the same sample extract. In addition, the extract can be subjected to chromatography, allowing the separation and measurement of different steroids, for example DHT, androstenedione, etc.

Some disadvantages should be listed as well. First, without doubt it is a challenging, time-consuming and costly assay and it requires high technical competence and accurate monitoring of the extraction efficiency. Sometimes it may be difficult to obtain a large volume of sample, e.g. from children, and the RIA may be affected by matrix effect (matrix difference between serum samples, particularly hemolyzed and lipemic samples, and solution of standards used to prepare the standard curve) and by the presence of auto-antibodies leading to falsely high or low values, depending on the type of antibody interaction occurring. Finally, we should not forget the problems related to organic solvents and radioactive waste disposal and to safety concerns.

Because of these problems, traditional RIAs have been almost completely replaced by non-extraction methods for clinical use. These kinds of commercially available RIAs are either based on double antibody separation or are in solid phase; i.e. the antibody is fixed at the wall of the reaction tubes (coated tubes) so that no centrifugation is required, reducing the hands-on time and improving practicability. Serum testosterone is displaced from carrier proteins by chemical agents competing for protein binding, e.g. danazol, although the exact nature of the kit components is usually known only to the manufacturers and is protected by property rights. Well-validated non-extraction methods may work well for male serum samples; although inaccurate testosterone concentrations are occasionally measured in individual samples containing abnormal SHBG concentrations or substances (e.g. drugs) interfering with the kit components. However, results obtained with different RIA kits have been repeatedly reported to be poorly comparable (Jockenhövel et al. 1992; Boots et al. 1998).

There are a number of advantages of the direct RIA methodology. First of all it is relatively simple to carry out, it requires a small volume of samples (usually 0.1 ml or less) and it can be automated, resulting in a very fast turnaround time, rendering it particularly suitable to the large number of samples tested in a routine clinical laboratory. It is also relatively inexpensive and generally fairly accurate for levels above 300 ng/dl (healthy men). There is some evidence that a well chosen and performed RIA may offer equal precision to LC-MS assay (Legro et al. 2010). There are, however, downsides to direct RIAs: concentrations of testosterone can be often overestimated, especially when levels sink below 10 nmol/l. Moreover, they are poorly standardized, reference ranges vary between assays, and direct RIAs share with extractive RIAs the same problems of matrix effect, radioprotection and radioactive waste disposal.

4.3.3 Other immunoassays

The most popular alternatives to radioactive methods are immunoassays based on non-radioactively labeled tracers such as fluoroimmunoassay (FIA), chemiluminescent assay (CLIA) and enzyme-linked immunosorbent assay (EIA/ELISA). They can be in liquid or in solid phase, whereby solid phase, microtiter plate-based assays are preferred due to easy handling and proneness to automation. Also in these assays it is the antigen that is labeled and competes with the endogenous testosterone for

binding to the antiserum. The primary antibody can be poly- or monoclonal and is usually bound to the tube wall or to the plate well. In EIAs/ELISAs the tracer is represented by testosterone coupled to an enzyme (alkaline phosphatase, β-galactosidase, penicillinase, acetylcholinesterase or horse radish peroxidase) which starts a colorimetric reaction upon addition of the substrate at the end of the incubation time. This results in color development which is inversely proportional to the amount of unlabelled testosterone and can be read by a spectrophotometer. The sensitivity of EIA/ELISA is affected by the number of steroid molecules coupled to the enzyme, and the proper molar ratio between steroid and enzyme must be carefully validated (Rassaie et al. 1992). In FIA the tracer is testosterone coupled to a molecule (e.g. europium) which fluoresces upon stimulation. The fluorescence is measured by a fluorimeter and, again, is inversely related to the amount of cold testosterone contained in the sample. Critical in EIAs/ELISAs and FIAs are the washing steps, which should be carefully carried out in order to eliminate non-specifically bound substances which would result in poor precision and falsely elevated readouts.

Automatic multianalyzers, mainly based on non-radioactive methods requiring a low sample volume (usually less than 0.1 ml) are now available and widely used in diagnostic clinical laboratories for the direct and quick measurement of serum testosterone. Some of these systems have been evaluated against the reference method based on MS, showing acceptable results at least in male samples (Fitzgerald and Herold 1996; Levesque et al. 1998; Gonzalez-Sagrado et al. 2000). However, inconsistency of results obtained with different methods is reported as well, and some systems seem to suffer from systematic problems, resulting in over- or underestimation of serum testosterone and/or insufficient sensitivity, especially in female samples (Taieb et al. 2002). This is very evident when comparing the results of external quality control trials (Middle 2002).

The quality control program of the College of American Pathologists clearly demonstrates how great the inaccuracy of total testosterone measurement is, even though one-third of the clinical laboratories use the same automated platform and three of these platforms cover two-thirds of the market (Rosner et al. 2007). The comparison of results obtained by immunoassays with those derived from MS shows a variability in testosterone levels between −4.7 and 2.6 nmol/l in adult males and between 0.7 and 3.3 nmol/l in females (Taieb *et al.* 2003). In such conditions, it is sometimes difficult to distinguish hypo- and eugonadal males, unless the laboratory has optimized its own method and population-related reference intervals. In any case, the diagnosis of hypogonadism requires multiple determinations of testosterone levels during 24 hours, with the inherent costs.

Furthermore, it seems impossible to trust the testosterone levels detected in women and children with these immunoassays (Wang *et al.* 2004). When women's samples are processed, all automated immunoassays seem to be affected by the interference of other steroids, such as dehydroepiandrosterone sulfate (DHEAS) (Warner *et al.* 2006; Middle 2007), and of drugs, such as danazol and mifepristone (RU486), thus introducing more variability and difficulty in result interpretation. This lack of specificity seriously affects clinical management in the newborn period and early infancy, where poor clinical correlation to steroid test levels is very frequent and sensitivity is not adequate enough to differentiate prepubertal and pubertal secretion.

A practical approach, as suggested by Kane *et al.* 2007), is to adopt a commercial total testosterone assay only if it provides validation against an MS assay and the regression plot of the data obtained by the two methods is supplied. The slope would give information about its accuracy and the intercept about its reliability at low concentrations. It may also be a good laboratory strategy to analyze male and female samples for total testosterone with two different calibrated assays.

As for every other method, each laboratory should carefully validate the results obtained by the multianalyzer before it is implemented for routine testosterone measurement. In practice, however, validation is limited by the fact that most of the systems are based on a master calibration curve carried out by the manufacturer and not available to customers. Each assay then requires only one or two calibrators to adjust the master curve and parallelism tests cannot be performed. As in the non-automatic assays, differences observed between the kits can be ascribed to differences in the matrix of the calibrators and in the affinity, titer and specificity of the antibodies used.

4.3.4 Assessment of free testosterone

The direct measurement of free testosterone in serum is based on the same principles governing the assay of free thyroid hormones, and has been extensively considered and reviewed by R. Ekins in the past (Ekins 1990). Serum testosterone exists in an equilibrium between free and protein-bound fractions: an equilibrium which is invariably disturbed by all methods of free-hormone measurement; a factor that should be kept in mind when choosing a method and analyzing the data. The methods of reference for free-hormone analysis are equilibrium dialysis and ultrafiltration.

4.3.4.1 Equilibrium dialysis

In equilibrium dialysis, the serum (dialysand) is put in contact with a buffer (dialysate) through a membrane which allows the passage of low-molecular-weight compounds (e.g. free hormones) but retains the binding proteins. As a consequence of the passage of free hormone molecules to the dialysate, new hormone molecules will dissociate from the binding proteins until a new equilibrium is reached and the free-hormone concentration is the same on the two sides of the membrane. The free hormone can now be measured in the dialysate either directly (e.g. by RIA) or indirectly by knowing the total hormone concentration and assessing the percentage of added labeled hormone passed in the free fraction. Provided that the ion composition of the buffer does not interfere with the equilibrium constant (K), dialysis is thermodynamically equivalent to serum dilution and leads to a reduction of the free-hormone concentration and to dissociation of new hormone from the binding proteins until a new equilibrium is established in the system. At equilibrium the original free-hormone concentration is therefore only "approximately" maintained because, since the total hormone concentration is constant, the final, measured free-hormone concentration will be somewhat diluted and lower than that in the original sample. This effect can be regarded as negligible if the relative free-hormone concentration is low, as in the case of free thyroxin (0.02%), but might become relevant in the case of free testosterone (2%), so that the buffer volume against which the sample is dialyzed should be kept to a minimum. In this respect, it is the total volume of dialysand plus dialysate which determines the dilution factor; while the position of the dialysis membrane between the two compartments, i.e. the individual volume of the two compartments, is irrelevant for the free-hormone concentration, which, at equilibrium, will be the same on the two sides (Ekins 1990).

High technical competence is required for this methodology and represents an important limitation. Each assay step introduces a specific variability source that contributes to the total variability and increases the risk of error. The purity of the tracer is crucial, as the presence of a contaminant that does not link to proteins can enhance the concentration of detected free testosterone. Finally, accuracy is affected by the accuracy of the total testosterone assay used.

4.3.4.2 Ultrafiltration

The problem of sample dilution is avoided in the case of ultrafiltration of undiluted serum, the second reference method in free-hormone determination. In this procedure a serum sample is centrifuged through a membrane with an appropriate molecular-weight cutoff. Only free hormone and low-molecular-weight compounds will be collected in the ultrafiltrate at a concentration equal to that in the original sample. The free hormone can be directly assessed by RIA of the ultrafiltrate or by indirect measurement of the relative fraction of labeled hormone added to the original samples which is recovered in the ultrafiltrate (Vlahos *et al.* 1982). Direct measurement by RIA is preferable both in ultrafiltration and in equilibrium dialysis, since the impurities of the tracer can result in inaccurate estimation of the free fraction. Ultrafiltration devices are commercially available (e.g. Centrifree® micropartition system, Millipore).

Possibly ultrafiltration may be limited if non-filterable binding competitors are present in the sample, or if binding proteins interact with the membrane; this will result in progressive increase of the free-hormone concentration in the filtrate. In addition it is affected by temperature, so that a strict control of this parameter is necessary. However, since the ultrafiltration time is rather short (one hour or less) compared to dialysis (several hours), the possible changes in the equilibrium ensuing from these and other factors may be assumed to be negligible. As for equilibrium dialysis, the testosterone RIA's accuracy directly affects the accuracy of the methodology which is not trustable at low concentrations.

Recently, free testosterone has been measured by LC-MS/MS following ultrafiltration or equilibrium dialysis, demonstrating the superiority of such an approach compared to the more common methods based on analog free testosterone measurement or calculated free testosterone (Chen *et al.* 2010).

4.3.4.3 Direct free testosterone assays

The principles of the direct free testosterone methods have been described in detail in the previous edition of this book (Simoni 2004). In practice such assays are based on a labeled compound to be added to the sample, the "analog," which is totally non-reactive with serum proteins, but can be recognized by the solid phase antibody present in a limited amount and which competes for binding with the free hormone in the sample.

Several commercially available kits are based on this principle and are widely used to assess free testosterone in clinical samples. Unfortunately, there is evidence that these methods are totally inaccurate (Fritz *et al.* 2008; Chen *et al.* 2010). In fact, the direct measurement of free testosterone in serum based on the labeled hormone "analog" is valid only if the analog does not interact with the serum proteins: a condition which is currently not met by commercial kits. In fact, neither the identity of the analog tracer, nor the validation of the kit (showing the absence of interactions with the serum protein) is usually disclosed by the manufacturer. On the contrary, the "analog" principle is often not even mentioned or is misrepresented in the instructions accompanying the kits, which are often validated only against other kits and not against dialysis or ultrafiltration. It should be kept in mind that, in practice, finding a hormone analog totally unreactive with serum proteins is very difficult, and several studies have shown that such an interaction indeed occurs, resulting in inaccurate measurements of free testosterone. In this respect it is interesting that serum free testosterone measured by an "analog" method accounts for 0.5–0.65% of total testosterone, while equilibrium dialysis and ultrafiltration give values of 1.5–4%, revealing inconsistencies between the different approaches (Rosner 1997; Winters *et al.* 1998). In a direct comparison, free testosterone values measured by a bestseller "analog" kit were only 20–30% of those measured by equilibrium dialysis (Vermeulen *et al.* 1999).

For these reasons the kits for direct free testosterone measurement presently available do not measure what they claim and should not be used (Rosner 2001; Swerdloff and Wang 2008). If LC-MS/MS coupled to ultrafiltration becomes technically affordable, this approach is likely to become the method of choice for assessment of free testosterone in clinical serum samples.

4.3.4.4 Salivary testosterone

Salivary testosterone is considered to be a good index of serum free testosterone, and a highly significant correlation with serum total and free testosterone has long been known (Wang *et al.* 1981). Recently a strong correlation with bioavailable testosterone has been demonstrated (Morley *et al.* 2006). As with other steroid hormones, free testosterone enters saliva though passive diffusion across the acinar cells of the salivary glands and can be measured directly in saliva by RIA or EIA with or without extraction.

The advantages and disadvantages of saliva as a diagnostic medium have been extensively reviewed (Lewis 2006; Levine *et al.* 2007; Chiappin *et al.* 2007). Based on a non-invasive, stress-free and easily repeatable sampling technique even outside the clinical setting, the assay is well suited for pediatric applications, for screening male hypogonadism (Morley *et al.* 2006) and for investigating biosocial models and testosterone–behavior relationship (Dabbs 1990; Shirtcliff *et al.* 2001; 2002; Booth *et al.* 2003; Granger *et al.* 2004).

The manner in which saliva samples are collected and stored may influence testosterone measurement, more than other analytes such as cortisol and DHEA, because of substances that can be used to stimulate saliva flow, the presence of a transient rise in testosterone levels in the first few minutes after chewing the gum, and the presence of blood contamination from oral microinjuries (Granger *et al.* 2004; Atkinson *et al.* 2008). Storage temperature and time are two variables that dramatically influence salivary testosterone assays (Granger *et al.* 2004). The study of the effect of five different clean-up methods on salivary steroid and protein concentration demonstrated that testosterone and DHEA were the analytes more strongly affected by pretreatment methods, calling for a careful validation of saliva sampling procedures before their adoption in clinical laboratory routine (Atkinson *et al.* 2008).

Since salivary testosterone provides a measure of free testosterone, its assessment has been considered especially in those conditions in which an elevation of serum concentrations of SHBG can hinder the accurate diagnosis of hypogonadism, for example in male aging. Given the problems related to direct measurement in saliva, several authors attempted LC-MS/MS of salivary testosterone with very promising results (Matsui *et al.* 2009; Macdonald *et al.* 2011). With the diffusion of MS-based methodologies, this approach might offer an accurate and straightforward assessment of free testosterone in the near future.

4.3.4.5 Bioavailable testosterone

Several lines of evidence suggest that not only free testosterone but also albumin-bound testosterone is available to the target tissues for biological activity (Manni *et al.* 1985). Therefore, the non-SHBG-bound testosterone is called "bioavailable testosterone." This parameter can be measured based on the property of ammonium sulfate to precipitate SHBG together with the steroids bound to it. Trace amounts of labeled testosterone are added to the samples and, after allowing for equilibration with endogenous testosterone, an equal volume of a saturated solution of ammonium sulfate is added (final concentration 50%) and SHBG is separated by centrifugation. The percentage of labeled testosterone remaining in the supernatant represents an estimate of bioavailable testosterone, which can be calculated knowing the total testosterone concentration of the sample (Manni *et al.* 1985).

Alternatively, testosterone can be measured directly in the supernatant by RIA (Dechaud *et al.* 1989). The ammonium sulfate concentration is critical to proper precipitation of SHBG only, and this parameter should be accurately tested in each laboratory in order to avoid precipitation of albumin as well, and underestimation of bioavailable testosterone (Davies *et al.* 2002). In spite of the apparent simplicity of the assay, relevant technical differences in the methodology and in the algorithms applied in various laboratories are the cause of often inaccurate results (De Ronde *et al.* 2006). A possible way to circumvent this problem is represented by the immunocapture of SHBG and SHBG-testosterone complexes by monoclonal antibodies coupled to magnetic beads, followed by magnetic separation and measurement of non-SHBG-bound testosterone by RIA in the supernatant (Raverot *et al.* 2010).

When properly done, bioavailable testosterone correlates quite well with total testosterone and calculated free testosterone. However, it is unclear, at the moment, whether the estimation of bioavailable testosterone provides any superior diagnostic power over the accurate assessment of the latter parameters in clinical conditions of mild hypogonadism accompanied by increased SHBG and possibly reduced concentrations of serum albumin, such as in LOH.

4.3.4.6 Calculated free testosterone

Assessment of free testosterone is recommended by several national and international scientific societies in consensus guidelines for the evaluation of androgen deficiency when serum total testosterone levels are borderline. The classical methods for free and bioavailable testosterone measurement reported above (i.e. equilibrium dialysis, ultrafiltration and ammonium sulfate precipitation), however, are too cumbersome for clinical routine. This is the main reason why "analog" methods became so widespread despite their unreliability. A very popular alternative is provided by the calculation of free testosterone starting from measured concentrations of total testosterone and SHBG and based on equilibrium-binding theory or empirical equations. There are at least five published formulae for free testosterone calculation, some of them available online (e.g. www.issam.ch/freetesto.htm), even as downloadable applications for tablets and smart phones.

These formulae have been recently reviewed and validated for their accuracy against equilibrium dialysis in over 2000 serum samples. This study demonstrated that commonly used formulae systematically overestimate free testosterone compared to laboratory measurement (Ly *et al.* 2010). Interestingly, calculations based on equilibrium-binding equation methods performed even worse than assumption-free, empirical formulae, revealing that the equilibrium-binding approach relies on only partially correct hypotheses. For instance, the reported value of the Testosterone–SHBG affinity constant differs by up to fourfold between different authors; possibly because it is still not clear if this "constant" is age related. Therefore, if calculated free testosterone is used in clinical practice, the physician must be aware of the limitations of such an approach and should not draw therapeutic decisions based only on this parameter.

4.3.5 Bioassay

Immunological methods measure just the mass of circulating testosterone, not its bioactivity. Under the assumption that the overall androgenic bioactivity in serum and peripheral tissues results from

bioavailable testosterone and other androgens, several in-vitro androgen bioassays have been developed. Currently six cell-based androgenic bioassays, based on detection of intracellular, AR-dependent events, have been reported in the literature (Roy *et al.* 2008; Need *et al.* 2010 and references therein). Such bioassays are interesting especially for screening and detecting substances with androgenic activity; for example endocrine disruptors (Soto *et al.* 2006). They are usually based on reporter genes (e.g. luciferase), stimulated by the activation of the AR induced by the testosterone/androgens present in the test sample. Both permanent and transient transfection systems have been tried.

These bioassays have a sensitivity of about 0.8–1 nM testosterone equivalents and are specific for androgens, but it is unclear which portion of circulating testosterone they actually measure. In fact, when long incubation times are used, testosterone dissociates from SHBG, affecting the equilibrium between bound and free/biologically available fraction. Other factors influencing the neat, end effect are the influx of the hormone into the cell and the intracellular metabolism. In addition, bioassays do not consider the passage of the hormone from the capillary blood flow into the tissues/cells. Inevitably every bioassay represents a static system, as opposed to the very dynamic, in-vivo situation. Long-term incubation bioassays correlate better with free/bioavailable testosterone; while short-term incubation bioassays correlate better with total testosterone. Therefore, the question arises of whether bioassays are really able to measure a unique, physiologically relevant fraction of serum testosterone which cannot be detected and quantified by other methods and could be useful in a diagnostic setting. For the time being, this does not seem to be the case (Need *et al.* 2010).

4.4 Measurement of dihydrotestosterone

The principles and the methods for testosterone assay are basically valid for DHT as well. The main problem in DHT measurement is the elevated cross-reactivity of all polyclonal antisera with testosterone, which renders the direct, accurate quantification of DHT in a male serum sample impossible. As a consequence, DHT has to be separated from testosterone before measurement or, alternatively, testosterone must be chemically modified so that it is not recognized by the antibody. At present there are only two ways of quantifying DHT in serum accurately: after chromatographic separation or after oxidation of testosterone. Both methods involve an extraction step.

The classical methods for chromatographic separation of DHT and testosterone are HPLC and celite chromatography, described in detail in the previous edition of this chapter (Simoni 2004). Recently, several authors applied GC-MS or LC-MS/MS to the measurement of DHT, and the simultaneous measurement of testosterone and DHT without derivatization in clinical samples has been validated (Shiraishi *et al.* 2008). This approach allows rapid, specific and accurate measurement, and it is conceivable that MS measurement of DHT will gain more popularity in the near future.

Several direct DHT kits using microtiter plate-based ELISA are commercially available, but no convincing evidence of their claimed specificity is provided by the manufacturer. The use of such methods cannot be recommended.

4.5   Quality control

Overall, commercially available kits for testosterone measurement perform fairly well in the male, eugonadal range; while inaccuracy and imprecision are a major problem at low concentrations. This prompted a group of stakeholders to convene a meeting to reach consensus about the urgent need for improvement in testosterone testing (Rosner *et al.* 2010). In essence, the recommendations acknowledged the lack of standardization of actual testosterone assays, pleading for definition of acceptable performance criteria, appropriate reference intervals and guidelines for patient preparation and sample handling. In addition, healthcare providers, research organizations and scientific journals are to be stimulated to promote, reimburse and accept only testosterone determinations performed with standardized methods; the latter to be developed with the active contribution of the manufacturers. Given the limitations of the current commercially available kits, the future seems to be irreversibly oriented towards adoption of MS-based methods, which, however, are still unaffordable for many small laboratories for both technical and budgetary reasons. In the meantime each laboratory should carefully revise the performance of its assay. Some suggestions are given hereunder.

4.5.1   Choice of the kit and assay validation

Presently most laboratories choose to measure serum testosterone and DHT by commercially available kits. In all cases the final adoption of a kit for routine determination should depend on an in-house re-validation of the candidate assay. This re-validation includes an assessment of the sensitivity, specificity, accuracy and intra-assay precision of the kit. The specificity and the accuracy of the assay are checked by performing cross-reactivity, parallelism and recovery tests. These tests are usually carried out by the kit manufacturer beforehand and the data are reported in the kit instructions, but it is good practice to repeat them in one's own laboratory, since experience shows that many systems fail to deliver what they promise. Parallelism and recovery tests are crucial and should be performed with several different individual serum samples, since, especially in direct, non-extraction methods, the matrix in which the calibrators are dissolved may be inappropriate, resulting in non-linearity. The serum–matrix effect can be avoided using extraction methods.

Commercial kits contain control sera. Kit controls usually perform quite well and provide results in the expected range. However, care should be taken to use independent, certified control sera, in which the testosterone concentration has been determined by MS. Quite often kit controls are in the expected range, while certified control sera are not. Such kits should not be used. Another criterion for choice is comparison of results in a sufficient number of patient sera to those obtained with a validated method. All these tests should be performed even if the candidate testosterone system is part of an automatic multianalyzer. Companies should be asked to contribute data on the calibrators and to allow complete validation before the choice to adopt that system is made. This is particularly relevant considering the overall poor performance in external quality control trials of most kits and automatic analyzers with sera containing low testosterone concentrations – i.e. from children, women and hypogonadal men.

Laboratories must often face the decision of whether to adopt a new methodology. This is due to the large number of kits competing for the market or to the launch of an "improved" kit version, to budgetary necessities calling for automation and/or adoption of a multianalyzer, or to more stringent regulatory

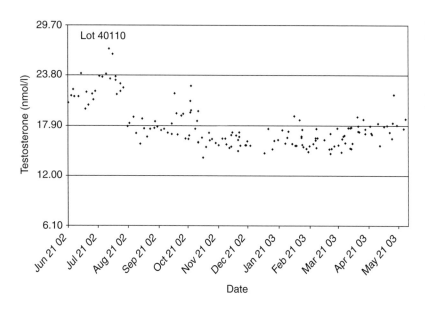

Fig. 4.1 Internal quality control. Results obtained measuring a certified control serum over one year by enzyme immunoassay (EIA). Shortly after introduction of this control serum it became evident that the assay had the tendency to overestimate the target value of this lot (17.9 nmol/l). After servicing of the pipettor/plate reader equipment and re-validation (August 2002), the results improved.

and environmental laws. All these aspects must be considered, but converting to a new methodology should never be at the cost of accuracy and reproducibility. Sometimes changes in reagent lots cause major differences in the results obtained with a kit; these become evident both from the clinical plausibility of the data and from internal quality control. In this case a full re-validation should be performed, the kit manufacturer approached and, if the problem persists, the methodology changed.

4.5.2   Internal quality control

Once a system has been adopted, some long-term parameters have to be kept under constant control. These parameters include intra- and inter-assay variability, assay drift, maximal and non-specific binding, and the standard curve characteristics, such as the slope and the dose at 50% curve displacement. Control charts have to be set up and constantly observed in order to distinguish between sporadic and systematic changes in some parameters; the latter being an indication of some modification in the kit (e.g. a change in a reagent lot) or some problem in the equipment. Intra-assay precision is evaluated by calculating the variability of the duplicate determinations. Measuring samples in singlicate does not allow evaluation of this parameter. In our experience testosterone and DHT should always be measured in

duplicate, since the intraduplicate variability at low concentrations is often >10%.

Another important parameter is assay drift. By measuring control sera at the beginning and at the end of the assay, it can be determined whether the results at the end of the assay have any tendency to be systematically over- or underestimated. This is particularly relevant in ELISAs and methods relying on colorimetric reactions. If such a tendency is discovered, the number of samples which can be measured in one assay should be reduced. As a general rule, if the assay embraces several microtiter plates, then calibrators or even entire standard curves should be run in each plate.

Inter-assay precision is checked by using certified control sera with three different testosterone concentrations (low, middle, high) in each assay. Changes in control sera lots have to be recorded. The results obtained in each assay must fall within a predetermined, allowed range, usually within ±2 standard deviations (SDs) of the target value, otherwise repeating the assay should be considered. Control sera can give results outside the allowed range sporadically, but ideally their variability should oscillate equally on the two sides of the target value. The persistence of results mainly on one side indicates a systematic problem, which, in the example of Fig. 4.1 was identified in the automatic pipettor.

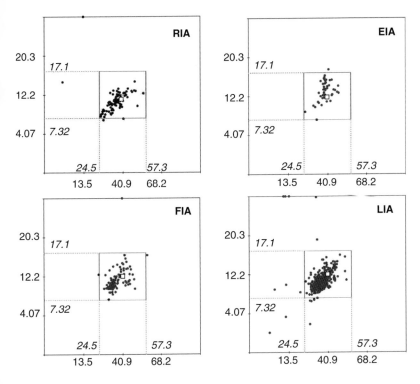

Fig. 4.2 External quality assessment. Results of two control sera with a testosterone concentration of 12.2 nmol/l (sample A, y-axis) and 40.9 nmol/l (sample B, x-axis), respectively as measured by MS in German laboratories participating in an EQA scheme. Results are grouped by radioimmunoassay (RIA), and methods based on enzymatic (EIA), fluorimetric (FIA) or luminescent (LIA) detection systems. Each dot represents results from one laboratory. Target values are indicated by the small white square at the center of each graph. According to current German guidelines the target is considered to be successfully met if the results fall within ±40% of the value measured by MS, indicated by the square defined by dotted lines. Results available online from the German Society of Clinical Chemistry (www.dgkc-online.de).

4.5.3   External quality assessment

In most western countries, successful participation in an external quality assessment (EQA) program is a prerequisite to obtain and maintain the license to perform diagnostic tests for many analytes, including testosterone. Participating laboratories receive samples with unknown testosterone concentrations and return the results to the scheme organizer. The results are then evaluated and the laboratory receives an assessment of its performance. An example of the results of the EQA survey in Germany, organized by the German Society of Clinical Chemistry is given in Fig. 4.2, showing the very high inter-laboratory variability of the results obtained from the measurement of two serum samples containing testosterone concentrations in the adult male range. Most of the laboratories manage to produce results falling within the allowed range, which, according to the actual German guidelines, permits variations of ±40% of the testosterone value measured by MS. This is, of course, a very wide range, such that the measurement of sample A of Fig. 4.2, which has a nominal value of 12.2 nmol/l, is considered successful if the laboratory obtains any value between 7.32 and 17.1 nmol/l. In

practice this means that a man with borderline serum testosterone concentrations has an equal probability of being classified as normal or hypogonadal (i.e. > or < 12 nmol/l), and both diagnoses are correct from the analytical point of view. The comparison between the four method groups shown in Fig. 4.2 does not reveal major differences among them.

In other countries, as in the USA, proficiency of testosterone assessment is not evaluated by comparing the results of the control sera distributed to those obtained by MS-based methods but just by assessing the consensus between all laboratories using the same methodology/instrument. An illustrative example of this is provided by Rosner *et al.* (2007), and highlights the consequences of this lack of standardization. Therefore, as long as commercially available kits are used, the accuracy of the serum testosterone determination is very much dependent on the in-house re-validation and on very strict *internal* quality control; both of which remain up to the individual laboratory.

External quality assessment for SHBG and free testosterone is much less advanced. The UK NEQAS (National External Quality Assessment Service) and US CAP (College of American Pathologists) offer schemes for SHBG, but only a few laboratories make use of them. The US CAP survey 2003 reports on 79 laboratories measuring SHBG and 9 laboratories measuring bioavailable testosterone by ammonium sulfate precipitation. As far as free testosterone is concerned, 6 laboratories were reported to use equilibrium dialysis, 3 laboratories centrifugal ultrafiltration and 70 laboratories used an "analog" method. In view of the analytical problem of the "analog" kits reported above, it is not surprising that these laboratories produce free testosterone results much too low compared to those obtained by free testosterone calculation, dialysis or ultrafiltration. No external quality assessment is presently available for DHT.

4.6 Key messages

- Serum testosterone is measured in clinical routine by immunological competitive methods based on polyclonal antisera and labeled hormone.
- The reference method for testosterone measurement is MS. A number of LC-MS/MS methods have been validated for accurate assessment of testosterone. Extraction methods should be used for accurate, reproducible testosterone measurements whenever MS-based methods are not possible.

- Non-extraction, direct methods based on non-radioactively labeled tracers are currently routinely used. Automatic multianalyzers are the systems mostly used for serum testosterone measurement. These methods show unacceptably high inaccuracy.
- Any testosterone measurement system, including those based on automatic analyzers, should be carefully validated in house against an extraction method before it is adopted for routine assays.
- Carefully validated immunological methods perform reasonably well in the male, eugonadal range.
- In general, all methods currently in use suffer from poor standardization.
- So-called "analog" free testosterone methods are unreliable. Calculated free testosterone is very popular, but the best estimation of free testosterone is given by dialysis or ultrafiltration.
- DHT should be measured by chromatographic or oxidative methods. Mass spectrometric methods are under development.
- Participation in external quality control programs is mandatory. Strict internal quality control is fundamental to ensure accurate measurements.

4.7   References

Anderson DC (1974) Sex-hormone-binding globulin. *Clin Endocrinol (Oxf)* **3**:69–96

Atkinson KR, Lo KR, Payne SR, Mitchell JS, Ingram JR (2008) Rapid saliva processing techniques for near real-time analysis of salivary steroids and protein. *J Clin Lab Anal* **22**:395–402

Booth A, Johnson DR, Granger DA, Crouter AC, McHale S (2003) Testosterone and child and adolescent adjustment: the moderating role of parent–child relationships. *Dev Psychol* **39**:85–98

Boots LR, Potter S, Potter D, Azziz R (1998) Measurement of total serum testosterone levels using commercially available kits: high degree of between-kit variability. *Fertil Steril* **69**:286–292

Borrey D, Moerman E, Cockx A, Engelrelst V, Langlois MR (2007)

Column-switching LC-MS/MS analysis for quantitative determination of testosterone in human serum. *Clin Chim Acta* **382**:134–137

Brandhorst G, Streit F, Kratzsch J, Schiettecatte J, Roth HJ, Luppa PB, Körner A, Kiess W, Binder L, Oellerich M, von Ahsen N (2011) Multicenter evaluation of a new automated electrochemiluminescence immunoassay for the quantification of testosterone compared to liquid chromatography tandem mass spectrometry. *Clin Biochem* **44**:264–247

Cawood ML, Field HP, Ford CG, Gillingwater S, Kicman A, Cowan D, Barth JH (2005) Testosterone measurement by isotope-dilution liquid chromatography-tandem mass spectrometry: validation of a method for routine clinical practice. *Clin Chem* **51**:1472–1479

Ceglarek U, Kortz L, Leichtle A, Fiedler GM, Kratzsch J, Thiery J (2009) Rapid quantification of steroid patterns in human serum by on-line solid-phase extraction combined with liquid chromatography-triple quadrupole linear ion trap mass spectrometry. *Clin Chim Acta* **401**:114–118

Chen Y, Yazdanpanah M, Hoffman BR, Diamandis EP, Wong PY (2009) Rapid determination of serum testosterone by liquid chromatography-isotope dilution tandem mass spectrometry and a split sample comparison with three automated immunoassays. *Clin Biochem* **42**:484–490

Chen Y, Yazdanpanah M, Wang XY, Hoffman BR, Diamandis EP, Wong PY (2010) Direct measurement of serum free testosterone by ultrafiltration followed by liquid chromatography tandem mass spectrometry. *Clin Biochem* **43**:490–496

Chiappin S, Antonelli G, Gatti R, De Palo EF (2007) Saliva specimen: a new laboratory tool for diagnostic and basic investigation. *Clin Chem Acta* **383**:30–40

Dabbs JM Jr (1990) Salivary testosterone measurements: reliability across hours, days, and weeks. *Physiol Behav* **48**:83–86

Davies R, Collier C, Raymond M, Heaton J, Clark A (2002) Indirect measurement of bioavailable testosterone with the Bayer Immuno 1 system. *Clin Chem* **48**:388–490

Dechaud H, Lejeune H, Garoscio-Cholet M, Mallein R, Pugeat M (1989) Radioimmunoassay of testosterone not bound to sex-steroid-binding protein in plasma. *Clin Chem* **35**:1609–1614

De Ronde W, van der Schouw YT, Pols HA, Gooren LJ, Muller M, Grobbee DE, de Jong FH (2006) Calculation of bioavailable and free testosterone in men: a comparison of 5 published algorithms. *Clin Chem* **52**:1777–1784

Dunn JF, Nisula BC, Rodbard D (1981) Transport of steroid hormones: binding of 21 endogenous steroids to both testosterone-binding globulin and corticosteroid-binding globulin in human plasma. *J Clin Endocrinol Metab* **53**:58–68

Dussault JH, Letarte J, Guyda H, Laberge C (1977) Serum thyroid hormone and TSH concentrations in newborn infants with congenital absence of thyroxine-binding globulin. *J Pediatr* **90**:264–265

Ekins R (1990) Measurement of free hormones in blood. *Endocr Rev* **11**:5–46

Fanelli F, Belluomo I, Di Lallo VD, Cuomo G, De Iasio R, Baccini M, Casadio E, Casetta B, Vicennati V, Gambineri A, Grossi G, Pasquali R, Pagotto U (2011) Serum steroid profiling by isotopic dilution-liquid chromatography-mass spectrometry: comparison with current immunoassays and reference intervals in healthy adults. *Steroids* **76**:244–253

Fitzgerald RL, Herold DA (1996) Serum total testosterone: immunoassay compared with negative chemical ionization gas chromatography-mass spectrometry. *Clin Chem* **42**:749–755

Fitzgerald RL, Griffin TL, Herold DA (2010) Analysis of testosterone in serum using mass spectrometry. *Methods Mol Biol* **603**:489–500

Fritz KS, McKean AJ, Nelson JC, Wilcox RB (2008) Analog-based free testosterone test results linked to total testosterone concentrations, not free testosterone concentrations. *Clin Chem* **54**:512–516

Furuyama S, Mayes DM, Nugent CA (1970) A radioimmunoassay for plasma testosterone. *Steroids* **16**:415–428

Gonzalez-Sagrado M, Martin-Gil FJ, Lopez-Hernandez S, Fernandez-Garcia N, Olmos-Linares A, Arranz-Pena ML (2000) Reference values and methods comparison of a new testosterone assay on the AxSYM system. *Clin Biochem* **33**:175–179

Granger DA, Shirtcliff EA, Booth A, Kivlighan KT, Schwartz EB (2004) The "trouble" with salivary testosterone. *Psychoneuroendocrinology* **29**:1229–1240

Guo T, Chan M, Soldin SJ (2004) Steroid profiles using liquid chromatography-tandem mass spectrometry with atmospheric pressure photoionization source. *Arch Pathol Lab Med* **128**:469–475

Guo T, Taylor RL, Singh RJ, Soldin SJ (2006) Simultaneous determination of 12 steroids by isotope dilution liquid chromatography-photospray ionization tandem mass spectrometry. *Clin Chim Acta* **372**:76–82

Harwood DT, Handelsman DJ (2009) Development and validation of a sensitive liquid chromatography-tandem mass spectrometry assay to simultaneously measure androgens and estrogens in serum without derivatization. *Clin Chim Acta* **409**:78–84

Janzen N, Sander S, Terhardt M, Peter M, Sander J (2008) Fast and direct quantification of adrenal steroids by tandem mass spectrometry in serum and dried blood spots. *J Chromatogr B Analyt Technol Biomed Life Sci* **861**:117–122

Jockenhövel F, Krüsemann C, Jaeger A, Olbricht T, Reinwein D (1992) Comparability of serum testosterone determination with the ten most commonly used commercial radioimmunoassays and with a new enzyme immunoassay. *Klin Lab* **38**:81–88

Kalhorn TF, Page ST, Howald WN, Mostaghel EA, Nelson PS (2007) Analysis of testosterone and dihydrotestosterone from biological fluids as the oxime derivatives using high-performance liquid chromatography/tandem mass spectrometry. *Rapid Commun Mass Spectrom* **21**:3200–3206

Kane J, Middle J, Cawood M (2007) Measurement of serum testosterone in women; what should we do? *Ann Clin Biochem* **44**:5–15

Krone N, Hughes BA, Lavery GG, Stewart PM, Arlt W, Shackleton CH (2010) Gas chromatography/mass spectrometry (GC/MS) remains a pre-eminent discovery tool in clinical steroid investigations even in the era of fast liquid chromatography tandem mass spectrometry (LC/MS/MS). *J Steroid Biochem Mol Biol* **121**:496–504

Kulle AE, Riepe FG, Melchior D, Hiort O, Holterhus PM (2010) A novel ultrapressure liquid chromatography tandem mass spectrometry method for the simultaneous determination of androstenedione, testosterone, and dihydrotestosterone in pediatric blood samples: age- and sex-specific reference data. *J Clin Endocrinol Metab* **95**:2399–2409

Kushnir MM, Rockwood AL, Roberts WL, Pattison EG, Bunker AM, Fitzgerald RL, Meikle AW (2006)

Performance characteristics of a novel tandem mass spectrometry assay for serum testosterone. *Clin Chem* **52**:120–128

Kushnir MM, Blamires T, Rockwood AL, Roberts WL, Yue B, Erdogan E, Bunker AM, Meikle AW (2010) Liquid chromatography-tandem mass spectrometry assay for androstenedione, dehydroepiandrosterone, and testosterone with pediatric and adult reference intervals. *Clin Chem* **56**:1138–1147

Kushnir MM, Rockwood AL, Roberts WL, Yue B, Bergquist J, Meikle AW (2011) Liquid chromatography tandem mass spectrometry for analysis of steroids in clinical laboratories. *Clin Biochem* **44**:77–88

Legro RS, Schlaff WD, Diamond MP, Coutifaris C, Casson PR, Brzyski RG, Christman GM, Trussell JC, Krawetz SA, Snyder PJ, Ohl D, Carson SA, Steinkampf MP, Carr BR, McGovern PG, Cataldo NA, Gosman GG, Nestler JE, Myers ER, Santoro N, Eisenberg E, Zhang M, Zhang H; Reproductive Medicine Network (2010) Total testosterone assay in women with polycystic ovary syndrome: precision and correlation with hirsutism. *J Clin Endocrinol Metab* **95**:5305–5313

Levesque A, Letellier M, Swirski C, Lee C, Grant A (1998) Analytical evaluation of the testosterone assay on the Bayer Immuno 1 system. *Clin Biochem* **31**:23–28

Levine A, Zagoory-Sharon O, Feldman R, Lewis JG, Weller A (2007) Measuring cortisol in human psycobiological studies. *Physiol Behav* **30**:43–53

Lewis JG (2006) Steroid analysis in saliva: an overview. *Clin Biochem Rev* **27**:139–146

Licea-Perez H, Wang S, Szapacs ME, Yang E (2008) Development of a highly sensitive and selective UPLC/MS/MS method for the simultaneous determination of testosterone and 5alpha-dihydrotestosterone in human

serum to support testosterone replacement therapy for hypogonadism. *Steroids* **73**:601–610

Ly LP, Sartorius G, Hull L, Leung A, Swerdloff RS, Wang C, Handelsman DJ (2010) Accuracy of calculated free testosterone formulae in men. *Clin Endocrinol (Oxf)* **73**:382–388

Macdonald PR, Owen LJ, Wu FC, Macdowall W, Keevil BG; NATSAL Team (2011) A liquid chromatography-tandem mass spectrometry method for salivary testosterone with adult male reference interval determination. *Clin Chem* **57**:774–775

Manni A, Pardridge WM, Cefalu W, Nisula BC, Bardin CW, Santner SJ, Santen RJ (1985) Bioavailability of albumin-bound testosterone. *J Clin Endocrinol Metab* **61**:705–710

Matsui F, Koh E, Yamamoto K, Sugimoto K, Sin HS, Maeda Y, Honma S, Namiki M (2009) Liquid chromatography-tandem mass spectrometry (LC-MS/MS) assay for simultaneous measurement of salivary testosterone and cortisol in healthy men for utilization in the diagnosis of late-onset hypogonadism in males. *Endocr J* **56**:1083–1093

Mendel CM (1992) The free hormone hypothesis. Distinction from the free hormone transport hypothesis. *J Androl* **13**:107–116

Mendel CM, Murai JT, Siiteri PK, Monroe SE, Inoue M (1989) Conservation of free but not total or non-sex-hormone-binding-globulin-bound testosterone in serum from Nagase analbuminemic rats. *Endocrinology* **124**:3128–3130

Middle JG (2002) *UK NEQAS for Steroid Hormones Annual Review 2002*. UK NEQAS, University Hospital Birmingham NHS Trust

Middle JG (2007) Dehydroepiandrosterone sulphate interferes in many direct immunoassays for testosterone. *Ann Clin Biochem* **44**:173–177

Moal V, Mathieu E, Reynier P, Malthièry Y, Gallois Y (2007) Low serum testosterone assayed by liquid chromatography-tandem mass spectrometry. Comparison with five immunoassay techniques. *Clin Chim Acta* **386**:12–19

Morley JE, Perry HM 3rd, Patrick P, Dollbaum CM, Kells JM (2006) Validation of salivary testosterone as a screening test for male hypogonadism. *Aging Male* **9**:165–169

Need EF, O'Loughlin PD, Armstrong DT, Haren MT, Martin SA, Tilley WD; the Florey Adelaide Male Aging Study, Witter GA, Buchanan G (2010) Serum testosterone bioassay evaluation in a large male cohort. *Clin Endocrinol* **72**:87–98

Nieschlag E, Loriaux DL (1972) Radioimmunoassay for plasma testosterone. *Z Klin Chem Klin Biochem* **10**:164–168

Rassaie MJ, Kumari LG, Pandey PK, Gupta N, Kochupillai N, Grover PK (1992) A highly specific heterologous enzyme-linked immunosorbent assay for measuring testosterone in plasma using antibody-coated immunoassay plates or polypropylene tubes. *Steroids* **57**:288–294

Raverot V, Lopez J, Grenot C, Pugeat M, Déchaud H (2010) New approach for measurement of non-SHBG-bound testosterone in human plasma. *Anal Chim Acta* **658**:87–90

Rauh M (2010) Steroid measurement with LC-MS/MS. Application examples in pediatrics. *J Steroid Biochem Mol Biol* **121**:520–527

Rauh M, Gröschl M, Rascher W, Dörr HG (2006) Automated, fast and sensitive quantification of 17 alpha-hydroxy-progesterone, androstenedione and testosterone by tandem mass spectrometry with on-line extraction. *Steroids* **71**:450–458

Rosner W (1997) Errors in the measurement of plasma free

testosterone. *J Clin Endocrinol Metab* 82:2014–2015

Rosner W (2001) An extraordinarily inaccurate assay for free testosterone is still with us. *J Clin Endocrinol Metab* 86:2903

Rosner W, Vesper H on behalf of the Endocrine Society and the endorsing organizations (2010) Toward excellence in testosterone testing: a consensus statement. *J Clin Endocrinol Metab* 95:4542–4548

Rosner W, Hryb DJ, Khan MS, Nakhla AM, Romas NA (1999) Sex hormone-binding globulin mediates steroid hormone signal transduction at the plasma membrane. *J Steroid Biochem Mol Biol* 69:481–485

Rosner W, Auchus RJ, Azziz R, Sluss PM, Raff H (2007) Position statement: utility, limitations and pitfalls in measuring testosterone: an Endocrine Society position statement. *J Clin Endocrinol Metab* 92:405–413

Roy P, Alevizaki M, Huhtaniemi I (2008) In vitro bioassays for androgens and their diagnostic applications. *Hum Reprod Update* 14:73–82

Salameh WA, Redor-Goldman MM, Clarke NJ, Reitz RE, Caulfield MP (2010) Validation of a total testosterone assay using high-turbulence liquid chromatography tandem mass spectrometry: total and free testosterone reference ranges. *Steroids* 75:169–175

Shackleton C (2010) Clinical steroid mass spectrometry: a 45-year history culminating in HPLC-MS/MS becoming an essential tool for patient diagnosis. *J Steroid Biochem Mol Biol* 121:481–490

Shiraishi S, Lee PW, Leung A, Goh VH, Swerdloff RS, Wang C (2008) Simultaneous measurement of serum testosterone and dihydrotestosterone by liquid chromatography-tandem mass spectrometry. *Clin Chem* 54:1855–1863

Shirtcliff EA, Granger DA, Schwartz E, Curran MJ (2001) Use of salivary biomarkers in biobehavioral research: cotton-based sample collection methods can interfere with salivary immunoassay results. *Psychoneuroendocrinology* 26:165–173

Shirtcliff EA, Granger DA, Likos A (2002) Gender differences in the validity of testosterone measured in saliva by immunoassay. *Horm Behav* 42:62–69

Simoni M (2004) Methodology for measuring testosterone, DHT and SHBG in a clinical setting. In: Nieschlag E, Behre HM (eds) *Testosterone: Action, Deficiency, Substitution*, 3rd edn. Cambridge University Press, Cambridge, pp 641–664

Simoni M, Nieschlag E (2010) Endocrine laboratory diagnosis. In: Nieschlag E, Behre HM, Nieschlag S (eds) *Andrology. Male Reproductive Health and Dysfunction*, 3rd edn. Springer-Verlag, Berlin, pp 109–118

Simoni M, Baraldi E, Baraghini GF, Boraldi V, Roli L, Seghedoni S, Verlardo A, Montanini V (1988) Twenty-four-hour pattern of plasma SHBG, total proteins and testosterone in young and elderly men. *Steroids* 52:381–382

Simoni M, Montanini V, Fustini MF, Del Rio G, Cioni K, Marrama P (1992) Circadian rhythm of plasma testosterone in men with idiopathic hypogonadotrophic hypogonadism before and during pulsatile administration of gonadotropin-releasing hormone. *Clin Endocrinol* 36:29–34

Singh RJ (2008) Validation of a high throughput method for serum/plasma testosterone using liquid chromatography tandem mass spectrometry (LC-MS/MS). *Steroids* 73:1339–1344

Soto AM, Maffini MV, Schaeberle CM, Sonnenschein C (2006) Strengths and weaknesses of in vitro assays for estrogenic and androgenic activity.

Best Pract Res Clin Endocrinol Metab 20:15–33

Swerdloff RS, Wang C (2008) Free testosterone measurement by the analog displacement direct assay: old concerns and new evidence. *Clin Chem* 54:458–460

Tai SS, Xu B, Welch MJ, Phinney KW (2007) Development and evaluation of a candidate reference measurement procedure for the determination of testosterone in human serum using isotope dilution liquid chromatography/tandem mass spectrometry. *Anal Bioanal Chem* 388:1087–1094

Taieb J, Benattar C, Birr AS, Lindenbaum A (2002) Limitations of steroid determination by direct immunoassay. *Clin Chem* 48:583–585

Taieb J, Mathian B, Millot F, Patricot MC, Mathieu E, Queyrel N, Lacroix I, Somma-Delpero C, Bouloux P (2003) Testosterone measured by 10 immunoassays and by isotope-dilution gas chromatography-mass spectrometry in sera from 116 men, women and children. *Clin Chem* 49:1381–1395

Thienpont LM, Van Uytfanghe K, Blincko S, Ramsay CS, Xie H, Doss RC, Keenl BG, Owen LS, Rockwood AL, Kushnir MM, Chun KY, Chandler DW, Field HP, Sluss PM (2008) State-of-the-art of serum testosterone measurement by isotope dilution-liquid chromatography-tandem mass spectrometry. *Clin Chem* 54:1290–1297

Turpeinen U, Linko S, Itkonen O, Hämäläinen E (2008) Determination of testosterone in serum by liquid chromatography-tandem mass spectrometry. *Scand J Clin Lab Invest* 68:50–57

Vaitukaitis J, Robbins JB, Nieschlag E, Ross GT (1971) A method for producing specific antisera with small doses of immunogen. *J Clin Endocrinol Metab* 33:988–991

Van Uytfanghe K, Stöckl D, Kaufman JM, Fiers T, Ross HA, De

Leenheer AP, Thienpont LM (2004) Evaluation of a candidate reference measurement procedure for serum free testosterone based on ultrafiltration and isotope dilution-gas chromatography-mass spectrometry. *Clin Chem* **50**:2101–2110

Vermeulen A, Verdonck L, Kaufman JM (1999) A critical evaluation of simple methods for the estimation of free testosterone in serum. *J Clin Endocrinol Metab* **84**:3666–3672

Vesper HW, Bhasin S, Wang C, Tai SS, Dodge LA, Singh RJ, Nelson G, Ohorodnik S, Clarke NJ, Salameh WA, Parker CR Jr, Razdan R, Mansell EA, Myers GL (2009) Interlaboratory comparison study of serum total testosterone [corrected] measurements performed by mass spectrometry methods. *Steroids* **74**:498–503

Vlahos I, MacMahon W, Sgoutas D, Bowers W, Thompson J, Trawick W (1982) An improved ultrafiltration method for determining free testosterone in serum. *Clin Chem* **28**:2286–2291

Wang C, Plymate S, Nieschlag E, Paulsen CA (1981) Salivary testosterone in men: further evidence of a direct correlation with free serum testosterone. *J Clin Endocrinol Metab* **53**:1021–1024

Wang C, Catlin DH, Demers LM, Starcevic B, Swerdloff RS (2004) Measurement of total serum testosterone in adult men: comparison of current laboratory methods versus liquid chromatography-tandem mass spectrometry. *J Clin Endocrinol Metab* **89**:534–543

Warner MH, Kane J, Atkin SL, Kilpatrick ES (2006) Dehydroepiandrosterone sulphate interferes with the Abbott Architect direct immunoassay for testosterone. *Ann Clin Biochem* **43**:196–199

Winters SJ, Kelley DE, Goodpaster B (1998) The "analog" free testosterone assay: are the results in men clinically useful? *Clin Chem* **44**:2178–2182

Wolthers BG, Kraan GP (1999) Clinical applications of gas chromatography and gas chromatography-mass spectrometry of steroids. *J Chromatogr A* **843**:247–274

Yamashita K, Miyashiro Y, Maekubo H, Okuyama M, Honma S, Takahashi M, Numazawa M (2009) Development of highly sensitive quantification method for testosterone and dihydrotestosterone in human serum and prostate tissue by liquid chromatography-electrospray ionization tandem mass spectrometry. *Steroids* **74**:920–926

The behavioral correlates of testosterone

John Bancroft

5.1 Introduction

When the two principal sex hormones, testosterone and estradiol, were first identified in the 1940s, they provided us with a simple distinction between a male hormone and a female hormone. Since then, as with most aspects of the human condition, scientific research has continued to uncover the complexity of sex hormone function, to the extent that our ability to comprehend is being challenged. In this chapter we will be focusing on the relationships between

Testosterone: Action, Deficiency, Substitution, ed. Eberhard Nieschlag and Hermann M. Behre, Assoc. ed. Susan Nieschlag.
Published by Cambridge University Press. © Cambridge University Press 2012.

testosterone and various aspects of our behavior; hence we will be principally concerned with hormone-related brain mechanisms that underlie those behaviors. We now know that testosterone and estradiol have an important role in both male and female brains, and that testosterone is converted to estradiol, leaving us unsure of how many correlates of testosterone are in fact primarily correlates of estradiol. There is now evidence to suggest that, much earlier in our phylogenetic history, testosterone was a precursor of estradiol (Thornton 2001). We have to grapple with the fact that if testosterone influences the behavior of women, it does so with levels of testosterone in the blood around a 10th of those found in men. We also have a variety of androgenic hormones in addition to testosterone to consider. In particular, DHEA and its sulfate, DHEAS, which are mainly produced by the adrenal glands, are present in the blood at levels substantially higher than testosterone or other androgens, yet their function is not well understood. There is relatively recent evidence of synthesis of androgenic hormones within brain cells, these being examples of what are now known as "neurosteroids," not derived from the classical hormones in the blood (e.g. King 2008). The original assumption that testosterone has direct effects only at genomic receptors is being challenged, and the genetic variability of ARs is now very evident. We will encounter most of these complexities as we progress through this chapter.

The evidence will be reviewed under three principal headings: (1) testosterone and gender differentiation; (2) activational effects of testosterone in men; and (3) activational effects of testosterone in women. Whereas the principal behaviors and associated physiologic responses to be considered relate to sex, the relevance of testosterone to mood and aggression, and how such relationships may interact with sex, will also be discussed.

5.2 Testosterone and gender differentiation

5.2.1 Gender differentiation of the brain

Whereas the role of testosterone, and its 5-α-reduced form, DHT, in determining the male anatomical development of the fetus, is reasonably clear (see Chapter 2), the impact of testosterone on gender differentiation of brain development is less well understood. Here we need to distinguish between "organizational" and "activational" effects of

hormones. Early exposure of the brain to hormones results in organization of its structure and responsiveness to the activational effects of the same hormones later in development. In lower animals, particularly rodents, there are clear differences between male and female brains determined by the organizational effects of both testosterone and estradiol. These effects are probably mediated mainly by hormonal influence on apoptosis, or programmed cell death, during brain development (Gorski 2000).

In the human, the picture is less clear and has resulted in much controversy (reviewed by Hines 2004). Gender differences in the size and shape of the corpus callosum, the main connecting pathway between the right and left hemispheres, have been found in some studies, but not all. In any case, such differences are probably most relevant to certain aspects of cognitive function, and not to gender-related or sexual behavior. The anterior hypothalamic/ preoptic area, which contains many testosterone and estradiol receptors, is of interest. This area has four sub-regions, called the interstitial nuclei of the anterior hypothalamus (INAH 1–4). Evidence of gender difference has only been found in INAH-3. This is consistently larger and contains more neurons in men than in women; though the behavioral significance of this is not yet clear. The central region of the bed nucleus of the stria terminalis (BNST), which also contains steroid-concentrating neurons (Hines 2004), is smaller in women than in men. This was also found to be smaller in six male-to-female transsexuals, leaving us uncertain as to whether this indicates a structural difference that may have contributed to their transgender identity, or whether it was a consequence of the administration of estradiol that is used by male-to-female transsexuals to produce feminizing bodily effects (Zhou et al. 1995). This raises the question of whether organizing effects of testosterone and estradiol on the brain are restricted to specific stages of human brain development, as they clearly are in rodents. These specific brain areas showing gender difference are too small to be examined functionally with brain imaging, and the evidence of their existence is so far based on post-mortem examination.

Our understanding of human brain development has, however, changed substantially in the past decade as a result of structural and functional brain imaging studies. It is now clear that there are major changes in the brain during the second decade of life (Weinberger et al. 2005). These are likely to be affected by hormonal changes around puberty, and hence will vary according to whether puberty is early, late or at the "normal" time. The timing of human puberty can vary substantially, with trends towards earlier puberty having occurred in certain parts of the world, and with evidence suggesting that this reflects an interaction between genetic factors and environmental conditions (Parent *et al.* 2003). It is also possible that adrenarche, which is confined to humans and primates, may also be involved in this longer-term brain organization by androgens, although this has not yet been studied.

Perrin *et al.* (2008), using magnetic resonance imaging (MRI) scanning in a cross-sectional study of adolescent boys and girls, found a clear sexual dimorphism in the increase of brain white matter, which was slight in girls and much more marked in boys. They also showed a relationship of this effect to functional polymorphism of the *AR* gene. It has previously been shown that a low number of CAG repeats in this gene (i.e. a short gene) is associated with a higher androgenic effect than *AR* genes with a high number of CAG repeats (a long gene) (e.g. Tut *et al.* 1997). Perrin *et al.* (2008) found the increase in white matter volume was greater in males with the short gene. This demonstrates the role of the *AR* gene in the organizational effects of testosterone.

The transcriptional function of the *AR* gene presents us with a puzzling gender difference. The short gene in the male, as it is more active than the long gene, results in a reduction in plasma testosterone levels; less testosterone is required to achieve the same effect. In contrast, in the female, whereas the short gene is also more active in its transcriptional function, it is associated with higher levels of plasma testosterone, reflecting the gender differences in control of androgen production. In the male this is mainly controlled via the hypothalamus. In the female there are probably direct effects of testosterone on the adrenal glands and the ovaries (Westberg *et al.* 2001). It is not clear what the implications of this are for the organizational effects of testosterone in female brain development. These issues about *AR* gene effects will be considered further later in this chapter.

5.2.2 The mode of action of androgens and estrogens in the brain

The current view is that there is one type of AR in the brain, which can be activated by either testosterone or DHT. Recent research with mice has revealed two estrogen receptors, ERα and ERβ. Male mice need at least one type of ER to show normal sexual function. The relevance of the ERs to the sexuality of female mice has not yet been clarified. In the human we have no directly comparable evidence.

The conventional wisdom is that testosterone acts in the brain via genomic effects (Rommerts 1990); whereas estradiol and progesterone, in addition to such intracellular genomic effects, can also have much more rapid effects by acting on the cell membrane – estradiol being excitatory and progesterone inhibitory. However, recent animal research has shown evidence of ARs in axons, dendrites and glial processes in the neocortex, hippocampus and amygdala. These may be involved in more rapid behavioral effects of androgens (Sarkey *et al.* 2008). Once again, we have no direct evidence of the relevance of this to humans.

Research on the site of action of testosterone in the non-human primate brain goes back more than thirty years, and we can assume more direct relevance to the human brain than with rodent research. Michael *et al.* (1989) used autoradiography to look at both androgen and estrogen activity in male rhesus monkeys. Activity of 5α-reductase, which converts testosterone into DHT, was fairly evenly distributed in the brain, whereas aromatase activity, which converts testosterone into estradiol, was much more localized. They concluded that testosterone acts by being converted to estradiol in the following areas: medial preoptic and ventromedial hypothalamic nuclei, the bed nucleus of the stria terminalis (BNST), and the cortical, medial and accessory amygdaloid nuclei. Testosterone activity, they concluded, was also mediated by ARs in the lateral septal, pre-mamillary and intercalated mamillary nuclei. Roselli *et al.* (2001), using in situ hybridization histochemistry to locate cytochrome P450 aromatase nRNA in the hypothalamus and amygdala of cynomolgus monkeys, reported broadly similar findings to those of Michael *et al.* (1989). Abdelgadir *et al.* (1999) used a ribonuclease protection assay to assess the distribution of AR mRNA in male rhesus monkeys. Again their findings were similar to those of Michael *et al.* (1989). They also compared intact with castrated males, and found little difference in the distribution of AR mRNA, concluding that, in the brain, AR is not regulated by androgen at the transcription level.

Two studies of AR distribution in the human male temporal cortex have been reported, both showing substantial amounts of AR (Sarrieau *et al.* 1990; Puy *et al.* 1995). In both studies, the temporal lobe was used simply because it was available from surgical interventions.

We have less evidence for the female brain. Finley and Kritzer (1999) found no difference between male and female rhesus monkeys in the amount of AR protein in the prefrontal cortex. There have been some post-mortem studies comparing the brains of men and women. Fernandez-Guasti *et al.* (2000) compared the hypothalami of five men and five women. They found AR immunoreactivity ranging from intense to relatively weak across several areas of the hypothalamus, and in general the level of receptor protein staining was less in the women. This gender difference was particularly marked in the lateral and medial mamillary nuclei; and in the paraventricular and supraoptic nuclei, staining was only found in the males. Overall, there was greater individual variability in the intensity of receptor staining in the women than in the men. Whereas most of this research has focused on the hypothalamus, those studies that have looked at other brain areas, such as the prefrontal cortex and temporal cortex, have indicated a wider distribution of ARs in the brain, which raises the possibility that effects of testosterone in the brain are not restricted to mechanisms relevant to sexuality and reproduction, and might include other activational effects (Kelly 1991).

5.3 Activational effects of testosterone and behavior in adult men

There are several types of information of relevance: (1) measurement of circulating levels of testosterone, in particular free testosterone, and their relationship to behavioral measures; (2) the consequences of reducing testosterone levels or blocking testosterone effects, either iatrogenically in the course of medical treatment, or experimentally; (3) the effects of exogenous testosterone administration, short term (single dose) and long term; (4) the impact of aging. The first category, relating circulating testosterone levels to behavioral parameters, is the most problematic. As Zitzmann and Nieschlag (2001) noted: "When interpreting testosterone levels, it is often overlooked that levels of the hormone in body fluids are only a small and transitory step in the cascade of hormone action from production to biological effect." It is therefore not surprising that correlations between plasma testosterone levels and specific behaviors vary not only across behaviors but also across studies.

An additional limitation is the tendency for testosterone levels in the blood to rise after relevant behaviors (e.g. after a man wins at a sporting activity), and usually we are left uncertain as to whether this has any functional relevance. The second and third categories of information allow us to assess the effects of sustained changes in testosterone availability. The fourth, the impact of aging in the male, presents a challenge as it faces us with complex interactions between different mechanisms and systems that are changing as a result of age. This is reviewed in Chapter 16, and also by Zitzmann *et al.* (2006), and will not be considered further in this chapter.

5.3.1 Sexual desire and response

In considering the sexual effects of testosterone, we need to identify four components of sexual arousal: information processing, incentive motivation, central arousal and genital response. The essence of sexual desire is incentive motivation linked to processing of sexually relevant information, with varying degrees of central arousal and genital response, which in the male is penile erection.

The normal range of total testosterone in men is large (10–35 nmol/l), and within this range there is little predictable relationship to measures of sexual desire or behavior (Raboch and Starka 1973; Kraemer *et al.* 1976). Two studies, in which erectile response to erotic stimuli was measured, found a correlation between plasma testosterone and latency but not degree of erectile response (Rubin *et al.* 1979; Lange *et al.* 1980). It is widely assumed that there is a level of testosterone or "threshold," above which increases in testosterone will make little or no difference to sexual desire or response. This "threshold" may vary across men but will be somewhere within the normal range, and it could increase with age.

5.3.1.1 Testosterone replacement in hypogonadal men

The effects of testosterone levels below the normal range are demonstrated in men with hypogonadism who receive TRT (testosterone replacement therapy). Most controlled studies have investigated hypogonadal men already on testosterone replacement for at least several months, who then have their exogenous testosterone withdrawn. The effects on sexual parameters during a period of this withdrawal are assessed and followed by administration of testosterone and placebo, using a double-blind, crossover design (Davidson *et al.* 1979; Luisi and Franchi 1980; Skakkebaek *et al.* 1981; Salmimies *et al.* 1982; Kwan *et al.* 1983; O'Carroll *et al.* 1985). Although most studies of this kind have been small, there has been a reassuring consistency in their findings. There is a decline in sexual interest within three to four weeks of androgen withdrawal, and if testosterone withdrawal lasts long enough, seminal emission will eventually be impaired. Placebo usually has little effect, but testosterone replacement restores sexual interest within one or two weeks. O'Carroll *et al.* (1985), comparing four doses of testosterone undecanoate (40, 80, 120 and 160 mg daily), showed a clear dose-response relationship in this respect. Effects on sexual activity with one's partner are less consistent, reflecting variable partner and relationship characteristics. Masturbation frequency more typically increases. Nocturnal penile tumescence (NPT) is predictably impaired during testosterone withdrawal and restored with testosterone replacement. Nocturnal penile tumescence occurs during REM sleep, which involves a "switching off" of noradrenergic cells in the locus coeruleus in the brainstem, which, via their spinal projections, are responsible for the inhibitory tone in the erectile tissues. Thus, in eugonadal men, this reduction in inhibitory tone resulting in erection indicates that there is normally some degree of "excitatory tone." The locus coeruleus has testosterone receptors (Parmeggiana and Morrison 1990), and this "excitatory tone" can be considered to be testosterone dependent.

A few studies of testosterone withdrawal and replacement have used psychophysiologic assessment of response to visual erotic stimuli. Interestingly, in the low testosterone state, erection to such stimuli can occur, but it is less rigid and more "stimulus bound" than during testosterone replacement. Thus, whereas some degree of erectile response to erotic stimuli can occur without testosterone, it is necessary for a full erection and also for a state of arousal that results in the erection continuing for a time after the sexual stimulus is "switched off" (Carani *et al.* 1995). This can be seen as a further manifestation of the central "excitatory tone."

These studies of testosterone withdrawal and replacement reviewed so far, involved hypogonadal men in Europe or North America. In the evaluation of a new androgen, 7α-methyl-19-nortestosterone or MENT, a similar placebo-controlled design was used, involving two small groups of hypogonadal men: one

from Scotland, the other from Hong Kong (Anderson *et al.* 1999). There were some interesting differences between the two groups. Although the effects on waking erections (i.e. NPT) were similar, the increase in sexual interest and, more strikingly, masturbation, was less in the Hong Kong men. This confronts us with the need to take cultural influences into account. Nocturnal penile tumescence is unlikely to be culturally sensitive, but masturbation and sexual interest, or at least the ways that they are reported and assessed, may well be.

Functional brain imaging has also been used to compare brain activity in response to sexual stimuli in hypogonadal men with and without testosterone replacement. Park *et al.* (2001), using functional MRI, reported on two such men. In both men, activation of the inferior frontal lobe, cingulate gyrus, insula and corpus callosum was greater with testosterone replacement. Redouté *et al.* (2005) used positron emission tomography (PET) scanning to compare brain response to sexual stimuli in nine hypogonadal (H) men, with (H+) and without (H−) testosterone replacement, and eight eugonadal men. They found greater activation in the right orbitofrontal cortex, insula and claustrum in the controls and H+ men than in the H− men. They also found deactivation of the left inferior frontal gyrus, suggestive of reduced inhibition of sexual arousal, but only in the controls and H+ men. Androgen receptors have been reported in the orbitofrontal cortex of primates (Finley and Kritzer 1999) and to a limited extent in the cingulate cortex (Abdelgadir *et al.* 1999). However, there is, as yet, no evidence of ARs in the insula or claustrum in primates or humans.

A further unresolved issue is whether men with primary hypogonadotropic hypogonadism respond in a similar way to those with secondary hypergonadotropic hypogonadism. The reported results have been inconsistent; Gooren (1988) compared two groups of six teenage males with delayed puberty aged between 14 and 18 years; one group hypogonadotropic (i.e. the primary problem being lack of gonadotropic stimulation of the testes), the other hypergonadotropic (i.e. the primary problem is failure of the testes to respond to gonadotropic stimulation). The hypogonadotropic group, while responding to testosterone replacement in a similar way in their erectile and ejaculatory responsiveness, showed less increase in sexual interest and frequency of sexual activity, and less positive change in mood and energy than the hypergonadotropic group. A crucial issue is whether a hypogonadal male has gone through normal pubertal development before the onset of hypogonadism. If he has not then there may be some residual abnormality of pubertal development that results in a deficient or altered brain response to testosterone. More research is needed on this issue.

5.3.1.2 Experimental reduction of testosterone in eugonadal men

In a study of normal men, aged 20–40, Bagatell *et al.* (1994a) lowered endogenous testosterone by means of a GnRH antagonist, NalGlu, on its own or in combination with 50 or 100 mg of intramuscular (im) testosterone enanthate or a placebo, each in a group of 9 or 10 men. This manipulation lasted for six weeks for each group. There was a clear reduction of sexual interest and activity when testosterone was reduced with NalGlu alone, consistent with the changes reported in withdrawal of testosterone replacement from hypogonadal men reviewed above. However, these changes were avoided with even the lowest dose of testosterone replacement (50 mg testosterone enanthate weekly), which resulted in testosterone levels well below the baseline levels. It is possible that if these low testosterone levels had been sustained over a longer period there may have been negative consequences. Comparable findings were reported by Behre *et al.* (1994), who used a different GnRH antagonist, cetrorelix. Overall, these findings indicate that for most men the normal range of testosterone is above that required for testosterone-dependent sexuality. We will return to possible explanations for this seemingly paradoxical fact later in this chapter.

The effects of increasing testosterone levels above the normal range for extended periods has become an issue with the recent interest in hormonal contraception for males. Although relatively high doses of exogenous testosterone suppress spermatogenesis, mainly by suppressing FSH, these effects are not well sustained over time, and side-effects are significant. Attention is therefore being given to combinations of testosterone, usually in a slow-release form, and a progestogen (e.g. dienogest). Progestogens, while effective in suppressing spermatogenesis, also have side-effects, and as yet no fully satisfactory regime for hormonal male contraception has been established or approved (Manetti and Honig 2010).

However, a number of studies have been published that give us information about the behavioral effects of increasing testosterone in eugonadal men. Anderson *et al.* (1992) carried out a placebo-controlled evaluation of 31 healthy men who were involved in an ongoing efficacy trial of hormonal male contraception. They were divided into two groups. One group had testosterone enanthate im injections of 200 mg weekly for eight weeks; in the other group weekly injections of placebo were given for four weeks followed by four, weekly injections of testosterone enanthate. Neither group showed any change in measures of sexual interactions with partners or masturbation. Both groups, however, showed an increase in subscale 2 of the Sexual Experience Scale (Frenken and Vennix 1981) during testosterone administration, but this did not happen with placebo. This subscale is an index of sexual interest independent of interaction with a partner. Bagatell *et al.* (1994b) administered testosterone enanthate 200 mg im to 19 eugonadal men. There were no effects on frequency of sexual activity, including masturbation, though there was a non-significant increase in reports of spontaneous erections. Yates *et al.* (1999) compared three dose levels of testosterone in eugonadal men over a 14-week period, using a placebo control. They found no increase in frequency of orgasm or daily ratings of sexual interest. Buena *et al.* (1993) recruited two groups of healthy men, aged 18–49 years, and suppressed testicular function with a GnRH analog (leuprorelin). One group was then given doses of testosterone replacement to achieve levels in the lower part of the normal range, and, in the other group, to achieve levels in the high part of the normal range.

They were assessed for nine weeks on this regime and, towards the end of this period, their NPT was assessed in a sleep laboratory. The two groups did not differ in measures of sexual interest or activity or in NPT (although rigidity of the NPT was not assessed).

There is therefore some inconsistency in this limited literature that may reflect differing levels of testosterone attained, and different methods of assessing their effects. It remains possible, however, that there is a "normal" range of testosterone which may vary to some extent across men, and that varying testosterone levels within the individual's "normal" range will produce no sexual effect, with levels below the individual's range resulting in impairment, and with levels above his range, an increase most predictably in sexual interest. Thus we can reasonably conclude that levels of testosterone in this "normal" range are necessary for the sexuality of men, which, given its fundamental role in reproduction, is not likely to show much genetic variability.

5.3.2 Testosterone, mood and aggression in men

5.3.2.1 Depression

Although reduction of sexual interest is more likely when testosterone levels are below the normal range, there is some evidence that depressed mood also may occur. This has received the most attention in older men. Barrett-Connor et al. (1999) studied 856 men, aged 50 to 89, who were attending a medical clinic. Depressed mood was assessed using the Beck Depression Inventory (BDI; Beck et al. 1961). Scores for the BDI were significantly and negatively associated with bioavailable testosterone and also, though less significantly, with DHT. Twenty-five of the men were diagnosed as clinically depressed, and their bioavailable testosterone was 17% lower than the remainder of the sample ($p < 0.01$). Shores et al. (2005) assessed 748 men aged 50 years or older without any previous history of diagnosed depressive illness. Men who at the outset had low testosterone levels were significantly more likely to become depressed over the next two years, independently of medical morbidity. Almeida et al. (2008), in an Australian community study, assessed 3987 men aged 71 to 89 years. Of these men, 203 (5.1%) were clinically depressed and they were significantly more likely to have total and free testosterone levels in the lowest quintile.

Amiaz and Seidman (2008) reviewed the relevant literature on testosterone and depression in men. They pointed out that in most of the earlier controlled studies of testosterone replacement in hypogonadal men, which focused on sexual effects, depressive mood was not systematically or adequately assessed. In several more recent randomized controlled trials of testosterone replacement, which have focused more on depressed mood, the results have been inconsistent. They concluded that there was no pervasive influence of testosterone on mood, but there might be a subgroup of depressed men who would benefit from testosterone therapy. This had been suggested by Schmidt et al. (2004). In an experimental study, 34 young, healthy volunteers (aged 23 to 46) had their endogenous testosterone levels reduced by leuprorelin, a GnRH analog that downregulates LH and FSH

secretion. In one group this was countered by testosterone replacement from the start ($n = 17$); the other group ($n = 17$) received leuprorelin alone for four weeks and then placebo was added. Mood was assessed by the BDI (Beck et al. 1961) plus daily self-ratings. Three men in the leuprorelin plus placebo group showed an increase in BDI score to 7 or higher, and one of these men met DSM-IV (Diagnostic and Statistical Manual of Mental Disorders) criteria for depressive disorder, his BDI score rising from 0 at baseline to 14. The authors concluded that "short-term hypogonadism is sufficient to precipitate depressive symptoms in only a small minority of younger men. The predictors of this susceptibility remain to be determined." Whether this susceptibility increases with age remains uncertain.

5.3.2.2 Aggression

The idea that testosterone is the "aggression hormone," accounting for why men are more aggressive than women, is a widely held myth often exploited by the media. Most of this chapter has focused on sexual behavior, and we have seen an unmistakable link between testosterone and male sexuality, although the precise nature of this link remains uncertain. With aggression, we are faced with a great deal of inconsistent evidence that is mainly based on attempts to correlate circulating levels of testosterone with personality characteristics related to aggression.

Harris (1999) provides an extensive review of the literature that vividly demonstrates this inconsistency. Various possibilities have been proposed. Testosterone may influence the aggressive personality either directly, as suggested by Christiansen and Knussman (1987), or indirectly through other aspects of the personality relevant to aggression. Thus testosterone may be related to irritability (Brown and Davis 1975); to the individual's level of frustration tolerance (Olweus et al. 1980; 1988); to dominance (Gray et al. 1991) or to impulsivity (Gladue 1991). Caprara et al. (1992) proposed that irritability plays a crucial role as a "bridge" construct between "emotional" and "cognitive" components of aggression.

Huesmann and Eron (1989) emphasized the developmental aspects of aggression. They proposed that severe, antisocial aggression usually emerges early in life, and that certain genetic characteristics and perinatal or traumatic events predispose a child to develop aggressive habits. Once established, these "cognitive structures" may be extremely resistant to change. "Through elaborative rehearsal of specific scripts, more general abstract scripts for social behavior are formed which are equally resistant to change." However, testosterone was not mentioned by Huesmann and Eron (1989). We might speculate that testosterone has an organizing role, or may activate established patterns of behavior, of the kind they described. Not surprisingly, in the conclusion to her review, Harris commented: "...it is still not clear what relationship testosterone has with aggression"!

A review of the literature on androgens and aggression across species was provided by Hines (2004). Whereas the relationship between testosterone and aggression may be more clear-cut in other non-primate species, gender difference is variable across species, and the aggressive potential of female mammals has been underestimated. Meta-analytic data from humans show that gender difference in physical aggression is moderate (effect size, $d = 0.50$), larger in children ($d = 0.58$) than in college students ($d = 0.27$) (Hyde 1984). This underlines the importance of the developmental process, with presumably an early organizational effect of testosterone on prepubertal aggressive behavior. There may also be a second organizational phase with puberty and associated brain development, though as yet it is not clear whether this moderates, or in any way influences the gender difference seen previously in childhood.

Book *et al.* (2001) reported a meta-analysis of published studies in humans that showed the average correlation between plasma testosterone levels and aggression to be small ($r = 0.14$). They suggested that this could also be an overestimate because of under reporting of negative findings.

In both human and non-human primates, experience of success in dominance encounters can cause a rise in testosterone, at least temporarily. Furthermore, in human studies, experience (e.g. of winning versus losing) and internal states (motivation and anticipation of certain types of competition) can influence testosterone levels (e.g. Neave and Wolfson 2003). However, the functional relevance of such short-term increase in circulating testosterone is not clear. It is sometimes assumed that it will increase behaviors relevant to aggression or dominance, but "there is little or no evidence to support this assumption" (Hines 2004). Overall, Hines concluded, the evidence points more to greater dominance resulting in higher testosterone than vice versa.

Hines (2004) made an important point about how testosterone might influence behavior by increasing arousal: "In terms of physiological states, it is thought that increased arousal strengthens behavioral proclivities that already exist, and so can amplify pre-existing inclinations to aggression. [...] arousal can sometimes be mislabeled as a different emotion, including anger or hostility. [...] arousal, either high or low, can be an aversive state and can increase the likelihood of aggression in a manner similar to that produced by situational factors."

In the previous section we saw "central arousal" as a complex state that we experience as "sexual arousal." However, the specifically sexual components are the genital response, and information processing that is focused on sexual meanings. The central arousal that occurs is not necessarily different to other types of arousal, although there is some suggestion that it might be influenced by testosterone receptors (ARs) in the noradrenergic system that, in general, determines central "arousal" in a non-specific way. What is not clear is whether these ARs allow an arousal response that is specific to sexual situations, or whether they allow testosterone to have a general arousal effect not restricted to sex.

So far, the literature has suggested there is a small minority of men who might show aggressive responses to changes in testosterone within the normal range. We have no clear evidence of aggression in hypogonadal men but no indication that they become more aggressive with testosterone replacement. Let us, therefore, focus on the six controlled studies that have assessed the effects of supraphysiological levels of testosterone on mood and aggression in eugonadal men.

In the placebo-controlled evaluation of sexuality and mood in 31 healthy men by Anderson *et al.* (1992), reported earlier, daily ratings of various aspects of mood were collected; these included "tense," "energetic," "unhappy," "irritable," "ready to fight," "easily angered." None of these showed any change with supraphysiological levels of testosterone compared to baseline or placebo.

Tricker *et al.* (1996) used a double-blind, placebo-controlled design, and administered 600 mg of im testosterone enanthate per week. The study was divided into a 4-week baseline period, a 10-week treatment period and a 16-week recovery period. Forty-three eugonadal men, 19–40 years of age, were randomized to one of four groups: Group 1, placebo, no exercise; Group 2, testosterone enanthate, no exercise; Group 3, placebo plus exercise; Group 4, testosterone enanthate plus exercise. Exercise consisted of thrice-weekly strength-training sessions. The Multidimensional Anger Inventory (MAI; Seigel 1986), which includes five different dimensions of anger (inward anger, outward anger, anger-arousal, hostile outlook and anger-eliciting situations), and a Mood Inventory (MI), were completed by subjects before, during and after the 10-week intervention. The man's significant other (e.g. spouse, or parent) answered the same questions about the subject's mood and mood-related behavior. There were no significant changes in any of the measures during the treatment period, and no differences in these variables between exercising and non-exercising or between placebo and testosterone enanthate–treated subjects. The authors concluded that supraphysiological doses of testosterone, when administered to normal men in a controlled setting, do not increase angry behavior. They did not, however, exclude the possibility that high doses might provoke angry behavior in men with a particular susceptibility to angry responses.

In the Yates *et al.* (1999) study reported earlier, mood was monitored throughout the study using the Buss–Durkee Hostility Inventory (BDHI; Buss and Durkee 1957), the Brief Psychiatric Rating Scale (BPRS: Overall and Gorham 1962), the Modified Mania Rating Scale (MMRS; Blackburn *et al.* 1977) and the Hamilton Depression Rating Scale (HDRS; Hamilton 1967). Only minimal effects on these measures of mood and behavior were observed during the 14-week testosterone administration and withdrawal phases for those who completed the study, and there was no evidence of a dose-dependent effect on any of the above measures. There were also no effects on psychosexual function. One participant on 500 mg of testosterone developed a brief state of agitated and irritable mania, and was therefore withdrawn from the study.

Pope *et al.* (2000) recruited 56 men, aged 20 to 50 (77% in the 20–29 year range), into a randomized, placebo-controlled crossover study. Participants were seen weekly for 25 weeks. This covered six weeks for treatment 1, six weeks for washout, six weeks for treatment 2 and seven weeks for final washout. In the active treatment, the first two, weekly injections contained 150 mg, the third and fourth weeks, 300 mg, and the fifth and sixth week, 600 mg of

testosterone cypionate. In the placebo condition, equivalent amounts of the sesame oil vehicle were injected. Assessment of mood and aggression involved the Young Mania Rating Scale (YMRS; Young *et al.* 1978), the 24 item Hamilton Depression Rating Scale (Hamilton 1960) and the Buss and Perry Aggression Questionnaire (Buss and Perry 1992), together with the Symptom Checklist-90-R (Derogatis 1994). In addition, daily diaries of manic and depressive symptoms, and how much he "liked" his current state, were completed by each participant, and a similar weekly diary was completed by a "significant other." During the second year of the study an additional measure was added: the Point Subtraction Aggression Paradigm (PSAP; Kouri *et al.* 1995). Each participant was seated in a booth equipped with a monitor screen and was told that he was playing against an unseen male opponent, which was actually a computer. The participant could accumulate points on the screen – exchangeable for money – by pressing one button, or he could deprive his "opponent" of points by pressing another button. During the session, the opponent provoked the participant by randomly depriving him of points. The participant's aggression score represented the total number of points that he subtracted from his opponent in retaliation to this provocation. Subjects who realized that the opponent was actually a computer were excluded from the analysis of this variable.

Manic scores on the YMRS increased significantly with testosterone treatment ($p = 0.002$). However, this effect resulted from a few participants reporting marked manic-type symptoms, whereas the majority showed little change. No participant reported violent behavior while receiving testosterone, but several described instances of uncharacteristic aggressiveness; one participant was withdrawn from the study after the fifth week because he became "alarmingly hypomanic and aggressive." Aggression scores on the PSAP increased significantly with testosterone treatment ($p = 0.03$) in spite of the smaller number of participants in this analysis ($n = 27$). Again, however, this effect depended on a few showing marked changes whereas most participants showed little change. The "manic" and "liking" scores on participants' daily diaries also showed a significant testosterone treatment effect. Diaries from "significant others" did not show a significant testosterone effect; although, at the end of the testosterone treatment period, the diary manic scores from participants and their "significant others" correlated significantly (Spearman $\rho = 0.59$; $p < 0.001$).

O'Connor *et al.* (2004) used a double-blind, placebo-controlled crossover design in a study of 28 healthy eugonadal men (mean age 32.3 years). This involved three eight-week periods; the middle period being "washout." A single im injection of testosterone undecanoate 1000 mg was compared to a single placebo injection, with randomization to one of two sequences (i.e. testosterone undecanoate – placebo, or placebo –testosterone undecanoate). Following testosterone undecanoate administration the testosterone levels were substantially raised for two weeks, though the LH levels remained suppressed for longer. The Profile of Mood States (POMS; McNair *et al.* 1992) was used to monitor mood. Various aspects of aggression, including both feelings and behavior, were monitored with the Aggression Questionnaire (AQ; Buss and Perry 1992), which was also completed by the partner (Partner Aggression Questionnaire or AQ-P; O'Connor *et al.* 2001), the Aggressive Provocation Questionnaire (APQ; O'Connor *et al.* 2001) and the Irritability subscale from the Buss–Durkee Hostility Inventory (Buss and Durkee 1957). In addition, the Rathus Assertiveness Schedule (Rathus 1973) and the State Self-Esteem Scale (Heatherton and Polivy 1991) were used. There were significant increases in anger/hostility scores for the first two weeks after testosterone undecanoate injection, but at levels that stayed within the normal range for US college samples. This was accompanied by a significant reduction in fatigue/inertia. There was no increase in aggressive behavior.

The final controlled study is unique in that testosterone was increased for only three days, and hence allows us to assess short-term effects of testosterone on mood. Su *et al.* (1993) reported a fixed-order, placebo-controlled, double-blind study. Twenty healthy men (mean age 27.5 years), with no prior history of anabolic steroid use, were admitted to the National Institute of Mental Health inpatient research ward for 14 days. This therefore involved another unique feature; all subjects were kept in the same environment during their participation in the study. After two days settling in, they experienced four consecutive three-day conditions. The first three days were a placebo baseline, then oral methyltestosterone 40 mg daily (the normal prescribed dose) was given for three days, followed by methyltestosterone 240 mg daily for three days, followed by placebo for three

days. There were subtle and statistically significant ($p < 0.05$) increases in positive mood (euphoria, energy and sexual arousal), negative mood (irritability, mood swings, violent feelings and hostility), although no aggressive behavior, and some cognitive impairment (distractibility, forgetfulness and confusion). As with the previous studies, these group changes concealed considerable individual variability. One subject, for example, had an acute manic episode. These variable reactions were not predicted by baseline characteristics or family psychiatric history.

The overall conclusion from these six controlled studies is that for the majority of eugonadal healthy men, temporary increases of plasma testosterone to supraphysiological levels do not increase aggressive feelings or behavior. But there is a minority who are affected, though in most such cases the effects have been more manic than aggressive. Such effects are suggestive of a relatively non-specific arousal mechanism, the manifestations of which may depend on personality characteristics or the particular circumstances at the time. It is possible that the relevant personality characteristics are the same as those that result in depressive reactions to lowered testosterone levels, as discussed above. It remains uncertain as to what extent these short-term effects of supraphysiological plasma testosterone levels are based on the same hormone-behavior mechanisms that result from normal levels.

5.3.2.3 Testosterone and sleep

If "arousal" is the essence of testosterone effects in the brain, how might it affect sleep? It has been recognized for some time that testosterone administration can induce sleep apnea (e.g. Sandblom *et al.* 1983). Conversely, sleep apnea is known to reduce testosterone as a result of dysfunction of the pituitary-gonadal axis (Luboshitzky *et al.* 2002). Sleep deprivation also reduces circulating testosterone levels in healthy men (e.g. Cortés-Gallegos *et al.* 1983).

Leibenluft *et al.* (1997) explored the effects of testosterone on sleep by inducing transient hypogonadism with leuprorelin, a GnRH analog. This was given for three months to 10 normal healthy male volunteers with an average age of 29 years. In the second and third months, at two week intervals, either testosterone enanthate 200 mg or placebo were given in a double-blind, randomized order, crossover design. Although no differences in timing or duration of sleep were observed, there was a significant reduction in the proportion of stage 4 sleep, and reduction of 24-hour prolactin levels, in the hypogonadal state compared with testosterone replacement. The authors concluded that testosterone "has relatively specific and discrete effects on sleep and hormonal rhythms in men."

Liu *et al.* (2003) carried out a placebo-controlled crossover evaluation of the effects of testosterone administration on sleep in older men. In the active phase, three, weekly im injections of Sustanon (a mixture of three testosterone esters) were given: 500 mg in the first week, and 250 mg in the second and third weeks. In the placebo condition, weekly injections of the excipient oil were given. In between treatments there was an eight-week washout period. Sleep and breathing were assessed by polysomnography at baseline, and at the end of each treatment period. Seventeen healthy men over the age of 60 participated. Total sleep time was reduced by an average of one hour, and disrupted breathing increased; both significant differences ($p < 0.05$). There was, however, no evidence of change in upper airway dimensions, making it unlikely that the sleep disruption was due to airway obstruction. The question arises of whether this negative effect of testosterone administration is more likely in older men. In the six studies of supraphysiological testosterone administration in eugonadal men, all less than 60 years of age, reviewed above, negative effects on sleep were only mentioned in two reports. Su *et al.* (1993) included a rating of insomnia in their daily diaries. They found a dose-related trend towards more insomnia with testosterone administration ($p < 0.1$). As each dose was only for three days, one wonders whether this may have become more marked with longer usage. Yates *et al.* (1999) described one participant who withdrew from the study because of an acute onset of distress, associated with marked irritability and sleep-onset insomnia. Clearly, testosterone is related to sleep in ways that may be important in states of testosterone deficiency and during testosterone replacement. But as yet we have an incomplete and somewhat confused picture of this relationship.

While the research reviewed here has indicated that a minority of men are susceptible to the hyper-arousing effects of testosterone administration, it has not yet enabled us to identify relevant characteristics of these responders. Future research should focus on potential predictors that might help to explain this minority response, and, if at all possible, to assess its heritability.

5.3.3 Summary of evidence in the male

There is consistent evidence of a relationship between testosterone and both sexual interest and NPT in younger men. This suggests that the main central effects of testosterone are on central arousal associated with response to sexual stimuli (Bancroft 1995). As a consequence, thoughts about sex, accompanied by central arousal, are experienced as manifestations of "sexual interest." The association with NPT is suggestive of a testosterone-dependent "excitatory tone" based on central arousal mechanisms, which is allowed expression through penile erection when the inhibitory tone maintaining the normally flaccid penis is reduced or "switched off" during REM sleep.

The relevance of testosterone to erectile function is more subtle or complex. There is recent evidence of testosterone-dependent mechanisms in the spinal cord and penis that are relevant (Montorsi and Oettel 2005). We can assume that testosterone-dependent arousal mechanisms will augment erectile response. But other mechanisms, including cognitive processing of sexual stimuli, as well as age and disease-related increases in erectile inhibitory tone, which are not testosterone dependent, have an equal or greater influence on erectile response.

Whereas the picture is comparatively clear during young adulthood and midlife, developmental processes involved both around puberty and with aging are less well understood. With the recent awareness of important brain development during the second decade, it is possible that testosterone is having an organizing as well as an activating effect around puberty. With aging, there are complex changes in testosterone receptor number and sensitivity, as well as other changes both centrally and peripherally, which makes the physiologic function of testosterone more obscure.

The concept of a threshold below which androgen deficiency occurs, and above which increasing androgen levels have little effect, is fairly consistently supported by the evidence. However, our ability to identify "the threshold level" remains limited. The level is likely to vary across individuals, and it may possibly change with age and exposure to sustained and different levels of testosterone. At present, we can only speculate on this issue. A number of studies have suggested that subtle effects may arise from increasing testosterone to supra-threshold levels.

We have little systematic evidence on the timing of testosterone effects on sexual responsiveness. The hormone replacement studies discussed above suggest that, after a period of testosterone withdrawal, it is several days or even two-to-three weeks before replacement testosterone has its maximum effects. On the other hand, short-term administration of testosterone to eugonadal men has apparently produced effects, albeit subtle, within three days (e.g. Carani *et al.* 1990; Su *et al.* 1993). Further research is required on this basic issue.

Whereas testosterone effects on sexuality are relatively universal in men, testosterone effects on mood and aggression, observed only in a minority of men studied, suggest that some men are more sensitive to such effects.

5.4 Activational effects of testosterone and behavior in adult women

The role of testosterone, at least in relation to sexuality, is better understood in men than in women, despite the fact that there is much more evidence in the literature relating to hormones and female sexuality, and more opportunities to study variations of hormones in the female (e.g. menstrual cycle, lactation, menopause). This reflects the complexity and greater inconsistency of the evidence in women. Later in this chapter, direct comparisons of the role of testosterone in men and women will be made.

Paradoxically, in research on the sexuality of women, more attention has been paid to testosterone than to estradiol. As mentioned earlier, one crucial and unresolved issue is the extent to which testosterone produces its effects, in both male and female, by conversion to estradiol.

5.4.1 Sexual desire and response

As in men, the essence of women's sexual desire is incentive motivation linked to processing of sexually relevant information, with varying degrees of central arousal and genital response. However, there is little evidence of what is being desired in women, and there may be important gender differences, or at least greater variability in women than in men (Bancroft and Graham 2011). In particular, is it desire for sexual

pleasure and/or orgasm, is it desire for emotional intimacy or closeness to one's partner, is it desire to give one's partner pleasure, or is it a combination of these? And how do these vary across women, and within the same woman dependent on context, and at different stages of life?

In the male, genital response, or penile erection, is obvious to him and hence there tends to be a high correlation between sexual desire and awareness of some degree of erection in men. The homologous form of genital response in the woman is clitoral tumescence, and this is less obvious to her and hence less central to her experience of sexual arousal. Women, in their experience of sexual desire, consequently focus more on whether they are feeling aroused in a more subjective sense (Graham 2010). In women there are two aspects of genital response which are uniquely female; the increased blood flow and pulse amplitude in the vaginal wall (as measured by vaginal pulse amplitude (VPA; Laan and Everaerd 1995), and the reduced sensitivity to pain from vaginal or cervical stimulation (Komisaruk and Sansone 2003), both of which are crucial to allow vaginal penetration without discomfort. But these two mechanisms may not otherwise contribute to the woman's experience of sexual arousal or desire.

Most women experience orgasm, but the hormonal regulation of this complex and ill-understood phenomenon remains unclear in both women and men. Seminal emission in men, which is linked to orgasm in some way that is also not well understood, is testosterone dependent. There is no equivalent of seminal emission in women.

The relevance of testosterone and other androgens to women's sexuality will be reviewed under the following headings: (1) circulating androgen levels in women; (2) iatrogenic lowering of androgens and (3) exogenous androgen administration.

5.4.1.1 Circulating androgen levels and their relation to the sexuality of women

Plasma total testosterone in women is on average less than 3.5 nmol/l; i.e. around 10% of levels in the male. Given the problems with assaying low levels of testosterone, there is no clear bottom of the normal range. Consistent with that is the absence of any recognizable testosterone deficiency in women, except when there has been an iatrogenic lowering (see below). Dehydroepiandrosterone and DHEAS are present in the plasma at levels as high as in men, at least in premenopausal women.

To what extent do plasma levels of testosterone relate to the sexuality of women? Davis *et al.* (2005) asked a community-based sample of 1021 Australian women, aged 18 to 75 years, to complete the Profile of Female Sexual Function (PFSF; Derogatis *et al.* 2004), and a measure of general well-being. One fasting morning blood sample was collected. In premenopausal women this was collected between day 8 of the cycle and onset of the next menses. (This is likely to obscure the modest but significant mid-cycle rise in testosterone that typically occurs.) Blood was assayed for testosterone (total and free), androstenedione and DHEAS.

The PFSF provides seven domain scores (desire, arousal, orgasm, pleasure, sexual concerns, responsiveness and self-image). These scores were not normally distributed in this sample, and were related to age. The sample was therefore divided into two age groups (younger, 18–44 years, $n = 339$; older, 45–75 years, $n = 646$). For each domain these two age groups were divided into those with low scores (zero for the older; the lowest 5% for the younger group) and the rest. The low scorers and the rest for each domain were then compared for plasma levels of androgens. Neither total nor free testosterone discriminated between these groups for any domain of sexual function, in either the younger or older women. Dehydroepiandrosterone sulfate, however, was significantly lower in the "low" scorers in three domains for each age group. For the younger group, the three domains were "desire," "arousal" and "responsiveness"; for the older group: "arousal," "responsiveness" and "pleasure." In addition, androstenedione was significantly lower for the older "low" responders in the "pleasure" domain.

This study by Davis *et al.* (2005) is by far the largest of its kind. However, their comparison of the low scorers on the PFSF with the rest leaves us with some unanswered questions. Many of the women in the "low" scorer groups may have seen themselves as having "a sexual problem." In an early and small study of oral contraceptive users, we found that women who defined themselves as having a "sexual problem" did not show any correlation between testosterone levels and a measure of sexual interest; whereas women who did not regard themselves as having a sexual problem showed a significant correlation (Bancroft *et al.* 1980; see below). One possible

explanation for this is that the establishment of a "sexual problem," with its various repercussions in the relationship, may serve to obscure subtle hormone–behavior relationships. It would therefore be interesting to know whether there was any correlation between testosterone levels and PFSF scores across the large non-problem component of the Davis *et al.* sample.

Few studies have investigated testosterone levels in women presenting specifically with problems of low sexual desire. Stuart *et al.* (1987) and Schreiner-Engel *et al.* (1995) found no difference in testosterone levels between women with low sexual interest and controls; on the other hand, Riley and Riley (2000) found a lower Free Androgen Index (FAI) in women complaining of lifelong absence of sexual drive compared to controls. These were all small studies, with numbers in each group ranging from 11 to 17.

Compared with men, there are natural variations of testosterone in women of reproductive age that warrant attention.

The menstrual cycle

Testosterone levels typically rise during the follicular phase and are at a maximum approximately for the middle third of the cycle, declining during the final third of the cycle to reach the lowest levels for the first few days of the next follicular phase. In some women, this mid-cycle rise in testosterone is a more discrete periovulatory peak. In a study of 37 women with normal ovulatory cycles, testosterone levels were highest during the mid-third of the cycle (Bancroft *et al.* 1983). In the 21 women who masturbated, frequency of masturbation was significantly correlated with mid-cycle testosterone levels; there was no correlation between testosterone and frequency of sexual activity with partner. There is now an extensive literature on variations of sexual interest and behavior through the menstrual cycle, though the findings are somewhat inconsistent (see Hedricks 1994 for a review). Sexual activity tends to be lowest during the menstrual phase, and sexual interest to be highest during the follicular phase or around ovulation, though there is considerable individual variability. Although mid-cycle increases in testosterone could be contributing to this pattern, other hormonal and non-hormonal explanations also have to be considered.

Lactation is associated with a lowering of plasma testosterone as well as estradiol, and often with reduced sexual interest. One small study (Alder *et al.* 1986) showed that breast-feeding women with low sexual interest had significantly lower plasma testosterone levels than breast feeders with normal sexual interest; however, this finding still awaits replication.

5.4.1.2 Aging and the menopause

Adrenal androgens, particularly DHEA and DHEAS, show an age-related decline in women over a relatively wide age span (Orentreich *et al.* 1984; Bancroft and Cawood 1996; Sulcová *et al.* 1997; Burger *et al.* 2000; Davison *et al.* 2005). This was most convincingly demonstrated in a study of ovariectomized women where ovarian androgens could not obscure the picture (Crilly *et al.* 1979). Ovarian androgens present a more complex picture. Decline in testosterone starts a few years before the menopausal transition, probably due to a reduction in the mid-cycle rise of testosterone (Roger *et al.* 1980; Zumoff *et al.* 1995; Mushayandebvu *et al.* 1996). The menopause *per se* has less predictable effects on ovarian androgens. In a longitudinal study of 172 women who made the transition from premenopausal to postmenopausal during the seven years of the study (Burger *et al.* 2000), total testosterone did not change, whereas free testosterone *increased* from pre- to postmenopausal. In the large Australian cross-sectional study, described above, a steady decline in testosterone (both total and free), androstenedione and DHEAS was found across age groups, with menopausal status having no influence on this decline (Davison *et al.* 2005), and there was no age-related change in SHBG.

The function of the interstitial cells of the ovary changes with the menopause. In premenopausal women, gonadotropic stimulation of the interstitial cells is regulated by the negative feedback of ovarian steroids. However, the rise in LH that accompanies the menopausal transition, resulting from the reduction in estrogen-induced negative feedback, may stimulate the interstitial cells to produce testosterone and androstenedione, sometimes excessively. In addition, factors such as body weight and insulin resistance influence this ovarian androgen production (see Cawood and Bancroft (1996) for a brief review of the evidence). Some researchers, however, have questioned whether the postmenopausal ovary is a significant source of androgens (e.g. Couzinet *et al.* 2001).

The variability of women's sexuality, striking enough in younger women, becomes even more marked in older women, when psychosocial factors

and the importance of fertility, amongst other things, influence the picture. As yet, no predictable association between the age-related decline in androgens and changes in the sexuality of older women has been demonstrated.

5.4.1.3 Effects of iatrogenic lowering of testosterone in women

There are three principal iatrogenic procedures that happen to reduce testosterone in women: oral contraceptive use, use of antiandrogens, and bilateral ovariectomy.

Oral contraceptives

It has been known for some time that oral contraceptives reduce free testosterone (Jung-Hoffman and Kuhl, 1987; Van der Vange *et al.* 1990; Janaud *et al.* 1992; Darney 1995; Thorneycroft *et al.* 1999; Boyd *et al.* 2001). Mid-cycle rises in testosterone and androstenedione are blocked by suppression of ovulation and the normal pattern of gonadal steroid production. In addition, the estrogen in the oral contraceptive increases SHBG levels and hence reduces the free testosterone available. There is more limited evidence of a reduction in DHEA and DHEAS (Coenen *et al.* 1996; Graham *et al.* 2007).

In spite of this consistent evidence, it is striking how little attention has been paid to the possible effects of this decline in androgens on women's sexuality (Bancroft and Sartorius, 1990; Davis and Castano 2004). In an early study (Bancroft *et al.* 1980), we compared 20 established oral contraceptive users complaining of sexual problems that they attributed to the oral contraceptive, with 20 oral contraceptive users without sexual problems, matched for oral contraceptive and age. The total testosterone levels were low in both groups (free testosterone was not estimated) and did not differ significantly. As mentioned earlier, we found a significant correlation between our measure of sexual interest ("frequency of sexual thoughts") and the testosterone level in the "no problem" group ($r = 0.65$; $p < 0.01$) but not in the "problem" group ($r = 0.02$; non-significant). A significant correlation between plasma testosterone and sexual interest was found in two other studies of oral contraceptive users (Bancroft *et al.* 1991; Alexander and Sherwin 1993). These three studies of women on oral contraceptives, and without sexual problems, are so far the only studies to show significant correlations between plasma testosterone and sexual interest in women. Thus these correlations are with testosterone levels in the lower part of the physiological range. This led Alexander and Sherwin (1993) to postulate a "threshold" effect in women, comparable to that in men, but at a much lower level of plasma testosterone; i.e. correlations between plasma testosterone level and measures of sexual interest will only become apparent when the testosterone levels are around or below this threshold level, which is presumably in the lower part of the normal range.

Most of the relevant literature on oral contraceptive use and sexuality has involved cross-sectional studies, where women who experienced negative sexual effects are likely to have discontinued oral contraceptive use, and hence "selected" themselves out of the study. Recently, we reported the first study to measure change in free testosterone *and* in measures of sexuality and mood in 61 women starting on oral contraceptives (Graham et al. 2007). Sexuality was assessed by the Interviewer Ratings of Sexual Function (IRSF), and mood by the Beck Depression Inventory (BDI; Beck et al. 1961). Highly significant reductions in free testosterone and DHEAS were found after three months on oral contraceptive, though there was considerable individual variability in the degree of reduction. As in previous studies, there was also considerable variability in the measures of sexuality and mood. Thus the "frequency of sexual thoughts," the principal measure of sexual interest, increased in 33% of women and decreased in 23%, with the remainder showing no change. On the BDI, while showing on average very little change, 39% of women showed improvement in mood and 29% worsened. Some support was found for the hypothesis that reduction in sexual interest (and other sexuality measures) is related to the reduction in free testosterone. Direct correlations between the change scores for both behavioral and hormonal measures were not significant, but when we correlated change in hormone level with the actual level of sexuality after three months on oral contraceptive, we found significant correlations between reduction in free testosterone and two behavioral variables; frequency of sexual thoughts ($r = 0.35$; $p = 0.006$), and percentage of occasions of sexual activity with partner when the woman felt sexually aroused or excited ($r = 0.28$; $p = 0.03$). We found no significant correlations with other aspects of sexual enjoyment or response, or involving change in DHEAS, or between hormonal change and mood scores. In some women, therefore,

a decline in testosterone after starting the oral contraceptive was associated with low levels of sexual interest. But there were other women who experienced a substantial decline in free testosterone and no apparent reduction, or even an increase in sexual interest. We have to keep in mind the varied psychological effects that an effective contraceptive may have on a woman's sexuality. In some women the freedom from concern about pregnancy may have a sexually liberating effect. We thus have to balance the effects of such inhibition reduction with the possible negative effects of testosterone reduction on sexual interest. Cultural factors influencing women's sexuality also need to be considered.

A range of factors may contribute to the complex effects of oral contraceptives on sexuality, but the possibility that a substantial minority of women are dependent sexually on testosterone, and experience negative sexual changes, particularly in sexual interest, because of the oral contraceptive–induced reduction in free testosterone, remains a distinct possibility. In comparison to the limited evidence in relation to oral contraceptives, there is virtually no systematically collected evidence of the effects of long-acting hormonal implants (e.g. Norplant) or injections (e.g. depot medroxyprogesterone acetate, DMPA) on women's sexuality. Given that DMPA is used in the United States to control male sex offenders (Walker 1978), it is disturbing that an official UK Government report (National Institute for Health and Clinical Excellence; NICE 2005) recommended the use of DMPA for contraception by young women when we have no idea what effects such long-acting methods have on women's sexuality or mood.

Antiandrogens in women

Antiandrogens work by blocking androgen effects at the receptor and also by reducing testosterone levels by means of negative feedback effects. Cyproterone acetate (CPA) is an antiandrogen that has been used for many years, at least in Europe, for treatment of androgen-dependent conditions such as acne and hirsutism in women. Little attention has been given to the possible sexual side-effects of such treatment. One study systematically assessed such effects. Appelt and Strauss (1986) studied 36 women who had not had sexual problems before starting on CPA, and, of these, 16 (44%) reported negative effects on their sex life; this rose to 61% if women not in sexual relationships were excluded.

Bilateral ovariectomy

With surgical removal of the ovaries, there is an immediate and substantial drop in circulating androgens. There have been a number of studies evaluating the effects of hormone replacement in women who present with sexual problems after ovariectomy, and these are considered below. What proportion of women experience sexual problems as a consequence of having their ovaries removed has received less attention. The following studies present a somewhat inconsistent picture.

Nathorst-Böös *et al.* (1993) compared the sexuality of women who had had bilateral ovariectomy and hysterectomy without any hormone replacement, with two groups of age-matched hysterectomized women, one having received ovariectomy plus estrogen replacement, the other hysterectomy alone. They found little difference between the ovariectomized women with and without estrogen replacement, about a half of whom reported a decrease in sexual interest. In contrast, 82% of those with intact ovaries reported an increase in sexual interest post-operatively. Comparable findings were presented by Bellerose and Binik (1993).

Farquhar *et al.* (2002) compared 57 women who had hysterectomy with both ovaries removed ("O&H") and 266 women who had hysterectomy alone ("H only"). They found no deterioration sexually in either group at six months post-operatively; however, the "hysterectomy alone" group reported a significant increase in sexual interest and frequency of sexual intercourse, presumably reflecting the health benefits of the surgery. The women who had both ovaries removed showed no such benefits.

Aziz *et al.* (2005) compared 217 women who had "H only" and 106 women who had "O&H." Estrogen replacement therapy was recommended for all the ovariectomized women and those in the "H only" group who had menopausal symptoms. Sexuality and well-being were assessed pre-operatively and at one year post-operatively. The "O&H" group showed no change in sexuality or well-being; whereas the "H only" group showed some worsening in 3 of the 14 sexuality variables. None of the group comparisons was significant. Both groups showed improvement in well-being. There were no correlations between the observed changes pre- to one year post-operation in androgen levels and any aspect of sexuality or well-being.

Teplin *et al.* (2007) compared 49 women who had "O&H" with 112 women who had "H only." The "H only" group was significantly younger at the time of surgery (40 vs. 45 years; $p < 0.001$). Assessment was carried out at six months and two years post-operatively. There were no differences in sexual functioning between the two groups.

Removal of both ovaries, in producing a substantial reduction of ovarian androgens in most women, should provide us with a test of the importance of androgens in women. The evidence reviewed above, however, gives us no clear or consistent answer. One reasonable conclusion is that there is no predictable decline in sexual functioning as a result of ovariectomy, and, as with oral contraceptive use, a substantial proportion of women can experience a reduction in androgens without obvious adverse effects on sexuality or well-being. There are, however, a number of limitations to this source of evidence:

1. Women undergoing such surgery, whether involving bilateral ovariectomy or only hysterectomy, are having the surgery because of some gynecological health problem likely to have an adverse effect on both their sexuality and well-being. Taking the immediate pre-operative period as the baseline, the expected outcome of the surgery is an improvement. In contrast with a woman starting on a steroidal contraceptive, therefore, there is the problem of a lack of a suitable baseline to evaluate the effects of androgen reduction following ovariectomy.

2. Women are not randomly assigned to "H only" or "O&H," and the decision is made partly on clinical indications, age and/or the woman's personal preference. This introduces the potential for confounding individual differences.

3. Studies vary in the extent to which hormone replacement therapy (HRT) was involved following surgery, and in only one of the cited studies (Bellerose and Binik 1993) was there comparison of HRT involving estrogen only and a combination of estrogen and testosterone.

4. None of the studies reviewed above has taken into consideration the possible negative effects of hysterectomy on women's sexual response. These have been observed to occur to a variable extent in other studies of hysterectomy (Komisaruk *et al.* 2011).

5. With the exception of the first two studies cited, results analyzed were presented as group averages. As is the case when assessing the effects of oral

contraceptives, a group average indicating no change may conceal the fact that some women have experienced improvement and some worsening. If, as the evidence from oral contraceptive use suggests, some women are dependent on testosterone for their sexuality and others are not, then using group averages, in which these two types of women are combined, will serve to obscure this distinction.

The studies of Nathorst-Böös *et al.* (1993) and Bellerose and Binik (1993) suggest that approximately a half of women experience a decline in sexuality following ovariectomy, and the other half do not, which may make it more likely that they will report improvements from the surgery.

5.4.1.4 The effects of exogenous androgen administration on the sexuality of women

Testosterone administration to healthy premenopausal women

In a psychophysiologic study, Tuiten *et al.* (2000) explored the timing of effects of an increase in testosterone in eight healthy women without sexual problems, who were given a single sublingual dose of testosterone in a placebo-controlled experiment. There was a rapid rise in plasma total testosterone after testosterone administration, reaching at least a 10-fold increase in baseline levels within the first 15 minutes, returning to baseline within 90 minutes. Subjective and VPA responses to erotic films were measured just before testosterone administration, 15 minutes after and on four further occasions 90 minutes apart. An enhanced VPA response to erotic stimuli was observed three to four hours after the peak increase in plasma testosterone, significantly correlated with an increase in subjective reports of "sexual lust" and "genital sensations." This is the only study to date that assessed the effects of an acute dosage of testosterone on sexual responsiveness of women. This indicates a latency in testosterone effect of three to four hours. There are no comparable data for men.

Premenopausal women with sexual problems

There was a phase in the 1970s and 1980s when the use of testosterone as a treatment for women's sexual problems was explored. Carney *et al.* (1978) assessed the combination of sexual counseling with either testosterone or diazepam administration, for couples in which the woman was sexually unresponsive. The testosterone group showed significantly greater improvement than the diazepam group in satisfaction with sexual intercourse, frequency of orgasm, sexual arousal and frequency of sexual thoughts. These results raised the question of whether this was a positive result of testosterone or a negative effect of diazepam on the effectiveness of the counseling. Mathews *et al.* (1983) attempted to replicate these findings with a similar design, but using placebo instead of diazepam. They found no difference between testosterone and placebo. Dow and Gallagher (1989) questioned whether the combination of counseling with testosterone therapy might have obscured the effects of testosterone therapy alone. They therefore carried out a further study, adding a third group, who received testosterone therapy alone. They found significant improvement in both of the combined groups (i.e. sex therapy plus testosterone or placebo) at the end of treatment and at four months follow-up, with no group difference, and significantly less improvement with testosterone alone. In each of these three studies, 10 mg or 20 mg of testosterone was administered sublingually (Testoral; Organon) once daily. This was shown to produce substantial increases in testosterone above the physiologic range, for four to five hours after administration (Bancroft 1989).

Bancroft *et al.* (1980) explored androgen administration in 15 women with sexual problems attributed to oral contraceptive use. Androstenedione was the androgen administered. This was well absorbed when taken orally, and produced increases in plasma testosterone as well as androstenedione. A double-blind, placebo-controlled crossover design was used, with each woman taking androstenedione and placebo, each for two months. Daily diary and interview ratings were used to assess behavioral change. Significant increases in plasma testosterone occurred in the androstenedione-treated group, but no significant differences in sexuality variables resulted. One woman, however, showed a clear improvement in sexual interest and response following the androstenedione administration, which was subsequently replicated, with administration of androstenedione followed by withdrawal, on three occasions following the study. It is noteworthy that, as a result of treatment, she differed hormonally from the other 14 women, not in terms of increased levels of testosterone, but of estradiol and of the estradiol : testosterone ratio.

Perhaps because of the largely negative findings from these first four studies, there followed a long period with no further research of this kind. The next comparable study in premenopausal women was not published until 2003 (Goldstat *et al.* 2003). In a double-blind crossover study in Australia, 31 women with low libido (mean age, 39.7 ± 4.2 years) used testosterone cream (10 mg/day) and placebo, each for 12 weeks (with a 4-week washout period between). Testosterone administration, which resulted in plasma testosterone levels at the high end of the normal range, was associated with significant improvements in general well-being and measures of sexuality (Sabbatsberg Sexual Self-Rating Scale; Garratt *et al.* 1995). This was followed by a larger Australian study (Davis *et al.* 2008) in which 261 premenopausal women, aged 35 to 46 years, who reported a decline in satisfying sexual events, and also had low serum free testosterone, were randomly assigned to one of three dose levels of transdermal testosterone or placebo. Free testosterone levels (normal range 3.8 to 21.8 pmol/l) were increased in the three testosterone groups, although least with the middle dose (6.4 to 10.5 pmol/l) and most with the high dose (7.8 to 18.7 pmol/l). All four groups showed an increase in satisfying sexual events, but it was only in the middle dose group, which showed the lowest increase in free testosterone, that this behavioral increase was significantly greater than in the placebo group.

Two explanations were offered to explain the lack of dose-response relationship: (1) there may be no benefit beyond the medium dose – though this doesn't explain why the high dose was less significant in its effects than the medium dose; (2) the higher dose may have produced more side-effects which could counteract positive effects. There is a third explanation that was not considered. If it is the case that only a proportion of women are sensitive to the behavioral effects of testosterone, then there may have been more of these women in the middle-dose group. It is noteworthy that there were more oral contraceptive users in the middle-dose group. As with most of the earlier literature, this study does not attempt to identify characteristics of testosterone-sensitive women, and results were presented only as group means (though with a substantial amount of variance).

Premenopausal women with endocrine abnormalities

Miller *et al.* (2001) reported on the abnormally low androgen levels in women with hypopituitarism. In a

later study, they assessed the effects of testosterone administration in such women, using a placebo-controlled, randomized design, with 24 women receiving 300 µg testosterone daily in a transdermal patch, and 27 women receiving placebo, each group for 12 months (Miller *et al.* 2006). In comparison with the placebo group, women in the testosterone group showed significant improvement in mood, measured by the Beck Depression Inventory (BDI), and in sexuality, as measured by the combined score from the Derogatis Interview for Sexual Function (Derogatis 1997), and the subscales for "arousal" and "behavior/experience."

Tuiten *et al.* (1996) studied eight young amenorrheic women with low weight, although none had the diagnosis of anorexia nervosa. They showed lower levels of sexual interest and activity, and lower testosterone levels than an age-matched comparison group of normally menstruating women. The amenorrheic group was given testosterone undecanoate, 40 mg daily for eight weeks, and placebo for eight weeks, in a double-blind crossover study. The two treatments did not differ in effects of daily ratings of sexuality or mood. The women were also evaluated psycho-physiologically with measurement of VPA in response to erotic fantasies and erotic films. They showed a significantly greater VPA response to film during testosterone administration, but this effect was not reflected in subjective ratings of arousal or mood.

Naturally postmenopausal women

Although the natural menopause has little direct effect on androgen levels (see Section 5.4.1.2), estrogen replacement (HRT) for menopausal symptoms increases SHBG and consequently reduces free testosterone. Conversely, testosterone administration will reduce SHBG levels and also, because of competitive binding with SHBG, increase the amount of free estradiol. Hence, it is of some interest to evaluate the effects of adding testosterone to the estrogen replacement.

Burger *et al.* (1987) reported on 20 postmenopausal women whose menopausal symptoms had been relieved by oral estrogen replacement but whose lack of sexual desire had persisted. Fourteen of these women had gone through natural menopause. They were randomly assigned to either estrogen implant (40 mg) or estrogen-plus-testosterone implant (estrogen 40 mg and testosterone 50 mg). The mean peak serum total testosterone levels following implant slightly exceeded the upper limit of the normal range (i.e. 3 nmol/l). On average, the combined implant group showed improvement in sexual desire and sexual enjoyment within the first six weeks. The "estrogen only" group did not report improvement, but when subsequently given an additional testosterone implant, they showed the same improvement as the original combined group. No information was given about the effects on mood or energy.

Myers *et al.* (1990) studied 40 naturally postmenopausal women who were randomly assigned to four groups of 10 subjects each: P (Premarin only), PP (Premarin plus Provera), PT (Premarin plus methyltestosterone), and PL (placebo), and assessed over a 10-week period with both self-ratings and laboratory measurement of VPA response to erotic stimuli. There were no group differences in treatment effects on any of the sexuality variables, including VPA, except for masturbation. This showed a trend towards higher frequency and a significant increase in enjoyment of masturbation in the PT group. There was a trend ($p = 0.06$) towards group differences in mood but, unfortunately, no further details were given of this measure.

Davis *et al.* (1995) studied 34 postmenopausal women, all but 2 of whom had gone through a natural menopause. All had shown intolerance of or inadequate response to oral HRT. They were randomly assigned to either estradiol implant or estradiol plus testosterone implants, administered every three months for two years. Women with specific complaints of low sexual desire were excluded because it was considered unethical to randomly assign them to estradiol only! Women in both groups showed significant improvement in sexuality measures, and, for most of the variables, the estradiol plus testosterone group improved significantly more than the estradiol group, except that towards the end of the two-year study period there was a decline in their measures of sexuality. This was attributed to a reduced frequency of implants because of continuing supraphysiological levels of testosterone. This suggests that some degree of desensitization to the testosterone had occurred.

More recently, Shifren *et al.* (2006) reported a large placebo-controlled trial of testosterone patches (300 μg) in naturally postmenopausal women meeting the DSM-IV criteria for hypoactive sexual desire disorder; 273 women received placebo and 276 testosterone. The average age was 54 years. Women showed significant improvement from testosterone administration in the primary outcome measure, the number of satisfying sexual episodes, and in a number of other measures including sexual desire. In contrast to earlier studies using im injection of testosterone, the use of transdermal testosterone administration produced plasma levels of free testosterone and bioactive testosterone that remained within the physiological range for women. Modest but significant correlations were found between increase in free testosterone and improvements in several aspects of sexual function.

Surgical menopause

Two studies will be considered closely (for a more comprehensive review of the earlier literature, see Bancroft 2003). In the first study, Sherwin *et al.* (1985) investigated women who were about to undergo hysterectomy and bilateral ovariectomy. A one-month baseline assessment preceded the surgery: an unusual feature in the now extensive literature on surgical menopause. Post-operatively, women were assigned randomly to one of four treatment groups: estrogen only (E), testosterone only (T), estrogen plus testosterone (E+T), or placebo. These were given in monthly injections for three months. All subjects then received one month of placebo, following which they were crossed over to one of the other three treatment groups. Women reported significantly higher levels of sexual desire, sexual fantasies and sexual arousal during the E+T and T conditions than during either the E or placebo conditions. They did not differ in measures of sexual activity with partner or orgasm. This is the only study in which testosterone administration on its own has been evaluated in ovariectomized women. It is also noteworthy because it focused on the immediate postoperative period in women who were not reporting significant sexual or mood problems pre-operatively.

Shifren *et al.* (2000) studied women who had undergone hysterectomy and bilateral ovariectomy from 1 to 10 years previously. In contrast to the previous study, all had impaired sexual function and all had been on Premarin, at least 0.625 mg daily for at least two months when recruited for the study. All subjects continued on the same dose of oral estrogen through the study. After a 4-week baseline assessment, they were given daily transdermal patches with placebo, 150 μg, or 300 μg of testosterone as the daily dose, each for 12 weeks, with the order of presentation randomized. Sexuality was assessed using the

Brief Index of Sexual Functioning for Women (BISF-W; Taylor *et al.* 1994). In spite of a substantial placebo response, there was significantly more improvement with the higher testosterone dose than with placebo on measures of frequency of sexual activity, and pleasure/orgasm, though not for sexual desire or arousal (the opposite pattern to that reported by Sherwin *et al.* 1985). Mood was significantly improved with the higher testosterone dose for ratings of both depression and "positive well-being." The transdermal route used in this study has the advantage of producing more physiological and more stable serum testosterone levels than the im routes used in most earlier studies, where supraphysiological peaks soon after injection are followed by gradual decline.

Although the design of these two studies was crucially different in a number of ways, there are some interesting contrasts in the findings. A more substantial placebo effect was reported by Shifren *et al.* (2000) than by Sherwin *et al.* (1985), and this was more marked in the younger women. Thus, Shifren *et al.* found no difference between placebo and active treatment on any variable in women younger than 48 years; the overall significant effects depended on the older women. The explanation for this age effect is not clear. It may reflect that for younger women loss of sexual interest or enjoyment is more problematic and hence the expectation of, or need for improvement, greater. In the study by Sherwin *et al.*, the less striking placebo effect may reflect the fact that women were recruited before they had established any post-operative decline in sexual interest. In contrast, such decline was an inclusion criterion for the Shifren *et al.* study. This emphasizes the importance of placebo control in studies where subjects are seeking a therapeutic effect.

Since the report by Shifren *et al.* (2000), there have been four further studies of similar size, one involving European and Australian women (Davis *et al.* 2006), and three in the USA (Braunstein *et al.* 2005; Buster *et al.* 2005; Simon *et al.* 2005). These are considered further in Chapter 23. Here again, in all these studies the results are presented only as mean change per treatment group, thus obscuring the proportion of women who were successfully treated. It is of crucial importance to the field, from both a theoretical and clinical perspective, to identify those women who respond to testosterone therapy, and establish in what ways they differ from those women who do not respond.

Until recently, little research attention has been paid to identifying different patterns of sexual desire and response in women. Of particular relevance is the question of what it is that is desired, which was considered earlier (in Section 5.4.1). Variations in the importance of these patterns may account for much of the variability in women's sexuality. It is also conceivable that certain patterns of sexual desire (e.g. desire for pleasure) may be more influenced by testosterone than others (e.g. desire to be desired). (See Bancroft and Graham 2011 for further discussion of this issue.)

5.4.2 Testosterone, mood and aggression in women
5.4.2.1 Mood

In premenopausal women there is the impact of the menstrual cycle, and many women experience a cycle-related variation in mood, which in its more problematic form is referred to as "premenstrual syndrome" or PMS. There is limited and inconsistent evidence that the cyclical variation in testosterone, which tends to be at its highest during the middle third of the cycle, may be associated with this cyclical mood pattern. In a small study of 11 women with severe premenstrual irritability and dysphoria (PMS) and 11 age-matched controls with no premenstrual problems, free testosterone levels were significantly higher in the PMS group in the follicular phase, around ovulation and in the luteal phase. Dehydroepiandrosterone levels were higher in the PMS group around ovulation (Erikkson *et al.* 1992). In contrast, Bloch *et al.* (1998) compared 10 women with PMS and 10 controls. The women with PMS had significantly *lower* total and free testosterone plasma levels with a blunting of the normal periovulatory peak. Premenstrual syndrome is a complex condition, resulting from a variety of mechanisms which vary in importance from one woman to another (Bancroft 1993). We should, therefore, not be surprised by inconsistencies of this kind, although it might be informative to identify the relevant differences between the two samples.

In women the perimenopause is a time of increased vulnerability to depression. In the large longitudinal Study of Women's Health Across the Nation (or SWAN), 3302 women entered the study aged 42 to 52, when premenopausal or early perimenopausal (Bromberger *et al.* 2010). Assays of most reproductive steroids, including testosterone, and assessment of depression, using the CES-D (Radloff 1977), were carried out annually for the next eight years. A logistic regression, accounting for most of the key variables assessed, showed that higher testosterone levels were significantly associated with higher odds of a CES-D score over 16. However, the significance of this testosterone effect was less than that found for menopausal status, ethnicity, age, education level, social support and occurrence of upsetting life events. Two small studies of women diagnosed with major depression have shown increased testosterone compared with controls. Baischer *et al.* (1995) assessed 20 women (mean age 32.5) diagnosed with major depressive disorder, and compared them with an age-matched control group. They were assessed twice; before and during treatment with clomipramine. Before treatment, plasma testosterone was significantly higher in the depressed women than the controls; after treatment testosterone levels were still higher than controls but the difference was no longer significant. Weber *et al.* (2000) reported on 11 severely depressed women (aged 28–77, mean 48.1) who were compared with 11 age-matched controls. Testosterone, androstenedione and DHT, together with cortisol, were all significantly higher in the depressed women. The authors concluded that their findings were best explained as a consequence of over-stimulation of the adrenal glands. Other studies were briefly reviewed by Bromberger *et al.* (2010), and they concluded that overall there has been considerable inconsistency on this issue.

Let us look briefly at the relation between androgens and mood in those studies we have already reviewed in relation to sexuality. In the large Australian survey (Davis *et al.* 2005), the relevant findings were published in a separate paper (Bell *et al.* 2006). This reported, in the younger age group, a significant association between DHEAS and "vitality." So far, this group has not indicated whether there was any association between "vitality" and sexual function or sexual well-being in this sample. Cawood and Bancroft (1996), in a comparatively small study of women aged 40–60 years, found that the only hormone significantly correlated to well-being was DHEA. No significant associations between DHEA, DHEAS, androstenedione or testosterone and measures of sexuality were found; however, one of the best predictors of quality of sexual life was the woman's state

of well-being. In a more recent national survey of women in heterosexual relationships, one of the best predictors of sexual distress was a marker of general emotional well-being (Bancroft *et al.* 2003). This underlines the importance of mood to sexuality, and the importance of sexuality to mood, particularly in women. Although it is well known in the psychiatric field that sexual interest tends to be low in depressive illness, this relationship in a more general sense has only recently started to receive attention (e.g. Davison *et al.* 2009).

The next source of evidence comes from iatrogenic lowering of testosterone in women. Oral contraceptive use is commonly associated with negative mood change, and this change, together with the negative sexual effects considered earlier, has been shown to be the most important predictor of discontinuation of oral contraceptives (Sanders *et al.* 2001). Oral contraceptives also predictably lower testosterone levels, though to a variable extent. However, in the study of women starting on oral contraceptives, considered earlier, in which some association between reduced testosterone levels and sexual interest was observed, there was no correlation between reduction in testosterone and negative mood change (Graham *et al.* 2007).

Bilateral ovariectomy, as considered earlier, produces substantial reductions in plasma testosterone. But there is no consistent evidence of the effect that this has on well-being or mood; the surgical procedure is likely to produce improvements in well-being in so far as it resolves the pre-operative health problems. In the study reported by Aziz *et al.* (2005) in which 106 women had ovariectomy and hysterectomy followed by estrogen replacement therapy, well-being was assessed pre-operatively and at one year post-operatively. There was no correlation between post-operative levels of androgens and well-being. Bellerose and Binik (1993) compared five groups of women aged 35–55 years: three groups of ovariectomized women, one group with no hormone replacement, one with estrogen only and one with estrogen plus testosterone; the fourth group had hysterectomy only; and the fifth was a control group of women with no surgery. Although there were differences in sexual interest and response, there were no differences in mood across the five groups.

Sherwin's prospective study of women undergoing hysterectomy and ovariectomy, considered earlier (in Section 5.4.1.4), gives us more controlled evidence of hormonal effects. This showed that testosterone, but not estrogen administration, countered negative effects of the surgery on sexual desire (Sherwin *et al.* 1985). The effects of testosterone and estradiol on mood and energy were reported in two additional papers. Sherwin and Gelfand (1985a) showed that mood was significantly better with all three hormone regimes (T, E+T, and E) compared to placebo. The testosterone-only group also had significantly higher hostility scores than the other three groups. In the third paper (Sherwin and Gelfand 1985b), it was reported that energy level, well-being and appetite were significantly higher in the two groups receiving testosterone than in the estrogen-only or placebo groups. Here again, the relations between these mood and energy effects and sexual effects have not been reported, and we cannot therefore judge the extent to which sexual improvement may have been secondary to mood improvement or vice versa.

Shifren *et al.* (2000) in their study, considered earlier (in Section 5.4.1.4), of women presenting with impaired sexual function after bilateral ovariectomy and hysterectomy, found that in addition to improvements in sexual function, there were significant improvements in both depression and "positive well-being" with the higher testosterone dose. Goldstat *et al.* (2003), in assessing the effects of testosterone administration for the treatment of low sexual desire, found significant improvements in general well-being as well as sexuality.

A number of placebo-controlled studies have evaluated the effects of DHEA administration on mood; the earlier studies were reviewed by Buvat (2003). The most consistent benefit observed has been improved energy and well-being, with less consistent effects on sexuality. Schmidt *et al.* (2005) reported a double-blind, placebo-controlled, crossover study of DHEA (for six weeks) in the treatment of 23 women and 23 men presenting with midlife onset of depression. In comparison to placebo, there was a significant improvement in mood and sexuality in both women and men. In a more recent review, Panjari and Davis (2010) concluded that there was no consistent benefit from DHEA administration for either mood or sexuality across the various studies. However, they confined their attention to postmenopausal women.

Apart from the SWAN study, none of these studies gave any indication that testosterone might increase the likelihood of depression, and there is no obvious mechanism by which it would do so. It is

possible that plasma testosterone levels might reflect other aspects of the woman's life, such as increased stress. But this should be more apparent in levels of adrenal androgens, such as androstenedione or DHEA. In the SWAN study these were not significant predictors of depression. Hopefully, further research will resolve this issue.

5.4.2.2 Aggression and assertiveness

Not surprisingly, the literature on testosterone and aggression in women is much more limited than in men. Only one of the studies involving testosterone administration to women, considered earlier, reported any effect relevant to aggression. Sherwin and Gelfand (1985a) found that ovariectomized women who received testosterone only, rather than testosterone plus estrogen, estrogen or placebo, had significantly higher hostility scores than the other three groups.

Two studies assessed women who had shown violent behavior. Ehlers *et al.* (1980) compared young female clinic attendees with a history of violence with a non-violent control group attending the same clinic. Those with a history of violence had significantly higher plasma testosterone levels. Dabbs *et al.* (1988) compared inmates in a women's prison with convictions for different types of crime. They divided them into five groups: Unprovoked Violence (UV) ($n = 15$), Defensive Violence (DV) ($n = 5$), Theft ($n = 40$), Drugs ($n = 14$) and Other ($n = 10$). Those convicted of Unprovoked Violence had the highest mean salivary testosterone (2.63 ng/100 ml) whereas the Defensive Violence group had the lowest (1.48 ng/100 ml). This was significantly higher in the UV group than the DV group and also the Theft group (1.94 ng/100 ml). Apart from the UV group, the other four groups did not differ significantly from each other.

Gladue (1991) measured testosterone, free testosterone and estradiol in samples of male and female students, and aggressive tendencies were assessed by a modification of the Olweus Multifaceted Aggression Inventory (Olweus 1975), originally designed for use with adolescents. He found significantly higher aggression scores in the men than in the women, with women being more likely to avoid confrontation. Testosterone and estradiol were positively correlated with several indices of aggressive behavior in men, but were *negatively* correlated with those same indices in women.

Harris *et al.* (1996) measured salivary testosterone in male and female students, and used a number of questionnaires to assess two personality factors, an aggression factor and a pro-social factor. The men scored higher than the women on the aggression factor and lower on the pro-social factor. In contrast to Gladue's (1991) findings, the aggression factor was positively correlated, and the pro-social factor negatively correlated, with testosterone in both men and women.

Van der Pahlen et al. (2002) studied 33 healthy women, mean age 28.3, with regular cycles. Each woman had one blood sample taken mid-cycle at 6 p.m. This was assayed for total and free testosterone, androstenedione, DHT and DHEA. Their aggressive propensities were assessed with the Buss–Perry Aggression Questionnaire (Buss and Perry 1992). This has four subscales: "physical aggression," "verbal aggression," "anger" and "hostility." A composite "aggression" score derived from the four subscales was compared to the hormone levels. Three hormones accounted for a significant proportion of the variance: free testosterone 24%, DHT 16% and androstenedione 14%. Two of the subscales showed significant correlations with hormones: "verbal aggression" with free testosterone ($r = 0.49$; $p < 0.004$), and "anger" with DHT ($r = 0.38$, $p = 0.03$). The authors concluded that other androgens in addition to testosterone were relevant to aggression.

Cashdan (2003) studied women students, with regular menstrual cycles and not using hormonal contraception, who were asked to complete a form on a total of 10 occasions on days when they felt that they had behaved in a competitive manner. For this purpose "competition" was defined very broadly: e.g. trying to improve one's position relative to someone else's. On the form they were asked to describe how they had felt and behaved. Blood samples were taken on one day early in the follicular phase, and were assayed for total and free testosterone, estradiol, androstenedione and cortisol. Women with low levels of androstenedione and total testosterone were less likely to express their competitive feelings overtly, while women with high levels of androstenedione were more likely to show their competitiveness with verbal aggression.

In an earlier study, involving women students from the same university (Utah), Cashdan (1995) compared women's ranking of themselves within the student group, with how they were ranked by other students participating in the study. She found that those women who "over-ranked" themselves in comparison to how they were ranked by others had higher testosterone and estradiol levels. The number of sexual partners was also correlated with testosterone and estradiol. In contrast, high ranking by one's peers was negatively correlated with androgens, particularly with androstenedione. Cashdan made an interesting interpretation, based on the fact that 62% of her sample were practicing Mormons. She distinguished between women who sought success and achievement through their own actions, and were hence more competitive with both men and women, and women who sought high "parental investment" from their sexual partners, traditional family values and premarital chastity. Apparently, practicing Mormons at Utah University are more likely to fit the second pattern; hence their tendency to devalue the women with higher androgen-related behaviors.

An intriguing situation in which to consider the effects of testosterone on aggression in genetic females is in the transition of female to male transgendered individuals. Part of this process involves administration of testosterone at dosages that would typically be used for treating hypogonadal males. Van Goozen et al. (1995) reported a study in which 35 female-to-male and 15 male-to-female transgendered individuals were assessed shortly before and three months after the start of cross-gender hormonal treatment. The female-to-male individuals showed an increase in aggression proneness, sexual arousability and spatial ability. The male-to-female individuals, who received an antiandrogen (cyproterone acetate) and estrogen, showed reduced aggression proneness and sexual arousability and improved verbal ability. Overall, however, self-ratings of mood and well-being showed little negative change, perhaps reflecting their welcome for these crucial hormonal treatments in the transgender process.

In summary, in women, we have little evidence that testosterone and estradiol have direct effects on mood, and somewhat inconsistent evidence that testosterone can enhance aggression.

5.4.3 Summary of evidence in the female

There are good reasons for thinking that testosterone has a role in the sexuality of women, but the evidence is inconsistent and confusing. There are a number of possible explanations for this:

1. Women may vary in the extent to which their sexuality is influenced by testosterone. There is much indirect evidence to support this: the possibility that oral contraceptives reduce sexual

interest by lowering free testosterone but only in a proportion of women; the negative sexual effects that antiandrogens have in a proportion of women; the finding that sexual interest is lowered in many but not all women after ovariectomy (approximately 50%). Sherwin (1988), who has conducted some of the most important research in this area, commented on the considerable inter-subject variability in ovariectomized women's responses to testosterone in her studies. It is striking that, in the extensive literature on hormone replacement in women, virtually no attention has been paid to individual variability. Without any attempt to control for such variability we should expect the kind of inconsistency across studies that we have encountered, particularly when sample sizes are small. Given that testosterone effects in the male are essential for reproduction, we should expect less variability in men. In women, however, such testosterone effects are probably irrelevant to reproduction, and hence genetic variability would not be surprising.

The variability in the association between testosterone and mood and aggression in women is not fundamentally different from that found in men. Hence we need to consider whether there are basic differences in the testosterone-dependent mechanisms involved in sexual response and mood/aggression responses.

2. We remain uncertain about the extent to which observed behavioral effects of exogenous testosterone are direct androgen effects or indirect effects resulting from increased availability of bioactive estrogen, resulting both from the conversion of testosterone to estradiol, and reduced binding of estradiol in the presence of increased testosterone.

3. The sexuality of women is powerfully influenced by mood, energy and well-being, and these aspects are affected by a wide variety of factors. Although possible effects of testosterone on mood, as well as sexuality, have been assessed in many of the studies considered, very few have directly considered the extent to which mood influences sexuality. In addition to depression, the sexuality of women is powerfully influenced by other psychological mechanisms. As in an early study of oral contraceptive users (Bancroft et al. 1980), the

relationship between testosterone and sexuality may be more apparent in women who are not experiencing significant relationship problems.

5.5 Comparison of testosterone effects in men and women

What are the principal points that emerge from a comparison of testosterone effects in men and women?

1. The evidence for an activating effect of testosterone on sexual interest and response is more consistent for men than for women. It has been proposed that this reflects greater individual variability of behavioral responsiveness to androgens among women. There obviously is variability among men but it appears to be of a much smaller magnitude.

2. Those women who are behaviorally responsive to testosterone respond to levels of testosterone that would be totally ineffective in men. This greater sensitivity to testosterone in women is apparent in behavioral and other CNS responses. It is less clear whether it is as apparent in the anabolic and skin effects of testosterone. The limited evidence we have about the distribution of testosterone receptors or ARs in the brain only adds to this puzzle. It so far indicates many more ARs in the male than the female brain, with some brain areas where the gender difference is particularly marked (see Section 5.2.2). Why do men, who need so much more testosterone for their sexually-relevant brain effects, have so many more testosterone receptors? The distribution of ARs, while overall at a much lower level, is more variable among women. This in itself is consistent with the idea of variable testosterone responsiveness in women. But this does not resolve the basic mystery.

3. Men and women may differ in the relationship between affect and sexuality. Although studies of androgen withdrawal and replacement in men show that mood, energy and well-being are affected, the impact on these variables appears to be more influential and predictable in women than in men. The reasons for this are poorly understood. In general, the relationship between mood and sexuality has received very little attention until recently, and we still have a lot to learn.

4. A fundamental difference between male and female mechanisms of androgen production may be relevant. More than 90% of testosterone in the male is produced by the testes. By contrast, a substantial proportion of androgen production in women is from the adrenal glands, and hence increased adrenal androgens can be expected in states associated with increased adrenal activity, such as anxiety, stress or depression. No evidence of increased testosterone in negative mood states in men has been found.

5. In the male, the evidence supports the idea of a threshold above which increased testosterone levels have little additional effect relevant to sexuality, and below which signs of androgen deficiency are likely to occur. It is possible that a small minority of men are sensitive to higher levels in terms of manic or aggressive response, but this does not seem to apply to male sexuality. In women we are faced with a dilemma. As yet, the only studies showing a significant correlation between plasma testosterone and sexual interest have involved women using oral contraceptives, whose testosterone levels are substantially lowered. If this has general validity, it would suggest that most women have much more testosterone than they need. It is already remarkable that testosterone can have effects in women at levels that are no more than a 10th of male levels: a gender difference that requires explanation. If in fact women need only a small proportion of that 10% then it is even more remarkable. Set against this is the evidence that supraphysiological levels of testosterone in women, that often result from im injection of testosterone esters, are associated with activational effects; though it is not clear whether such effects are specifically sexual or more non-specifically arousing, or a mixture of both. Furthermore, such effects are typically of limited duration, with the need for increasing frequency of testosterone injections to maintain them. This suggests the development of "tolerance," and points to a desensitization effect.

How does our increasing knowledge of the androgen and estrogen receptors help in our attempts to understand the role of testosterone in men and women? The starting point is the condition of complete androgen insensitivity syndrome (CAIS), possibly the most extreme example of abnormality in the *AR* gene, although it may involve a variety of mutations (see Chapter 3). Interviews with 15 women with CAIS were reported recently (Bancroft 2009), along with a review of other studies of women with CAIS; Money and Ehrhardt (1972; 10 women), Vague (1983; 7 women), Wisniewski *et al.* (2000; 14 women) and, the largest study, Minto *et al.* (2003; 59 women). Across these studies, apart from an increased likelihood of experiencing difficulties with a small or tight vagina early in their first sexual relationship, these women present a varied picture of female sexuality, not clearly different from "normal" women, although shifted towards the less responsive end of the range. Many of them experienced orgasm, often without difficulty. Thus it would seem that orgasm is not testosterone dependent. Unfortunately, this evidence does not give us any clear guidance towards testosterone-dependent aspects of women's sexuality.

What other effects do polymorphisms of the *AR* gene have in men and women? The *AR* gene is located on chromosome Xq11–12, a polymorphic polyglutamate in the *AR* encoded by the nucleotides cysteine, adenine and guanine; hence CAG (Westberg *et al.* 2001; see Chapter 3).

In the male, abnormalities range from severe conditions, such as X-linked spinobulbar muscular atrophy, to varying degrees of hypogonadism, and in some cases impaired spermatogenesis (Zitzmann and Nieschlag 2003). However, in a recent Brazilian study (Andersen *et al.* 2010), CAG *AR* repeats were genotyped in 79 men with erectile dysfunction (ED) and 340 controls. There was no association between the *AR* CAG repeat polymorphism and ED. An important point that is emerging is that rather than consider the effects of plasma testosterone levels *per se*, we should be looking at the interaction between plasma testosterone and the length of the CAG repeat on the *AR* gene. As an example, the effects of testosterone replacement on prostate growth in hypogonadal men are potentially problematic in men with the short CAG repeats, and hence lower doses of testosterone would be advised in such cases.

Various behavioral patterns, which are clearly different in males and females, have nevertheless shown inconsistent correlations with plasma testosterone levels, which may reflect differences in CAG length. In an interesting study of 301 adolescent males (mean age 14.4 years) in which non-aggressive and aggressive risk taking, dominance, depression, and self-esteem were among the variables assessed, Vermeersch *et al.* (2010) found that free testosterone was more strongly related to both non-aggressive and aggressive risk taking in boys with shorter CAG repeat lengths, and was only related to dominance in boys with short CAG lengths. They also found that free testosterone was negatively associated with depressive symptoms and self-esteem in boys with longer CAG lengths. Simmons and Roney (2011) considered the contrast between "mating effort" and "survival" in men and commented that "an expanding body of research suggests that circulating androgens regulate the allocation of energy between mating and survival effort in human males, with higher androgen levels promoting greater investment in mating effort." They studied 138 undergraduate students, measuring upper body strength, BMI, measures of dominance (a subscale of the Self-Perceived Social Status Scale; N. R. Buttermore and L. A. Kirkpatrick (unpublished) "Distinguishing dominance and prestige: two distinct pathways to status") and the Sociosexual Orientation Inventory (SOI; Simpson and Gangestad 1991), which gives a measure of propensity for casual sex. Subjects with shorter CAG repeat lengths had greater upper body strength and scored higher on measures of dominance and prestige. Plasma testosterone levels were not predictive of any of these measures, nor of SOI. The authors suggested that long-term testosterone exposure interacting with the *AR* gene polymorphisms would account for more of the variance in these measures than current testosterone levels, and concluded that such effects related to long-term mating effort rather than casual sex.

Thus we are starting to understand and hopefully find a solution for much of the variability in the literature on testosterone and male sexuality and mood. However, as we have already encountered, the variability in the relation between testosterone, sexuality and mood is substantially greater in women. To what extent will assessment of *AR* polymorphisms help us grapple with this?

Interestingly, there are important gender differences in this respect. Westberg *et al.* (2001) carried out genotyping and hormone assays in 270 women from a large population-based Swedish cohort. They observed associations between serum androgen levels and CAG repeats, but with some striking differences from those observed in men. The major influence of ARs on testosterone production in women is stimulatory, rather than inhibitory as in men. Short repeats

were associated with higher testosterone levels. Whereas in men the inhibitory effect is mediated via the hypothalamus and LH secretion, in women the stimulation is due to a direct effect of ARs in the adrenal gland and ovaries. For some reason, which Westberg *et al.* could not explain, this stimulatory effect was not relevant to DHEAS (or presumably DHEA which they did not assay), and this is the principal androgen secreted by the adrenal glands. The mystery of DHEA is further deepened! The polymorphisms of the two estrogen receptors, ERα and ERβ were also explored. Short CAG repeats of the ERβ were associated with high levels of serum testosterone and free testosterone. Westberg *et al.* suggested "The possibility that a relatively pronounced influence of androgens during development leads to an increase in serum androgen levels in adult women should be considered." As yet, however, gene polymorphisms have not helped us to explain any of the major variations in female sexuality.

5.5.1 Some hypothetical ideas about testosterone and gender differences

Two possible explanatory models of the role of testosterone in women can be considered. The first is that women vary in their sensitivity to testosterone, and for most women a high sensitivity is associated with a very low "threshold" level, sufficient to maintain the testosterone effects. In addition there could be women who have much lower sensitivity to testosterone, possibly as a result of some degree of desensitization in early development along "male" lines. They will experience a decline in testosterone-dependent responses when the testosterone level is lowered, as by oral contraceptives or ovariectomy. In contrast, the high-sensitivity women will still have enough testosterone after such iatrogenic reductions.

The second model is that some women are responsive to testosterone effects on their sexuality, whereas others are not. That would assume that for many women, possibly the majority, sexuality is not testosterone dependent, whereas for some there is a testosterone-dependent component added. This requires consideration of how the sexuality of the non-testosterone-dependent woman differs from that of the testosterone-dependent woman.

In the next section I will propose two hypotheses which have the potential to be tested and may lead to a better understanding of the complex role of testosterone. In the second hypothesis that focuses on women, I will be using the second of the two explanatory models I have just described.

5.5.1.1 The Desensitization hypothesis

Men have far more testosterone than they need for activational effects in the brain. On the other hand, they need high levels to establish and maintain the masculinizing effects in the rest of the body, including spermatogenesis. How much they need for maintaining peripheral sexual responses, such as erection, is not clear. But it could possibly be higher than needed for the brain effects. It is therefore postulated that, at some stage of development, a desensitization of ARs in the brain occurs. This allows high levels of testosterone to be maintained in the circulation without excessive and maladaptive activation of the testosterone-dependent system in the brain. As this is necessary for normal male sexual function and hence reproduction, which can be called the *"basic pattern"* of male sexuality, we would not expect much genetic variation in the determinants of this desensitization process.

Exposure to substantially higher levels of testosterone during fetal development and also during the first few weeks postnatally could be responsible for desensitizing the CNS to testosterone effects in the male. Although, as we have already considered, there are crucial differences in the control of androgens in women, it may be relevant to consider conditions in which females are exposed to high androgen levels during fetal development. The best example is congenital adrenal hyperplasia (CAH), particularly the salt-losing variety that is associated with higher levels of testosterone during fetal development. This is not only associated with some degree of masculinization of behavior, but also low levels of sexual interest and activity and low fertility (Meyer-Bahlburg *et al.* 2003). Although in such cases there are a number of factors which could impair normal sexual development, this evidence is consistent with there being some degree of desensitization to the high fetal levels of testosterone, which fall and remain in the normal female range once the CAH is treated.

An interesting question is whether this hypothetical desensitization mechanism is an "organizing effect" of high testosterone levels, which is only operative during early development, or whether such suppression is possible if exposure to high levels occurs later in development. Evidence of "tolerance" to

supraphysiological levels of testosterone was reported in several of the HRT studies in women reviewed earlier. This suggests that such desensitization might occur later in life also, at least to some extent. If there is any validity in this "desensitization hypothesis," it is important that we know about it, as it could be highly relevant to long-term effects of sustained supraphysiological levels of testosterone in older women. However, we should also keep in mind the possibility that there may be a decline in testosterone receptor sensitivity in women as they age, comparable to that found in men.

I first wrote about this "desensitization hypothesis" in 2002 (Bancroft 2002), and have written about it several times since. However, I have not yet encountered any reaction to it in the literature, either positive or negative. I am aware that the hypothesis is crude, as I am unable to provide any plausible explanation of how such desensitization might occur. But I must leave that to those who have a better understanding of receptor physiology. This takes us to the second hypothesis.

5.5.1.2 The "By-product" hypothesis

This assumes that there is a *"basic pattern"* of women's sexuality which, as with the "basic pattern" in the male, is necessary for reproduction, and hence is of fundamental importance. This may depend on the woman's motivation to be sexually desired by her partner and to accept his wish for vaginal intercourse. It may also involve the desire for the emotional intimacy that is typically associated with penile-vaginal intercourse. Awareness of its fundamental reproductive purpose may also be a contributory factor. This "basic pattern" is helped by the woman's relatively automatic vaginal lubrication response and specialized pain reduction mechanisms that result in vaginal penetration being painless. The vaginal response is dependent on estradiol, although the determinants of the woman's desire for this type of interaction are not yet understood.

Thus I am proposing that there are two "basic patterns" essential for reproduction; the male pattern is testosterone dependent and involves insertion of the erect penis into the female partner, rewarded by the associated pleasure, in particular with the orgasm that accompanies seminal emission. I would assume that both "basic patterns" are sufficiently fundamental to reproduction that there will be little genetic variation in their determinants. In addition, I am proposing that, as examples of "by-products" using the concept introduced by Symons (1979), components of the male pattern are evident in some women, presumably reflecting variable genetic determination. This concept has been persuasively argued by Lloyd (2005), amid much controversy, to explain the occurrence of orgasm in women. I am proposing that testosterone-dependent effects, mainly in the motivation for sexual pleasure, are other "by-products." It is also feasible that there are aspects of male sexuality that are "by-products" of the female "basic pattern."

However, finding aspects of female sexual experience that can be shown to be dependent on testosterone is not going to be easy.

5.5.1.3 One way forward

While by no means simple, this theoretical model, based on two principal hypotheses, is open to testing in observational and clinical studies. It is possible that receptor polymorphisms, which are being intensively studied, will be of relevance. At this point it is not clear how we would use the recently acquired knowledge in this respect.

One way forward, at this point in time, is to focus first on developing a typology of women's sexuality, which aims to characterize at least two different types, which would then allow groups of women, who fit the characteristics of each type, to be compared on variables that relate to testosterone effects, which would include *AR* gene polymorphisms, levels of plasma testosterone and other androgens, and other possible indicators of androgen effects. This approach to a typology of women's sexuality has recently been considered at more length(Bancroft and Graham 2011).

5.6 Key messages

- We have little understanding of how and where testosterone works within the brain, either in organization of brain development or as activational effects. There is limited evidence of the distribution of ARs and ERs in the human brain. Evidence from non-human primates suggests certain areas in the subcortical brain where testosterone works principally by being aromatized to estradiol and other areas where it acts directly via ARs. There is also limited evidence of ARs in the brain being less frequent and more variable across women than in men.
- There is reasonably consistent evidence that testosterone is necessary for normal sexual desire and sexual arousal in men, and also contributes to normal erectile function, spermatogenesis and the capacity for seminal emission. Decline in testosterone with age can contribute to the complex effects of aging on male sexual function.
- Variability in the relationship between plasma testosterone and male sexual function is attributable in part to the length of CAG repeats in the *AR* gene. The effects of specific testosterone levels in the male need to be assessed in interaction with CAG repeat length.
- Whereas there is little evidence of a correlation between plasma testosterone levels and mood or aggression in men, effects of supraphysiological levels of testosterone indicate that a small minority of men may be sensitive to the arousing effects of testosterone, either as manic mood or aggression. This presumably reflects a genetic variability not relevant to the effects of physiological testosterone levels on male sexuality.
- As with men, there is no consistent evidence of a correlation between plasma testosterone levels and sexual interest or response in women. The effects of iatrogenic lowering of testosterone, e.g. by use of oral contraceptives, or bilateral ovariectomy, indicate that a proportion of women, but not all, experience a decline in sexual interest and responsiveness. This has raised the possibility that women vary markedly in their sensitivity to testosterone, or that some are responsive to testosterone and others are not. Administration of testosterone to women with lowered sexual interest often produces improvement.
- The majority of the relevant literature on women ignores the possibility of individual variability in testosterone sensitivity and presents results as group means. There has been no attempt to identify potential markers of testosterone responsiveness in women.
- The main difference between men and women in relation to testosterone is that plasma levels of testosterone in women are around 10% of those in the male, and testosterone administration can produce behavioral effects in women with dosages that would be totally ineffective in men. The basis for this gender difference in sensitivity to testosterone has not yet been explained.
- The sources of testosterone and other androgens and the control of their synthesis are clearly different in men and women. Ninety percent of testosterone in the male comes from the testes. In the female around 25% comes from the ovary

and 25% from the adrenal glands, with the remainder derived from peripheral conversion of androstenenedione or DHEA. Control of testosterone production in the male is via the hypothalamus and LH secretion. In the female it is via ARs in the adrenal glands and ovaries.

- There is also a striking gender difference in the impact of the CAG repeat length of the *AR* gene.

Whereas in men the short gene inhibits testosterone synthesis, in women it stimulates it.

- Hypotheses have been proposed in this chapter to account for the major gender difference in testosterone levels and for the possible variability of testosterone responsiveness in women.

5.7 References

Abdelgadir SE, Roselli CE, Choate JVA, Resko JA (1999) Androgen receptor messenger ribonucleic acid in brains and pituitaries of male rhesus monkeys: studies on distribution, hormonal control, and relationship to luteinizing hormone secretion. *Biol Reprod* **60**:1251–1256

Alder E, Cook A, Davidson D, West C, Bancroft J (1986) Hormones, mood and sexuality in lactating women. *Brit J Psychiat* **148**:74–79

Alexander GM, Sherwin BB (1993) Sex steroids, sexual behavior, and selection attention for erotic stimuli in women using oral contraceptives. *Psychoneuroendocrinology* **18**:91–102

Almeida OP, Yeap BB, Hankey GJ, Jamrozik K, Flicker L (2008) Low free testosterone concentration as a potentially treatable cause of depressive symptoms in older men. *Arch Gen Psychiatry* **65**:283–289

Amiaz R, Seidman SN (2008) Testosterone and depression in men. *Curr Opin Endocrinol Diabet Obes* **15**:278–28

Andersen ML, Guindalini C, Santos-Silva R, Bittencourt LRA, Tufik S (2010) Androgen receptor CAG repeat polymorphism is not associated with erectile dysfunction complaints, gonadal steroids and sleep parameters: data from a population-based survey. *J Androl* **32**:524–529

Anderson RA, Bancroft J, Wu FCW (1992) The effects of exogenous testosterone on sexuality and mood of normal men. *J Clin Endocr Metab* **75**:1503–1507

Anderson RA, Martin CW, Kung A, Everington D, Pun TC, Tan KCB, Bancroft J, Sundaram K, Moo-Young AJ, Baird DT (1999) 7α-Methyl-19-Nortestosterone (MENT) maintains sexual behavior and mood in hypogonadal men. *J Clin Endocr Metab* **84**:3556–3562

Appelt H, Strauss B (1986) The psychoendocrinology of female sexuality: a research project. *German J Psychol* **10**:143–156

Aziz A, Bramstrom M, Bergquist C, Silverstolpe G (2005) Perimenopausal androgen decline after oophorectomy does not influence sexuality or psychological wellbeing. *Fert Steril* **83**:1021–1028

Bagatell CJ, Heiman JR, Rivier JE, Bremner WJ (1994a) Effects of endogenous testosterone and estradiol on sexual behavior in normal young men. *J Clin Endocr Metab* **78**:711–716

Bagatell CJ, Heiman JR, Matsumoto AM, Rivier JE, Bremner WJ (1994b) Metabolic and behavioral effects of high-dose exogenous testosterone in healthy men. *J Clin Endocr Metab* **79**:561–567

Baischer W, Koinig G, Hartmann B, Huber J, Langer G (1995) Hypothalamic-pituitary-gonadal axis in depressed premenopausal women: elevated blood testosterone concentrations compared to normal controls. *Psychoneuroendocrinology* **20**:553–559

Bancroft J (1989) *Human Sexuality and its Problems*, 2nd edn. Churchill Livingstone, Edinburgh

Bancroft J (1993) The premenstrual syndrome – a reappraisal of the concept and the evidence. *Psychol Med* Suppl **24**:1–47

Bancroft J (1995) Are the effects of androgens on male sexuality noradrenergically mediated? Some consideration of the human. *Neurosci Biobehav Rev* **19**:325–330

Bancroft J (2002) Sexual effects of androgens in women: Some theoretical considerations. *Fert Steril* **77** (Suppl 4):S55–S59

Bancroft J (2003) Androgens and sexual function in men and women. In: Bremner W, Bagatell C (eds) *Androgens in Health and Disease*. Humana Press, Totowa, NJ, pp 259–290

Bancroft J (2009) *Human Sexuality and its Problems*, 3rd edn. Churchill Livingstone, Edinburgh

Bancroft J, Cawood EHH (1996) Androgens and the menopause: a study of 40 to 60 year old women. *Clin Endocrinol* **45**:577–587

Bancroft J, Graham CA (2011) The varied nature of women's sexuality: unresolved issues and a theoretical approach. *Horm Behav* **59**:717–729

Bancroft J, Sartorius N (1990) The effects of oral contraceptives on well-being and sexuality. *Oxford Rev Reprod Biol* **12**:57–92

Bancroft J, Davidson DW, Warner P, Tyrer G (1980) Androgens and sexual behaviour in women using oral contraceptives. *Clin Endocrinol* **12**:327–340

Bancroft J, Sanders D, Davidson D, Warner P (1983) Mood, sexuality, hormones and the menstrual cycle III. Sexuality and the role of androgens. *Psychosom Med* 45:509–516

Bancroft J, Sherwin B, Alexander GM, Davidson DW, Walker A (1991) Oral contraceptives, androgens, and the sexuality of young women. II. The role of androgens. *Arch Sex Behav* 20:121–135

Bancroft J, Loftus J, Long JS (2003) Distress about sex: a national survey of women in heterosexual relationships. *Arch Sex Behav* 32:193–208

Barrett-Connor E, von Mühlen DG, Kritz-Silverstein D (1999) Bioavailable testosterone and depressed mood in older men: the Rancho Bernardo Study. *J Clin Endocr Metab* 84:573–577

Beck AT, Ward CH, Mendelson M, Mock J, Erbaugh J (1961) An inventory for measuring depression. *Arch Gen Psychiatry* 4:561–571

Behre HM, Böckers A, Schlingheider A, Nieschlag E (1994) Sustained suppression of serum LH, FSH and testosterone and increase of high-density lipoprotein cholesterol by daily injections of the GnRH antagonist cetrorelix over 8 days in normal men. *Clin Endocrinol* 40:241–248

Bell RJ, Donath S, Davison SL, Davis SR (2006) Endogenous androgen levels and well-being: differences between premenopausal and postmenopausal women. *Menopause* 13:65–71

Bellerose SB, Binik YM (1993) Body image and sexuality in oophorectomized women. *Arch Sex Behav* 22:435–460

Blackburn IM, Loudon JB, Ashworth CM (1977) A new scale for measuring mania. *Psychol Med* 7:453–458

Bloch M, Schmidt PJ, Su T-P, Tobin MB, Rubinow DR (1998) Pituitary-adrenal hormones and testosterone across the menstrual cycle in women with premenstrual

syndrome and controls. *Biol Psychiat* 43:897–903

Book AS, Starzyk KB, Quinsey VL (2001) The relationship between testosterone and aggression: a meta-analysis. *Aggress Violent Behav* 6:579–599

Boyd RA, Zegarac EA, Posvar EL, Flack MR (2001) Minimal androgenic activity of a new oral contraceptive containing norethindrone acetate and graduated doses of ethinyl estradiol. *Contraception* 63:71–76

Braunstein GD, Sundwall DA, Katz M, Shifren JL, Buster JE, Simon JA, Bachman G, Aguirre OA, Lucas JD, Rodenberg C, Buch A, Watts NB (2005) Safety and efficacy of a testosterone patch for the treatment of hypoactive sexual desire disorder in surgically menopausal women. *Arch Intern Med* 165:1582–1589

Bromberger JT, Schott LL, Kravitz HM, Sowers M, Avis NE, Gold EB, Randolph JF Jr, Matthews KA (2010) Longitudinal change in reproductive hormones and depressive symptoms across the menopausal transition. *Arch Gen Psychiatry* 67:598–607

Brown WA, Davis GH (1975) Serum testosterone and irritability in man. *Psychosom Med* 37:87

Buena F, Swerdloff RS, Steiner BS, Lutchmansingh P, Peterson MA, Pandian MR, Galmarini M, Bhasin S (1993) Sexual function does not change when serum testosterone levels are pharmacologically varied within the normal male range. *Fertil Steril* 59:1118–1123

Burger H, Hailes J, Nelson J, Menelaus M (1987) Effect of combined implants of oestradiol and testosterone on libido in postmenopausal women. *Brit Med J* 294:936–937

Burger HG, Dudley EC, Cui J, Dennerstein L, Hopper JL (2000) A prospective longitudinal study of serum testosterone, dehydroepiandrosterone sulfate, and sex hormone-binding globulin levels through the menopause

transition. *J Clin Endocr Metab* 85:2832–2838

Buss AH, Durkee A (1957) An inventory for assessing different kinds of hostility. *J Consult Psychol* 21:343–349

Buss AH, Perry M (1992) The Aggression Questionnaire. *J Personal Soc Psychol* 63:452–459

Buster JE, Kingsberg SA, Aguirre O, Brown C, Breaux JG, Buch A, Rodenberg CA, Wekselman K, Casson P (2005) Testosterone patch for low sexual desire in surgically menopausal women: a randomized trial. *Obstet Gynecol* 105:944–952

Buvat J (2003) Androgen therapy with dehydroepiandrosterone. *World J Urol* 21:346–355

Caprara GV, Barbaranelli C, Comrey AL (1992) A personological approach to the study of aggression. *Personality Individ Diff* 13:77–84

Carani C, Scuteri A, Marrama P, Bancroft J (1990) The effects of testosterone administration and visual erotic stimuli on nocturnal penile tumescence in normal men. *Horm Behav* 24:435–441

Carani C, Granata ARM, Bancroft J, Marrama P (1995) The effects of testosterone replacement on nocturnal penile tumescence and rigidity and erectile response to visual erotic stimuli in hypogonadal men. *Psychoneuroendocrinology* 20:743–753

Carney A, Bancroft J, Mathews A (1978) Combination of hormonal and psychological treatment for female sexual unresponsiveness: a comparative study. *Brit J Psychiat* 132:339–356

Cashdan E (1995) Hormones, sex and status in women. *Horm Behav* 29:354–366

Cashdan E (2003) Hormones and competitive aggression in women. *Aggress Behav* 29:107–115

Cawood EHH, Bancroft J (1996) Steroid hormones, the menopause, sexuality and well-being of women. *Psychol Med* 26:925–936

Christiansen K, Knussman R (1987) Androgen levels and components of aggression in men. *Horm Behav* **21**:170–180

Coenen CMH, Thomas CMG, Borm GF, Hollanders JMG, Rolland R (1996) Changes in androgens during treatment with four low-dose contraceptives. *Contraception* **53**:171–176

Cortés-Gallegos V, Castaneda G, Alonso R, Sojo I, Carranco A, Cervantes C, Parra A (1983) Sleep deprivation reduces circulating androgens in healthy men. *Arch Androl* **10**:33–37

Couzinet B, Meduri G, Lecce MG, Young J, Brailly S, Loosfelt H, Milgrom E, Schaison G (2001) The postmenopausal ovary is not a major androgen-producing gland. *J Clin Endocr Metab* **86**:5060–5066

Crilly RG, Marshall DH, Nordin BE (1979) The effect of age on plasma androstenedione concentration in oophorectomised women. *Clin Endocrinol* **10**:199–201

Dabbs JM Jr, Ruback RB, Frady Rl, Hopper CH, Sgoutas DS (1988) Saliva testosterone and criminal violence among women. *Pers Indiv Differ* **9**:269–275

Darney PD (1995) The androgenicity of progestins. *Am J Med* **98** (Suppl 1A):104S–110S

Davidson JM, Carmago CA, Smith ER (1979) Effects of androgens on sexual behavior of hypogonadal men. *J Clin Endocr Metab* **48**:955–958

Davis AR, Castano PM (2004) Oral contraceptives and libido in women. *Annu Rev Sex Res* **15**:297–320

Davis S, Papalia MA, Norman RJ, O'Neill S, Redelman M, Williamson M, Stuckey BG, Wlodarczyk J, Gard'ner K, Humberstone A (2008) Safety and efficacy of a testosterone metered-dose transdermal spray for treating decreased sexual satisfaction in pre-menopausal women: a randomized trial. *Ann Intern Med* **148**:569–577

Davis SR, McCloud P, Strauss BJG, Burger H (1995) Testosterone enhances estradiol's effects on postmenopausal bone density and sexuality. *Maturitas* **21**:227–236

Davis SR, Davison SL, Donath S, Bell RJ (2005) Circulating androgen levels and self-reported sexual function in women. *JAMA* **294**:91–96

Davis SR, van der Mooren MJ, van Lunsen RH, Lopes P, Ribot C, Rees M, Moufarege A, Rodenberg C, Buch A, Purdie DW (2006) Efficacy and safety of a testosterone patch for the treatment of hypoactive sexual desire disorder in surgically menopausal women: a randomized, placebo-controlled trial. *Menopause* **13**:387–396

Davison SL, Bell R, Donath S, Montalto JG, Davis SR (2005) Androgen levels in adult females: changes with age, menopause and oophorectomy. *J Clin Endocr Metab* **90**:3847–3853

Davison SL, Bell RJ, LaChina M, Holden SL, Davis SR (2009) The relationship between self-reported sexual satisfaction and general well-being in women. *J Sex Med* **6**:2690–2697

Derogatis L, Rust J, Golombok S, Bouchard C, Nachtigall L, Rodenberg C, Kuznicki J, McHorney CA (2004) Validation of the profile of female sexual function (PFSF) in surgically and naturally menopausal women. *J Sex Marital Ther* **30**:25–36

Derogatis LR (1994) *Symptom Checklist-90-R: Administration, Scoring, and Procedures Manual.* National Computer Systems Inc, Minneapolis, MN

Derogatis LR (1997) The Derogatis Interview for Sexual Functioning (DISF/DISFSR): an introductory report. *J Sex Mar Ther* **231**:291–304

Dow MGT, Gallagher J (1989) A controlled study of combined hormonal and psychological treatment for sexual unresponsiveness in women. *Brit J Clin Psychol* **28**:201–212

Ehlers CL, Rickler KC, Hovey JE (1980) A possible relationship between plasma testosterone and aggressive behavior in a female outpatient population. In: Girgis M, Kiloh LG (eds) *Limbic Epilepsy and Dyscontrol Syndrome.* North Holland Biomedical Press, New York, pp 183–194

Erikkson E, Sundblad C, Lisjö P, Modigh K, Andersch B (1992) Serum levels of androgens are higher in women with premenstrual irritability and dysphoria than in controls. *Psychoneuroendocrinology* **17**:195–204

Farquhar CM, Sadler L, Harvey S, McDoudall J, Yazdi G, Meuli K (2002) A prospective study of the short-term outcomes of hysterectomy with and without oophorectomy. *Aust N Z J Obstet Gynaecol* **42**:197–204

Fernandez-Guasti A, Kruijver FPM, Fodor M, Swaab DF (2000) Sex differences in the distribution of androgen receptors in the human hypothalamus. *J Comp Neurol* **425**:422–435

Finley SK, Kritzer MF (1999) Immuno-reactivity for intracellular androgenreceptors in identified subpopulations of neurons, astrocytes and oligodendrocytes in primate prefrontal cortex. *J Neurobiol* **40**:446–457

Frenken J, Vennix P (1981) *Sexuality Experience Scales Manual.* Swets and Zeitlinger BV, Zeist, the Netherlands

Garratt A, Torgerson D, Wyness J, Hall M, Reid DM (1995) Measuring sexual function in pre menopausal women. *Br J Obstet Gynaecol* **102**:311–316

Gladue BA (1991) Aggressive behavioral characteristics, hormones, and sexual orientation in men and women. *Aggress Behav* **17**:313–326

Goldstat R, Briganti E, Tran J, Wolfe R, Davis SR (2003) Transdermal testosterone therapy improves well-being, mood and sexual function in pre-menopausal women. *Menopause* 10:390–398

Gooren LJG (1988) Hypogonadotropic hypogonadal men respond less well to androgen substitution treatment than hypergonadotropic hypogonadal men. *Arch Sex Behav* 17:265–270

Gorski RA (2000) Sexual differentiation of the nervous system. In: Kandel ER, Schwartz JH, Jesell TM (eds) *Principles of Neural Science*, 4th edn. McGraw-Hill, New York, pp 1131–1148

Graham CA (2010) The DSM diagnostic criteria for Female Sexual Arousal Disorder. *Arch Sex Behav* 39:240–255

Graham CA, Bancroft J, Doll HA, Greco T, Tanner A (2007) Does oral-contraceptive-induced reduction in free testosterone adversely affect the sexuality or mood of women? *Psychoneuroendocrinology* 32:246–255

Gray A, Jackson DN, McKinlay JB (1991) The relation between dominance, anger, and hormones in normally aging men: results from the Massachusetts male aging study. *Psychosom Med* 53:375–385

Hamilton M (1960) A rating scale for depression. *J Neurol Neurosurg Psychiatry* 23:56–62

Hamilton M (1967) Development of a rating scale for primary depressive illness. *Br J Soc Clin Psychol* 6:278–296

Harris JA (1999) Review and methodological considerations in research on testosterone and aggression. *Aggress Viol Behav* 4:273–291

Harris JA, Rushton JP, Hampson E, Jackson DN (1996) Salivary testosterone and self-report aggressive and prosocial personality characteristics in men and women. *Aggress Behav* 22:313–331

Heatherton TF, Polivy J (1991) Development and validation of a scale for measuring state self-esteem. *J Pers Soc Psychol* 60:895–910.

Hedricks CA (1994) Female sexual activity across the human menstrual cycle: a biopsychosocial approach. *Annu Rev Sex Res* 5:122–172

Hines M (2004) *Brain Gender*. Oxford University Press, Oxford

Huesmann LR, Eron LD (1989) Individual differences and the trait of aggression. *Europ J Personal* 3:95–106

Hyde JS (1984) How large are gender differences in aggression? A developmental meta-analysis. *Develop Psychol* 20:722–736

Janaud A, Rouffy J, Upmalis D, Dain M-P (1992) A comparison of lipid and androgen metabolism with triphasic oral contraceptive formations containing norgestimate or levonorgestrel. *Acta Obstet Gynecol Scand Suppl* 156:33–38

Jung-Hoffman C, Kuhl H (1987) Divergent effects of two low-dose oral contraceptives on sex hormone-binding globulin and free testosterone. *Amer J Obs Gynecol* 156:199–203

Kelly DD (1991) Sexual differentiation of the nervous system. In: Kandel ER, Schwartz JH, Jessell TM (eds) *Principles of Neural Science*. Appleton & Lange, Norwalk, pp 959–973

King SR (2008) Emerging roles for neurosteroids in sexual behavior and function. *Andrologia* 29:524–533

Komisaruk BR, Sansone G (2003) Neural pathways mediating vaginal function: the vagus nerve and spinal cord oxytocin. *Scandinav J Psychol* 44:241–250

Komisaruk BR, Frangos E, Whipple B (2011) Hysterectomy improves sexual response? Addressing a crucial omission in the literature. *J Minim Invas Gyn* 18:288–295

Kouri EM, Lukas SE, Pope HG Jr, Oliva PS (1995) Increased aggressive responding in male volunteers following the administration of gradually increasing doses of testosterone cypionate [published correction appears in Drug Alcohol Depend 1998; 50:255]. *Drug Alcohol Depend* 40:73–79

Kraemer HC, Becker HB, Brodie HTH, Doering CH, Moos RH, Hamburg DA (1976) Orgasmic frequency and plasma testosterone levels in normal human males. *Arch Sex Behav* 5:125

Kwan M, Greenleaf WJ, Mann J, Crapo L, Davidson JM (1983) The nature of androgen action on male sexuality: a combined laboratory-self-report study on hypogonadal men. *J Clin Endocr Metab* 57:557–562

Laan E, Everaerd W (1995) Determinants of sexual arousal: psychophysiological theory and data. *Annu Rev Sex Res* 6:32–76

Lange JD, Brown WA, Wincze JP, Zwick W (1980) Serum testosterone concentration and penile tumescence changes in men. *Horm Behav* 14:267

Leibenluft E, Schmidt PJ, Turner EH, Danaceau MA, Ashman SB, Wehr TA, Rubinow DR (1997) Effects of leuprolide-induced hypogonadism and testosterone replacement on sleep, melatonin and prolactin secretion in men. *J Clin Endocr Metab* 82:3203–3207

Liu PY, Yee B, Wishart SM, Jimenez M, Jung DG, Grunstein RR, Handelsman DJ (2003) The short-term effects of high-dose testosterone on sleep, breathing, and function in older men. *J Clin Endocr Metab* 88:3605–3613

Lloyd EA (2005) *The Case of the Female Orgasm: Bias in the Science of Evolution*. Harvard University Press, Cambridge, MA

Luboshitzky R, Aviv A, Hefetz A, Herer P, Shen-Orr Z, Lavie L, Lavie P (2002) Decreased pituitary-gonadal secretion in men with obstructive sleep apnea. *J Clin Endocr Metab* 87:3394–3398

Luisi M, Franchi F (1980) Double-blind group comparative study of testosterone undecanoate and mesterolone in hypogonadal male patients. *J Endocrinol Invest* 3:305–308

Manetti GJ, Honig SC (2010) Update on male hormonal contraception: is the vasectomy in jeopardy? *Internat J Impot Res* 22:159–170

Mathews A, Whitehead A, Kellett J (1983) Psychological and hormonal factors in the treatment of female sexual dysfunction. *Psychol Med* 13:83–92

McNair DM, Lorr M, Droppleman LF (1992) *EdITS Manual for the Profile of Mood States.* Educational and Industrial Testing Service, San Diego

Meyer-Bahlburg HFL, Baker SW, Dolezal C, Carlson AD, Obeid JSD, New MI (2003) Long-term outcome in congenital adrenal hyperplasia: gender and sexuality. *Endocrinologist* 13:227–232

Michael RP, Rees HD, Bonsall RW (1989) Sites in the male primate brain at which testosterone acts as an androgen. *Brain Res* 502:11–20

Miller KK, Sesmilo G, Schiller A, Schoenfeld D, Burton S, Klibanski A (2001) Androgen deficiency in women with hypopituitarism. *J Clin Endocr Metab* 86:561–567

Miller KK, Biller BM, Beauregard C, Lipman JG, Jones J, Schoenfeld D, Sherman JC, Swearingen B, Loeffler J, Klibanski A (2006) Effects of testosterone replacement in androgen-deficient women with hypopituitarism: a randomized, double-blind, placebo-controlled study. *J Clin Endocr Metab* 91:1683–1690

Minto CL, Liao KL-M, Conway GS, Creighton SM (2003) Sexual function in women with complete androgen insensitivity syndrome. *Fert Steril* 80:157–164

Money J, Ehrhardt A (1972) *Man and Woman: Boy and Girl.* Johns Hopkins Press, Baltimore

Montorsi F, Oettel M (2005) Testosterone and sleep-related

erections: an overview. *J Sex Med* 2:771–784

Mushayandebvu T, Castracane VD, Gimpel T, Adel T, Santoro N (1996) Evidence for diminished mid-cycle ovarian androgen production in older reproductive aged women. *Fert Steril* 65:721–723

Myers LS, Dixen J, Morrissette D, Carmichael M, Davidson JM (1990) Effects of estrogen, androgen, and progestin on sexual psychophysiology and behavior in postmenopausal women. *J Clin Endocr Metab* 70:1124–1131

Nathorst-Böös J, von Schoultz B, Carlström K (1993) Elective ovarian removal and estrogen replacement therapy – effects on sexual life, psychological wellbeing and androgen status. *J Psychosom Obstet Gynaecol* 14:283–293

National Institute for Health and Clinical Excellence (NICE) (2005) *Long-Acting Reversible Contraception: The Effective and Appropriate Use of Long-Acting Reversible Contraception.* RCOG Press, London

Neave N, Wolfson S (2003) Testosterone, territoriality, and the 'home advantage'. *Physiol Behav* 78:269–275

O'Carroll RE, Shapiro C, Bancroft J (1985) Androgens, behaviour and nocturnal erections in hypogonadal men: the effect of varying the replacement dose. *Clin Endocrinol* 23:527–538

O'Connor DB, Archer J, Wu FCW (2001) Measuring aggression: self-reports, partner reports and responses to provoking scenarios. *Aggress Behav* 27:79–101

O'Connor DB, Archer J, Wu FCW (2004) Effects of testosterone on mood, aggression, and sexual behavior in young men: a double-blind, placebo-controlled, cross-over study. *J Clin Endocri Metab* 89:2837–2845

Olweus D (1975) *Development of a Multi-Faceted Aggression Inventory*

for Boys. Report No. 6. University of Bergen, Bergen, Norway

Olweus D, Mattsson A, Schalling D, Low H (1980) Testosterone, aggression, physical, and personality dimensions in normal adolescent males. *Psychosom Med* 42:253–269

Olweus D, Mattsson A, Schalling D, Low H (1988) Circulating testosterone levels and aggression in adolescent males: a causal analysis. *Psychosom Med* 42:253–269

Orentreich N, Brind JL, Rizer RL, Vogelman JH (1984) Age changes and sex differences in serum dehydroepiandrosterone sulfate concentrations throughout adulthood. *J Clin Endocr Metab* 59:551–555

Overall JE, Gorham DR (1962) The Brief Psychiatric Rating Scale. *Psychol Res* 10:799–812

Panjari M, Davis SR (2010) DHEA for postmenopausal women: a review of the evidence. *Maturitas* 66:172–179

Parent AS, Teilmann G, Juul A, Skakkebaek NE, Toppari J, Bourguignon J-P (2003) The timing of normal puberty and the age limits of sexual precocity: variations around the world, secular trends, and changes after migration. *Endocr Rev* 24:668–693

Park K, Kang HK, Seo JJ, Kim HJ, Ryu SB, Jeong GW (2001) Blood-oxygenation level-dependent functional magnetic resonance imaging for evaluating cerebral regions of female sexual arousal response. *Urology* 57:1189–1194

Parmeggiana PL, Morrison AR (1990) Alterations in autonomic functions during sleep. In: Loewy AD, Spyer KM (eds) *Central Regulation of Autonomic Functions.* Oxford University Press, New York, pp 367–386

Perrin JS, Hervé PY, Leonard G, Perron M, Pike GB, Pittiot A, Richer L, Veillette S, Pausova Z, Paus T (2008) Growth of white matter in the adolescent brain: role of testosterone and androgen receptor. *J Neurosci* **28**:9519–9524

Pope HG Jr, Kouri EM, Hudson JI (2000) Effects of supraphysiological doses of testosterone on mood and aggression in normal men. *Arch Gen Psychiatry* **57**:133–140

Puy L, MacLusky NJ, Becker L, Karsan N, Trachtenberg J, Brown TJ (1995) Immuno-cytochemical detection of androgen receptor in human temporal cortex: characterization and application of polyclonal androgen receptor antibodies in frozen and paraffin-embedded tissues. *J Steroid Biochem Mol Biol* **55**:197–209

Raboch J, Starka L (1973) Reported coital activity of men and levels of plasma testosterone. *Arch Sex Behav* **2**:309

Radloff LS (1977) The CES-D Scale. A self-report depression scale for research in the general population. *App Psych Meas* **1**:385–401

Rathus SA (1973) A 30-item schedule for assessing assertive behavior. *Behav Ther* **4**:398–406

Redouté J, Stoléru S, Pugeat M, Costes N, Lavenne F, Le Bars D, Dechaud H, Cinotti L, Pujol JF (2005) Brain processing of visual sexual stimuli in treated and untreated hypogonadal patients. *Psychoneuroendocrinology*, **30**:461–482

Riley A, Riley E (2000) Controlled studies on women presenting with sexual drive disorder: I. Endocrine status. *J Sex Marital Ther* **26**:269–283

Roger M, Nahoul K, Scholler R, Bagrel D (1980) Evolution with ageing of four plasma androgens in postmenopausal women. *Maturitas* **2**:171–177

Rommerts FFG (1990) Testosterone: an overview of biosynthesis, transport, metabolism and action. In: Nieschlag E, Behre HM (eds) *Testosterone: Action, Deficiency, Substitution.* Springer-Verlag, Berlin, pp 1–22

Roselli CE, Klosterman S, Resko JA (2001) Anatomic relationships between aromatase and androgen receptor mRNA expression in the hypothalamus and amygdala of adult male cynomolgus monkeys. *J Comp Neurol* **439**:208–223

Rubin H, Henson D, Falvo R, High R (1979) The relationship between men's endogenous levels of testosterone and their penile responses to erotic stimuli. *Behav Res Ther* **17**:305

Salmimies P, Kockott G, Pirke KM, Vogt HJ, Schill WB (1982) Effects of testosterone replacement on sexual behavior in hypogonadal men. *Arch Sex Behav* **11**:345–353

Sandblom RE, Matsumoto AM, Scoene RB, Lee KA, Giblin EC, Bremner WJ, Pierson DJ (1983) Obstructive sleep apnoea induced by testosterone administration. *N Engl J Med* **308**:508–510

Sanders SA, Graham CA, Bass J, Bancroft J (2001) A prospective study of the effects of oral contraceptives on sexuality and well-being and their relationship to discontinuation. *Contraception* **64**:51–58

Sarkey S. Azcoita I, Garcia-Segura LM, Garcia-Ovejero D, DonCarlos LL (2008) Classical androgen receptors in non-classical sites in the brain. *Horm Behav* **53**:753–764

Sarrieau A, Mitchell JB, Lal S, Olivier A, Quirion E, Meaney MJ (1990) Androgen binding sites in human temporal cortex. *Neuroendocrinology* **51**:713–716

Schmidt PJ, Berlin KL, Danaceau MA, Neeren A, Haq MA, Roca CA, Rubinow DR (2004) The effects of pharmacologically induced hypogonadism on mood in healthy men. *Arch Gen Psychiat* **61**:997–1004

Schmidt PJ, Daly RC, Bloch M, Smith MJ, Danaceau MA, Simpson St.CL, Murphy JH, Haq N, Rubinow DR (2005) Dehydroepiandrosterone monotherapy in midlife-onset

major and minor depression. *Arch Gen Psychiat* **62**:154–162

Schreiner-Engel P, Schiavi RC, White D, Ghizzani A (1995) Low sexual desire in women: the role of reproductive hormones. *Horm Behav* **23**:221–234

Seigel JM (1986) The multi-dimensional anger inventory. *J Personality Soc Psych* **51**:191–200

Sherwin BB (1988) A comparative analysis of the role of androgen in human male and female sexual behavior: behavioral specificity, critical thresholds, and sensitivity. *Psychobiology* **16**:416–425

Sherwin BB, Gelfand MM (1985a) Sex steroids and affect in the surgical menopause: a double-blind, cross-over study. *Psychoneuroendocrinol* **10**:325–335

Sherwin BB, Gelfand MM (1985b) Differential symptom response to parenteral estrogen and/or androgen administration in the surgical menopause. *Am J Obstet Gynecol* **151**:153–160

Sherwin BB, Gelfand MM, Brender W (1985) Androgen enhances sexual motivation in females: a prospective, crossover study of sex steroid administration in the surgical menopause. *Psychosom Med* **47**:339–351

Shifren JL, Braunstein GD, Simon JA, Casson PR, Buster JE, Redmond GP, Burki RE, Ginsberg ES, Rosen RC, Leiblum SR, Caramelli KE, Mazer NA (2000) Transdermal testosterone treatment in women with impaired sexual function after oophorectomy. *N Engl J Med* **343**:682–688

Shifren JL, Davis SR, Moreau M, Waldbaum A, Bouchard C, Derogatis L, Derzco C, Bearnson P, Kakos N, O'Neill S, Levine S, Wechselman K, Buch A, Rodenberg C, Kroll R (2006) Testosterone patch for the treatment of hypoactive sexual desire disorder in naturally menopausal women: results from the INTIMATE NM1 Study. *Menopause* **13**:770–779

Shores MM, Moceri VM, Sloan KL, Alvin M, Matsumoto MD, Kivlahan DR (2005) Low testosterone levels predict incident depressive illness in older men: effects of age and medical morbidity. *J Clin Psychiat* **66**:7–14

Simmons ZL, Roney JR (2011) Variation in CAG repeat length of the androgen receptor gene predicts variables associated with intrasexual competitiveness in human males. *Horm Behav* **60**:306–312

Simon J, Braunstein G, Nachtigall L, Utian W, Katz M, Miller S, Waldbaum A, Bouchard C, Derzko C, Buch A, Rodenberg C, Lucas J, Davis S (2005) Testosterone patch increases sexual activity and desire in surgically menopausal women with hypoactive sexual desire disorder. *J Clin Endocrinol Metab* **90**:5226–5233

Simpson JA, Gangestad SW (1991) Individual differences in sociosexuality – evidence for convergent and discriminant validity. *J Pers Soc Psychol* **60**:870–883

Skakkebaek NE, Bancroft J, Davidson DW, Warner P (1981) Androgen replacement with oral testosterone undecanoate in hypogonadal men: a double blind controlled study. *Clin Endocrinol* **14**:49–61

Stuart FM, Hammond DC, Pett MA (1987) Inhibited sexual desire in women. *Arch Sex Behav* **16**:91–106

Su TP, Pagliaro M, Schmidt PJ, Pickar D, Wolkowitz O, Rubinow DR (1993) Neuropsychiatric effects of anabolic steroids in male normal volunteers. *JAMA* **269**:2760–2764

Sulcová J, Hill M, Hampl R, Stárka L (1997) Age and sex related differences in serum levels of unconjugated dehydroepiandrosterone and its sulphate in normal subjects. *J Endocrinol* **154**:57–62

Symons D (1979) *The Evolution of Human Sexuality*. Oxford University Press, New York

Taylor JF, Rosen RC, Leiblum SR (1994) Self-report assessment of female sexual function: psychometric evaluation of the Brief Index of Sexual Functioning for Women. *Arch Sex Behav* **23**:627–643

Teplin V, Vittinghoff E, Lin F, Learman LA, Richter HE, Kuppermann M (2007) Oophorectomy in premenopausal women. Health-related quality of life and sexual functioning. *Obstet Gynecol* **109**:347–354

Thorneycroft IH, Stanczyk FZ, Bradshaw KD, Ballagh SA, Nichols M, Weber ME (1999) Effect of low-dose oral contraceptives on androgenic markers and acne. *Contraception* **60**:255–262

Thornton JW (2001) Evolution of vertebrate steroid receptors from an ancestral estrogen receptor by ligand exploitation and serial genome expansions. *PNAS* **98**:5671–5676

Tricker R, Casaburi R, Storer TW, Clevenger B, Berman N, Shirazi A, Bhasin S (1996) The effect of supraphysiological doses of testosterone on angry behavior in healthy eugonadal men – a clinical research center study. *J Clin Endocr Metab* **81**:3754–3758

Tuiten A, Laan E, Panhuysen G, Everaerd W, de Haan E, Koppeschaar H, Vroon P (1996) Discrepancies between genital responses and subjective sexual function during testosterone substitution in women with hypothalamic amenorrhea. *Psychosom Med* **58**:234–241

Tuiten A, Van Honk J, Koppeschaar H, Bernaards C, Thijssen J, Verbaten R (2000) Time course of effects of testosterone administration on sexual arousal in women. *Arch Gen Psychiat* **57**:149–153

Tut TG, Ghadessy FJ, Trifiro MA, Pinsky I, Yong EL (1997) Long polyglutamine tracts in the androgen receptor are associated with reduced transactivation, impaired sperm production, and male infertility. *J Clin Endocr Metab* **82**:3777–3782

Vague J (1983) Testicular feminization syndrome: an experimental model for the study of hormone action on sexual behavior. *Horm Res* **18**:62–68

Van der Pahlen B, Lindman R, Sarkola T, Mäkisalo H, Eriksson CJP (2002) An exploratory study on self-evaluated aggression and androgens in women. *Aggress Behav* **28**:273–280

Van der Vange N, Blankenstein MA, Kloosterboer HJ, Haspels AA, Thijssen JH (1990) Effects of seven low-dose combined oral contraceptives on sex hormone binding globulin, corticosteroid binding globulin, total and free testosterone. *Contraception* **41**:345–352

Van Goozen SHM, Cohen-Kettenis PT, Gooren LJG, Frijda NH, Van de Poll NE (1995) Gender differences in behaviour: activating effects of cross-sex hormones. *Psychoneuroendocrinology* **20**:343–363

Vermeersch H, T'Sjoen G, Kaufman JM, Vincke J, Van Houtte M (2010) Testosterone, androgen receptor gene CAG repeat length, mood and behaviour in adolescent males. *Europ J Endocrinol* **163**:319–328

Walker PA (1978) The role of antiandrogens in the treatment of sex offenders. In: Qualls CB, Wincze JP, Barlow DH (eds) *The Prevention of Sexual Disorders*. Plenum, New York, pp 117–136

Weber B, Lewicka S, Deuschle M, Colla M, Heuser I (2000) Testosterone, androstenedione and dihydrotestosterone concentrations are elevated in female patients with major depression. *Psychoneuroendocrinology* **25**:765–771

Weinberger DR, Elvevag B, Giedd JN (2005) *The Adolescent Brain: A Work in Progress*. The National Campaign to Prevent Teen Pregnancy, Washington, DC.

Available at: www.teenpregnancy. org/resources/reading/pdf/BRAIN. pdf (accessed Jan 16, 2012)

Westberg L, Baghaei F, Rosmond R, Hellstrand M, Landén M, Jansson M, Holm G, Björntorp P, Eriksson E (2001) Polymorphisms of the androgen receptor gene and the estrogen receptor β gene are associated with androgen levels in women. *J Clin Endocr Metab* **86**:2562–2568

Wisniewski AB, Migeon CJ, Meyer-Bahlburg HFL, Gearhart JP, Berkowitz GD, Brown TR (2000) Complete androgen insensitivity syndrome: long-term medical, surgical and psychosexual outcome. *J Clin Endocr Metab* **85**:2664–2669

Yates WR, Perry PJ, MacIndoe J, Holman T, Ellingrod V (1999) Psychosexual effects of three doses of testosterone cycling in normal men. *Biol Psychiat* **45**:254–260

Young RC, Biggs JT, Ziegler VE, Meyer DA (1978) A rating scale for mania: reliability, validity, and sensitivity. *Br J Psychiat* **133**:429–435

Zhou J, Hofman MA, Gooren LJG, Swaab DF (1995) A sex difference in the human brain and its relation to transexuality. *Nature* **378**:68–70

Zitzmann M, Nieschlag E (2001) Testosterone levels in healthy men and the relation to behavioural and physical characteristics: facts and constructs. *Europ J Endocrinol* **144**:183–197

Zitzmann M, Nieschlag E (2003) The CAG repeat polymorphism within the androgen receptor gene and maleness. *Int J Androl* **26**:76–83

Zitzmann M, Faber S, Nieschlag E (2006) Association of specific symptoms and metabolic risks with serum testosterone in older men. *J Clin Endocr Metab* **91**:4335–4343

Zumoff B, Strain GW, Miller LK, Rosner W (1995) Twenty-four-hour mean plasma testosterone concentration declines with age in normal premenopausal women. *J Clin Endocr Metab* **80**:1429–1430

The role of testosterone in spermatogenesis

Liza O'Donnell and Robert I. McLachlan

6.1   Introduction

Testosterone production and action is critical for male fertility. An absence of androgen signaling during fetal life results in failure of the urogenital tract to virilize, inhibition of testicular descent, abnormalities in accessory organs, such as the epididymis, prostate and seminal vesicles, and an inability to produce sperm. This chapter focuses on the role of testosterone in the initiation and maintenance of germ cell development, known as spermatogenesis.

Much of what we know about testosterone and spermatogenesis is based on studies in which testosterone levels are experimentally manipulated in rodents, non-human primates and men. In recent times,

transgenic models have also been utilized extensively and provide important information on the sites and mechanisms of androgen action in spermatogenesis. Luteinizing hormone from the pituitary stimulates the Leydig cells of the testis to produce testosterone, from fetal life through to adulthood. Testosterone is essential for many aspects of spermatogenesis, including meiosis and differentiation of haploid germ cells (a process known as spermiogenesis). Androgen action is primarily mediated by ARs within Sertoli cells; however, AR-mediated action on Leydig cells and peritubular myoid cells is also important. The specific molecular pathways of androgen action are not yet well characterized, with both genomic and non-genomic pathways thought

Testosterone: Action, Deficiency, Substitution, ed. Eberhard Nieschlag and Hermann M. Behre, Assoc. ed. Susan Nieschlag.
Published by Cambridge University Press. © Cambridge University Press 2012.

to be involved. While androgen-dependent genes have been discovered, there are surprisingly few. Evidence is emerging that androgens may modulate spermatogenesis by the coordination of transcriptional and translational events, including the regulation of small RNA species that modulate protein expression.

In this chapter, we review the current information on the roles of testosterone in the initiation and maintenance of spermatogenesis in rodents, monkeys and men. While testosterone has independent effects on spermatogenesis, it also cooperates with FSH to facilitate quantitatively normal sperm production, and thus we will briefly cover the role of FSH and its synergy with testosterone. Because testosterone can be metabolized to estradiol in the testis, and estrogenic actions can influence male fertility, we will briefly review the role of estrogen in spermatogenesis. Our primary focus will be on the sites and mechanisms of androgen action that are essential for germ cell development. This information will be explored in terms of the clinical importance of androgens in normal and disordered gonadal development, how deficiency states are best managed to restore fertility, and what strategies can be used for the withdrawal of testicular androgenic support for the purposes of contraception.

6.2 Organization and kinetics of spermatogenesis

6.2.1 Basic and common features

The testis contains the seminiferous tubules and interstitial tissue, enclosed by a capsule called the tunica. Male gamete development, or spermatogenesis, occurs within the seminiferous tubules (Fig. 6.1). The interstitial tissue contains the steroidogenic Leydig cells which produce testosterone, as well as the blood and lymphatic vessels that are essential for the movement of hormones and nutrients into, and out of, the testis, and a population of resident macrophages. The seminiferous tubules are surrounded by peritubular myoid cells and layers of basement membrane.

Spermatogenesis comprises the development of sperm from spermatogonia. Spermatogonial stem cells divide and self-renew before becoming committed to differentiation. Differentiating spermatogonia undergo a series of mitoses to amplify the pool of cells that enter meiosis. Once primary spermatocytes enter meiosis, they undergo a long (several weeks) prophase where chromosomes are replicated and homologous

recombination occurs to ensure the genetic diversity of the gametes. Cells then undergo two meiotic divisions in rapid succession to produce haploid round spermatids. These spermatids undergo a major and complex morphological, structural and functional maturation and development process (spermiogenesis), resulting in the production of mature elongated spermatids that are released into the seminiferous epithelium (spermiation), yet these cells do not exhibit progressive motility but are capable of fertilization following injection into oocytes in vitro.

Germ cell development occurs in close contact with the somatic cells of the epithelium, the Sertoli cells (Fig. 6.1). These cells possess highly specialized cytological and structural features enabling them to functionally and physically support the development of germ cells as they move within the epithelium from the basement membrane (spermatogonia) to the luminal edge prior to the release of sperm. Sertoli cells divide during the fetal and early pubertal period to produce a fixed population of cells that determines the size and sperm output of the adult testis (De Franca et al. 1995). At the end of their proliferative period, Sertoli cells undergo a terminal differentiation and form a series of tight and occluding junctions that provide the basis of the blood–testis barrier, an exclusion barrier that allows the Sertoli cell to determine the microenvironment of the meiotic and post-meiotic germ cells.

Among mammals, germ cell development is not randomly distributed within the seminiferous epithelium, but is arranged in strictly defined cellular associations (Fig. 6.1; reviewed in de Kretser and Kerr 1988; Russell et al. 1990). A particular association of germ cells is referred to as a stage, and the number of stages of spermatogenesis in a particular species is defined by the number of morphologically recognizable germ cell associations. Every stage is thought to derive from one stem cell and hence represents a cell clone, with intercellular bridges remaining that allow continued cellular communication (Ren and Russell 1991). The seminiferous epithelium is staged based upon the morphology of the developing acrosome in spermatids (Clermont and Leblond 1955), and the number of spermatogenic stages varies between species. For example, there are 12 stages in mice, 14 in rats and 6 in humans (Russell et al. 1990). Dividing the spermatogenic process into stages is critical because many processes and actions occur physiologically in a stage-specific manner. Conversely, disturbances of spermatogenesis imposed by endocrine

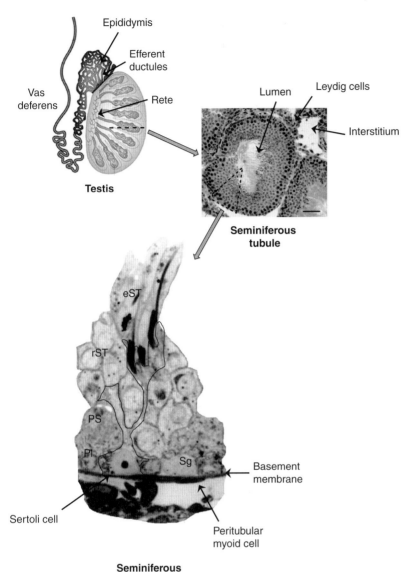

Fig. 6.1 The organization of the testis and seminiferous epithelium. Diagram of the testis and epididymis is shown, along with a cross-section of rat testis (bar = 50 μm). The seminiferous tubules have a well-defined lumen, into which the mature sperm are released prior to their passage to the epididymis via the rete testis and then efferent ductules. The interstitium contains the steroidogenic Leydig cells that produce testosterone, as well as the blood and lymphatic tissues which allow for the exchange of hormones and nutrients between the testis and the circulation. A cross-section through adult rat seminiferous epithelium shows a Sertoli cell (with prominent nucleolus) with its cytoplasmic extensions outlined as they encompass germ cells at various stages of development. This particular cross-section shows the typical cellular associations seen at stage VII of the rat spermatogenic cycle. Basement membrane and peritubular myoid cells encircle the outside of the tubule. Abbreviations: Sg, spermatogonia; Pl, preleptotene spermatocyte; PS, pachytene spermatocyte; rST, round spermatid; eST, elongated spermatid.

deficiencies or exposure to toxicants – at least initially – frequently manifest in a stage-specific pattern. Each stage of spermatogenesis exhibits species-specific timing, and the length of time for a complete cycle (i.e. all stages in succession) also differs; for example, the duration of one cycle is 7–9 days for the mouse, 12–14 days for the rat, and 16 days for man (Russell *et al.* 1990). The different kinetics of spermatogenesis result in the time taken for spermatogonia to develop into sperm differing; e.g. 35 days in mice and 64 days in men. The kinetics of spermatogenesis are unlikely to be affected by gonadotropin manipulation (reviewed in O'Donnell *et al.* 2006).

Whereas it was previously believed that the Sertoli cells govern the kinetics of the spermatogenic process, it is now thought that this ability resides within the germ cell itself. Germ cell transplantation from rat to mouse testes revealed that rat germ cell development could be supported by mouse Sertoli cells and that the transplanted rat germ cells developed according to the kinetics of rat spermatogenesis (Franca *et al.* 1998). This suggests that germ cells develop according to their own predetermined timing, which will then influence stage-related morphological and functional changes within the Sertoli cells. However, stage-related changes occurred in embryonic Sertoli cells in the absence of mature germ cells (Timmons *et al.* 2002), indicating that these cells possess an ability to undergo time-dependent functional changes well before spermatogenesis is established.

Evaluation of the spermatogenic process can be qualitative or quantitative. Qualitatively normal spermatogenesis refers to the presence of all germ cell types and spermatogenic stages; whereas quantitatively normal spermatogenesis refers to the production of all germ cell types in normal numbers. This distinction is very important for the discussion of the relative role of testosterone and FSH in spermatogenesis and for the assessment of toxic actions on spermatogenesis. Elongated spermatids possess tightly compacted heads which, unlike all other testicular cells, are resistant to homogenization in detergent-based buffers. Accordingly the number of homogenization-resistant spermatids per testis has long been used to quantitatively assess spermatogenesis. The use of stereology to accurately enumerate specific germ cell populations in thick (25 µm) sections of testis along with Sertoli cells (Wreford 1995) allows an assessment of the kinetics of spermatogenic response to various experimental settings, and facilitates a better understanding of how specific germ cells and cellular processes respond to endocrine manipulation.

6.2.2 Species-specific features

Although the spermatogenic process has many common features, substantial differences must also be kept in mind when considering its hormonal regulation. For the purpose of this chapter, the discussion of species-specific aspects is largely confined to a comparison between rodents (mouse, rat, hamster) and primates (non-human primates and man).

The system of spermatogonial renewal is quite different between rodents and primates. Rodent stem spermatogonial development is well described, and several generations of differentiating and dividing type A spermatogonia exist prior to formation of type B spermatogonia (de Rooij and Grootegoed 1998). In the primate, $A_{d(dark)}$ spermatogonia are considered to be the "resting" or reserve stem cell population, $A_{p(pale)}$ spermatogonia are considered to be the proliferative spermatogonia, and B spermatogonia are considered to be committed to differentiation. The precise relationship between A_d and A_p spermatogonia and their kinetics are still under investigation.

Type A_p spermatogonia undergo mitosis and provide daughter cells to enter the spermatogenic process and to renew the spermatogonial stem cell population. Type A_d spermatogonia rarely divide in the intact testis and are considered to replenish the A_p spermatogonial population in the case of severe spermatogonial depletion; e.g. following testicular irradiation (van Alphen *et al.* 1989). Conversely, there may be a transition of A_p into A_d spermatogonia as a protective mechanism during various onslaughts, such as gonadotropin suppression or irradiation (van Alphen *et al.* 1988; O'Donnell *et al.* 2001a).

Among rodents, a tubule cross-section is occupied by a single spermatogenic stage (single-stage arrangement); however, in primates more complex, multi-stage arrangements are seen (Wistuba *et al.* 2003). In New World monkeys, hominoids and humans, tubules are predominantly multi-stage but are single stage in macaques and intermediate in baboon. The human multi-stage arrangement has been suggested to derive from a helical arrangement of spermatogenic stages (Schulze and Rehder 1984), but this view has also been challenged (Johnson *et al.* 1996). Alternatively, it might be the size of each clone (see Section 6.2.1) that determines whether or not a particular spermatogenic stage entirely occupies a tubule cross-section (Wistuba *et al.* 2003).

6.3 The hypothalamo-hypophyseal-testicular axis

The hypothalamic-pituitary-testicular (HPT) axis ensures the establishment and maintenance of testicular function, specifically androgen secretion (for virilization) and spermatogenesis (for fertility). Gonadotropin-releasing hormone is secreted in a pulsatile fashion from hypothalamic neurons into the hypophyseal portal circulation to stimulate the synthesis and release of the gonadotropin hormones, LH and FSH from the pituitary (Fig. 6.2). Luteinizing hormone stimulates testicular Leydig cells to synthesize and secrete testosterone. Testosterone levels within the testis are exceedingly high (50–100-fold serum levels) and act on the peritubular cells that surround the seminiferous tubules and, most importantly, on the somatic Sertoli cells within their walls, thereby providing critical support for spermatogenesis. It must be recognized that testosterone exerts pleiotropic effects on reproductive and non-reproductive tissues; ARs are widely distributed, and androgens play major

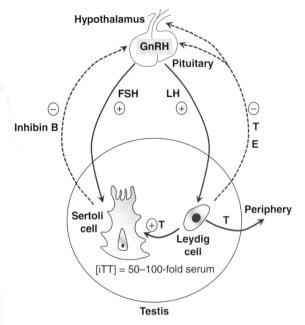

Fig. 6.2 The hypothalamic-pituitary-testicular (HPT) axis in primates. Gonadotropin-releasing hormone (GnRH) is secreted in a pulsatile fashion from hypothalamic neurons into the hypophyseal portal circulation to stimulate the synthesis and release of the gonadotropic hormones, luteinizing hormone (LH) and follicle-stimulating hormone (FSH) from the pituitary which have positive effects (solid arrows) on testicular functions. Luteinizing hormone acts on receptors within the Leydig cell plasma membrane to stimulate the synthesis and release of testosterone (T), resulting in an intratesticular testosterone concentration ([iTT]) approximately 50–100-fold that of serum testosterone concentrations. Testosterone acts on testicular somatic cells, including the Sertoli cells, to regulate spermatogenesis, and is also secreted into the peripheral circulation to maintain androgen-dependent functions. Testosterone exerts a negative feedback effect (dashed arrows) on the pituitary release of LH, but it predominantly acts via negative regulation of hypothalamic GnRH secretion. The inhibitory effects of testosterone in the brain are mediated in part via its aromatization to estradiol (E). Follicle-stimulating hormone acts directly on Sertoli cells of the testis to mediate spermatogenesis. Feedback regulation of FSH is effected by the Sertoli cell product, inhibin B and by sex steroid, predominately estradiol at the pituitary level.

roles in metabolism, adipose tissue and hematopoietic, muscle and brain function (Dankbar *et al.* 1995). Interference with these testosterone actions (or those of its derivative steroid hormones) must be considered with strategies that manipulate testicular androgen secretion or action. Testosterone is both a hormone acting directly on androgen receptors but also serves as a "prohormone" via its conversion to other steroids; specifically 5α-reduction to DHT or aromatization to estradiol (Handelsman 2008). Follicle-stimulating hormone acts directly on Sertoli

cells via G-protein-mediated surface receptors to support spermatogenesis.

The secretion of GnRH and gonadotropin hormones is controlled by testicular steroid and protein factors. Testosterone is the major steroid eliciting a negative feedback effect on LH at the pituitary level, but it predominantly acts at the hypothalamic level (Veldhuis *et al.* 1997; Fingscheidt *et al.* 1998). The regulation of FSH is more complex: in terms of steroid feedback, estradiol appears to be the main regulator in the adult male (Pitteloud *et al.* 2008). However, the primary endocrine regulator of serum FSH is the Sertoli cell product, inhibin B, which exerts a negative feedback signal at the gonadotrope level and reflects the adequacy of spermatogenesis (Fingscheidt *et al.* 1998; Ramaswamy *et al.* 1998; Pitteloud *et al.* 2008). Activin and follistatin are also involved in FSH feedback regulation, but act more as local regulators within the pituitary cell rather than as endocrine factors (de Kretser *et al.* 2004; Bernard *et al.* 2010). Activins selectively stimulate FSH secretion, and follistatin binds to activin and presumably determines and regulates activin-associated effects through this mechanism (McConnell *et al.* 1998). The physiological relevance of activin for spermatogenesis is strongly indicated by the observation that over-expression of follistatin is associated with spermatogenic defects, reduced testis size and reduced fertility in mice (Guo *et al.* 1998; de Kretser *et al.* 2001).

6.4 Testosterone and spermatogenesis

6.4.1 Neonatal androgen secretion

Activation of the HPT axis occurs at three times during human development: transiently during fetal life, in the first three to six months of postnatal life (Gendrel *et al.* 1980; Grumbach 2005) and then continually from puberty. A distinct peak of testosterone synthesis and secretion occurs for variable durations in the perinatal phase in other species, but the physiological significance of the accompanying rise in testosterone production is not entirely clear.

Inhibition of gonadotropin release by GnRH antagonist treatment delayed puberty and testicular development in rats, but eventually fertility reverted to normal (Kolho and Huhtaniemi 1989a; 1989b);

while in primates no untoward effects on adult testicular function and fertility were evident (Lunn *et al.* 1997). These data cannot be taken to mean that the perinatal gonadotropin androgen surge has no role in all non-human primates or humans. A deficiency in the fetal and perinatal gonadotropin surge may have profound consequence in adulthood; for example in congenital GnRH deficiency, permanent effects on penile size (micropenis) and a reduced Sertoli cell proliferative phase that may limit adult testis size and spermatogenic potential (Sharpe *et al.* 2003; Grumbach 2005; Sykiotis *et al.* 2010).

6.4.2 Role of androgens in the initiation and maintenance of spermatogenesis

The LH-induced rise in intratesticular testosterone (iTT) at puberty is the primary stimulus for the initiation of spermatogenesis, which itself has an absolute requirement for androgen action. In both immature animals and those made experimentally gonadotropin deficient, spermatogenesis can be established and maintained by a direct action of testosterone on the seminiferous tubules (see Section 6.5). Rat models have been used extensively to explore minimal and optimal iTT levels required for the initiation, restoration or maintenance of spermatogenesis. Increases in iTT can be induced by administration of exogenous testosterone in high dose (passive diffusion) or by hCG/LH administration (Leydig cell stimulation). An excellent model is the hypogonadal (hpg) mouse that lacks endogenous gonadotropin secretion, in which exogenous testosterone treatment induced spermatogenesis and sperm capable of in-vitro fertilization (Singh *et al.* 1995).

In immature non-human primates, the administration of very high doses of testosterone will induce complete spermatogenesis, albeit to a limited degree (Marshall *et al.* 1984). A remarkable clinical corollary is the finding of spermatogenesis in regions adjacent to Leydig cell tumors, presumably due to locally high iTT (Weinbauer and Nieschlag 1996). In boys with activating mutations of the LH receptor, testosterone alone (in the absence of measurable FSH) can initiate precocious puberty and maturation of the testis (Shenker *et al.* 1993; Gromoll *et al.* 1998). Conversely, patients with inactivating mutations of the LH receptor are both poorly virilized and have small testes, suggesting an impairment of germ cell development in association

with reduced/absent local iTT production (Kremer *et al.* 1995; Gromoll *et al.* 2000).

These data clearly demonstrate the ability of testosterone to initiate the spermatogenic process; yet these data cannot prove that testosterone is indispensable. For example, "fertile eunuchs" have atrophied Leydig cells and complete spermatogenesis (Behre *et al.* 2010), yet one cannot prove iTT levels are zero or that very low (unmeasurable) iTT levels are not providing support for limited spermatogenesis. This consideration may also account for the observation that spermatogenesis becomes established later in the life of the LH receptor knock-out mouse (Zhang *et al.* 2003). One can conclude that spermatogenesis can be induced by testosterone levels that are substantially lower than in normal puberty.

During pubertal initiation, testosterone also stimulates GH secretion and GH-dependent growth factor levels. While body and organ size in general are reduced in GH-deficient and IGF-1/2-deficient mice, spermatogenesis is complete in these small testes, suggesting no direct involvement of GH and growth factors in initiation of spermatogenesis (Sjogren *et al.* 1999).

An interesting pathway for stimulating testosterone production by Leydig cells has apparently developed in the common marmoset (*Callithrix jacchus*). In the intact and normal marmoset, LH receptor exon 10, although genomically present, is not expressed (Zhang *et al.* 1997). For the human LH receptor, this exon is necessary for the expression of receptor protein (Zhang *et al.* 1998). Interestingly, a clinical case lacking LH receptor exon 10 has been described (Gromoll *et al.* 2000). This boy had developed a male phenotype but presented with retarded pubertal development, small testes and delayed bone maturation, all indicative of androgen deficiency. Given the similarity to marmoset LH receptor status, this patient was successfully treated with hCG, indicating that exon 10 is involved in differential LH/hCG recognition. More recently it was found that marmoset pituitary expresses hCG (Gromoll *et al.* 2003), raising the possibility that marmoset Leydig cells are driven by hCG rather than LH. It would be interesting to know the dependence of marmoset spermatogenesis on iTT. In any case, it is obvious that the control of Leydig cell function and testosterone production by LH is entirely different in humans and marmosets (Michel *et al.* 2007).

6.4.3 Adult spermatogenesis: maintenance and reinitiation

There are many animal, non-human and human model studies establishing that testosterone alone can maintain sperm production in adulthood. Testosterone, in the absence of FSH, can maintain at least *qualitatively* normal spermatogenesis in adult rats (Huang *et al.* 1987; Zirkin *et al.* 1989; Awoniyi *et al.* 1992; McLachlan *et al.* 1994a) and monkeys (Marshall *et al.* 1983; 1986) (see Section 6.6 for a discussion on the likely requirement for FSH in combination with testosterone to maintain *quantitatively* normal spermatogenesis). While LH is the primary driver of testosterone secretion, LH-independent production of small amounts of androgen appears able to maintain low levels of sperm production in mice (Zhang *et al.* 2003).

Suppression of LH/FSH secretion followed by selective LH/testosterone replacement has been used to demonstrate that testosterone alone can maintain or restore qualitatively normal spermatogenesis. Suppression of gonadotropins can be achieved by GnRH immunization or antagonist administration (Chandolia *et al.* 1991a; Awoniyi *et al.* 1992; McLachlan *et al.* 1994b), removal of the pituitary (Huang *et al.* 1987) or by the administration of sex steroids (testosterone ± estradiol) (Awoniyi *et al.* 1989; Zirkin *et al.* 1989; McLachlan *et al.* 1994a; O'Donnell *et al.* 1994). It is worthwhile noting that sex steroid administration in rats causes marked decreases in LH with only minor changes in FSH, but suppresses both LH and FSH in monkeys and men. The subsequent restoration of iTT levels can be achieved by LH or hCG in primates, or in rodents by the administration of large doses of exogenous androgen which diffuse into the testis from the circulation (LH or hCG cannot be chronically administered to rodents due to antibody formation). This administration of high-dose testosterone in rodents likely has systemic effects, and in the case of the GnRH-immunized rodent, can stimulate the pituitary to secrete FSH (McLachlan *et al.* 1994b), necessitating the use of alternate strategies, such as immunoneutralization of FSH (Meachem *et al.* 1998), to explore the specific role of testosterone.

The maintenance or reinitiation of adult spermatogenesis by testosterone occurs over a narrow dose range (Zirkin 1998). For example in rats, low-dose testosterone and estradiol administration suppresses LH secretion, iTT levels fall to ~3% of normal, and elongated spermatid production ceases (O'Donnell *et al.* 1994; 1999). When larger doses of exogenous testosterone are given, elongated spermatid production recommences; however, iTT concentrations do not always show a significant rise (O'Donnell *et al.* 1996a; 1999). Hence small changes in iTT levels result in large changes in sperm output. In adult rats with slightly suppressed FSH, spermatid production was suppressed when iTT was reduced to 4.2–4.6% of normal, but was maintained when the testosterone level was held at 7.4–8.8% of normal (Sun *et al.* 1990). The level of testosterone needed to maintain spermatogenesis is at least fourfold lower than the concentration present in the normal testis (Huang *et al.* 1987). An iTT level of approx 20 ng/ml (~70 nmol/l) is sufficient for the maintenance of complete spermatogenesis in rats (Awoniyi *et al.* 1989; Zirkin 1998). This threshold concentration of testosterone is still approximately four to eightfold greater than serum testosterone levels, and greatly exceeds the dissociation constant of the testicular AR (3 nmol/l). How the seminiferous epithelium responds to such small changes in androgen concentrations in a setting where the AR is likely fully saturated is unclear. It is also intriguing to note that the threshold dose of testosterone required to *initiate* spermatogenesis in the mouse is about an order of magnitude greater than that needed for the *maintenance* of adult spermatogenesis, suggesting that two different mechanisms of androgen action may exist in the testis (Handelsman *et al.* 1999) depending on maturational status. Again, the mechanism of this effect is unknown.

In patients with hypogonadotropic hypogonadism, hCG (as an LH substitute) is used to stimulate Leydig cell androgen secretion and elevate iTT levels to initiate or restore spermatogenesis in pre- or postpubertal onset cases, respectively. In brief, in prepubertal cases the initiation of spermatogenesis adequate for fertility often requires the addition of FSH (by pulsatile GnRH or administration of hMG or urinary/recombinant human FSH) after several months of initial hCG therapy (Büchter *et al.* 1998); while in men with adult onset hypogonadotropic hypogonadism, hCG alone will often suffice (Finkel *et al.* 1985; Burris *et al.* 1988; Hayes and Pitteloud 2004). However, in patients with hypogonadotropic hypogonadism in whom spermatogenesis had been induced with hCG/hMG, when continuing on hCG alone to maintain normal peripheral testosterone levels, the sperm output persisted but waned over time (Depenbusch *et al.* 2002). Earlier reports also show that hCG maintained spermatogenesis in men with hypogonadotropic hypogonadism (Johnsen 1978; Vicari *et al.* 1992) but to a submaximal extent. In support is the classic series of studies by Matsumoto and Bremner, where hypogonadotropic hypogonadism was experimentally induced in normal men, and the ability of hCG and/or FSH to maintain or restore spermatogenesis was examined (Matsumoto *et al.* 1983; Matsumoto and Bremner 1985; Matsumoto *et al.* 1986). These studies concluded that while qualitatively normal spermatogenesis was maintained by either hormone, quantitatively normal sperm output required both gonadotropins.

Thus, maintenance and reinitiation of spermatogenesis by testosterone/hCG in patients with hypogonadotropic hypogonadism is possible (Nieschlag *et al.* 1999) with some difference in outcome likely to result from patient differences – variable etiology, time of onset (pre- and post-pubertal), preceding therapy, prior history of cryptorchidism and pre-therapy testicular volume (Liu *et al.* 2002; 2009). Comparing doses, the reinitiation of spermatogenesis seems to require more testosterone – either higher doses or longer duration of exposure – than does the maintenance of spermatogenesis. This became particularly evident from studies using GnRH analog treatment and testosterone substitution in a hormonal contraceptive context; wherein concomitant testosterone supplementation prevented the induction of azoospermia, but delayed substitution with the same dose of testosterone failed to do so (Weinbauer and Nieschlag 1996).

In summary, data from animal and human models in a wide variety of settings support the following concepts:

- In adulthood iTT levels are 50–100-fold higher than serum levels.
- Intratesticular testosterone levels at 5–20% of normal can support spermatogenesis, and even low levels (e.g. 2% of normal adult levels) can support a degree of spermatogenesis in some species/individuals.
- A narrow dose-response range exists between iTT levels and sperm output; small changes in iTT concentrations can produce large changes in sperm output (see Section 6.5.4 for further discussion).

6.5 Androgen action on spermatogenesis

6.5.1 Testicular androgen production and metabolism

Testosterone is produced by the interstitial Leydig cells under LH stimulation, resulting in iTT levels vastly greater than serum levels in all species examined. In man they are 50–200-fold higher but vary over a 5–10-fold range amongst healthy men (Morse *et al.* 1973; Jarow *et al.* 2001; McLachlan *et al.* 2002a; Matthiesson *et al.* 2005). Recently Roth *et al.* (2010a) confirmed the relationship between serum LH and iTT.

The concentration gradient between the testis and circulation is maintained even when Leydig cell steroidogenesis is experimentally suppressed (Zirkin *et al.* 1989). In rodents, it has been suggested that the testis acts as a "reservoir" through testosterone binding with high affinity to androgen binding protein (ABP), a Sertoli cell product under androgen and FSH control (Jarow and Zirkin 2005). Transgenic over-expression of testicular ABP, which could theoretically reduce testosterone bioavailability, causes germ cell apoptosis (Jeyaraj *et al.* 2003). However, the molar concentrations of iTT far exceed that of ABP, and thus the extent to which ABP modulates testosterone bioavailability and action is unclear. Also its relevance to the human is moot as ABP is not made within the testis, with the sex-steroid binding protein, SHBG, being produced by the liver and entering the circulation.

In man the alternative possibility for the continued excess of iTT relative to serum testosterone in the presence of immeasurably low serum LH (<0.5% baseline using supersensitive methods (Robertson *et al.* 2001)) is the existence of LH-independent "constitutive" androgen secretion. While low iTT levels (~2–3% baseline) are often associated with a complete failure of spermatogenesis, in some settings they may support a limited degree of spermatogenesis. This provides a potential explanation for the failure of androgen-based male hormonal contraceptive strategies (that rely exclusively on gonadotropin withdrawal) to be universally effective, with ~5% of normal men maintaining sperm densities >1 million/ml (Liu *et al.* 2008). Establishing the absence of androgen action in any model is essentially impossible due to constraints of assay methods.

Yet several indirect lines of evidence for continued androgen action following "shutdown" of the HPT axis can be found in both animals and man. For example, a further deterioration in spermatogenesis is seen with the addition of the androgen receptor inhibitor, flutamide, to GnRH antagonist-treated rats (Kangasniemi *et al.* 1996). This concept provides a ready explanation for the eventual establishment of spermatogenesis in the LH receptor knock-out mouse (Zhang *et al.* 2003). In a human androgen–progestin contraceptive context, support comes from the finding of significant (13–55 nM) iTT levels in men with spermatogenic suppression (Jarow *et al.* 2001; McLachlan *et al.* 2002a), and evidence that high doses of exogenous testosterone may allow sufficient back diffusion to reduce contraceptive efficacy (Meriggiola *et al.* 2002; Liu *et al.* 2008). Finally, data suggest an improved contraceptive effect with the inclusion of CPA, a progestin with AR-inhibiting activity, in a hormonal contraceptive regimen (Meriggiola *et al.* 1998). The use of high-dose CPA in men with prostate cancer has been reported to severely inhibit spermatogenesis (Re *et al.* 1979), an effect that one could speculate relates to more complete loss of androgen action that goes above and beyond that due to gonadotropin withdrawal.

While one can hypothesize that the complete elimination of androgen action from the human seminiferous epithelium would ensure universal azoospermia, it is a difficult notion to pursue as it must specifically target the testis whilst maintaining non-gonadal actions essential for physical and psychological health. Potential strategies might be to target testis androgen synthesis and/or AR-responsivity, for example an inhibitor of the 17β-hydroxysteroid dehydrogenase type 3, or alternatively, a testis-specific inhibitor of the AR or its coactivators. A much better understanding of testosterone–AR signaling in the testis is clearly needed.

Testosterone is the major androgen found within the testis, with levels far exceeding that of other metabolites (Jarow and Zirkin 2005; O'Donnell *et al.* 2006). Testicular testosterone is synthesized from precursors, androstenedione and DHEA. A recent study using testicular fluid aspiration in normal and GnRH antagonist-treated normal men has shown that their baseline concentrations are about 25% that of testosterone, implying rapid conversion to testosterone, and vastly in excess of their serum levels. Androstenedione levels fell markedly with LH suppression, while DHEA less so; the 50% fall in serum androstenedione shows the testis to be a major source of this steroid, but unchanged serum DHEA suggests this is predominantly of adrenal origin (Roth *et al.* 2011).

Testosterone is metabolized by the 5α-reductase enzyme to DHT which is a potent androgen. Dihydrotestosterone is further metabolized in the testis by 3α-hydroxysteroid dehydrogenase to 5α-androstane-3α,17β-diol (3α-adiol). This metabolite interacts only weakly with the AR; however, it can be readily converted back to DHT and thus can act as an androgenic precursor, at least in some species (Wilson *et al.* 2003). In many peripheral tissues where testosterone levels are comparatively low, the 5α-reduction of testosterone to the more potent androgen DHT is necessary for the full expression of androgen action (Deslypere *et al.* 1992). This is because, at equimolar concentrations, DHT binds with higher affinity to, and forms a more stable complex with, the AR than testosterone, and is consequently much more potent in inducing an androgenic response in various assays and reporter systems (Grino *et al.* 1990; Deslypere *et al.* 1992; Zhou *et al.* 1995; Jarow and Zirkin 2005). In the normal testis DHT levels are much lower than testosterone on a molar basis and thus unlikely to be a "player" in androgenic stimulation of spermatogenesis under normal settings, despite its higher potency.

However, the 5α-reduction of testosterone may be important for androgen action on spermatogenesis in situations where iTT levels are low. During the pubertal initiation of spermatogenesis in rodents, DHT and 3α-adiol are the predominant androgens present in the testis (Corpechot *et al.* 1981), and there is a peak in the testicular activity of both 5α-reductase isoenzymes (Killian *et al.* 2003). Investigation of whether 5α-reduction to DHT is required during the initiation of spermatogenesis is hampered by the fact that inhibition of 5α-reductase causes an increase in testosterone to levels that are likely able to act directly on the AR without amplification (George *et al.* 1989; Killian *et al.* 2003). Nevertheless, it seems likely that the 5α-reduction of testosterone is important for the ability of testosterone to initiate spermatogenesis during puberty (O'Donnell *et al.* 2006).

In adult rodents, 5α-reduction to DHT is important for spermatogenesis when iTT levels are experimentally lowered, since the androgen-dependent restoration of germ cell numbers by a suboptimal dose of testosterone was impaired by the co-administration of a 5α-reductase inhibitor (O'Donnell *et al.* 1996a; 1999). This data, along with observations in men (Anderson *et al.* 1996), point to a potential role for 5α-reductase in maintaining androgen action during male hormonal contraception when iTT levels are decreased. This concept has proved difficult to explore in clinical studies, and to date no additive effects have been seen from the inclusion of 5α-reductase inhibitors in a small number of men undergoing hormonal contraception (McLachlan *et al.* 2000; Kinniburgh *et al.* 2001; Matthiesson *et al.* 2005). In summary, testosterone is the major androgen acting on the AR during spermatogenesis, but the 5α-reduction of testosterone to DHT may contribute at lower testosterone concentrations.

Within the testis, testosterone is aromatized to estradiol catalyzed by the aromatase cytochrome P450 enzyme (P450arom, the product of the *CYP19* gene). The testis is the major site of estrogen production in the male, and prodigious levels of estradiol are present within testicular fluids and much higher than in the circulation in many species (Hess 2003). In normal men, the concentration of testicular estradiol is surprisingly high, with levels of 11 000–58 000 pmol/l (Zhao *et al.* 2004; Matthiesson *et al.* 2005), and the testis : serum estradiol concentration gradient (407-fold) is even larger than that of testosterone (120-fold) (Matthiesson *et al.* 2005). The aromatase enzyme is expressed in various testicular cell types including Sertoli cells; while germ cells themselves are an important source of estrogen (Hess 2003; Carreau and Hess 2010; Carreau *et al.* 2011). Estrogen receptors, like ARs, are members of the steroid hormone family of receptors, and bind to estrogen response elements (EREs) in the promoter region of estrogen-responsive genes to modulate transcription. The ER subtypes form homo- and heterodimers, and the relative expression of each subtype within a particular cell determines the cell's ability to respond to particular ligands (Hall and McDonnell 1999). Both ER genes (*ERα* and *ERβ*) are widely expressed in the testis, with conflicting immunohistochemical data reported for various species (reviewed in O'Donnell *et al.* 2001b; Carreau and Hess 2010). The general consensus is that ERα predominates in Leydig cells and ERβ in the seminiferous epithelium, as reviewed in Carreau and Hess (2010). Germ cells are also capable of responding to rapid, non-genomic actions

of estradiol via a membrane-bound receptor (Carreau and Hess 2010; Carreau *et al.* 2011). The role of testosterone metabolism to estradiol in spermatogenesis is discussed in Section 6.6.3.

6.5.2 Testicular androgen receptor and sites of androgen action

The AR is expressed in Sertoli cells, Leydig cells and peritubular myoid cells (Bremner *et al.* 1994; Van Roijen *et al.* 1995). The general consensus is that germ cells lack AR, despite some conflicting immunohistochemical studies, reviewed in O'Donnell *et al.* (2006). In any case, it seems that AR in germ cells is not essential for their development, since germ cells without AR develop normally in testes which contain functional AR (Johnston *et al.* 2001; Tsai *et al.* 2006). Sertoli cells in the neonatal period show weak AR immunoreactivity which progressively increases after day 14, when Sertoli cells cease proliferating and commence terminal differentiation, to reach adult levels at day 45. In the adult, the expression of the AR varies in relation to the stage of spermatogenesis. The mid-spermatogenic stages (VII–VIII in the rat and mouse, and II–III in the human) are considered the most androgen responsive (Walker and Cheng 2005; O'Donnell *et al.* 2006). Consistent with these findings, immunohistochemical studies show that AR protein is maximal in these stages in rats (Bremner *et al.* 1994), monkeys (McKinnell *et al.* 2001) and man (Suarez-Quian *et al.* 1999).

In recent years, data from transgenic mouse models have provided important information on the sites of testosterone and androgen action in spermatogenesis, reviewed in Wang *et al.* (2009). Ablation of AR in all tissues results in an androgen insensitivity syndrome and failure of the urogenital tract to develop normally (Wilson 1992), making it difficult to study the role of the AR in the initiation of spermatogenesis. The dependence of spermatogenesis on androgen was highlighted by studies in which androgen (both testosterone and DHT), in the absence of FSH, was able to initiate spermatogenesis in mice congenitally deficient in GnRH (hpg mice) (Singh *et al.* 1995). Using a Cre-lox conditional knock-out strategy, two mouse lines were created in which functional AR was selectively ablated from Sertoli cells (Chang *et al.* 2004; De Gendt *et al.* 2004). The resultant spermatogenic arrest in Sertoli cell androgen

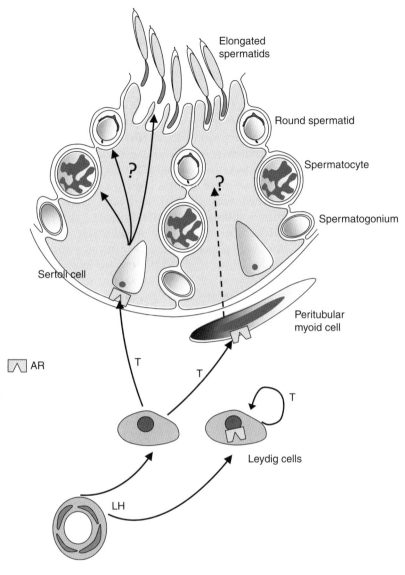

Fig. 6.3 Diagram of sites of androgen action in the testis. Luteinizing hormone from the circulation stimulates Leydig cells to synthesize and secrete testosterone (T). Testosterone acts on androgen receptors (ARs) within testicular somatic cells. Testosterone can be further metabolized to DHT, which also acts via the ARs in a setting of reduced iTT (not shown), primarily when testosterone levels are low (see Section 6.5.1). Androgens act on nuclear ARs in Sertoli cells to modulate their function. Unknown signals (solid arrows) from the Sertoli cells impact on androgen-dependent germ cell processes, particularly spermatocyte survival and progression through meiotic division, as well as progression through spermiogenesis. Unknown androgen-regulated signals also modulate the ability of the Sertoli cell to release elongated spermatids at spermiation. Androgen also acts on ARs in peritubular myoid cells (dashed arrow) to modulate Sertoli cell functions and, in turn, support germ cell development though unknown mechanisms. An autocrine action of androgen on AR in Leydig cells is required for optimal steroidogenesis, which in turn is important for quantitatively normal spermatogenesis.

receptor knock-out (SCARKO) mice proved that the initiation of spermatogenesis required androgen action on the Sertoli cell. The ability of androgen to stimulate spermatogenesis involves a direct action on Sertoli cell AR, because the androgen-mediated induction of spermatogenesis in hpg mice requires the presence of AR in Sertoli cells (O'Shaughnessy *et al.* 2010a). The effects of androgen on spermatogenesis rely on the classic, genomic AR pathway within Sertoli cells, because Sertoli cell expression of a mutant AR protein, which is unable to bind to androgen response elements in DNA, causes spermatogenic arrest (Lim *et al.* 2009). Interestingly, however, at least some of the effects of androgen on spermatogenesis

are mediated by AR in peritubular myoid cells (Welsh *et al.* 2009). The ablation of AR from many, but not all, peritubular cells results in azoospermia and infertility, and suggests that androgens act on AR within peritubular cells which in turn modulate Sertoli cell function and their ability to support spermatogenesis (Welsh *et al.* 2009). Within Leydig cells, AR is also required for optimal steroidogenesis to produce intratesticular androgens necessary for germ cell development (Tsai *et al.* 2006). Therefore androgen action on AR within the somatic cells of the testis is essential for spermatogenesis (Fig. 6.3).

In terms of androgen regulation of germ cell development, the initiation and maintenance of meiosis is well known to be particularly androgen sensitive (Handelsman *et al.* 1999). In the absence of androgen action, spermatogonia can enter meiosis; however, spermatocyte survival during the long meiotic prophase, and their subsequent meiotic division, relies on androgen action on Sertoli cell AR. This is evidenced by the phenotype of SCARKO mice, which displayed meiotic arrest, with very few haploid spermatids produced (Chang *et al.* 2004; De Gendt *et al.* 2004). Although spermatogonial numbers were normal, SCARKO mice displayed elevated apoptosis and a progressive loss of pachytene spermatocytes after stage VII, indicating that testosterone acts via the Sertoli cell AR to support spermatocyte survival (De Gendt *et al.* 2004). The final meiotic division was also markedly compromised, with observations suggesting a failure of diplotene spermatocytes to enter the first meiotic division (Chang *et al.* 2004). These studies demonstrate that the completion of meiosis is absolutely dependent on androgen action via the Sertoli cell AR; however, the precise androgen-dependent signals from the Sertoli cells and how they regulate survival and division of spermatocytes remain unknown.

Androgen action is also well known to be required for the initiation, maintenance and restoration of haploid germ cell development (spermiogenesis; reviewed in O'Donnell *et al.* 2006; Ruwanpura *et al.* 2010). In adult rats, the suppression of iTT to ∼3% of normal causes the premature detachment of round spermatids from Sertoli cells at the beginning of the elongation phase, thereby preventing the production of elongating and elongated spermatids (O'Donnell *et al.* 1996b). This premature detachment can be completely restored within four days of testosterone replacement (O'Donnell *et al.* 1994). These observations, along with others (Cameron and Muffly 1991), suggest that androgens act to modulate intercellular adhesion between Sertoli cells and spermatids, specifically at a time when the spermatid forms specialized adhesion junctions with the Sertoli cell (McLachlan *et al.* 2002b). Androgen also maintains round spermatid survival, particularly in stage VII and VIII (O'Donnell *et al.* 2006). Spermiogenic arrest is also seen in various transgenic models where androgen action is reduced (e.g. Holdcraft and Braun 2004a; Pakarainen *et al.* 2005; Lim *et al.* 2009).

The final release of sperm from the Sertoli cell at the end of spermatogenesis occurs via a process known as spermiation. Spermiation is well known to be sensitive to androgen withdrawal, with various suppression regimes resulting in the failure of Sertoli cells to release spermatids (O'Donnell *et al.* 2011). Spermatids that are not released are instead rapidly phagocytosed by the Sertoli cell. Spermiation failure is an acute response to androgen and gonadotropin suppression (Russell and Clermont 1977), and sperm release from the testis is reduced by 50–90% within the first week (Saito *et al.* 2000; O'Donnell *et al.* 2009). Spermiation failure is a major factor in the rapid (within four to six weeks) suppression of sperm counts seen in men with reduced intratesticular androgen levels resulting from androgen-based hormonal contraception (McLachlan *et al.* 2002a; Matthiesson *et al.* 2006). Androgen suppression alone can cause spermiation failure (Saito *et al.* 2000), and we have noted that the addition of an AR antagonist to an androgen suppression regime results in more profound spermiation failure (Saito *et al.* 2000; O'Donnell *et al.* 2009). Observations in mice expressing AR with reduced function highlight that spermiation is sensitive to reduced AR signaling (Holdcraft and Braun 2004a). Sperm release in vitro can be reduced by the administration of an AR antagonist (Shupe *et al.* 2011). However, this process is unlikely to rely solely upon androgens, as various other endocrine disturbances also induce acute spermiation failure (reviewed in O'Donnell *et al.* 2011), and numerous kinase and phosphatase modulators can modulate sperm release in vitro (Chapin *et al.* 2001).

It is generally considered that androgens are not required for the development of spermatogonial populations in rodents (e.g. Haywood *et al.* 2003; De Gendt *et al.* 2004). Spermatogonia are highly responsive to changes in FSH (Haywood *et al.* 2003); thus the decreased numbers seen in gonadotropin-suppressed in men are likely a consequence of reduced FSH, rather than androgenic support (McLachlan *et al.* 2002a; Ruwanpura *et al.* 2010). However, androgens may be able to maintain adult spermatogonial populations in men when FSH levels are reduced, at least in the short term (Matthiesson *et al.* 2006). Although direct action on the Sertoli cell AR does not seem to be required for spermatogonial development (De Gendt *et al.* 2004), spermatogonia were reduced in mice with total testicular AR ablation (Tan *et al.* 2005). This latter observation may be a consequence of the abdominal location of the testes in these mice, leading to compromised Sertoli cell function, or may reflect a role for androgen support of spermatogonia outside of the seminiferous epithelium, such as via peritubular myoid cells (Tan *et al.* 2005). Consistent with this, ablation of AR from most, but not all, peritubular cells (PTM-ARKO mice) leads to a reduced number of spermatogonia in adult mice (Welsh *et al.* 2009). This may reflect an androgen-mediated effect on peritubular myoid cell secretion of growth factors and/or basement membrane deposition, which may in turn influence spermatogonial development (Welsh *et al.* 2009). However, high iTT levels were observed in PTM-ARKO mice, which may inhibit spermatogonial development. An inhibitory effect of high serum/intratesticular testosterone on spermatogonia has been observed in adult rodents (Meachem *et al.* 1998; Shetty *et al.* 2001), but whether this phenomenon occurs in primates is unclear.

As evidenced throughout this section, many effects of androgens on spermatogenesis are mediated via Sertoli cells. Androgens, acting on the AR, modulate the expression of various genes and proteins within Sertoli cells (De Gendt *et al.* 2004; Tan *et al.* 2005), which in turn mediate the Sertoli cell's ability to support germ cell development; see Section 6.5.3. Observations in transgenic mice indicate that neonatal Sertoli cell proliferation, and hence the attainment of a normal Sertoli cell population, is unaffected by an absence of AR signaling via the Sertoli cell (De Gendt *et al.* 2004; Tan *et al.* 2005; Lim *et al.* 2009), but is dependent on FSH action (Allan *et al.* 2004). However, androgen action via the genomic AR pathway *outside* the Sertoli cell may be important for the FSH-mediated effects on Sertoli cell populations (Schauwaers *et al.* 2007; Lim *et al.* 2008; 2009); a mechanism which may explain the reduced Sertoli cell numbers in certain models with ablation of AR from all testicular cells, but no reduction when AR is ablated from Sertoli cells only (De Gendt *et al.* 2004; Johnston *et al.* 2004; Tan *et al.* 2005). This mechanism may be mediated in part by androgens acting on peritubular myoid cells to modulate paracrine factor secretion and/or basement membrane deposition important for Sertoli cell proliferation (Welsh *et al.* 2009). It is clear from many studies that androgens are essential for the differentiation and maturation of Sertoli cells and for their ability to support germ cell development. The ability of Sertoli cells to form tight junctions

and hence create a permeability barrier and to maintain testicular immune privilege has recently been shown to be androgen dependent (Meng *et al.* 2005; Kaitu'u-Lino *et al.* 2007; Meng *et al.* 2011).

Finally it is worth noting that studies in non-human primates revealed that testosterone induced the appearance of α-smooth muscle actin in the peritubular cells of the testis (Schlatt *et al.* 1993). These results are supported by observations in peritubular cells which lack AR in a transgenic mouse line (Welsh *et al.* 2009). These observations suggest that testosterone initiates the contractile function of these cells, which may be important for movement of sperm along the seminiferous tubules. Recent studies in mice in which AR was ablated from testicular arteriole (SMC) suggest a role for androgens in the control of vasomotion and fluid dynamics in the testis (Welsh *et al.* 2010).

6.5.3 Mechanisms of androgen action in the testis

Androgens act on intracellular receptors and can activate different pathways to modulate cellular function during spermatogenesis (Walker 2009). The "classic" or genomic pathway of AR action involves androgen (testosterone or DHT) diffusing through the plasma membrane and interacting with AR which have previously been bound to heat shock proteins in the cytoplasm. Androgen binding to the AR causes a conformational change, or activation, of the ligand-receptor complex such that it attains high affinity for specific binding sites within DNA. The activated receptor translocates to the nucleus and binds to sequences, known as androgen response elements (AREs), in the promoter region of androgen-responsive genes. The DNA binding initiates the recruitment of coactivators or co-repressor proteins that modulate gene transcription. This genomic action of AR causes changes in gene transcription in 30–40 min, and changes to cellular proteins several hours later (Walker 2009). Androgen response elements can be non-selective, in that they can respond to progesterone or glucocorticoid receptors, or selective, in that they respond to AR only. That selective vs. non-selective AREs drive different biological processes in spermatogenesis was recently demonstrated by the finding of reduced germ cell numbers in the male SPARKI (Specificity-Affecting AR knockIn) mouse (Schauwaers *et al.* 2007). In this model, the second zinc finger of the AR DNA-binding domain was replaced with that of the glucocorticoid receptor, resulting in an AR that binds non-selective AREs but is unable to recognize selective AREs. Spermatogenesis was compromised in these mice, but the spermatogenic phenotype differed from SCARKO mice, in which both selective and non-selective ARE responses are impaired. Therefore studies in the SPARKI mice show that androgen responses during spermatogenesis are mediated by both selective and non-selective AREs.

At least two non-genomic pathways of androgen action have been proposed to participate in the response of Sertoli cells to androgen stimulation (reviewed in Walker 2010). One involves the rapid (20–40 s) and transient influx of calcium into Sertoli cells, which appears to involve K(+)ATP channels, activation of an unknown G-protein-coupled receptor and the phospholipase C pathway (Loss et al. 2004), reviewed by Walker (2010). The second is an AR-dependent pathway involving ligand-bound AR in the plasma membrane. Although studies suggest that a small population of ARs exists near the plasma membrane, there is as yet no definitive evidence of AR within the membrane (Walker 2010), and no immunohistochemical evidence of membrane AR localization in the seminiferous epithelium. In this model of non-genomic AR action, ligand-bound AR recruits and activates Src kinase, which in turn activates the EGF receptor. These events activate the ERK-MAP-kinase pathway and ultimately, phosphorylation of the transcription factor CREB. Phosphorylated CREB then modulates the transcription of CREB-regulated genes (reviewed by Walker 2010).

Investigation into the different androgen-dependent molecular pathways and their specific roles in spermatogenesis is hampered by the fact that such studies largely rely on observations in isolated Sertoli cells. As such it has been difficult to determine the relative contributions of the genomic and non-genomic pathways to androgen-dependent processes such as meiosis and spermiogenesis. In-vitro studies suggest that the non-genomic AR pathway may contribute to the regulation of Sertoli cell–germ cell adhesion and spermiation (Shupe et al. 2011). Genomic AR actions were assessed by the selective disruption of the AR DNA-binding domain in Sertoli cells, thus theoretically eliminating genomic AR mechanisms but preserving non-genomic mechanisms (Lim

et al. 2009). The resulting phenotype recapitulated the phenotype of SCARKO mice (i.e. predominant meiosis defect), suggesting that genomic AR mechanisms are essential for the androgen-mediated initiation of spermatogenesis, and providing indirect evidence that non-genomic AR pathways play no major role (Lim et al. 2009). However, the generation of transgenic mouse models or pharmacological strategies in which the non-genomic AR pathway is specifically affected in vivo is needed to elucidate the role of non-genomic androgen actions in spermatogenesis.

The precise genes and proteins regulated by androgens in Sertoli cells, and other testicular cells, are not well understood. The best characterized androgen-responsive gene in Sertoli cells is *Rhox5*, formerly known as *Pem* (Lindsey and Wilkinson 1996), which may act as a key intermediate in modulating androgen action on Sertoli cells (Hu et al. 2010). Other androgen-induced genes have been discovered in the SCARKO model, including *Tubb3* and *Spinlw* (*Eppin*) (O'Shaughnessy et al. 2010b). While some genes are directly modulated by an ARE-dependent mechanism, many other genes are modulated indirectly, via androgen-induced changes in transcription or paracrine factors (O'Shaughnessy et al. 2010b). Microarray analysis of androgen-dependent seminiferous tubules undergoing acute androgen and FSH suppression revealed transcriptional changes in both Sertoli cells and germ cells, with cohorts of genes being up- or downregulated in a cell- and stage-specific manner (O'Donnell et al. 2009), supporting the concept that androgen action in the testis regulates a cascade of transcriptional changes within the seminiferous epithelium.

We recently demonstrated that androgens can modulate miRNAs within Sertoli cells (Fig. 6.4), and that these miRNAs in turn influence protein translation (Nicholls et al. 2011). We have also observed changes in germ cell proteins in response to androgen suppression and replacement (O'Donnell and Stanton, unpublished data). Taken together, androgen action in vivo mediates spermatogenesis by modulating, directly and indirectly, gene and protein expression within Sertoli cells and germ cells. How the germ cells respond to this androgenic stimulus is unclear, but likely involves androgen-induced changes in cell surface receptors or paracrine factor production by Sertoli cells.

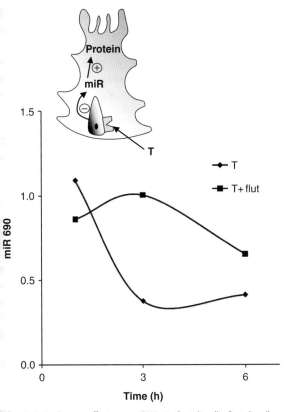

Fig. 6.4 Androgen effects on miRNAs in Sertoli cells. Sertoli cells were isolated from 20-day-old rats and cultured in the absence of hormones for four days, prior to the addition of FSH and testosterone (T), with or without the androgen receptor antagonist flutamide (flut) for 0–6 hours. Levels of one miRNA species (miR 690) were measured by quantitative PCR and normalized to GAPDH (glyceraldehyde 3-phosphate dehydrogenase). Data is shown as mean of three separate experiments, adapted from (Nicholls *et al.* 2011). In this instance, T treatment rapidly suppresses this miRNA, and the T-mediated inhibition is blocked by the AR antagonist. Since miRNAs typically act by suppressing translation of their target protein, this T-mediated inhibition of miR 690 would be expected to result in increased translation of its target protein(s). Acute regulation of miRNA species in Sertoli cells may be one mechanism by which androgens can modulate cellular responses.

6.5.4 Relationship between testicular androgen concentrations and spermatogenic progression

As discussed in Section 6.4.3, spermatogenesis can be supported by levels of androgen that are about one-quarter of the levels present in the normal adult testis, and a very narrow dose-response range exists in rodents between testicular androgens and sperm production. This latter observation may in part reflect the involvement of 5α-reduction of testosterone at lower doses (O'Donnell *et al.* 1996a); however, there is currently no explanation for why small changes in testicular androgen concentration have dramatic consequences for spermatogenesis. What is certain, though, is that different processes in spermatogenesis have different sensitivities to, or requirements for, androgens. This concept has been demonstrated consistently in transgenic mouse models and in rat suppression and replacement models.

When promoting spermatogenesis in the congenitally GnRH-deficient hpg mouse, the survival of spermatocytes and their entry into meiotic division was stimulated by comparatively low doses of androgens that are unable to restore spermatid elongation (Singh *et al.* 1995; Handelsman *et al.* 1999). Higher levels of androgen will promote spermatid elongation (Handelsman *et al.* 1999), probably via the androgen-dependent effects on mid-spermiogenesis (O'Donnell *et al.* 1994). These observations are supported by the phenotypes of transgenic mouse lines with variable inactivation of AR action within Sertoli cells. Ablation of AR function in Sertoli cells causes meiotic arrest and very limited spermiogenesis (Chang *et al.* 2004; De Gendt *et al.* 2004; Lim *et al.* 2009); whereas reduced (but not ablated) androgen signaling or production can support meiosis but spermiogenesis is disrupted (Zhang *et al.* 2001; Holdcraft and Braun 2004a; Lim *et al.* 2009). Thus the completion of meiosis requires less androgen action on the Sertoli cell than does the completion of spermiogenesis. In our rat studies, levels of testosterone around 3% of normal will maintain meiosis; whereas levels 12% of normal are required for elongated spermatid production (O'Donnell *et al.* 1994; 1999).

There is also a dose effect of androgen on different processes within spermiogenesis, at least in rodents. When testosterone levels are reduced to about 3% of normal, the survival of step 7 round spermatids is maintained, but the adhesion of step 8 round spermatids to Sertoli cells is not supported; further withdrawal of androgenic support, by an AR antagonist or 5α-reductase inhibitor, induces apoptosis of step 7 round spermatids (O'Donnell *et al.* 1996a; 1999). The release of sperm from Sertoli cells at the end of spermiogenesis also requires considerable androgenic support, and we have noted that levels of testosterone (8% of normal in adult rats) that support elongated spermatid production at ~50% of normal do not fully support spermiation, with many spermatids being retained by Sertoli cells, and thus reducing the sperm output from the testis (O'Donnell *et al.* 1999 and unpublished data).

Inhibition of androgen action will first result in the failure of spermatid release (Russell and Clermont 1977; Saito *et al.* 2000), followed by a more gradual decline in germ cell populations (Saito *et al.* 2000). This indicates that spermiation in the adult is acutely sensitive to a loss of androgen (and/or gonadotropin) action (reviewed in O'Donnell *et al.* 2011). This concept explains why spermiation failure is seen in men undergoing acute gonadotropin withdrawal (McLachlan *et al.* 2002a). In these men, LH and FSH are undetectable by highly sensitive assays (Robertson *et al.* 2001; McLachlan *et al.* 2002a), and iTT and DHT are reduced to ~2.5% and ~65% of normal, respectively. The maintenance of some testicular androgen action in these men likely explains why their germ cells progressed through meiosis and spermiogenesis (McLachlan *et al.* 2002a); however, the number of cells entering meiosis was reduced as a consequence of FSH suppression resulting in lower numbers of meiotic precursor cells (spermatogonia) (see Section 6.6.2).

In summary, it is clear that some aspects of spermatogenesis, particularly the completion of meiosis, can be maintained by very low levels of androgen action in the testis, and that different androgen-dependent processes within spermatogenesis have different thresholds for androgen action. There may be considerable between-subject variation in the specific androgenic requirement for each androgen-dependent process, as is suggested by studies in humans (Zhengwei *et al.* 1998; McLachlan *et al.* 2002a; Matthiesson *et al.* 2005). Spermiation failure, which has a major influence on sperm output from the testis, also shows a highly variable response to androgen suppression in monkeys (O'Donnell *et al.* 2001a), men (Matthiesson *et al.* 2005) and even in rodents (Saito *et al.* 2000; O'Donnell *et al.* 2009). Thus individual variations in the sensitivities of different spermatogenic processes to androgens may explain why a correlation between iTT levels and sperm output has been so difficult to establish in gonadotropin-suppressed monkeys and men (Zhengwei *et al.* 1998; Weinbauer *et al.* 2001; Narula *et al.* 2002; Matthiesson *et al.* 2006). In these models, the extent of FSH suppression in response to exogenous androgen administration and the ability to support spermatogonial populations (see Section 6.6) likely adds further complexity to the correlation between

testicular androgens and sperm counts (Weinbauer *et al.* 2001; Narula *et al.* 2002). Because of the ability of low levels of androgen action to support some aspects of spermatogenesis, it is likely that novel approaches will be needed to diminish intratesticular androgen action to the extent required for complete spermatogenic suppression in a contraceptive setting.

6.6 Other endocrine factors in the control of spermatogenesis

6.6.1 Follicle-stimulating hormone and spermatogenesis

The specific roles for FSH in spermatogenesis have been reviewed extensively elsewhere (Nieschlag *et al.* 1999; Holdcraft and Braun 2004b; O'Donnell *et al.* 2006; O'Shaughnessy *et al.* 2009; Ruwanpura *et al.* 2010) and therefore will only briefly be considered here. Follicle-stimulating hormone receptors are present only on Sertoli cells (Heckert and Griswold 1993), reflecting the importance of this gonadotropin for Sertoli cell function. Testicular FSH receptor expression in the rat is highest in stages XIII–II (Heckert and Griswold 1993; Rannikko *et al.* 1996); e.g. when type A spermatogonia proliferate and the meiotic division is being completed. In the human testis, FSH receptor expression could not be clearly associated with a particular spermatogenic stage(s) but was unequivocally confined to Sertoli cells (Böckers *et al.* 1994). There has been considerable confusion in the literature over the specific roles of FSH, independent of androgens, in spermatogenesis. This is in part probably due to the fact that FSH can support a low level of LH-independent androgen production by Leydig cells (e.g. Haywood *et al.* 2002; 2003; reviewed in O'Shaughnessy *et al.* 2009), making it more difficult to study the effects of FSH in a complete absence of androgen action.

Follicle-stimulating hormone has a key role in regulating the proliferation and function of Sertoli cells (Means *et al.* 1980; Wreford *et al.* 2001; Allan *et al.* 2004; Grover *et al.* 2004; Abel *et al.* 2008; reviewed in O'Shaughnessy *et al.* 2009; Ruwanpura *et al.* 2010). Follicle-stimulating hormone regulates postnatal, but not fetal, Sertoli cell proliferation to establish a quantitatively normal, functional population of Sertoli cells. Given that the number of Sertoli cells is a key determinant of adult sperm output, this function of FSH is important for quantitatively normal spermatogenesis. This is evidenced by transgenic mouse models lacking FSH action that show reduced sperm counts due to a smaller Sertoli cell population and various defects in the ability of Sertoli cells to support germ cell development (Wreford et al. 2001; Allan et al. 2004; Grover et al. 2004). Follicle-stimulating hormone also has a key role in spermatogonial development as evidenced by studies in rodents (Haywood et al. 2003; Abel et al. 2008) and primates (Weinbauer et al. 1991; Marshall et al. 1995). Follicle-stimulating hormone regulates spermatogonial populations by preventing apoptosis and possibly by supporting proliferation (reviewed in Ruwanpura et al. 2010). In monkeys and men, type A and B spermatogonia are highly sensitive to gonadotropin withdrawal; although there are differences between the sensitivity of spermatogonial subtypes depending on the experimental context. Follicle-stimulating hormone maintained spermatogonial populations and their progression into meiosis in gonadotropin-suppressed humans (Matthiesson et al. 2006), and stimulated spermatogonial numbers in gonadotropin-suppressed monkeys (Weinbauer et al. 1991; Marshall et al. 1995).

Observations on various transgenic mouse models reveal that FSH supports other aspects of spermatogenesis that, when combined with testosterone action, are essential for quantitatively normal spermatogenesis (also see Section 6.6.2). Such aspects include a possible FSH-mediated paracrine factor(s) from Sertoli cells that influences Leydig cell number, maturation and steroidogenesis (O'Shaughnessy et al. 2009). Although meiosis and spermiogenesis are regarded as androgen-dependent processes, FSH likely has some permissive role in these processes via its effects on Sertoli cell function (e.g. Abel et al. 2008; reviewed in Ruwanpura et al. 2010).

Follicle-stimulating hormone is clearly important for spermatogenesis in non-human primates and humans, as reviewed elsewhere (Nieschlag et al. 1999). For example, in the GnRH antagonist-treated non-human primate model, human FSH was able to qualitatively maintain and restore spermatogenesis (Weinbauer et al. 1991). Immunization against FSH in rhesus and bonnet monkeys provoked marked testicular involution and even infertility (Moudgal et al. 1997; Nieschlag et al. 1999). Studies in gonadotropin-suppressed cynomolgus monkeys (Narula et al. 2002; Weinbauer et al. 2001) reveal correlations between spermatogenesis and FSH. The ability of monkeys to achieve azoospermia as opposed to oligospermia was associated with lower FSH levels which in turn likely resulted in lower numbers of B spermatogonia (O'Donnell et al. 2001a). Therefore the degree of FSH suppression, as well as androgen suppression, is likely important for the induction of azoospermia in a gonadotropin-suppressed, contraceptive setting. Follicle-stimulating hormone alone can maintain human germ cell development for six weeks during gonadotropin suppression, further emphasizing FSH's permissive role in human spermatogenesis, and the fact that optimal contraceptive suppression requires suppression of both LH and FSH (Matthiesson et al. 2006). In considering threshold serum levels of FSH, or LH, action on human spermatogenesis, highly sensitive assay methods should be used as these may reveal interesting relationships (Robertson et al. 2001). For example, in the context of androgen–progestin-based male hormonal contraception (the efficacy of which depends upon profound gonadotropin suppression), men with sperm concentrations below 0.1 million/ml had significantly lower gonadotropin levels (serum FSH ∼ 0.12 IU/l; serum LH ∼ 0.05 IU/l) than oligozoospermic men (sperm concentrations, 0.1–5 million/ml; serum FSH, 0.23–0.5 IU/l; serum LH, 0.05–0.56 IU/l). In multivariate analysis, the suppression of serum LH to less than 5% of baseline values (<0.15 IU/l) was found to be a consistent and highly significant predictor of suppression to below 1 million/ml; while that was not true for serum FSH (McLachlan et al. 2004).

Finally, it is interesting to note that seasonally breeding animals seem to have a greater dependence on FSH than non-seasonal animals. In the Djungarian hamster, the testes undergo marked involution when the light : dark exposure is shifted from 16 : 8 to 8 : 16; LH administration is unable to restore spermatogenesis; however, FSH reinitiates the entire process (Lerchl et al. 1993). Similarly in another seasonally breeding mammal, the prairie dog (Cynomys ludovicanus), FSH but not LH/testosterone induced germ cell activation when given during the seasonal involution phase (Foreman 1998).

In summary, FSH-independent actions are essential for quantitatively normal sperm output. Important FSH-specific actions include the development of a full complement of functional Sertoli cells with an optimal ability to support germ cell development, and the ability to support spermatogonial populations and their entry into meiosis.

6.6.2 Androgen and follicle-stimulating hormone; cooperative effects on spermatogenesis

It is apparent from the above discussion that androgens and FSH have distinct roles in spermatogenesis. However, overall these hormones act cooperatively to promote maximal spermatogenic output (summarized in Fig. 6.5). Androgen and FSH have synergistic, additive, and redundant effects on spermatogenesis and Sertoli cell activity, as demonstrated in transgenic mouse models (Abel *et al.* 2008). Androgen and FSH appear to cooperate by acting independently to support different processes within spermatogenesis; for example FSH's ability to support spermatogonial development and testosterone's ability to support spermatid development. There is also the potential for androgen and FSH to cooperate in some metabolic pathways (Walker and Cheng 2005), in which setting either hormone may support a process to a qualitative degree, but both hormones combined are required for a maximal response. The cooperative effects of androgens and FSH on rodent and human spermatogenesis have been reviewed recently elsewhere (Ruwanpura *et al.* 2010), and will be considered only briefly here.

There is good evidence that androgen or FSH act on spermatogenesis at a lower dose when the other is present (Zirkin 1998; McLachlan *et al.* 2002b; O'Donnell *et al.* 2006). In particular there appears to be a strong case for a potentiating effect of FSH on androgen action, as in many experimental settings the androgen requirements of spermatogenesis are lower in the presence of circulating FSH (reviewed in O'Donnell *et al.* 2006). Conversely, studies suggest that even very low levels of androgen may facilitate FSH action on spermatogenesis (e.g. Chandolia *et al.* 1991b; Spiteri-Grech *et al.* 1993). Therefore the ability of either hormone to stimulate or maintain spermatogenesis is greatly enhanced when even low levels of the other are present.

A major site of androgen and FSH cooperativity is likely to be the prevention of apoptosis/promotion of germ cell survival, particularly of spermatocytes and round spermatids (reviewed in Ruwanpura *et al.* 2010). During gonadotropin suppression, germ cell apoptosis is first seen in the mid-spermatogenic stages (VII and VIII in rodents), with spermatocytes and round spermatids being the most susceptible (Sinha

Hikim and Swerdloff 1999). Germ cell survival during gonadotropin withdrawal could be maintained by either hormone alone, but the combination of both androgen and FSH had a synergistic effect (El Shennawy *et al.* 1998). The ability of either hormone to prevent germ cell apoptosis likely explains why both FSH and hCG maintained germ cell populations in gonadotropin-suppressed humans (Matthiesson *et al.* 2006).

When considering combined androgen and FSH suppression, there are species-dependent differences in the response of spermatogenesis (Fig. 6.6). In rodents, gonadotropin suppression induced by GnRH immunization causes a decline in spermatogonial populations (Fig. 6.6), with spermatogenesis primarily arrested during meiosis (Meachem *et al.* 1998). In contrast, in primates, spermatogenesis primarily shows a defect in spermatogonial development, with meiotic and spermatid populations largely maintained until they undergo a gradual attrition (Zhengwei *et al.* 1998; O'Donnell *et al.* 2001a; McLachlan *et al.* 2002a; Matthiesson *et al.* 2005). There are slight differences between monkeys and man in terms of the spermatogonial subtype first affected by gonadotropin suppression; however, in both species there is evidence for an inhibition of the mitosis of A_p spermatogonia, and for the transition of A_p to "resting" A_d spermatogonia during gonadotropin suppression (McLachlan *et al.* 2002b; Fig. 6.6). These gonadotropin suppression paradigms do not allow a dissection of the sensitivity of primate spermatogonia to androgen or FSH, making it difficult to ascribe hormone-specific roles. The fact that the response of type B spermatogonia to gonadotropin suppression correlates more closely with FSH than iTT in both monkeys and men (O'Donnell *et al.* 2001a; McLachlan *et al.* 2002a), together with the FSH-specific effects in rodents (see Section 6.6.1), suggests that these cells are particularly FSH sensitive (Fig. 6.6).

Postnatal Sertoli cells are a major target for androgen and FSH action, and both hormones have major effects on Sertoli cell morphology, function and gene expression (O'Shaughnessy *et al.* 2009). Sertoli cell morphology and ability to support germ cells was impaired in mice in which the Sertoli cells lacked either active FSH or androgen receptors, but was more markedly impaired in mice lacking both (Abel *et al.* 2008). These results suggest that androgen and FSH act in a cooperative manner to directly modulate Sertoli cell function, morphology and the ability to support germ cells. The ability of androgen and FSH

Sertoli cells

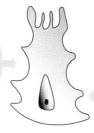

FSH
- Essential for a full complement of Sertoli cells

FSH and T
- Potentiate one another's action on Sertoli cell function and germ cell development
- Likely have complementary, redundant, additive and synergistic functions within Sertoli cells

T
- Action on Sertoli cell AR essential for normal function
- Action on PTM AR supports Sertoli cell number

Germ cells

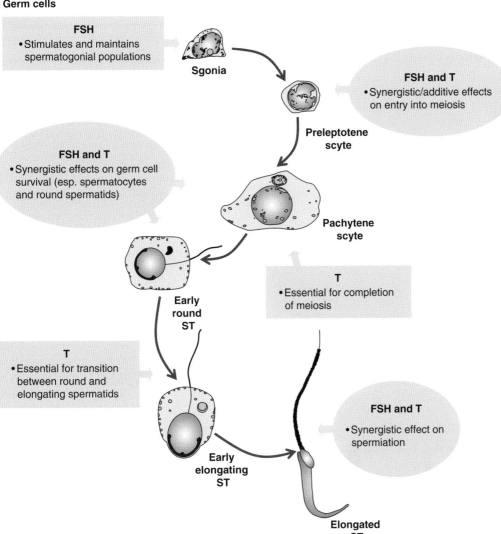

FSH
- Stimulates and maintains spermatogonial populations

Sgonia

FSH and T
- Synergistic/additive effects on entry into meiosis

Preleptotene scyte

FSH and T
- Synergistic effects on germ cell survival (esp. spermatocytes and round spermatids)

Pachytene scyte

Early round ST

T
- Essential for completion of meiosis

T
- Essential for transition between round and elongating spermatids

FSH and T
- Synergistic effect on spermiation

Early elongating ST

Elongated ST

Fig. 6.5 Roles of androgen and FSH in spermatogenesis as assessed in rodent models. The action of both androgen and FSH is required for quantitatively normal spermatogenesis. This diagram briefly summarizes the likely independent and additive/synergistic effects of androgen and FSH on spermatogenesis in rodents. Androgen and FSH act on receptors in Sertoli cells to support spermatogenesis, but androgen also acts on other testicular somatic cells including peritubular myoid cells (PTM) and Leydig cells. The precise sites of action of androgen and FSH in spermatogenesis have been primarily elucidated in transgenic mouse models and adult rat suppression and reinitiation/maintenance models. Abbreviations: T, testosterone; sgonia, spermatogonia; scyte, spermatocyte; ST, spermatid.

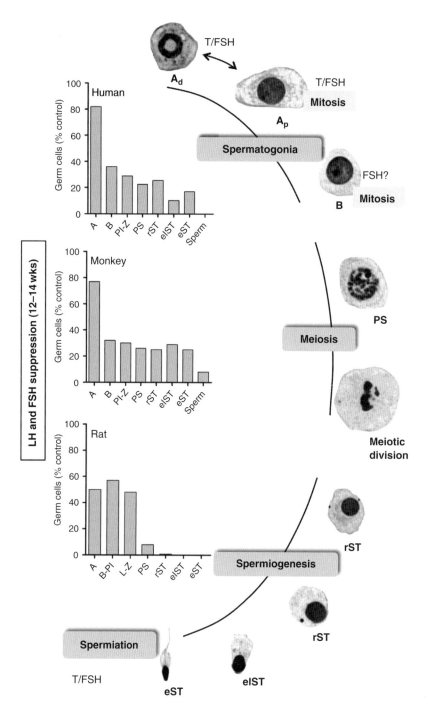

Fig. 6.6 Response of spermatogenesis to androgen and FSH withdrawal in rodents and primates. Graphs show germ cell populations in humans, monkeys and rats undergoing 12–14 weeks of gonadotropin suppression. Gonadotropin suppression was induced by 12 weeks of testosterone plus progestin treatment in humans (see McLachlan *et al.* 2002a), 14 weeks of testosterone treatment in monkeys (see O'Donnell *et al.* 2001a) and 12 weeks of immunization against GnRH in rats (see Meachem *et al.* 1998). See the cited papers for details of enumeration of germ cells. Humans and monkeys show similar patterns of suppression, with a major block between A and B spermatogonia, yet maintenance of some meiotic and spermiogenic populations; whereas rat spermatogenesis shows a major block during meiosis. The cells shown to the right are human germ cells, indicating the process of spermatogenesis in man. The specific spermatogenic processes that are impaired by 12–14 weeks of gonadotropin suppression in humans (and monkeys) are indicated (T/FSH). In this setting of reduced FSH and iTT, some maintenance of meiosis and spermiogenesis occurs (see graphs); however, based on studies in rodents (see Section 6.5.2), it is possible that more profound suppression of intratesticular androgens could impair these processes. The mitoses of A_p spermatogonia are thought to be impaired by gonadotropin withdrawal, with the transition of A_p spermatogonia to "resting" A_d spermatogonia seen during acute gonadotropin suppression (reviewed in McLachlan *et al.* 2002b). Correlations between type B spermatogonia numbers and FSH, but not iTT, suggest that the mitosis of these cells may be more sensitive to FSH. The release of mature elongated spermatids from the Sertoli cells during spermiation is also highly sensitive to gonadotropin suppression in men (as well as in monkeys and rats). Abbreviations: A_d, type A dark spermatogonia; A_p, type A pale spermatogonia; B, type B spermatogonia; Pl, preleptotene spermatocytes; L, leptotene spermatocytes; Z, zygotene spermatocytes; PS, pachytene spermatocytes; rST, round spermatids; elST, elongating spermatids; eST, elongated spermatids.

to cooperate in modulating Sertoli cell function is also highlighted by studies investigating the process of spermiation. When either androgen or FSH was suppressed in adult rats, Sertoli cells failed to release approximately 10% of elongated spermatids. However, the suppression of both hormones in combination had a synergistic effect, such that approximately 50% of the spermatids failed to be released (Saito *et al.* 2000). Taken together, it seems likely that androgen and FSH regulate distinct and overlapping functions in Sertoli cells which cooperate to support different aspects of germ cell development.

In summary, it can be concluded that, in rodents and primates, the combination of androgen and FSH consistently produces a better stimulatory effect on spermatogenesis than either factor alone. For quantitatively normal spermatogenesis and fertility, the action of both androgen and FSH is required.

6.6.3 Aromatization of testosterone to estradiol; role in spermatogenesis

The metabolism of testosterone to estradiol by the aromatase enzyme and its role in spermatogenesis has been the subject of intensive review, and we refer the reader to previous reviews on this topic (O'Donnell et al. 2001b; Hess 2003; Carreau and Hess 2010; Carreau et al. 2011). There is a variety of evidence to suggest that exogenous estrogens and phytoestrogens can exert effects during testicular development which can have adverse consequences for male fertility (reviewed in O'Donnell et al. 2001b); however this section will focus on the potential role of the metabolism of testosterone to estradiol in normal spermatogenesis.

Mice lacking the aromatase gene (Robertson et al. 1999; Robertson et al. 2002; Carreau and Hess 2010) and ERα are infertile (Eddy et al. 1996; Hess et al. 1997), highlighting a critical role for estrogen in male fertility. The disturbed spermatogenesis observed in the ERα knock-out (ERαKO) mouse was a consequence of disturbed efferent ductule function, whereby the failure of the efferent ductules to resorb seminiferous tubule fluid resulted in fluid accumulation in the testis and secondary defects to spermatogenesis (Eddy et al. 1996; Hess et al. 1997). Estrogen receptor-α regulates epithelial cell morphology as well as ion channel and aquaporin water channel function in the efferent ductules (reviewed in Carreau and Hess 2010). Conversely, there was no evidence of disturbed efferent ductule function in the aromatase knock-out mouse (ArKO), but the spermatogenesis phenotype observed was consistent with an effect on Sertoli cells and/or germ cells, and worsened with age (Robertson et al. 1999; 2002). How this action was mediated was unclear since ERβKO mice were fertile (Dupont et al. 2000) despite ERβ being widely expressed in the seminiferous epithelium.

Several recent advances have shed light on how estradiol and its receptors influence spermatogenesis. First, it has been established that estradiol can act directly on testicular germ cells via a non-genomic pathway mediated by a G-protein-coupled receptor known as GPR30 (Chimento et al. 2010; Carreau et al. 2011). Second, efferent ductule development and function was shown to be regulated by estradiol-independent activation of ERα (Sinkevicius et al. 2009), explaining why efferent ductule function was not compromised in aromatase-deficient mice. Third, mice expressing a mutated ERα which is unable to bind estradiol (ENERKI mice) had a spermatogenic phenotype almost identical to the ArKO mouse, including a late-onset phenotype (Sinkevicius et al. 2009), suggesting that estradiol signaling via ERα is important for the progression of spermatogenesis. This latter proposition was proven by the fact that the administration of a selective agonist capable of activating the mutant ERα in ENERKI mice rescued the spermatogenic phenotype (Sinkevicius et al. 2009). Intriguingly, activation of ERα during the neonatal period, but not after puberty, was required to rescue the phenotype, suggesting that estradiol-dependent activation of ERα in the neonatal testis is required for fertility in adulthood. It is not yet known what cells/processes in the neonatal testis rely on estradiol–ERα action, and how they can influence the maintenance of spermatogenesis in adulthood. Taken together, these new findings suggest that spermatogenesis relies on estradiol-dependent and independent activation of the classic estrogen receptors during development, and that estradiol can exert effects on spermatogenesis via non-classic estrogen receptors (reviewed in Carreau and Hess 2010; Carreau et al. 2011).

The ability of estradiol to stimulate spermatogenesis during gonadotropin deficiency has been the subject of some debate. Treatment of postnatal hypogonadal (hpg) mice with estradiol stimulated qualitatively normal spermatogenesis, but was also associated with a stimulation of FSH (Ebling et al. 2000). Spermatogenesis (and FSH) was able to be stimulated by an ERα, but not ERβ, agonist (Allan et al. 2010). Since FSH in the absence of androgen can only stimulate pre-meiotic germ cell development in these mice (Haywood et al. 2003), the induction of spermatogenesis observed during estradiol treatment is unlikely to be solely due to circulating FSH, although an FSH effect is possible (Baines et al. 2008). The ability of estradiol to stimulate spermatogenesis relies on the presence of a functional AR, despite no detectable increase in iTT (Baines et al. 2005; Lim *et al.* 2008). The stimulatory effects of estradiol required a functional ERα, but not ERβ, and were associated with changes in Sertoli cell morphology and gene expression, including the expression of Sertoli cell androgen-dependent genes (Allan *et al.* 2010). Thus, estradiol stimulates spermatogenesis via mechanisms that require both ERα and AR in a setting of circulating FSH. It is possible that estrogen acts directly on ERα and/or on hetereodimers of ERα/AR in Sertoli cells (Allan *et al.* 2010) to modulate key Sertoli cell functions which, in concert with FSH, facilitate germ cell development. While iTT levels are very low in this model (Baines *et al.* 2005; Lim *et al.* 2008), DHT levels were not measured, and thus it is possible that low levels of androgen action could be preserved via an FSH-mediated upregulation of 5α-reductase (Pratis *et al.* 2003).

In summary, estradiol likely has a permissive/supportive role in spermatogenesis, although the precise estradiol-dependent processes are unknown.

6.7   Implications for treatment of secondary hypogonadism and for male hormonal contraception

The pivotal role of androgen action in supporting spermatogenesis underscores certain aspects of approaches to fertility control. First, hCG as an LH substitute has proven effective when given at doses of 1500 IU two to three times per week. These doses appear supraphysiological when one looks at reports of iTT level with graded hCG exposure, wherein 500 IU twice weekly would seem more than adequate (Roth *et al.* 2010b). Yet conventional (likely excess) hCG doses do not appear to adversely affect the therapeutic effect, despite the provision of excess substrate for aromatization to estradiol. The hCG does need to be titrated to avoid excessive androgen levels with clinical side-effects, and co-suppression of endogenous FSH (if present). Those issues aside, there appears to be "no downside" to supraphysiological iTT levels induced by conventional hCG doses. Finally, it must be emphasized that, in some men, hCG treatment must be protracted (one to two years), especially for the initial induction of spermatogenesis in Kallmann syndrome, but this seems only reasonable given the time course of normal puberty.

Conversely in the male hormonal contraception paradigm, the complete abolition of androgen effect does not appear achievable with strategies based on pituitary gonadotropin inhibition using GnRH analogs and/or sex steroid administration, presumably because of LH-independent androgen secretion maintaining low iTT levels (1–2% baseline) and some spermatogenesis in a minority (∼5%) of men. This so-called "non-responder" group may well represent the extreme end of a normal distribution for androgen action threshold on spermatogenesis wherein "a little bit of androgen goes a long way." As argued above, the true elimination of androgen action, perhaps through testis-specific enzyme inhibition or targeted blockade of testicular AR or its co-modulators, may well achieve the long-held goal of universal azoospermia. However, this demands a better understanding of these underlying processes and the generation of novel therapeutic tools; this will be a long road and demands the continued partnership between basic and clinical scientists, and industry.

6.8   Key messages

- Testosterone is essential for spermatogenesis and able to act alone to qualitatively initiate, maintain and reinitiate spermatogenesis and formation of spermatozoa.
- Full, quantitatively normal spermatogenesis requires the combined action of testosterone and FSH.
- Testosterone and FSH cooperate in the regulation of spermatogenesis via redundant, additive, complementary and synergistic actions.
- Androgen actions on receptors in Sertoli cells, peritubular myoid cells and Leydig cells, but not germ cells, are essential for spermatogenesis.
- Key androgen-dependent processes in rodent spermatogenesis include the completion of meiosis and the progression through spermiogenesis.
- A very narrow dose-response range exists between iTT levels and sperm output; this "hair trigger" effect combined with interindividual differences leads to difficulties in correlating the two parameters.
- Testosterone metabolism to DHT may play a role in maintaining androgen action when testosterone concentrations are low.
- Testosterone metabolism to estradiol has a supportive role in spermatogenesis, though the precise cellular processes involved are unclear.

- Several androgen-dependent genes have been identified in the testis, but the cellular pathways by which androgens mediate somatic and germ cell functions are unclear.
- For male hormonal contraception, withdrawal of androgen action is essential to achieving maximal effect. In some men, LH-independent Leydig cell androgen secretion apparently maintains spermatogenesis, pointing to the need for alternative approaches.
- In the setting of hypogonadotropic hypogonadism, hCG (as an LH substitute) restores iTT, but treatment may take months–years to be

effective, and co-administration with FSH takes advantage of the well-known synergies at multiple points in germ cell development and spermiation.

Acknowledgements

The authors were supported by a NHMRC Australia Program Grant no. 494802 and by the Victorian Government's Operational Infrastructure Support Program. R. I. McLachlan was supported by a NHMRC Australia Research Fellowship no. 441103.

6.9   References

Abel MH, Baker PJ, Charlton HM, Monteiro A, Verhoeven G, De Gendt K, Guillou F, O'Shaughnessy PJ (2008) Spermatogenesis and Sertoli cell activity in mice lacking Sertoli cell receptors for follicle-stimulating hormone and androgen. *Endocrinology* **149**:3279–3285

Allan CM, Garcia A, Spaliviero J, Zhang FP, Jimenez M, Huhtaniemi I, Handelsman DJ (2004) Complete Sertoli cell proliferation induced by follicle-stimulating hormone (FSH) independently of luteinizing hormone activity: evidence from genetic models of isolated FSH action. *Endocrinology* **145**:1587–1593

Allan CM, Couse JF, Simanainen U, Spaliviero J, Jimenez M, Rodriguez K, Korach KS, Handelsman DJ (2010) Estradiol induction of spermatogenesis is mediated via an estrogen receptor-alpha mechanism involving neuroendocrine activation of follicle-stimulating hormone secretion. *Endocrinology* **151**:2800–2810

Anderson RA, Wallace AM, Wu FC (1996) Comparison between testosterone enanthate-induced azoospermia and oligozoospermia in a male contraceptive study. III. Higher 5 alpha-reductase activity in oligozoospermic men administered supraphysiological doses of

testosterone. *J Clin Endocrinol Metab* **81**:902–908

Awoniyi CA, Santulli R, Sprando RL, Ewing LL, Zirkin BR (1989) Restoration of advanced spermatogenic cells in the experimentally regressed rat testis: quantitative relationship to testosterone concentration within the testis. *Endocrinology* **124**:1217–1223

Awoniyi CA, Zirkin BR, Chandrashekar V, Schlaff WD (1992) Exogenously administered testosterone maintains spermatogenesis quantitatively in adult rats actively immunized against gonadotropin-releasing hormone. *Endocrinology* **130**:3283–3288

Baines H, Nwagwu MO, Furneaux EC, Stewart J, Kerr JB, Mayhew TM, Ebling FJ (2005) Estrogenic induction of spermatogenesis in the hypogonadal (hpg) mouse: role of androgens. *Reproduction* **130**:643–654

Baines H, Nwagwu MO, Hastie GR, Wiles RA, Mayhew M, Ebling FJ (2008) Effects of estradiol and FSH on maturation of the testis in the hypogonadal (hpg) mouse. *Reprod Biol Endocrinol* **6**:4

Behre HM, Nieschlag E, Weiacker P, Simoni M, Partsch CJ (2010) Diseases of the hypothalamus and the pituitary gland. In: Nieschlag E, Behre HM, Nieschlag S (eds) *Andrology. Male Reproductive*

Health and Dysfunction, 3rd edn. Springer-Verlag, Berlin, pp 169–192

Bernard DJ, Fortin J, Wang Y, Lamba P (2010) Mechanisms of FSH synthesis: what we know, what we don't, and why you should care. *Fertil Steril* **93**:2465–2485

Böckers TM, Nieschlag E, Kreutz MR, Bergmann M (1994) Localization of follicle-stimulating hormone (FSH) immunoreactivity and hormone receptor mRNA in testicular tissue of infertile men. *Cell Tissue Res* **278**:595–600

Bremner WJ, Millar MR, Sharpe RM, Saunders PT (1994) Immunohistochemical localization of androgen receptors in the rat testis: evidence for stage-dependent expression and regulation by androgens. *Endocrinology* **135**:1227–1234

Büchter D, Behre HM, Kliesch S, Nieschlag E (1998) Pulsatile GnRH or human chorionic gonadotropin/human menopausal gonadotropin as effective treatment for men with hypogonadotropic hypogonadism: a review of 42 cases. *Eur J Endocrinol* **139**:298–303

Burris AS, Rodbard HW, Winters SJ, Sherins RJ (1988) Gonadotropin therapy in men with isolated hypogonadotropic hypogonadism: the response to human chorionic gonadotropin is predicted by initial testicular size. *J Clin Endocrinol Metab* **66**:1144–1151

Cameron DF, Muffly KE (1991) Hormonal regulation of spermatid binding. *J Cell Sci* **100**:623–633

Carreau S, Hess RA (2010) Oestrogens and spermatogenesis. *Philos Trans R Soc Lond B Biol Sci* **365**:1517–1535

Carreau S, Bois C, Zanatta L, Silva FR, Bouraima-Lelong H, Delalande C (2011) Estrogen signaling in testicular cells. *Life Sci* **89**:584–587

Chandolia RK, Weinbauer GF, Behre HM, Nieschlag E (1991a) Evaluation of a peripherally selective antiandrogen (Casodex) as a tool for studying the relationship between testosterone and spermatogenesis in the rat. *J Steroid Biochem Mol Biol* **38**:367–375

Chandolia RK, Weinbauer GF, Fingscheidt U, Bartlett JM, Nieschlag E (1991b) Effects of flutamide on testicular involution induced by an antagonist of gonadotrophin-releasing hormone and on stimulation of spermatogenesis by follicle-stimulating hormone in rats. *J Reprod Fertil* **93**:313–323

Chang C, Chen YT, Yeh SD, Xu Q, Wang RS, Guillou F, Lardy H, Yeh S (2004) Infertility with defective spermatogenesis and hypotestosteronemia in male mice lacking the androgen receptor in Sertoli cells. *Proc Natl Acad Sci USA* **101**:6876–6881

Chapin RE, Wine RN, Harris MW, Borchers CH, Haseman JK (2001) Structure and control of a cell-cell adhesion complex associated with spermiation in rat seminiferous epithelium. *J Androl* **22**:1030–1052

Chimento A, Sirianni R, Delalande C, Silandre D, Bois C, Ando S, Maggiolini M, Carreau S, Pezzi V (2010) 17 beta-estradiol activates rapid signaling pathways involved in rat pachytene spermatocytes apoptosis through GPR30 and ER alpha. *Mol Cell Endocrinol* **320**:136–144

Clermont Y, Leblond CP (1955) Spermiogenesis of man, monkey, ram and other mammals as shown by the periodic acid-Schiff technique. *Am J Anat* **96**:229–253

Corpechot C, Baulieu EE, Robel P (1981) Testosterone, dihydrotestosterone and androstanediols in plasma, testes and prostates of rats during development. *Acta Endocrinol (Copenh)* **96**:127–135

Dankbar B, Brinkworth MH, Schlatt S, Weinbauer GF, Nieschlag E, Gromoll J (1995) Ubiquitous expression of the androgen receptor and testis-specific expression of the FSH receptor in the cynomolgus monkey (Macaca fascicularis) revealed by a ribonuclease protection assay. *J Steroid Biochem Mol Biol* **55**:35–41

De Franca LR, Hess RA, Cooke PS, Russell LD (1995) Neonatal hypothyroidism causes delayed Sertoli cell maturation in rats treated with propylthiouracil: evidence that the Sertoli cell controls testis growth. *Anat Rec* **242**:57–69

De Gendt K, Swinnen JV, Saunders PT, Schoonjans L, Dewerchin M, Devos A, Tan K, Atanassova N, Claessens F, Lecureuil C, Heyns W, Carmeliet P, Guillou F, Sharpe RM, Verhoeven G (2004) A Sertoli cell-selective knockout of the androgen receptor causes spermatogenic arrest in meiosis. *Proc Natl Acad Sci USA* **101**:1327–1332

de Kretser DM, Kerr JB (1988) The cytology of the testis. In: Knobil E, Neill JD (eds) *The Physiology of Reproduction*. Raven Press Ltd, New York, pp 837–932

de Kretser DM, Loveland KL, Meehan T, O'Bryan MK, Phillips DJ, Wreford NG (2001) Inhibins, activins and follistatin: actions on the testis. *Mol Cell Endocrinol* **180**:87–92

de Kretser DM, Buzzard JJ, Okuma Y, O'Connor AE, Hayashi T, Lin SY,

Morrison JR, Loveland KL, Hedger MP (2004) The role of activin, follistatin and inhibin in testicular physiology. *Mol Cell Endocrinol* **225**:57–64

Depenbusch M, von Eckardstein S, Simoni M, Nieschlag E (2002) Maintenance of spermatogenesis in hypogonadotropic hypogonadal men with human chorionic gonadotropin alone. *Eur J Endocrinol* **147**:617–624

de Rooij DG, Grootegoed JA (1998) Spermatogonial stem cells. *Curr Opin Cell Biol* **10**:694–701

Deslypere JP, Young M, Wilson JD, McPhaul MJ (1992) Testosterone and 5 alpha-dihydrotestosterone interact differently with the androgen receptor to enhance transcription of the MMTV-CAT reporter gene. *Mol Cell Endocrinol* **88**:15–22

Dupont S, Krust A, Gansmuller A, Dierich A, Chambon P, Mark M (2000) Effect of single and compound knockouts of estrogen receptors alpha (ERalpha) and beta (ERbeta) on mouse reproductive phenotypes. *Development* **127**:4277–4291

Ebling FJ, Brooks AN, Cronin AS, Ford H, Kerr JB (2000) Estrogenic induction of spermatogenesis in the hypogonadal mouse. *Endocrinology* **141**:2861–2869

Eddy EM, Washburn TF, Bunch DO, Goulding EH, Gladen BC, Lubahn DB, Korach KS (1996) Targeted disruption of the estrogen receptor gene in male mice causes alteration of spermatogenesis and infertility. *Endocrinology* **137**:4796–4805

El Shennawy A, Gates RJ, Russell LD (1998) Hormonal regulation of spermatogenesis in the hypophysectomized rat: cell viability after hormonal replacement in adults after intermediate periods of hypophysectomy. *J Androl* **19**:320–334; discussion:341–342

Fingscheidt U, Weinbauer GF, Fehm HL, Nieschlag E (1998) Regulation of gonadotrophin secretion by inhibin, testosterone and gonadotrophin-releasing hormone in pituitary cell cultures of male monkeys. *J Endocrinol* **159**:103–110

Finkel DM, Phillips JL, Snyder PJ (1985) Stimulation of spermatogenesis by gonadotropins in men with hypogonadotropic hypogonadism. *N Engl J Med* **313**:651–655

Foreman D (1998) Effects of exogenous hormones on spermatogenesis in the male prairie dog (Cynomys ludovicianus). *Anat Rec* **250**:45–61

Franca LR, Ogawa T, Avarbock MR, Brinster RL, Russell LD (1998) Germ cell genotype controls cell cycle during spermatogenesis in the rat. *Biol Reprod* **59**:1371–1377

Gendrel D, Chaussain JL, Roger M, Job JC (1980) Simultaneous postnatal rise of plasma LH and testosterone in male infants. *J Pediatr* **97**:600–602

George FW, Johnson L, Wilson JD (1989) The effect of a 5 alpha-reductase inhibitor on androgen physiology in the immature male rat. *Endocrinology* **125**:2434–2438

Grino PB, Griffin JE, Wilson JD (1990) Testosterone at high concentrations interacts with the human androgen receptor similarly to dihydrotestosterone. *Endocrinology* **126**:1165–1172

Gromoll J, Partsch CJ, Simoni M, Nordhoff V, Sippell WG, Nieschlag E, Saxena BB (1998) A mutation in the first transmembrane domain of the lutropin receptor causes male precocious puberty. *J Clin Endocrinol Metab* **83**:476–480

Gromoll J, Eiholzer U, Nieschlag E, Simoni M (2000) Male hypogonadism caused by homozygous deletion of exon 10 of the luteinizing hormone (LH) receptor: differential action of human chorionic gonadotropin and LH. *J Clin Endocrinol Metab* **85**:2281–2286

Gromoll J, Wistuba J, Terwort N, Godmann M, Muller T, Simoni M (2003) A new subclass of the luteinizing hormone/chorionic gonadotropin receptor lacking exon 10 messenger RNA in the New World monkey (Platyrrhini) lineage. *Biol Reprod* **69**:75–80

Grover A, Sairam MR, Smith CE, Hermo L (2004) Structural and functional modifications of Sertoli cells in the testis of adult follicle-stimulating hormone receptor knockout mice. *Biol Reprod* **71**:117–129

Grumbach MM (2005) A window of opportunity: the diagnosis of gonadotropin deficiency in the male infant. *J Clin Endocrinol Metab* **90**:3122–3127

Guo Q, Kumar TR, Woodruff T, Hadsell LA, DeMayo FJ, Matzuk MM (1998) Overexpression of mouse follistatin causes reproductive defects in transgenic mice. *Mol Endocrinol* **12**:96–106

Hall JM, McDonnell DP (1999) The estrogen receptor beta-isoform (ERbeta) of the human estrogen receptor modulates ERalpha transcriptional activity and is a key regulator of the cellular response to estrogens and antiestrogens. *Endocrinology* **140**:5566–5578

Handelsman DJ (2008) Androgen physiology, pharmacology and abuse. In: de Groot L, McLachlan RI (eds) *Endocrinology of Male Reproduction*. www.endotext.org/male/male2/maleframe2.htm (MDText.com, Inc), South Dartmouth, MA, Chapter 2

Handelsman DJ, Spaliviero JA, Simpson JM, Allan CM, Singh J (1999) Spermatogenesis without gonadotropins: maintenance has a lower testosterone threshold than initiation. *Endocrinology* **140**:3938–3946

Hayes F, Pitteloud N (2004) Hypogonadotropic hypogonadism and gonadotropin therapy. In: de Groot L, McLachlan RI (eds) *Endocrinology of Male Reproduction*.

www.endotext.org/male/male2/maleframe2.htm (MDText.com, Inc), South Dartmouth, MA, Chapter 5

Haywood M, Tymchenko N, Spaliviero J, Koch A, Jimenez M, Gromoll J, Simoni M, Nordhoff V, Handelsman DJ, Allan CM (2002) An activated human follicle-stimulating hormone (FSH) receptor stimulates FSH-like activity in gonadotropin-deficient transgenic mice. *Mol Endocrinol* **16**:2582–2591

Haywood M, Spaliviero J, Jimemez M, King NJ, Handelsman DJ, Allan CM (2003) Sertoli and germ cell development in hypogonadal (hpg) mice expressing transgenic follicle-stimulating hormone alone or in combination with testosterone. *Endocrinology* **144**:509–517

Heckert L, Griswold MD (1993) Expression of the FSH receptor in the testis. *Recent Prog Horm Res* **48**:61–77

Hess RA (2003) Estrogen in the adult male reproductive tract: a review. *Reprod Biol Endocrinol* **1**:52

Hess RA, Bunick D, Lee KH, Bahr J, Taylor JA, Korach KS, Lubahn DB (1997) A role for oestrogens in the male reproductive system. *Nature* **390**:509–512

Holdcraft RW, Braun RE (2004a) Androgen receptor function is required in Sertoli cells for the terminal differentiation of haploid spermatids. *Development* **131**:459–467

Holdcraft RW, Braun RE (2004b) Hormonal regulation of spermatogenesis. *Int J Androl* **27**:335–342

Hu Z, Dandekar D, O'Shaughnessy PJ, De Gendt K, Verhoeven G, Wilkinson MF (2010) Androgen-induced Rhox homeobox genes modulate the expression of AR-regulated genes. *Mol Endocrinol* **24**:60–75

Huang HF, Marshall GR, Rosenberg R, Nieschlag E (1987) Restoration of spermatogenesis by high levels of testosterone in hypophysectomized rats after long-term regression. *Acta Endocrinol (Copenh)* **116**:433–444

Jarow JP, Zirkin BR (2005) The androgen microenvironment of the human testis and hormonal control of spermatogenesis. *Ann N Y Acad Sci* **1061**:208–220

Jarow JP, Chen H, Rosner TW, Trentacoste S, Zirkin BR (2001) Assessment of the androgen environment within the human testis: minimally invasive method to obtain intratesticular fluid. *J Androl* **22**:640–645

Jeyaraj DA, Grossman G, Petrusz P (2003) Dynamics of testicular germ cell apoptosis in normal mice and transgenic mice overexpressing rat androgen-binding protein. *Reprod Biol Endocrinol* **1**:48

Johnsen SG (1978) Maintenance of spermatogenesis induced by HMG treatment by means of continuous HCG treatment in hypogonadotrophic men. *Acta Endocrinol (Copenh)* **89**:763–769

Johnson L, McKenzie KS, Snell JR (1996) Partial wave in human seminiferous tubules appears to be a random occurrence. *Tissue Cell* **28**:127–136

Johnston DS, Russell LD, Friel PJ, Griswold MD (2001) Murine germ cells do not require functional androgen receptors to complete spermatogenesis following spermatogonial stem cell transplantation. *Endocrinology* **142**:2405–2408

Johnston H, Baker PJ, Abel M, Charlton HM, Jackson G, Fleming L, Kumar TR, O'Shaughnessy PJ (2004) Regulation of Sertoli cell number and activity by follicle-stimulating hormone and androgen during postnatal development in the mouse. *Endocrinology* **145**:318–329

Kaitu'u-Lino TJ, Sluka P, Foo CF, Stanton PG (2007) Claudin-11 expression and localisation is regulated by androgens in rat Sertoli cells in vitro. *Reproduction* **133**:1169–1179

Kangasniemi M, Dodge K, Pemberton AE, Huhtaniemi I, Meistrich ML (1996) Suppression of mouse spermatogenesis by a gonadotropin-releasing hormone antagonist and antiandrogen: failure to protect against radiation-induced gonadal damage. *Endocrinology* **137**:949–955

Killian J, Pratis K, Clifton RJ, Stanton PG, Robertson DM, O'Donnell L (2003) 5alpha-reductase isoenzymes 1 and 2 in the rat testis during postnatal development. *Biol Reprod* **68**:1711–1718

Kinniburgh D, Anderson RA, Baird DT (2001) Suppression of spermatogenesis with desogestrel and testosterone pellets is not enhanced by addition of finasteride. *J Androl* **22**:88–95

Kolho KL, Huhtaniemi I (1989a) Neonatal treatment of male rats with a gonadotropin-releasing hormone antagonist results in altered function of the pituitary-testicular axis in adult age. *Biol Reprod* **41**:1084–1090

Kolho KL, Huhtaniemi I (1989b) Suppression of pituitary-testis function in rats treated neonatally with a gonadotrophin-releasing hormone agonist and antagonist: acute and long-term effects. *J Endocrinol* **123**:83–91

Kremer H, Kraaij R, Toledo SP, Post M, Fridman JB, Hayashida CY, van Reen M, Milgrom E, Ropers HH, Mariman E (1995) Male pseudohermaphroditism due to a homozygous missense mutation of the luteinizing hormone receptor gene. *Nat Genet* **9**:160–164

Lerchl A, Sotiriadou S, Behre HM, Pierce J, Weinbauer GF, Kliesch S, Nieschlag E (1993) Restoration of spermatogenesis by follicle-stimulating hormone despite low intratesticular testosterone in photoinhibited hypogonadotropic Djungarian hamsters

(Phodopus sungorus). *Biol Reprod* **49**:1108–1116

Lim P, Allan CM, Notini AJ, Axell AM, Spaliviero J, Jimenez M, Davey R, McManus J, MacLean HE, Zajac JD, Handelsman DJ (2008) Oestradiol-induced spermatogenesis requires a functional androgen receptor. *Reprod Fertil Dev* **20**:861–870

Lim P, Robson M, Spaliviero J, McTavish KJ, Jimenez M, Zajac JD, Handelsman DJ, Allan CM (2009) Sertoli cell androgen receptor DNA binding domain is essential for the completion of spermatogenesis. *Endocrinology* **150**:4755–4765

Lindsey JS, Wilkinson MF (1996) Pem: a testosterone- and LH-regulated homeobox gene expressed in mouse Sertoli cells and epididymis. *Dev Biol* **179**:471–484

Liu PY, Gebski VJ, Turner L, Conway AJ, Wishart SM, Handelsman DJ (2002) Predicting pregnancy and spermatogenesis by survival analysis during gonadotrophin treatment of gonadotrophin-deficient infertile men. *Hum Reprod* **17**:625–633

Liu PY, Swerdloff RS, Anawalt BD, Anderson RA, Bremner WJ, Elliesen J, Gu YQ, Kersemaekers WM, McLachlan RI, Meriggiola MC, Nieschlag E, Sitruk-Ware R, Vogelsong K, Wang XH, Wu FC, Zitzmann M, Handelsman DJ, Wang C (2008) Determinants of the rate and extent of spermatogenic suppression during hormonal male contraception: an integrated analysis. *J Clin Endocrinol Metab* **93**:1774–1783

Liu PY, Baker HW, Jayadev V, Zacharin M, Conway AJ, Handelsman DJ (2009) Induction of spermatogenesis and fertility during gonadotropin treatment of gonadotropin-deficient infertile men: predictors of fertility outcome. *J Clin Endocrinol Metab* **94**:801–808

Loss ES, Jacobsen M, Costa ZS, Jacobus AP, Borelli F, Wassermann GF (2004) Testosterone modulates K(+) ATP channels in Sertoli cell membrane via the PLC-PIP2 pathway. *Horm Metab Res* **36**:519–525

Lunn SF, Cowen GM, Fraser HM (1997) Blockade of the neonatal increase in testosterone by a GnRH antagonist: the free androgen index, reproductive capacity and postmortem findings in the male marmoset monkey. *J Endocrinol* **154**:125–131

Marshall GR, Wickings EJ, Lüdecke DK, Nieschlag E (1983) Stimulation of spermatogenesis in stalk-sectioned rhesus monkeys by testosterone alone. *J Clin Endocrinol Metab* **57**:152–159

Marshall GR, Wickings EJ, Nieschlag E (1984) Testosterone can initiate spermatogenesis in an immature nonhuman primate, Macaca fascicularis. *Endocrinology* **114**:2228–2233

Marshall GR, Jockenhövel F, Lüdecke D, Nieschlag E (1986) Maintenance of complete but quantitatively reduced spermatogenesis in hypophysectomized monkeys by testosterone alone. *Acta Endocrinol (Copenh)* **113**:424–431

Marshall GR, Zorub DS, Plant TM (1995) Follicle-stimulating hormone amplifies the population of differentiated spermatogonia in the hypophysectomized testosterone-replaced adult rhesus monkey (Macaca mulatta). *Endocrinology* **136**:3504–3511

Matsumoto AM, Bremner WJ (1985) Stimulation of sperm production by human chorionic gonadotropin after prolonged gonadotropin suppression in normal men. *J Androl* **6**:137–143

Matsumoto AM, Karpas AE, Paulsen CA, Bremner WJ (1983) Reinitiation of sperm production in gonadotropin-suppressed normal men by administration of follicle-stimulating hormone. *J Clin Invest* **72**:1005–1015

Matsumoto AM, Karpas AE, Bremner WJ (1986) Chronic human chorionic gonadotropin

administration in normal men: evidence that follicle-stimulating hormone is necessary for the maintenance of quantitatively normal spermatogenesis in man. *J Clin Endocrinol Metab* **62**:1184–1192

Matthiesson KL, Stanton PG, O'Donnell L, Meachem SJ, Amory JK, Berger R, Bremner WJ, McLachlan RI (2005) Effects of testosterone and levonorgestrel combined with a 5alpha-reductase inhibitor or gonadotropin-releasing hormone antagonist on spermatogenesis and intratesticular steroid levels in normal men. *J Clin Endocrinol Metab* **90**:5647–5655

Matthiesson KL, McLachlan RI, O'Donnell L, Frydenberg M, Robertson DM, Stanton PG, Meachem SJ (2006) The relative roles of follicle-stimulating hormone and luteinizing hormone in maintaining spermatogonial maturation and spermiation in normal men. *J Clin Endocrinol Metab* **91**:3962–3969

McConnell DS, Wang Q, Sluss PM, Bolf N, Khoury RH, Schneyer AL, Midgley AR Jr, Reame NE, Crowley WF Jr, Padmanabhan V (1998) A two-site chemiluminescent assay for activin-free follistatin reveals that most follistatin circulating in men and normal cycling women is in an activin-bound state. *J Clin Endocrinol Metab* **83**:851–858

McKinnell C, Saunders PT, Fraser HM, Kelnar CJ, Kivlin C, Morris KD, Sharpe RM (2001) Comparison of androgen receptor and oestrogen receptor beta immunoexpression in the testes of the common marmoset (Callithrix jacchus) from birth to adulthood: low androgen receptor immunoexpression in Sertoli cells during the neonatal increase in testosterone concentrations. *Reproduction* **122**:419–429

McLachlan RI, Wreford NG, Meachem SJ, De Kretser DM, Robertson DM (1994a) Effects of testosterone on spermatogenic cell populations

in the adult rat. *Biol Reprod* **51**:945–955

McLachlan RI, Wreford NG, Tsonis C, De Kretser DM, Robertson DM (1994b) Testosterone effects on spermatogenesis in the gonadotropin-releasing hormone-immunized rat. *Biol Reprod* **50**:271–280

McLachlan RI, McDonald J, Rushford D, Robertson DM, Garrett C, Baker HW (2000) Efficacy and acceptability of testosterone implants, alone or in combination with a 5alpha-reductase inhibitor, for male hormonal contraception. *Contraception* **62**:73–78

McLachlan RI, O'Donnell L, Stanton PG, Balourdos G, Frydenberg M, de Kretser DM, Robertson DM (2002a) Effects of testosterone plus medroxyprogesterone acetate on semen quality, reproductive hormones, and germ cell populations in normal young men. *J Clin Endocrinol Metab* **87**:546–556

McLachlan RI, O'Donnell L, Meachem SJ, Stanton PG, de Kretser DM, Pratis K, Robertson DM (2002b) Identification of specific sites of hormonal regulation in spermatogenesis in rats, monkeys, and man. *Recent Prog Horm Res* **57**:149–179

McLachlan RI, Robertson DM, Pruysers E, Ugoni A, Matsumoto AM, Anawalt BD, Bremner WJ, Meriggiola C (2004) Relationship between serum gonadotropins and spermatogenic suppression in men undergoing steroidal contraceptive treatment. *J Clin Endocrinol Metab* **89**:142–149

Meachem SJ, Wreford NG, Stanton PG, Robertson DM, McLachlan RI (1998) Follicle-stimulating hormone is required for the initial phase of spermatogenic restoration in adult rats following gonadotropin suppression. *J Androl* **19**:725–735

Means AR, Dedman JR, Tash JS, Tindall DJ, van Sickle M, Welsh MJ (1980) Regulation of the testis

Sertoli cell by follicle stimulating hormone. *Annu Rev Physiol* **42**:59–70

Meng J, Holdcraft RW, Shima JE, Griswold MD, Braun RE (2005) Androgens regulate the permeability of the blood-testis barrier. *Proc Natl Acad Sci USA* **102**:16696–16700

Meng J, Greenlee AR, Taub CJ, Braun RE (2011) Sertoli cell-specific deletion of the androgen receptor compromises testicular immune privilege in mice. *Biol Reprod* **85**:254–260

Meriggiola MC, Bremner WJ, Costantino A, Di Cintio G, Flamigni C (1998) Low dose of cyproterone acetate and testosterone enanthate for contraception in men. *Hum Reprod* **13**:1225–1229

Meriggiola MC, Costantino A, Bremner WJ, Morselli-Labate AM (2002) Higher testosterone dose impairs sperm suppression induced by a combined androgen-progestin regimen. *J Androl* **23**:684–690

Michel C, Gromoll J, Chandolia R, Luetjens CM, Wistuba J, Simoni M (2007) LHR splicing variants and gene expression in the marmoset monkey. *Mol Cell Endocrinol* **279**:9–15

Morse HC, Horike N, Rowley MJ, Heller CG (1973) Testosterone concentrations in testes of normal men: effects of testosterone propionate administration. *J Clin Endocrinol Metab* **37**:882–886

Moudgal NR, Sairam MR, Krishnamurthy HN, Sridhar S, Krishnamurthy H, Khan H (1997) Immunization of male bonnet monkeys (M. radiata) with a recombinant FSH receptor preparation affects testicular function and fertility. *Endocrinology* **138**:3065–3068

Narula A, Gu YQ, O'Donnell L, Stanton PG, Robertson DM, McLachlan RI, Bremner WJ (2002) Variability in sperm suppression during testosterone administration to adult monkeys is related to follicle stimulating hormone suppression and not to intratesticular androgens. *J Clin Endocrinol Metab* **87**:3399–3406

Nicholls PK, Harrison CA, Walton KL, McLachlan RI, O'Donnell L, Stanton PG (2011) Hormonal regulation of Sertoli cell micro-RNAs at spermiation. *Endocrinology* **152**:1670–1683

Nieschlag E, Simoni M, Gromoll J, Weinbauer GF (1999) Role of FSH in the regulation of spermatogenesis: clinical aspects. *Clin Endocrinol (Oxf)* **51**:139–146

O'Donnell L, McLachlan RI, Wreford NG, Robertson DM (1994) Testosterone promotes the conversion of round spermatids between stages VII and VIII of the rat spermatogenic cycle. *Endocrinology* **135**:2608–2614

O'Donnell L, Stanton PG, Wreford NG, Robertson DM, McLachlan RI (1996a) Inhibition of 5 alpha-reductase activity impairs the testosterone-dependent restoration of spermiogenesis in adult rats. *Endocrinology* **137**:2703–2710

O'Donnell L, McLachlan RI, Wreford NG, de Kretser DM, Robertson DM (1996b) Testosterone withdrawal promotes stage-specific detachment of round spermatids from the rat seminiferous epithelium. *Biol Reprod* **55**:895–901

O'Donnell L, Pratis K, Stanton PG, Robertson DM, McLachlan RI (1999) Testosterone-dependent restoration of spermatogenesis in adult rats is impaired by a 5alpha-reductase inhibitor. *J Androl* **20**:109–117

O'Donnell L, Narula A, Balourdos G, Gu YQ, Wreford NG, Robertson DM, Bremner WJ, McLachlan RI (2001a) Impairment of spermatogonial development and spermiation after testosterone-induced gonadotropin suppression in adult monkeys (Macaca fascicularis). *J Clin Endocrinol Metab* **86**:1814–1822

O'Donnell L, Robertson KM, Jones ME, Simpson ER (2001b) Estrogen and spermatogenesis. *Endocr Rev* **22**:289–318

O'Donnell L, Meachem SJ, Stanton PG, McLachlan RI (2006) Endocrine regulation of spermatogenesis. In: Neill JD (ed) *Knobil and Neill's Physiology of Reproduction*, 3rd edn. Elsevier, San Diego, CA, pp 1017–1069

O'Donnell L, Pratis K, Wagenfeld A, Gottwald U, Muller J, Leder G, McLachlan RI, Stanton PG (2009) Transcriptional profiling of the hormone-responsive stages of spermatogenesis reveals cell-, stage-, and hormone-specific events. *Endocrinology* **150**:5074–5084

O'Donnell L, Nicholls PK, O'Bryan MK, McLachlan RI, Stanton PG (2011) Spermiation: the process of sperm release. *Spermatogenesis* **1**:14–35

O'Shaughnessy PJ, Morris ID, Huhtaniemi I, Baker PJ, Abel MH (2009) Role of androgen and gonadotrophins in the development and function of the Sertoli cells and Leydig cells: data from mutant and genetically modified mice. *Mol Cell Endocrinol* **306**:2–8

O'Shaughnessy PJ, Verhoeven G, De Gendt K, Monteiro A, Abel MH (2010a) Direct action through the Sertoli cells is essential for androgen stimulation of spermatogenesis. *Endocrinology* **151**:2343–2348

O'Shaughnessy PJ, Monteiro A, Verhoeven G, De Gendt K, Abel MH (2010b) Effect of FSH on testicular morphology and spermatogenesis in gonadotrophin-deficient hypogonadal mice lacking androgen receptors. *Reproduction* **139**:177–184

Pakarainen T, Zhang FP, Makela S, Poutanen M, Huhtaniemi I (2005) Testosterone replacement therapy induces spermatogenesis and partially restores fertility in luteinizing hormone receptor knockout mice. *Endocrinology* **146**:596–606

Pitteloud N, Dwyer AA, DeCruz S, Lee H, Boepple PA, Crowley WF Jr, Hayes FJ (2008) The relative role of gonadal sex steroids and gonadotropin-releasing hormone pulse frequency in the regulation of follicle-stimulating hormone secretion in men. *J Clin Endocrinol Metab* 93:2686–2692

Pratis K, O'Donnell L, Ooi GT, Stanton PG, McLachlan RI, Robertson DM (2003) Differential regulation of rat testicular 5alpha-reductase type 1 and 2 isoforms by testosterone and FSH. *J Endocrinol* 176:393–403

Ramaswamy S, Pohl CR, McNeilly AS, Winters SJ, Plant TM (1998) The time course of follicle-stimulating hormone suppression by recombinant human inhibin A in the adult male rhesus monkey (Macaca mulatta). *Endocrinology* 139:3409–3415

Rannikko A, Penttila TL, Zhang FP, Toppari J, Parvinen M, Huhtaniemi I (1996) Stage-specific expression of the FSH receptor gene in the prepubertal and adult rat seminiferous epithelium. *J Endocrinol* 151:29–35

Re M, Micali F, Santoro L, Cuomo M, Racheli T, Scapellato F, Iannitelli M (1979) Histological characteristics of the human testis after long-term treatment with cyproterone acetate. *Arch Androl* 3:263–268

Ren HP, Russell LD (1991) Clonal development of interconnected germ cells in the rat and its relationship to the segmental and subsegmental organization of spermatogenesis. *Am J Anat* 192:121–128

Robertson DM, Pruysers E, Stephenson T, Pettersson K, Morton S, McLachlan RI (2001) Sensitive LH and FSH assays for monitoring low serum levels in men undergoing steroidal contraception. *Clin Endocrinol (Oxf)* 55:331–339

Robertson KM, O'Donnell L, Jones ME, Meachem SJ, Boon WC, Fisher CR, Graves KH, McLachlan RI,

Simpson ER (1999) Impairment of spermatogenesis in mice lacking a functional aromatase (cyp 19) gene. *Proc Natl Acad Sci USA* 96: 7986–7991

Robertson KM, O'Donnell L, Simpson ER, Jones ME (2002) The phenotype of the aromatase knockout mouse reveals dietary phytoestrogens impact significantly on testis function. *Endocrinology* 143: 2913 2921

Roth MY, Lin K, Amory JK, Matsumoto AM, Anawalt BD, Snyder CN, Kalhorn TF, Bremner WJ, Page ST (2010a) Serum LH correlates highly with intratesticular steroid levels in normal men. *J Androl* 31:138–145

Roth MY, Page ST, Lin K, Anawalt BD, Matsumoto AM, Snyder CN, Marck BT, Bremner WJ, Amory JK (2010b) Dose-dependent increase in intratesticular testosterone by very low-dose human chorionic gonadotropin in normal men with experimental gonadotropin deficiency. *J Clin Endocrinol Metab* 95:3806–3813

Roth MY, Page ST, Lin K, Anawalt BD, Matsumoto AM, Marck B, Bremner WJ, Amory JK (2011) The effect of gonadotropin withdrawal and stimulation with human chorionic gonadotropin on intratesticular androstenedione and DHEA in normal men. *J Clin Endocrinol Metab* 96:1175–1181

Russell LD, Clermont Y (1977) Degeneration of germ cells in normal, hypophysectomized and hormone treated hypophysectomized rats. *Anat Rec* 187:347–366

Russell LD, Ettlin RA, Sinha Hikim AP, Clegg ED (1990) *Histological and Histopathological Evaluation of the Testis*. Cache River Press, Clearwater, FL

Ruwanpura SM, McLachlan RI, Meachem SJ (2010) Hormonal regulation of male germ cell development. *J Endocrinol* 205:117–131

Saito K, O'Donnell L, McLachlan RI, Robertson DM (2000) Spermiation failure is a major contributor to early spermatogenic suppression caused by hormone withdrawal in adult rats. *Endocrinology* 141:2779–2785

Schauwaers K, De Gendt K, Saunders PT, Atanassova N, Haelens A, Callewaert L, Moehren U, Swinnen JV, Verhoeven G, Verrijdt G, Claessens F (2007) Loss of androgen receptor binding to selective androgen response elements causes a reproductive phenotype in a knockin mouse model. *Proc Natl Acad Sci USA* 104:4961–4966

Schlatt S, Weinbauer GF, Arslan M, Nieschlag E (1993) Appearance of alpha-smooth muscle actin in peritubular cells of monkey testes is induced by androgens, modulated by follicle-stimulating hormone, and maintained after hormonal withdrawal. *J Androl* 14:340–350

Schulze W, Rehder U (1984) Organization and morphogenesis of the human seminiferous epithelium. *Cell Tissue Res* 237:395–407

Sharpe RM, McKinnell C, Kivlin C, Fisher JS (2003) Proliferation and functional maturation of Sertoli cells, and their relevance to disorders of testis function in adulthood. *Reproduction* 125:769–784

Shenker A, Laue L, Kosugi S, Merendino JJ Jr, Minegishi T, Cutler GB Jr (1993) A constitutively activating mutation of the luteinizing hormone receptor in familial male precocious puberty. *Nature* 365:652–654

Shetty G, Wilson G, Huhtaniemi I, Boettger-Tong H, Meistrich ML (2001) Testosterone inhibits spermatogonial differentiation in juvenile spermatogonial depletion mice. *Endocrinology* 142:2789–2795

Shupe J, Cheng J, Puri P, Kostereva N, Walker WH (2011) Regulation of Sertoli-germ cell adhesion and sperm release by FSH and nonclassical testosterone signaling. *Mol Endocrinol* **25**:238–252

Singh J, O'Neill C, Handelsman DJ (1995) Induction of spermatogenesis by androgens in gonadotropin-deficient (hpg) mice. *Endocrinology* **136**:5311–5321

Sinha Hikim AP, Swerdloff RS (1999) Hormonal and genetic control of germ cell apoptosis in the testis. *Rev Reprod* **4**:38–47

Sinkevicius KW, Laine M, Lotan TL, Woloszyn K, Richburg JH, Greene GL (2009) Estrogen-dependent and-independent estrogen receptor-alpha signaling separately regulate male fertility. *Endocrinology* **150**:2898–2905

Sjogren K, Liu JL, Blad K, Skrtic S, Vidal O, Wallenius V, LeRoith D, Tornell J, Isaksson OG, Jansson JO, Ohlsson C (1999) Liver-derived insulin-like growth factor I (IGF-I) is the principal source of IGF-I in blood but is not required for postnatal body growth in mice. *Proc Natl Acad Sci USA* **96**:7088–7092

Spiteri-Grech J, Weinbauer GF, Bolze P, Chandolia RK, Bartlett JM, Nieschlag E (1993) Effects of FSH and testosterone on intratesticular insulin-like growth factor-I and specific germ cell populations in rats treated with gonadotrophin-releasing hormone antagonist. *J Endocrinol* **137**:81–89

Suarez-Quian CA, Martinez-Garcia F, Nistal M, Regadera J (1999) Androgen receptor distribution in adult human testis. *J Clin Endocrinol Metab* **84**:350–358

Sun YT, Wreford NG, Robertson DM, de Kretser DM (1990) Quantitative cytological studies of spermatogenesis in intact and hypophysectomized rats: identification of androgen-dependent stages. *Endocrinology* **127**:1215–1223

Sykiotis GP, Hoang XH, Avbelj M, Hayes FJ, Thambundit A, Dwyer A, Au M, Plummer L, Crowley WF Jr, Pitteloud N (2010) Congenital idiopathic hypogonadotropic hypogonadism: evidence of defects in the hypothalamus, pituitary, and testes. *J Clin Endocrinol Metab* **95**:3019–3027

Tan KA, De Gendt K, Atanassova N, Walker M, Sharpe RM, Saunders PT, Denolet E, Verhoeven G (2005) The role of androgens in Sertoli cell proliferation and functional maturation: studies in mice with total or Sertoli cell-selective ablation of the androgen receptor. *Endocrinology* **146**:2674–2683

Timmons PM, Rigby PW, Poirier F (2002) The murine seminiferous epithelial cycle is pre-figured in the Sertoli cells of the embryonic testis. *Development* **129**:635–647

Tsai MY, Yeh SD, Wang RS, Yeh S, Zhang C, Lin HY, Tzeng CR, Chang C (2006) Differential effects of spermatogenesis and fertility in mice lacking androgen receptor in individual testis cells. *Proc Natl Acad Sci USA* **103**:18975–18980

van Alphen MM, van de Kant HJ, de Rooij DG (1988) Repopulation of the seminiferous epithelium of the rhesus monkey after X irradiation. *Radiat Res* **113**:487–500

van Alphen MM, van de Kant HJ, de Rooij DG (1989) Protection from radiation-induced damage of spermatogenesis in the rhesus monkey (*Macaca mulatta*) by follicle-stimulating hormone. *Cancer Res* **49**:533–536

Van Roijen JH, Van Assen S, Van Der Kwast TH, De Rooij DG, Boersma WJ, Vreeburg JT, Weber RF (1995) Androgen receptor immunoexpression in the testes of subfertile men. *J Androl* **16**:510–516

Veldhuis JD, Iranmanesh A, Samojlik E, Urban RJ (1997) Differential sex steroid negative feedback regulation of pulsatile follicle-stimulating hormone secretion in healthy older men: deconvolution analysis and steady-state sex-steroid hormone infusions in frequently sampled healthy older individuals. *J Clin Endocrinol Metab* **82**:1248–1254

Vicari E, Mongioi A, Calogero AE, Moncada ML, Sidoti G, Polosa P, D'Agata R (1992) Therapy with human chorionic gonadotrophin alone induces spermatogenesis in men with isolated hypogonadotrophic hypogonadism – long-term follow-up. *Int J Androl* **15**:320–329

Walker WH (2009) Molecular mechanisms of testosterone action in spermatogenesis. *Steroids* **74**:602–607

Walker WH (2010) Non-classical actions of testosterone and spermatogenesis. *Philos Trans R Soc Lond B Biol Sci* **365**:1557–1569

Walker WH, Cheng J (2005) FSH and testosterone signaling in Sertoli cells. *Reproduction* **130**:15–28

Wang RS, Yeh S, Tzeng CR, Chang C (2009) Androgen receptor roles in spermatogenesis and fertility: lessons from testicular cell-specific androgen receptor knockout mice. *Endocr Rev* **30**:119–132

Weinbauer GF, Nieschlag E (1996) The Leydig cell as a target for male contraception. In: Payne AH, Hardy MP, Russell LD (eds). *The Leydig Cell.* Cache River Press, Vienna, IL, pp 629–662

Weinbauer GF, Behre HM, Fingscheidt U, Nieschlag E (1991) Human follicle-stimulating hormone exerts a stimulatory effect on spermatogenesis, testicular size, and serum inhibin levels in the gonadotropin-releasing hormone antagonist-treated nonhuman primate (*Macaca fascicularis*). *Endocrinology* **129**:1831–1839

Weinbauer GF, Aslam H, Krishnamurthy H, Brinkworth MH, Einspanier A, Hodges JK (2001) Quantitative analysis of spermatogenesis and apoptosis in the common marmoset (*Callithrix jacchus*) reveals high rates of spermatogonial turnover and high spermatogenic efficiency. *Biol Reprod* **64**:120–126

Welsh M, Saunders PT, Atanassova N, Sharpe RM, Smith LB (2009) Androgen action via testicular peritubular myoid cells is essential for male fertility. *FASEB J* 23: 4218–4230

Welsh M, Sharpe RM, Moffat L, Atanassova N, Saunders PT, Kilter S, Bergh A, Smith LB (2010) Androgen action via testicular arteriole smooth muscle cells is important for Leydig cell function, vasomotion and testicular fluid dynamics. *PLoS One* 5:e13632

Wilson JD (1992) Syndromes of androgen resistance. *Biol Reprod* 46:168–173

Wilson JD, Leihy MW, Shaw G, Renfree MB (2003) Unsolved problems in male physiology: studies in a marsupial. *Mol Cell Endocrinol* 211:33–36

Wistuba J, Schrod A, Greve B, Hodges JK, Aslam H, Weinbauer GF, Luetjens CM (2003) Organization of seminiferous epithelium in primates: relationship to spermatogenic efficiency, phylogeny, and mating system. *Biol Reprod* 69:582–591

Wreford NG (1995) Theory and practice of stereological techniques applied to the estimation of cell number and nuclear volume in the testis. *Microsc Res Tech* 32: 423–436

Wreford NG, Rajendra Kumar T, Matzuk MM, de Kretser DM (2001)

Analysis of the testicular phenotype of the Follicle-Stimulating Hormone β-subunit knockout and the activin type II receptor knockout mice by stereological analysis. *Endocrinology* 142:2916–2920

Zhang FP, Rannikko AS, Manna PR, Fraser HM, Huhtaniemi IT (1997) Cloning and functional expression of the luteinizing hormone receptor complementary deoxyribonucleic acid from the marmoset monkey testis: absence of sequences encoding exon 10 in other species. *Endocrinology* 138:2481–2490

Zhang FP, Kero J, Huhtaniemi I (1998) The unique exon 10 of the human luteinizing hormone receptor is necessary for expression of the receptor protein at the plasma membrane in the human luteinizing hormone receptor, but deleterious when inserted into the human follicle-stimulating hormone receptor. *Mol Cell Endocrinol* 142:165–174

Zhang FP, Poutanen M, Wilbertz J, Huhtaniemi I (2001) Normal prenatal but arrested postnatal sexual development of luteinizing hormone receptor knockout (LuRKO) mice. *Mol Endocrinol* 15:172–183

Zhang FP, Pakarainen T, Poutanen M, Toppari J, Huhtaniemi I (2003) The low gonadotropin-independent

constitutive production of testicular testosterone is sufficient to maintain spermatogenesis. *Proc Natl Acad Sci USA* 100:13692–13697

Zhao M, Baker SD, Yan X, Zhao Y, Wright WW, Zirkin BR, Jarow JP (2004) Simultaneous determination of steroid composition of human testicular fluid using liquid chromatography tandem mass spectrometry. *Steroids* 69:721–726

Zhengwei Y, Wreford NG, Royce P, de Kretser DM, McLachlan RI (1998) Stereological evaluation of human spermatogenesis after suppression by testosterone treatment: heterogeneous pattern of spermatogenic impairment. *J Clin Endocrinol Metab* 83:1284–1291

Zhou ZX, Lane MV, Kemppainen JA, French FS, Wilson EM (1995) Specificity of ligand-dependent androgen receptor stabilization: receptor domain interactions influence ligand dissociation and receptor stability. *Mol Endocrinol* 9:208–218

Zirkin BR (1998) Spermatogenesis: its regulation by testosterone and FSH. *Semin Cell Dev Biol* 9:417–421

Zirkin BR, Santulli R, Awoniyi CA, Ewing LL (1989) Maintenance of advanced spermatogenic cells in the adult rat testis: quantitative relationship to testosterone concentration within the testis. *Endocrinology* 124:3043–3049

Androgens and hair: a biological paradox with clinical consequences

Valerie Anne Randall

7.1 Introduction

Hair growth plays important roles in human social and sexual communication. People throughout the world classify a person's state of health, sex, sexual maturity and age, often subconsciously, by assessing their scalp and body hair. Hair's importance is seen in many social customs in different cultures. Hair removal generally has a strong depersonalizing effect, such as shaving the heads of soldiers, prisoners and Buddhist or Christian monks. In contrast, long hair often has positive connotations, like Samson's strength in the Bible and the uncut hair of Sikhs. Body hair is also involved; for example, the widespread customs of daily shaving of men's beards and women's axillary hair in Northern Europe and the USA. Therefore, we should not be surprised that hair growth abnormalities, either more or less than "normal," even common male pattern baldness, cause widespread psychological distress.

Androgens are the most obvious regulators of human hair growth. Although hair with a major protective role, such as the eyelashes, eyebrows and scalp hair, is produced by children in the absence of androgens, the formation of long pigmented hair on the axillae, pubis, face etc. needs androgens in both

Testosterone: Action, Deficiency, Substitution, ed. Eberhard Nieschlag and Hermann M. Behre, Assoc. ed. Susan Nieschlag. Published by Cambridge University Press. © Cambridge University Press 2012.

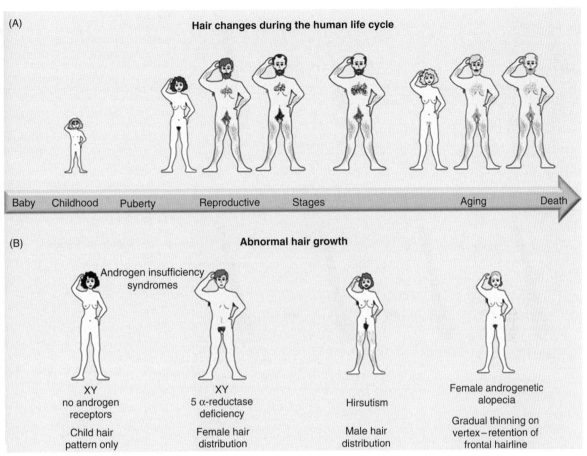

Fig. 7.1 Human hair varies with life stage and endocrine state. (A) Changes in hair distribution and color signal a person's age, state of maturity and sex. Visible (i.e. terminal) hair with protective functions normally develops in children on the scalp, eyelashes and eyebrows. Once puberty occurs, more terminal hair develops on the axilla and pubis in both sexes, and on the face, chest, limbs and often back in men. Androgens also stimulate hair loss from the scalp in men with the appropriate genes in a patterned manner, causing androgenetic alopecia. As age increases hair follicles lose their ability to make pigment, causing graying (canities). (B) People with various androgen insufficiency syndromes demonstrate that none of this occurs without functional androgen receptors and that only axillary and female pattern of lower pubic triangle hairs are formed in the absence of 5α-reductase type 2. Male pattern hair growth (hirsutism) occurs in women with abnormalities of plasma androgens or from idiopathic causes, and women may also develop a different form of hair loss, female androgenetic alopecia or female pattern hair loss (FPHL). See plate section for color version.

sexes. In contrast, androgens may also inhibit hair growth on the scalp, causing baldness (Figs. 7.1 and 7.2). How one type of hormone can simultaneously cause these contradictory effects in the same tissue in different body sites within one person is a unique endocrinological paradox. The hair follicle has another exciting characteristic. It is the only tissue in the adult body which can regenerate itself, often producing a new hair with different features. This is how androgens can cause such major changes.

Over the last 20 years, there has been much interest in the hair follicle, promoted by the discovery that the antihypertensive drug, minoxidil, could

sometimes stimulate hair growth, and the recognition of its regenerative capacity. However, we still know relatively little about the precise functioning of this complex cell biological system. On the other hand, our increased understanding of how androgens work in the follicle has enabled the treatment of female hirsutism with antiandrogens, such as cyproterone acetate, and the 5α-reductase type 2 inhibitor, finasteride, developed to regulate prostate disorders, is now available in many countries for use in male pattern baldness. Greater understanding of hair follicle biology may also enable the development of further approaches to treatment in the future.

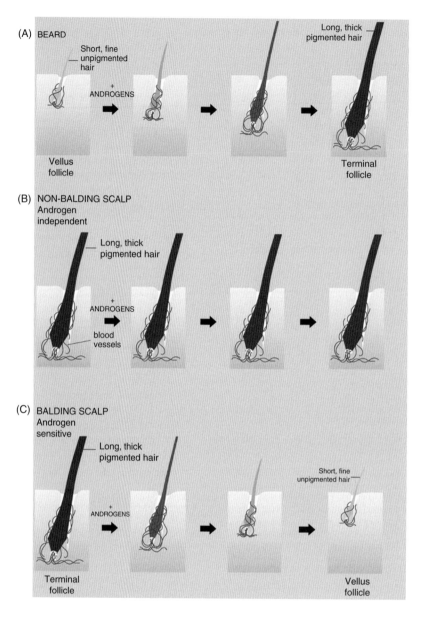

Fig. 7.2 Androgens have paradoxically different effects on human hair follicles depending on their body site. (A) During and after puberty, androgens stimulate the gradual transformation of small follicles producing tiny, virtually colorless, *vellus* hairs, to terminal follicles producing longer, thicker and more pigmented hairs. These changes involve passing through the hair cycle (see Fig. 7.3). (B) At the same time, many follicles on the scalp and eyelashes continue to produce the same type of hairs, apparently unaffected by androgens. (C) In complete contrast, androgens may inhibit follicles on specific areas of the scalp in genetically susceptible individuals, causing the reverse transformation of terminal follicles to *vellus* ones, and androgenetic alopecia. (Diagram reproduced from Randall 2000a.) See plate section for color version.

People have been intrigued by the changes in hair growth during a person's life (see Fig. 7.1) for thousands of years, with Aristotle first recognizing the connection between beard growth and the testes (reviewed by Randall 2003). This chapter will cover our current knowledge of the structure and function of hair follicles, their responses to androgens, the mechanism of action of androgens in the follicle, and current modes of controlling androgen-potentiated hair disorders.

7.2 Structure and function of the hair follicle

7.2.1 The roles of human hair

Hairs cover almost the entire body surface of human beings except for the soles of the feet, palms of the hands and the lips. They are fully keratinized tubes of dead epithelial cells where they project outside the skin. They taper to a point, but otherwise are

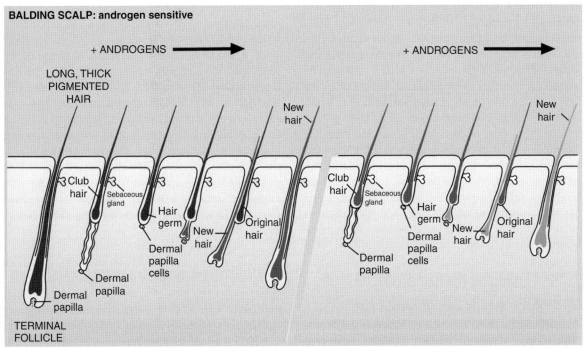

Fig. 7.3 Androgen inhibition of hair size on the scalp leads to balding. Hair follicles pass through regular cycles of growth (anagen), regression (catagen), rest (telogen) and hair shedding during which the lower part of the follicle is regenerated. This enables the follicle to produce a different type of hair in response to hormonal stimuli to coordinate to changes in the body's development, e.g. sexual maturity or seasonal climate changes. Androgens inhibit follicles on specific areas of the scalp in genetically susceptible individuals, causing the regenerated follicles to be smaller, protrude less into the dermis and produce smaller, less-pigmented hairs. Eventually the terminal hairs of childhood and early adulthood are replaced by the vellus hairs of androgenetic alopecia, and the area appears bald. Follicles must pass through a full hair cycle, probably a succession of cycles, to accomplish major changes. (Diagram reproduced from Randall 2010.) See plate section for color version.

extremely variable in length, thickness, color and cross-sectional shape. These differences occur between individuals, e.g. blonde, red or dark haired people, and between specific body areas within one individual, such as the long, thick scalp and beard hairs and the short, fine ones on the back of the hand. Changes also occur in some areas within an individual at different stages of their life; e.g. darker, thicker and longer beard hairs replace the fine, short, almost colorless hairs on a boy's face after puberty (Fig. 7.1).

The main functions of mammalian hair are insulation and camouflage. These are no longer necessary for the "naked ape," although vestiges remain in the seasonal patterns of our hair growth (Randall and Ebling 1991) and the erection of our body hairs when shivering with cold (goosebumps). Mammals often have hairs specialized as neuroreceptors, e.g. whiskers, and this remains, slightly, in human body hair, with its good nerve supply. However, the main functions of human hair are protection and communication.

Eyelashes and eyebrow hairs prevent substances entering the eyes, and head hair protects the scalp and back of the neck from sun damage during our upright posture. During puberty the development of axillary and pubic hair signals the beginning of sexual maturity in both sexes (Marshall and Tanner 1969; Winter and Faiman 1972; 1973), while a man's beard readily distinguishes the sexes (Jansen and Van Baalen 2006), like the mane of the lion (Fig. 7.1).

7.2.2 Structure of the hair follicle

Each hair is produced by a hair follicle; the biology of the hair follicle was reviewed recently by Randall and Botchkareva (2009). Hair follicles are cylindrical, epithelial down-growths from the epidermis into the dermis and subcutaneous fat, which enlarge at the base into a hair bulb surrounding the tear-shaped, mesenchyme-derived dermal papilla (Fig. 7.3). The dermal papilla, containing specialized fibroblast-like cells in an extracellular matrix, regulates many aspects of hair growth (Reynolds and Jahoda 2004). Hairs are produced by epithelial cell division in the hair bulb; the keratinocytes move upwards, differentiating into the various layers of the follicle. The central portion forms the hair itself, the color of which is produced by pigment donated by the follicular melanocytes in the hair bulb. By the time it reaches the surface the cells are fully keratinized and dead. Each hair is surrounded by two multi-layered epithelial sheaths: the inner root sheath, which helps it move through the skin and which disintegrates when level with the sebaceous gland, and the outer root sheath, which becomes continuous with the epidermis, completing the skin's protective barrier (Fig. 7.3). Cell division continues until the hair reaches the appropriate length for its body site.

7.2.3 Changing the hair produced by a follicle via the hair growth cycle

To fulfill all its roles, the type of hair produced by a follicle often needs to change. Follicles possess a unique mechanism for this: the hair growth cycle (Kligman 1959; Fig. 7.3). This involves destruction of the original lower follicle and its regeneration to form another which can produce a hair with different characteristics. Thus postnatal follicles retain the ability to recapitulate the later stages of follicular embryogenesis throughout life, a unique characteristic in adults. Exactly how differently sized a hair can be to its immediate predecessor is currently unclear because many changes, like producing a full beard (Hamilton 1958) or androgenetic alopecia (Hamilton 1951a), take several years.

Hairs are produced in *anagen*, the growth phase. Once a hair reaches its full length, a short apoptosis-driven involution phase, *catagen*, occurs, where cell division and pigmentation stops, and the hair becomes fully keratinized with a swollen "club" end and moves up in the skin with the regressed dermal papilla. After a period of rest, *telogen*, the dermal papilla cells and associated keratinocyte stem cells reactivate, and a new lower follicle develops downwards, guided by the dermal sheath which surrounded the previous follicle. The new hair then grows up into the original upper follicle (Fig. 7.3). The existing hair is generally lost; although previously believed due to the new hair's upward movement, a further active shedding stage, *exogen*, is now recognized (Higgins *et al.* 2009).

Hair follicle regeneration is characterized by dramatic changes in microanatomy and cellular activity which are still not fully understood. Hair follicle transition between the hair cycle stages is governed by epithelial–mesenchymal interactions between the follicular keratinocytes and the dermal papilla cells. Cell fate during hair follicle growth and involution is controlled by numerous growth regulators. During active growth and hair production, factors promoting proliferation, differentiation and survival predominate, including WNT5a, SCF, HGF, FGF7 and IGF-1, while hair follicle regression is characterized by activation of various signaling pathways that induce apoptosis (Botchkareva and Kishimoto 2003; Botchkareva *et al.* 2006).

The epithelial stem cells necessary to synthesize a new hair have been identified in the bulge region of the outer root sheath below the sebaceous gland (Cotsarelis *et al.* 1990; Hsu *et al.* 2011). The bulge contains stem cells with a wide potency, which are able to replace cells of the epidermis and sebaceous glands as well as the hair follicle (Waters *et al.* 2007; Shimomura and Christiano 2010), and is also associated with the melanocyte stem cells (Nishimura 2011) and nestin-expressing stem cells which can produce nerve cell lineages (Lui *et al.* 2011). Recently Rabbani *et al.* (2011) have shown coordinated activation of epithelial and melanocyte stem cells in the bulge. Our understanding of this aspect of hair follicle activity has expanded dramatically and is the focus of much attention with the aim of developing the hair follicle as a stem cell source for regenerative medicine.

The processes of the hair growth cycle allow the follicle to replace the hair with a new one which may resemble the original or may be larger, smaller and/or a different color depending on the environment or stage of a mammal's maturity (Fig. 7.3). Changes in hair length involve alterations in the length of *anagen*. This can range from two to three years or more on the head, to produce long scalp hair (Kligman 1959), to only about two months for the short hairs on the finger (Saitoh and Sakamoto 1970). These changes are coordinated by the pineal-hypophysis-pituitary system (Ebling *et al.* 1991; Randall 2007). Coordination to the environment is particularly important for some mammals, such as mountain hares, which need a longer, warmer and white coat in the snowy winter, but a shorter, brown coat in the summer to increase their chances of survival (Flux 1970). Human beings from temperate regions also exhibit seasonal changes n both scalp (Orentreich 1969; Randall and Ebling 1991; Courtois *et al.* 1996) and body hair (Randall and Ebling 1991), in line with seasonal changes in melatonin, prolactin and cortisol secretion (Wehr 1998; Wehr *et al.* 2001). The main change in human hair growth is the production of adult patterns of body hair growth after puberty, like the male lion's mane, in response to androgen (Fig. 7.2); some seasonal fluctuations in human body hair growth may also coordinate at least in part to those of androgens (Randall and Ebling 1991; Randall 2008).

These annual seasonal changes are important for any investigations of androgen-dependent or scalp hair growth, particularly in individuals living in temperate zones. For example, scalp hair loss may be exacerbated during the increased autumnal shedding in both male and female patients. This has particularly important implications for any assessments of new therapies or treatments to stimulate, inhibit or remove hair; to be accurate, measurements need to be carried out over a year to avoid natural seasonal variations (Randall 2008).

7.3 The paradoxical effects of androgens on human hair growth

7.3.1 Human hair growth before and after puberty

In utero the human body is covered with quite long, colorless *lanugo* hairs. These are shed before birth and at birth, or shortly after; babies normally exhibit pigmented, quite thick protective hairs on the eyebrows and eyelashes and variable amounts on the scalp, and by the age of three or four the scalp hair is usually quite well developed, though it will not yet have reached its maximum length. These readily visible pigmented hairs are known as *terminal* hairs and are formed by large deep *terminal* follicles (Fig. 7.2). This emphasizes that terminal hair growth on the scalp, eyelashes and eyebrows is not androgen dependent. The "hairless" rest of the body is normally covered with fine, short almost colorless *vellus hairs* produced by small, short *vellus* follicles (Fig. 7.2). The molecular mechanisms involved in the distribution and formation of the different types of follicles during embryogenesis are not clear, but secreted signaling factors such as Sonic hedgehog, WNT and growth factors (e.g. the EGF and FGF families), nuclear factors including various homeobox genes and others

such as *Hairless* and *Tabby*, plus transmembrane molecules and extracellular matrix molecules have all been implicated in the mesenchymal–epithelial interactions (Rendl *et al.* 2005).

One of the first signs of puberty is the gradual appearance of a few larger and more pigmented *intermediate* hairs, first in the pubic region and later in the axillae. Intermediate-sized hair follicles have recently been characterized on the face (Miranda *et al.* 2010). These are replaced by longer and darker terminal hairs (Fig. 7.2), and the area spreads. In boys, similar changes occur gradually on the face starting above the mouth and on the central chin, eventually generally spreading over the lower part of the face and parts of the neck, readily distinguishing the adult male (Marshall and Tanner 1969; 1970). Adult men's pubic hair distribution also differs from women's, extending in a diamond shape up to the navel in contrast to women's inverted triangle. Terminal hair on the chest and sometimes the back is also normally restricted to men, though both sexes may also develop intermediate terminal hairs on their arms and legs, with terminal hairs normally restricted to the lower limbs in women (Fig. 7.1). In all areas the responses are gradual, often taking many years. Beard weight increases dramatically during puberty, but continues to rise until the mid-thirties (Hamilton 1958); while terminal hair growth on the chest and in the external ear canal may be first seen many years after puberty (Hamilton 1946).

The amount of body hair is very variable and differs both between families within one race and between races, with Caucasians generally exhibiting more than Japanese (Hamilton 1958). This implicates a genetically determined response to circulating triggers. The responses of the follicles themselves also vary, with female hormone levels being sufficient to stimulate terminal hair growth in the pubis and axillae, but male hormones being required for other areas, such as the beard and chest. Beard hair growth also remains high, even after 70, while axillary growth is maximal in the mid-twenties and falls quite rapidly then in both sexes (Hamilton 1958). This also seems paradoxical; markedly different responses in the two areas, although both respond to apparently similar stimulation by androgens.

During early puberty the frontal hair line is usually straight across the top of the forehead. With increasing age there is frequently a progressive regression of the frontal hair line in a prescribed

(A)

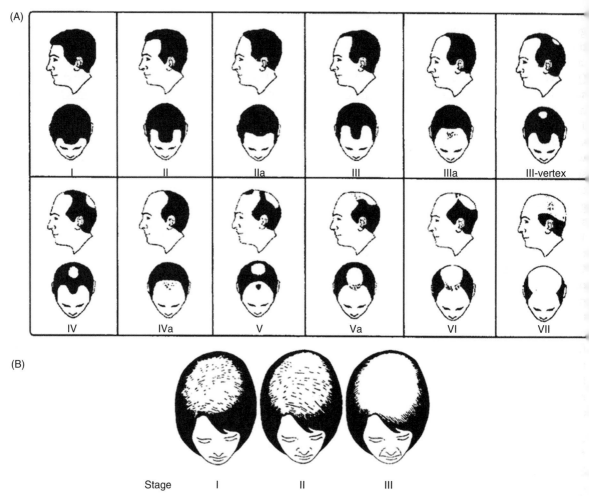

(B)

Stage   I   II   III

Fig. 7.4 Patterns of hair loss in androgenetic alopecia in men and women differ. Androgens cause a gradual inhibition of hair growth on the scalp in genetically predisposed individuals. This is much more common in men than in women, and the pattern of the hair loss in men (A Hamilton 1951a) differs from that in women (B; Ludwig 1977). In men, the first signs are generally temporal regression, which spreads backwards and joins thinning regions on the vertex to give a bald crown. In women, the front hairline is normally retained, and a general thinning on the vertex gradually becomes more pronounced until the vertex becomes bald. It is also less clear whether androgens are actually involved in women.

manner (described below in Section 7.5.1), accompanied by progressive thinning of terminal hair on the vertex (Fig. 7.4). This is characterized by a gradual inhibition of terminal follicles to smaller vellus follicles (Fig. 7.3), with the length of anagen decreasing and that of telogen increasing. This is an example of a much more dramatic biological paradox. How does one hormone stimulate hair growth in many areas such as the face, have no effect in others, e.g. eyelashes, while inhibiting follicles on the scalp? These contrasts are presumably due to differential gene expression within follicles from the various body sites. The intrinsic response of individual follicles is

retained when follicles are transplanted to other skin sites (Ebling and Johnson 1959), the basis of corrective hair follicle transplant surgery (Orentreich and Durr 1982; Gokrem *et al.* 2008).

7.3.2 Evidence for the role of androgens

Although androgens are the clearest regulators of human hair growth unlike most other mammals (Ebling *et al.* 1991), various other circulating factors have an effect (reviewed in Randall 2007). These include adequate nutritional supplies, due to the follicles' high metabolic demands (Bradfield 1971), the hormones of pregnancy, which cause a prolonged anagen resulting in a synchronized shedding of a proportion of scalp hairs post-partum (Lynfield 1960), and lack of thyroid hormone which restricts hair growth (Jackson *et al.* 1972). Growth hormone is also necessary in combination with androgens for normal body hair development in boys (Zachmann and Prader 1970; Zachmann *et al.* 1976). There is much evidence supporting androgens' importance, which fits in well with the concept of much terminal hair growth being a secondary sexual characteristic. Terminal hair appearance in puberty parallels the rise in circulating androgen levels and occurs later in boys than girls (Marshall and Tanner 1969; 1970; Winter and Faiman 1972; 1973). Testosterone also stimulates beard growth in eunuchs and elderly men (Chieffi 1949). An extensive US study also showed that castration before puberty prevented beard and axillary hair growth and after puberty reduced them (Hamilton 1951b; 1958). Nevertheless, the strongest evidence for the essential nature of androgens is the lack of any body hair, even the female pubic and axillary pattern, or evidence of any male pattern baldness, in adult XY androgen insensitivity patients with absent or dysfunctional androgen receptors, despite normal or raised circulating levels of androgens (Fig. 7.1, B) (see Chapter 3).

7.4 The mechanism of androgen action in the hair follicle

7.4.1 Hair growth in androgen insufficiency syndromes

As described in Chapter 2 of this book, androgens from the blood stream enter the cell and bind to specific, intracellular androgen receptors, usually in the form of testosterone or its more potent metabolite, 5α-dihydrotestosterone. The hormone-receptor complex, generally in combination with transcriptional regulators, then activates the appropriate gene transcription for that cell type. Androgen insufficiency patients without functional androgen receptors demonstrate the absolute requirement for androgen receptors within hair follicles for the development of the hair growth ascribed in Section 7.3.2 to androgens (see Chapter 3). These individuals produce no body hair at puberty, even with high circulating androgen levels, nor do they go bald (Fig. 7.1).

Men with 5α-reductase deficiency also contribute to our understanding because they exhibit axillary and female pattern pubic hair, but very little beard growth; they are also not reported to show male pattern baldness (Griffin and Wilson 1989; Fig. 7.3). Although the identification of two forms of 5α-reductase (type 1 and type 2) makes the situation complex, all individuals with 5α-reductase deficiency so far are deficient in 5α-reductase type 2, confirming its importance for much androgen-dependent hair growth. A role for 5α-reductase in baldness is also supported by the ability of oral finasteride, a 5α-reductase type 2 inhibitor (Kaufman *et al.* 1998; Shapiro and Kaufman 2003) and the dual 5α-reductase inhibitor, dutasteride (Olsen *et al.* 2006), to promote hair regrowth. This suggests that the formation of terminal pubic and axillary hair can be mediated by testosterone itself, while that of the secondary sexual hair of men requires the presence of 5α-dihydrotestosterone. This demonstrates a third paradox in androgen effects on hair follicles. Why does the stimulation of increasing size in some follicles like beard require 5α-dihydrotestosterone formation, while follicles in the axillary and pubic regions carry out the same changes in the absence of 5α-dihydrotestosterone? Since androgens are stimulating the same transformation, presumably via the same receptor, this is currently difficult to understand, although it is further evidence of the intrinsic differences within hair follicles. It suggests that some less well-known aspect of androgen action is involved in hair follicles normally specific to men, which requires 5α-dihydrotestosterone, such as interaction with a specific transcription factor. Interestingly, androgen-dependent sebum production by the sebaceous glands attached to hair follicles is also normal in 5α-reductase deficiency type 2 (Imperato-McGinley *et al.* 1993).

7.4.2 The current model for androgen action in the hair follicle

7.4.2.1 The role of the dermal papilla

The mesenchyme-derived dermal papilla plays a major role in determining the type of hair produced by a follicle, as shown by an elegant series of experiments involving the rat whisker by Oliver, Jahoda, Reynolds and colleagues (Reynolds and Jahoda 2004). Whisker dermal papillae transplanted into ear or glabrous skin initiated the production of whisker follicles, and hair growth could also be stimulated by

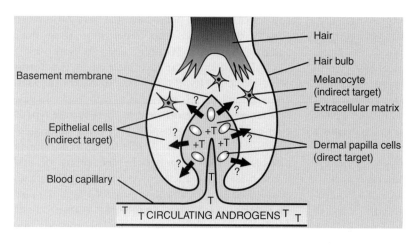

Fig. 7.5 Current model of androgen action in the hair follicle: in the current, well-accepted hypothesis, androgens from the blood enter the hair follicle via the dermal papilla's blood supply. If appropriate, they are metabolized to 5α-dihydrotestosterone. They bind to androgen receptors in the key regulatory cells of the follicle, the dermal papilla cells causing changes in their production of regulatory paracrine factors; these then alter the activity of dermal papilla cells, follicular keratinocytes and melanocytes. T = testosterone; ? = unknown paracrine factors. (Modified from Randall 2000b.) See plate section for color version.

cultured dermal papilla cells reimplanted in vivo (Jahoda *et al.* 1984).

In many embryonic steroid-regulated tissues, including the prostate and the breast, steroids act via the mesenchyme (Thomson *et al.* 1997). Since hair follicles recapitulate the stages of embryogenesis during their growth cycles to reform a new lower hair follicle, they may behave like an embryonic tissue in the adult. Studies on testosterone metabolism in vitro by plucked hair follicles, which leave the dermal papilla behind in the skin, from different body sites, did not reflect the requirements for 5α-reductase in vivo (reviewed in Randall 1994; Randall *et al.* 1991), leading to the hypothesis that androgens would act on the other components of the hair follicle via the dermal papilla (Randall *et al.* 1991; Randall 2007). In this hypothesis androgens would alter the ability of the dermal papilla cells to synthesize, or release, controlling factors which would affect follicular keratinocytes, melanocytes and connective tissue sheath cells, and also probably the dermal endothelial cells, to alter the follicle's blood supply in proportion to its change in size (Fig. 7.5). These factors could be growth factors and/or extracellular matrix proteins. This model would facilitate a mechanism for precise control during the complex changes needed to alter a follicle's size in response to androgens.

This hypothesis has now received a great deal of experimental support. Androgen receptors have been localized by immunohistochemistry in the dermal papilla and not the keratinocyte cells (Choudhry *et al.* 1992; Itami *et al.* 1995a). Cultured dermal papilla cells derived from androgen-sensitive follicles

such as beard (Randall *et al.* 1992) and balding scalp (Hibberts *et al.* 1998) contain higher levels of specific, saturable androgen receptors than androgen-insensitive non-balding scalp in vitro; this has been confirmed by studies using RT-PCR (reverse transcription polymerase chain reaction) (Ando *et al.* 1999). Most importantly, metabolism of testosterone by cultured dermal papilla cells also reflects hair growth in 5α-reductase deficiency patients with beard, but not pubic or non-balding scalp, cells forming 5α-dihydrotestosterone in vitro (Itami *et al.* 1990; Thornton *et al.* 1993; Hamada *et al.* 1996); similar results have been obtained examining gene expression of 5α-reductase type 2 by RT-PCR (Ando *et al.* 1999). This has led to wide acceptance of the hypothesis (Randall 2007; 2008).

However, some more recent observations suggest minor modifications. The lower part of the connective tissue sheath, or dermal sheath, which surrounds the hair follicle and isolates it from the dermis, can form a new dermal papilla and stimulate new human hair follicle development in another person (Reynolds *et al.* 1999). Cultured dermal sheath cells from beard follicles contain similar levels of androgen receptors to beard dermal papilla cells (unpublished data: Merrick AE, Randall VA, Messenger AG, Thornton MJ. Beard dermal sheath cells contain androgen receptors: implications for future inductions of human hair follicles.), and balding scalp dermal sheath expresses the mRNA for 5α-reductase type 2 like the dermal papilla (Asada *et al.* 2001), indicating that the dermal sheath can respond to androgens without the dermal papilla acting as an intermediary. Clearly the dermal sheath also plays an important role in the hair follicle. This may be as a reserve to replace the key inductive and controlling role of the dermal papilla cells if they are lost, to ensure follicles are not lost. Alternatively, or in addition, the dermal sheath cells may respond directly to androgens to facilitate the increase or decrease in size of the sheath or even the dermal papilla in the development of a new anagen follicle; this would enable the new hair follicle to be larger or smaller depending on the follicle's specific response to androgens.

In addition, studies on the beard hair medulla, a central structure only seen in the middle of large human hairs, showed coexpression of a specialized keratin, hHa7, and the androgen receptor (Jave-Suarez et al. 2004). Since the hHa7 gene promoter also contained sequences with high homology to the androgen response element (ARE), keratin hHa7 expression may be androgen regulated. However, no stimulation occurred when the promoter was transfected into prostate cells, and keratin hHa7, with the same promoter, is also expressed in androgen-insensitive body hairs of chimpanzees, making the significance unclear. Nevertheless, the current model needs modification to include possible specific, direct action of androgens on lower dermal sheath and medulla cells.

7.4.2.2 Paracrine factors implicated in mesenchyme–epithelial interactions in the hair follicle

The production of growth factors by cultured dermal papilla cells derived from human and rat hair follicles has been investigated by several groups on the basis of the primary role of the dermal papilla, its potential probable role in androgen action and the retention of hair growth-promoting ability by cultured rat cells (discussed above). Cultured dermal papilla cells secrete both extracellular matrix factors and soluble, proteinaceous growth factors (Randall 2007). Bioassays demonstrate that human dermal papilla cells secrete factors which stimulate the growth of other dermal papilla cells (Randall et al. 1991; Thornton et al. 1998), outer root sheath cells (Itami et al. 1995a), transformed epidermal keratinocytes (Hibberts and Randall 1996) and endothelial cells (Hibberts et al. 1996a). Importantly, testosterone in vitro stimulated greater mitogenic capacity of beard cells to affect beard, but not scalp, dermal papilla cells (Thornton et al. 1998), outer root sheath cells (Itami

et al. 1995a) and keratinocytes (Hibberts and Randall 1996). In contrast, testosterone decreased the mitogenic capacity of androgenetic alopecia dermal papilla cells from both men (Hibberts and Randall 1996) and stump-tailed macaques (Obana et al.1997). Interestingly, conditioned media from balding cells inhibited not only the growth of other human dermal papilla cells but also mouse hair growth in vivo (Hamada and Randall 2006). This implies that an autocrine mechanism is involved in androgen-mediated hair follicle changes; a view which is supported by the actual changes that occur in dermal papilla cell numbers and size (Elliott et al. 1999). As well as supporting the hypothesis for the mechanism of action, these results demonstrate that the paradoxical effects of androgen on hair follicles observed in vivo are reflected in vitro, strengthening the use of cultured dermal papilla cells as a model system for studying androgen action in vitro.

The main emphasis of research now lies in identifying specific factors whose production by dermal papilla cells is altered by androgens (reviewed by Randall 2007). To date only insulin-like growth factor (IGF-1), a potent mitogen, is identified as androgen-stimulated in beard cells in vitro (Itami et al. 1995b). DNA microarray methods also revealed that three genes, SFRP2, MN1, and ATP1B1, were expressed at significantly higher levels in beard than normal scalp cells, but no changes were detected due to androgen in vitro (Rutberg et al. 2006). However, stem cell factor (SCF), the ligand for the melanocyte receptor c-kit, is secreted in greater quantities by dermal papilla cells derived from beard hair follicles (with generally darker hairs) than non-balding scalp cells (Hibberts et al. 1996b), while cells from balding follicles (which have pale hairs) produce significantly less. However, the concentration and distribution of the melanocytes in the balding scalp follicles remain unchanged (Randall et al. 2008). Since SCF plays important roles in hair pigmentation (reviewed in Randall et al. 2008), the dermal papilla probably provides local SCF for follicular melanocytes. Androgens in vivo appear to alter SCF expression by facial dermal papilla cells to change melanocyte activity and thus hair color.

Androgens also inhibit balding dermal papilla cells' gene expression of protease nexin-1, a potent inhibitor of serine proteases which regulate cellular growth and differentiation in many tissues (Sonoda et al. 1999). This may act by altering the amount of extracellular matrix components produced and therefore the size of the follicle and hair produced (Elliott *et al.* 1999).The inhibitory effects of media conditioned by balding dermal papilla cells on dermal papilla cell growth in vitro and mouse hair growth in vivo (Hamada and Randall 2006) suggest the active secretion of an inhibitory factor(s). The recent demonstration that bald scalp from men with androgenetic alopecia retains hair follicle stem cells but lacks CD200-rich and CD34+ hair pigmentor cells also suggests that inhibitory factors are involved (Garza *et al.* 2011). Androgens do stimulate the production of transforming growth factor beta1 (TGF-β1) in balding dermal papilla cells with transfected androgen receptors (Inui *et al.* 2002) and TGF-β2 (Hibino and Nishiyama 2004) in natural balding cells. Transforming growth factor beta is a strong candidate for an inhibitor of keratinocyte activity in alopecia, as it inhibits hair follicle growth in vitro (Philpott 2000), and a probable suppressor of TGF-β1 delayed catagen progression in mice in vivo (Tsuji *et al.* 2003), although TGF-β2 and TNF-α were actually slightly reduced in balding cells in a limited DNA macroarray analysis (Midorikawa *et al.* 2004). In addition, 5α-dihydrotestosterone did increase the production of dickkopf 1 (DKK1), which stimulated apoptosis in keratinocytes (Kwack *et al.* 2008), and inhibited keratinocyte growth by modifying WNT signaling in balding dermal papilla cells (Kitagawa *et al.* 2009).

Thus, studying dermal papilla cells already implicates several factors: IGF-1 in enlargement; SCF in altered pigmentation; and nexin-1, TGF-β, and DKK1 in miniaturization. Alterations in several factors are probably necessary to precisely control the major cell biological rearrangements required when follicles change size. Further study of this area should increase our understanding of the complex hair follicle and lead to better treatments for hair follicle disorders.

7.5 Androgen-dependent hair growth conditions

7.5.1 Androgenetic alopecia in men

A generalized loss of hair follicles from the scalp known as *senescent balding* has been reported in both sexes by the seventh or eighth decade (Kligman 1988; Courtois *et al.* 1995). This differs from the progressive baldness seen in *androgenetic alopecia*, also known as *male pattern baldness, male pattern alopecia, common baldness* or *androgen-dependent alopecia*. As androgenetic alopecia develops, anagen becomes shorter, resulting in shorter hairs and an increasing percentage of hairs in telogen (see Section 7.2.3); follicle miniaturization is also seen histologically, and the hairs become thinner (Braun-Falco and Christophers 1968; Kligman 1988; Rushton *et al.* 1991; Whiting 1993). The connective tissue sheath left in the dermis when the follicle becomes miniaturized may become subject to chronic inflammation; this may prevent terminal hair regrowth in long-term baldness (Kligman 1988).

Balding occurs in men in a precise pattern described by Hamilton (1951a), starting with regression of the frontal hairline in two wings and balding in the center of the vertex. Hamilton graded this progression from type I, prepubertal scalp with terminal hair on the forehead and all over the scalp, through gradual regression of the frontal hairline and thinning on the vertex, to type VII, where the bald areas became fully coalesced to leave hair only around the back and sides of the head (Fig. 7.4). Norwood modified Hamilton's classification, including variations for the middle grades; this scale is used extensively during clinical trials (Norwood 1975). The physiology and pathophysiology of androgenetic alopecia is reviewed more fully by Randall (2000b; 2005; 2010), and an approach to its diagnosis was recently reported by the European Consensus Group (Blume-Peytavi *et al.* 2011a).

7.5.1.1 Incidence, role and consequences

The incidence of androgenetic alopecia in Caucasians is high, with estimates varying widely, but progression to type II is detected in 95% of men (Hamilton 1951a). It is also seen in other primates, being well studied in the stump-tailed macaque. This suggests a natural progression of a secondary sexual characteristic rather than the malfunction of a disease. Marked androgenetic alopecia would obviously highlight the surviving older man as a leader, like the silver back of the chief male gorilla and the larger antlers of the mature deer stags. Others have speculated that the flushed bald skin would look aggressive to an opponent (Goodhart 1960) or mean there was less hair for the opposition to pull (Ebling 1985), giving the bald man important advantages. The lower incidence of androgenetic alopecia amongst men from African races (Setty 1970) suggests that any advantages did not outweigh the evolutionary survival advantages of the hairs' protection of the scalp from the hot tropical sun.

In the current youth-orientated culture of industrialized societies, the association of increasing hair loss with age combined with the major role of hair in human communication means that androgenetic alopecia has strong negative connotations. It often causes well-documented psychological distress and reduction in the quality of life, even though it is not life-threatening or physically painful, in both men (e.g. Franzoi *et al.* 1990; Girman *et al.* 1998) and women (Van der Donk *et al.*1991; Cash 1993). Other people perceive men with visible hair loss as older, less physically and socially attractive, weaker and duller. In parallel, people with androgenetic alopecia have a poor self-image, feel older and are lacking in self-confidence, even those who seem accepting of their condition and have never sought treatment (Girman *et al.*1998), and this has recently been shown to apply to men from many countries (Cash 2009). Male pattern baldness primarily causes concern amongst those who develop marked loss before their forties, and early balding has been linked to myocardial infarction (Lesko *et al.* 1993). Whether this indicates a dual end-organ sensitivity or reflects the psychological stress early balding induces in the youth-orientated American culture is unknown. No relationship between the incidence of balding and prostatic carcinoma was detected in men aged between 50 and 70 by Demark-Wahnefried *et al.* (1997), while others report both an increased (Giles *et al.* 2002; Yassa *et al.* 2011) and a reduced relative risk (Wright *et al.* 2010). Since both conditions have very high incidence in Caucasians, it would be unlikely that there would be a specific clear-cut relationship that could be useful clinically to predict cancer risk from hair loss.

7.5.1.2 Roles of androgens and genes

Male pattern baldness is androgen dependent, since it does not occur in castrates, unless they are given testosterone (Hamilton 1942), nor in XY individuals with androgen insensitivity due to non-functional androgen receptors (see Chapter 3). The genetic involvement in androgenetic alopecia is also pronounced. It runs in families, there are racial differences, and androgen replacement stimulated balding only in castrated men with a family history (Hamilton 1942). Although androgenetic alopecia has historically been accepted as an autosomal dominant trait with variable penetrance (Bergfeld 1955), this is based on a familial analysis in 1916 (Osbourn 1916), and a more complex, polygenic inheritance is more likely

(Ellis and Harrap 2001). Interestingly, a very strong correlation in incidence was found in 54 sets of sons and fathers, with 81.5% of balding sons having balding fathers (Hamilton–Norwood scale III or higher) (Ellis and Harrap 2001; Ellis *et al.* 2001a). This is greater than expected from an autosomal dominant inheritance and could imply a paternally inherited gene, e.g. on the Y chromosome, or the involvement of a gene that is capable of being paternally imprinted (i.e. preferentially inactivated by methylation of DNA, etc.).

Several genes have been investigated for association with androgenetic alopecia. No association was detected with neutral polymorphic markers for either type 1 (SRD5A1) or type 2 (SRD5A2) 5α-reductase genes in case–control association studies of Australian (Ellis *et al.* 1998) or Korean (Asian) men (Ha *et al.* 2003). A later study found an association with a mutant allele (A49T) of 5α-reductase type 2, but this decreased the incidence of alopecia, although increasing that of prostate cancer (Hayes *et al.* 2006)! Known dimorphic and polymorphic markers within the androgen receptor gene are more linked to balding in Caucasian men (Ellis *et al.* 2001b). The *Stu* I restriction fragment length polymorphism (RFLP) in exon 1 was present in 98% of 54 young balding men and 92% of 392 older balding men, but was also found in 77% of their older, non-balding controls. Analysis of triplet repeat polymorphisms, CAG and GAC, revealed significantly higher incidence of short/short polymorphic CAG/GGC haplotypes in balding subjects and lower short/long, although no significance was provided. Interestingly, shorter triplet repeat lengths are associated with precocious puberty, i.e. appearance of pubic hair before age eight (Hoffmann and Happle 2000) and androgen-dependent prostate cancer (Stanford *et al.* 1997). Whether this has functional significance, such as increased androgen sensitivity, or simply reflects linkage disequilibrium with a causative mutation, is not clear. However, when the binding capacity for a range of steroids was compared between androgen receptors from balding and non-balding follicle dermal papilla cells, no differences were detected (Hibberts *et al.* 1998), and no link was seen with increased copy number variations of the androgen receptor gene (Cobb *et al.* 2009).

Recently, genetic variability in a 1 Mb region within and centromeric to the androgen receptor gene was found associated with androgenetic alopecia

(Hillmer *et al.* 2008), and the strongest risk was associated with a variant in the flanking ectodysplasin A2 receptor gene (*EDA2R*) (Hillmer *et al.* 2009). Links with a locus on chromosome 20 (20 pll) have also been reported in several populations (Hillmer *et al.* 2008; Richards *et al.* 2008). Other genes have also been implicated, including a link to one allele of the steroid metabolism gene, *CYP17*, to both women with polycystic ovaries and their brothers with early onset androgenetic alopecia (Carey *et al.* 1993). An interesting connection is severe, early onset androgenetic alopecia in men with the X-linked gene for adrenoleukodystrophy, who tend to have low testosterone levels (Konig *et al.* 2000). The gene for *hairless*, which results in a complete loss of hair (Ahmad *et al.* 1998), also showed a marginally significant correlation with androgenic alopecia with two mutations, but these became insignificant after correction for multiple testing (Hillmer *et al.* 2002). The situation is still not fully clear, but is moving forward rapidly.

7.5.2 Androgenetic alopecia in women

Androgenetic alopecia has also been described in women, but the pattern of expression is normally different and the incidence less. Post-pubertal recession to type II was found in about 25% of Caucasian women by age 50 (Hamilton 1951a), although this did not develop further. Although women can exhibit the "male" pattern, they generally do not show the frontal recession and usually exhibit a different pattern, retaining the frontal hair line but having a progressive diffuse loss or thinning on the vertex which may lead to balding (Ludwig 1977) (Fig. 7.4). This type of balding is frequently termed female pattern hair loss (FPHL) rather than androgenetic alopecia. Venning and Dawber (1988) found that 80% of premenopausal women had thinning in Ludwig stages I–III; while 13% had Hamilton types II–IV. After the menopause, 37% exhibited the "male" pattern with some showing marked templar M-shaped recession, although not progressing beyond Hamilton stage IV.

The progression of balding in women is normally slow, and a full endocrinological investigation is generally recommended if a rapid onset is seen. Although female pattern hair loss is seen frequently in association with hyperandrogenism, other women frequently have no other symptoms of androgen

abnormality (reviewed by Cousen and Messenger 2010). Recent report of an XY individual with complete androgen insensitivity and no other androgen-dependent characteristics who exhibits female pattern hair loss (Cousen and Messenger 2010) does suggest that sometimes at least there may be an androgen-independent, or androgen receptor-independent, mechanism. Overall, there is some debate about whether androgen is essential for this hair loss in women (Birch *et al.* 2002), though this is still generally assumed. If, as occurs in men, the changes develop due to the genetically influenced, specific follicular responses within the scalp follicles themselves, it is not surprising that circulating androgen abnormalities are often absent.

7.5.3 Hirsutism

Hirsutism is the development of male pattern body hair growth in women. This normally benign condition causes marked psychological distress because the person erroneously feels that they are changing sex. The extent of body hair growth which causes a problem varies and depends on the amount of normal body hair amongst her race or subgroup. Normally hirsutism would include terminal hair on the face, chest or back. Ferriman and Gallwey (1961) introduced a scale for grading hirsutism which is widely used, especially to monitor hirsutism progression with, or without, treatment. An approach for the evaluation of hirsutism has recently been established as a European consensus (Blume-Peytavi *et al.* 2009).

Hirsutism is often associated with an endocrine abnormality of the adrenal or ovary which causes raised androgens and is very frequently (over 70% of cases) associated with polycystic ovarian syndrome (PCOS). It can also be caused by Cushing syndrome, acromegaly, hyperprolactinemia and drugs (Azziz 2003; Alsantali and Shapiro 2009). Some women have no obvious underlying clinical or biochemical disorder and are termed "idiopathic." The proportion of these is larger in older papers as modern methods increase the range of abnormalities that can be detected, e.g. low SHBG. The assumption that idiopathic hirsutism is due to a greater sensitivity of the follicles to normal androgens is given credence by hirsutism occurring asymmetrically on only one side of a woman (Jenkins and Ash 1973).

7.6 Treatment of androgen-potentiated hair disorders

7.6.1 Androgenetic alopecia

Mainly because the pathogenic mechanisms of androgenetic alopecia are not fully understood, the treatments available are limited and vary in effectiveness. Over the centuries, a wide range of remedies has been suggested (Lambert 1961), and current treatments include wigs and hairpieces, surgery and medical therapies including hormone action modifiers and non-hormonal therapy (Ross and Shapiro 2005; Rogers and Avram 2008). Several of these are based on our understanding of the mechanisms of androgen action within the follicle. Recently some investigators have also started looking into the application of lasers for androgenetic alopecia based on the low levels of visible or near infrared light used to reduce inflammation etc. (Leavitt *et al.* 2009; Kim *et al.* 2011).

7.6.1.1 Surgery

All surgical methods capitalize on the different intrinsic responses to androgens by spreading "non-balding," i.e. occipital and parietal, terminal follicles over the androgen-sensitive scalp regions (Orentreich and Durr 1982). Originally involving the transplant of small biopsies with several follicles, this usually now involves micro-grafts with one or two follicles. Once established, these expensive and painful treatments are long-lasting; however, the effect can be marred by the continual natural progression of balding, which may well require further transplants to avoid isolation of the transplanted region. Future modifications may include culturing dermal papilla cells to expand the non-balding follicular material before replanting into balding regions (Randall 2010; Aoi *et al.* 2012).

7.6.1.2 Non-hormonal therapy

The ideal treatment for alopecia is an externally applied (topical) substance which would act locally to stimulate hair growth only in specific target areas, with no side-effects. Minoxidil, a vasodilator used for hypertension, stimulated excessive hair growth as a side-effect. This provoked major interest in hair follicle biology because it demonstrated that vellus follicles could be stimulated to form terminal hairs. Topical application of minoxidil has been used in both male and female androgenetic alopecia for over

25 years. However, its mechanism of action has been very uncertain (Messenger and Rundegren 2004). Recent detection of appropriate ATP-sensitive potassium (K_{ATP}) channels in the dermal papilla of human hair follicles, and appropriate responses in human hair follicles in organ culture (Shorter *et al.* 2008) has confirmed a probable action via these channels. Minoxidil stimulates regrowth in up to 30%, with only about 10% obtaining complete regrowth; most success occurs with younger men and with the early stages of balding, i.e. Hamilton stage V or less (Dawber and Van Neste 1995). A stronger topical application of a 5% solution is now licensed for use in men in many countries (Olsen *et al.* 2002), and recently a more acceptable, user-friendly, foam-based application has been developed (Blume-Peytavi 2011b).

Recently, prostaglandin $F_{2\alpha}$ ($PGF_{2\alpha}$) analogs, such as latanoprost and bimatoprost, used as eye drops to reduce intraocular pressure in glaucoma, have been reported to stimulate eyelashes to lengthen, thicken and darken (Curran 2009). Bimatoprost (Latisse), a prostamide $F_{2\alpha}$ analog, was licensed for the treatment of hypotrichosis of the eyelashes by the FDA in December 2008 (NDA 022369). No other drugs have caused such a dramatic stimulation of hair growth after a local application as these prostaglandin analogs have on eyelashes; minoxidil's effect topically is much less than via the original oral ingestion (Messenger and Rundegren 2004). The eyelashes are highly specialized, short hairs which have evolved to protect the eyes from foreign objects. They have marked differences to scalp hairs, and their follicles lack the normal arrector pili muscle found in scalp follicles (Thibaut *et al.* 2009). Although specialized, eyelashes are produced by hair follicles and are replaced regularly via the hair cycle (Thibaut *et al.* 2009), like all other hair follicles. However, human hair follicles also exhibit markedly different behaviors depending on their body site, including the major differences in response to androgens discussed above, and hair graying with age occurs first above the ears before gradually spreading over the scalp (Keogh and Walsh 1965). We have carried out a range of studies on scalp hair follicles and shown that bimatoprost can stimulate hair follicle growth in organ culture and that scalp follicles contain appropriate receptors to respond in vivo (unpublished data: Khidhir KG, Woodward DF, Farjo NP, Farjo BK, Tang ES, Wang JW, Picksley SM, Randall VA. A prostaglandin-related glaucoma therapy offers a novel approach for treating alopecia). Based on this, clinical trials of bimatoprost applied topically in both men and women are now beginning in the USA and Germany. A short study of another glaucoma drug, latanoprost, a $PGF_{2\alpha}$ analog, has reported some effects on androgenetic alopecia in men (Blume-Peytavi *et al.* 2011c).

7.6.1.3 Endocrine-based treatments

Antiandrogen therapy is not a practical option for men due to the side-effects, but cyproterone acetate, in combination with estrogen to ensure contraception and prevent potential feminization of a male fetus, has been used in women. It increased the percentage of hair follicles in anagen and may cause some regrowth, but is probably most effective in preventing further progression (Dawber and Van Neste 1995; Vexiau *et al.* 2002). Since cyproterone acetate is unavailable in the USA, spironolactone and high-dose cimetidine have been used as alternative antiandrogens.

Finasteride, a 5α-reductase type 2 inhibitor, was developed to treat androgen-potentiated prostate disorders and is now available as an oral treatment for androgenetic alopecia in men in many countries at a lower dose of 1 mg/d. Clinical trials demonstrated significant effects on stimulating hair regrowth in younger men with mild to moderate hair loss (Kaufman *et al.* 1998). More recently effects have also been seen in older men (Kaufman *et al.* 2008a; 2008b). Even if hair did not regrow, balding progression was frequently halted and no significant adverse effects have been reported. Unfortunately, no effects of finasteride have been seen in postmenopausal women with androgenetic alopecia (Price *et al.* 2000); use in premenopausal women requires ensuring against contraception as for antiandrogens. Topical routes of application of finasteride in liposomes have also been studied but are not yet available clinically (Kumar *et al.* 2007). Interestingly, response to finasteride in women has recently been shown to depend on genetic variations in the androgen receptor gene, bringing in a whole new area of epigenetics to alopecia treatment (Keene and Goren 2011). Previously, Tang *et al.* (2003) reported that response to finasteride in men was correlated to the ability of their follicle dermal papilla cells to produce IGF-1. Both these results show how important it is to understand the mechanism of androgen action in hair follicles to develop new treatments. A short trial of dutasteride, a dual inhibitor of both 5α-reductase types 1 and 2

showed similar, possibly better effects than finasteride in men (Olsen *et al.* 2006).

Although a range of treatments is now available, all medications need to be used continually because they are opposing a natural process which, if treatment is discontinued, retains all the components to continue to progress.

7.6.2 Hirsutism

Once a serious underlying pathology has been eliminated, a range of treatments is available for hirsutism (Azziz 2003; Martin *et al.* 2008; Alsantali and Shapiro 2009; Lapidoth *et al.* 2010). These range from simple cosmetic treatments to oral pharmaceutical medication.

7.6.2.1 Non-hormonal approaches

Cosmetic treatments such as bleaching and depilatory measures, such as shaving, waxing or depilatory creams, are common, but only remove hair or reduce the amount or appearance of hair temporarily. Electrolysis, with the aim of permanent removal by killing the dermal papilla and germinative epithelium/stem cells is the most established long-lasting treatment, but it is expensive, time consuming and may cause scarring. Photoepilation, using laser or intense pulse light (IPL) treatment, is a more recently introduced alternative to electrolysis (Sanchez *et al.* 2002; Alsantali and Shapiro 2009). A Cochrane review of photoepilation found that alexandrite and diode lasers were more useful, while there was little evidence of effectiveness with IPL, longer wavelength (Nd:YAG) or ruby lasers (Haedersdal and Gotzsche 2006).

A hair growth inhibitor, eflornithine hydrochloride, is available by prescription as a topical cream as Vaniqa®, or under other names around the world. It is an irreversible inhibitor of the enzyme ornithine decarboxylase which is approved by the FDA (USA) for the reduction of unwanted facial hair in women. It is used alone or as an adjuvant to laser therapy (Lapidoth *et al.* 2010).

7.6.2.2 Endocrine-based treatments

Oral contraceptives are generally considered the first-line therapy for hirsutism in premenopausal women (Martin *et al.* 2008), in the form of an estrogen, frequently ethinyl estradiol, in combination with a progestin. The progestin used should not have androgenic properties, and a combination with an antiandrogenic form, which should compete for the androgen receptor in the follicle, such as cyproterone acetate or drospirenone, is recommended (Alsantali and Shapiro 2009). Oral contraceptives act by suppressing luteinizing hormone secretion and thereby inhibiting ovarian androgen biosynthesis, increasing SHBG production (which decreases serum free androgens), and causing some reduction in androgen synthesis by the adrenals.

If the oral contraceptives are insufficient, antiandrogens are recommended (Martin *et al.* 2008). The most common antiandrogen treatment, outside the USA, is cyproterone acetate, given with estrogen if the woman is premenopausal. It is used at higher doses, but must still be balanced with estrogens if pregnancy is a possibility. Spironolactone, an aldosterone antagonist, known to have antiandrogen activity, or flutamide, a pure non-steroidal antiandrogen, can be used as alternatives (Swiglo *et al.* 2008); flutamide is not recommended as a front-line therapy due to hepatotoxicity (Martin *et al.* 2008; Alsantali and Shapiro 2009). Patients have to be well motivated because hair growth on the face generally takes at least nine months before a noticeable effect occurs, although any acne will be cleared in a couple of months and effects on thigh hair growth will be seen in four to six months (Sawers *et al.* 1982). Facial responses are seen first on the sides of the face and last on the upper lip, in reverse order to the appearance of facial hair in men (personal observations).

Finasteride (see Section 7.6.2.1) has also been used for hirsutism with some success (Lakryc *et al.* 2003; Alsantali and Shapiro 2009). This seems logical, as 5α-reductase type 2 is necessary for male pattern body hair growth (see Section 7.4.1). Contraception is still required, as with all endocrine treatments, due to the potential to affect the development of a male fetus.

Metformin, insulin-sensitizing therapy, aimed at altering the insulin resistance and hence the hyperandrogenism often associated with polycystic ovarian disease, has been used clinically (Harborne *et al.* 2003). However, insulin-sensitizing drugs including the thiazolidinediones (e.g. rosiglitazone and pioglitazone) do not appear effective (Cosma *et al.* 2008).

Overall, there have been major changes in the treatment of androgen-potentiated disorders over the last 10 years. The ideal therapy of a uniformly effective, topical treatment which is inactivated on contact with the blood or is specific for hair follicles is not yet available. Further research on the biology of androgen action in the hair follicle may facilitate its development.

7.7 Key messages

- Androgens are the main regulator of human hair growth and responsible for initiating clinical conditions including androgenetic alopecia and hirsutism.
- Androgens have paradoxically different effects on hair follicles depending on their body site. They can stimulate the formation of large hairs, e.g. beard, axilla; have no effect, e.g. eyelashes; or inhibit follicles on the scalp.
- All effects are gradual.
- Common androgen-potentiated disorders of hair growth, including hirsutism in women and androgenetic alopecia in both sexes, particularly in men, cause widespread psychological distress due to the importance of hair in human communication.
- Androgen receptors are necessary for all androgen-dependent growth and 5α-reductase type 2 for most hair, except for female patterns of axillary and pubic hair, even in men.
- The action of androgens on human hair follicles demonstrates several paradoxes: contrasting effects in different sites; major differences in the persistence of stimulatory effects depending on body region; a varying requirement for the formation of 5α-dihydrotestosterone even amongst follicles exhibiting increased growth. Since these are all site-related and retained on transplantation, these indicate intrinsic differences within follicles, presumably determined during embryonic development.
- The current model for androgen action in the hair follicle proposes that androgens act via the cells of the dermal papilla, altering their production of regulatory paracrine factors such as growth factors, which then influence the activity of other follicular components, e.g. keratinocytes, melanocytes and endothelial cells. The dermal sheath may also play a role as a direct androgen target.
- Treatment for androgen-dependent hair disorders involves cosmetic, surgical, endocrine and non-endocrine related therapies.
- A 5α-reductase type 2 inhibitor, finasteride, and antiandrogens, generally cyproterone acetate, are being used to control androgenetic alopecia and hirsutism. Such treatments of

premenopausal women require combination with estrogens to ensure contraception to avoid possible feminization of a male fetus.

- Treatments may need several months to show their effects and will need to be used continually as long as the source of androgens is present.
- Non-endocrine treatments for hair loss include minoxidil; prostaglandin-related glaucoma drugs are under investigation.

- Further understanding of the mechanism of androgens in the hair follicle is necessary to enable the development of better treatments, preferably working topically and specific to the hair follicle.

Acknowledgements

I should like to acknowledge the assistance in preparation of this manuscript by Lucy Scott, and Chris Bowers and Jenny Braithwaite for the figures.

7.8   References

Ahmad W, Faiyaz ul Haque M, Brancolini V, Tsou HC, ul Haque S, Lam H, Aita VM, Owen J, deBlaquiere M, Frank J, Cserhalmi-Friedman PB, Leask A, McGrath JA, Peacocke M, Ahmad M, Ott J, Christiano AM (1998) Alopecia universalis associated with a mutation in the human hairless gene. *Science* **279**:720–724

Alsantali A, Shapiro J (2009) Management of hirsutism. *Skin Therapy Lett* **14**:1–3

Ando Y, Yamaguchi Y, Hamada K, Yoshikawa K, Itami S (1999) Expression of mRNA for androgen receptor, 5α-reductase and 17β-hydroxysteroid dehydrogenase in human dermal papilla cells. *Br J Dermatol* **141**:840–845

Aoi N, Inoue K, Kato H, Suga H, Higashino T, Eto H, Doi K, Araki J, Iida T, Katsuta T, Yoshimura KJ (2012) Clinically applicable transplantation procedure of dermal papilla cells for hair follicle regeneration. *J Tissue Eng Regen Med* **6**:85–95. DOI 10.1002/term.400

Asada Y, Sonoda T, Ojiro M, Kurata S, Sato T, Ezaki T, Takayasu S (2001) 5α-reductase type 2 is constitutively expressed in the dermal papilla and connective tissue sheath of the hair follicle in vivo but not during culture in vitro. *J Clin Endocr Metab* **86**:2875–2880

Azziz R (2003) The evaluation and management of hirsutism. *Obstet Gynaecol* **101**:995–1007

Bergfeld WF (1955) Androgenetic alopecia: an autosomal dominant disorder. *Am J Med* **98**:955–985

Birch MP, Lalla SC, Messenger AG (2002) Female pattern hair loss. *Clin Exp Dermatol* **27**:383–388

Blume-Peytavi U, Atkin S, Shapiro J, Lavery S, Grimalt R, Hoffmann R, Gieler U, Messenger A (2009) European Consensus on the evaluation of women presenting with excessive hair growth. *Eur J Dermatol* **19**:597–602

Blume-Peytavi U, Blumeyer A, Tosti A, Finner A, Marmol V, Trakatelli M, Reygagne P, Messenger A; European Consensus Group (2011a) S1 guideline for diagnostic evaluation in androgenetic alopecia in men, women and adolescents. *Br J Dermatol* **164**:5–15

Blume-Peytavi U, Hillmann K, Dietz E, Canfield D, Garcia Bartels N (2011b) A randomized, single-blind trial of 5% minoxidil foam once daily versus 2% minoxidil solution twice daily in the treatment of androgenetic alopecia in women. *J Am Acad Dermatol* **65**:1126–1134.e2

Blume-Peytavi U, Lönnfors S, Hillmann K, Garcia Bartels N (2011c) A randomized double-blind placebo-controlled pilot study to assess the efficacy of a 24-week topical treatment by latanoprost 0.1% on hair growth and pigmentation in healthy volunteers with androgenetic alopecia. *J Am Acad Dermatol* Aug 27 [Epub ahead of print]

Botchkareva NV, Ahluwalia G, Shander D (2006) Apoptosis in the hair follicle. *J Invest Dermatol* **126**:258–264

Botchkareva VA, Kishimoto J (2003) Molecular control of epithelial-mesenchymal interactions during hair follicle cycling. *J Invest Dermatol Symp Proc* **8**:46–55

Bradfield RB (1971) Protein deprivation: comparative response of hair roots, serum protein and urinary nitrogen. *Amer J Clin Nutrit* **24**:405–410

Braun-Falco O, Christophers E (1968) Hair root patterns in male pattern alopecia. In: Baccareda-Boy A, Moretti G, Fray JR (eds) *Biopathology of Pattern Alopecia*. Karger, Basel, pp 141–145

Carey AH, Chan KL, Short F, White D, Williamson R, Franks S (1993) Evidence for a single gene effect causing polycystic ovaries and male pattern baldness. *Clin Endocrinol* **38**:653–658

Cash TF (1993) Psychological effects of androgenetic alopecia on women: comparisons with balding men and with female control subjects. *J Am Acad Dermatol* **29**:568–575

Cash TF (2009) Attitudes, behaviors, and expectations of men seeking medical treatment for male pattern hair loss: results of a multinational survey. *Curr Med Res Opin* **25**:1811–1820

Chieffi M (1949) Effect of testosterone administration on the beard growth of elderly males. *J Geront* **4**:200–204

Choudhry R, Hodgins MB, Van Der Kwast TH, Brinkman AO, Boersma WJA (1992) Localisation of androgen receptors in human skin by immunohistochemistry: implications for the hormonal regulation of hair growth, sebaceous glands and sweat glands. *J Endocrinol* **133**:467–475

Cobb JE, White SJ, Harrap SB, Ellis JA (2009) Androgen receptor copy number variation and androgenetic alopecia: a case-control study. *PLoS One* **4**:e5081

Cosma M, Swiglo BA, Flynn DN, Kurtz DM, Labella ML, Mullan RJ, Elamin MB, Erwin PJ, Montori VM (2008) Clinical review: insulin sensitizers for the treatment of hirsutism: a systematic review and metaanalyses of randomized controlled trials. *J Clin Endocr Metab* **93**:1135–1142

Cotsarelis C, Sun T, Lavker R (1990) Label-retaining cells reside in the bulge area of the pilosebaceous unit; implications for follicular stem cells, hair cycle and skin carcinogenesis. *Cell* **61**:1329–1337

Courtois M, Loussouarn G, Hourseau C, Grollier JF (1995) Ageing and hair cycles. *Br J Dermatol* **132**:86–93

Courtois M, Loussouarn G, Hourseau S, Grollier JF (1996) Periodicity in the growth and shedding of hair. *Br J Dermatol* **134**:47–54

Cousen P, Messenger A (2010) Female pattern hair loss in complete androgen insensitivity syndrome. *Br J Dermatol* **162**:1135–1137

Curran, MP (2009) Bimatoprost: a review of its use in open angle glaucoma and ocular hypertension. *Drugs Aging* **26**:1049–1071

Dawber R, Van Neste D (1995) *Hair and Scalp Disorders*. Martin Dunitz, London

Demark-Wahnefried W, Lesko SM, Conaway MR, Robertson CN, Clark RV, Lobaugh B, Mathias BJ, Strigo TS, Paulsa DF (1997) Serum androgens: associations with prostate cancer risk and hair pattening. *J Androl* **18**:495–450

Ebling FJG (1985) Age changes in cutaneous appendages. *J Appl Cosmetol* **3**:243–250

Ebling FJG, Johnson E (1959) Hair growth and its relation to vascular supply in rotated skin grafts and transposed flaps in the albino rat. *J Embry Exp Morph* **9**:285–293

Ebling FJG, Hale PA, Randall VA (1991) Hormones and hair growth. In: Goldsmith LA (ed) *Biochemistry and Physiology of the Skin*, 2nd edn. Clarenden Press, Oxford, pp 660–696

Elliott K, Stephenson TJ, Messenger AG (1999) Differences in hair follicle dermal papilla volume are due to extracellular matrix volume and cell number: implications for the control of hair follicle size and androgen responses. *J Invest Dermatol* **113**:873–877

Ellis JA, Harrap SB (2001) The genetics of androgenetic alopecia. *Clin Dermatol* **19**:149–154

Ellis JA, Stebbing M, Harrap SB (1998) Genetic analysis of male pattern baldness and the 5α-reductase genes. *J Invest Dermatol* **110**:849–853

Ellis JA, Stebbing M, Harrap SB (2001a) Male pattern baldness is not associated with established cardiovascular risk factors in the general population. *Clin Sci* **100**:401–404

Ellis JA, Stebbing M, Harrap SB (2001b) Polymorphism of androgen receptor gene is associated with male pattern baldness. *J Invest Dermatol* **116**:452–455

Ferriman D, Gallwey JD (1961) Clinical assessment of body hair growth in women. *J Clin Endocr Metab* **21**:1440–1447

Flux JEC (1970) Colour change of mountain hares (Lepus timidus scoticus) in north-east Scotland. *Zool* **162**:345–358

Franzoi SL, Anderson J, Frommelt S (1990) Individual differences in men's perceptions of and reactions to thinning hair. *J Soc Psychol* **130**:209–218

Garza LA, Yang CC, Zhao T, Blatt HB, Lee M, He H, Stanton DC, Carrasco L, Spiegel JH, Tobias JW, Cotsarelis G (2011) Bald scalp in men with androgenetic alopecia retains hair follicle stem cells but lacks CD200-rich and CD34-positive hair follicle progenitor cells. *J Clin Invest* **121**:613–622

Giles GG, Severi G, Sinclair R, English DR, McCredie MR, Johnson W, Boyle P, Hopper JL (2002) Androgenetic alopecia and prostate cancer: findings from an Australian case-control study. *Can Epidemiol* **11**:549–553

Girman CJ, Rhodes T, Lilly FRW Guo SS, Siervogel RM, Patrick DL, Chumlea WC (1998) Effects of self-perceived hair loss in a community sample of men. *Dermatology* **197**:223–229

Gokrem S, Baser NT, Aslan G (2008) Follicular unit extraction in hair transplantation: personal experience. *Ann Plast Surg* **60** (2):127–133

Goodhart DB (1960) The evolutionary significance of human hair patterns and skin coloring. *Adv Sci* **17**:53–59

Griffin JE, Wilson JD (1989) The resistance syndromes: 5α-reductase deficiency, testicular feminisation and related disorders. In: Scriver CR, Baudet AL, Sly WS, Valle D (eds) *The Metabolic Basis of Inherited Disease*. McGraw-Hill, New York, pp 1919–1944

Ha SJ, Kim JS, Myung JW, Lee HJ, Kim JW (2003) Analysis of genetic polymorphisms of steroid 5α-reductase type 1 and 2 genes in Korean men with androgenetic alopecia. *J Dermatol Sci* **31**:135–141

Haedersdal M, Gotzsche PC (2006) Laser and photoepilation for unwanted hair growth. *Cochrane Database Syst Rev* **4**:CD004684

Hamada K, Randall VA (2006) Inhibitory autocrine factors produced by the mesenchyme-derived hair follicle dermal papilla may be a key to male pattern baldness. *Br J Dermatol* **154**:609–618

Hamada K, Thornton MJ, Liang I, Messenger AG, Randall VA (1996) Pubic and axillary dermal papilla cells do not produce 5α-dihydrotestosterone in culture. *J Invest Dermatol* **106**:1017–1022

Hamilton JB (1942) Male hormone stimulation is a prerequisite and an incitant in common baldness. *Amer J Anat* **71**:451–480

Hamilton JB (1946) A secondary sexual character that develops in men but not in women upon aging of an organ present in both sexes. *Anat Rec* **94**:466–467

Hamilton JB (1951a) Patterned loss of hair in man; types and incidence. *Ann N Y Acad Sci* **53**:708–728

Hamilton JB (1951b) Quantitative measurement of a secondary sex character and axillary hair. *Ann N Y Acad Sci* **53**:585–599

Hamilton JB (1958) Age, sex and genetic factors in the regulation of hair growth in man: a comparison of Caucasian & Japanese populations. In: Montagna W, Ellis RA (eds) *The Biology of Hair Growth*. Academic Press, New York, pp 399–433

Harborne L, Fleming R, Lyall H, Norman J, Sattar N (2003) Descriptive review of the evidence for the use of metformin in polycystic ovary syndrome. *Lancet* **361**:1894–1901

Hayes VM, Saveri G, Padilla E, Morris H, Tilley W, Southey M, English D, Sutherland R, Hopper J, Boyle P, Giles G (2006) 5α-reductase type 2 gene variant associations with prostate cancer risk, circulating hormone levels and androgenetic alopecia. *Int J Cancer* **120**:776–780

Hibberts NA, Randall VA (1996) Testosterone inhibits the capacity of cultured balding scalp dermal papilla cells to produce keratinocyte mitogenic factors. In: Van Neste D,

Randall VA (eds) *Hair Research for the Next Millennium*. Elsevier Science, Amsterdam, pp 303–306

Hibberts NA, Sato K, Messenger AG, Randall VA (1996a) Dermal papilla cells from human hair follicles secrete factors (eg VEGF) mitogenic for endothelial cells. *J Invest Dermatol* **106**:341

Hibberts NA, Messenger AG, Randall VA (1996b) Dermal papilla cells derived from beard hair follicles secrete more stem cell factor (SCF) in culture than scalp cells or dermal fibroblasts. *Biochem Biophys Res Commun* **222**:401–405

Hibberts NA, Howell AE, Randall VA (1998) Dermal papilla cells from human balding scalp hair follicles contain higher levels of androgen receptors than those from non-balding scalp. *J Endocrinol* **156**:59–65

Hibino T, Nishiyama T (2004) Role of TGF-b2 in the human hair cycle. *J Dermatol Sci* **35**:9–18

Higgins CA, Richardson, GD, Westagte GE, Jahoda CA (2009) Exogen involves gradual release of the hair club fiber in the vibrissa follicle model. *Exp Dermatol* **18**:793–795

Hillmer AM, Kruse R, Macciardi F, Heyn U, Betz RC, Ruzicka T, Propping P, Nothen MM, Cichon S (2002) The hairless gene in androgenetic alopecia: results of a systematic mutation screening and a family-based association approach. *Br J Dermatol* **146**:601–608

Hillmer AM, Brockschmidt FF, Hanneken S, Eigelshoven S, Steffens M, Flaquer A, Herms S, Becker T, Kortüm AK, Nyholt DR, Zhao ZZ, Montgomery GW, Martin NG, Mülenisen TW, Alblas MA, Moebus S, Jöckel KH, Bröcker-Preuss M, Erbel R, Reinartz R, Betz RC, Cichon S, Propping P, Baur MP, Wienker TF, Kruse R, Nöthen MM (2008) Susceptibility variants for male pattern baldness on chromosome 20p11. *Nat Genet* **40**:1279–1281

Hillmer AM, Freudenberg J, Myles S, Herms S, Tang K, Hughes DA, Brockschmidt FF, Ruan Y, Stonkeking M, Nöthen MM (2009) Recent positive selection of a human androgen receptor/ectodysplasin A2 receptor haplotype and its relationship to male pattern baldness. *Hum Genet* **126**:255–264

Hoffmann R, Happle R (2000) Current understanding of androgenetic alopecia. Part II: clinical aspects and treatment. *Eur J Dermatol* **10**:410–417

Hsu YC, Pasolli HA, Fuchs E (2011) Dynamics between stem cells, niche, and progeny in the hair follicle. *Cell* **144**:92–105

Imperato-McGinley J, Gautier T, Cai L, Yee B, Epstein J, Pochi P (1993) The androgen control of sebum production. Studies of subjects with dihydrotestosterone deficiency and complete androgen insensitivity. *J Clin Endocr Metab* **76**:524–528

Inui S, Fukuzato Y, Nakasima T, Yoshikawa (2002) Androgen-inducible TGF-beta1 from balding dermal papilla cells inhibits epithelial cell growth: a clue to understand paradoxical effects of androgen on human hair growth. *FASEB J* **16** (14):1967–1969

Itami S, Kurata S, Takayasu S (1990) 5α-reductase activity in cultured human dermal papilla cells from beard compared with reticular dermal fibroblasts. *J Invest Dermatol* **94**:150–152

Itami S, Kurata S, Sonada T, Takayasu S (1995a) Interactions between dermal papilla cells and follicular epithelial cells in vitro: effect of androgen. *Br J Dermatol* **132**:527–532

Itami S, Kurata S, Takayasu S (1995b) Androgen induction of follicular epithelial cell growth is mediated via insulin-like growth factor I from dermal papilla cells. *Biochem Biophys Res Commun* **212**:988–994

Jackson D, Church RE, Ebling FJG (1972) Hair diameter in female baldness. *Br J Dermatol* **87**:361–367

Jahoda CA, Horne KA, Oliver RF (1984) Induction of hair growth by implantation of cultured dermal papilla cells. *Nature* **311** (5986):560–562

Jansen VA, Van Baalen M (2006) Altruism through beard chromodynamics. *Nature* **440**:663–666

Jave-Suarez LF, Langbein L, Winter H, Praetzel S, Rogers MA, Schweizer J (2004) Androgen regulation of the human hair follicle: the type 1 hair keratin hHa7 is a direct target gene in trichocytes. *J Invest Dermatol* **122**:555–564

Jenkins JS, Ash S (1973) The metabolism of testosterone by human skin in disorders of hair growth. *J Endocrinol* **59**:345–351

Kaufman KD, Olsen EA, Whiting D, Savi R, De Villez R, Bergfeld W; Finasteride Male Pattern Hair Loss Study Group (1998) Finasteride in the treatment of men with androgenetic alopecia. *J Am Acad Dermatol* **39**:578–589

Kaufman KD, Rotonda J, Shah AK, Meehan AG (2008a) Long-term treatment with finasteride 1 mg decreases the likelihood of developing further visible hair loss in men with androgenetic alopecia (male pattern hair loss). *Eur J Dermatol* **18**:400–406

Kaufman KD, Girman CJ, Round EM, Johnson-Levonas AO, Shah AK, Rotonda J (2008b) Progression of hair loss in men with androgenetic alopecia (male pattern hair loss): long-term (5-year) controlled observational data in placebo-treated patients. *Eur J Dermatol* **18**:407–411

Keene S, Goren (2011) A therapeutic hotline. Genetic variations in the androgen receptor gene and finasteride response in women with androgenetic alopecia mediated by epigenetics. *Dermatol Ther* **24**:296–300

Keogh EV, Walsh RJ (1965) Rate of greying of human hair. *Nature* **207**:877–878

Kim WS, Lee HI, Lee JW, Lim YY, Lee SJ, Kim BJ, Kim MN, Song KY, Park WS (2011) Fractional photothermolysis laser treatment of male pattern hair loss. *Dermatol Surg* **37**:41–51

Kitagawa T, Matsuda KI, Inui S, Takenaka H, Katoh N, Itami S, Kishimoto S, Kawata M (2009) Keratinocyte growth inhibition through the modification of Wnt signaling by androgen in balding dermal papilla cells. *J Clin Endocrinol Metab* **94**:1288–1294

Kligman AM (1959) The human hair cycle. *J Invest Dermatol* **33**:307–316

Kligman AM (1988) The comparative histopathology of male-pattern baldness and senescent baldness. *Clin Dermatol* **6**:108–118

Konig A, Happle R, Tchitcherina E, Schaefer JR, Sokolowski P, Kohler W, Hoffmann R (2000) An X-linked gene involved in androgenetic alopecia: a lesson to be learned from adrenoleukodystrophy. *Dermatology* **200**:213–218

Kumar R, Singh B, Bakshi G, Katare OP (2007) Development of liposomal systems of finasteride for topical applications: design, characterization, and in vitro evaluation. *Pharm Dev Technol* **12**:591–601

Kwack, MH, Sung YK, Chung EJ (2008) Dihydrotestosterone-inducible dickkopf 1 from balding dermal papilla cells causes apoptosis in follicular keratinocytes. *J Invest Dermat* **128**:262–269

Lakryc EM, Motta EL, Soares JM Jr, Haider MA, de Lima GR, Baracat EC (2003) The benefits of finasteride for hirsute women with polycystic ovary syndrome or idiopathic hirsutism. *Gynaecol Endocrinol* **17**:57–63

Lambert G (1961) *The Conquest of Baldness. The Wonderful Story of Hair*. Souvenir Press, London

Lapidoth M, Dierickx C, Lanigan S, Paasch U, Campo-Voegeli A, Dahan S, Marini L, Adatto M (2010) Best practice options for hair removal in patients with unwanted facial hair using combination therapy with laser: guidelines drawn up by an expert working group. *Dermatology* **221**:34–42

Leavitt M, Charles G, Heyman E, Michaels D (2009) HairMax LaserComb laser phototherapy device in the treatment of male androgenetic alopecia: a randomized, double-blind, sham device-controlled, multicentre trial. *Clin Drug Investig* **29**:283–292

Lesko SM, Rosenberg L, Shapiro S (1993) A case-control study of baldness in relation to myocardial infarction in men. *JAMA* **269**:998–1003

Ludwig E (1977) Classification of the types of androgenetic alopecia (common baldness) occurring in the female sex. *Br J Dermatol* **97**:247–254

Lui F, Uchugonova A, Kimura H, Zhang C, Zhao M, Zhang L, Koenig K, Duong J, Aki R, Saito N, Mii S, Amoh Y, Katsuoka K, Hoffman RM (2011) The bulge area is the major hair follicle source of nestin-expressing pluripotent stem cells which can repair the spinal cord compared to the dermal papilla. *Cell Cycle* **10**:830–839

Lynfield YL (1960) Effect of pregnancy on the human hair cycle. *J Invest Dermatol* **35**:323–327

Marshall WA, Tanner JM (1969) Variations in pattern of pubertal change in girls. *Arch Dis Child* **44**:291–303

Marshall WA, Tanner JM (1970) Variations in the pattern of pubertal changes in boys. *Arch Dis Child* **45**:13–23

Martin KA, Chang RJ, Ehrmann DA, Ibanez L, Lobo RA, Rosenfield RL, Shapiro J, Montori VM, Swiglo BA (2008) Evaluation and treatment of hirsutism in premenopausal women: an Endocrine Society clinical practice guideline. *J Clin Endocrinol Metab* **93**:1105–1120

Messenger AG, Rundegren J (2004) Minoxidil: mechanisms of action on hair growth. *Br J Dermatol* **150**:186–194

Midorikawa T, Chikazawa T, Yoshino T, Takada K, Arase S (2004) Different gene expression profile observed in dermal papilla cells related to androgenic alopecia by DNA macroarray analysis. *J Dermatol Sci* **36**:25–32

Miranda BH, Tobin DJ, Sharpe DT, Randall VA (2010) Intermediate hair follicles: a new more clinically relevant model for hair growth investigations. *Br J Dermatol* **163**:287–295

Nishimura EK (2011) Melanocyte stem cells: a melanocyte reservoir in hair follicles for hair and skin pigmentation. *Pigment Cell Melanoma Res* **24**:401–410

Norwood OT (1975) Male pattern baldness, classification and incidence. *South Med J* **68**:1359–1365

Obana N, Chang C, Uno H (1997) Inhibition of hair growth by testosterone in the presence of dermal papilla cells from the frontal bald scalp of the post-pubertal stump-tailed macaque. *Endocrinology* **138**:356–361

Olsen EA, Dunlap FE, Funicella T, Koperski JA, Swinehart JM, Tschen EH, Trancik RJ (2002) A randomized clinical trial of 5% topical minoxidil versus 2% topical minoxidil and placebo in the treatment of androgenetic alopecia in men. *J Am Acad Dermatol* **47**:377–385

Olsen EA, Hordinsky M, Whiting D, Stough D, Hobbs S, Ellis ML, Wilson T, Rittmaster RS (2006) The importance of dual 5alpha-reductase inhibition in the treatment of male pattern hair loss: results of a randomized placebo-controlled study of dutasteride versus finasteride. *J Am Acad Dermatol* **55**:1014–1023

Orentreich N (1969) Scalp hair replacement in man. In: Montagna

W, Dobson RL (eds) *Hair Growth*, Advances in Biology of Skin, Vol. 9. Pergamon Press, Oxford, pp 99–108

Orentreich N, Durr NP (1982) Biology of scalp hair growth. *Clin Plas Surg* **9**:197–205

Osbourn D (1916) Inheritance of baldness. *J Hered* **7**:347–355

Philpott MP (2000) The roles of growth factors in hair follicles: investigations using cultured hair follicles. In: Camacho F, Randall VA, Price VH (eds) *Hair and its Disorders: Biology, Research and Management*. Martin Dunitz, London, pp 103–113

Price VH, Roberts JL, Hordinsky M, Olsen EA, Savin R, Bergfeld W, Fiedler V, Lucky A, Whiting DA, Pappas F, Culbertson J, Kotey P, Meehan A, Waldstreicher J (2000) Lack of efficacy of finasteride in postmenopausal women with androgenetic alopecia. *J Am Acad Dermatol* **43**:768–776

Rabbani P, Takeo M, Chou W, Myung P, Bosenberg M, Chin L, Taketo MM, Ito M (2011) Coordinated activation of Wnt in epithelial and melanocyte stem cells initiates pigmented hair regeneration. *Cell* **10** (145):941–955

Randall VA (1994) Androgens and human hair growth. *Clin Endocrinol* **40**:439–457

Randall VA (2000a) Androgens: the main regulator of human hair growth. In: Camacho F, Randall VA, Price VH (eds) *Hair and its Disorders: Biology, Research and Management*. Martin Dunitz, London, pp 69–82

Randall VA (2000b) The biology of androgenetic alopecia. In: Camacho F, Randall VA, Price VH (eds) *Hair and its Disorders: Biology, Research and Management*. Martin Dunitz, London, pp 123–136

Randall VA (2003) Biological effects of androgens on the hair follicle: experimental approaches. In: Van Neste D (ed) *Hair Science and*

Technology, Skinterface, Brussels, pp 75–92

Randall VA (2005) Physiology and pathophysiology of androgenetic alopecia. In:Degroot LJ, Jameson JL (eds)*Endocrinology*, 5th edn. W B Saunders Co, Philadelphia, Section XIV, Burger HG (ed) Male Reproduction, Chapter 178, pp 3295–3309

Randall VA (2007) Hormonal regulation of hair follicles exhibits a biological paradox. *Semin Cell Dev Biol* **18**:274–285

Randall VA (2008) Androgens and hair growth. *Dermatol Ther* **21**:314–328

Randall VA (2010) Molecular basis of androgenetic alopecia In: Trüeb RM, Tobin DJ (eds) *Aging Hair*. Springer-Verlag, Berlin, Chapter 2, pp 9–24

Randall VA, Botchkareva NV (2009) The biology of hair growth. In: Ahluwalia GA (ed) *Cosmetic Applications of Laser and Light Based Systems*. William Andrew, Norwich, NY, pp 3–35

Randall VA, Ebling FJG (1991) Seasonal changes in human hair growth. *Br J Dermatol* **124**:146–151

Randall VA, Thornton MJ, Hamada K, Redfern CPF, Nutbrown M, Ebling FJG, Messenger AG (1991) Androgens and the hair follicle: cultured human dermal papilla cells as a model system. *Ann N Y Acad Sci* **642**:355–375

Randall VA, Thornton MJ, Messenger AG (1992) Cultured dermal papilla cells from androgen-dependent human follicles (e.g. beard) contain more androgen receptors than those from non-balding areas. *J Endocrinol* **133**:141–147

Randall VA, Jenner T, Hibberts N, De Oliveira I, Vafaee T (2008) Stem cell factor/c-kit signalling in normal and androgenetic alopecia hair follicles. *J Endocrinol* **197**:1–14

Rendl M, Lewis L, Fuchs E (2005) Molecular dissection of mesenchymal-epithelial interactions in the hair follicle. *PLoS Biol* **3**:331

Reynolds AJ, Jahoda CAB (2004) Cultured human and rat tooth papilla cells induce hair follicle regeneration and fiber growth. *Differentiation* 72:566–575

Reynolds AJ, Lawrence C, Cserhalmi-Friedman PB, Christiano AM, Jahoda CAB (1999) Trans-gender induction of hair follicles. *Nature* 402:33–34

Richards JB, Yuan X, Geller F, Waterworth D, Bataille V, Glass D, Song K, Waeber G, Vollenweider P, Aben KK, Kiemeney LA, Walters B, Soranzo N, Thorsteinsdottir U, Kong A, Rafnar T, Deloukas P, Sulem P, Stefansson H, Stefansson K, Spector TD, Mooser V (2008) Male pattern baldness susceptibility locus at 20p11. *Nat Genet* 40:1282–1284

Rogers NE, Avram MR (2008) Medical treatments for male and female pattern hair loss. *J Am Acad Dermatol* 59:547–566; quiz 5675–5686

Ross EK, Shapiro J (2005) Management of hair loss. *Dermatol Clin* 23:227–243

Rushton DH, Ramsay ID, Norris MJ, Gilkes JJH (1991) Natural progression of male pattern baldness in young men. *Clin Exp Dermatol* 16:188–192

Rutberg SE, Kolpak ML, Gourley JA, Tan G, Henry JP, Shander D (2006) Differences in expression of specific biomarkers distinguish human beard from scalp dermal papilla cells. *J Invest Dermatol* 126:2583–2595

Saitoh M, Sakamoto M (1970) Human hair cycle. *J Invest Dermatol* 54:65–81

Sanchez LA, Perez M, Azziz R (2002) Laser hair reduction in the hirsute patient: a critical assessment. *Hum Reprod Update* 8:169–181

Sawers RA, Randall VA, Iqbal MJ (1982) Studies on the clinical and endocrine aspects of antiandrogens. In: Jeffcoate SL (ed) *Androgens and Antiandrogen Therapy*, Current topics in Endocrinology. John Wiley & Sons, Ltd., Chichester, pp 145–168

Setty LR (1970) Hair patterns of the scalp of white and Negro males. *Amer J Phys Anthrop* 33:49–55

Shapiro J, Kaufman KD (2003) Use of finasteride in the treatment of men with androgenetic alopecia (male pattern hair loss). *J Invest Dermatol Symp Proc* 8:20–23

Shimomura Y, Christiano AM (2010) Biology and genetics of hair. *Ann Rev Genomics Hum Genet* 11:109–132

Shorter K, Farjo NP, Picksley SM, Randall VA (2008) Human hair follicles contain two forms of ATP sensitive potassium channels, only one of which is sensitive to minoxidil. *FASEB* 22:1725–1736

Sonoda T, Asada Y, Kurata S, Takayasu S (1999) The mRNA for protease nexin-1 is expressed in human dermal papilla cells and its level is affected by androgen. *J Invest Dermatol* 113:308–313

Stanford JL, Just JJ, Gibbs M, Wicklund KG, Neal CL, Blumenstein BA, Ostrander EA (1997) Polymorphic repeats in the androgen receptor gene: molecular markers of prostate cancer risk. *Cancer Res* 57:1194–1198

Swiglo BA, Cosma M, Flynn DN, Kurtz DM, Labella ML, Mullan RJ, Erwin PJ, Montori VM (2008) Clinical review: antiandrogens for the treatment of hirsutism: a systematic review and metaanalyses of randomized controlled trials. *J Clin Endocr Metab* 93:1153–1160

Tang L, Bernardo O, Bolduc C, Lui H, Madani S, Shapiro J (2003) The expression of insulin-like growth factor 1 in follicular dermal papillae correlates with therapeutic efficacy of finasteride in androgenetic alopecia. *J Am Acad Dermatol* 49:229–233

Thibaut S, De Becker E, Caisey L, Baras D, Karatas S, Jammayrac O, Pisella PJ, Bernard BA (2009) Human eyelash characterization. *Br J Dermatol* 162:304–310

Thomson AA, Foster BA, Cunha GR (1997) Analysis of growth factor and receptor mRNA levels during development of the rat seminal vesicle and prostate. *Development* 124:2431–2439

Thornton MJ, Laing I, Hamada K, Messenger AG, Randall VA (1993) Differences in testosterone metabolism by beard and scalp hair follicle dermal papilla cells. *Clin Endocrinol* 39:633–639

Thornton MJ, Hamada K, Messenger AG, Randall VA (1998) Beard, but not scalp, dermal papilla cells secrete autocrine growth factors in response to testosterone in vitro. *J Invest Dermatol* 111:727–732

Tsuji Y, Denda S, Soma T, Raferty L, Momoi T, Hibino T (2003) A potential suppressor of TGF-β delays catagen progression in hair follicles. *J Invest Dermatol Symp Proc* 8:65–68

Van der Donk J, Passchier J, Knegt-Junk C, Wegen-Keijser MH, Nieboer C, Stolz E, Verhage F (1991) Psychological characteristics of women with androgenetic alopecia: a controlled study. *Br J Dermatol* 125:248–252

Venning VA, Dawber R (1988) Patterned androgenic alopecia. *J Amer Acad Dermatol* 18:1073–1077

Vexiau P, Chaspoux C, Boudou P, Fiet J, Jouanique C, Hardy N, Reygagne P (2002) Effects of minoxidil 2% vs. cyproterone acetate treatment on female androgenetic alopecia: a controlled, 12-month randomized trial. *Br J Dermatol* 146:992–999

Waters JM, Richardson GD, Jahoda CA (2007) Hair follicle stem cells. *Semin Cell Dev Biol* 18:245–254

Wehr TA (1998) Effects of seasonal changes in daylength on human neuroendocrine function. *Horm Res* 49:118–124

Wehr TA, Duncan WC Jr, Sher L, Aeschbach D, Schwartz PJ, Turner

EH, Postolache TT, Rosenthal NE (2001) A circadian signal of change of season in patients with seasonal affective disorder. *Arch Gen Psychiatry* **58**:1115–1116

Whiting DA (1993) Diagnostic and predictive value of horizontal sections of scalp biopsy specimens in male pattern androgenetic alopecia. *J Am Acad Dermatol* **28**:755–763

Winter JSD, Faiman C (1972) Pituitary-gonadal relations in male children and adolescents. *Paed Res* **6**:125–135

Winter JSD, Faiman C (1973) Pituitary-gonadal relations in female children and adolescents. *Paed Res* **7**:948–953

Wright JL, Page ST, Lin DW, Stanford JL (2010) Male pattern baldness and prostate cancer risk in a population-based case-control study. *Can Epidemiol* **34**:131–135

Yassa M, Saliou M, De Rycke Y, Hemery C, Henni M, Bachaud JM, Thiounn N, Cosset JM, Giraud P (2011) Male pattern baldness and the risk of prostate cancer. *Ann Oncol* **22**:1824–1827

Zachmann M, Prader A (1970) Anabolic and androgenetic effect of testosterone in sexually immature boys and its dependency on GH. *J Clin Endocr Metab* **30**:85–95

Zachmann M, Aynsley-Green A, Prader A (1976) Interrelations of the effects of growth hormone and testosterone in hypopituitarism. In: Pecile A, Muller EE (eds) *Growth Hormone and Related Peptides*. Excerpta Medica, Amsterdam, pp 286–290

Testosterone and bone

Dirk Vanderschueren, Mieke Sinnesael, Evelien Gielen,
Frank Claessens, and Steven Boonen

8.1 Introduction

Osteoporosis is an important and increasing health problem, especially in the elderly: fractures are a considerable burden for society because of associated economic costs, morbidity as well as mortality (Center et al. 1999; Ensrud et al. 2000; Empana et al. 2004; Fechtenbaum et al. 2005; Lippuner et al. 2005; Maravic et al. 2005; Orsini et al. 2005). Osteoporosis is also a gender-related disease: although age-adjusted mortality after hip fracture is higher in men than in women, fewer men are affected by osteoporosis (Center et al. 1999; Kanis et al. 2000; Johnell and Kanis 2006). Possible explanations for this gender difference in fracture risk are that men have broader and therefore stronger bones than women and also – in contrast to postmenopausal women – do not experience accelerated estrogen deficiency related to bone loss (Seeman 2003). In this context, a question arises: to what extent does higher male lifelong androgen secretion contribute to these gender-related differences of bone development and loss? Androgens are traditionally considered to protect against osteoporosis and may therefore potentially explain – at least partly – the lower male fracture risk (Khosla et al. 2008). In 1947, Fuller Albright already demonstrated that administration of testosterone induced a positive calcium balance in both postmenopausal women and eugonadal men (Reifenstein and Albright 1947). Moreover, animal studies support this concept of anabolic as well as antiresorptive skeletal action of androgens: androgens for instance stimulate bone formation during growth and inhibit bone resorption after growth in orchidectomized male rodents (Vanderschueren et al. 2004). In hypogonadal men testosterone replacement inhibits bone resorption (Basaria and Dobs 2001). Therefore, potential beneficial skeletal effects of androgen and/or SARM replacement in elderly men with low-normal or borderline low testosterone concentrations have received growing attention during the last decades, as illustrated by a rising number of publications on testosterone and bone in Pubmed (1970–1990: 818 publications; 1990–2011: 2421 publications).

Testosterone: Action, Deficiency, Substitution, ed. Eberhard Nieschlag and Hermann M. Behre, Assoc. ed. Susan Nieschlag.
Published by Cambridge University Press. © Cambridge University Press 2012.

However, testosterone is also a prohormone of estradiol. Many, if not all bone-sparing actions of testosterone may therefore be explained by conversion of androgens into estrogens and subsequent stimulation of the estrogen receptors, which are also – in addition to androgen receptors – present in male bone cells. Indeed, since 1994 several case reports of men suffering from severe osteoporosis despite normal or high testosterone concentrations have been reported (Lanfranco *et al.* 2008; Smith *et al.* 2008; Zirilli *et al.* 2008). Low bone mass in these men was explained by estrogen – not testosterone – deficiency, either caused by an inactivating mutation in the principal ERα (Smith *et al.* 1994) and/or in the aromatase enzyme that converts androgens into estrogens (Morishima *et al.* 1995; Carani *et al.* 1997; Bilezikian *et al.* 1998; Bouillon *et al.* 2004). Thus, estrogens appear to be involved also in male, and not only in female, skeletal homeostasis. These observations have fueled the more recent assumption that estrogen and not androgen receptor-mediated androgen action is necessary for male skeletal maintenance.

Little is known about the role of endogenous testosterone in elderly women. However, older postmenopausal women with higher circulating concentrations of testosterone also have significantly greater bone mineral density (BMD), independently of body mass index (BMI), suggesting that circulating testosterone may play a role in the maintenance of bone density, even in postmenopausal women with low serum estradiol concentrations (Rariy *et al.* 2011).

In this chapter, the role of testosterone for male bone health will be reviewed. We will also try to indicate to what extent testosterone action depends on direct activation of the AR or, alternatively, on indirect activation of the ER after aromatization into estrogens. Finally, we will briefly address some of the potential underlying mechanisms of testosterone action on bone.

8.2 Testosterone deficiency and male osteoporosis

The role of testosterone deficiency in the development of osteoporosis in men remains controversial. Some of the controversy is due to the confusing use of the term "osteoporosis in men." Osteoporosis in men – in contrast to postmenopausal osteoporosis which is largely explained by estrogen deficiency – indeed represents not a single, but a number of disorders. The impact of changes in serum testosterone on the pathophysiology may therefore differ according to the etiology of these different forms of male osteoporosis.

8.2.1 Testosterone deficiency and senile osteoporosis

Senile osteoporosis is characterized by fragility fractures which occur in very old men (Boonen *et al.* 1997). Recently the relationship between testosterone and age-related bone loss, bone turnover and fractures has been studied very extensively in large cohorts of elderly community-dwelling men (Barrett-Connor *et al.* 2000; Goderie-Plomp *et al.* 2004; Amin *et al.* 2006; Bjornerem *et al.* 2007; Meier *et al.* 2008). Most of these studies found either no or a weak association between age-related changes in serum testosterone and bone loss as well as occurrence of fractures (see Table 8.1). However, according to most of these studies, the age-related rise of SHBG appears to be related to bone loss in men. Moreover, serum estradiol predicts bone loss as well as fractures in elderly men. These observations further strengthened the concept that skeletal action of testosterone is indirectly mediated by estrogens. Indeed, in the Osteoporotic Fractures in Men Study (MrOS), low estrogen concentrations appeared to increase fracture risk even in men with high testosterone concentrations (Mellstrom *et al.* 2008). In this study, the relationship between serum estrogen and fracture risk is not linear. The threshold for estrogen is around a very low concentration of only 16 pg/ml. These low concentrations can only be measured precisely by mass spectrometry, which probably explains why the role of estrogens was not established previously in other studies using less precise immunoassay methods (Goderie-Plomp *et al.* 2004; Bjornerem *et al.* 2007).

Many other risk factors for senile osteoporosis have currently been identified. A FRAX score, which calculates the absolute risk for major osteoporotic as well as hip fractures in men, has been developed similarly as in women, since many of the risk factors for senile osteoporosis are not gender specific (Kanis *et al.* 2008). In this FRAX score, estradiol concentrations are not included. Neither

Table 8.1 Overview of cohort studies in men which used fracture as an end-point in relation to serum sex steroid concentrations at start of the study. The average age at start of the study, the duration of the study, the method of measurement of sex steroid and the main results are given.

Study	Average age	Number	Duration (years)	LC-MS/MS	Immunoassay	Main result
Rancho Bernardo (Barrett-Connor et al. 2000)	66	352	12		X	E: inverse correlation with fractures T: no correlation with fractures
Dubbo (Meier et al. 2008)	>60	609	16	X		T: no correlation with fractures E: inverse correlation with fractures
Tromso (Bjornerem et al. 2007)	50–84	1364	8.4		X	T, E, SHBG: no correlation with fractures
Rotterdam (Goderie-Plomp et al. 2004)	67.6 ± 6.8	178	6.5		X	T, E, SHBG: no correlation with fractures
Framingham (Amin et al. 2006)	71	793	18		X	E: inverse correlation with fractures T + E: inverse correlation with fractures
MrOS (Mellstrom et al. 2008)	75	2639	3.3	X		E, SHBG: inverse correlation with fractures

Abbreviations: LC-MS/MS, liquid chromatography–tandem mass spectrometry; E, estrogen; T, testosterone; SHBG, sex hormone-binding globulin.

is frailty, as measured by the frailty index of Rockwood (Rockwood and Mitnitski 2007) or the operational definition of Fried (Fried *et al.* 2001), taken into account in this fracture risk assessment of elderly men. Yet, especially in less-healthy elderly men, in whom there is a higher prevalence of hypogonadism, lower testosterone and especially lower free testosterone are associated with loss of muscle strength and may increase the risk for sarcopenia, frailty, falls and fractures (Schatzl *et al.* 2003; Auyeung *et al.* 2011; O'Connell *et al.* 2011). In these less-healthy men, the relative contribution of age-related changes in serum testosterone to the risk for osteoporosis and the loss of muscle mass and strength remains to be further investigated (see also Chapter 16). Indeed, most studies only include relatively healthy community-dwelling men of whom only a low percentage is suffering from late-onset male hypogonadism.

8.2.2 Testosterone deficiency and idiopathic male osteoporosis

Idiopathic male osteoporosis is much less frequent than senile osteoporosis, and is characterized by fragility fractures, mainly at the spine, occurring in middle-aged men (Khosla *et al.* 1994; Kelepouris *et al.* 1995). By definition, the cause of this entity is still unknown (therefore the term "idiopathic" is used) but it is speculated that low bone mass and fragility in these men is caused primarily by low bone formation at the level of the individual bone remodeling unit, as evidenced by low wall thickness shown by bone histomorphometry (Pernow *et al.* 2006; 2009). In contrast to postmenopausal osteoporosis, the total number of bone remodeling units on the inner bone surfaces does not appear to be increased in these men. Although it cannot be excluded that deficient action and/or secretion of estrogens and IGF-1 may be involved in the pathophysiology of idiopathic male osteoporosis, in case control studies serum testosterone concentrations are not different in men suffering from idiopathic osteoporosis (Kurland *et al.* 1997; Pernow *et al.* 2009).

8.2.3 Testosterone deficiency and secondary osteoporosis

Like postmenopausal women, men with hypogonadal osteoporosis – in contrast to men suffering from senile or idiopathic osteoporosis – do have high bone turnover (Jackson *et al.* 1987). High bone turnover is characterized by an increased number of bone remodeling units on the bone surface as well as by a relative imbalance of bone formation versus bone resorption in these units. Therefore, hypogonadal osteoporosis clearly is a distinct entity of secondary osteoporosis. Hypogonadal osteoporosis may occur following chemical or surgical castration in men suffering from prostatic carcinoma or sexual delinquency (Stepan *et al.* 1989; Daniell 1997; Wei *et al.* 1999). It is well established that chemical and surgical castration induces rapid bone loss as well as fractures. The fracture risk in these men is very high and increases early after castration (Melton *et al.* 2011). Therefore, hypogonadal osteoporosis clearly illustrates that sex steroids are essential for the maintenance of skeletal integrity in men as well as in women. However, this does not answer the question of to what extent bone loss is related to either testosterone or estrogen deficiency, or both. Testosterone deficiency may also occur in other secondary forms of osteoporosis such as steroid-induced osteoporosis, but its relative contribution to the pathophysiology of bone loss in these men is less well established (Reid 1998).

8.3 Testosterone deficiency and areal bone density

Areal bone density, measured by dual-emission X-ray absorptiometry (DXA), is used as a proxy for osteoporosis in men as in women. Indeed, low areal bone density is associated with fracture risk in both sexes (De Laet *et al.* 1997; 1998). Areal bone density is greater in men than in women because it reflects not only volumetric bone density but also bone geometry. Areal bone density is indeed a two-dimensional projection obtained by DXA of the three-dimensional bone, which reflects bone size as well as bone density

per volume (or volumetric bone density). Therefore, broader male bones are denser bones on DXA. Denser bones are stronger bones and may explain – at least partly – the lower number of fractures in men later in life.

Areal bone density is expressed as T-scores, which are standard deviations compared to the mean areal bone density of a young reference group. Male reference values are higher than female reference values, because a young male reference group has a higher bone size, whereas volumetric bone density does not appear to be different between sexes (Seeman 2001). Since higher references of areal bone density reflect lower fracture risk, most authors advocate the more conservative use of female instead of male references in men, in order not to overestimate fracture risk in men based on DXA measurements (Kanis and Gluer 2000; Kanis 2002). Other authors still consider male references appropriate in men, as well as a T-score of -1 and -2.5 for the respective diagnoses of osteopenia and osteoporosis as in postmenopausal women (Kamel 2005; Baim *et al.* 2008). The use of female versus male references has an impact on the number of men being diagnosed as having either osteopenia or osteoporosis (Holt *et al.* 2002). In the recent FRAX scores the same absolute density measurements for the femoral neck are used for men and women.

Low areal bone density in men may result from deficient peak bone mass acquisition. There is a strong genetic component related to the interindividual variation of bone mineral gain during growth, as shown in twin studies and comparative studies of bone density of father and sons as well as brothers (Pelat *et al.* 2007). Besides genetic factors, androgens are also involved in the increase of bone size during puberty (see animal data or preclinical studies (Callewaert *et al.* 2010a; 2010b)). Bone size and therefore strength and area are relatively higher in men compared to women which – at least partially – may account for skeletal sexual dimorphism. Therefore, although age-related changes in testosterone in elderly men may not contribute to fracture risk later in life, normal secretion and action of testosterone at younger age is required for the relative gender-specific protection against osteoporosis in the elderly. Nevertheless, most men with decreased bone density do not have lower testosterone concentrations in case control studies (Meier *et al.* 1987; Khosla *et al.* 1998; Rapado *et al.* 1999; Araujo *et al.* 2008). In contrast, lower average estradiol – not testosterone –

concentrations are reported in some (Khosla *et al.* 1998; Araujo *et al.* 2008) but not all of these studies (Meier *et al.* 1987). Indeed, not only testosterone but also estradiol is important for the acquisition of areal bone density and/or maintenance (Callewaert *et al.* 2010a). Lower estradiol concentrations in men seem to be associated with wider medullary inner bone area and thinner cortices, suggesting that estradiol may inhibit net endocortical bone resorption during growth (Vermeulen *et al.* 2002). Estrogen replacement in one adult patient suffering from androgen insensitivity increased cortical bone area by reducing the inner endocortical surface, without effect on trabecular bone parameters, as shown by peripheral computerized tomography (pQCT) (Taes *et al.* 2009). Interestingly, also in one aromatase-deficient adolescent man the increase of areal bone density following estrogen replacement was related to an increase of cortical – not trabecular – bone pQCT parameters, but this increase was explained by an increase of the outer and not of the inner cortical bone surface (Bouillon *et al.* 2004). Therefore, these few case reports suggest that estrogen has more effect on cortical than on trabecular growing bone in men. Nevertheless, the relative contribution of AR-mediated versus estrogen action on bone acquisition remains not fully established in humans, in contrast to animal studies (see Section 8.9).

8.4 Skeletal effects of testosterone replacement in hypogonadal men

Not only the terminology of osteoporosis, but also of that of hypogonadism, is somewhat confusing in the literature on androgens and bones. Many hypogonadal men included in studies looking at associations between bone density and testosterone replacement still have significant residual testosterone secretion, which is in contrast to the more severe estradiol deficiency in postmenopausal women or to the sharp decline of testosterone observed in men following chemical or surgical castration. The threshold of testosterone and/or estradiol concentrations below which bone resorption is increased is not well defined in hypogonadal men, but may be below the traditional testosterone threshold of two standard deviations below the mean concentration in young adult men.

Patients with isolated hypogonadotropic hypogonadism (IHH) represent the most severe and complete model of hypogonadism since they have very low residual testosterone concentrations (Finkelstein *et al.* 1987). Moreover, in these patients, hypogonadism occurs during puberty, which is a very critical period for skeletal growth and development (Finkelstein *et al.* 1999). Severe sex steroid deficiency – testosterone, estradiol or both – may inhibit their peak bone mass acquisition, thereby explaining the severe deficit of areal bone density, especially in those men with open epiphyses at time of diagnosis. Areal bone density in these adolescent men is also low because it reflects mainly a two-dimensional projection of their small growth-delayed bones. Moreover, not only secretion but even timing of testosterone secretion during puberty may impact on areal bone density, as shown in studies in patients with delayed puberty (Finkelstein *et al.* 1992; Bertelloni *et al.* 1995). These patients also have lower areal bone density at adult age. Their lower areal bone density may again be explained by growth failure, since volumetric in contrast to areal bone density was not different from controls at least in one study (Bertelloni *et al.* 1998). The potential impact of early low-dose testosterone replacement on future areal bone density has not been well documented in these patients suffering from delayed puberty. Some studies have advocated the use of aromatase inhibitors in combination with low-dose testosterone replacement in order to further adult height in boys suffering from delayed puberty, but this may be at a cost and risk of normal peak bone mass acquisition due to induction of estrogen deficiency (Dunkel and Wickman 2002).

The impact of testosterone deficiency on bone in patients with less severe and complete types of hypogonadism is not well established. Klinefelter syndrome represents one of the most frequent forms of hypergonadotropic hypogonadism in men. Patients with Klinefelter syndrome frequently have important residual testosterone secretion, and may also have higher estradiol concentrations which may impact on their skeletal development as well. Moreover, some of the skeletal deficit reported in Klinefelter patients may not be related to hormonal but directly to the underlying chromosomal abnormality (Ferlin *et al.* 2011).

Nevertheless, testosterone replacement clearly increases and/or maintains areal bone density in hypogonadal men with well-documented underlying testicular or hypothalamic-pituitary dysfunction (Katznelson *et al.* 1996; Behre *et al.* 1997). Areal bone density is therefore considered as a well-accepted and efficient measurement to evaluate the long-term impact of testosterone replacement in these patients. However, testosterone replacement studies are uncontrolled because of obvious ethical reasons. Moreover, these studies include hypogonadal men with mixed causes of hypogonadism as well as more or less severe forms of hypogonadism. In addition, long-term bone data on testosterone replacement in hypogonadal men are retrospective. Finally, different modes of androgen replacement (intramuscular versus transdermal) may have differing impacts on bone. For instance, im testosterone replacement increases both estradiol and testosterone concentrations, and often above the average physiological range (Anderson et al. 1997). Therefore, effects of testosterone replacement on bone may be related to estradiol and/or (higher) testosterone concentrations.

8.5 Skeletal effects of testosterone replacement in elderly men

The potential benefit of testosterone replacement on bone in elderly men remains a matter of debate. The administration of testosterone to hypogonadal men (especially after chemical and surgical castration) inhibits bone resorption and maintains bone mass, whereas its effect in elderly men with borderline low testosterone or low-normal testosterone concentrations is more controversial (Isidori et al. 2005). Recent studies by Kenny et al. (2001; 2002) and Crawford et al. (2003) for instance showed no to minor effects on areal bone density after 12 months of treatment. One of the problems which may explain some of this controversy is the inclusion of elderly men with only minor or no testosterone deficiency. Baseline testosterone concentrations of these elderly men are often only borderline and frequently above 200 ng/dl. Furthermore, studies that have investigated bone end-points mainly focused on areal bone density. None of these studies were powered to investigate fracture risk, which requires much greater numbers of patients. Indeed, sample size of most of these studies was small, and duration of follow-up during testosterone therapy relatively short. In addition, different modes of testosterone replacement were used, which makes it difficult to compare studies. As mentioned before, im testosterone replacement induces higher concentrations of testosterone and estradiol than transdermal testosterone substitution, which may explain a greater effect of the former administration

especially in the elderly (Anderson et al. 1997). In accordance with this assumption, the effect of testosterone on bone density was only significant for im and not for transdermal replacement in a meta-analysis of studies in elderly men (Fabbri et al. 2007). Moreover, in this meta-analysis, the effect of im replacement only significantly increased lumbar and not femoral density. The only study that reported an increase of both lumbar and femoral density following testosterone replacement (with or without finasteride) included elderly men with lower testosterone at baseline, which may explain its greater effect (Page et al. 2005). Another study could not show a significant increase of lumbar and femoral bone density following transdermal testosterone in elderly men with low testosterone concentrations at baseline; however, a positive trend towards a significant improvement of bone density was found in those men with the lowest testosterone levels at inclusion (below 200 ng/dl) (Snyder et al. 1999). Inclusion of elderly men with concentrations above this threshold may therefore explain the limited benefit of testosterone on bone density in these studies.

8.6 Skeletal effects of other hormonal agents such as SERMs, SARMs, non-aromatizable androgens and aromatase inhibitors in men

Given the potential effect of estradiol action on male bone, selective estrogen receptor modulators (SERMs) may be considered as osteoporosis therapy. However, only limited data are available with respect to the action of SERMs in men. Raloxifene significantly lowered the decrease in bone density in prostate carcinoma patients following chemical castration (Smith et al. 2004). Raloxifene also had significant effects on bone turnover markers in elderly men, however without data on bone density (Doran et al. 2001).

Selective androgen receptor modulators (SARMs), which are the counterpart of SERMs, are another potential alternative for testosterone but so far only evaluated in preclinical animal studies (Gao et al. 2005; Kearbey et al. 2009).

Administration of the non-aromatizable androgen dihydrotestosterone (DHT) gel to elderly men did not significantly affect the bone turnover marker osteocalcin, but other more relevant bone end-points such as areal bone density are not available (Ly et al. 2001).

Administration of the aromatase inhibitor anastrozole does increase testosterone levels, but decreases both estradiol concentrations and areal bone mineral density in elderly men (Burnett-Bowie *et al.* 2009). Therefore, the use of an aromatase inhibitor as alternative strategy to increase testosterone levels in elderly men may have unwanted side-effects on bone.

8.7 Skeletal effects of other non-hormonal anti-osteoporotic drugs in hypogonadal men

Antiresorptive, anti-osteoporotic drugs such as the bisphosphonates alendronic acid (Ringe *et al.* 2002), risedronic acid (Boonen *et al.* 2009) and zoledronic acid (Smith *et al.* 2003), as well the RANKL (receptor activator of nuclear factor-κB ligand) antagonist denosumab (Smith *et al.* 2009), that have a well-documented anti-fracture efficacy in postmenopausal osteoporosis, also increase bone density in osteoporotic male patients with concomitant low testosterone levels. Two-year treatment with zoledronic acid also decreased vertebral fracture risk overall in the patient group with osteoporosis (Brown *et al.* 2007).

An anabolic agent such as parathyroid hormone (PTH), approved for treatment of osteoporosis in postmenopausal women, also increases bone density to a similar extent in men and women (Misiorowski 2010).

Therefore, physicians currently have a choice between different treatment modalities for efficient prevention of fracture risk, even in hypogonadal patients not receiving testosterone replacement.

8.8 Preclinical studies of sex steroid replacement in male rodents

As discussed, the relative contribution of non-aromatizable versus aromatizable androgen action on bone development and maintenance remains not well defined in humans. However, in male orchidectomized rats, both non-aromatizable (Venken *et al.* 2005) and aromatizable androgens (Vanderschueren *et al.* 2000) increase bone formation during skeletal growth and decrease bone resorption after growth.

During growth, testosterone increases cortical bone size (periosteal bone formation) and length (longitudinal bone formation). These actions are partly related to a direct action of androgens via the AR and partly to an indirect action of androgens through aromatization

into estrogen and activation of the ERα. For instance, periosteal bone formation is clearly mediated by the AR, as shown by lack of effect of high-dose testosterone in androgen-resistant mice, in contrast to a stimulatory action in corresponding wild types (Venken *et al.* 2006). A lower concentration of estrogens stimulates GH-IGF-1 and thereby also periosteal as well as longitudinal bone formation; whereas higher concentrations of estrogens induce growth plate closure in both sexes (Vanderschueren *et al.* 2005).

The dual mode of action of testosterone on trabecular bone is also confirmed during and after growth (Callewaert *et al.* 2009; 2010a). The number of trabeculae is only maintained in the presence of sufficient androgen and/or estrogen concentrations which require androgen and estrogen receptor alpha (not beta) respectively. Cortical bone medullary expansion also increases in the elderly rodent, which is insufficiently counterbalanced by periosteal bone formation. Estrogen inhibits net endocortical bone resorption, and testosterone may stimulate periosteal bone formation but its effect is weaker compared to younger bones (Vanderschueren *et al.* 2004).

An important finding from animal studies is that the effect of testosterone on bone may occur at subphysiological concentrations in these elderly non-growing rodents (Vanderschueren *et al.* 2000). In a comparative study, the effect of non-aromatizable androgens is significant but less potent than testosterone in this animal model (Vandenput *et al.* 2002).

If translated to humans, this preclinical observation may explain why extensive and rapid bone loss at both cortical and trabecular sites is only observed when testosterone concentrations are very low, as is the case after orchidectomy. Bone loss observed in elderly men with normal and/or borderline low testosterone is indeed much slower than the rapid bone loss observed after orchidectomy. Bone loss in aging men is also mainly caused by trabecular thinning and less by trabecular disruption, as observed following castration. Therefore, the mechanism of age-related bone loss in the human is clearly different from the bone loss observed after orchidectomy in the rodent. Lower estrogen concentrations in aging men may, even in the presence of normal testosterone concentrations, enhance endosteal bone resorption (Falahati-Nini *et al.* 2000; Vanderschueren *et al.* 2004; Reim *et al.* 2008). The relative and potentially important role of estrogen in the maintenance of human bone is, however, much more difficult to address in preclinical models because of lower serum estrogen concentration in rodents compared to men (Falahati-Nini *et al.* 2000).

8.9 Potential mechanism of androgen receptor-mediated androgen action

Three major types of mature bone cells are present within the bone matrix: osteocytes, osteoblasts and osteoclasts.

Osteoblasts are responsible for the synthesis of matrix constituents and bone formation, and arise from multipotential mesenchymal stem cells (Manolagas 2000; Harada and Rodan 2003). The osteodifferentiation originates from a progenitor cell, the osteoprogenitor, and progresses through a number of precursor stages to the mature osteoblast (Harada and Rodan 2003). In this regard, an essential event in osteoblast differentiation is the activation of runt-related transcription factor 2 (Runx2) and osterix (Osx), as mice deficient in one of these transcription factors completely lack osteoblasts (Ducy 2000; Harada and Rodan 2003).

Osteocytes are terminally differentiated osteoblasts that are fully embedded in the secreted matrix (Bonewald and Johnson 2008).

Osteoclasts, the exclusive bone resorbing cells, are multinucleated cells that arise from hematopoietic stem cells of the monocyte/macrophage lineage (Manolagas 2000; Boyle *et al.* 2003). Two cytokines are essential for the commitment of hematopoietic stem cells to the myeloid lineage: receptor activator of nuclear factor-κB ligand (RANKL) and macrophage-colony stimulating factor (M-CSF). These proteins are produced by marrow stromal cells and osteoblasts. Binding of RANKL to its receptor RANK, expressed on osteoclasts and its hematopoietic precursor cells, is necessary for osteoclast formation and differentiation. These stimulating effects on osteoclastogenesis are counterbalanced by osteoprotegerin (OPG), which is secreted by stromal cells and osteoblasts, by acting as a soluble inhibitor of RANKL (Boyle *et al.* 2003).

Androgens may inhibit bone resorption, but the mechanism of AR-mediated action on bone cells is not well established. One of the open questions is which bone cell constitutes the principal target for androgen action. Indeed, both osteoblasts and osteoclasts, as well as their respective precursor cells, may be a target for androgen action.

Androgens may have a direct effect on the preosteoclasts/osteoclasts. Pederson *et al.* (1999) have

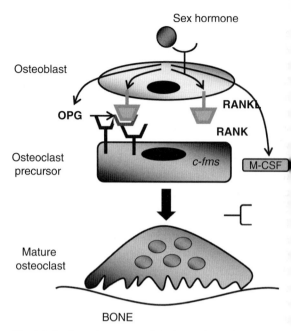

Fig. 8.1 A schematic overview of the RANKL/RANK/OPG system. Receptor activator of nuclear factor-κB ligand mediates a signal for osteoclast formation through RANK expressed on osteoclast progenitors. Osteoprotegerin counteracts this effect by competing for and neutralizing RANKL. Osteoclast differentiation factor is a ligand for osteoprotegerin/osteoclastogenesis-inhibitory factor. M-CSF is an essential factor for osteoclast proliferation and differentiation, which is produced by osteoblasts in osseous tissues and acts through its receptor c-fms. See plate section for color version.

demonstrated that osteoclasts express ARs and that DHT directly inhibits the resorptive capacity of isolated human, murine and avian osteoclasts in vitro. Furthermore, androgens may also directly modulate RANKL-induced osteoclast formation, independently of bone marrow cells (Fig. 8.1) (Huber *et al.* 2001). The impact of AR-mediated androgen action was illustrated by the study of Kawano *et al.*, who showed that the suppressive function of the AR system on *RANKL* gene expression mediates the protective effects of androgens on bone remodeling through the inhibition of bone resorption (Kawano *et al.* 2003). Analysis of primary osteoblasts and osteoclasts from global AR knock-out mice indeed revealed that AR function was required for the suppressive effects of androgens on osteoclastogenesis and that this AR function was mediated by osteoblasts (Kawano *et al.* 2003).

Besides the RANKL–OPG pathway, AR-mediated action may be involved in other aspects of function and interaction of osteoblasts and osteoclasts.

It is well established that estrogens affect generation and survival of osteoblasts and osteoclasts. According to Nakamura *et al.* (2007), estrogens reduce number and survival of osteoclasts, and therefore bone resorption, in female but not in male mice, hereby again suggesting that the AR function may be more important in the male. Possibly, the AR also acts via Runx2, an osteoblast master transcription factor which promotes osteoblast-mediated osteoclastogenesis and bone resorption via stimulation of genes which encode for M-CSF and RANKL. The binding of the AR to Runx2 inhibits Runx2 functioning in osteoblasts during later stages of their development. In mice, this AR-mediated repression of Runx2 in osteoblasts resulted in restrained osteoclastogenesis (Baniwal *et al.* 2009). Accumulation of ROS during the aging process was also suggested as a potential mechanism of senile as well as hypogonadal osteoporosis: ROS indeed appear to influence both generation and survival of osteoclasts, osteoblasts and osteocytes. Declining levels of estrogens or androgens decrease the defense mechanisms against oxidative stress in bone, and this may account for the increased bone resorption associated with the acute loss of both of these hormones (Manolagas 2010).

8.10 Key messages

- Hypogonadism and therefore sex steroid deficiency is a well-established cause of high turnover osteoporosis, but most osteoporotic male patients do not suffer from hypogonadism.
- Testosterone replacement maintains bone in hypogonadal men, but its anti-fracture efficacy is not well documented.
- The extent to which the effect of testosterone replacement in men is due to either AR-mediated action or to conversion of estrogens is not fully understood.
- A dual mode of action of testosterone is, however, clearly established in animal model studies, but the underlying mechanism of the aforementioned actions and bone target cells are still unclear.
- Both androgens and estrogens may have an effect on osteoclast and osteoblast generation and survival as well as cross-talk between osteoblasts and osteoclasts.
- Many of the agents used for the treatment of postmenopausal women also appear to be effective in men suffering from osteoporosis.

8.11 References

Amin S, Zhang Y, Felson DT, Sawin CT, Hannan MT, Wilson PW, Kiel DP (2006) Estradiol, testosterone, and the risk for hip fractures in elderly men from the Framingham Study. *Am J Med* **119**:426–433

Anderson FH, Francis RM, Peaston RT, Wastell HJ (1997) Androgen supplementation in eugonadal men with osteoporosis: effects of six months' treatment on markers of bone formation and resorption. *J Bone Miner Res* **12**:472–478

Araujo AB, Travison TG, Leder BZ, Mckinlay JB (2008) Correlations between serum testosterone, estradiol, and sex hormone-binding globulin and bone mineral density in a diverse sample of men. *J Clin Endocrinol Metab* **93**:2135–2141

Auyeung TW, Lee JS, Kwok T, Leung J, Ohlsson C, Vandenput L, Leung PC, Woo J (2011) Testosterone but not estradiol level is positively related to muscle strength and physical performance independent of muscle mass: a cross-sectional study in 1489 older men. *Eur J Endocrinol* **164**:811–817

Baim S, Leonard MB, Bianchi ML, Hans DB, Kalkwarf HJ, Langman CB, Rauch F (2008) Official positions of the International Society for Clinical Densitometry and executive summary of the 2007 ISCD Pediatric Position Development Conference. *J Clin Densitom* **11**:6–21

Baniwal SK, Khalid O, Sir D, Buchanan G, Coetzee GA, Frenkel B (2009) Repression of Runx2 by androgen receptor (AR) in osteoblasts and prostate cancer cells: AR binds Runx2 and abrogates its recruitment to DNA. *Mol Endocrinol* **23**:1203–1214

Barrett-Connor E, Mueller JE, Von Muhlen DG, Laughlin GA, Schneider DL, Sartoris DJ (2000) Low levels of estradiol are associated with vertebral fractures in older men, but not women: the Rancho Bernardo Study. *J Clin Endocrinol Metab* **85**:219–223

Basaria S, Dobs AS (2001) Hypogonadism and androgen replacement therapy in elderly men. *Am J Med* **110**:563–572

Behre HM, Kliesch S, Leifke E, Link TM, Nieschlag E (1997) Long-term effect of testosterone therapy on bone mineral density in hypogonadal men. *J Clin Endocrinol Metab* **82**:2386–2390

Bertelloni S, Baroncelli GI, Battini R, Perri G, Saggese G (1995) Short-term effect of testosterone treatment on reduced bone density in boys with constitutional delay of puberty. *J Bone Miner Res* **10**:1488–1495

Bertelloni S, Baroncelli GI, Ferdeghini M, Perri G, Saggese G (1998) Normal volumetric bone mineral density and bone turnover in young men with histories of constitutional delay of puberty. *J Clin Endocrinol Metab* **83**:4280–4283

Bilezikian JP, Morishima A, Bell J, Grumbach MM (1998) Increased bone mass as a result of estrogen therapy in a man with aromatase deficiency. *N Engl J Med* **339**:599–603

Bjornerem A, Ahmed LA, Joakimsen RM, Berntsen GK, Fonnebo V, Jorgensen L, Oian P, Seeman E, Straume B (2007) A prospective study of sex steroids, sex hormone-binding globulin, and non-vertebral fractures in women and men: the Tromso Study. *Eur J Endocrinol* **157**:119–125

Bonewald LF, Johnson ML (2008) Osteocytes, mechanosensing and Wnt signaling. *Bone* **42**:606–615

Boonen S, Vanderschueren D, Geusens P, Bouillon R (1997) Age-associated endocrine deficiencies as potential determinants of femoral neck (type II) osteoporotic fracture occurrence in elderly men. *Int J Androl* **20**:134–143

Boonen S, Orwoll ES, Wenderoth D, Stoner KJ, Eusebio R, Delmas PD (2009) Once-weekly risedronate in men with osteoporosis: results of a 2-year, placebo-controlled, double-blind, multicenter study. *J Bone Miner Res* **24**:719–725

Bouillon R, Bex M, Vanderschueren D, Boonen S (2004) Estrogens are essential for male pubertal periosteal bone expansion. *J Clin Endocrinol Metab* **89**:6025–6029

Boyle WJ, Simonet WS, Lacey DL (2003) Osteoclast differentiation and activation. *Nature* **423**:337–342

Brown JE, Ellis SP, Lester JE, Gutcher S, Khanna T, Purohit OP, Mccloskey E, Coleman RE (2007) Prolonged efficacy of a single dose of the bisphosphonate zoledronic acid. *Clin Cancer Res* **13**:5406–5410

Burnett-Bowie SA, Mckay EA, Lee H, Leder BZ (2009) Effects of aromatase inhibition on bone mineral density and bone turnover in older men with low testosterone levels. *J Clin Endocrinol Metab* **94**:4785–4792

Callewaert F, Venken K, Ophoff J, De Gendt K, Torcasio A, Van Lenthe GH, Van Oosterwyck H, Boonen S, Bouillon R, Verhoeven G, Vanderschueren D (2009) Differential regulation of bone and body composition in male mice with combined inactivation of androgen and estrogen receptor-alpha. *FASEB J* **23**:232–240

Callewaert F, Boonen S, Vanderschueren D (2010a) Sex steroids and the male skeleton: a tale of two hormones. *Trends Endocrinol Metab* **21**:89–95

Callewaert F, Sinnesael M, Gielen E, Boonen S, Vanderschueren D (2010b) Skeletal sexual dimorphism: relative contribution of sex steroids, GH-IGF1, and mechanical loading. *J Endocrinol* **207**:127–134

Carani C, Qin K, Simoni M, Faustini-Fustini M, Serpente S, Boyd J, Korach KS, Simpson ER (1997) Effect of testosterone and estradiol in a man with aromatase deficiency. *N Engl J Med* **337**:91–95

Center JR, Nguyen TV, Schneider D, Sambrook PN, Eisman JA (1999) Mortality after all major types of osteoporotic fracture in men and women: an observational study. *Lancet* **353**:878–882

Crawford BA, Liu PY, Kean MT, Bleasel JF, Handelsman DJ (2003) Randomized placebo-controlled trial of androgen effects on muscle and bone in men requiring long-term systemic glucocorticoid treatment. *J Clin Endocrinol Metab* **88**:3167–3176

Daniell HW (1997) Osteoporosis after orchiectomy for prostate cancer. *J Urol* **157**:439–444

De Laet CE, Van Hout BA, Burger H, Hofman A, Pols HA (1997) Bone density and risk of hip fracture in men and women: cross sectional analysis. *BMJ* **315**:221–225

De Laet CE, Van Hout BA, Burger H, Weel AE, Hofman A, Pols HA (1998) Hip fracture prediction in elderly men and women: validation in the Rotterdam study. *J Bone Miner Res* **13**:1587–1593

Doran PM, Riggs BL, Atkinson EJ, Khosla S (2001) Effects of raloxifene a selective estrogen receptor modulator, on bone turnover markers and serum sex steroid and lipid levels in elderly men. *J Bone Miner Res* **16**:2118–2125

Ducy P (2000) Cbfa1: a molecular switch in osteoblast biology. *Dev Dyn* **219**:461–471

Dunkel L, Wickman S (2002) Novel treatment of delayed male puberty with aromatase inhibitors. *Horm Res* **57** (Suppl 2):44–52

Empana JP, Dargent-Molina P, Breart G (2004) Effect of hip fracture on mortality in elderly women: the EPIDOS prospective study. *J Am Geriatr Soc* **52**:685–690

Ensrud KE, Thompson DE, Cauley JA, Nevitt MC, Kado DM, Hochberg MC, Santora AC 2nd, Black DM (2000) Prevalent vertebral deformities predict mortality and hospitalization in older women with low bone mass. Fracture Intervention Trial Research Group. *J Am Geriatr Soc* **48**:241–249

Fabbri A, Giannetta E, Lenzi A, Isidori AM (2007) Testosterone treatment to mimic hormone physiology in androgen replacement therapy. A view on testosterone gel and other preparations available. *Expert Opin Biol Ther* **7**:1093–1106

Falahati-Nini A, Riggs BL, Atkinson EJ, O'fallon WM, Eastell R, Khosla S (2000) Relative contributions of testosterone and estrogen in regulating bone resorption and formation in normal elderly men. *J Clin Invest* **106**:1553–1560

Fechtenbaum J, Cropet C, Kolta S, Horlait S, Orcel P, Roux C (2005) The severity of vertebral fractures and health-related quality of life in osteoporotic postmenopausal women. *Osteoporos Int* 16:2175–2179

Ferlin A, Schipilliti M, Vinanzi C, Garolla A, Di Mambro A, Selice R, Lenzi A, Foresta C (2011) Bone mass in subjects with Klinefelter syndrome: role of testosterone levels and androgen receptor gene CAG polymorphism. *J Clin Endocrinol Metab* 96:E739–E745

Finkelstein JS, Klibanski A, Neer RM, Greenspan SL, Rosenthal DI, Crowley WF Jr (1987) Osteoporosis in men with idiopathic hypogonadotropic hypogonadism. *Ann Intern Med* 106:354–361

Finkelstein JS, Neer RM, Biller BM, Crawford JD, Klibanski A (1992) Osteopenia in men with a history of delayed puberty. *N Engl J Med* 326:600–604

Finkelstein JS, Klibanski A, Neer RM (1999) Evaluation of lumber spine bone mineral density (BMD) using dual energy X-ray absorptiometry (DXA) in 21 young men with histories of constitutionally-delayed puberty. *J Clin Endocrinol Metab* 84:3400–3401; author reply:3403–3404

Fried LP, Tangen CM, Walston J, Newman AB, Hirsch C, Gottdiener J, Seeman T, Tracy R, Kop WJ, Burke G, Mcburnie MA (2001) Frailty in older adults: evidence for a phenotype. *J Gerontol A Biol Sci Med Sci* 56:M146–M156

Gao W, Reiser PJ, Coss CC, Phelps MA, Kearbey JD, Miller DD, Dalton JT (2005) Selective androgen receptor modulator treatment improves muscle strength and body composition and prevents bone loss in orchidectomized rats. *Endocrinology* 146:4887–4897

Goderie-Plomp HW, Van Der Klift M, De Ronde W, Hofman A, De Jong FH, Pols HA (2004) Endogenous sex hormones, sex hormone-binding globulin, and the risk of incident vertebral fractures in elderly men and women: the Rotterdam Study. *J Clin Endocrinol Metab* 89:3261–3269

Harada S, Rodan GA (2003) Control of osteoblast function and regulation of bone mass. *Nature* 423:349–355

Holt G, Khaw KT, Reid DM, Compston JE, Bhalla A, Woolf AD, Crabtree NJ, Dalzell N, Wardley-Smith B, Lunt M, Reeve J (2002) Prevalence of osteoporotic bone mineral density at the hip in Britain differs substantially from the US over 50 years of age: implications for clinical densitometry. *Br J Radiol* 75:736–742

Huber DM, Bendixen AC, Pathrose P, Srivastava S, Dienger KM, Shevde NK, Pike JW (2001) Androgens suppress osteoclast formation induced by RANKL and macrophage-colony stimulating factor. *Endocrinology* 142:3800–3808

Isidori AM, Giannetta E, Greco EA, Gianfrilli D, Bonifacio V, Isidori A, Lenzi A, Fabbri A (2005) Effects of testosterone on body composition, bone metabolism and serum lipid profile in middle-aged men: a meta-analysis. *Clin Endocrinol (Oxf)* 63:280–293

Jackson JA, Kleerekoper M, Parfitt AM, Rao DS, Villanueva AR, Frame B (1987) Bone histomorphometry in hypogonadal and eugonadal men with spinal osteoporosis. *J Clin Endocrinol Metab* 65:53–58

Johnell O, Kanis JA (2006) An estimate of the worldwide prevalence and disability associated with osteoporotic fractures. *Osteoporos Int* 17:1726–1733

Kamel HK (2005) Male osteoporosis: new trends in diagnosis and therapy. *Drugs Aging* 22:741–748

Kanis JA (2002) Diagnosis of osteoporosis and assessment of fracture risk. *Lancet* 359:1929–1936

Kanis JA, Gluer CC (2000) An update on the diagnosis and assessment of osteoporosis with densitometry. Committee of Scientific Advisors, International Osteoporosis Foundation. *Osteoporos Int* 11:192–202

Kanis JA, Johnell O, Oden A, Sembo I, Redlund-Johnell I, Dawson A, De Laet C, Jonsson B (2000) Long-term risk of osteoporotic fracture in Malmo. *Osteoporos Int* 11:669–674

Kanis JA, Johnell O, Oden A, Johansson H, Mccloskey E (2008) FRAX and the assessment of fracture probability in men and women from the UK. *Osteoporos Int* 19:385–397

Katznelson L, Finkelstein JS, Schoenfeld DA, Rosenthal DI, Anderson EJ, Klibanski A (1996) Increase in bone density and lean body mass during testosterone administration in men with acquired hypogonadism. *J Clin Endocrinol Metab* 81:4358–4365

Kawano H, Sato T, Yamada T, Matsumoto T, Sekine K, Watanabe T, Nakamura T, Fukuda T, Yoshimura K, Yoshizawa T, Aihara K, Yamamoto Y, Nakamichi Y, Metzger D, Chambon P, Nakamura K, Kawaguchi H, Kato S (2003) Suppressive function of androgen receptor in bone resorption. *Proceedings of the National Academy of Sciences of the United States of America* 100:9416–9421

Kearbey JD, Gao W, Fisher SJ, Wu D, Miller DD, Dalton JT (2009) Effects of selective androgen receptor modulator (SARM) treatment in osteopenic female rats. *Pharm Res* 26:2471–2477

Kelepouris N, Harper KD, Gannon F, Kaplan FS, Haddad JG (1995) Severe osteoporosis in men. *Ann Intern Med* 123:452–460

Kenny M, Prestwood KM, Gruman CA, Marcello KM, Raisz LG (2001) Effects of transdermal testosterone on bone and muscle in older men with low bioavailable testosterone levels. *J Gerontol A Biol Sci Med Sci* 56:M266–M272

Kenny M, Prestwood KM, Gruman CA, Fabregas G, Biskup B, Mansoor G (2002) Effects of transdermal testosterone on lipids and vascular reactivity in older men with low bioavailable testosterone levels. *J Gerontol A Biol Sci Med Sci* **57**:M460–M465

Khosla S, Lufkin EG, Hodgson SF, Fitzpatrick LA, Melton LJ 3rd (1994) Epidemiology and clinical features of osteoporosis in young individuals. *Bone* **15**:551–555

Khosla S, Melton LJ 3rd, Atkinson EJ, O'fallon WM, Klee GG, Riggs BL (1998) Relationship of serum sex steroid levels and bone turnover markers with bone mineral density in men and women: a key role for bioavailable estrogen. *J Clin Endocrinol Metab* **83**:2266–2274

Khosla S, Amin S, Orwoll E (2008) Osteoporosis in men. *Endocr Rev* **29**:441–464

Kurland ES, Rosen CJ, Cosman F, Mcmahon D, Chan F, Shane E, Lindsay R, Dempster D, Bilezikian JP (1997) Insulin-like growth factor-I in men with idiopathic osteoporosis. *J Clin Endocrinol Metab* **82**:2799–2805

Lanfranco F, Zirilli L, Baldi M, Pignatti E, Corneli G, Ghigo E, Aimaretti G, Carani C, Rochira V (2008) A novel mutation in the human aromatase gene: insights on the relationship among serum estradiol, longitudinal growth and bone mineral density in an adult man under estrogen replacement treatment. *Bone* **43**:628–635

Lippuner K, Golder M, Greiner R (2005) Epidemiology and direct medical costs of osteoporotic fractures in men and women in Switzerland. *Osteoporos Int* **16** Suppl 2:S8–S17

Ly LP, Jimenez M, Zhuang TN, Celermajer DS, Conway J, Handelsman DJ (2001) A double-blind, placebo-controlled, randomized clinical trial of transdermal dihydrotestosterone gel on muscular strength, mobility, and quality of life in older men with partial androgen deficiency. *J Clin Endocrinol Metab* **86**:4078–4088

Manolagas SC (2000) Birth and death of bone cells: basic regulatory mechanisms and implications for the pathogenesis and treatment of osteoporosis. *Endocr Rev* **21**:115–137

Manolagas SC (2010) From estrogen-centric to aging and oxidative stress: a revised perspective of the pathogenesis of osteoporosis. *Endocr Rev* **31**:266–300

Maravic M, Le Bihan C, Landais P, Fardellone P (2005) Incidence and cost of osteoporotic fractures in France during 2001. A methodological approach by the national hospital database. *Osteoporos Int* **16**:1475–1480

Meier C, Nguyen TV, Handelsman DJ, Schindler C, Kushnir MM, Rockwood AL, Meikle W, Center JR, Eisman JA, Seibel MJ (2008) Endogenous sex hormones and incident fracture risk in older men: the Dubbo Osteoporosis Epidemiology Study. *Arch Intern Med* **168**:47–54

Meier DE, Orwoll ES, Keenan EJ, Fagerstrom RM (1987) Marked decline in trabecular bone mineral content in healthy men with age: lack of association with sex steroid levels. *J Am Geriatr Soc* **35**:189–197

Mellstrom D, Vandenput L, Mallmin H, Holmberg AH, Lorentzon M, Oden A, Johansson H, Orwoll ES, Labrie F, Karlsson MK, Ljunggren O, Ohlsson C (2008) Older men with low serum estradiol and high serum SHBG have an increased risk of fractures. *J Bone Miner Res* **23**:1552–1560

Melton LJ 3rd, Lieber MM, Atkinson EJ, Achenbach SJ, Zincke H, Therneau TM, Khosla S (2011) Fracture risk in men with prostate cancer: a population-based study. *J Bone Miner Res* **26**:1808–1815

Misiorowski W (2010) Parathyroid hormone and its analogues – molecular mechanisms of action and efficacy in osteoporosis therapy. *Endokrynol Pol* **62**:73–78

Morishima A, Grumbach MM, Simpson ER, Fisher C, Qin K (1995) Aromatase deficiency in male and female siblings caused by a novel mutation and the physiological role of estrogens. *J Clin Endocrinol Metab* **80**:3689–3698

Nakamura T, Imai Y, Matsumoto T, Sato S, Takeuchi K, Igarashi K, Harada Y, Azuma Y, Krust A, Yamamoto Y, Nishina H, Takeda S, Takayanagi H, Metzger D, Kanno J, Takaoka K, Martin TJ, Chambon P, Kato S (2007) Estrogen prevents bone loss via estrogen receptor alpha and induction of Fas ligand in osteoclasts. *Cell* **130**:811–823

O'Connell M, Tajar A, Roberts S, Wu F (2011) Do androgens play any role in the physical frailty of ageing men? *J Androl* **34**:17

Orsini LS, Rousculp MD, Long SR, Wang S (2005) Health care utilization and expenditures in the United States: a study of osteoporosis-related fractures. *Osteoporos Int* **16**:359–371

Page ST, Amory JK, Bowman FD, Anawalt BD, Matsumoto M, Bremner WJ, Tenover JL (2005) Exogenous testosterone (T) alone or with finasteride increases physical performance, grip strength, and lean body mass in older men with low serum T. *J Clin Endocrinol Metab* **90**:1502–1510

Pederson L, Kremer M, Judd J, Pascoe D, Spelsberg TC, Riggs BL, Oursler MJ (1999) Androgens regulate bone resorption activity of isolated osteoclasts in vitro. *Proc Natl Acad Sci USA* **96**:505–510

Pelat C, Van Pottelbergh I, Cohen-Solal M, Ostertag A, Kaufman JM, Martinez M, De Vernejoul MC (2007) Complex segregation analysis accounting for GxE of bone mineral density in European pedigrees selected through a male proband with low BMD. *Ann Hum Genet* **71**:29–42

Pernow Y, Granberg B, Saaf M, Weidenhielm L (2006) Osteoblast dysfunction in male idiopathic osteoporosis. *Calcif Tissue Int* **78**:90–97

Pernow Y, Hauge EM, Linder K, Dahl E, Saaf M (2009) Bone

histomorphometry in male idiopathic osteoporosis. *Calcif Tissue Int* **84**:430–438

Rapado A, Hawkins F, Sobrinho L, Diaz-Curiel M, Galvao-Telles A, Arver S, Melo Gomes J, Mazer N, Garcia E, Costa J, Horcajada C, Lopez-Gavilanes E, Mascarenhas M, Papapietro K, Lopez Alvarez MB, Pereira MC, Martinez G, Valverde I, Garcia JJ, Carballal JJ, Garcia I (1999) Bone mineral density and androgen levels in elderly males. *Calcif Tissue Int* **65**:417–421

Rariy CM, Ratcliffe SJ, Weinstein R, Bhasin S, Blackman MR, Cauley JA, Robbins J, Zmuda JM, Harris TB, Cappola R (2011) Higher serum free testosterone concentration in older women is associated with greater bone mineral density, lean body mass, and total fat mass: the cardiovascular health study. *J Clin Endocrinol Metab* **96**:989–996

Reid IR (1998) Glucocorticoid-induced osteoporosis: assessment and treatment. *J Clin Densitom* **1**:65–73

Reifenstein EC Jr, Albright F (1947) The metabolic effects of steroid hormones in osteoporosis. *J Clin Invest* **26**:24–56

Reim NS, Breig B, Stahr K, Eberle J, Hoeflich A, Wolf E, Erben RG (2008) Cortical bone loss in androgen-deficient aged male rats is mainly caused by increased endocortical bone remodeling. *J Bone Miner Res* **23**:694–704

Ringe JD, Orwoll E, Daifotis A, Lombardi A (2002) Treatment of male osteoporosis: recent advances with alendronate. *Osteoporos Int* **13**:195–199

Rockwood K, Mitnitski A (2007) Frailty in relation to the accumulation of deficits. *J Gerontol A Biol Sci Med Sci* **62**:722–727

Schatzl G, Madersbacher S, Temml C, Krenn-Schinkel K, Nader A, Sregi G, Lapin A, Hermann M, Berger P, Marberger M (2003) Serum androgen levels in men: impact of health status and age. *Urology* **61**:629–633

Seeman E (2001) Clinical review 137: Sexual dimorphism in skeletal size, density, and strength. *J Clin Endocrinol Metab* **86**:4576–4584

Seeman E (2003) Periosteal bone formation – a neglected determinant of bone strength. *N Engl J Med* **349**:320–323

Smith EP, Boyd J, Frank GR, Takahashi H, Cohen RM, Specker B, Williams TC, Lubahn DB, Korach KS (1994) Estrogen resistance caused by a mutation in the estrogen-receptor gene in a man. *N Engl J Med* **331**:1056–1061

Smith EP, Specker B, Bachrach BE, Kimbro KS, Li XJ, Young MF, Fedarko NS, Abuzzahab MJ, Frank GR, Cohen RM, Lubahn DB, Korach KS (2008) Impact on bone of an estrogen receptor-alpha gene loss of function mutation. *J Clin Endocrinol Metab* **93**:3088–3096

Smith MR, Eastham J, Gleason DM, Shasha D, Tchekmedyian S, Zinner N (2003) Randomized controlled trial of zoledronic acid to prevent bone loss in men receiving androgen deprivation therapy for nonmetastatic prostate cancer. *J Urol* **169**:2008–2012

Smith MR, Fallon MA, Lee H, Finkelstein JS (2004) Raloxifene to prevent gonadotropin-releasing hormone agonist-induced bone loss in men with prostate cancer: a randomized controlled trial. *J Clin Endocrinol Metab* **89**:3841–3846

Smith MR, Egerdie B, Hernandez Toriz N, Feldman R, Tammela TL, Saad F, Heracek J, Szwedowski M, Ke C, Kupic A, Leder BZ, Goessl C (2009) Denosumab in men receiving androgen-deprivation therapy for prostate cancer. *N Engl J Med* **361**:745–755

Snyder PJ, Peachey H, Hannoush P, Berlin JA, Loh L, Holmes JH, Dlewati A, Staley J, Santanna J, Kapoor SC, Attie MF, Haddad JG Jr, Strom BL (1999) Effect of testosterone treatment on bone mineral density in men over 65

years of age. *J Clin Endocrinol Metab* **84**:1966–1972

Stepan JJ, Lachman M, Zverina J, Pacovsky V, Baylink DJ (1989) Castrated men exhibit bone loss: effect of calcitonin treatment on biochemical indices of bone remodeling. *J Clin Endocrinol Metab* **69**:523–527

Taes Y, Lapauw B, Vandewalle S, Zmierczak H, Goemaere S, Vanderschueren D, Kaufman JM, T'sjoen G (2009) Estrogen-specific action on bone geometry and volumetric bone density: longitudinal observations in an adult with complete androgen insensitivity. *Bone* **45**:392–397

Vandenput L, Boonen S, Van Herck E, Swinnen JV, Bouillon R, Vanderschueren D (2002) Evidence from the aged orchidectomized male rat model that 17beta-estradiol is a more effective bone-sparing and anabolic agent than 5alpha-dihydrotestosterone. *J Bone Miner Res* **17**:2080–2086

Vanderschueren D, Vandenput L, Boonen S, Van Herck E, Swinnen JV, Bouillon R (2000) An aged rat model of partial androgen deficiency: prevention of both loss of bone and lean body mass by low-dose androgen replacement. *Endocrinology* **141**:1642–1647

Vanderschueren D, Vandenput L, Boonen S, Lindberg MK, Bouillon R, Ohlsson C (2004) Androgens and bone. *Endocr Rev* **25**:389–425

Vanderschueren D, Vandenput L, Boonen S (2005) Reversing sex steroid deficiency and optimizing skeletal development in the adolescent with gonadal failure. *Endocr Dev* **8**:150–165

Venken K, Boonen S, Van Herck E, Vandenput L, Kumar N, Sitruk-Ware R, Sundaram K, Bouillon R, Vanderschueren D (2005) Bone and muscle protective potential of the prostate-sparing synthetic androgen 7alpha-methyl-19-nortestosterone: evidence from the aged orchidectomized male rat model. *Bone* **36**:663–670

Venken K, De Gendt K, Boonen S, Ophoff J, Bouillon R, Swinnen JV, Verhoeven G, Vanderschueren D (2006) Relative impact of androgen and estrogen receptor activation in the effects of androgens on trabecular and cortical bone in growing male mice: a study in the androgen receptor knockout mouse model. *J Bone Miner Res* **21**:576–585

Vermeulen A, Kaufman JM, Goemaere S, Van Pottelberg I (2002) Estradiol in elderly men. *Aging Male* **5**:98–102

Wei JT, Gross M, Jaffe CA, Gravlin K, Lahaie M, Faerber GJ, Cooney KA (1999) Androgen deprivation therapy for prostate cancer results in significant loss of bone density. *Urology* **54**:607–611

Zirilli L, Rochira V, Diazzi C, Caffagni G, Carani C (2008) Human models of aromatase deficiency. *J Steroid Biochem Mol Biol* **109**: 212–218

Androgen effects on the skeletal muscle

Shalender Bhasin, Ravi Jasuja, Carlo Serra, Rajan Singh, Thomas W. Storer, Wen Guo, Thomas G. Travison, and Shezad Basaria

9.1   Introduction

The idea that androgens have anabolic effects on the muscle is not novel; humans have known since antiquity that the removal of the testes depletes men's vigor. In modern times, shortly after the synthesis of testosterone, Kochakian at the University of Rochester and Kenyon *et al.* at the University of Chicago provided unequivocal evidence of the anabolic effects of testosterone by demonstrating that androgen administration increases nitrogen retention in castrated males of many mammalian species, and in eunuchoidal men and women (Kochakian and Murlin 1935; Kochakian 1937; 1950; Kenyon *et al.* 1940). The decades of 1940 and 1950 witnessed the synthesis of novel steroidal androgen receptor modulators, mostly

with an intent to produce more selective androgens with enhanced anabolic activity. These androgenic-anabolic steroids were first used in professional sports by Russian weightlifters; however, the use of androgens spread widely to athletes in other parts of the world and to other sports (Yesalis *et al.* 1993; Yesalis and Bahrke 1995; Freeman *et al.* 2001). In the early 1980s, with the availability of underground steroid handbooks, the use of androgens spilled over from the athletes into the general community of recreational bodybuilders. In spite of the wide empiric evidence of anabolic activity of androgens emerging from the experience of athletes and bodybuilders, the academic community continued to maintain a puritanical denial; the Endocrine Society

Testosterone: Action, Deficiency, Substitution, ed. Eberhard Nieschlag and Hermann M. Behre, Assoc. ed. Susan Nieschlag. Published by Cambridge University Press. © Cambridge University Press 2012.

issued a position statement declaring that anabolic steroids do not enhance muscle mass or strength. In the mid-1990s, the publication of well-conducted, randomized clinical trials finally put this controversy to rest, demonstrating unequivocally that when energy and protein intake, and exercise stimulus are standardized, the administration of a supraphysiological dose of testosterone increases fat-free mass and maximal voluntary strength, and that the concomitant administration of a standardized resistance exercise program augments the anabolic effects of androgens on muscle mass and maximal voluntary strength (Bhasin et al. 1996). Since then, substantial pharmaceutical and academic research effort has focused on the development of androgens as function-promoting anabolic therapies. This chapter will review the large body of epidemiological and clinical trial evidence of the anabolic effects of androgens on skeletal muscle, and explore the hypothesis that testosterone-induced increases in muscle mass and strength can translate into improved physical function and health outcomes in older men with mobility limitation or sarcopenia. The chapter will also describe the mechanisms by which androgens increase skeletal muscle mass, and strategies that can be used to enhance the selectivity of androgen action to improve the risk-to-benefit ratio.

9.2 The association of circulating testosterone concentrations and muscle mass, muscle performance and physical function: epidemiological evidence

Prepubertal boys and girls have similar muscle mass; however, during the pubertal transition, the boys accrue on average 4.5 kg greater muscle mass than girls, largely due to the interactive effects of testosterone and GH. Healthy, hypogonadal men have lower fat-free mass (Katznelson et al. 1996; 1998) and higher fat mass than age-matched eugonadal men. Circulating testosterone levels have been associated with appendicular muscle mass and the strength of upper and lower extremity muscles in men (Morley et al. 1997; Baumgartner et al. 1998; Melton et al. 2000a; 2000b; Baumgartner 2000; Roy et al. 2002). In epidemiological studies of community-dwelling older men, lower testosterone concentrations are associated with reduced physical function, assessed using performance-based as well as self-reported measures of physical function (van den

Beld et al. 2000; Schaap et al. 2005; Orwoll et al. 2006; Krasnoff et al. 2009; Cawthon et al. 2009). In the Osteoporotic Fractures in Men Study (MrOS), low bioavailable testosterone levels were associated with lower levels of physical performance and increased risk of falls (Orwoll et al. 2006). The association of bioavailable testosterone level with fall risk in the MrOS study persisted even after adjusting for measures of physical performance, suggesting that testosterone levels may reduce fall propensity through other mechanisms (Orwoll et al. 2006). Low free testosterone levels have also been associated with increased risk of incident mobility limitations and progression of mobility limitation in men in the Framingham Heart Study (Krasnoff et al. 2009).

Epidemiological studies have demonstrated an inverse relationship between serum testosterone levels and measures of obesity and visceral fat mass (Seidell et al. 1990; Khaw and Barrett-Connor 1992). Total and free testosterone concentrations have been negatively correlated with waist/hip circumference ratio, visceral fat area, glucose, insulin and C-peptide concentrations (Seidell et al. 1990; Khaw and Barrett-Connor 1992).

9.3 The effects of experimental lowering of endogenous testosterone concentrations on body composition

The suppression of endogenous testosterone levels in men by administration of a long-acting GnRH agonist analog is associated with loss of fat-free mass, an increase in fat mass, and a decrease in fractional muscle protein synthesis (Mauras et al. 1998). Testosterone suppression is also associated with a decrease in whole body leucine oxidation as well as non-oxidative leucine disappearance rates (Mauras et al. 1998).

9.4 The effects of physiological testosterone replacement in models of androgen deficiency

In all models of androgen deficiency that have been examined, testosterone replacement has been shown consistently to exert anabolic effects. For example, in pioneering studies conducted by Kochakian, testosterone replacement increased nitrogen retention in castrated males of several mammalian species (Kochakian and Murlin 1935; Kochakian 1937; 1950). Other studies reported nitrogen retention in eunuchoidal men, boys before puberty, and in women after testosterone supplementation (Kenyon *et al.* 1940). Several recent studies have re-examined the effects of testosterone on body composition and muscle mass in hypogonadal men in more detail (Brodsky *et al.* 1996; Wang *et al.* 1996a; 2000; Bhasin *et al.* 1997; Snyder *et al.* 2000; Steidle *et al.* 2003). These studies are in agreement that replacement doses of testosterone, when administered to healthy, androgen-deficient men, increase fat-free mass, muscle size, and maximal voluntary strength (Brodsky *et al.* 1996; Wang *et al.* 1996a; 2000; Bhasin *et al.* 1997; Snyder *et al.* 2000; Steidle *et al.* 2003). The muscle accretion during testosterone treatment has been reported to increase in fractional muscle protein synthesis in some studies (Brodsky *et al.* 1996; Mauras *et al.* 1998).

9.5 Testosterone dose-response relationships in young and older men

Testosterone administration increases skeletal muscle mass in healthy men; these anabolic effects of testosterone are related to the dose administered and the circulating testosterone concentrations (Bhasin *et al.* 2001; 2005; Storer *et al.* 2003; Woodhouse *et al.* 2003; 2004). In a randomized, masked study of testosterone dose-response relationships, healthy young and older men were treated with a long-acting GnRH agonist to suppress endogenous testosterone production and given concurrently with one of several graded doses of testosterone enanthate, ranging from 25 mg intramuscularly weekly to 600 mg intramuscularly weekly (Bhasin *et al.* 2001; 2005; Storer *et al.* 2003; Woodhouse *et al.* 2003; 2004). Testosterone administration was associated with dose-dependent increments in fat-free mass, appendicular muscle mass and maximal voluntary strength in the leg press exercise in healthy young as well as older men (Bhasin *et al.* 2001; 2005; Storer *et al.* 2003; Woodhouse *et al.* 2003; 2004). In multivariate models, the gains in lean body mass and muscle size during testosterone administration could largely be explained by testosterone dose and the circulating testosterone concentrations (Woodhouse *et al.* 2003). Changes in whole-body, appendicular, truncal, and intermuscular fat mass were inversely associated with testosterone dose and circulating testosterone concentrations (Woodhouse *et al.* 2004). Unlike resistance exercise training, testosterone administration does not improve the contractile properties of skeletal muscle; thus specific force, that is, the maximal voluntary strength per unit muscle volume, does not change during testosterone administration (Storer *et al.* 2003).

Plasma clearance rates of testosterone are lower in older men than in young men; consequently the increments in serum testosterone concentrations at any given testosterone dose are higher in older men than in young men (Coviello *et al.* 2006). Older men also experience greater increments in hemoglobin and hematocrit in response to testosterone administration, even after adjusting for the higher testosterone levels (Calof *et al.* 2005; Coviello *et al.* 2008; Fernández-Balsells *et al.* 2010). These age-related differences in hematocrit response to testosterone cannot be explained easily on the basis of changes in erythropoietin or transferring receptor levels (Coviello *et al.* 2008). We have shown recently that testosterone suppresses hepcidin, an important regulator of iron availability for hematopoiesis, suggesting that testosterone might stimulate erythropoiesis by increasing iron availability (Bachman *et al.* 2010).

9.6 Randomized controlled trials of testosterone and other androgens in men with chronic diseases

The course of many chronic illnesses, such as chronic obstructive lung disease, end-stage renal disease, congestive heart failure, many types of cancers, tuberculosis and HIV infection, are associated with loss of lean body mass and strength, and increased risk of functional limitations, disability and poor disease outcomes (MacAdams *et al.* 1986; Reid 1987; Coodley *et al.* 1994; Dobs *et al.* 1996; Grinspoon *et al.* 1996; 2000; Arver *et al.* 1999; Salehian *et al.* 1999; Rietschel *et al.* 2000; Bhasin *et al.* 2006). Accordingly, there has been considerable interest in the application of androgens as anabolic therapy to improve physical function and exercise capacity.

Several randomized trials have examined the effects of androgen supplementation in men with chronic illness (Buchwald *et al.* 1977; Berns *et al.* 1992; Schols *et al.* 1995; Reid *et al.* 1996; Coodley and Coodley 1997; Grinspoon *et al.* 1998; Bhasin *et al.* 1998; 2000; Dobs *et al.* 1999; Johansen 1999; Johansen *et al.* 1999; Painter and Johansen 1999; Sattler *et al.* 1999; Strawford *et al.* 1999a; 1999b; Crawford *et al.* 2003; Casaburi *et al.* 2004). Meta-analyses of placebo-controlled randomized trials of testosterone replacement in HIV-infected men with weight loss are in agreement that men assigned to the testosterone arm of these trials experienced greater gains in body weight and fat-free mass than those randomized to the placebo arm (Kong and Edmonds 2002; Johns *et al.* 2005; Bhasin *et al.* 2006). However, the trials included in these meta-analyses were characterized by heterogeneous patient populations, small sample sizes and differences in testosterone dose and regimens. The three studies that showed gains in fat-free mass selected patients with low testosterone levels (Grinspoon *et al.* 1998; Bhasin *et al.* 1998; 2000). In a placebo-controlled, randomized trial (Bhasin *et al.* 2000), we demonstrated that testosterone replacement in HIV-infected men with low testosterone levels is associated with significant gains in fat-free mass and maximal voluntary strength in the leg press, leg curls, bench press and latissimus dorsi pull-downs. Thus, when the confounding influence of the learning effect is minimized and appropriate androgen-responsive measures of muscle strength are selected, testosterone replacement is associated with demonstrable increase in maximal voluntary strength in HIV-infected men with low testosterone levels. We do not know whether androgen replacement improves well-being, physical function, or other health-related outcomes in HIV-infected men.

The patients with *end-stage renal disease* who are on maintenance hemodialysis experience loss of skeletal muscle mass, and decreased physical function and exercise capacity (Johansen 1999; Johansen *et al.* 1999; Painter and Johansen 1999). Nandrolone decanoate has been reported to increase hemoglobin levels and fat-free mass in men with end-stage renal disease (Buchwald *et al.* 1977; Berns *et al.* 1992; Johansen *et al.* 1999). Testosterone replacement is associated with a greater increase in fat-free mass, bone density, muscle strength, and quality of life than placebo in men receiving glucocorticoids (Reid *et al.* 1996; Crawford *et al.* 2003). Schols *et al.* (1995) have reported modest increases in lean body mass and respiratory muscle strength with a low dose of nandrolone in men and women with chronic obstructive pulmonary disease (COPD). In a placebo-controlled, randomized trial, Casaburi *et al.* (2004) demonstrated that testosterone therapy in men with COPD who have low testosterone levels increases fat-free mass, muscle size and maximal muscle strength to a greater extent than placebo. The effects of the combined testosterone and resistance exercise training on muscle strength were greater than those of testosterone alone (Casaburi *et al.* 2004).

9.7 Randomized trials of testosterone in healthy older men

Meta-analyses of randomized clinical trials in community dwelling, healthy, middle-aged and older men have confirmed that testosterone therapy is associated with greater increments in fat-free mass and grip strength, and greater reductions in fat mass than those associated with placebo administration alone (Fig. 9.1) (Tenover 1992; Morley *et al.* 1993; Urban *et al.* 1995; Sih *et al.* 1997; Ferrando *et al.* 1998; 2002; Clague *et al.* 1999; Snyder *et al.* 1999a; Tenover 1999; 2000; Kenny *et al.* 2001; Blackman *et al.* 2002; Johns *et al.* 2005; Page *et al.* 2005; Bhasin *et al.* 2006; Nair *et al.* 2006; Emmelot-Vonk *et al.* 2008; LeBrasseur *et al.* 2009; Basaria *et al.* 2010; Travison *et al.* 2011). Testosterone therapy improves self-reported physical function, such as that measured using the physical function domain of the MOS SF-36 (Snyder *et al.* 1999a). However, testosterone administration has not been shown to improve performance-based measures of physical function in healthy older men, in spite of remarkable gains in muscle mass and strength (Storer *et al.* 2008). The first generation studies of testosterone were characterized generally by their small sample size, inclusion of healthy men without any functional limitations, and varying testosterone doses and regimens. The measures of physical function used in many trials had a low ceiling (Bhasin *et al.* 2006).

The doses of testosterone used in some of the trials were relatively low and were associated with either small or no significant increments in testosterone levels (Bhasin *et al.* 2006). As testosterone effects on the skeletal muscle are related to testosterone dose and circulating concentrations, it is possible that these doses were insufficient to produce clinically meaningful changes in muscle mass and strength.

A major reason for the failure to demonstrate improvements in physical function is that testosterone trials of the first generation were conducted in healthy older men and used measures of physical function that had a relatively low ceiling (Bhasin *et al.* 2006). The widely used measures such as 0.625 m stair climb, standing up from a chair, and 20 m walk are tasks that require only a small fraction of an individual's maximal voluntary strength. In most healthy, older men, the baseline maximal voluntary strength is far higher than the threshold below which these measures would detect impairment. Given the low intensity of the tasks used, it is not surprising that

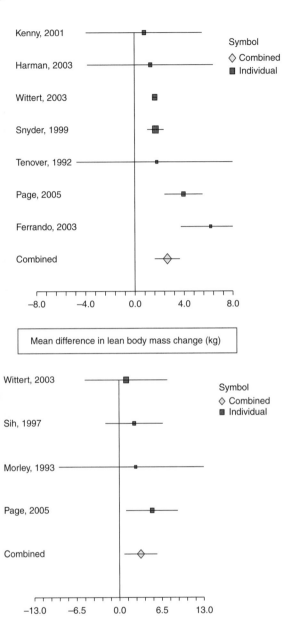

Fig. 9.1 A meta-analysis of the randomized trials of testosterone in middle-aged and older men. The names of the first authors are listed. Overall, the men assigned to testosterone arms of the trials had greater gains in lean body mass than those assigned to the placebo arms of the trial. Reproduced with permission from Bhasin et al. (2006).

relatively healthy older individuals recruited in these initial testosterone trials showed neither impairment in these threshold-dependent measures of physical function at baseline, nor an improvement in

performance on these tasks during testosterone administration. It also is possible that translation of muscle mass and strength gains into functional improvements may require functional training or cognitive and behavioral intervention. We do not know whether task-specific training is necessary to induce the types of neuromuscular adaptations that are necessary for improvements in physical function. The subjects recruited in the first generation trials of testosterone were healthy community-dwelling men who did not have any functional limitations.

Several recent testosterone trials aimed at determining whether testosterone therapy improves physical function in older men with mobility limitations or one or more frailty characteristics (Kenny *et al.* 2001; Basaria *et al.* 2010; Srinivas-Shankar *et al.* 2010; Travison *et al.* 2011). In a placebo-controlled trial (Srinivas-Shankar *et al.* 2010), prefrail or frail older men were randomized to either 50 mg testosterone gel or placebo gel for six months. The men randomized to the testosterone arm experienced greater improvements in isometric knee extension peak torque, lean body mass, and somatic and sexual symptoms than those randomized to the placebo arm. Although measures of physical function did not differ significantly between the two arms, they improved in the subgroup of older and frail men (Srinivas-Shankar *et al.* 2010). In a testosterone trial in older men with mobility limitation (the TOM Trial; Basaria *et al.* 2010; Travison *et al.* 2011), the subjects were randomized to either placebo or 10 g testosterone gel daily for six months. The testosterone dose was adjusted to achieve testosterone levels between 500 and 1000 ng/dl. The men randomized to the testosterone arm experienced greater improvements in leg-press strength, chest-press strength and power, and loaded stair-climbing speed and power than those assigned to the placebo arm (Fig. 9.2). A greater proportion of men in the testosterone arm improved more than the minimal clinically important difference for leg-press and chest-press strength and stair-climbing speed than did in the placebo arm. The men in the testosterone arm also experienced a higher frequency of adverse events and cardiovascular-related events than those in the placebo arm, leading the trial's Data and Safety Monitoring Board to recommend enrollment cessation and no further administration of study medication (Basaria *et al.* 2010; Travison *et al.* 2011). Clinical trial data on the effects of testosterone on cardiovascular events are limited. The participants

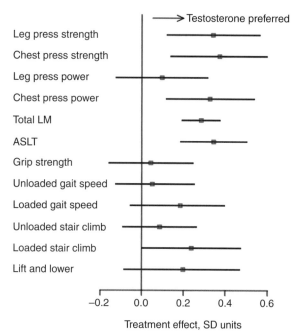

Fig. 9.2 The effects of testosterone on measures of muscle mass, muscle performance and physical function in the Testosterone in Older Men with Mobility Limitations Trial (the TOM Trial). Absolute treatment differences (testosterone vs. placebo arms) are plotted for the primary and secondary outcomes in units normalized to the baseline standard deviation (SD) of measurement; point estimates (red) are accompanied by 95% confidence intervals. Abbreviations: ASLT, appendicular skeletal lean tissue mass; LM, lean mass. Reproduced with permission from Travison et al. 2011.

in the TOM trial were older men (mean age 74) with high prevalence of chronic conditions, such as heart disease, diabetes, obesity, hypertension, and hyperlipidemia (Basaria et al. 2010; Travison et al. 2011). The men assigned to the testosterone arm experienced significantly higher frequencies of total adverse events, and cardiac, respiratory, and dermatological events than those assigned to the placebo group; these differences persisted after adjustment for baseline risk factors (Basaria et al. 2010; Travison et al. 2011). Men 75 years of age or older and men with higher on-treatment testosterone levels appeared to be at greater risk of cardiovascular events. Meta-analyses of randomized testosterone trials have reported numerically greater number of cardiovascular events in the testosterone arms than in the placebo arms of trials, but these differences have not been statistically significant presumably because of the small number of subjects enrolled in these trials (Calof et al. 2005; Fernández-Balsells et al. 2010). However, these meta-

analyses are limited by the small size of most trials, heterogeneity of subject populations, poor quality of adverse event reporting, and short treatment duration in many trials. Most trials recruited healthy older men.

Thus, the randomized trials are in agreement that testosterone increases muscle mass and strength. However, substantial increases in lean body mass and leg-press strength during testosterone administration have not been associated with consistent improvements in measures of physical function, such as walking speed (Bhasin et al. 2006; Storer et al. 2008). Additionally, the findings of the TOM Trial have raised concern that frail older persons with a high burden of chronic disease may be susceptible to increased risk of adverse events during testosterone administration, especially at high testosterone concentrations (Basaria et al. 2010; Travison et al. 2011). Therefore, the therapeutic application of testosterone as a function-promoting anabolic therapy is predicated crucially upon the development of strategies which facilitate the translation of muscle mass and strength gains into functional improvements at lower testosterone concentrations that can be administered safely. Such adjunctive strategies might include physical exercise interventions that emphasize cognitive and behavioral training, or combined administration of testosterone with other anabolic agents such as recombinant human growth hormone. Empiric experience in athletes suggests that task-specific training is necessary for translating the muscle mass and strength gains induced by androgen administration into improvements in performance. Further studies are needed to determine whether physical activity interventions can facilitate the translation of testosterone-induced increases in muscle mass and strength into clinically meaningful gains in physical function and health-related outcomes at lower testosterone doses that can be administered safely.

9.8 Testosterone's effects on mood, fatigue/energy, sense of well-being and quality of life

Epidemiological studies have reported an inconsistent association of testosterone levels with mood indices (Barrett-Connor et al. 1999; Margolese 2000; Seidman et al. 2001; 2002). Low bioavailable testosterone has been weakly associated with depression in men (Barrett-Connor et al. 1999; Margolese 2000; Seidman *et al.* 2002). Testosterone appears to be associated more with dysthymic mood than with major depressive disorder (Seidman *et al.* 2002). Testosterone trials in men with refractory depression taking antidepressants have revealed conflicting results (Seidman and Rabkin 1998; Pope *et al.* 2003).

In open-label trials, androgen administration in androgen-deficient men has been reported to improve positive aspects of mood and reduce negative aspects of mood (Wang *et al.* 1996b). Similar improvements in mood and sense of well-being have been reported with testosterone replacement in surgically menopausal women and women with adrenal insufficiency (Arlt *et al.* 1999; 2000; Shifren *et al.* 2000).

In HIV-infected men with low testosterone levels, testosterone supplementation has been reported to restore libido and energy, and alleviate depressed mood (Rabkin *et al.* 1995; 2000a; 2000b). There is additional evidence that androgen improves energy and reduces sense of fatigue in HIV-infected men (Wagner *et al.* 1998; Knapp *et al.* 2008).

The effects of short-term testosterone therapy on overall quality-of-life (QoL) scores using generic QoL questionnaires have been inconsistent (Morley 2000; Reddy *et al.* 2000; Novak *et al.* 2002; Kenny *et al.* 2002). However, these studies did not have sufficient power. Also, the QoL questionnaires used (e.g. SF-36) in previous studies are multidimensional and include several domains that are not androgen responsive. Testosterone administration has been reported to improve self-reported physical function (Snyder *et al.* 1999a).

9.9 Reaction time

Testosterone improves neuromuscular transmission and reaction time in a frog hind leg model (Leslie *et al.* 1991; Blanco *et al.* 1997). It is possible that testosterone may influence fall propensity by reducing reaction time.

9.10 Strategies for achieving selectivity of testosterone action: dissociating the beneficial effects of testosterone from its adverse effects

First, it is apparent that very substantial gains in skeletal muscle mass and strength are achievable with supraphysiological doses of testosterone, and that the administration of higher doses is limited by the potential for adverse events, especially in older men with high burdens of chronic conditions. Therefore, strategies to achieve greater selectivity of action are necessary to realize the beneficial anabolic effects without the undesirable adverse effects. Second, remarkable gains in skeletal muscle mass and strength induced by testosterone administration have not been associated consistently with improvements in physical function measures. Therefore, adjunctive strategies, such as physical activity interventions, or cognitive and behavioral training, might be needed to induce neuromuscular and behavioral adaptations that are necessary for translating muscle strength gains into clinically meaningful improvements in physical function.

Historically, three approaches have been used to achieve selectivity of hormone action: the elucidation of molecular targets in the signaling cascade of hormone action that might provide greater tissue selectivity, the development of selective hormone receptor modulators, and the tissue-specific delivery of hormone. We will focus on the mechanism-based discovery of more selective function-promoting anabolic therapies.

9.10.1 Mechanisms by which testosterone increases skeletal muscle mass

There is general agreement that testosterone's anabolic effects on the skeletal muscle are mediated through the AR (Fig. 9.3); the evidence for non-genomic effects is weak. Testosterone-induced increase in muscle mass is associated with hypertrophy of both type I and type II skeletal muscle fibers (Sinha-Hikim *et al.* 2002). However, testosterone does not affect the absolute number or the relative proportion of type I and II muscle fibers (Sinha-Hikim *et al.* 2002). Testosterone administration also is associated with a dose-related increase in the number of satellite cells and myonuclei (Sinha-Hikim *et al.* 2003; 2006). However, the myonuclear domain – the ratio of muscle fiber cross-sectional area to myonuclear number – does not change during testosterone administration.

Several hypotheses have been proposed to explain the anabolic effects of testosterone on the skeletal muscle, and they are not mutually exclusive: stimulation of muscle protein synthesis, stimulation of the GH/IGF-1 axis, and the regulation of mesenchymal muscle progenitor cell differentiation.

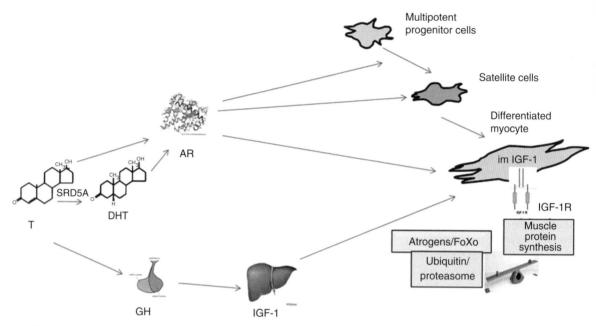

Fig. 9.3 Potential mechanisms of the anabolic effects of testosterone on the skeletal muscle. Testosterone (T) could potentially increase muscle mass through multiple mechanisms. The vast majority of evidence suggests that testosterone's effects are mediated through the AR. It does not appear that 5-alpha reduction of testosterone is essential for mediating testosterone's effects on the muscle. Testosterone stimulates GH secretion and increases IGF-1 levels, but circulating GH and IGF-1 are not essential for mediating testosterone's effects on the muscle. Testosterone promotes the differentiation of mesenchymal multipotent progenitor cell into the myogenic lineage. Whether testosterone has direct effects on muscle protein synthesis, muscle protein degradation or atrophy pathways remains to be investigated. Testosterone's effect on proliferation and differentiation of skeletal muscle progenitor cells requires the mediation of IGF-1R signaling. See plate section for color version.

The observation that testosterone and other androgens increase nitrogen retention in androgen-deficient men (Kochakian and Murlin 1935; Kochakian 1937; 1950; Kenyon *et al.* 1940) led to the hypothesis that testosterone stimulates muscle protein synthesis. Several investigators using stable isotopes have shown that testosterone therapy improves fractional muscle protein synthesis and reutilization of amino acids (Brodsky *et al.* 1996; Mauras *et al.* 1998; Sheffield-Moore *et al.* 1999; 2006; Bhasin *et al.* 2003). The effects of testosterone on muscle protein degradation are less clear.

The muscle protein synthesis hypothesis does not easily explain the reciprocal change in fat mass or the increased number of satellite cells in testosterone-treated men (Sinha-Hikim *et al.* 2003; 2004; 2006). Therefore, we considered the alternate hypothesis that testosterone might regulate the differentiation of mesenchymal multipotent cells, promoting their differentiation into the myogenic lineage and inhibiting adipogenic differentiation. Androgen receptor protein is expressed in mesenchymal progenitor cells in

the skeletal muscle, predominantly in the satellite cells, identified by their location outside the sarcolemma but inside the lamina, and by c-MET, and CD34 staining (Sinha-Hikim *et al.* 2004). Androgen receptor protein expression is also observed in many myonuclei, and in CD34+ cells outside the lamina, vascular endothelial cells and myofibroblasts (Sinha-Hikim *et al.* 2004).

We determined the effects of testosterone and DHT on the differentiation of multipotent, mesenchymal C3H10T1/2 cells (Singh *et al.* 2003; 2009). Although untreated cells express low levels of AR protein, DHT and testosterone upregulate AR expression in these cells. Incubation with testosterone and DHT increases the number of MyoD+ myogenic cells and MHC+ myotubes (Singh *et al.* 2003; 2009). Testosterone and DHT upregulate the expression of MyoD, and MHC mRNA and protein levels increased dose dependently. Both testosterone and DHT also decrease the number of oil red O positive adipocytes and downregulate the expression of PPARγ2 mRNA and PPARγ2 and C/EBPα proteins that are markers of adipogenic differentiation (Singh *et al.* 2003; 2009; Gupta *et al.* 2009). The effects of testosterone and DHT on myogenesis and adipogenesis are blocked by bicalutamide, an androgen receptor antagonist (Singh *et al.* 2003; 2009). Hence, testosterone and DHT regulate the differentiation of mesenchymal multipotent cells by promoting their differentiation into the myogenic lineage and inhibiting their differentiation into adipocytes through an AR-mediated pathway (Singh *et al.* 2003; 2009).

In separate studies, we have shown that DHT also regulates the differentiation of human marrow-derived, mesenchymal stem cells (hMSCs) from adult men (Gupta *et al.* 2009). Dihydrotestosterone upregulates AR expression and inhibits lipid accumulation in adipocytes differentiated from hMSCs and downregulates the expression of aP2, PPARγ, leptin and C/EBPα (Gupta *et al.* 2009). Bicalutamide attenuates DHT's inhibitory effects on adipogenic differentiation of hMSCs. Adipocytes differentiated in the presence of DHT accumulate smaller oil droplets, suggesting reduced extent of maturation. Dihydrotestosterone decreases the incorporation of labeled fatty acid into triglyceride, and downregulates acetyl CoA carboxylase and DGAT2 expression in adipocytes derived from hMSCs. Thus, DHT inhibits adipogenic differentiation of hMSCs through an AR-mediated pathway (Gupta *et al.* 2009)).

WNT signaling plays an important role in regulating the differentiation of mesenchymal progenitor cells, and testosterone and DHT promote the association of liganded androgen receptor with β-catenin, stabilizing the latter and causing the androgen receptor–β-catenin complex to translocate into the nucleus and activate a number of WNT target genes (Singh *et al.* 2006; 2009). Double immunofluorescence and immunoprecipitation studies have revealed that AR, β-catenin, and TCF-4 are colocalized in the nucleus in both testosterone-treated (100 nM) and DHT-treated (10 nM) cells (Singh *et al.* 2006; 2009), suggesting that they interact to form a complex. Both β-catenin and TCF-4 play an essential role in mediating androgen effects on the differentiation of C3H10T1/2 cells (Singh *et al.* 2009).

Testosterone regulates the expression of several WNT target genes, including follistatin, which plays an essential role in mediating testosterone's effects on myogenesis (Singh *et al.* 2003; 2006; 2009). The androgen signal is cross-communicated to the TGF-β/SMAD pathway through follistatin (Singh *et al.* 2009), which blocks TGF-β/SMAD signaling in vivo and in vitro. When administered to castrated mice, follistatin increases skeletal muscle mass and decreases fat mass without affecting the prostate. Thus, follistatin, a mediator of androgen action, may have potential as a selective function-promoting anabolic therapy that might increase skeletal muscle mass without affecting the prostate.

In a myocyte-specific AR knock-out (mARKO) mouse, lean body mass is lower in the mARKO than in control mice (Ophoff *et al.* 2009). The weight of the androgen-sensitive levator ani is significantly reduced (−46%); whereas the weights of other muscle groups were slightly reduced (Reddy *et al.* 2000), suggesting that in addition to its effects on muscle progenitor cells, testosterone affects post-mitotic myocytes.

9.10.2 The role of circulating growth hormone and IGF-1, and intramuscular IGF-1 signaling in mediating testosterone's effects on the muscle

Testosterone stimulates pulsatile GH secretion and increases serum IGF-1 concentrations in peripubertal boys and in boys with constitutional delay of puberty (Eakman *et al.* 1996; Giustina *et al.* 1997; Bondanelli *et al.* 2003). Androgen administration has also been shown to increase circulating IGF-1 levels and upregulate intramuscular IGF-1 mRNA expression in men (Ferrando *et al.* 2002). However, in castrated, hypophysectomized mice, testosterone increases muscle mass, indicating that circulating GH and IGF-1 are not essential for mediating the anabolic effects of testosterone on the muscle (Serra *et al.* 2011).

Testosterone stimulates the proliferation of human skeletal muscle cells in vitro: an effect blocked by small interference RNA targeting human IGF-1 receptor (IGF-1R) (sihIGF-1R) (Serra *et al.* 2011). In differentiation conditions, testosterone promotes the fusion of human skeletal muscle cells into larger myotubes, an effect attenuated by sihIGF-1R (Serra *et al.* 2011). Thus, intramuscular IGF-1 signaling plays an important role in mediating testosterone's effects on skeletal muscle progenitor cell growth and differentiation (Serra *et al.* 2011)).

9.11 Perspective on the future of testosterone as a function-promoting therapy

Strong clinical trial data support the view that androgens increase skeletal muscle mass and maximal voluntary strength. However, we do not know whether testosterone administration improves physical function and health outcomes and reduces disability in older individuals with functional limitations. Additionally, there are unresolved concerns about the potential long-term adverse effects of testosterone on cardiovascular events and the prostate. Strategies to increase the selectivity of androgen action are needed to achieve a higher risk-to-benefit ratio. Additionally, it is possible that risk-factor-based multimodality interventions that include physical activity interventions or combination of anabolic therapies might be needed to improve physical function at testosterone doses that can be safely administered. Given the uncertainty about the regulatory approval pathway and concerns about long-term safety, the initial efficacy trials are likely to be conducted in the treatment mode rather than in the prevention mode and for short-term indications in conditions associated with grievous outcomes, such as cancer cachexia and hip fracture, and to promote rehabilitation after an acute illness.

9.12 Key messages

- There is an enormous unmet need for function-promoting anabolic therapies for functional limitations associated with aging and acute and chronic illnesses.
- Randomized trials are in agreement that testosterone administration increases skeletal muscle mass and maximal voluntary strength; these effects are related to testosterone dose and concentrations.

- Testosterone acts through multiple mechanisms to increase skeletal muscle mass; it promotes the differentiation of mesenchymal multipotent cells into myogenic lineage and inhibits their differentiation into adipogenic lineage through an AR-mediated pathway that involves cross-communication between the WNT-β-catenin and TGF-β signaling pathways. Testosterone stimulates GH and IGF-1 secretion, but circulating GH and IGF-1 are not essential for mediating the anabolic effects of testosterone on the muscle. Intramuscular IGF-1 receptor signaling plays an important role in mediating the anabolic effects of testosterone on the muscle.
- In spite of unequivocal increases in muscle mass and strength, testosterone has not been shown to improve performance-based measures of physical function and health outcomes. Physical activity interventions that incorporate cognitive and behavioral therapy, or multimodality interventions that include one or more anabolic therapies based on risk-factor identification might be needed to translate testosterone-induced muscle mass and strength gains into functional improvements.
- Neither the clinical benefits nor the long-term risks of testosterone therapy are known. Frail elderly most in need of anabolic therapy may also be at increased risk of cardiovascular adverse events. Strategies to dissociate the beneficial anabolic effects of testosterone from its adverse effects are needed. Such strategies might include the development of selective androgen receptor modulators, mechanism-specific therapies and tissue-specific delivery.

9.13 References

Arlt W, Callies F, van Vlijmen JC, Koehler I, Reincke M, Bidlingmaier M, Huebler D, Oettel M, Ernst M, Schulte HM, Allolio B (1999) Dehydroepiandrosterone replacement in women with adrenal insufficiency. *N Engl J Med* **341**:1013–1020

Arlt W, Callies F, Allolio B (2000) DHEA replacement in women with adrenal insufficiency – pharmacokinetics, bioconversion and clinical effects on well-being, sexuality and cognition. *Endocr Res* **26**:505–511

Arver S, Sinha-Hikim I, Beall G, Guerrero M, Shen R, Bhasin S (1999) Serum dihydrotestosterone and testosterone concentrations in human immunodeficiency virus-infected men with and without weight loss. *J Androl* **20**:611–618

Bachman E, Feng R, Travison T, Li M, Olbina G, Ostland V, Ulloor J, Zhang A, Basaria S, Ganz T, Westerman M, Bhasin S (2010) Testosterone suppresses hepcidin in men: a potential mechanism for testosterone-induced erythrocytosis. *J Clin Endocrinol Metab* **95**:4743–4747

Barrett-Connor E, von Muhlen DG, Kritz-Silverstein D (1999) Bioavailable testosterone and depressed mood in older men: the Rancho Bernardo Study. *J Clin Endocrinol Metab* **84**:573–577

Basaria S, Coviello AD, Travison TG, Storer TW, Farwell WR, Jette AM, Eder R, Tennstedt S, Ulloor J, Zhang A, Choong K, Lakshman KM, Mazer NA, Miciek R, Krasnoff J, Elmi A, Knapp PE, Brooks B, Appleman E, Aggarwal S, Bhasin G, Hede-Brierley L, Bhatia A, Collins L, LeBrasseur N, Fiore LD, Bhasin S (2010) Adverse events associated with testosterone administration. *N Engl J Med* **363**:109–122

Baumgartner RN (2000) Body composition in healthy aging. *Ann N Y Acad Sci* **904**:437–448

Baumgartner RN, Koehler KM, Gallagher D, Romero L, Heymsfield SB, Ross RR, Garry PJ, Lindeman RD (1998) Epidemiology of sarcopenia among the elderly in New Mexico. *Am J Epidemiol* **147**:755–763

Berns JS, Rudnick MR, Cohen RM (1992) A controlled trial of recombinant human erythropoietin and nandrolone decanoate in the treatment of anemia in patients on chronic hemodialysis. *Clin Nephrol* **37**:264–267

Bhasin S, Storer TW, Berman N, Callegari C, Clevenger B, Phillips J, Bunnell TJ, Tricker R, Shirazi A, Casaburi R (1996) The effects of supraphysiologic doses of testosterone on muscle size and strength in normal men. *N Engl J Med* **335**:1–7

Bhasin S, Storer TW, Berman N, Yarasheski KE, Clevenger B, Phillips J, Lee WP, Bunnell TJ, Casaburi R (1997) Testosterone replacement increases fat-free mass and muscle size in hypogonadal men. *J Clin Endocrinol Metab* **82**:407–413

Bhasin S, Storer TW, Asbel-Sethi N, Kilbourne A, Hays R, Sinha-Hikim I, Shen R, Arver S, Beall G (1998)

Effects of testosterone replacement with a nongenital, ransdermal system, Androderm, in human immunodeficiency virus-infected men with low testosterone levels. *J Clin Endocrinol Metab* **83**: 3155–3162

Bhasin S, Storer TW, Javanbakht M, Berman N, Yarasheski KE, Phillips J, Dike M, Sinha-Hikim I, Shen R, Hays RD, Beall G (2000) Testosterone replacement and resistance exercise in HIV-infected men with weight loss and low testosterone levels. *JAMA* **283**: 763–770

Bhasin S, Woodhouse L, Casaburi R, Singh AB, Bhasin D, Berman N, Chen X, Yarasheski KE, Magliano L, Dzekov C, Dzekov J, Bross R, Phillips J, Sinha-Hikim I, Shen R, Storer TW (2001) Testosterone dose-response relationships in healthy young men. *Am J Physiol Endocrinol Metab* **281**:E1172–E1181

Bhasin S, Taylor WE, Singh R, Artaza J, Sinha-Hikim I, Jasuja R, Choi H, Gonzalez-Cadavid NF (2003) The mechanisms of androgen effects on body composition: mesenchymal pluripotent cell as the target of androgen action. *J Gerontol A Biol Sci Med Sci* **58**: M1103–M1110

Bhasin S, Woodhouse L, Casaburi R, Singh AB, Mac RP, Lee M, Yarasheski KE, Sinha-Hikim I, Dzekov C, Dzekov J, Magliano L, Storer TW (2005) Older men are as responsive as young men to the anabolic effects of graded doses of testosterone on the skeletal muscle. *J Clin Endocrinol Metab* **90**:678–688

Bhasin S, Calof OM, Storer TW, Lee ML, Mazer NA, Jasuja R, Montori VM, Gao W, Dalton JT (2006) Drug insight: testosterone and selective androgen receptor modulators as anabolic therapies for chronic illness and aging. *Nat Clin Pract Endocrinol Metab* **2**:146–159

Blackman MR, Sorkin JD, Munzer T, Bellantoni MF, Busby-Whitehead J,

Stevens TE, Jayme J, O'Connor KG, Christmas C, Tobin JD, Stewart KJ, Cottrell E, St Clair C, Pabst KM, Harman SM (2002) Growth hormone and sex steroid administration in healthy aged women and men: a randomized controlled trial. *JAMA* **288**: 2282–2292

Blanco CE, Popper P, Micevych P (1997) Anabolic-androgenic steroid induced alterations in choline acetyltransferase messenger RNA levels of spinal cord motoneurons in the male rat. *Neuroscience* **78**:873–882

Bondanelli M, Ambrosio MR, Margutti A, Franceschetti P, Zatelli MC, degli Uberti EC (2003) Activation of the somatotropic axis by testosterone in adult men: evidence for a role of hypothalamic growth hormone-releasing hormone. *Neuroendocrinology* **77**:380–387

Brodsky IG, Balagopal P, Nair KS (1996) Effects of testosterone replacement on muscle mass and muscle protein synthesis in hypogonadal men-a clinical research center study. *J Clin Endocrinol Metab* **81**:3469–3475

Buchwald D, Argyres S, Easterling RE, Oelshlegel FJ Jr, Brewer GJ, Schoomaker EB, Abbrecht PH, Williams GW, Weller JM (1977) Effect of nandrolone decanoate on the anemia of chronic hemodialysis patients. *Nephron* **18**:232–238

Calof OM, Singh AB, Lee ML, Kenny AM, Urban RJ, Tenover JL, Bhasin S (2005) Adverse events associated with testosterone replacement in middle-aged and older men: a meta-analysis of randomized, placebo-controlled trials. *J Gerontol A Biol Sci Med Sci* **60**:1451–1457

Casaburi R, Bhasin S, Cosentino L, Porszasz J, Somfay A, Lewis MI, Fournier M, Storer TW (2004) Effects of testosterone and resistance training in men with chronic obstructive pulmonary disease. *Am J Respir Crit Care Med* **170**:870–878

Cawthon PM, Ensrud KE, Laughlin GA, Cauley JA, Dam TT, Barrett-Connor E, Fink HA, Hoffman AR, Lau E, Lane NE, Stefanick ML, Cummings SR, Orwoll ES; Osteoporotic Fractures in Men (MrOS) Research Group (2009) Sex hormones and frailty in older men: the osteoporotic fractures in men (MrOS) study. *J Clin Endocrinol Metab* **94**:3806–3815

Clague JE, Wu FC, Horan MA (1999) Difficulties in measuring the effect of testosterone replacement therapy on muscle function in older men. *Int J Androl* **22**:261–265

Coodley GO, Coodley MK (1997) A trial of testosterone therapy for HIV-associated weight loss. *Aids* **11**:1347–1352

Coodley GO, Loveless MO, Nelson HD, Coodley MK (1994) Endocrine function in the HIV wasting syndrome. *J Acquir Immune Defic Syndr* **7**:46–51

Coviello AD, Lakshman K, Mazer NA, Bhasin S (2006) Differences in the apparent metabolic clearance rate of testosterone in young and older men with gonadotropin suppression receiving graded doses of testosterone. *J Clin Endocrinol Metab* **91**:4669–4675

Coviello AD, Kaplan B, Lakshman KM, Chen T, Singh AB, Bhasin S (2008) Effects of graded doses of testosterone on erythropoiesis in healthy young and older men. *J Clin Endocrinol Metab* **93**:914–919

Crawford BA, Liu PY, Kean MT, Bleasel JF, Handelsman DJ (2003) Randomized placebo-controlled trial of androgen effects on muscle and bone in men requiring long-term systemic glucocorticoid treatment. *J Clin Endocrinol Metab* **88**:3167–3176

Dobs AS, Few WL 3rd, Blackman MR, Harman SM, Hoover DR, Graham NM (1996) Serum hormones in men with human immunodeficiency virus-associated

wasting. *J Clin Endocrinol Metab* **81**:4108–4112

Dobs AS, Cofrancesco J, Nolten WE, Danoff A, Anderson R, Hamilton CD, Feinberg J, Seekins D, Yangco B, Rhame F (1999) The use of a transscrotal testosterone delivery system in the treatment of patients with weight loss related to human immunodeficiency virus infection. *Am J Med* **107**:126–132

Eakman GD, Dallas JS, Ponder SW, Keenan BS (1996) The effects of testosterone and dihydrotestosterone on hypothalamic regulation of growth hormone secretion. *J Clin Endocrinol Metab* **81**:1217–1223

Emmelot-Vonk MH, Verhaar HJ, Nakhai Pour HR, Aleman A, Lock TM, Bosch JL, Grobbee DE, van der Schouw YT (2008) Effect of testosterone supplementation on functional mobility, cognition, and other parameters in older men: a randomized controlled trial. *JAMA* **299**:39–52

Fernández-Balsells MM, Murad MH, Lane M, Lampropulos JF, Albuquerque F, Mullan RJ, Agrwal N, Elamin MB, Gallegos-Orozco JF, Wang AT, Erwin PJ, Bhasin S, Montori VM (2010) Clinical review 1: adverse effects of testosterone therapy in adult men: a systematic review and meta-analysis. *J Clin Endocrinol Metab* **95**:2560–2575

Ferrando AA, Tipton KD, Doyle D, Phillips SM, Cortiella J, Wolfe RR (1998) Testosterone injection stimulates net protein synthesis but not tissue amino acid transport. *Am J Physiol* **275**:E864–E871

Ferrando AA, Sheffield-Moore M, Yeckel CW, Gilkison C, Jiang J, Achacosa A, Lieberman SA, Tipton K, Wolfe RR, Urban RJ (2002) Testosterone administration to older men improves muscle function: molecular and physiological mechanisms. *Am J Physiol Endocrinol Metab* **282**:E601–E607

Freeman ER, Bloom DA, McGuire EJ (2001) A brief history of

testosterone. *J Urol* **165**: 371–373

Giustina A, Scalvini T, Tassi C, Desenzani P, Poiesi C, Wehrenberg WB, Rogol AD, Veldhuis JD (1997) Maturation of the regulation of growth hormone secretion in young males with hypogonadotropic hypogonadism pharmacologically exposed to progressive increments in serum testosterone. *J Clin Endocrinol Metab* **82**:1210–1219

Grinspoon S, Corcoran C, Lee K, Burrows B, Hubbard J, Katznelson L, Walsh M, Guccione A, Cannan J, Heller H, Basgoz N, Klibanski A (1996) Loss of lean body and muscle mass correlates with androgen levels in hypogonadal men with acquired immunodeficiency syndrome and wasting. *J Clin Endocrinol Metab* **81**:4051–4058

Grinspoon S, Corcoran C, Askari H, Schoenfeld D, Wolf L, Burrows B, Walsh M, Hayden D, Parlman K, Anderson E, Basgoz N, Klibanski A (1998) Effects of androgen administration in men with the AIDS wasting syndrome. A randomized, double-blind, placebo-controlled trial. *Ann Intern Med* **129**:18–26

Grinspoon S, Corcoran C, Stanley T, Baaj A, Basgoz N, Klibanski A (2000) Effects of hypogonadism and testosterone administration on depression indices in HIV-infected men. *J Clin Endocrinol Metab* **85**:60–65

Gupta V, Bhasin S, Guo W, Singh R, Miki R, Chauhan P, Choong K, Tchkonia T, Lebrasseur NK, Flanagan JN, Hamilton JA, Viereck JC, Narula NS, Kirkland JL, Jasuja R (2009) Effects of dihydrotestosterone on differentiation and proliferation of human mesenchymal stem cells and preadipocytes. *Mol Cell Endocrinol* **296**:32–40

Johansen KL (1999) Physical functioning and exercise capacity in patients on dialysis. *Adv Ren Replace Ther* **6**:141–148

Johansen KL, Mulligan K, Schambelan M (1999) Anabolic effects of nandrolone decanoate in patients receiving dialysis: a randomized controlled trial. *Jama* **281**:1275–1281

Johns K, Beddall MJ, Corrin RC (2005) Anabolic steroids for the treatment of weight loss in HIV-infected individuals. *Cochrane Database Syst Rev* **19**:CD005483

Katznelson L, Finkelstein JS, Schoenfeld DA, Rosenthal DI, Anderson EJ, Klibanski A (1996) Increase in bone density and lean body mass during testosterone administration in men with acquired hypogonadism. *J Clin Endocrinol Metab* **81**:4358–4365

Katznelson L, Rosenthal DI, Rosol MS, Anderson EJ, Hayden DL, Schoenfeld DA, Klibanski A (1998) Using quantitative CT to assess adipose distribution in adult men with acquired hypogonadism. *Am J Roentgenol* **170**:423–427

Kenny AM, Prestwood KM, Gruman CA, Marcello KM, Raisz LG (2001) Effects of transdermal testosterone on bone and muscle in older men with low bioavailable testosterone levels. *J Gerontol A Biol Sci Med Sci* **56**:M266–M272

Kenny AM, Bellantonio S, Gruman CA, Acosta RD, Prestwood KM (2002) Effects of transdermal testosterone on cognitive function and health perception in older men with low bioavailable testosterone levels. *J Gerontol A Biol Sci Med Sci* **57**:M321–M325

Kenyon A, Knowlton K, Sandiford I, Koch FC, Lotwin G (1940) A comparative study of the metabolic effects of testosterone propionate in normal men and women and in eunuchoidism. *Endocrinology* **26**:26–45

Khaw KT, Barrett-Connor E (1992) Lower endogenous androgens predict central adiposity in men. *Ann Epidemiol* **2**:675–682

Knapp PE, Storer TW, Herbst KL, Singh AB, Dzekov C, Dzekov J, LaValley M, Zhang A, Ulloor J, Bhasin S (2008) Effects of a supraphysiological dose

of testosterone on physical function, muscle performance, mood, and fatigue in men with HIV-associated weight loss. *Am J Physiol Endocrinol Metab* **294**:E1135–E1143

Kochakian C (1937) Testosterone and testosterone acetate and the protein and energy metabolism of castrate dogs. *Endocrinology* **21**:750–755

Kochakian C (1950) Comparison of protein anabolic property of various androgens in the castrated rat. *Am J Physiol* **60**:53–58

Kochakian C, Murlin J (1935) The effect of male hormone on the protein and energy metabolism of castrate dogs. *J Nutrition* **10**:437–459

Kong A, Edmonds P (2002) Testosterone therapy in HIV wasting syndrome: systematic review and meta-analysis. *Lancet Infect Dis* **2**:692–699

Krasnoff J, Basaria S, Pencina M, Kaur G, Coviello A, Vasan R, Bhasin S, Murabito JM (2009) Free testosterone levels are associated with mobility limitation and physical performance in community-dwelling men: the Framingham Offspring Study. *J Clin Endocrinol Metab* **95**:2790–2799

LeBrasseur NK, Lajevardi N, Miciek R, Mazer N, Storer TW, Bhasin S (2009) Effects of testosterone therapy on muscle performance and physical function in older men with mobility limitations (The TOM Trial): design and methods. *Contemp Clin Trials* **30**:133–140

Leslie M, Forger NG, Breedlove SM (1991) Sexual dimorphism and androgen effects on spinal motoneurons innervating the rat flexor digitorum brevis. *Brain Res* **561**:269–273

MacAdams MR, White RH, Chipps BE (1986) Reduction of serum testosterone levels during chronic glucocorticoid therapy. *Ann Intern Med* **104**:648–651

Margolese HC (2000) The male menopause and mood: testosterone decline and depression in the aging

male—is there a link? *J Geriatr Psychiatry Neurol* **13**:93–101

Mauras N, Hayes V, Welch S, Rini A, Helgeson K, Dokler M, Veldhuis JD, Urban RJ (1998) Testosterone deficiency in young men: marked alterations in whole body protein kinetics, strength, and adiposity. *J Clin Endocrinol Metab* **83**:1886–1892

Melton LJ 3rd, Khosla S, Crowson CS, O'Connor MK, O'Fallon WM, Riggs BL (2000a) Epidemiology of sarcopenia. *J Am Geriatr Soc* **48**:625–630

Melton LJ 3rd, Khosla S, Riggs BL (2000b) Epidemiology of sarcopenia. *Mayo Clin Proc* **75** (Suppl):S10–S12; discussion:S12–S13

Morley JE (2000) Andropause, testosterone therapy, and quality of life in aging men. *Cleve Clin J Med* **67**:880–882

Morley JE, Perry HM 3rd, Kaiser FE, Kraenzle D, Jensen J, Houston K, Mattammal M, Perry HM Jr (1993) Effects of testosterone replacement therapy in old hypogonadal males: a preliminary study. *J Am Geriatr Soc* **41**:149–152

Morley JE, Kaiser FE, Perry HM 3rd, Patrick P, Morley PM, Stauber PM, Vellas B, Baumgartner RN, Garry PJ (1997) Longitudinal changes in testosterone, luteinizing hormone, and follicle-stimulating hormone in healthy older men. *Metabolism* **46**:410–413

Nair KS, Rizza RA, O'Brien P, Dhatariya K, Short KR, Nehra A, Vittone JL, Klee GG, Basu A, Basu R, Cobelli C, Toffolo G, Dalla Man C, Tindall DJ, Melton LJ 3rd, Smith GE, Khosla S, Jensen MD (2006) DHEA in elderly women and DHEA or testosterone in elderly men. *N Engl J Med* **355**:1647–1659

Novak A, Brod M, Elbers J (2002) Andropause and quality of life: findings from patient focus groups and clinical experts. *Maturitas* **43**:231–237

Ophoff J, Van Proeyen K, Callewaert F, De Gendt K, De Bock K, Vanden

Bosch A, Verhoeven G, Hespel P, Vanderschueren D (2009) Androgen signaling in myocytes contributes to the maintenance of muscle mass and fiber type regulation but not to muscle strength or fatigue. *Endocrinology* **150**:3558–3566

Orwoll E, Lambert LC, Marshall LM, Blank J, Barrett-Connor E, Cauley J, Ensrud K, Cummings SR (2006) Endogenous testosterone levels, physical performance, and fall risk in older men. *Arch Intern Med* **166**:2124–2131

Page ST, Amory JK, Bowman FD, Anawalt BD, Matsumoto AM, Bremner WJ, Tenover JL (2005) Exogenous testosterone (T) alone or with finasteride increases physical performance, grip strength, and lean body mass in older men with low serum T. *J Clin Endocrinol Metab* **90**:1502–1510

Painter P, Johansen K (1999) Physical functioning in end-stage renal disease. Introduction: a call to activity. *Adv Ren Replace Ther* **6**:107–109

Pope HG Jr, Cohane GH, Kanayama G, Siegel AJ, Hudson JI (2003) Testosterone gel supplementation for men with refractory depression: a randomized, placebo-controlled trial. *Am J Psychiatry* **160**:105–111

Rabkin JG, Rabkin R, Wagner G (1995) Testosterone replacement therapy in HIV illness. *Gen Hosp Psychiatry* **17**:37–42

Rabkin JG, Ferrando SJ, Wagner GJ, Rabkin R (2000a) DHEA treatment for HIV+ patients: effects on mood, androgenic and anabolic parameters. *Psychoneuroendocrinology* **25**:53–68

Rabkin JG, Wagner GJ, Rabkin R (2000b) A double-blind, placebo-controlled trial of testosterone therapy for HIV-positive men with hypogonadal symptoms. *Arch Gen Psychiatry* **57**:141–147; discussion:155–146

Reddy P, White CM, Dunn AB, Moyna NM, Thompson PD (2000) The effect of testosterone on health-related quality of life in elderly males – a pilot study. *J Clin Pharm Ther* **25**:421–426

Reid IR (1987) Serum testosterone levels during chronic glucocorticoid therapy. *Ann Intern Med* **106**:639–640

Reid IR, Wattie DJ, Evans MC, Stapleton JP (1996) Testosterone therapy in glucocorticoid-treated men. *Arch Intern Med* **156**:1173–1177

Rietschel P, Corcoran C, Stanley T, Basgoz N, Klibanski A, Grinspoon S (2000) Prevalence of hypogonadism among men with weight loss related to human immunodeficiency virus infection who were receiving highly active antiretroviral therapy. *Clin Infect Dis* **31**:1240–1244

Roy TA, Blackman MR, Harman SM, Tobin JD, Schrager M, Metter EJ (2002) Interrelationships of serum testosterone and free testosterone index with FFM and strength in aging men. *Am J Physiol Endocrinol Metab* **283**:E284–E294

Salehian B, Jacobson D, Swerdloff RS, Grafe MR, Sinha-Hikim I, McCutchan JA (1999) Testicular pathologic changes and the pituitary-testicular axis during human immunodeficiency virus infection. *Endocr Pract* **5**:1–9

Sattler FR, Jaque SV, Schroeder ET, Olson C, Dube MP, Martinez C, Briggs W, Horton R, Azen S (1999) Effects of pharmacological doses of nandrolone decanoate and progressive resistance training in immunodeficient patients infected with human immunodeficiency virus. *J Clin Endocrinol Metab* **84**:1268–1276

Schaap LA, Pluijm SM, Smit JH, van Schoor NM, Visser M, Gooren LJ, Lips P (2005) The association of sex hormone levels with poor mobility, low muscle strength and incidence of falls among older men and women. *Clin Endocrinol (Oxf)* **63**:152–160

Schols AM, Soeters PB, Mostert R, Pluymers RJ, Wouters EF (1995) Physiologic effects of nutritional support and anabolic steroids in patients with chronic obstructive pulmonary disease. A placebo-controlled randomized trial. *Am J Respir Crit Care Med* **152**:1268–1274

Seidell JC, Bjorntorp P, Sjostrom L, Kvist H, Sannerstedt R (1990) Visceral fat accumulation in men is positively associated with insulin, glucose, and C-peptide levels, but negatively with testosterone levels. *Metabolism* **39**:897–901

Seidman SN, Rabkin JG (1998) Testosterone replacement therapy for hypogonadal men with SSRI-refractory depression. *J Affect Disord* **48**:157–161

Seidman SN, Araujo AB, Roose SP, McKinlay JB (2001) Testosterone level, androgen receptor polymorphism, and depressive symptoms in middle-aged men. *Biol Psychiatry* **50**:371–376

Seidman SN, Araujo AB, Roose SP, Devanand DP, Xie S, Cooper TB, McKinlay JB (2002) Low testosterone levels in elderly men with dysthymic disorder. *Am J Psychiatry* **159**:456–459

Serra C, Bhasin S, Tangherlini F, Barton ER, Ganno M, Zhang A, Shansky J, Vandenburgh HH, Travison TG, Jasuja R, Morris C (2011) The role of GH and IGF-I in mediating anabolic effects of testosterone on androgen-responsive muscle. *Endocrinology* **152**:193–206

Sheffield-Moore M, Urban RJ, Wolf SE, Jiang J, Catlin DH, Herndon DN, Wolfe RR, Ferrando AA (1999) Short-term oxandrolone administration stimulates net muscle protein synthesis in young men. *J Clin Endocrinol Metab* **84**:2705–2711

Sheffield-Moore M, Paddon-Jones D, Casperson SL, Gilkison C, Volpi E, Wolf SE, Jiang J, Rosenblatt JI, Urban RJ (2006) Androgen therapy induces muscle protein anabolism in older women. *J Clin Endocrinol Metab* **91**:3844–3849

Shifren JL, Braunstein GD, Simon JA, Casson PR, Buster JE, Redmond GP, Burki RE, Ginsburg ES, Rosen RC, Leiblum SR, Caramelli KE, Mazer NA (2000) Transdermal testosterone treatment in women with impaired sexual function after oophorectomy. *N Engl J Med* 343:682–688

Sih R, Morley JE, Kaiser FE, Perry HM 3rd, Patrick P, Ross C (1997) Testosterone replacement in older hypogonadal men: a 12-month randomized controlled trial. *J Clin Endocrinol Metab* 82:1661–1667

Singh R, Artaza JN, Taylor WE, Gonzalez-Cadavid NF, Bhasin S (2003) Androgens stimulate myogenic differentiation and inhibit adipogenesis in C3H 10T1/2 pluripotent cells through an androgen receptor-mediated pathway. *Endocrinology* 144:5081–5088

Singh R, Artaza JN, Taylor WE, Braga M, Yuan X, Gonzalez-Cadavid NF, Bhasin S (2006) Testosterone inhibits adipogenic differentiation in 3T3-L1 cells: nuclear translocation of androgen receptor complex with beta-catenin and T-cell factor 4 may bypass canonical Wnt signaling to down-regulate adipogenic transcription factors. *Endocrinology* 147:141–154

Singh R, Bhasin S, Braga M, Artaza JN, Pervin S, Taylor WE, Krishnan V, Sinha SK, Rajavashisth TB, Jasuja R (2009) Regulation of myogenic differentiation by androgens: cross-talk between androgen receptor/β-catenin and follistatin/TGF-β signaling pathways. *Endocrinology* 150:1259–1268

Sinha-Hikim I, Artaza J, Woodhouse L, Gonzalez-Cadavid N, Singh AB, Lee MI, Storer TW, Casaburi R, Shen R, Bhasin S (2002) Testosterone-induced increase in muscle size in healthy young men is associated with muscle fiber hypertrophy. *Am J Physiol Endocrinol Metab* 283: E154–E164

Sinha-Hikim I, Roth SM, Lee MI, Bhasin S (2003) Testosterone-induced muscle hypertrophy is associated with an increase in satellite cell number in healthy, young men. *Am J Physiol Endocrinol Metab* 285:E197–E205

Sinha-Hikim I, Taylor WE, Gonzalez-Cadavid NF, Zheng W, Bhasin S (2004) Androgen receptor in human skeletal muscle and cultured muscle satellite cells: up-regulation by androgen treatment. *J Clin Endocrinol Metab* 89:5245–5255

Sinha-Hikim I, Cornford M, Gaytan H, Lee ML, Bhasin S (2006) Effects of testosterone supplementation on skeletal muscle fiber hypertrophy and satellite cells in community-dwelling older men. *J Clin Endocrinol Metab* 91:3024–3033

Snyder PJ, Peachey H, Hannoush P, Berlin JA, Loh L, Lenrow DA, Holmes JH, Dlewati A, Santanna J, Rosen CJ, Strom BL (1999a) Effect of testosterone treatment on body composition and muscle strength in men over 65 years of age. *J Clin Endocrinol Metab* 84:2647–2653

Snyder PJ, Peachey H, Hannoush P, Berlin JA, Loh L, Holmes JH, Dlewati A, Staley J, Santanna J, Kapoor SC, Attie MF, Haddad JG Jr, Strom BL (1999b) Effect of testosterone treatment on bone mineral density in men over 65 years of age. *J Clin Endocrinol Metab* 84:1966–1972

Snyder PJ, Peachey H, Berlin JA, Hannoush P, Haddad G, Dlewati A, Santanna J, Loh L, Lenrow DA, Holmes JH, Kapoor SC, Atkinson LE, Strom BL (2000) Effects of testosterone replacement in hypogonadal men. *J Clin Endocrinol Metab* 85:2670–2677

Srinivas-Shankar U, Roberts SA, Connolly MJ, O'Connell MD, Adams JE, Oldham JA, Wu FC (2010) Effects of testosterone on muscle strength, physical function, body composition, and quality of life in intermediate-frail and frail elderly men: a randomized, double-

blind, placebo-controlled study. *J Clin Endocrinol Metab* 95:639–650

Steidle C, Schwartz S, Jacoby K, Sebree T, Smith T, Bachand R (2003) AA2500 testosterone gel normalizes androgen levels in aging males with improvements in body composition and sexual function. *J Clin Endocrinol Metab* 88:2673–2681

Storer TW, Magliano L, Woodhouse L, Lee ML, Dzekov C, Dzekov J, Casaburi R, Bhasin S (2003) Testosterone dose-dependently increases maximal voluntary strength and leg power, but does not affect fatigability or specific tension. *J Clin Endocrinol Metab* 88: 1478–1485

Storer TW, Woodhouse L, Magliano L, Singh AB, Dzekov C, Dzekov J, Bhasin S (2008) Changes in muscle mass, muscle strength, and power but not physical function are related to testosterone dose in healthy older men. *J Am Geriatr Soc* 56:1991–1999

Strawford A, Barbieri T, Van Loan M, Parks E, Catlin D, Barton N, Neese R, Christiansen M, King J, Hellerstein MK (1999a) Resistance exercise and supraphysiologic androgen therapy in eugonadal men with HIV-related weight loss: a randomized controlled trial. *JAMA* 281:1282–1290

Strawford A, Barbieri T, Neese R, Van Loan M, Christiansen M, Hoh R, Sathyan G, Skowronski R, King J, Hellerstein M (1999b) Effects of nandrolone decanoate therapy in borderline hypogonadal men with HIV-associated weight loss. *J Acquir Immune Defic Syndr Hum Retrovirol* 20:137–146

Tenover JL (1999) Testosterone replacement therapy in older adult men. *Int J Androl* 22:300–306

Tenover JL (2000) Experience with testosterone replacement in the elderly. *Mayo Clin Proc* 75 (Suppl): S77–S81; discussion:S82

Tenover JS (1992) Effects of testosterone supplementation in the aging male. *J Clin Endocrinol Metab* **75**:1092–1098

Travison TG, Basaria S, Storer TW, Jette AM, Miciek R, Farwell WR, Choong K, Lakshman K, Mazer NA, Coviello AD, Knapp PE, Ulloor J, Zhang A, Brooks B, Nguyen AH, Eder R, Lebrasseur N, Elmi A, Appleman E, Hede-Brierley L, Bhasin G, Bhatia A, Lazzari A, Davis S, Ni P, Collins L, Bhasin S (2011) Clinical meaningfulness of the changes in muscle performance and physical function associated with testosterone administration in older men with mobility limitation. *J Gerontol A Biol Sci Med Sci* **66**:1090–1099

Urban RJ, Bodenburg YH, Gilkison C, Foxworth J, Coggan AR, Wolfe RR, Ferrando A (1995) Testosterone administration to elderly men increases skeletal muscle strength and protein synthesis. *Am J Physiol* **269**:E820–E826

van den Beld AW, de Jong FH, Grobbee DE, Pols HA, Lamberts SW (2000) Measures of bioavailable serum testosterone and estradiol and their relationships with muscle strength, bone density, and body composition in elderly men. *J Clin Endocrinol Metab* **85**:3276–3282

Wagner GJ, Rabkin JG, Rabkin R (1998) Testosterone as a treatment for fatigue in HIV+ men. *Gen Hosp Psychiatry* **20**:209–213

Wang C, Eyre DR, Clark R, Kleinberg D, Newman C, Iranmanesh A, Veldhuis J, Dudley RE, Berman N, Davidson T, Barstow TJ, Sinow R, Alexander G, Swerdloff RS (1996a) Sublingual testosterone replacement improves muscle mass and strength, decreases bone resorption, and increases bone formation markers in hypogonadal men – a clinical research center study. *J Clin Endocrinol Metab* **81**: 3654–3662

Wang C, Alexander G, Berman N, Salehian B, Davidson T, McDonald V, Steiner B, Hull L, Callegari C, Swerdloff RS (1996b) Testosterone replacement therapy improves mood in hypogonadal men – a clinical research center study. *J Clin Endocrinol Metab* **81**: 3578–3583

Wang C, Swerdloff RS, Iranmanesh A, Dobs A, Snyder PJ, Cunningham G, Matsumoto AM, Weber T, Berman N (2000) Transdermal testosterone gel improves sexual function, mood, muscle strength, and body composition parameters in hypogonadal men. Testosterone Gel Study Group. *J Clin Endocrinol Metab* **85**:2839–2853

Woodhouse LJ, Reisz-Porszasz S, Javanbakht M, Storer TW, Lee M, Zerounian H, Bhasin S (2003) Development of models to predict anabolic response to testosterone administration in healthy young men. *Am J Physiol Endocrinol Metab* **284**: E1009–E1017

Woodhouse LJ, Gupta N, Bhasin M, Singh AB, Ross R, Phillips J, Bhasin S (2004) Dose-dependent effects of testosterone on regional adipose tissue distribution in healthy young men. *J Clin Endocrinol Metab* **89**:718–726

Yesalis CE, Bahrke MS (1995) Anabolic-androgenic steroids. Current issues. *Sports Med* **19**:326–340

Yesalis CE, Kennedy NJ, Kopstein AN, Bahrke MS (1993) Anabolic-androgenic steroid use in the United States. *JAMA* **270**:1217–1221

Testosterone and cardiovascular disease

Kevin S. Channer and T. Hugh Jones

10.1 Epidemiology

Coronary heart disease remains the most important cause of death in the western world, and is increasingly prevalent in the developing world because of changes in risk factor profile. However, there remain large differences in the prevalence of ischemic heart disease between different geographical areas of the world. For example, Japan has a low prevalence and Scotland a high prevalence (www.heartstats.org; Fig. 10.1). Despite these differences there is one epidemiological fact that is consistent between populations; more than twice as many men are affected compared to women. This relationship persists at all ages, so that at any age coronary death rates are higher in men than women. This male predominance is not explained by differences in the standard risk factor profiles between men and women. Data from the British Heart Foundation show that there is little difference between the frequencies of smoking, hypertension, diabetes and hypercholesterolemia between men and women in the UK population. The observed difference in gender prevalence of

Testosterone: Action, Deficiency, Substitution, ed. Eberhard Nieschlag and Hermann M. Behre, Assoc. ed. Susan Nieschlag.
Published by Cambridge University Press. © Cambridge University Press 2012.

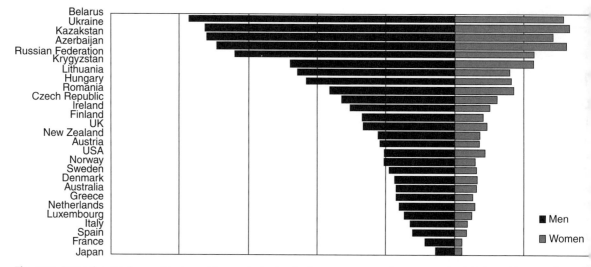

Fig. 10.1 Figure showing the consistent sex difference in death rates for coronary artery disease across both high- and low-prevalence communities. Data are for men and women aged 35–74 for 1998, from the BHF coronary statistics database released in 2002. See plate section for color version.

coronary heart disease led to two theories – that females are in some way protected by virtue of their sex hormone profile or that testosterone exerts a detrimental influence on the cardiovascular system.

10.2 Is estrogen cardio-protective?

Epidemiologically, coronary events are very rare in pre-menopausal women and only increase after the menopause, being more common in those with an early menopause. Experimental data in animals do suggest that estrogens reduce the development of atherosclerosis (see later). Similarly, coronary plaque burden has been shown to be lower in women who use hormone replacement therapy and in those who are taking the oral contraceptive pill. This led to the widespread view that female hormones were protective and led to studies of hormone replacement therapy in postmenopausal women with the expectation that this would reduce the incidence of cardiovascular disease.

However, two large randomized placebo-controlled clinical trials did not show this. In the HERS study (Hulley *et al.* 1998), postmenopausal women, of average age 66.7 years with a previous history of coronary heart disease, were randomly assigned to combination estrogen and progestogen treatment or placebo. Over the four years of the study there was no difference in the incidence of cardiovascular events between the groups. However, in the first year of treatment there was an excess of thrombotic events attributed to the thrombogenic effects of estrogens. This was

offset by a reduction in events in the latter years (years four and five) of the trial, leading the investigators to consider whether, in the long term, female combination HRT is beneficial. An open-label, three-year follow-up study (Grady *et al.* 2002) of the participants in the HERS study, which included 93% of the original cohort, also showed no difference in cardiovascular events. These data show that HRT does not reduce the risk of further cardiovascular events in women.

A second large, randomized controlled trial (Rossouw *et al.* 2002), of combination estrogen and progestogen versus placebo in over 16 000 postmenopausal women aged between 50 and 79 years, the Women's Health Initiative (WHI) study, was stopped early after 5.2 years because of an excess of breast cancers. The data showed an excess cardiovascular risk although there was no overall difference in all-cause mortality.

These clinical trial data have categorically demonstrated that female HRT is not cardio-protective. But what about testosterone in men?

10.3 Is testosterone cardio-protective?

High doses of exogenous anabolic steroids are undoubtedly associated with cardiac disease, sudden cardiac death and liver disease, but there is no evidence that high endogenous testosterone levels, within the normal range, are harmful. More importantly, coronary atherosclerosis increases with age coincident with a fall in serum testosterone levels

(Simon *et al*. 1992). This in itself suggests that testosterone does not induce atheroma formation.

10.4 Low testosterone and cardiovascular events

There is one clinical scenario where the effect of a reduction in circulating testosterone on cardiac disease can be seen. In men with prostate cancer, androgen deprivation therapy (ADT), including castration, has been used for years for palliation. In 1998, Satariano *et al*. (1998) first reported the observation that cardiovascular deaths were second only to death from the cancer in these men. The size of the excess cardiovascular detriment in this setting is significant. In one observational study of 73 196 men aged 66 years or older with prostate cancer, followed for 10 years, those treated with androgen deprivation therapy experienced a 44% increase in the risk of diabetes and a 16% increase in the risk of coronary heart disease events (death or myocardial infarction) (Keating *et al*. 2006). Orchidectomy was associated with a 34% increase in diabetes but no increased risk of coronary heart disease. In a study of over 22 000 men with prostate cancer, those who received ADT had a 20% increased risk of cardiovascular morbidity in the first year of treatment (Saigal *et al*. 2007) compared with those who did not. Another study showed that men over the age of 65 years treated with ADT had a two-fold increased risk of a fatal cardiovascular event over a 10-year follow-up period (Tsai *et al*. 2007). Several studies have now shown that ADT causes increased cardiovascular co-morbidity, probably through an increase in insulin resistance (reviewed in Shahani *et al*. 2008 and Taylor *et al*. 2009), which is an associated consequence of hypotestosteronemia. There are studies which have not shown an effect of cardiovascular mortality, like the small EORTC (European Organisation for Research and Treatment of Cancer) 226863 trial (Bolla *et al*. 2010), but the totality of the evidence has led to a science advisory statement from the American Heart Association, American Cancer Society and the American Urological Association to recommend that all patients receiving ADT have cardiovascular risk factor assessment on a regular basis, and that those with coexistent cardiovascular disease have their secondary prevention treatment optimized (Levine *et al*. 2010).

These studies show that manipulation of the individual prevailing hormonal profile to produce a hypogonadal state results in an excess of cardiovascular events and death.

It would be expected, therefore, that population-based follow-up studies would also show that a low prevailing testosterone level is a marker of an increased risk of cardiovascular events. The literature on this has been previously reviewed up to 2001 by Wu and von Eckardstein (2003). At that time there were 39 studies which examined the relationship between testosterone blood level and coronary artery disease (CAD). Of 32 cross-sectional studies, half found that subjects with CAD had lower levels of testosterone than controls, and half found no difference. Of the seven prospective, nested, case control studies, none showed that low testosterone was associated with an increased risk of developing overt symptomatic CAD.

This inconsistency can be explained by a number of factors. There is a biological and diurnal variation in testosterone blood level which none of these studies took into account, as most were not conducted specifically to address this question. All the prospective studies looked at a number of risk factors, and testosterone blood level was often an afterthought. The influence of the timing of sampling, type of assay, storage, and effect of co-morbidities on testosterone blood level effectively dilutes the power of these studies. More importantly, it is increasingly recognized that the sensitivity of the AR is very important in translating the biological effects of the prevailing testosterone blood level. Without knowledge of the receptor sensitivity in individuals it is very difficult to understand the biological consequence of a particular level of testosterone in the circulating blood.

An alternative method of assessing the influence of testosterone on atherosclerosis is to use prospective cohort studies of actual markers of atherosclerosis, with individuals acting as their own controls. These studies are all consistent in demonstrating that low testosterone in an individual increases atherogenesis.

10.5 Low testosterone and accelerated atherosclerosis

There are a number of observational models of atheroma development in humans.

10.5.1 Coronary atheroma

There have been a number of relatively small studies of the relationship between CAD and testosterone blood level, dating from 1985. Some have been positive (Chute *et al.* 1987; English *et al.* 2000a; Dobr-zycki *et al.* 2003; Rosano *et al.* 2007; Malkin *et al.* 2010), and some negative (Hauner *et al.* 1991; Kabakci *et al.* 1999; Davoodi *et al.* 2007). Phillips *et al.* (1994) published the first study, of men with CAD identified at coronary angiography, to demonstrate a relationship between the prevailing free testosterone blood level and the degree of atherosclerosis. The findings showed a negative correlation even after adjusting for body mass index and age. Moreover, these authors also demonstrated later (Phillips *et al.* 2004) that standard accepted cardiovascular risk factors (smoking, hypertension, diabetes, hypercholesterolemia and obesity) did not closely correlate with the degree of atherosclerotic coronary artery stenosis at angiography, whereas age, free testosterone level and HDL-cholesterol level did.

A large study of 930 men with angiographically proven coronary artery disease found that 16.3% had total testosterone levels < 8.1 nmol/l and 20.9% had bioavailable testosterone below the normal range (<2.6 nmol/l) (Malkin *et al.* 2010).

There are many potential confounding factors which influence testosterone level, including acute inflammation and illness, technical assay differences and the relative importance of bioavailable testosterone compared with total testosterone. In a case control study of men having coronary angiography, total and bioavailable testosterone was significantly lower in men with CAD compared to those with normal arteries (English *et al.* 2000a). In this careful study men were excluded from the study if they suffered an acute illness or acute infarction within the previous three months, and blood samples were taken in the early morning period (before 08.30–09.30). Moreover, the strongest association was seen with bioavailable testosterone rather than either total or free testosterone.

10.5.2   Carotid artery atheroma

Carotid atherosclerosis as identified by an increase in the intima-media thickness in the carotid artery, using Doppler ultrasound scanning, is more common in men with a lower level of testosterone (Makinen *et al.* 2005). In a large cross-sectional population study in Sweden of over 1400 men (Svartberg *et al.* 2006), there was a negative correlation between carotid intima-media thickness and total testosterone level, even after adjustment for age, smoking, systolic blood pressure and use of lipid-lowering medication.

However, in a further study from the same group, there was no correlation between the change in plaque area, measured seven years apart in over 1000 men, and testosterone levels (Vikan *et al.* 2009). By comparison, two other serial studies have shown that men with lower levels of testosterone develop a greater increase in the intima-media thickness over time, indicating accelerated atherogenesis (Muller *et al.* 2004). Men with clinically significant carotid artery stenosis also appear to have lower than normal levels of testosterone. In a case control study, 124 men having carotid endarterectomy had significantly lower total testosterone and SHBG levels than controls (Debing *et al.* 2008). A multivariate analysis including relevant clinical and physiological factors showed a significant inverse correlation between total testosterone and the degree of internal carotid artery stenosis.

In one small treatment study, carotid intima-media thickness appeared to be reduced following physiological replacement therapy in men with low baseline testosterone levels (Mathur *et al.* 2009). These interventional data need to be repeated in a larger cohort to satisfactorily answer the question of whether TRT does ameliorate the age-related progression of atherosclerosis in men.

10.5.3   Peripheral arterial disease

Similarly, atherosclerosis identified as calcified aortic plaques on lateral abdominal X-rays was shown to be significantly more advanced in individuals who had a low testosterone level over a follow-up period of seven years (Hak *et al.* 2002). Thoracic aortic intima-media thickness has been studied by trans-esophageal echocardiography in a small study of 42 men who had no clinical evidence of vascular disease (Demirbag *et al.* 2005). These authors demonstrated an inverse relationship between total testosterone level and aortic intima-media thickness.

Atherosclerosis in another vascular bed has been studied. Retinal atherosclerosis has been associated with a low DHEA blood level but not with a low total testosterone level (Tedeschi-Reiner *et al.* 2009). In a Swedish cross-sectional study involving nearly 3000 men, a multivariate analysis showed that low free testosterone and high free estradiol were independently associated with a reduction in ankle-brachial index, which is a marker of peripheral vascular disease (Tivesten *et al.* 2007). Arterial stiffness of large arteries is a surrogate marker for atherosclerosis and can be measured non-invasively by the carotid-femoral pulse wave velocity. In a cross-sectional study of 376 subjects, a low pulse wave velocity was inversely related to total and bioavailable testosterone levels, although the statistical strength of the association was lost when age was included (Pour *et al.* 2007). In a recent Japanese study, however, although low testosterone blood level predicted cardiovascular events it appeared to be independent of changes in flow-mediated brachial reactivity (Akishita *et al.* 2010).

Men with end-stage kidney disease on maintenance hemodialysis have a high incidence of hypogonadal levels of blood testosterone. In one study of 100 non-diabetic men of whom half had low blood levels of testosterone, vascular reactivity was reduced and carotid intima-media thickness increased compared to men with normal testosterone levels (Karakitsos *et al.* 2006).

The mechanism underlying the observed excess cardiovascular events may be explained by accelerated atherosclerosis as a consequence of changes in the cardiovascular risk factor profile that occur as testosterone blood level falls.

10.6 Testosterone in animal models of atherosclerosis

There are a number of animal models showing that castration or hypogonadism is associated with increased atherosclerosis. Moreover, supplemental testosterone therapy to physiological levels ameliorates or prevents the aortic accumulation of cholesterol, with a reduction in plaque size in models of atherosclerosis. Larsen *et al.* (1993) published the first study examining the effects of testosterone replacement in orchidectomized male rabbits fed a pro-atherogenic diet. Animals received supplemental testosterone enanthate (100 µl of 250 mg/ml concentrated solution), for a period of 17 weeks via twice-weekly im injection. Following cholesterol feeding, aortic cholesterol accumulation was significantly retarded in the testosterone-treated, compared to the placebo-treated, group (Larsen *et al.* 1993). Comparable to these findings, Bruck *et al.* (1997) demonstrated gender-specific anti-atherogenic effects of testosterone and estradiol in orchidectomized male and female rabbits fed a pro-atherogenic diet for a 12-week period. Rabbits received either testosterone enanthate (25 mg/kg·wk) or estradiol (1 mg/kg·wk), alone or in combination via weekly im injection, or

no treatment. Testosterone administration significantly inhibited atheroma formation in male rabbits, whilst an increase in plaque size was noted in females; no protective effect was seen in male rabbits given estradiol, although it significantly inhibited atheroma in females. Interestingly, simultaneous administration of both testosterone and estradiol reduced atheroma formation in both sexes. Alexandersen *et al.* (1999) examined the effects of testosterone and DHEA on atheroma formation in sexually mature male rabbits. Rabbits were randomized to bilateral castration or sham operation, with the castrated animals subsequently assigned to four study groups: (1) 500 mg oral DHEA daily, (2) 80 mg oral testosterone undecanoate daily; (3) 25 mg im injection of testosterone enanthate, twice weekly; or (4) placebo. The sham-operated group received no treatment. Animals were fed a pro-atherogenic diet for 35 weeks to induce aortic atherosclerosis. Alexandersen *et al.* reported a doubling of aortic plaque formation in castrated compared to sham-operated animals. Treatment with oral testosterone or DHEA prevented this increase in atheroma formation; whilst treatment with im testosterone was associated with a significant reduction in plaque formation. Others also report that DHEA inhibits plaque formation in this model (Gordon *et al.* 1988; Arad *et al.* 1989; Eich *et al.* 1993); whilst testosterone is also reported to inhibit neo-intimal plaque development in endothelial denuded rabbit aortic rings (Hanke *et al.* 2001).

Physiological testosterone supplementation has also been shown to reduce atherosclerosis in orchidectomized LDL receptor knock-out mice fed a cholesterol-enriched diet for a period of eight weeks (Nathan *et al.* 2001). Increased aortic lesion formation was reported in orchidectomized male mice; whilst a reduction in plaque development was demonstrated in orchidectomized animals receiving physiological testosterone supplementation. However, this effect was not observed in animals treated simultaneously with testosterone and the aromatase inhibitor anastrozole. In contrast to Bruck *et al.* (1997), this study demonstrated that conversion to estradiol was responsible for the testosterone-mediated attenuation of lesion formation. However, more recently Qui *et al.* (2010) showed that the non-aromatized natural androgen 5α-dihydrotestosterone (DHT), when used as androgen replacement in castrated rabbits, reduced the fatty streak development in the aorta by reducing foam cell formation from macrophages.

These studies show that the mechanism underpinning the effect on atherosclerosis remains controversial. Does testosterone exert its anti-atherosclerotic effect through conversion to estrogen, or is it an independent effect? Another controversial area concerns the relative importance of the nuclear AR in the mechanism of this effect.

In one animal model of hypogonadism in mice, in which the blood testosterone level is only 10% of littermate controls, and which also has an absent nuclear AR (the testicular feminized mouse), physiological testosterone supplementation reduces fatty streak formation (Nettleship *et al.* 2007a). This study utilized Tfm (testicular feminized) mice ($n = 31$) and XY littermates ($n = 8$) which were separated into five experimental groups. Each group received saline (Tfm, $n = 8$; XY littermates, $n = 8$), physiological testosterone alone (Tfm, $n = 8$), physiological testosterone in conjunction with the ERα antagonist fulvestrant (Tfm, $n = 8$), or physiological testosterone in conjunction with the aromatase inhibitor anastrozole (Tfm, $n = 7$). All groups were fed a cholesterol-enriched diet for 28 weeks. Serial sections from the aortic root were examined for fatty streak formation, and whole blood was collected for measurement of total cholesterol, high-density lipoprotein cholesterol (HDL-C), non-HDL-C, testosterone and 17β-estradiol. This study demonstrated that physiological testosterone replacement significantly reduced fatty streak formation in Tfm mice compared with placebo-treated controls; an effect that was independent of the androgen receptor. The effect persisted even in the presence of an ER blocker and an aromatase inhibitor. Serum HDL-C was also significantly increased following physiological testosterone replacement; however co-treatment with either fulvestrant (an ER blocker) or anastrozole (an aromatase inhibitor) demonstrated that the observed increase in HDL-C was consistent with conversion to 17β-estradiol (Nettleship *et al.* 2007a).

In an AR knock-out, apolipoprotein E deficient mouse model which is also testosterone deficient, Bourghardt *et al.* (2010) also showed that fatty streak development was increased when they were fed a high lipid diet, and this effect was reduced by the addition of testosterone. They also showed that fatty streak was increased in orchidectomized mice and reduced with testosterone replacement. The authors suggested that these results implied that low testosterone states are associated with accelerated atherosclerosis by both an AR dependent and independent mechanisms.

In a castrated rabbit model (Li *et al.* 2008), aortic plaque growth was reduced by TRT, but this effect was lost when flutamide (a nuclear AR blocker) was given concurrently. Castration increased inflammatory cytokine levels; an effect blocked by TRT but only in the absence of flutamide. These data also suggest that the nuclear AR is important in modulating the effect of testosterone on atheroma formation.

10.7 What is the evidence for accelerated atherosclerosis in hypogonadal states?

In order to better understand how changes in testosterone blood level may influence vascular function and structure, it is necessary to understand the pathophysiology of atherosclerosis.

Atherosclerosis is a disease of the intima of the medium and large arteries including the aorta, carotid and cerebral arteries. Coronary artery disease is characterized pathologically by the atherosclerotic plaque, which is described as a focal inflammatory fibro-proliferative response to multiple forms of endothelial injury, in which a number of distinct but overlapping pathways of pathogenesis are involved.

It is thought that the principal event initiating atheromatous lesion formation is endothelial cell injury. This encourages monocyte attachment, via the expression of adhesion molecules and chemokines on the endothelial cell surface. When activated by injury, endothelial cells and the attached monocytes and macrophages generate free radicals, which oxidize LDL, resulting in lipid peroxidation and destruction of the receptor needed for normal receptor-mediated clearance of LDL. Consequently, oxidized LDL (ox-LDL) accumulates in the sub-endothelial space, where it is taken up by macrophages via scavenger receptors to form foam cells (Ross 1999). Oxidized LDL is proposed to exacerbate the local inflammatory response, and has other effects, such as inhibiting the production of nitric oxide, an important chemical mediator with multiple anti-atherogenic properties, including vasorelaxation. After taking up LDL, these macrophages (now foam cells) migrate sub-endothelially. Sub-endothelial collections of foam cells and to a lesser extent T-lymphocytes form the "fatty streaks," which presage atherosclerosis.

Although the "fatty streaks" themselves are not clinically significant, they are now accepted to be the precursors of more advanced lesions, which may go on to become the sites of thrombosis (Lusis 2000).

Advanced atheroma is characterized by the following histological criteria: accumulations of lipid, SMC, T-lymphocytes, macrophages, necrotic cell debris and matrix components (including minerals), associated with structural disorganization and thickening of the intima, with deformity of the arterial wall. The advanced lesion is contained within a fibrous cap, formed by SMC proliferation and vascular remodeling, the result of the unabated response to endothelial injury. The cap consists of SMC surrounded by collagen, elastic fibers and proteoglycans (Tedgui and Mallat 2001).

Rupture of the fibrous cap results in the spillage of the contents of the advanced lesion into the vessel lumen. This results in the formation of a thrombus, which either heals, causing further lesion progression and further compromising flow at the local site, or occludes the coronary artery completely resulting in myocardial infarction and sudden death. Plaque rupture and thrombosis are the primary complications of the advanced lesion, which cause unstable coronary syndromes (Ross 1999).

Over recent years increasing evidence has emerged that a number of the cellular mechanisms intimate to the atherosclerotic process are modulated beneficially by testosterone.

10.7.1 Effects on serum cytokine levels

Cytokines are key players in the atherosclerotic process. Pro-inflammatory cytokines such as interleukin 1-beta (IL-1β) and tumor necrosis factor alpha (TNF-α) are known to increase adhesion molecule expression, promote SMC proliferation and induce matrix metalloproteinase activity, which are critical mechanisms in the initiation of plaque development and rupture. Observational evidence suggests that inflammatory cytokines and serum testosterone levels are interconnected. In one study of men with CAD, it was shown that serum levels of IL-1β increased significantly in a step-wise manner in line with the atherosclerotic burden (Nettleship et al. 2007b). Moreover, when patients were classified by their serum testosterone level, being either eugonadal, "borderline" hypogonadal or hypogonadal, a step-wise increase in IL-1β with lower testosterone status was observed. These data suggest that the underlying testosterone status may modulate IL-1β production in men with CAD.

Testosterone appears capable of modulating both pro- and anti-inflammatory cytokine production by leukocytes in vitro (Li et al. 1993; Kanda et al. 1996; 1997; Bebo et al. 1999; D'Agostino et al. 1999; Liva and Voskuhl 2001; Corrales et al. 2006). Castrated male mice are reported to have increased TNF-α production, following administration of bacterial endotoxin; an effect which was suppressed by subsequent testosterone replacement (Spinedi et al. 1992). Similarly, young hypogonadal men with delayed puberty caused by IHH are reported to exhibit elevated serum levels of inflammatory cytokines compared to healthy controls, which can be corrected by TRT (Yesilova et al. 2000). Elderly, hypogonadal men have also been found to have raised serum levels of TNF-α and interleukin 6 (Khosla et al. 2002).

Testosterone replacement therapy reduces cytokine activation in hypogonadal men. Malkin et al. (2004a) completed a randomized, single-blind, placebo-controlled crossover study of physiological testosterone therapy (one month of Sustanon100® via fortnightly im injection) in 10 men with CAD and hypotestosteronemia. This level of TRT was sufficient to significantly reduce serum levels of TNF-α. The investigators repeated their work in a larger study using the same testosterone dosing regimen, but using a randomized, placebo-controlled crossover protocol in 27 hypogonadal men with concomitant cardiovascular disease (Malkin et al. 2004b). Physiological TRT was again shown to significantly lower serum levels of TNF-α, and also induced a significant decrease in serum levels of IL-1β. As well as the reduction in pro-inflammatory cytokines following physiological testosterone administration, a significant elevation was observed in serum levels of the anti-inflammatory cytokine interleukin 10 (IL-10).

10.7.2 Effects on adhesion molecule expression

Testosterone is reported to have a modulatory effect upon endothelial cell adhesion molecule expression. Dihydrotestosterone has been shown to increase monocyte adhesion to IL-1β-stimulated human umbilical vein endothelial cells (HUVECs) and human umbilical artery endothelial cells (HUVACs) obtained from male donors, and also to increase IL-1β-induced vascular cell adhesion molecule 1 (VCAM-1) expression in these cells (McCrohon et al. 1999), via activation of nuclear factor kappa B (NF-κB) transcription factor. Similarly, Zhang et al. (2002) reported an increase in TNF-α-induced expression of VCAM-1 and the cell adhesion molecule (E-selectin), which mediates monocyte adhesion to cytokine-activated endothelial cells, by testosterone in HUVECs. In both studies the action of testosterone was abolished by AR antagonism. In contrast, testosterone reduced TNF-α-induced VCAM-1 expression in HUVECs of female origin, an activity blocked by ER antagonism and aromatase inhibition (Mukherjee et al. 2002). These data suggest that testosterone may have a detrimental influence upon adhesion molecule expression in males via an interaction with the AR, but induces potentially beneficial reductions in adhesion molecule expression in females via aromatization to 17β-estradiol.

However, vascular specificity is also apparent. Importantly, testosterone is reported to reduce TNF-α-induced VCAM-1 expression in human aortic endothelial cells (Hatakeyama et al. 2002). This cell line is more relevant in terms of atherosclerosis, compared to umbilical cells. Evidently further study is warranted, but these data suggest that testosterone could potentially exert a beneficial effect upon adhesion molecule expression.

Neo-intimal proliferation occurs after vessel wall injury, for example during angioplasty, and is a cause for early re-stenosis. One novel study in pigs, which have anatomically and functionally similar coronary arteries to humans, has shown that testosterone also influences vascular repair mechanisms. In this study, pigs were castrated and then either given TRT or placebo. Those pigs given TRT had reduced neo-intimal proliferation compared to those with a prevailing low testosterone level (Tharp et al. 2009). By comparison, when exogenous additional testosterone or dihydrotestosterone is given to normal animals, arterial calcification is increased (McRobb et al. 2009).

10.7.3 Effects on vascular reactivity

Maintenance of a correct response to vasoconstrictive and vasodilatory agents is essential in the control of vascular tone. This is especially important in atherosclerosis within the coronary circulation, where reduced vasodilatation and enhanced vasoconstriction causes further restriction of coronary blood flow through the partially occluded atherosclerotic vessel, and can also lead to vasospasm, thereby exacerbating anginal symptoms. In both human and animals models testosterone has been shown to elicit marked coronary vasodilatation, both in vivo and in vitro

(Yue et al. 1995; Chou et al. 1996; Webb et al. 1999a; Crews and Khalil 1999a; English et al. 2000b; 2001; Deenadayalu et al. 2001; Pugh et al. 2002a; Jones et al. 2004a); an action which diminishes with aging (English et al. 2000b). Testosterone-induced vasodilatation is rapid in onset and is unaffected by AR blockade (Yue et al. 1995; English et al. 2000b; Tep-areenan et al. 2002; Jones et al. 2002; 2004b) or deficiency (Jones et al. 2003a), and is preserved in endothelial-denuded vessels (Perusquia et al. 1996; Perusquia and Villalon 1999; Murphy and Khalil 1999; Crews and Khalil 1999b; Honda et al. 1999) and in the presence of nitric oxide synthase inhibitors (Yue et al. 1995; Honda et al. 1999; Deenadayalu et al. 2001; Jones et al. 2004a; 2004b), guanylate cyclase or cyclooxygenase (Yue et al. 1995; Chou et al. 1996; Jones et al. 2004a; 2004b; Crews and Khalil 1999a; 1999b). These observations clearly demonstrate that the vasodilatory action of testosterone is mediated directly via an interaction at the level of the vascular smooth muscle.

Furthermore, the observation that testosterone-induced dilatation is not attenuated by covalent linkage to albumin, which prevents its endocytosis into the SMC (Ding and Stallone 2001; Jones et al. 2004a), implies that the dilatory signaling process is initiated at the smooth muscle cell membrane, which has been demonstrated to contain testosterone binding sites (Jones et al. 2003b; 2004a; 2004b). The proposed underlying mechanism of action of testosterone is thought to occur via activation of calcium-sensitive potassium channels (K_{Ca}) (Deenadayalu et al. 2001; Tep-areenan et al. 2002). Alternatively a number of studies report an agonist-dependent variance in the vasodilatory efficacy of testosterone (Yue et al. 1995; Crews and Khalil 1999a; 1999b; Perusquia and Villalon 1999; Murphy and Khalil 1999; Ding and Stallone 2001; English et al. 2002; Jones et al. 2002), consistent with calcium antagonistic action upon voltage-gated calcium channels (VGCCs) (Jones et al. 2003c), although an inhibitory action upon store-operated calcium channels (SOCCs) also occurs in the systemic vasculature (Jones et al. 2003a). Endogenous testosterone has been shown to increase the expression of L-type calcium channels by a direct action on the gene promoter in porcine coronary smooth muscle cells (Bowles et al. 2004). Electrophysiological studies have demonstrated that testosterone in physiological concentrations inhibits both L-type and T-type VGCCs in vascular SMC (Scragg et al. 2004). These findings are supported by microfluorimetric studies in the rat smooth muscle cell line A7r5 which showed that DHT as well as testosterone inhibited the L-type calcium channel (Hall *et al.* 2006). The effects of physiological testosterone concentrations were absent in the presence of nifedipine, an L-type calcium channel blocker, but not the T-type calcium channel blocker pimozide. This is likely to be mediated via direct binding to the main α_{1C} subunit of the VGCC, since a similar inhibitory action is observed in HEK293 cells transfected with this channel protein. This is supported by the finding that a single point mutation at the nifedipine binding site renders the effect of testosterone inactive (Scragg *et al.* 2007). This evidence strongly demonstrates that testosterone is a natural ligand for the nifedipine binding site on L-type calcium channels.

Testosterone also beneficially modulates responses induced by other vasoactive stimuli. Both chronic exposure to physiological testosterone therapy (Kang *et al.* 2002) and acute exposure to supraphysiological doses of testosterone (Ong *et al.* 2000) are reported to increase flow-mediated brachial artery vasodilatation, occurring as a result of increased nitric oxide release from the endothelium in response to changes in sheer stress in men with CAD. Long-term physiological testosterone therapy also improves nitrate-mediated brachial artery vasodilatation in these patients (Kang *et al.* 2002). Brachial artery reactivity correlates closely with coronary arterial responsiveness (Anderson *et al.* 1995a), which would support a beneficial long-term effect for testosterone upon atherosclerotic coronary vasomotion. By contrast, hypogonadal men without cardiovascular disease exhibit elevated flow- and nitrate-mediated brachial artery vasodilation (Zitzmann *et al.* 2002), which is restored to control levels following testosterone replacement. Similarly flow-mediated, but not nitrate-mediated, brachial artery vasodilatation has been shown to be increased in men in whom testosterone levels have been therapeutically or surgically lowered, as a treatment for prostate carcinoma (Herman *et al.* 1997). Discrepancies may be due to the residual density of the ARs, which are upregulated in hypogonadal men in response to lower endogenous testosterone (Malkin *et al.* 2006a). In circumstances where there is combined testosterone and AR deficiency in the testicular feminized mouse, there is reduced endothelial-dependent vasodilatation (Jones *et al.* 2003a). These data implicate an interaction between testosterone acting at the cell membrane and the nuclear AR in the long-term regulation of vascular tone (reviewed in Jones *et al.* 2004b).

Hypotestosteronemia is associated with hypertension and arterial stiffening. Androgen deprivation therapy for prostate carcinoma leads to increased vascular stiffness assessed after three months (Smith *et al.* 2001). There have been several trials of TRT in eugonadal, hypogonadal and obese men which have observed impressive reductions in both systolic and diastolic blood pressure over periods as short as six months and for as long as 10 years (Mårin *et al.* 1993; Anderson *et al.* 1996; Zitzmann and Nieschlag 2007).

10.7.4   Effects on hemostatic factors

In the majority of cases, myocardial infarction occurs as a result of coronary thrombosis, triggered by atherosclerotic plaque rupture and disruption of the vascular endothelium. The thrombotic process is complex, and dependent upon a variety of intrinsic pro- and anti-thrombotic mediators which determine the coagulation status. The anti-coagulation agents tissue plasminogen activator (tPA) and tissue factor pathway inhibitor (TFPI), and the pro-thrombotic factor plasminogen activator inhibitor 1 (PAI-1) are integral to this process. Plasminogen activator inhibitor 1 is a predictor of myocardial infarction and progression of atherosclerosis in patients with stable CAD (Thogerson *et al.* 1998; Bavenholm *et al.* 1998). Evidence suggests that low serum testosterone is associated with a hyper-coagulable state. Indeed, serum testosterone levels and tPA are reported to be positively correlated, whilst a negative correlation exists between serum levels of testosterone and PAI-1 and clotting factor VII (the levels of which are reduced by TFPI) (Glueck *et al.* 1993; Phillips *et al.* 1994; 1995; Pugh *et al.* 2002b). Moreover, both testosterone replacement in hypogonadal men, and androgen treatment in healthy men, leads to reduced PAI-1 levels (Caron *et al.* 1989; Beer *et al.* 1996). Similarly, a number of cross-sectional studies have shown that hypotestosteronemia is associated with high levels of the acute phase protein, fibrinogen (Yang *et al.* 1993; De Pergola *et al.* 1997), and that testosterone replacement can reduce fibrinogen levels (Anderson *et al.* 1995b. This beneficial effect on coagulation status appears to be lost in men who have developed CAD, as physiological TRT in men with CAD has recently been reported to have no effect on serum fibrinogen levels, tPA or PAI-1 (Smith *et al.* 2005).

In a long-term clinical study from Sweden (Svartberg *et al.* 2009), of 1350 men followed up for 10 years, androgen levels in men were not associated with risk of venous thromboembolism. This is an important observation, since an increased risk of arterial and venous thromboembolism is associated with both female hormone replacement therapy (HRT) and use of the oral contraceptive pill (WHO 1997). This is thought to account for the increased incidence in vascular events and death associated with HRT in the recent Women's Health Initiative study (Rossouw *et al.* 2002; see above). This adverse effect on coagulation is not a property shared by testosterone.

10.7.5 Effects on erythropoiesis

Testosterone treatment may increase erythropoiesis, and, as a consequence, increase hematocrit. There is a dose-related effect on erythropoiesis which is more striking in older rather than younger men (Coviello *et al.* 2008). The effect is seen within a month of replacement therapy and peaks by 12 months, but is not associated with a change in either erythropoietin or soluble transferrin receptor (Coviello *et al.* 2008). The mechanism whereby testosterone increases erythropoiesis remains unknown. This in itself may pose a threat by theoretically increasing thrombotic risk. Guidelines recognize this potential issue and recommend that when TRT is initiated that the hematocrit is monitored after 3 and 12 months and then annually. It is suggested that treatment be interrupted if the hematocrit rises above 55%, and/or venesection be offered to maintain this level (Wang *et al.* 2008).

Earlier studies suggested that this effect is seen mainly when replacement therapy is given in high dosage or when the mode of delivery exposes the individual to transient high levels.

In the latest study of topical treatment with a 2% gel applied daily to the axilla in androgen-deficient men with symptoms of hypogonadism, the treatment was discontinued in four men (2.6%) after three months of treatment because of a high hematocrit above 0.54% (Wang *et al.* 2011). A previous study, involving 227 men who used a 1% gel, had shown significant changes in hemoglobin or hematocrit, with 11.3% exceeding the upper normal range for hematocrit at 50 mg/day and none at this dose needing to stop therapy (Wang *et al.* 2000). In another large study of 220 men with type 2 diabetes or metabolic syndrome and hypogonadism (Jones *et al.* 2011), gel replacement therapy was associated with a non-significant increase in hemoglobin of, on

average, 1.42 ± 1.55 g/dl, and hematocrit increased by 0.03 ± 0.04 g/dl.

In long-term studies of injectable TRT, hemoglobin and hematocrit have been shown to increase, but not above the acceptable normal ranges (Minnemann *et al.* 2007).

Although there is potential for adverse effects on the circulation of a higher than normal hematocrit, there is also the potential for benefit. Chronic heart failure is associated with persistent inflammatory activation, and chronic anemia is part of the syndrome especially in cachectic patients.

10.7.6 Effects on total and LDL cholesterol

Elevated serum cholesterol, especially LDL cholesterol, is a powerful risk factor for the premature development of atherosclerosis. It is the sub-endothelial accumulation of LDL cholesterol that provokes a local inflammatory response, that results in the generation of "fatty streaks" (smooth raised plaques located beneath the endothelium), which represent the initial phase of atherosclerosis.

Low endogenous serum levels of testosterone have been reported, in a number of cross-sectional studies, to be correlated with higher serum levels of total and LDL cholesterol (Barrett-Connor and Khaw 1988; Barrett-Connor 1992; Haffner *et al.* 1993; Simon *et al.* 1997; Isidori *et al.* 2005; Mäkinen *et al.* 2008). These data suggest that hypogonadal men may exhibit an adverse pro-atherogenic lipid profile. Moreover, TRT causes significant reductions in total and LDL cholesterol in hypogonadal men (Tenover 1992; Tripathy *et al.* 1998; Howell *et al.* 2001; Ly *et al.* 2001); an effect which is maintained in eugonadal individuals (Thompson *et al.* 1989; Bagatell *et al.* 1994; Uyanik *et al.* 1997). Serum total cholesterol levels have been shown to decline following physiological testosterone replacement in hypogonadal men with CAD, despite these patients already being treated with statin drugs (HMG-CoA reductase inhibitors) (Malkin *et al.* 2004a).

Although LDL cholesterol is associated with an adverse cardiovascular profile, so HDL cholesterol is associated with a reduced risk profile. Testosterone has been shown to reduce HDL-C in some (Bagatell *et al.* 1994; Rossouw *et al.* 2002), but not all (Gliczynski *et al.* 1996; Uyanik *et al.* 1997) studies. However, reductions in HDL-C are generally smaller and less pronounced than those of other lipid fractions (Whitsel *et al.* 2001; Jones and Saad 2009).

In animal models, serum levels of total cholesterol are raised in the testosterone-deficient testicular feminized (Tfm) mouse. Furthermore, following testosterone supplementation in the Tfm mouse, HDL-C was demonstrated to be significantly raised compared to placebo controls (Nettleship *et al.* 2007a).

Triglycerides have also been implicated in atherogenesis, particularly in diabetic populations. In a large study of middle-aged men with hypogonadal symptoms, low testosterone was associated with high triglycerides as well as low HDL-C (Mäkinen *et al.* 2008). In one clinical study (Agledahl *et al.* 2008), elderly men with low testosterone levels had higher BMI, waist circumference and triglyceride levels after fatty meals.

10.8 Treatment studies in men with atherosclerosis

10.8.1 Angina pectoris

The observational studies and animal experiments described above indicate that men with a low level of circulating testosterone have an increased atherogenic profile, and demonstrably more atherosclerosis. The process of atherosclerosis in humans results in various clinical manifestations. First, sudden thrombotic occlusion of arteries at the site of atherosclerotic plaques causes acute coronary syndromes (myocardial infarction) and stroke. Epidemiological studies (described above) do suggest that these events are more common in men with lower levels of testosterone, especially, for example, after prostate surgery. A study of men attending a urology clinic for ED (Corona *et al.* 2010) showed that men with a low testosterone level were more likely to have fatal cardiovascular events during a relatively short follow-up period of just over four years. These authors found no statistical relationship between testosterone levels and major cardiovascular events.

Second, progressive atherosclerosis causes fixed narrowing of arteries which results in reduced blood flow to vital organs, and tissue ischemia. The classical clinical manifestation of this is angina pectoris.

In men with hypogonadism, does TRT improve symptoms of angina?

Testosterone therapy has been used in men with angina since the 1940s, with observational evidence of improvement. In one study of 100 patients with angina (including eight women), Lesser (1946) showed clinical improvement with testosterone in 91%, with no change in 9%.

The first randomized controlled trial was conducted in 1977. Jaffe (1977) published the results of the effects of weekly injections of testosterone cypionate or placebo on post-exercise ST segment changes on the 12-lead electrocardiograph (ECG) after the two-step test (an early form of exercise testing). He showed statistically significant reductions in the sum of ST segment change by 31.7% at the end of four weeks and 51.2% by eight weeks of treatment. The only other positive finding was an increase in hemoglobin concentration of 0.7–1.4 g/dl by the end of the trial. However, Jaffe found no correlation between the change in hemoglobin concentration and the degree of ST change. He postulated that the effect may have been mediated by an increase in coronary artery blood flow consequent upon vasodilation. The dose of testosterone used in this study was probably supraphysiological. Webb *et al.* (1999) used quantitative coronary angiography to show that increasing doses of intra-coronary infusions of testosterone caused progressive coronary vasodilatation. Rosano *et al.* (1999) and Webb *et al.* (1999b) studied the effect of intravenous testosterone on angina threshold using standard exercise testing, and showed that time to 1 mm ST segment depression was prolonged after intravenous testosterone compared with both baseline and placebo.

Our group showed for the first time in a randomized, placebo-controlled clinical trial that physiological doses of testosterone improved angina threshold but only significantly in those men with a low baseline level of testosterone (English *et al.* 2000c). In this study men were selected only if they had a reproducibly positive treadmill exercise test. They were treated with low dose physiological replacement therapy by skin patches delivering 5 mg testosterone daily in a slow-release form. This dose is sufficient to raise testosterone levels to normal in 93% of hypogonadal patients. Treatment did increase total testosterone levels but not outside the normal range. There was no measurable difference in hemoglobin levels with this formulation. Exercise duration and time to 1 mm ST segment depression was prolonged in those men taking testosterone, but the effect was most marked in those men with low starting levels. In a repeat study in men with hypogonadism and angina, and using a crossover methodology, we found much more marked improvements (Malkin *et al.*

217

Table 10.1 Review of all published studies of testosterone in men with angina

Author	Drug dosage	Primary outcome	n	Result
Hamm (1942)	Variable		7	Decreased frequency of angina
Walker (1942)	Variable		9	Increased exercise tolerance
Sigler (1943)	Low		16	Increased exercise duration
Lesser (1946)	Low		92	Improvement in 85
Jaffe (1977)	Physiological	Exercise test	50	Decreased ST depression
Wu and Weng (1993)	Variable	Holter	62	Decreased ischemia on Holter
Rosano et al. (1999)	High	Exercise test	14	Increased time to ischemia
Webb et al. (1999b)	High	Exercise test	14	Increased time to ischemia
English et al. (2000c)	Physiological	Exercise test	46	Increased time to ischemia
Thompson et al. (2002)	High and physiological	Exercise test SPECT scan	32	Neutral
Malkin et al. (2004a)	Physiological	Exercise test	10	Increased time to ischemia
Mathur et al. (2009)	Physiological	Exercise test	13	Increased time to ischemia

Abbreviations: SPECT, single photon emission computed tomography.

2004a) in all men despite concomitant anti-anginal therapy. All these clinical studies report improvements over the short-term (three months). The durability of the response was tested in a long-term study of 12 months duration using depot injections every 3 months (testosterone undecanoate – Nebido®—) in men with chronic stable angina and reproducibly low early morning testosterone blood level (<12 nmol/l) (Mathur et al. 2009). This randomized, placebo-controlled, parallel-group study showed significant and persistent improvement in exercise duration and time to 1mm ST segment depression on treadmill testing with active treatment.

In all there have been 12 studies of the use of testosterone therapy in men with angina with consistently positive results. An overview of these trials has shown that the size of the clinical benefit is greater in those men with low baseline levels of testosterone (<12 nmol/l), and the effect lasts for at least one year (see Table 10.1).

The mechanism underpinning the improvement in exercise duration and the direct anti-ischemic effect seen in these clinical studies is probably coronary artery vasodilatation. In vitro, isolated human arteries from hypogonadal men show an augmented vasodilatation to testosterone compared with control arteries from eugonadal men (Malkin et al. 2006a). After three months of physiological replacement therapy this augmented response was less obvious. This

suggests downregulation of the dilatory response after replacement therapy, which was not seen in the clinical study where the improvement in angina threshold was persistent at 12 months. Laboratory studies indicate that testosterone causes vasodilatation by interaction with the L-type calcium channel in the smooth muscle cell membrane of vessels, which is the site of action for the drug nifedipine, which is also a known anti-anginal agent (Scragg et al. 2004).

Additional clinical benefits that have been seen in these men treated with replacement doses of testosterone include favorable modifications to standard accepted risk factors including:

- total cholesterol (see Chapter 11 for further details) and LDL (Malkin et al. 2004b);
- obesity and insulin resistance (Malkin et al. 2007);
- improved fibrinolysis (Smith et al. 2005);
- reduced inflammation/cytokine activation (Malkin et al. 2004b);
- improved diabetic control (Kapoor et al. 2006; Jones et al. 2011).

10.9 Testosterone and heart failure

Chronic heart failure (CHF) can best be described as a syndrome characterized by impairment of cardiac function associated with a maladaptive metabolic and neuro-hormonal axis. Chronic heart failure is a common clinical problem and a major public health

Table 10.2 Metabolic changes in heart failure

Metabolic axis	Specific compounds	Relationship with chronic heart failure	Clinical effect in heart failure	Effect of pharmacological modification	Available therapies
Renin-angiotensin	Angiotensin II	Relates to severity of CHF and predicts deterioration and mortality	Vasoconstriction, fluid retention, myocardial fibrosis	Improves symptoms and reduces mortality	ACE-I ARBs
	Aldosterone		Myocardial fibrosis	Improves symptoms and reduces mortality	Spironolactone Eplerenone
Catecholamines	Adrenalin Noradrenalin	Relate to severity of CHF and predict deterioration, mortality and sudden death	Increase risk of sudden death, worsen cardiac function	Improve symptoms and reduce mortality	β-Blockers
Glucocorticoid	Cortisol	Elevated	Catabolic	Unknown	None
Insulin		Resistance to insulin action in proportion to severity of CHF	Impaired glucose delivery, catabolic	Unknown	
Growth hormone		Reduced in heart failure, resistance at receptor level	Catabolic		Recombinant growth hormone
Androgens	Testosterone	Reduced in heart failure	Catabolic	Improves endurance	Testosterone
	Dehydroepiandrosterone	Reduced in heart failure	Catabolic	Unknown	
Immune/ cytokine	Tumor necrosis factor	Elevated	Catabolic	None	Monoclonal antibodies
	Interleukin 1	Elevated	Catabolic	None	Monoclonal antibodies

Abbreviations: ACE-I, angiotensin-converting enzyme inhibitor; ARB, angiotensin receptor blocker; β-blocker, beta-adrenoceptor blocker.

issue. The prevalence of CHF in the UK is 1% and in Europe alone it is thought that around 10 million people are affected by CHF (Swedberg *et al.* 2005), imposing a financial burden in the UK accounting for 4–5% of the National Health Service budget. In most patients the clinical condition is characterized by relentlessly progressive breathlessness, worsening exercise tolerance and overwhelming fatigue. Modern heart failure drug therapy uses combinations of angiotensin-converting enzyme inhibitors, beta-adrenergic receptor blockers and direct aldosterone antagonists which improve symptoms and prolong life, but do not prevent eventual decompensation to progressive heart failure. Other widely used therapies such as loop diuretics, digoxin and other anti-arrhythmics may improve symptoms and keep patients from unwanted hospital admission but have no demonstrable effect on mortality (Swedberg *et al.* 2005).

Despite modern advances in the detection, diagnosis and treatment of CHF, the prognosis of this condition is still poor and is no better than the prognosis of most malignancies. Severe heart failure which is characterized by breathlessness at rest or on minimal exertion has an annualized mortality of 50% (Swedberg *et al.* 2005).

10.9.1 Pathophysiology

In order to appreciate the potential role for testosterone in the treatment of men with heart failure, it is necessary to understand some background pathophysiology of the condition. Chronic heart failure is a unique metabolic syndrome characterized by perturbation of numerous endocrine and inflammatory parameters. These changes are important since they relate to the severity of heart failure and directly contribute to deterioration and prognosis. A summary of the heart failure metabolic syndrome is displayed in Table 10.2.

The physiological consequence of inadequate cardiac pumping action is reduced cardiac output, resulting in low organ perfusion pressure. This results in neuro-humeral activation of systems causing fluid retention and vasoconstriction, which aim to return the cardiac output and blood pressure to normal. However, many of these adaptive changes are ultimately detrimental and cause worsening of cardiac function and eventually lead to deterioration in the severity of heart failure. Strategies to simply increase cardiac muscle contraction – with inotropes, for example – merely accelerate the decline in function leading to a worse outcome. The mainstay of modern drug therapy is to interfere pharmacologically with these adaptive changes and so to delay the inevitable cardiac decline. Symptoms are controlled and deterioration slowed by inhibition of the renin-angiotensin-aldosterone axis and blockade of catecholamine receptors, as summarized in Table 10.2. Disordered and excess immune activation has been explored with small trials of immunoglobulin and also pentoxifylline, with varying benefit. The possibility of reducing pro-inflammatory cytokines has been intensively investigated, and although initial studies of anti-TNF "biological" drugs were promising, definitive benefit has not been borne out in major clinical trials (Anker and Coats 2002).

10.9.2 Androgen status in heart failure

Patients with heart failure have been shown to have a clear anabolic–catabolic imbalance, with an excess of catabolic hormones and a deficiency of many anabolic hormones, which is associated with a poorer prognosis and significant morbidity (Anker *et al.* 1997). Jankowska *et al.* (2006) showed that hormonal deficiencies in gonadal, adrenal and somatotropic hormones in men with heart failure were independent markers of poor prognosis, but it is not clear whether these changes are the cause or the result of heart failure. Whether cause or effect, when testosterone levels are low in men with heart failure then this is a poor prognostic marker (Guder *et al.* 2010; Wehr *et al.* 2011). About a quarter to a third of men with moderate-severity heart failure have biochemical evidence of testosterone deficiency (Kontoleon *et al.* 2003; Malkin *et al.* 2006b). One of the most important features of severe heart failure is a severe anabolic–catabolic imbalance resulting in cardiac cachexia (Anker *et al.* 1997), which is defined clinically as the non-intentional loss of 6 kg lean mass over a six-month period. Cachexia is the most extreme symptom of heart failure, and most subjects experience a more gradual catabolic decline. Cardiac cachexia is strongly associated with testosterone deficiency. The clinical characteristics of muscular wasting and weakness in heart failure show that the condition is not simply a disease of the heart: there are multi-system effects. Many of the cardinal symptoms of heart failure such as breathlessness and fatigue are due to abnormal muscle function, impaired mobilization of energy and ultimately loss of lean muscle mass (Coats 2001). It is these features of heart failure, intuitively similar to a state of frank androgen deficiency, which led to the idea of using testosterone treatment as a catabolic antagonist.

10.9.3 Theoretical basis for testosterone as a treatment for heart failure

Testosterone is a logical choice as a treatment for heart failure, as the condition is characterized by anabolic deficiency, low-grade inflammation and a loss of muscle mass and strength. These are effects that testosterone treatment, even at physiological doses, may improve. In addition, in heart failure there is systemic peripheral vasoconstriction resulting in increased systemic vascular resistance. As discussed above, since testosterone is also a direct coronary and peripheral vasodilator, this action should improve cardiac output and function.

10.9.4 Cardiac effects of testosterone treatment

Within the boundaries of the normal physiological range, testosterone therapy seems to have relatively little effect on myocardial morphology and function. There are animal data that profound testosterone depletion (castration) results in reduced left ventricular mass, reduced cardiac output and reduced ejection fraction (Scheuer et al. 1987), possibly through the expression of certain calcium ion channels and protein synthesis. In Klinefelter syndrome, echocardiographic data indicate that systolic function is impaired and systolic velocities correlate with testosterone levels (Andersen et al. 2008). There are considerably more data on the effects of supraphysiological testosterone treatment on the myocardium. There is general uniformity in cell culture studies, intact animal treatment studies and observational studies of power athletes known to abuse anabolic androgens, showing that a very high dose damages the myocardium. The important specific findings from the human observational studies include increased left ventricular mass and hypertrophy, smaller ventricular cavity dimensions and evidence of early diastolic dysfunction due to stiffening and loss of left ventricular compliance (Urhausen et al. 2004).

10.9.5 Non-cardiac effects of testosterone treatment

There have been numerous clinical trials of androgen therapy on the effects of body composition and voluntary physical strength. The trials can be broadly divided into those using physiological or non-physiological testosterone therapy and those testing the effects in morbid populations, androgen-deficient males and normal subjects. There is a general consistency within the literature, with well-conducted, prospective randomized controlled trials showing that testosterone improves anabolic function. This improvement in function is characterized by increased voluntary muscle strength, increased lean (muscle) mass and reduced fat mass (Isidori et al. 2005). These effects are seen in all patient groups and with testosterone preparations within the physiological replacement range. The morbid populations studied include patients with weight loss and cachexia due to malignancy, HIV infection and inflammatory autoimmune disease.

In one recent interventional study of frail hypogonadal men, supraphysiological dosages of TRT were used in an attempt to improve muscle strength (Basaria et al. 2010). The study was positive in showing significant increases in muscle strength but was stopped early because of an excess of cardiovascular side-effects. The authors reported that 23 patients taking testosterone had cardiovascular complications compared with 5 in the placebo group, and on this basis stopped the trial. Critical review of this paper shows that in fact there were only 6 hard end-points in the treatment group compared with 1 in the placebo group. About half of the group had a history of cardiovascular disease, and the rest had significant cardiovascular risk factors. If this study shows anything it is that men with hypogonadism should be treated only with physiological doses of testosterone for true replacement therapy. The literature shows that testosterone replacement should be managed in the same way that thyroid hormone replacement is. Replacement dosages should aim to maintain normal physiological levels. If the Basaria trial had been conducted in hypothyroid patients with high cardiovascular risk and replacement had aimed at supraphysiological levels, the same (or worse) result would have been seen.

In patients with heart failure, skeletal muscle is abnormal with muscle fiber atrophy and a shift from oxidative to glycolytic metabolism. Some authorities believe that these muscle changes result in autonomic and ventilatory responses which contribute to symptoms of breathlessness and fatigue. These changes can be temporarily reversed by exercise training. At the cellular level, a potential site of action for testosterone treatment has been identified which involves the local expression of IGF-1 and the nuclear accumulation of pro-myogenic, anti-adipogenic stem cell regulator, β-catenin (Gentile et al. 2010). These findings strongly suggest that the anabolic effect of physiological doses of testosterone is likely to be beneficial for patients with heart failure.

10.9.6 Insulin resistance

One of the major hormonal derangements in heart failure is resistance to the action of insulin, which is another example of a maladaptive humeral change in the complex syndrome of heart failure. The severity of heart failure is related to the severity of the insulin resistance, and impaired insulin-mediated glucose uptake is a powerful independent prognostic marker (Anker *et al.* 1997). The mechanism underlying insulin resistance in heart failure is obscure, though it appears functionally different from insulin resistance in other morbid populations, which in general are characterized by reduced phosphorylation of intracellular post-insulin receptor proteins. It is likely that the cause is multifactorial and involves impaired post-receptor signaling and other neuro-hormonal and immune alterations present in severe heart failure (Kemppainen *et al.* 2003). It is notable that insulin resistance can be improved by both conventional heart failure treatments such as angiotensin converting enzyme inhibitors and β-adrenergic receptor blockers as well as non-pharmacological treatments such as graded exercise. Testosterone treatment has a positive effect on insulin sensitivity both in normal subjects and morbid populations such as obese men and diabetics (Kapoor *et al.* 2005; Jones *et al.* 2011). In a small placebo-controlled crossover study in men with chronic heart failure (see Chapter 11), testosterone improved fasting glucose and insulin levels, and insulin resistance as measured by HOMA (Homeostatic Model Assessment), and this was associated with increased lean mass and reduced fat mass (Malkin *et al.* 2007).

10.9.7   Inflammation

There is low-grade, subclinical inflammatory activation in chronic heart failure. Inflammatory mediators such as tumor necrosis factor (TNF-α) and interleukins such as IL-1 and IL-6 are elevated in patients with heart failure, and contribute to cachexia and insulin resistance (Anker *et al.* 1997). Testosterone replacement therapy reduces blood levels of inflammatory cytokines in hypogonadal men with co-morbid disease such as diabetes and coronary disease (Malkin *et al.* 2004b). However, significant clinical effects in men with heart failure have not been detected in vivo (Pugh *et al.* 2005), although clinical trials at present are limited and under-powered.

10.9.8   Hemodynamics in heart failure

Testosterone therapy has beneficial effects on the hemodynamics of heart failure. Experimental human data have confirmed that testosterone in vitro is a dilator of pre-constricted systemic vessels (isolated from subcutaneous fat) (Malkin *et al.* 2006a). Furthermore, an important in-vivo crossover study, using invasive hemodynamic monitoring in 12 patients with chronic heart failure randomized to six hours of acute testosterone therapy or placebo in random order, has confirmed the thesis that testosterone reduces systemic vascular resistance and consequently increases cardiac index (Fig. 10.2) (Pugh *et al.* 2003). The levels of testosterone in the treatment phase of this study were in the high physiological range and show that, in the short term at least, testosterone increases cardiac output as a result of reducing vascular resistance and increasing myocardial stroke volume. Further analysis of these data demonstrates that the patients with the lowest baseline testosterone levels (patients below the median) derived a greater hemodynamic effect. Pulmonary vascular resistance is frequently elevated in men with chronic left ventricular failure, due in part to dysregulation of smooth muscle tone. There is in vitro evidence in human pulmonary arteries and veins that physiological levels of testosterone act as a vasodilator. Potentially this effect of testosterone could contribute to the beneficial effect of testosterone observed in clinical trials (Jones *et al.* 2002; Smith *et al.* 2008; Rowell *et al.* 2009).

10.9.9   Erythropoietic effects of testosterone

As discussed above, one of the consequences of chronic heart failure is persistent chronic anemia. This is usually mild, but in some patients (particularly those with cardiac cachexia) it can be an intractable problem. Indeed, the problem of anemia has prompted studies of the role of erythropoietin in patients with heart failure. A meta-analysis of the available randomized, controlled trial evidence does show a small benefit when erythropoietin is given to patients with heart failure, compared with placebo (Kotecha *et al.* 2011). Testosterone increases hemoglobin in a dose-responsive way, and this effect is beneficial in these patients.

In the treatment trials in heart failure (Malkin *et al.* 2006b; Caminiti *et al.* 2009), men given TRT had a small but statistically significant increase in hematocrit by about 1.5% over placebo, but no change in hemoglobin level.

10.9.10   Clinical trials of testosterone therapy in heart failure

There are few trials of androgen treatment in heart failure. A single animal study using a low dose of

(A)

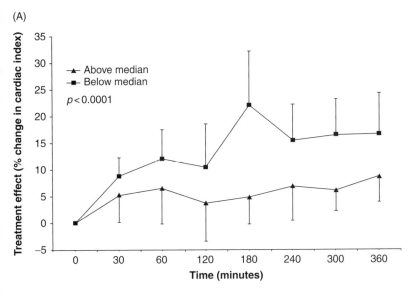

(B)

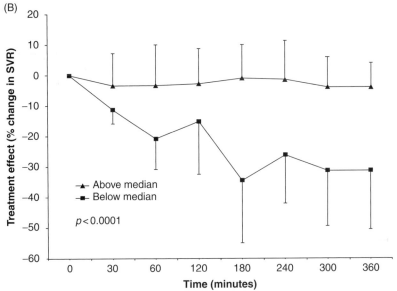

Fig. 10.2 Figure showing the acute hemodynamic changes seen on (A) cardiac index and (B) systemic vascular resistance (SVR) after high-dose buccal testosterone in men with heart failure. The data show the effect of testosterone in men with baseline bioavailable testosterone above or below the median of 4.6 nmol/l. From Pugh *et al.* (2003).

nandrolone decanoate improved survival in male hamsters with an inherited cardiomyopathy. An unblinded descriptive study of 12 male patients found improvements in echocardiographic parameters (reduced left ventricular diameter, reduced left ventricular mass) and reductions in brain natriuretic peptide (a serum marker of heart failure severity).

The first prospective, double-blind studies of testosterone treatment in heart failure were from the same scientific research group. In a pilot study using injections of im testosterone (Sustanon 100) every fortnight, Pugh *et al.* (2004) found testosterone to improve mood, symptom scores and endurance (using an incremental shuttle walk test). In the larger follow-up study to this pilot (Malkin *et al.* 2006b), using low-dose daily transdermal testosterone patches (Androderm 5 mg or placebo), the effect on endurance was confirmed. Testosterone was found to increase exercise capacity as measured with an incremental shuttle walk test. The improvement in exercise capacity in this study was less than observed in the pilot, in which larger doses of testosterone were given, suggesting that there may be a dose-response relationship. Examination of the pooled data confirms that the patients treated with im testosterone achieved higher serum levels of testosterone and greater increases in functional capacity. These data suggest that the biological effects of testosterone on functional exercise capacity are related to the serum levels reached in vivo. Furthermore, consistent with this notion, there was a positive correlation with the increase in exercise capacity and serum bioavailable testosterone at three and six months. Other secondary outcomes from this study included improved physician-assigned symptom scores, increased voluntary muscle strength, increased left ventricular cavity length by echocardiography, and a trend to a reduction in left ventricular mass. Systolic blood pressure fell in the placebo group over the 12 months follow-up, which is a recognized part of the natural history of heart failure and is an adverse prognostic sign; systolic blood pressure in the testosterone group was maintained.

There have been two further studies of TRT in patients with heart failure – one in men and one in women. In a short-term study of three-months duration, Caminiti et al. (2009) examined the effects of TRT or placebo using a long-acting depot testosterone in 70 men (average age 70 years) with heart failure in association with reduced systolic function on echocardiography (<40% mean ejection fraction 32%). Only 30% were clinically and biochemically hypogonadal. They used cardio-pulmonary exercise test and six-minute walk tests to assess functional improvement, which improved in those men taking TRT, in relation to the change in testosterone blood level.

They examined the relationship between oxygen consumption and ventilation which is deranged in men with heart failure, and showed that TRT reduced the gradient of the ventilation/CO_2 elimination rate slope, which implies a beneficial effect of testosterone on ventilatory efficiency. Effectively this means that men treated with TRT felt less breathless per unit of exercise compared with their peers on placebo. These authors also showed that TRT improved baroreceptor sensitivity, which is a novel finding in humans. As baroreceptor sensitivity is decreased in heart failure (and associated with an adverse prognosis), such a change has theoretical advantages. The greatest benefits were seen in men with lower baseline levels of testosterone.

This research group has also used low-level TRT in a six-month study of women with heart failure and showed similar effects. The safety of testosterone therapy in women with heart failure in the long term has not been assessed (Iellamo et al. 2010).

Heart failure is a condition of high mortality, chronic debilitating symptoms and recurrent hospitalization. Novel therapies should either improve morbidity or survival or both; ideally therapy should be widely applicable, inexpensive and show benefit in the presence of coexisting heart-failure therapies. Although TRT cannot be advocated for women, testosterone treatment is indicated in at least 25% of men with heart failure who will have a low testosterone blood level. These men all have symptoms compatible with hypogonadism, so there is no reason to withhold therapy, once prostate malignancy had been excluded. In those men with a testosterone blood level within the normal range it can be argued that, within the context of the hormonal imbalance of heart failure, this represents a relative androgen deficiency. However, as discussed above it is important to only use physiological doses of replacement therapy to avoid potential complications.

10.10 Testosterone levels and mortality

The disadvantage of having a low blood testosterone level is not only related to the development of accelerated atherosclerosis. Ruige et al. (2011) have reviewed the published literature on overall mortality and testosterone level up to 2009. There does appear to be an excess mortality in elderly men (>70 years of age) who have a low testosterone level, which is especially marked in studies published since 2007. Five recent studies have demonstrated that lower baseline testosterone levels are a significant predictive marker for mortality even after controlling for the effects of co-morbid conditions. In 2004, Shores et al. (2004) reported that hypotestosteronemia was a marker for mortality in a group of 44 geriatric inpatients within a six-month period. In a follow-on study, the same group performed a computerized analysis of the Veteran's Affair's clinical database (Shores et al. 2006), including 850 men followed up over a four- to eight-year period. After controlling for co-morbid conditions which would affect mortality, e.g. concurrent cancer, they found that men with low testosterone levels had an 88% (20.1 vs. 34.9%, $p < 0.001$) relative increase in all-cause mortality risk when compared with those with normal testosterone levels at baseline. In 2007, the InCHIANTI study demonstrated that an age-associated fall in bioavailable testosterone was associated with increased risk of death (Maggio et al.

(A)

Survival by testosterone status. Bio-T/all-cause mortality (adjusted)

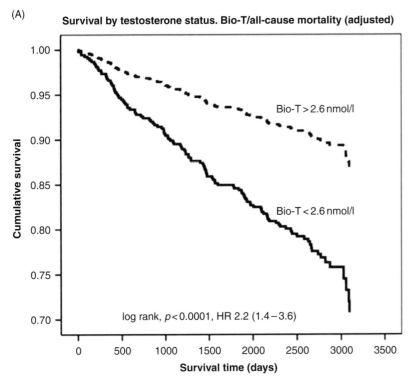

Fig. 10.3 Survival curves for mortality based on baseline bioavailable testosterone (bio-T). (A) All-cause mortality; (B) vascular mortality. The solid line represents patients with baseline bio-T less than 2.6 nmol/l; the broken line represents patients with bio-T greater than 2.6 nmol/l. HR, hazard ratio (From Malkin *et al.* 2010).

(B)

Survival by testosterone status. Bio-T/vascular mortality (adjusted)

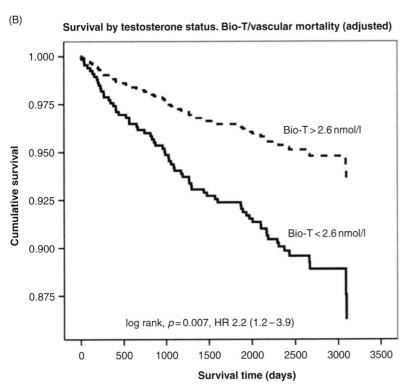

2007). In a six-year follow-up study of 410 men aged over 65 years, they found that this effect was made more pronounced and more statistically significant when low testosterone was associated with similar declines in IGF and DHEAS. In contrast to men with all three hormones above the lowest quartiles, men with one, two or three hormones in the lowest quartiles were increasingly at more risk of death.

In 2008, Laughlin *et al.* studied an older group (mean age of 71 years) of 794 men over a period of up to 20 years (Laughlin *et al.* 2008). They found a significant fall in bioavailable testosterone but not total testosterone with age. The risk of death was greater for men in the lowest baseline quartile of both total and bioavailable testosterone compared with those in the highest quartile. After adjusting for age, adiposity, and lifestyle choices, the risk of death was 44% greater for the lowest compared to the highest quartile of total testosterone (hazard ratio (HR): 1.44; 95% CI: 1.12–1.84) and 50% higher for the lowest compared to the highest quartile of bioavailable testosterone (HR: 1.50; CI: 1.15–1.96).

In the largest study to date investigating the effects of endogenous testosterone levels and mortality, the European Prospective Investigation into Cancer Norfolk study (EPIC-Norfolk) (Khaw *et al.* 2007) prospectively investigated all-cause and cardiovascular mortality in 11 606 healthy men between the ages of 40 and 79 years at baseline. Over a 6–10-year follow-up period, they observed a statistically significant association between baseline serum testosterone level and all-cause (HR: 0.75; CI: 0.55–1.00), cardiovascular (HR: 0.62; CI: 0.45–0.84) and cancer-related (HR: 0.59; CI: 0.42–0.85) deaths ($p < 0.001$) for each association after controlling for co-morbid conditions and behaviors. They found that a 1 SD increase in baseline testosterone (~6 nmol/l) was associated with an approximate 14% risk reduction in mortality over the study period.

In 2010, two more long-term epidemiological studies showing that a low serum testosterone is associated with an excess mortality were published (Haring *et al.* 2010; Malkin *et al.* 2010). Most of these studies have been in populations of normal men without overt vascular disease. However, in the recently published study by Malkin *et al.* (2010), 930 men with angiographically proven CAD were prospectively followed up over a seven-year period. These authors observed baseline prevalence of hypogonadism in this group (by a strict criterion) to be 24%. In this androgen-deficient group the mortality was 21% versus only 12% in the eugonadal group ($p = 0.002$). Low bioavailable testosterone but not total testosterone significantly influenced the all-cause and cardiovascular mortality after the multivariate analysis (Fig. 10.3), suggesting that this is the more sensitive assay in detecting pathological deficiency and risk. Low testosterone, therefore, appears to be a marker for increased mortality.

The effect of TRT on survival in men with or without cardiovascular disease is unknown, as clinical trials have not been sufficiently powered or protracted to detect any change. Nevertheless, the current evidence base on physiological TRT in some morbid populations is compelling. Hypogonadal men with type 2 diabetes, angina pectoris and heart failure have been shown to derive benefit. Given the costs of large, long-term randomized controlled trials, a registry of treated and untreated patients with any or all of these conditions in association with biochemical testosterone deficiency could provide useful data.

10.11 Key messages

- Men have a higher cardiovascular risk than women.
- Low testosterone is associated with accelerated atherosclerosis in both animal and human studies.
- Low testosterone is associated with an adverse atherogenic risk profile.
- Replacement testosterone therapy to normal physiological levels improves symptoms of angina and heart failure in men with hypogonadism.
- Low testosterone is a marker of increased cardiovascular and all-cause mortality.
- Large, randomized controlled trials are needed to test the hypothesis that physiological testosterone replacement will reduce this adverse effect on mortality.

10.12 References

Agledahl I, Hansen JB, Svartberg J (2008) Postprandial triglyceride metabolism in elderly men with subnormal testosterone levels. *Asian J Androl* **10**:542–549

Akishita M, Hashimoto M, Ohike Y, Ogawa S, Iijima K, Eto M, Ouchi Y (2010) Low testosterone level as a predictor of cardiovascular events in Japanese men with coronary risk factors. *Atherosclerosis* **210**:232–236

Alexandersen P, Haarbo J, Byrjalsen I, Lawaetz H, Christiansen C (1999) Natural androgens inhibit male atherosclerosis: a study in castrated, cholesterol-fed rabbits. *Circ Research* **84**:813–819

Andersen NH, Bojesen A, Kristensen K, Birkebaek NH, Fedder J, Bennett P, Christiansen JS, Gravholt CH (2008) Left ventricular dysfunction in Klinefelter syndrome is associated to insulin resistance, abdominal adiposity and hypogonadism. *Clin Endocrinol (Oxf)* **69**:785e91

Anderson FH, Francis RM, Faulkner K (1996) Androgen supplementation in eugonadal men with osteoporosis – effects of 6 months of treatment on bone mineral density and cardiovascular risk factors. *Bone* **18**:171–177

Anderson RA, Ludlam CA, Wu FCW (1995b) Haemostatic effects of supraphysiological levels of testosterone in normal men. *Thromb Haemostasis* **74**:693–697

Anderson TJ, Uehata A, Gerhard MD, Meredith IT, Knab S, De La Grange D, Lieberman EH, Ganz P, Creager MA, Yeung AC, Selwyn AP (1995a) Close relation of endothelial function in the human coronary and peripheral circulations. *J Am Coll Cardiol* **26**:1235–1241

Anker SD, Coats AJ (2002) How to RECOVER from RENAISSANCE? The significance of the results of RECOVER, RENAISSANCE, RENEWAL and ATTACH. *Int J Cardiol* **86**:123–130

Anker SD, Chua TP, Ponikowski P, Harrington D, Swan JW, Kox WJ, Poole-Wilson PA, Coats AJ (1997) Hormonal changes and catabolic/anabolic imbalance in chronic heart failure and their importance for cardiac cachexia. *Circulation* **96**:526–534

Arad Y, Badimon JJ, Badimon L, Hembree WC, Ginsberg HN (1989) Dehydroepiandrosterone feeding prevents aortic fatty streak formation and cholesterol accumulation in the cholesterol-fed rabbit. *Arteriosclerosis* **9**:159–166

Bagatell CJ, Heiman JR, Matsumoto AM, Rivier JE, Bremner WJ (1994) Metabolic and behavioral effects of high dose exogenous testosterone in healthy men. *J Clin Endocrinol Metab* **79**:561–567

Barrett-Connor E (1992) Lower endogenous androgen levels and dyslipidemia in men with non-insulin-dependent diabetes mellitus. *Ann Int Med* **117**:807–811

Barrett-Connor E, Khaw KT (1988) Endogenous sex hormones and cardiovascular disease in men. A prospective population-based study. *Circulation* **78**:539–545

Basaria S, Coviello AD, Travison TG, Storer TW, Farwell WR, Jette AM, Eder R, Tennstedt S, Ulloor J, Zhang A, Choong K, Lakshman KM, Mazer NA, Miciek R, Krasnoff J, Elmi A, Knapp PE, Brooks B, Appleman E, Aggarwal S, Bhasin G, Hede-Brierley L, Bhatia A, Collins L, LeBrasseur N, Fiore LD, Bhasin S (2010) Adverse events associated with testosterone administration. *N Engl J Med* **363**:109–122

Bavenholm P, de Faire U, Landou C, Efendic S, Nilsson J, Wilman B, Hamsten A (1998) A progression of coronary artery disease in young male post-infarction patients is linked to disturbances of carbohydrate and lipoprotein metabolism and to impaired fibrinolytic function. *Eur Heart J* **19**:402–410

Bebo BF, Schuster JC, Vandenbark AA, Offner H (1999) Androgens alter the cytokine profile and reduce encephalitogenicity of myelin-reactive T cells. *J Immunol* **162**:35–40

Beer NA, Jakubowicz DJ, Matt DW, Beer RM, Nestler JE (1996) Dehydroepiandrosterone reduces plasma plasminogen activator inhibitor type 1 and tissue plasminogen activator antigen in men. *Am J Med Sci* **311**:205–210

Bolla M, Van Tienhoven G, Warde P, Dubois JB, Mirimanoff RO, Storme G, Bernier J, Kuten A, Sternberg C, Billiet I, Torrecilla JL, Pfeffer R, Cutajar CL, Van der Kwast T, Collette L (2010) External irradiation with or without long-term androgen suppression for prostate cancer with high metastatic risk: 10-year results of an EORTC randomised study. *Lancet Oncol* **11**:1066–1073

Bourghardt J, Wilhelmson AS, Alexanderson C, De Gendt K, Verhoeven G, Krettek A, Ohlsson C, Tivesten A (2010) Androgen receptor-dependent and independent atheroprotection by testosterone in male mice. *Endocrinology* **151**:5428–5437

Bowles DK, Maddali KK, Ganjam VK, Rubin LJ, Tharp DL, Turk JR, Heaps CL (2004) Endogenous testosterone increases L-type Ca^{2+} channel expression in porcine coronary smooth muscle. *Am J Physiol* **287**:H2091–H2098

Bruck B, Brehme U, Gugel N, Hanke S, Finking G, Lutz C, Benda N, Schmahl FW, Haasis R, Hanke H (1997) Gender-specific differences in the effects of testosterone and estrogen on the development of atherosclerosis in rabbits. *Arterioscler Thromb Vasc Biol* **17**:2192–2199

Caminiti G, Volterrani, M, Iellamo F, Marazzi G, Massaro R, Miceli M, Mammi C, Piepoli M, Fini M, Rosano GMC (2009) Effect of long-acting testosterone treatment on functional exercise capacity, skeletal muscle performance, insulin resistance, and baroreflex sensitivity in elderly patients with chronic heart failure. A double-blind, placebo-controlled, randomized study. *J Am Coll Cardiol* **54**:919–927

Caron P, Bennet A, Camare R, Louvet JP, Boneu B, Sie P (1989) Plasminogen activator inhibitor in plasma is related to testosterone in men. *Metab Clin Exper* **38**:1010–1015

Chou TM, Sudhir K, Hutchison SJ, Ko E, Amidon TM, Collins P, Chatterjee K (1996) Testosterone induces dilation of canine coronary conductance and resistance arteries in vivo. *Circulation* **94**:2614–2619

Chute CG, Baron JA, Plymate SR, Kiel DP, Pavia AT, Lozner EC, O'Keefe T, MacDonald GJ (1987) Sex hormones and coronary artery disease. *Am J Med* 83:853–859

Coats AJ (2001) Heart failure: what causes the symptoms of heart failure? *Heart* 86:574–578

Corona G, Monami M, Boddi V, Cameron-Smith M, Fisher A, de Vita G, Melani C, Balzi D, Sforza A, Forti G, Mannucci E, Maggi M (2010) Low testosterone is associated with an increased risk of MACE lethality in subjects with erectile dysfunction. *J Sex Med* 7:1557–1564

Corrales JJ, Almeida M, Burgo R, Mories MT, Miralles JM, Orfao A (2006) Androgen-replacement therapy depresses the ex vivo production of inflammatory cytokines by circulating antigen-presenting cells in aging type-2 diabetic men with partial androgen deficiency. *J Endocrinol* 189:595–604

Coviello AD, Kaplan B, Lakshman KM, Chen T, Singh AB, Bhasin S (2008) Effects of graded doses of testosterone on erythropoiesis in healthy young and older men. *J Clin Endocrinol Metab* 93:914–919

Crews JK, Khalil RA (1999a) Antagonistic effects of 17 beta-estradiol, progesterone, and testosterone on Ca^{2+} entry mechanisms of coronary vasoconstriction. *Art Thromb Vasc* 19:1034–1040

Crews JK, Khalil RA (1999b) Gender-specific inhibition of Ca^{2+} entry mechanisms of arterial vasoconstriction by sex hormones. *Clin Exp Pharmacol & Physiol* 26:707–715

D'Agostino P, Milano S, Barbera C, Di Bella G, La Rosa M, Ferlazzo V, Farruggio R, Miceli DM, Miele M, Castagnetta L, Cillari E (1999) Sex hormones modulate inflammatory mediators produced by macrophages. *Ann NY Acad Sci* 876:426–429

Davoodi G, Amirezadegan A, Borumand MA, Dehkori MR, Kazemisaeid A, Yaminisharif A (2007) The relationship between level of androgenic hormones and coronary artery disease in men. *Cardiovasc J Africa* 18:362–366

Debing E, Peeters E, Duquet W, Poppe K, Velkeniers B, Van Den Brande P (2008) Men with atherosclerotic stenosis of the carotid artery have lower testosterone levels compared with controls. *Int Angiol* 27:135–141

Deenadayalu VP, White RE, Stallone JN, Gao X, Garcia AJ (2001) Testosterone relaxes coronary arteries by opening the large-conductance, calcium-activated potassium channel. *Am J Physiol – Heart C* 281:H1720–H1727

Demirbag R, Yilmaz R, Ulucay A, Unlu D (2005) The inverse relationship between thoracic aortic intima media thickness and testosterone level. *Endocr Res* 31:335–344

De Pergola G, De Mitrio V, Sciaraffia M, Pannacciulli N, Minenna A, Giorgino F, Petronelli M, Laudadio E, Giorgino R (1997) Lower androgenicity is associated with higher plasma levels of pro-thrombotic factors irrespective of age, obesity, body fat distribution, and related metabolic parameters in men. *Metabolism* 46:1287–1293

Ding AQ, Stallone JN (2001) Testosterone-induced relaxation of rat aorta is androgen structure specific and involves K+ channel activation. *J Appl Physiol* 91:2742–2750

Dobrzycki S, Serwatka W, Nadlewski S, Korecki J, Jackowski R, Paruk J, Ladny JR, Hirnle T (2003) An assessment of correlations between endogenous sex hormone levels and the extensiveness of coronary heart disease and the ejection fraction of the left ventricle in males. *Med Invest* 50:162–169

Eich DM, Nestler JE, Johnson DE, Dworkin GH, Ko D, Wechsler AS, Hess ML (1993) Inhibition of

accelerated coronary atherosclerosis with dehydroepiandrosterone in the heterotopic rabbit model of cardiac transplantation. *Circulation* 87:261–269

English KM, Mandour O, Steeds RP, Diver MJ, Jones TH, Channer KS (2000a) Men with coronary artery disease have lower levels of androgens than men with normal coronary angiograms. *Eur Heart J* 21:890–894

English KM, Jones RD, Jones TH, Morice AH, Channer KS (2000b) Aging reduces the responsiveness of coronary arteries from male Wistar rats to the vasodilatory action of testosterone. *Clin Sci* 99:77–82

English KM, Steeds RP, Jones TH, Diver MJ, Channer KS (2000c) Low-dose transdermal testosterone therapy improves angina threshold in men with chronic stable angina: a randomized, double-blind, placebo-controlled study. *Circulation* 102:1906–1911

English KM, Jones RD, Jones TH, Morice AH, Channer KS (2001) Gender differences in the vasomotor effects of different steroid hormones in rat pulmonary and coronary arteries. *Horm Metab Res* 33:645–652

English KM, Jones RD, Jones TH, Morice AH, Channer KS (2002) Testosterone acts as a coronary vasodilator by a calcium antagonistic action. *J Endocrinol Invest* 25:455–458

Gentile MA, Nantermet PV (2010) Androgen mediated improvement of body composition and muscle function involves a novel early transcriptional program including IGF-1, MGF and induction of beta-catenin. *J Mol Endocrinol* 44:55e73

Gliczynski S, Ossowski M, Slowinska-Srzednicka J, Brzezinska A, Zgliczynski W (1996) Effect of testosterone replacement therapy on lipids and lipoproteins in hypogonadal and elderly men. *Atherosclerosis* 121:35–43

Glueck CJ, Glueck HI, Stroop D, Speirs J, Hamer T, Tracy T (1993) Endogenous testosterone, fibrinolysis, and coronary heart disease risk in hyperlipidemic men. *J Lab Clin Med* **122**:412–420

Gordon GB, Bush DE, Weisman HF (1988) Reduction of atherosclerosis by administration of dehydroepiandrosterone. A study in hypercholesterolaemic New Zealand White rabbits with aortic intimal injury. *J Clin Invest* **82**:712–720

Grady D, Herrington D, Bittner V, Blumenthal R, Davidson M, Hlatky M, Hsia J, Hulley S, Herd A, Khan S, Newby LK, Waters D, Vittinghoff E, Wenger N; HERS Research Group (2002) Cardiovascular disease outcomes during 6.8 years of hormone therapy (HERS II). *JAMA* **288**:49–57

Guder G, Fratz S, Bauersach SJ, Allolio B, Ertl G, Angermann CE, Stork S (2010) Low serum androgens and mortality in heart failure. *Heart* **96**:504–509

Haffner SM, Mykkanen L, Valdez RA, Katz MS (1993) Relationship of sex hormones to lipids and lipoproteins in non-diabetic men. *J Clin Endocrinol Metab* **77**:1610–1615

Hak AE, Witteman JC, de Jong FH, Geerlings MI, Hofman A, Pols HA (2002) Low levels of endogenous androgens increase the risk of atherosclerosis in elderly men: the Rotterdam study. *J Clin Endocrinol Metab* **87**:3632–3639

Hall J, Jones RD, Jones TH, Channer KS, Peers C (2006) Selective inhibition of L-type Ca^{2+} channels in A7r5 cells by physiological levels of testosterone. *Endocrinology* **147**:2675–2680

Hamm L (1942) Testosterone propionate in the treatment of angina pectoris. *J Clin Endocrinol* **2**:325–328

Hanke H, Lenz C, Spindler KD, Weidemann W (2001) Effect of testosterone on plaque development and androgen receptor expression in the arterial vessel wall. *Circulation* **103**:1382–1385

Haring B, Volzke H, Steveling A, Krebs A, Felix SB, Schofl C, Dorr M, Nauck M, Wallaschofski H (2010) Low serum testosterone levels are associated with increased risk of mortality in a population-based cohort of men aged 20–79. *Eur Heart J* **31**:1491–1501

Hatakeyama H, Nishizawa M, Nakagawa A, Nakano S, Kigoshi T, Uchida K (2002) Testosterone inhibits tumor necrosis factor-alpha-induced vascular cell adhesion molecule-1 expression in human aortic endothelial cells. *FEBS Letters* **530**:129–132

Hauner H, Stangl K, Burger K, Busch U, Blömer H, Pfeiffer EF (1991) Sex hormone concentrations in men with angiographically assessed coronary artery disease – relationship to obesity and body fat distribution. *Klin Wsch* **69**:664–668

Herman SM, Robinson JC, McCredie RJ, Adams MR, Boyer MJ, Celermajer DS (1997) Androgen deprivation is associated with enhanced endothelium-dependent dilatation in adult men. *Arterioscler Thromb Vasc Biol* **17**:2004–2009

Honda H, Unemoto T, Kogo H (1999) Different mechanisms for testosterone-induced relaxation of aorta between normotensive and spontaneously hypertensive rats. *Hypertension* **34**:1232–1236

Howell SJ, Radford JA, Adams JE, Smets EM, Warburton R, Shalet SM (2001) Randomized placebo-controlled trial of testosterone replacement in men with mild Leydig cell insufficiency following cytotoxic chemotherapy. *Clin Endocrinol* **55**:315–324

Hulley S, Grady D, Bush T, Furberg C, Herrington D, Riggs B, Vittinghof E (1998) Randomized trial of estrogen plus progestin for secondary prevention of coronary heart disease in postmenopausal women. Heart and Estrogen/progestin Replacement Study (HERS) Research Group. *JAMA* **280**:605–613

Iellamo F, Volterrani M, Caminiti G, Karam R, Massaro R, Fini M, Collins P, Rosano GMC (2010) Testosterone therapy in women with chronic heart failure. A pilot double-blind, randomized, placebo-controlled study. *J Am Coll Cardiol* **256**:1310–1316

Isidori AM, Giannetta E, Greco EA, Gianfrilli D, Bonifacio V, Isidori A, Lenzi A, Fabbri A (2005) Effects of testosterone on body composition, bone metabolism and serum lipid profile in middle-aged men: a meta-analysis. *Clin Endocrinol (Oxf)* **63**:280–293

Jaffe MD (1977) Effect of testosterone cypionate on postexercise ST segment depression. *Br Heart J* **39**:1217–1222

Jankowska EA, Biel B, Majda J, Szklarska A, Lopuszanska M, Medras M, Anker SD, Banasiak W, Poole-Wilson PA, Ponikowski P (2006) Anabolic deficiency in men with chronic heart failure: prevalence and detrimental impact on survival. *Circulation* **114**:1829–1837

Jones RD, English KM, Pugh PJ, Morice AH, Jones TH, Channer KS (2002) Pulmonary vasodilatory action of testosterone: evidence of a calcium antagonistic action. *J Cardiovasc Pharmacol* **39**:814–823

Jones RD, Pugh PJ, Hall J, Channer KS, Jones TH (2003a) Altered circulating hormone levels, endothelial function and vascular reactivity in the testicular feminised mouse. *Eur J Endocrinol* **148**:111–120

Jones RD, Pugh PJ, Jones TH, Channer KS (2003b) The vasodilatory action of testosterone: a potassium channel opening or a calcium antagonistic action? *Br J Pharm* **138**:733–744

Jones RD, Ruban LN, Morton IE, Roberts SA, English KM, Channer KS, Jones TH (2003c) Testosterone inhibits the prostaglandin F-2-alpha mediated increase in intracellular calcium in A7r5 aortic smooth muscle cells: evidence of an antagonistic action upon store-operated calcium channels. *J Endocrinol* **178**:381–393

Jones RD, English KM, Jones TH, Channer KS (2004a) Testosterone-induced coronary vasodilatation occurs via a non-genomic mechanism: evidence of a direct calcium antagonistic action. *Clin Sci* **107**:149–158

Jones RD, Jones TH, Channer KS (2004b) The influence of testosterone upon vascular reactivity. *Eur J Endocrinol* **151**:29–37

Jones TH, Saad F (2009) The effects of testosterone on risk factors for, and mediators of, the atherosclerotic process. *Atherosclerosis* **207**:308–327

Jones TH, Arver S, Behre H, Buvat J, Meuleman E, Irribarren IM, Morales A, Volterrani M, Yellowlees A, Howell JD, Channer KS (2011) Testosterone replacement in hypogonadal men with type 2 diabetes and/or metabolic syndrome (the TIMES2 study). *Diabetes Care* **34**:828–837

Kabakci G, Yildirir A, Can I, Unsal I, Erbas B (1999) Relationship between endogenous sex hormone levels, lipoproteins and coronary atherosclerosis in men undergoing coronary angiography. *Cardiology* **92**:221–225

Kanda N, Tsuchida T, Tamaki K (1996) Testosterone inhibits immunoglobulin production by human peripheral blood mononuclear cells. *Clin Exper Immunol* **106**:410–415

Kanda N, Tsuchida T, Tamaki K (1997) Testosterone suppresses anti-DNA antibody production in peripheral blood mononuclear cells from patients with systemic lupus erythematosus. *Arthritis Rheum* **40**:1703–1711

Kang SM, Jang Y, Kim JY, Chung N, Cho SY, Chae JS, Lee JH (2002) Effect of oral administration of

testosterone on brachial arterial vasoreactivity in men with coronary artery disease. *Am J Cardiol* **89**:862–864

Kapoor D, Malkin CJ, Channer KS, Jones TH (2005) Androgens, insulin resistance and vascular disease in men. *Clin Endocrinol (Oxf)* **63**:239–250

Kapoor D, Goodwin E, Channer KS, Jones TH (2006) Testosterone replacement therapy improves insulin resistance, glycaemic control, visceral adiposity and hypercholesterolaemia in hypogonadal men with type 2 diabetes. *Eur J Endocrinol* **154**:899–906

Karakitsos D, Patrianakos AP, De Groot E, Boletis J, Karabinis A, Kyriazis J, Samonis G, Parthenakis FI, Vardas PE, Daphnis E (2006) Androgen deficiency and endothelial dysfunction in men with end-stage kidney disease receiving maintenance hemodialysis. *Am J Nephrol* **26**:536–543

Keating NL, O'Malley AJ, Smith MR (2006) Diabetes and cardiovascular disease during androgen deprivation therapy for prostate cancer. *J Clin Onc* **24**:4448–4456

Kemppainen J, Tsuchida H, Stolen K, Karlsson H, Bjornholm M, Heinonen OJ, Nuutila P, Krook A, Knuuti J, Zierath JR (2003) Insulin signalling and resistance in patients with chronic heart failure. *J Physiol* **550** (Pt 1):305–315

Khaw KT, Dowsett M, Folkerd E, Bingham S, Wareham N, Luben R, Welch A, Day N (2007) Endogenous testosterone and mortality due to all causes, cardiovascular disease, and cancer in men: European prospective investigation into cancer in Norfolk (EPIC-Norfolk) Prospective Population Study. *Circulation* **116**:2694–2701

Khosla S, Atkinson EJ, Dunstan CR, O'Fallon WM (2002) Effect of estrogen versus testosterone on circulating osteoprotegerin and other cytokine levels in normal

elderly men. *J Clin Endocrinol Metab* **87**:1550–1554

Kontoleon PE, Anastasiou-Nana MI, Papapetrou PD, Alexopoulos G, Ktenas V, Rapti AC, Tsagalou EP, Nanas JN (2003) Hormonal profile in patients with congestive heart failure. *Int J Cardiol* **87**:179–183

Kotecha D, Ngo K, Walters JA, Manzano L, Palazzuoli A, Flather MD (2011) Erythropoietin as a treatment of anemia in heart failure: systematic review of randomized trials. *Am Heart J* **161**:822–831.e2

Larsen BA, Nordestgaard BG, Stender S, Kjeldsen K (1993) Effect of testosterone on atherogenesis in cholesterol-fed rabbits with similar plasma cholesterol levels. *Atherosclerosis* **99**:79–86

Laughlin GA, Barrett-Connor E, Bergstrom J (2008) Low serum testosterone and mortality in older men. *J Clin Endocrinol Metab* **93**:68–75

Lesser MA (1946) Testosterone propionate therapy in one hundred cases of angina pectoris. *J Clin Endocrinol* **6**:549–557

Levine GN, D'Amico AV, Berger P, Clark PE, Eckel RH, Keating NL, Milani RV, Sagalowsky AI, Smith MR, Zakai N; American Heart Association Council on Clinical Cardiology and Council on Epidemiology and Prevention, the American Cancer Society, and the American Urological Association (2010) Androgen-deprivation therapy in prostate cancer and cardiovascular risk: a science advisory from the American Heart Association, American Cancer Society and American Urological Association: endorsed by the American Society for Radiation Oncology. *Circulation* **121**:833–840

Li S, Li X, Li Y (2008) Regulation of atherosclerotic plaque growth and stability by testosterone and its receptor via influence of inflammatory reaction. *Vascul Pharmacol* **49**:14–18

.i Z, Danis V, Brooks P (1993) Effect of gonadal steroids on the production of IL-1 and IL-6 by blood mononuclear cells in vitro. *Clin Exp Rheumatol* **11**:157–162

.iva SM, Voskuhl RR (2001) Testosterone acts directly on CD4(+) T lymphocytes to increase IL-10 production. *J Immunol* **167**:2060–2067

.usis A (2000) Atherosclerosis. *Nature* **407**:233–241

.y LP, Jimenez M, Zhuang TN, Celermajer DS, Conway AJ, Handelsman DJ (2001) A double-blind, placebo-controled, randomized clinical trial of transdermal dihydrotestosterone gel on muscular strength, mobility, and quality of life in older men with partial androgen deficiency. *J Clin Endocrinol Metab* **86**:4078–4088

Maggio M, Lauretani F, Ceda GP, Bandinelli S, Ling SM, Metter EJ, Artoni A, Carassale L, Cazzato A, Ceresini G, Guralnik JM, Basaria S, Valenti G, Ferrucci L (2007) Relationship between low levels of anabolic hormones and 6-year mortality in older men: the aging in the Chianti area (InCHIANTI) study. *Arch Intern Med* **167**:2249–2254

Makinen J, Jarvisalo MJ, Pollanen P, Perheentupa A, Irjala K, Koskenvuo M, Makinen J, Huhtaniemi I, Raitakari OT (2005) Increased carotid atherosclerosis in andropausal middle-aged men. *J Am Coll Cardiol* **45**:1603–1608

Mäkinen JI, Perheentupa A, Irjala K, Pöllänen P, Mäkinen J, Huhtaniemi I, Raitakari OT (2008) Endogenous testosterone and serum lipids in middle-aged men. *Atherosclerosis* **197**:688–693

Malkin CJ, Pugh PJ, Morris PD, Kerry KE, Jones RD, Jones TH, Channer KS (2004a) Testosterone replacement in hypogonadal men with angina improves ischaemic threshold and quality of life. *Heart* **90**:871–876

Malkin CJ, Pugh PJ, Jones RD, Kapoor D, Channer KS, Jones TH (2004b)

The effect of testosterone replacement on endogenous inflammatory cytokines and lipid profiles in hypogonadal men. *J Clin Endocrinol Metab* **89**:3313–3318

Malkin CJ, Jones RD, Jones TH, Channer KS (2006a) Effect of testosterone on ex vivo vascular reactivity in man. *Clin Sci (Lond)* **111**:265–274

Malkin CJ, Pugh PJ, West JN, van Beek EJ, Jones TH, Channer KS (2006b) Testosterone therapy in men with moderate severity heart failure: a double-blind randomized placebo controlled trial. *Eur Heart J* **27**:57–64

Malkin CJ, Jones TH, Channer KS (2007) The effect of testosterone on insulin sensitivity in men with heart failure. *Eur J Heart Fail* **9**:44–50

Malkin CJ, Pugh PJ, Morris PD, Asif S, Jones TH, Channer KS (2010) Low serum testosterone and increased mortality in men with coronary heart disease. *Heart* **96**:1821–1825

Mårin P, Holmäng S, Gustafsson C, Jönsson L, Kvist H, Elander A, Eldh J, Sjöström L, Holm G, Björntorp P (1993) Androgen treatment of abdominally obese men. *Obes Res* **1**:245–251

Mathur A, Malkin C, Saeed B, Muthasamy S, Jones TH, Channer KS (2009) The long term effect of testosterone replacement therapy on angina threshold and atheroma in patients with chronic stable angina. *Eur J Endocrinol* **161**:443–449

McCrohon JA, Jessup W, Handelsman DJ, Celermajer DS (1999) Androgen exposure increases human monocyte adhesion to vascular endothelium and endothelial cell expression of vascular cell adhesion molecule-1. *Circulation* **99**:2317–2322

McRobb L, Handelsman DJ, Heather AK (2009) Androgen-induced progression of arterial calcification in apolipoprotein E-null mice is uncoupled from plaque growth and lipid levels. *Endocrinology* **150**:841–848

Minnemann T, Schubert M, Hübler D, Gouni-Berthold I, Freude S, Schumann C, Oettel M, Ernst M, Mellinger U, Sommer F, Krone W, Jockenhövel F (2007) A four-year efficacy and safety study of the long-acting parenteral testosterone undecanoate *Aging Male* **10**:155–158

Mukherjee TK, Dinh H, Chaudhuri G, Nathan L (2002) Testosterone attenuates expression of vascular cell adhesion molecule-1 by conversion to estradiol by aromatase in endothelial cells: implications in atherosclerosis. *Natl Acad Sci USA* **99**:4055–4060

Muller M, van den Beld AW, Bots ML, Grobbee DE, Lamberts SW, van der Schouw YT (2004) Endogenous sex hormones and progression of carotid atherosclerosis in elderly men. *Circulation* **109**:2074–2079

Murphy JG, Khalil RA (1999) Decreased [Ca(2+)](i) during inhibition of coronary smooth muscle contraction by 17beta-estradiol, progesterone, and testosterone. *J Pharmacol Exp Ther* **291**:44–52

Nathan L, Shi WB, Dinh H, Mukherjee TK, Wang XP, Lusis AJ, Chaudhuri G (2001) Testosterone inhibits early atherogenesis by conversion to estradiol: critical role of aromatase. *Natl Acad Sci USA* **98**:3589–3593

Nettleship JE, Jones TH, Channer KS, Jones RD (2007a) Physiological testosterone replacement therapy attenuates fatty streak formation and improves high-density lipoprotein cholesterol in the Tfm mouse: an effect that is independent of the classic androgen receptor. *Circulation* **116**:2427–2434

Nettleship JE, Pugh PJ, Channer KS, Jones T, Jones RD (2007b) Inverse relationship between serum levels of interleukin-1beta and testosterone in men with stable coronary artery disease. *Horm Metab Res* **39**:366–371

Ong PJ, Patrizi G, Chong WC, Webb CM, Hayward CS, Collins P (2000)

Testosterone enhances flow-mediated brachial artery reactivity in men with coronary artery disease. *Am J Cardiol* **85**:269–272

Perusquia M, Villalon CM (1999) Possible role of Ca^{2+} channels in the vasodilating effect of 5 beta-dihydrotestosterone in rat aorta. *Eur J Pharmacol* **371**:169–178

Perusquia M, Hernandez R, Morales MA, Campos MG, Villalon CM (1996) Role of endothelium in the vasodilating effect of progestins and androgens on the rat thoracic aorta. *Gen Pharmacol* **27**:181–185

Phillips GB, Pinkernell BH, Jing TY (1994) The association of hypotestosteronemia with coronary artery disease in men. *Arterioscler Thromb* **14**:701–706

Phillips GB, Jing TY, Laragh JH, Sealey JE (1995) Serum sex hormone levels and renin-sodium profile in men with hypertension. *Am J Hypertens* **8**:626–629

Phillips GB, Pinkernell BH, Jing TY (2004) Are major risk factors for myocardial infarction the major predictors of degree of coronary artery disease in men? *Metabolism* **53**:324–359

Pour HRN, Grobbee DE, Bots ML, Verhaar HJJ, Muller M, van der Schouw YT (2007) Circulating sex hormone levels and aortic stiffness in men. *JAGS* **55**:621–637

Pugh PJ, Jones RD, Jones TH, Channer KS (2002a) Intrinsic responses of rat coronary arteries in vitro: influence of testosterone, calcium and effective transmural pressure. *Endocrine* **19**:155–162

Pugh PJ, Channer KS, Parry H, Downes T, Jones TH (2002b) Bio-available testosterone levels fall acutely following myocardial infarction in men: association with fibrinolytic factors. *Endocrine Res* **28**:161–173

Pugh PJ, Jones TH, Channer KS (2003) Acute haemodynamic effects of testosterone in men with chronic heart failure. *Eur Heart J* **24**:909–915

Pugh PJ, Jones RD, West JN, Jones TH, Channer KS (2004) Testosterone treatment for men with chronic heart failure. *Heart* **90**:446–447

Pugh PJ, Jones RD, Malkin CJ, Hall J, Nettleship JE, Kerry KE (2005) Physiologic testosterone therapy has no effect on serum levels of tumour necrosis factor-alpha in men with chronic heart failure. *Endocr Res* **31**:271–283

Qiu Y, Yanase T, Hu H, Tanaka T, Nishi Y, Liu M, Sueishi K, Sawamura T, Nawata H (2010) Dihydrotestosterone suppresses foam cell formation and attenuates atherosclerosis development. *Endocrinology* **151**:3307–3316

Rosano GM, Sheiban I, Massaro R, Pagnotta P, Marazzi G, Vitale C, Mercuro G, Volterrani M, Aversa A, Fini M (2007) Low testosterone levels are associated with coronary artery disease in male patients with angina. *Int J Impot Res* **19**:176–182

Rosano GMC, Leonardo F, Pagnotta P, Pelliccia F, Panina G, Cerquetani E, della Monica PL, Bonfigli B, Volpe M, Chierchia SL (1999) Acute anti-ischemic effect of testosterone in men with coronary artery disease. *Circulation* **99**:1666–1670

Ross R (1999) Atherosclerosis: an inflammatory disease. *N Engl J Med* **340**:115–126

Rossouw JE, Anderson GL, Prentice RL, LaCroix AZ, Kooperberg C, Stefanick ML, Jackson RD, Beresford SA, Howard BV, Johnson KC, Kotchen JM, Ockene J; Writing Group for the Women's Health Initiative Investigators (2002) Risks and benefits of estrogen plus progestin in healthy postmenopausal women: principal results. *JAMA* **288**:321–333

Rowell KO, Hall J, Pugh PJ, Jones TH, Channer KS, Jones RD (2009) Mechanisms of agonist-induced constriction in isolated human pulmonary arteries. *Vasc Pharmacol* **51**:8–12

Ruige JB, Mahmoud AM, De Bacquer D, Kaufman JM (2011) Endogenous testosterone and cardiovascular disease in healthy men: a meta-analysis. *Heart* **97**:870–875

Saigal CS, Gore JL, Krupski TL, Hanley J, Schonlau M, Litwin MS (2007) Androgen deprivation therapy increases cardiovascular morbidity in men with prostate cancer. *Cancer* **110**:1493–1500

Satariano WA, Ragland KE, Van Den Eeden SK (1998) Cause of death in men diagnosed with prostate carcinoma. *Cancer* **83**:1180–1188

Scheuer J, Malhotra A, Schaible TF, Capasso J (1987) Effects of gonadectomy and hormonal replacement on rat hearts. *Circ Res* **61**:12–19

Scragg JL, Jones RD, Channer KS, Jones TH, Peers C (2004) Testosterone is a potent inhibitor of L-type Ca^{2+} channels. *Biochem Bioph Res Comm* **318**:503–506

Scragg JL, Dallas ML, Peers C (2007) Molecular requirements for L-type Ca^{2+} channel blockade by testosterone. *Cell Calcium* **42**:11–15

Shahani S, Braga-Basaria M, Basaria S (2008) Androgen deprivation therapy in prostate cancer and metabolic risk for atherosclerosis. *J Clin Endocrinol Metab* **93**:2042–2049

Shores MM, Moceri VM, Gruenewald DA, Brodkin KI, Matsumoto AM, Kivlahan DR (2004) Low testosterone is associated with decreased function and increased mortality risk: a preliminary study of men in a geriatric rehabilitation unit. *J Am Geriatr Soc* **52**:2077–2081

Shores MM, Matsumoto AM, Sloan KL, Kivlahan DR (2006) Low serum testosterone and mortality in male veterans. *Arch Intern Med* **166**:1660–1665

Sigler LHTJ (1943) Treatment of angina pectoris by testosterone propionate. *NY J Med* **43**:1424–1428

Simon D, Preziosi P, Barrett-Connor E, Roger M, Saint-Paul M, Nahoul K,

Papoz L (1992) The influence of aging on plasma sex hormones in men: the Telecom Study. *Am J Epidemiol* **135**:783–791

Simon D, Charles MA, Nahoul K, Orssaud G, Kremski J, Hully V, Joubert E, Papoz L, Eschwege E (1997) Association between plasma total testosterone and cardiovascular risk factors in healthy adult men: the Telecom Study. *J Clin Endocrinol Metab* **82**:682–685

Smith A, English K, Malkin C, Jones R, Jones T, Channer K (2005) Testosterone does not adversely affect fibrinogen or tissue plasminogen activator (tPA) and plasminogen activator inhibitor-1 (PAI-1) levels in 46 men with chronic stable angina. *Eur J Endocrinol* **152**:285–291

Smith AM, Bennett RT, Jones TH, Cowen ME, Channer KS, Jones RD (2008) Characterisation of the vasodilatory action of testosterone in the human pulmonary circulation. *Vasc Health Risk Management* **4**:1459–1466

Smith JC, Bennett S, Evans LM, Kynaston HG, Parmar M, Mason MD, Cockcroft JR, Scanlon MF, Davies JS (2001) The effects of induced hypogonadism on arterial stiffness, body composition and metabolic parameters in males with prostate cancer. *J Clin Endocrinol Metab* **86**:4261–4267

Spinedi E, Suescun MO, Hadid R, Daneva T, Gaillard RC (1992) Effects of gonadectomy and sex hormone therapy on the endotoxin-stimulated hypothalamo-pituitary-adrenal axis: evidence for a neuroendocrine-immunological sexual dimorphism. *Endocrinology* **131**:2430–2436

Svartberg J, von Muhlen D, Mathiesen E, Joakimsen O, Bonan KH, Stensland-Bugge E (2006) Low testosterone levels are associated with carotid atherosclerosis in men. *J Intern Med* **259**:576–582

Svartberg J, Braekkan SK, Laughlin GA, Hansen JB (2009) Endogenous

sex hormone levels in men are not associated with risk of venous thromboembolism: the Tromso study. *Eur J Endocrinol* **160**:833–838

Swedberg K, Cleland J, Dargie H, Drexler H, Follath F, Komajda M, Tavazzi L, Smiseth OA, Gavazzi A, Haverich A, Hoes A, Jaarsma T, Korewicki J, Lévy S, Linde C, Lopez-Sendon JL, Nieminen MS, Piérard L, Remme WJ; Task Force for the Diagnosis and Treatment of Chronic Heart Failure of the European Society of Cardiology (2005) Guidelines for the diagnosis and treatment of chronic heart failure: executive summary (update 2005): The Task Force for the Diagnosis and Treatment of Chronic Heart Failure of the European Society of Cardiology. *Eur Heart J* **26**:1115–1140

Taylor LG, Canfield SE, Du XL (2009) Review of major adverse effects of androgen-deprivation therapy in men with prostate cancer. *Cancer* **115**:2388–2399

Tedgui A, Mallat Z (2001) Anti-inflammatory mechanisms in the vascular wall. *Circ Res* **88**:877–887

Tedeschi-Reiner E, Ivekovic R, Novak-Laus K, Reiner Z (2009) Endogenous steroid sex hormones and atherosclerosis of retinal arteries in men. *Med Sci Monit* **15**:211–216

Tenover JS (1992) Effects of testosterone in the aging male. *J Clin Endocrinol Metab* **75**:1092–1098

Tep-areenan P, Kendall DA, Randall MD (2002) Testosterone-induced vasorelaxation in the rat mesenteric arterial bed is mediated predominantly via potassium channels. *Br J Pharmacol* **135**:735–740

Tharp DL, Masseau I, Ivey J, Ganjam VK, Bowles DK (2009) Endogenous testosterone attenuates neointima formation after moderate coronary balloon injury in male swine. *Cardiovasc Res* **82**:152–160

Thogerson AM, Jansson JH, Boman K, Nilsson TK, Weinehall L,

Huhtasaari F, Hallmans G (1998) High plasminogen activator inhibitor and tissue plasminogen activator levels in plasma precede a first myocardial infarction in both men and women: evidence for the fibrinolytic system as an independent primary risk factor. *Circulation* **98**:2241–2247

Thompson PD, Cullinane EM, Sady SP, Chenevert C, Saritelli AL, Sady MA, Herbert PN (1989) Contrasting effects of testosterone and stanozolol on serum lipoprotein levels. *JAMA* **261**:1165–1168

Thompson PD, Ahlberg AW, Moyna NM, Duncan B, Ferraro-Borgida M, White CM, McGill CC, Heller GV (2002) Effect of intravenous testosterone on myocardial ischaemia in men with coronary artery disease. *Am Heart J* **143**:249–256

Tivesten A, Mellström D, Jutberger H, Fagerberg B, Lernfelt B, Orwoll E, Karlsson MK, Ljunggren O, Ohlsson C (2007) Low serum testosterone and high serum estradiol associate with lower extremity peripheral arterial disease in elderly men. The MrOS Study in Sweden. *J Am Coll Cardiol* **50**:1070–1076

Tripathy D, Shah P, Lakshmy R, Reddy KS (1998) Effect of testosterone replacement on whole body glucose utilisation and other cardiovascular risk factors in males with idiopathic hypogonadotrophic hypogonadism. *Horm Metab Res* **30**:642–645

Tsai HK, D'Amico AV, Sadetsky N, Chen M-H, Carroll PR (2007) Androgen deprivation therapy for localised prostate cancer and the risk of cardiovascular mortality. *J Nat Cancer Inst* **99**:1516–1524

Urhausen A, Albers T, Kindermann W (2004) Are the cardiac effects of anabolic steroid abuse in strength athletes reversible? *Heart* **90**:496–501

Uyanik BS, Ari Z, Gumus B, Yigitoglu MR, Arslan T (1997) Beneficial effects of testosterone undecanoate on the lipoprotein profiles in healthy elderly men. *Jap Heart J* **38**:73–82

Vikan T, Johnsen SH, Schirmer H, Njolstad I, Svartberg J (2009) Endogenous testosterone and the prospective association with carotid atherosclerosis in men: the Tromso study. *Eur J Epidemiol* **24**:289–295

Walker TC (1942) The use of testosterone propionate and estrogenic substance in the treatment of essential hypertension, angina and peripheral vascular disease. *J Clin Endoc* **2**:560–568

Wang C, Swerdloff RS, Iranmanesh A, Dobs A, Snyder PJ, Cunningham G, Matsumoto AM, Weber T, Berman N; Testosterone Gel Study Group (2000) Transdermal testosterone gel improves sexual function, mood, muscle strength and body composition parameters in hypogonadal men. *J Clin Endocrinol Metab* **85**:2839–2853

Wang C, Nieschlag E, Swerdloff E, Behre HM, Hellstrom WJ, Gooren LJ, Kaufman JM, Legros J-J, Lunenfeld B, Morales A, Morely JE, Schulman C, Thompson IM, Weldner W, Wu FCW (2008) Investigation, treatment and monitoring of late-onset hypogonadism in males. Consensus statement. *Eur J Endocrinol* **159**:507–514

Wang C, Ilani N, Arver S, McLachlan RI, Soulis T, Watkinson A (2011) Efficacy and safety of the 2% formulation of testosterone topical solution applied to the axillae in androgen-deficient men. *Clin Endocrinol (Oxf)* **75**:836–843. DOI 10.1111/j.1365–2265.2011.04152.x

Webb CM, McNeill JG, Hayward CS, de Zeigler D, Collins P (1999a) Effects of testosterone on coronary vasomotor regulation in men with coronary heart disease. *Circulation* **100**:1690–1696

Webb CM, Adamson DL, de Zeigler D, Collins P (1999b) Effect of acute testosterone on myocardial ischemia in men with coronary artery disease. *Am J Cardiol* **83**:437–439

Wehr E, Pilz S, Boehm BO, Marz W, Grammer T, Obermayer-Pietsch B (2011) Low free testosterone is associated with heart failure mortality in older men referred for coronary angiography. *Eur J Heart Fail* **13**:482–488

Whitsel EA, Boyko EJ, Matsumoto AM, Anawalt BD (2001) Intramuscular testosterone esters and plasma lipids in hypogonadal men: a meta-analysis. *Am J Med* **111**:261–269

WHO (1997) Acute myocardial infarction and combined oral contraceptives: results of an international multi-centre case-control study: WHO collaborative study of cardiovascular disease and steroid hormone contraception. *Lancet* **349**:1202–1209

Wu FC, von Eckardstein A (2003) Androgens and coronary artery disease. *Endocr Rev* **24**:183–217

Wu SZ, Weng XZ (1993) Therapeutic effects of an androgenic preparation on myocardial ischemia and cardiac function in 62 elderly male coronary heart disease patients. *Chin Med J* **106**:415–418

Yang XC, Jing TY, Resnick LM, Phillips GB (1993) Relation of haemostatic risk factors to other risk factors for coronary heart disease and to sex hormones in men. *Arterioscler Thromb* **13**:467–471

Yesilova Z, Ozata M, Kocar IH, Turan M, Pekel A, Sengul A, Ozdemir IC (2000) The effects of gonadotropin treatment on the immunological features of male patients with idiopathic hypogonadotropic hypogonadism. *J Clin Endocrinol Metab* **85**:66–70

Yue P, Chatterjee K, Beale C, Poole-Wilson PA, Collins P (1995) Testosterone relaxes rabbit coronary arteries and aorta. *Circulation* **91**:1154–1160

Zhang X, Wang LY, Jiang TY, Zhang HP, Dou Y, Zhao JH, Zhao H, Qiao ZD, Qiao JT (2002) Effects of testosterone and 17-beta-estradiol on TNF-alpha-induced E-selectin and VCAM-1 expression in endothelial cells. Analysis of the underlying receptor pathways. *Life Sci* **71**:15–29

Zitzmann M, Nieschlag E (2007) Androgen receptor gene CAG repeat length and body mass index modulate the safety of long-term intramuscular testosterone undecanoate therapy in hypogonadal men. *J Clin Endocrino Metab* **92**:3844–3853

Zitzmann M, Brune M, Nieschlag E (2002) Vascular reactivity in hypogonadal men is reduced by androgen substitution. *J Clin Endocrinol Metab* **87**:5030–5037

Testosterone, obesity, diabetes and the metabolic syndrome

T. Hugh Jones and Kevin S. Channer

11.1   Introduction

Many epidemiological studies have found a high prevalence of low testosterone levels in men with obesity, metabolic syndrome and type 2 diabetes mellitus. A significant proportion of men with these conditions have been shown to have classical symptoms of testosterone deficiency, providing a diagnosis of hypogonadism. Obesity is a major risk factor for the development of the metabolic syndrome and eventually type 2 diabetes. Both metabolic syndrome and type 2 diabetes are associated with increased morbidity and mortality from cardiovascular disease. Indeed, three-quarters of men with type 2 diabetes die as a result of coronary heart disease or stroke. There is an accumulating volume of published research which links testosterone deficiency with important cardiovascular risk factors, especially those which comprise the key components of the metabolic syndrome.

Insulin resistance is the common biochemical abnormality between these conditions and is in itself a well-recognized cardiovascular risk factor. Understanding the link between testosterone and obesity and insulin resistance is fundamental to determining its role in the pathophysiology of these disorders. A question which is constantly asked is whether or not a low testosterone level is merely a consequence of obesity, which is a state of inflammation, and/or does it promote adiposity? A similar query addresses the low testosterone state associated with cardiovascular disease, cancer, HIV, chronic pulmonary disease and other inflammatory disorders, in that it could be a biomarker of illness, but does

Testosterone: Action, Deficiency, Substitution, ed. Eberhard Nieschlag and Hermann M. Behre, Assoc. ed. Susan Nieschlag. Published by Cambridge University Press. © Cambridge University Press 2012.

IDF

NCEP ATP III

Essential:

*Central obesity waist >94 cm

Three factors from:

*Central obesity waist >102 cm

Fasting glucose >5.6 mmol/l

Plus two from:

Blood pressure >130/85

Fasting triglycerides >1.7 mmol/l

Fasting glucose >5.6 mmol/l

HDL cholesterol <1.03 mmol/l

Blood pressure >130/85

Fasting triglycerides >1.7 mmol/l

HDL cholesterol <1.03 mmol/l

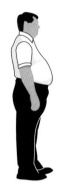

Fig. 11.1 Definitions of the metabolic syndrome which are in common usage. *These two definitions have recently been amalgamated, with agreement that three out of the five criteria are required for the diagnosis. As there are ethnic and population differences in the degree of elevated waist circumference, it is important that this is taken into account for country-specific measurements. In addition, drug treatment of elevated triglycerides, blood pressure and fasting glucose and reduced HDL-C, even if normalized for each criterion, are included (Alberti *et al.* 2009). See plate section for color version.

testosterone substitution have therapeutic benefits? Evidence from recent clinical intervention studies does support beneficial effects on certain cardiovascular risk end-points as well as relief of hypogonadal symptoms.

11.2 Association of low testosterone with obesity

Increased body fat is a well-known clinical feature of hypogonadism which is clearly manifest in eunuchoidal body habitus in men with overt hypogonadism (Allan and McLachlan 2010; MacDonald *et al.* 2010). Several epidemiological studies have demonstrated an inverse relationship of testosterone levels with BMI and central obesity (Seidell *et al.* 1990; Pasquali *et al.* 1991; Simon *et al.* 1992; Haffner *et al.* 1993; Couillard *et al.* 2000; Svartberg *et al.* 2004a). The gradual decline of testosterone with age has been shown to be associated with an increase in truncal obesity as demonstrated by measurement of waist circumference (Khaw and Barrett-Connor 1992). Furthermore, ADT in the treatment of prostate carcinoma leads to an increase in waist circumference and body fat mass.

Many studies have used waist circumference as a measure of central obesity that includes subcutaneous as well as visceral fat. Central adiposity, however, does not fully correlate with the degree of visceral fat. CT, MRI and DXA scanning provide more accurate methods of assessing visceral fat volume. Studies using these techniques have confirmed the inverse relationship of testosterone with visceral adiposity (Seidell *et al.* 1990; Couillard *et al.* 2000). Total testosterone levels correlate

inversely with the accumulation of visceral fat, but not other fat depots, on CT scan after 7.5 years follow-up in a group of 110 men (Tsai *et al.* 2000). The Quebec Family Study found negative correlations of total testosterone with waist circumference, body fat mass and visceral and subcutaneous fat in a group of 130 men (Blouin *et al.* 2005). The Tromso study of 1548 men aged 24–85 years showed that greater waist circumference was associated with low SHBG as well as testosterone (Svartberg *et al.* 2004a). There are only a small number of studies that have investigated the effect of weight loss on testosterone levels. One study found that a massive weight loss of between 26 and 129 kg over a period of between 5 and 39 months led to an increase in free and total testosterone and SHBG (Strain *et al.* 1988)

11.3 Metabolic syndrome and type 2 diabetes

11.3.1 The metabolic syndrome

The metabolic syndrome is a constellation of cardiovascular risk factors which together are strongly associated with the future development of coronary heart disease, myocardial infarction, stroke and sudden cardiac death. These risk factors include central obesity, impaired fasting glucose or glucose tolerance or known type 2 diabetes, hypertriglyceridemia, low HDL cholesterol and hypertension. There are several definitions of the metabolic syndrome, of which two are in common use: the International Diabetes Federation (IDF) (Zimmet *et al.* 2005) and the National Cholesterol Education Programme-Adult Treatment Panel III (NCEP ATP III)

(Grundy *et al.* 2004) (Fig. 11.1). The main difference between the definitions is that, in the IDF, central obesity is an essential component, whereas it is not in the NCEP ATP III. A joint statement has been released in which these two definitions have been amalgamated (see caption, Fig. 11.1; Alberti *et al.* 2009).

The central biochemical defect which is common between metabolic syndrome and type 2 diabetes is insulin resistance. It is recognized that men with metabolic syndrome and impaired glucose tolerance are at high risk of developing type 2 diabetes. Insulin resistance is the intermediary factor which promotes the development of hyperglycemia, hypertriglyceridemia, low HDL cholesterol and hypertension. Factors which contribute to the insulin resistance are central obesity, lack of exercise, genetic abnormalities and, more recently identified, testosterone deficiency in men. Insulin resistance is also associated with endothelial dysfunction (microalbuminuria), inflammation, small dense lipoproteins and a pro-thrombotic milieu.

11.3.2   Testosterone and the metabolic syndrome

Several epidemiological studies have shown that either low total and/or free testosterone and SHBG are all independent predictors for the subsequent clinical development of the metabolic syndrome and for type 2 diabetes (Haffner *et al.* 1996; Stellato *et al.* 2000; Oh *et al.* 2002; Svartberg *et al.* 2004a; Laaksonen *et al.* 2004; Selvin *et al.* 2007; Haring *et al.* 2009). These include the Massachusetts Male Aging Study (MMAS), the Multiple Risk Factor Intervention Trial (MRFIT), Third National Health and Nutrition Examination Survey (NHANES III), the Rancho Bernardo, Tromso and SHIP studies. The Rancho Bernardo Study, during an eight-year follow-up period, found an inverse correlation between baseline testosterone and fasting glucose and insulin levels as well as glucose tolerance.

Importantly, two studies, the MMAS (15-year follow-up) and NHANES III, have found that the increased risk for metabolic syndrome and diabetes is also relevant for initially non-obese men (Kupelian *et al.* 2006; Selvin *et al.* 2007). The NHANES III study reported a four-fold increased risk for the prevalence of diabetes in the lowest tertile of testosterone at baseline, when the data were corrected for adiposity, age and race/ethnicity. Conversely, when controlled for obesity, the Quebec family study showed that men with higher total and bioavailable testosterone and SHBG had a

reduced risk of developing the metabolic syndrome (Blouin *et al.* 2005). These studies are important in that they exclude obesity as a cause for the low testosterone state; thus demonstrating that testosterone deficiency may be a precursor to the development of obesity.

Total testosterone has been reported to be 19%, free testosterone 11% and SHBG 18% lower in patients with metabolic syndrome compared to those without it (Laaksonen *et al.* 2005). The association between low testosterone and metabolic syndrome has also been reported in other studies (Muller *et al.* 2005; Maggio *et al.* 2006). Furthermore, the greater the number of components of the metabolic syndrome, the lower the testosterone level and the greater the risk of clinical hypogonadism (Corona *et al.* 2006).

Men with metabolic syndrome have a higher prevalence of ED (26.7%) when compared to healthy controls (13%) (Isidori *et al.* 2005a). The coexistence of testosterone deficiency with ED in men with metabolic syndrome leads to more severe forms of ED (Corona *et al.* 2006).

11.3.3   Testosterone and type 2 diabetes

Numerous studies have consistently found that men with type 2 diabetes have a high prevalence of low circulating testosterone levels. A meta-analysis of 21 studies up until 2005, which included data from 3825 subjects, found that total testosterone levels were, on average, 2.66 nmol/l lower in men with diabetes compared to healthy controls (Ding *et al.* 2009). Until more recently it was assumed that this was mainly related to lower levels of SHBG that occur in men with states of insulin resistance, which include obesity, metabolic syndrome and type 2 diabetes. Ding and colleagues in their meta-analysis found no significant decrease in SHBG, only a non-significant reduction of 5.07 nmol/l ($p = 0.15$) in diabetic men.

A landmark study, where the authors measured free testosterone by equilibrium dialysis in 103 men with diabetes (mean age 55 years), reported that one-third had levels below the normal range (Dhindsa *et al.* 2004). Another study, which assayed bioavailable testosterone by ammonium sulfate precipitation, found that 14% had levels below the normal range, with a further 36% in the lower 16% of the normal range (Kapoor *et al.* 2007a). The Third National Health and Nutrition Survey (NHANES III) reported that men in the lower tertile of free or bioavailable testosterone were approximately four times more likely to have diabetes than those in the upper tertile with data adjusted for age, obesity and ethnicity (Selvin *et al.* 2007).

Guidelines for the clinical diagnosis of hypogonadism state that the patient should have symptoms as well as biochemical evidence of testosterone deficiency. The first study to evaluate the prevalence of hypogonadism in a population of men with type 2 diabetes was published in 2007 (Kapoor *et al.* 2007a). This was a cross-sectional study of 355 men with type 2 diabetes who were >30 years of age, recruited mainly from the district retinopathy screening service as well as the hospital diabetic clinic. The prevalence of hypogonadal men with a total testosterone level <8 nmol/l was 17%, with a further 25% with total testosterone between 8 and 12 nmol/l. The prevalence of hypogonadal men with a free testosterone level < 255 pmol/l was 42%; bioavailable testosterone < 2.5 nmol/l (lower limit of normal) was 14%, and 29% had levels between 2.5 and 4 nmol/l.

The most common form of classical hypogonadism is Klinefelter syndrome. It has been shown that 75% of men with this condition are undiagnosed in the general population (Bojesen *et al.* 2003). Furthermore, men with Klinefelter syndrome had a higher risk of developing metabolic syndrome and type 2 diabetes than the normal population (Bojesen *et al.* 2006). In addition, men with XSBMA, also called Kennedy disease, a genetic polymorphism with excess CAG repeats in exon 1 of the AR leading to a condition associated with a relatively insensitive AR, which is associated with the development of diabetes, provide further evidence of a link between impaired androgen status and diabetes.

11.3.4 Androgen deprivation therapy for prostate carcinoma

The link between low testosterone and the increased risk of developing diabetes is supported by the effects of ADT for prostatic carcinoma. A large follow-up study of 73 196 men treated with ADT, when compared to men with prostate cancer under surveillance, reported an increased risk of incident diabetes, myocardial infarction and cardiovascular disease (Keating *et al.* 2006).

Fasting insulin levels rise and insulin sensitivity falls, with an elevation in HbA1c, after initiation of ADT (Smith *et al.* 2006; Haider *et al.* 2007). A small study of men with type 2 diabetes on insulin therapy, treated with ADT for advanced prostate cancer, showed marked deterioration in their diabetic control and required significant increases in their insulin doses to maintain glycemic control (Haider *et al.* 2007). This implies that there should be extra vigilance, for those men with diabetes, in the early phase after commencing ADT (Levine *et al.* 2010). Androgen deprivation therapy for prostate cancer produces a severe state of hypogonadism which increases central adiposity and percentage body fat, and decreases lean mass (Smith *et al.* 2001; 2002; 2006). The change in body fat is mainly subcutaneous and not visceral fat, which is atypical for the metabolic syndrome (Faris and Smith 2010). These findings all suggest a specific role for testosterone in carbohydrate as well as fat metabolism.

11.4 Interactions between the hypothalamic-pituitary-testicular axis and adipose tissue

It is known that, first, a low testosterone state promotes an increase in fat deposition and that, second, obesity impairs testosterone secretion. These two important effects can lead to a vicious cycle between obesity and hypogonadism. Several mechanisms are involved in this cycle, which mainly include the effects of aromatase and adipocytokines. First, the Hypogonadal-Obesity Cycle was proposed to explain the suppressive effect of obesity on testosterone (Cohen 1999). More recently this has been developed to include the effects of adipocytokines known as the Hypogonadal-Obesity-Adipocytokine Hypothesis (Jones 2007). (Fig. 11.2).

Aromatase activity which converts testosterone to estradiol is primarily found in adipocytes and in particular central fat deposits. The greater the degree of adiposity, the higher the aromatase activity. Aromatase inhibitors have been shown to increase testosterone production in obese men (Zumoff *et al.* 2003; Loves *et al.* 2008). The fact that clomifene, an antiestrogen which works at the hypothalamic level, also increases testosterone confirms the importance of the inhibitory action of estrogens on the hypothalamic-pituitary-testicular axis (Guay *et al.* 1995).

Adipose tissue is the largest endocrine organ, which produces several hormones including pro-inflammatory cytokines. Metabolic syndrome and type 2 diabetes are recognized as pro-inflammatory states. Increased circulating free fatty acids activate NF-κB (nuclear factor kappa-light-chain-enhancer of activated B cells) pathways which then promote

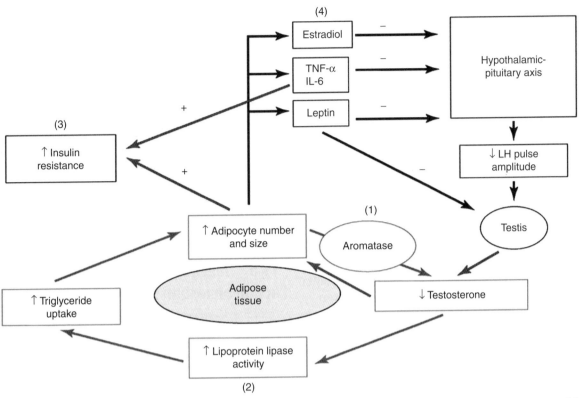

Fig. 11.2 The Hypogonadal-Obesity-Adipocytokine Hypothesis. (1) High aromatase activity in adipocytes converts testosterone to estradiol. Reduced tissue testosterone facilitates triglyceride storage in adipocytes by allowing (2) increased lipoprotein lipase activity and stimulating pluripotent stem cells to mature into adipocytes. (3) Increased adipocyte mass is associated with greater insulin resistance. (4) Estradiol and adipocytokines TNF-α, IL-6 and leptin (as a result of leptin resistance in human obesity) inhibit the hypothalamic-pituitary-testicular axis response to decreasing androgen levels (blue arrows). Orange arrow, hypogonadal obesity cycle; green arrow, low testosterone promotes the formation of adipocytes from pluripotent stem cells; +, positive effect; −, negative effect. See plate section for color version. (From Jones 2010).

cytokine release. Pro-inflammatory cytokines have a major pathological role in atherogenesis and plaque instability. The pro-inflammatory cytokines or adipocytokines involved are tumor necrosis factor α (TNF-α), interleukin 1 (IL-1), interleukin 6 (IL-6), IL-1β, plasminogen activator inhibitor 1 (PAI-1) and serum amyloid A. Tumor necrosis factor α, IL-1β and IL-6 are all known to suppress the hypothalamic-pituitary-testicular axis (Jones and Kennedy 1993). The hormone/cytokine leptin is exclusively synthesized and secreted by adipocytes. In human obesity, leptin inhibits the hypothalamic release of GnRH. Furthermore, leptin inhibits the action of hCG on the Leydig cell (Isidori et al. 1999). This explains why the commonest form of hypogonadism, hypogonadotropic hypogonadism with low or normal LH levels, is observed in men with central obesity. However, although weight loss can be associated with a rise in

testosterone, there is no reciprocal increase in LH levels (Strain et al. 1988; Zumoff et al. 2003). Men with insulin resistance and obesity have an impaired Leydig cell response to exogenous gonadotropins (Pitteloud et al. 2005a).

Kisspeptin is a peptide involved in the negative feedback of gonadal steroids on GnRH release from the hypothalamus (George et al. 2010). Kisspeptin is produced in the rat arcuate and anterior periventricular nuclei, and stimulates GnRH neurons via activation of the KISS1 receptor. Kisspeptin stimulates the release of LH, FSH and testosterone. There is evidence from animal studies that estrogens and also leptin resistance inhibit the neuronal release of kisspeptin. These combined actions impair the homeostatic response to upregulate testosterone production and in turn compensate for the increased breakdown of testosterone to estradiol by adipose tissue.

A persistent state of testosterone deficiency promotes an increase in the amount of fat. It has been shown that a low testosterone milieu results in favoring pluripotent stem cells to mature into adipocytes as opposed to myocytes (Singh *et al.* 2003). Evidence is also accruing that a low testosterone state facilitates the synthesis and storage of triglycerides in fat cells. Adipocytes are known to express ARs (Bjorntorp 1996). Testosterone has been shown to have a direct effect on cultured adipocytes and adipose tissue, which implies that it has effects on intracellular lipid metabolism and potentially also has effects on lipolysis and lipogenesis (Blouin *et al.* 2008). Testosterone may also increase lipolysis by increasing the number of β-adrenergic receptors (De Pergola 2000).

Lipoprotein lipase, which resides on the extracellular surface of adipocytes as well as being present in the circulation, breaks down circulating triglycerides to fat. Fatty acids are then taken up into the adipocyte and then converted back into triglycerides for storage. Testosterone inhibits lipoprotein lipase activity; therefore, when testosterone is reduced this promotes triglyceride storage. The increased rate of fat deposition also stimulates the transformation of immature pre-adipocytes into mature cells.

11.5   Role of the androgen receptor polymorphism

It has been demonstrated that the CAG repeat polymorphism in exon 1 of the androgen receptor influences the actions of testosterone in healthy men and those with Klinefelter syndrome (Zitzmann 2009). There is recent evidence that this polymorphism modulates the effect of testosterone in men with type 2 diabetes (Stanworth *et al.* 2008; 2011). Although men with type 2 diabetes had a distribution of CAG repeats similar to that found in a healthy population, testosterone and LH levels were found to be significantly increased in men with a more insensitive AR. Importantly, less sensitive ARs are associated with higher waist circumference, BMI, serum leptin and systolic blood pressure.

High-density lipoprotein cholesterol was found to be positively associated with increasing AR sensitivity. The difficulty in evaluating this as a close association is subject to a potential paradox. It is known that an atherogenic lipid profile is associated with low testosterone and estradiol. In healthy and diabetic men,

HDL-C is independently correlated positively with testosterone and estradiol (Van Pottelbergh *et al.* 2003; Stanworth *et al.* 2011). Animal work has shown that testosterone replacement in the testicular feminized mouse, which has an inactive AR, leads to an increase in HDL-C (Nettleship *et al.* 2007). This raises the hypothesis that HDL-C levels are related to estradiol and may be independent of the AR.

Androgen receptor sensitivity may be more important clinically in the presence of co-morbidities. As described, testosterone levels are lower in a diabetic population, so a fall in testosterone in an individual with an insensitive receptor could give rise to symptoms of hypogonadism, occurring with testosterone levels in the lower or even mid-normal range.

11.6   Mechanisms of testosterone action on insulin sensitivity/resistance

Insulin resistance is recognized as the central biochemical defect in men with metabolic syndrome and/or type 2 diabetes. The presence of insulin resistance in type 2 diabetes is also known to be a major cardiovascular risk factor, equivalent in degree to smoking (Bonora *et al.* 2002). In clinical practice the major cause of insulin resistance is central obesity; however, lack of exercise and genetic factors are also involved. The volume of central fat is directly proportional to the degree of insulin resistance; whereas there is no relationship with subcutaneous fat.

Population studies of healthy men have demonstrated an inverse relationship between insulin and testosterone levels (Simon *et al.* 1992; Tibblin *et al.* 1996). Androgen deprivation therapy for the treatment of prostate carcinoma results in an increase in fasting insulin levels within three months with GnRH therapy (Smith *et al.* 2001; Dockery *et al.* 2003) and orchidectomy (Xu *et al.* 2002). The Rancho Bernardo Study found a significant inverse relationship of low baseline testosterone with follow-up fasting and postchallenge glucose and insulin levels and HOMA-IR (Homeostatic Model Assessment of Insulin Resistance) eight years later (Oh *et al.* 2002).

Sex hormone-binding globulin levels are independently inversely correlated with insulin resistance (Birkeland *et al.* 1993). This led to the presumption that it was the mechanism by which testosterone levels were low in insulin-resistant states. Several studies have shown that the bioavailable and free-testosterone fractions, which are independent of

SHBG, correlate with insulin sensitivity (Andersson *et al.* 1994; Endre *et al.* 1996; Simon *et al.* 1997). It is important therefore to recognize that testosterone and SHBG are independently associated with insulin sensitivity (Kapoor *et al.* 2005, for review). Statin therapy decreases SHBG and total testosterone but has no effect on free or bioavailable levels (Stanworth *et al.* 2009). These findings underline the need to assess free or bioavailable testosterone status clinically, especially in borderline cases.

The mechanisms by which testosterone promotes insulin sensitivity are not fully elucidated. The three tissues which account for the majority of the body's insulin sensitivity are muscle, liver and fat (mainly central fat depots). Low testosterone states are associated with increased adiposity, which in turn leads to decreased insulin sensitivity. Changes in the sex steroid environment induced in healthy men by the aromatase inhibitor letrozole, with or without estradiol patches, demonstrated that testosterone increased insulin sensitivity and postprandial glucagon-like peptide 1 (GLP-1) and decreased the postprandial rise in triglycerides (Lapauw *et al.* 2010). Interleukin 6 and TNF-α are known to promote insulin resistance. Acute withdrawal of testosterone from men with hypogonadism led to a relatively rapid reduction in insulin sensitivity over a two-week period (Yialamas *et al.* 2007). This finding implies that other mechanisms apart from body fat are involved.

In human type 2 diabetes, evidence shows that insulin resistance is associated with a reduction in insulin-stimulated muscle glycogen synthesis, which occurs as a result of a defect in insulin-stimulated transport activity. Studies have found that this can be ascribed to increases in lipid metabolites, which include fatty acyl CoA and diacylglycerol, which lead to stimulation of a serine/threonine kinase cascade, which in turn produces defects in insulin signaling through serine/threonine phosphorylation of the insulin receptor substrate 1 (IRS-1) in muscle (Sato *et al.* 2008). In liver a similar mechanism occurs, where increased diacylglycerol activates protein kinase C, which results in reduced insulin-stimulated tyrosine phosphorylation of IRS-2. There are few published papers which have investigated potential mechanisms by which testosterone increases insulin sensitivity.

Glut-4 is the major glucose transporter in muscle and fat but is not present in liver. Testosterone and DHEA in muscle (the latter probably by local conversion to testosterone by 5α-reductase in rats) increased Glut-4 protein expression and translocation to the membrane (Sato *et al.* 2008). This study also found that testosterone increased phosphorylation of Akt and protein kinase C – both key steps in the regulation of Glut-4 signaling pathways. These effects were blocked by a DHT inhibitor, suggesting that local conversion of testosterone to DHT was essential for this effect to occur. In addition, they reported that testosterone increased activity of phosphofructokinase and hexokinase, key enzymes involved in glycolysis. Testosterone has also been shown to stimulate PI-3 kinase in osteoblasts, which increases Akt phosphorylation (Kang *et al.* 2004).

Mitochondrial dysfunction is also associated with insulin resistance. A study of 60 men using the hyperinsulinemic-euglycemic clamp compared insulin resistance with testosterone status (Pitteloud *et al.* 2005b). Testosterone levels correlated positively with insulin sensitivity, aerobic capacity (VO$_2$max) and expression of genes involved in mitochondrial oxidative phosphorylation from skeletal muscle biopsies. The largest difference in mitochondrial gene expression was found with ubiquinol cytochrome c reductase binding protein (UQCRB), showing a 20% reduction in tissue from men with type 2 diabetes and impaired glucose tolerance.

11.7 Effect of testosterone replacement on insulin sensitivity

11.7.1 Obesity

Marin and colleagues were the first to discover that testosterone administration lowered plasma insulin and glucose disposal over three months (Marin *et al.* 1992a). However, a supraphysiological dose of testosterone resulted in a reduction in glucose tolerance. The beneficial effects on insulin sensitivity were more pronounced in the men with lower testosterone levels. A decrease in waist/hip ratio was observed, but no effect on body mass. Muscle strength, the fractional velocity of glycogen synthase and the diameter of type IIB fibers increased. Another study followed 23 middle-aged abdominally obese men for eight months (Marin *et al.* 1992b). Testosterone therapy improved insulin resistance as demonstrated by using the euglycemic-hyperinsulinemic clamp. A fall in blood glucose, diastolic blood pressure and cholesterol was also detected.

11.7.2 Metabolic syndrome and/or type 2 diabetes

Kapoor and co-workers published the first study of TRT in hypogonadal men with type 2 diabetes in 2006 (Kapoor *et al.* 2006). This was a randomized, double-blind, placebo-controlled, crossover trial with subjects assigned to either 200 mg im mixed testosterone esters (24 mg testosterone propionate, 48 mg testosterone phenylpropionate, 48 mg testosterone isocaproate, 80 mg testosterone undecanoate – Sustanon®) every fortnight, or placebo every two weeks for three months, with a one-month washout phase before crossing over for the final three months. This study found that insulin resistance as assessed by HOMA-IR improved significantly with testosterone substitution.

A larger multicenter European study (the TIMES2 study) has confirmed that testosterone improved insulin resistance as assessed by HOMA-IR by 15% after 6 months and was maintained after 12 months in the total population (Jones *et al.* 2011) (Fig. 11.3). This study recruited 220 men with either metabolic syndrome and/or type 2 diabetes aged $\geq$ 40 years, with symptoms of hypogonadism and either a morning total testosterone <11 nmol/l and/or a free testosterone <255 pmol/l. Subjects received either 60 mg 2% testosterone gel or placebo. The testosterone dose was titrated to give a testosterone level >17 nmol/l (dose range 20–80 mg/day) with dummy dose adjustments in the placebo group. Changes in diabetes, lipid lowering, anti-obesity and hypertensive drugs were prohibited in the first 6 months unless crucial for clinical care. Between 6 and 12 months drug alterations were allowed for ethical reasons.

In the group of men with type 2 diabetes ($n = 130$), testosterone therapy significantly reduced insulin resistance by 15%, whereas a similar reduction was observed in those men with metabolic syndrome ($n = 162$), who showed a similar fall in insulin resistance but approached significance, $p = 0.0690$, after 6 months and with $p = 0.054$ after 12 months. It is important to recognize the high proportion of men with diabetes who were already treated with metformin. Metformin is known to improve insulin sensitivity by approximately 15%, so that the additional benefit of testosterone would be in addition to the effects of this drug.

The Moscow study examined the effect of depot im testosterone undecanoate on insulin resistance over 30 weeks in a randomized, double-blind, placebo-controlled trial in 184 men with metabolic syndrome and hypogonadism (Kalinchenko *et al.* 2010). Testosterone undecanoate 1000 mg was administered at 6 and 18 weeks by slow im injection. Although this study included approximately one-third of subjects with type 2 diabetes, results given were cumulated from the total study population. The study did find that HOMA-IR decreased ($p = 0.04$).

11.8 Effect of testosterone on components of the metabolic syndrome and type 2 diabetes

11.8.1 Central adiposity and body composition

Testosterone substitution in men with hypogonadism is well known to improve body composition, with a decrease in fat and an increase in lean mass (Wang *et al.* 2000). Testosterone replacement in metabolic syndrome and/or type 2 diabetes has been shown to reduce central adiposity in all but one trial, BMI in one (which involved an exercise component) and body fat content in another study (Kapoor *et al.* 2006; Heufelder *et al.* 2009; Kalinchenko *et al.* 2010; Jones *et al.* 2011). Testosterone decreases serum leptin, which reflects body fat content (Kapoor *et al.* 2007b).

11.8.2 Hyperglycemia

Hemoglobin A1c is the principal and gold standard test to assess glycemic control in people with type 2 diabetes. The UKPDS (United Kingdom Prospective Diabetes Study) in type 2 diabetes showed that a reduction in HbA1c had major benefits in reducing the risk of both the microvascular (retinopathy, nephropathy, neuropathy) and macrovascular (myocardial infarction, stroke, peripheral vascular disease and sudden death) complications of type 2 diabetes (Straton *et al.* 2000). Any intervention in lifestyle, pharmacological or other method, that lowers HbA1c would therefore have an important effect on outcomes in relation to these complications.

Two clinical trials have shown that testosterone replacement in diabetic men lowers HbA1c. The first was the study of Kapoor and co-workers which reported a fall of HbA1c of −0.37% over three months, with a fall in fasting blood glucose of −1.6 nmol/l (Kapoor *et al.* 2006). No other study has shown

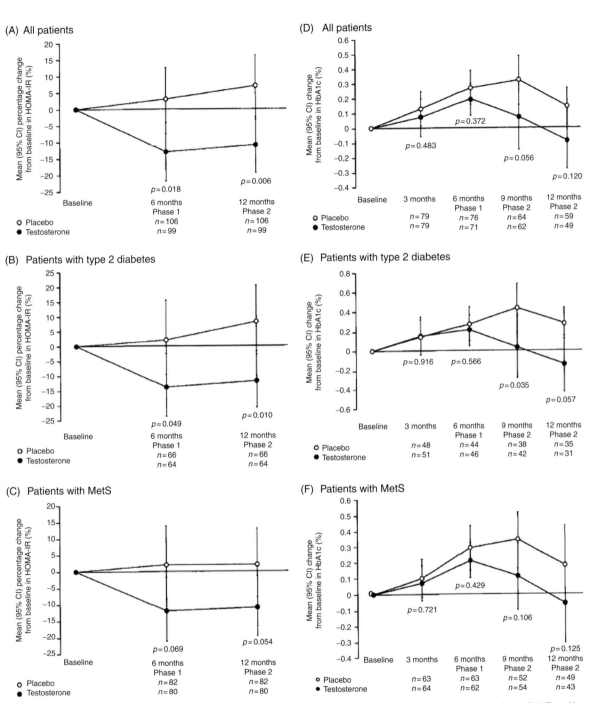

Fig. 11.3 Effect of TRT on insulin resistance (assessed by HOMA-IR) and HbA1c in hypogonadal men with metabolic syndrome (MetS) and/or type 2 diabetes. Mean (95% CI) percentage change from baseline in HOMA-IR (intention-to-treat population, last observation carried forward) and change from baseline HbA1c (intention-to-treat population, study completers) among all patients (A and D) and patients with type 2 diabetes (B and F), and with metabolic syndrome (C and F). The p-values are reported for comparisons between treatment and placebo groups. (From Jones et al. 2011).

a significant fall in fasting blood glucose, which may be due to the confounding issue of concomitant therapies in diabetic management. A second study compared diet and exercise with diet, exercise and testosterone substitution, which was non-placebo-controlled, in newly diagnosed drug-naïve men with type 2 diabetes. After 12 months, those men treated with testosterone had an HbA1c reduction of 1.3% compared to 0.5% for those treated with diet and exercise alone: a comparative benefit of 0.8% with testosterone (Heufelder *et al.* 2009).

The TIMES2 study reported a significant reduction in HbA1c (−0.45%) compared to placebo after nine months' treatment. This, however, was observed in phase 2 of the study where, for ethical reasons, primary care physicians were allowed, where clinically indicated, to alter hypoglycemic drugs. The fact that changes occurred in both treatment and placebo groups and were statistically significant does suggest a potential therapeutic effect, but this cannot be categorically stated. It is important however to recognize that the primary inclusion criterion for this study was hypogonadism, and subjects were not selected for poor diabetic control.

11.8.3   Dyslipidemia

The majority of cross-sectional studies have found that low testosterone is associated with an atherogenic lipid profile, with high total and LDL cholesterol and triglycerides and low HDL-C, although some studies disagree (Isidori *et al.* 2005b). The relationship between testosterone and HDL-C is complex and has not yet been fully elucidated. High-density lipoprotein cholesterol protects against atherosclerotic plaque progression, and levels are generally lower in men. The major function of HDL-C is the reverse transport of cholesterol from the periphery to the liver for excretion. In healthy and diabetic men testosterone positively correlates with HDL-C and its major constituent, apolipoprotein A1 (Van Pottelbergh *et al.* 2003; Stanworth *et al.* 2011). There is evidence from animal studies that supports a hypothesis that testosterone conversion to 17β-estradiol stimulates ERα-mediated production of HDL-C (Nettleship *et al.* 2007).

The majority of studies have either shown no effect or a small decrease in HDL-C with testosterone therapy. However, trials with testosterone undecanoate depot report an increase in HDL-C.

Longer-term studies have shown that, after an initial fall in HDL-C, levels return to baseline with time (Jones *et al.* 2011). The reasons for the differences between studies are unclear; however, it has been postulated that testosterone stimulation of reverse cholesterol transport may lead to increased consumption of HDL-C.

Although in many studies testosterone levels correlate inversely with triglycerides, trials of testosterone replacement have generally not shown a significant reduction in blood levels. The Heufelder study described above, in newly diagnosed drug-naïve hypogonadal men with diabetes treated over 12 months, reported lowering in triglycerides (Heufelder *et al.* 2009). No effect has been observed in other studies involving diabetes or metabolic syndrome.

11.8.4   Hypertension

Hypotestosteronemia is associated with hypertension, controlled or not (Khaw and Barrett-Connor 1988), but this could be related to a higher incidence of obesity in men with this condition (Svartberg *et al.* 2004b). Furthermore, an inverse relationship exists between testosterone and diastolic blood pressure (Bocchi *et al.* 2008; Jones and Saad 2009). Some studies have found that testosterone reduces diastolic and, less frequently, systolic blood pressure (Marin *et al.* 1993; Kalinchenko *et al.* 2010; Jones 2010). Testosterone and anabolic steroid, respectively, is known to increase blood pressure in animal studies and humans (Jones 2010). Hence blood pressure should be monitored in TRT.

11.8.5   Inflammation

Low testosterone is associated with increased circulating IL-6 and C-reactive protein (CRP) in type 2 diabetes (Kapoor *et al.* 2007b). Testosterone replacement failed to suppress IL-1β, IL-6 and TNF-α, but reduced adiponectin and leptin in this study. Testosterone has been shown to decrease TNF-α and increase IL-10 in men with coronary heart disease (Malkin *et al.* 2004). In the Moscow study, testosterone substitution reduced TNF-α, IL-1β and CRP, whereas a fall in IL-6 approached significance, but treatment had no effect on IL-10, an anti-atherogenic cytokine (Kalinchenko *et al.* 2010). Testosterone replacement has been shown to inhibit TNF-α, IL-1β and IL-6 from cultured peripheral blood monocytes in vitro, from androgen-deficient men with type 2 diabetes (Corrales *et al.* 2006).

11.9 Cholesterol and lipoproteins

Although cholesterol is not included in the definition of metabolic syndrome, this substance plays an important role in atherogenesis in men with these conditions. Total and LDL cholesterol are both independently and negatively correlated with testosterone (Isidori *et al.* 2005b). Meta-analyses of clinical trials have shown that testosterone replacement reduces total and LDL cholesterol. Intervention studies have found that testosterone replacement significantly lowers cholesterol and LDL cholesterol between 0.25 and 0.5 mmol/l even in men already treated with statins (Jones and Saad 2009).

Lipoprotein (a) (Lpa) is the strongest independent risk factor for cardiovascular disease. The function of Lpa is unknown. Recently the European Atherosclerosis Society has advised that Lpa, which is mainly genetically determined, be measured in men who have moderate or high cardiovascular risk. Testosterone substitution decreases Lpa in hypogonadal men with and without diabetes (Zmuda *et al.* 1996; Jones *et al.* 2011). There is currently no evidence that reducing Lpa has any effect on overall cardiovascular risk.

11.10 Erectile dysfunction

Erectile dysfunction is common in men with metabolic syndrome (26%) and in type 2 diabetes (up to 70%) (Wang *et al.* 2011). Erectile dysfunction is multifactorial in diabetic men, with vasculopathy, autonomic neuropathy, hypogonadism and psychological factors being involved. Erectile dysfunction may be the first clinical sign of cardiovascular disease and the herald of future cardiovascular events including myocardial infarction. Early diagnosis provides a "window of opportunity," to improve lifestyle issues and medication, to reduce cardiovascular risk and ultimately events and death.

The severity of ED is greater the lower the testosterone level in type 2 diabetes (Kapoor *et al.* 2007c). Low testosterone is associated with a failure to respond to sildenafil, and replacement can convert non-responders to responders. Testosterone substitution improves libido and the International Index of Erectile Function score in hypogonadal men with metabolic syndrome and/or type 2 diabetes (Jones *et al.* 2011).

11.11 Clinical implications

International clinical guidelines now recommend that "serum testosterone should be measured in men with type 2 diabetes mellitus with symptoms suggestive of testosterone deficiency" (Wang *et al.* 2008). The clinical diagnosis does need careful and rigorous assessment before a decision to treat can be made. There is now evidence that testosterone replacement can improve sexual health and the response to phosphodiesterase-5 inhibitors. Evidence is accumulating to support a beneficial action of testosterone on insulin sensitivity and cardiovascular risk factors (Wang *et al.* 2011). Larger randomized, placebo-controlled trials are still required to verify these benefits and to determine whether these effects persist over a longer period of time.

11.12 Key messages

- There is a high prevalence of hypogonadism in men with metabolic syndrome and type 2 diabetes.
- Low testosterone and SHBG in healthy men are independent risk factors for the future onset of metabolic syndrome and type 2 diabetes.
- The interrelationships between adipose tissue and the hypothalamic-pituitary axis suppress the homeostatic mechanism, leading to impaired testosterone production and eventually to a state of hypogonadotropic hypogonadism.
- Insulin resistance is the central biochemical defect in metabolic syndrome and type 2 diabetes, which adversely affects cardiovascular risk factors, resulting in the increased number of cardiovascular events and mortality in these conditions.
- Testosterone has a key role in promoting insulin sensitivity via actions on carbohydrate and fat metabolism as well as insulin signaling pathways.
- Short-term studies up to one year in duration have shown that TRT improves insulin resistance, but not all have had consistent benefits to other components of the metabolic syndrome.
- Erectile dysfunction may be the first symptom of vascular disease, and men should be treated to reduce cardiovascular risk. There is a high prevalence of testosterone deficiency in men with ED.

- Testosterone replacement in hypogonadal men with metabolic syndrome and/or type 2 diabetes improves sexual health.

- The clinical diagnosis of hypogonadism requires careful assessment of symptoms, and biochemical testosterone deficiency.

11.13 References

Alberti KGMM, Eckel RH, Grundy SM, Zimmet PZ, Cleeman JI, Donato KA, Fruchart J-C, James WPT, Loria CM, Smith SC (2009) Harmonizing the metabolic syndrome. *Circulation* **120**:1640–1645

Allan CA, McLachlan RI (2010) Androgens and obesity. *Curr Opin Endocrinol Diabetes Obes* **17**:224–232

Andersson B, Marin P, Lissner L, Vermeulen A, Bjorntorp P (1994) Testosterone concentrations in women and men with NIDDM. *Diabetes Care* **17**:405–411

Birkeland KI, Hanssen KF, Torjesen PA, Vaaler S (1993) Level of sex hormone binding globulin is positively correlated with insulin sensitivity in men with type 2 diabetes. *J Clin End Metab* **76**:275–278

Bjorntorp P (1996) The regulation of adipose tissue distribution in humans. *Int J Obes Relat Metab Disord* **20**:291–302

Blouin, K, Despres JP, Couillard C, Tremblay A, Prud'homme D, Bouchard C, Tchernuf A (2005) Contribution of age and declining androgen levels to features of the metabolic syndrome in men. *Metabolism* **54**:1034–1040

Blouin K, Boivin A, Tchernof A (2008) Androgens and body fat distribution. *J Steroid Biochem Mol Biol* **108**:272–280

Bocchi EA, Carvalho VO, Guimaraes GV (2008) Inverse correlation between testosterone and ventricle ejection fraction, hemodynamics and exercise capacity in heart failure patients with erectile dysfunction. *Int Braz J Urol* **34**:302–310

Bojesen A, Juul S, Gravholt CH (2003) Prenatal and postnatal prevalence of Klinefelter's syndrome: a national registry study. *J Clin Endocrinol Metab* **88**:622–628

Bojesen A, Kristensen K, Birkeback NH (2006) The metabolic syndrome is frequent in men with Klinefelter's Syndrome. *Diabetes Care* **29**:1591–1598

Bonora E, Formentini G, Calcaterra F, Lombardi S, Marini F, Zenari L, Saggiani F, Poli M, Perbellini S, Raffaelli A, Cacciatori V, Santi L, Targher G, Bonadonna R, Muggeo M (2002) HOMA-estimated insulin resistance is an independent predictor of cardiovascular disease in type 2 diabetic subjects: prospective data from the Verona Diabetes Complications Study. *Diabetes Care* **25**:1135–1141

Cohen P (1999) The hypogonadal-obesity-cycle. *Med Hypothesis* **52**:49–51

Corona G, Mannucci E, Schulman C, Petrone L, Mansani R, Cilotti A, Balercia G, Chiarini V, Forti G, Maggi M (2006) Psychobiologic correlates of the metabolic syndrome and associated sexual dysfunction. *Eur Urol* **50**:595–604

Corrales JJ, Almeida M, Burgo R, Mories MT, Miralles JM, Orfao A (2006) Androgen replacement therapy depresses the ex-vivo production on inflammatory cytokines by circulating antigen-presenting cells in aging type 2 diabetic men with partial androgen deficiency. *J Endocrinol* **189**:595–604

Couillard C, Gagnon J, Bergeron J, Leon AS, Rao DC, Skinner JS, Wilmore JH, Després JP, Bouchard C (2000) Contribution of body fatness and adipose tissue distribution to the age variation in plasma steroid hormone concemtrations in men: the HERITAGE Family Study. *J Clin Endocrinol Metab* **85**:1026–1031

De Pergola G (2000) The adipose tissue metabolism: role of testosterone and dehydroepiandrosterone. *Int J Obes Relat Metab Disord* **24** (Suppl 2): S59–S63

Dhindsa S, Prabhakar S, Sethi M, Bandyo Padhyay A, Chaudhuri A, Dandona P (2004) Frequent occurrence of hypogonadotrophic hypogonadism in type 2 diabetes. *J Clin Endocrinol Metab* **89**:5462–5468

Ding EL, Song Y, Manson JE, Hunter DJ, Lee CC, Rifai N, Buring JE, Gaziano JM, Liu S (2009) Sex hormone-binding globulin and risk of type 2 diabetes in women and men. *N Engl J Med* **361**: 1152–1163

Dockery F, Bulpitt CJ, Agarwal S, Donaldson M, Rajkumar C (2003) Testosterone suppression in men with prostate cancer leads to an increase in arterial stiffness and hyperinsulinaemia. *Clin Sci* **104**:195–201

Endre T, Mattiasson I, Berglund G, Hulthen UL (1996) Low testosterone and insulin resistance in hypertension prone men. *J Hum Hypertens* **10**:755–761

Faris JE, Smith MR (2010) Metabolic sequelae associated with androgen deprivation therapy for prostate cancer. *Curr Opin Endocrinol Diabetes Obes* **17**:240–246

George JT, Miller RP, Anderson RA (2010) Hypothesis: kisspeptin mediates male hypogonadism in obesity and type 2 diabetes. *Neuroendocrinology* **91**: 302–307

Grundy SM, Brewer HB Jr, Cleeman JI, Smith SC Jr, Lenfant C (2004) Definition of metabolic syndrome: report of the National Heart, Lung, and Blood Institute/American Heart Association conference on scientific issues related to definition. *Circulation* **109**:433–438

Guay AM, Bansal S, Heatley GJ (1995) Effect of raising endogenous testosterone levels in impotent men with secondary hypogonadism: double blind placebo-controlled trial with clomiphene citrate. *J Clin Endocrinol Metab* **80**:3546–3552

Haffner SM, Valdez RA, Stern MP, Katz MS (1993) Obesity, body fat distribution and sex hormones in men. *Int J Obes Relat Metab Disord* **17**:643–649

Haffner SM, Shaten J, Stern MP, Smith GD, Kuller L (1996) Low levels of sex hormone binding globulin and testosterone predict the development of non insulin dependent diabetes mellitus in men. *Am J Epidemiol* **143**:889–897

Haider A, Yassin A, Saad F, Shabsigh R (2007) Effect of androgen deprivation on glycaemic control and on cardiovascular risk factors in men with advanced prostate cancer with diabetes. *Aging Male* **10**:189–196

Haring R, Volzke H, Felix SB, Schipf S, Dorr M, Rosskopf D, Nauck M, Schofl C, Wallaschofski H (2009) Prediction of metabolic syndrome by low serum testosterone levels in men. Results from the study of health in Pomerania. *Diabetes Care* **58**:2027–2031

Heufelder AE, Saad F, Bunck MC, Gooren L (2009) Fifty-two-week treatment with diet and exercise plus transdermal testosterone reverses the metabolic syndrome and improves glycemic control in men with newly diagnosed type 2 diabetes and subnormal plasma testosterone. *J Androl* **30**:726–733

Isidori AM, Caprio M, Stroll F, Moretti C, Frajese G, Isidori A, Fabbri A (1999) Leptin and androgens in male obesity: evidence for leptin contribution to reduced androgen levels *J Clin Endocrinol Metab* **84**:3673–3680

Isidori AM, Giannetta E, Gianfrilli D, Greco EA, Bonifacio V, Aversa A, Isidori A, Fabbri A, Lenzi A (2005a) Effects of testosterone on sexual function in men: results of a meta-analysis. *Clin Endocrinol (Oxf)* **63**:381–394

Isidori AM, Gianetta E, Greco EA, Gianfrilli D, Bonifacio V, Isidori A, Lenzi A, Fabbri A (2005b) Effects of testosterone on body composition, bone metabolism and serum lipid profile in middle-aged men: a meta-analysis. *Clin Endocrinol (Oxf)* **63**:280–293

Jones TH (2007) Testosterone associations with erectile dysfunction, diabetes and the metabolic syndrome. *Eur Urol Suppl* **6**:847–857

Jones TH (2010) Testosterone deficiency: a risk factor for cardiovascular disease? *Trends Endocrinol Metab* **21**:496–503

Jones TH, Kennedy RL (1993) Cytokines and hypothalamic-pituitary function. *Cytokine* **5**:531–538

Jones TH, Saad F (2009) The effects of testosterone on risk factors for, and the mediators of, the atherosclerotic process. *Atherosclerosis* **207**:318–327

Jones TH, Arver S, Behre HM, Buvat J, Meuleman E, Moncada I, Morales AM, Volterrani M, Yellowlees A, Howell JD, Channer KS (2011) Testosterone replacement in hypogonadal men with type 2 diabetes and/or metabolic syndrome (The TIMES2 Study). *Diabetes Care* **34**:828–837

Kalinchenko SY, Tishova YA, Mskhalaya GJ, Gooren LJ, Giltay EJ, Saad F (2010) Effects of testosterone supplementation on markers of the metabolic syndrome and inflammation in hypogonadal men with the metabolic syndrome: the double-blinded placebo-controlled Moscow study. *Clin Endocrinol (Oxf)* **73**:602–612

Kang HY, Cho CL, Huang KL, Wang JC, Hu YC, Lin HK, Chang C, Huang KE (2004) Nongenomic androgen activation of phosphatidylinositol3-kinase/Akt signalling pathway in MC3T3-E1 osteoblasts. *J Bone Miner Res* **19**:1181–1190

Kapoor D, Malkin CJ, Channer KS, Jones TH (2005) Androgens, insulin resistance and vascular disease in men. *Clin Endocrinol (Oxf)* **63**:239–250

Kapoor D, Goodwin E, Channer KS, Jones TH (2006) Testosterone replacement therapy improves insulin resistance, glycaemic control, visceral adiposity and hypercholesterolaemia in hypogonadal men with type 2 diabetes. *Eur J Endocrinol* **154**:899–906

Kapoor D, Aldred H, Clark S, Channer KS, Jones TH (2007a) Clinical and biochemical assessment of hypogonadism in men with type 2 diabetes: correlations with bioavailable testosterone and visceral adiposity. *Diabetes Care* **30**:911–917

Kapoor D, Clarke S, Channer KS, Jones TH (2007b) The effect of testosterone replacement therapy on adipocytokines and C-reactive protein in hypogonadal men with type 2 diabetes. *Eur J Endocrinol* **156**:595–602

Kapoor D, Clarke S, Channer KS, Jones TH (2007c) Erectile dysfunction is associated with low bioactive testosterone levels and visceral adiposity in men with type 2 diabetes. *Int J Androl* **30**:500–507

Keating NL, O'Malley AJ, Freedland SJ, Smith MR (2006) Diabetes and cardiovascular disease during androgen deprivation therapy: observational study of veterans with prostate cancer. *J Natl Cancer Inst* **102**:39–46

Khaw KT, Barrett-Connor E (1988) Blood pressure and endogenous testosterone in men: an inverse relationship. *J Hypertens* **6**:329–332

Khaw KT, Barrett-Connor E (1992) Lower endogenous androgens predict central adiposity in men. *Am Epidemiol* **2**:675–682

Kupelian V, Page ST, Araujo AB, Travison TG, Bremner WJ, McKinlay JB (2006) Low sex hormone-binding globulin, total testosterone, and symptomatic androgen deficiency are associated with development of the metabolic syndrome in non-obese men. *J Clin Endocrinol Metab* **91**:843–850

Laaksonen DE, Niskanen L, Punnonen K, Nyyssonen K, Tuomainen TP, Valkonen VP, Salonen R, Salonen JT (2004) Testosterone and sex hormone-binding globulin predict the metabolic syndrome and diabetes in middle-aged men. *Diabetes Care* **27**: 1036–1041

Laaksonen DE, Niskanen L, Punnonen K, Nyyssonen K, Tuomainen TP, Valkonen VP, Salonen JT (2005) The metabolic syndrome and smoking in relation to hypogonadism in middle-aged men: a prospective cohort study. *J Clin Endocrinol Metab* **90**:712–719

Lapauw B, Ouwens M, Hart LM, Wuyts B, Holst JJ, T'Sjoen G, Kaufman JM, Ruige JB (2010) Sex steroids affect triglyceride handling, glucose-dependent insulinotropic polypeptide, and insulin sensitivity: a 1-week randomized clinical trial in healthy young men. *Diabetes Care* **33**:1831–1833

Levine GN, D'Amico AV, Berger P, Clark PE, Eckel RH, Keating NL, Milani RV, Sagalowsky AI, Smith MR, Zakai N (2010) Androgen-deprivation therapy in prostate cancer and cardiovascular risk: a science advisory from the American Heart Association, American Cancer Society and American Urological Association: endorsed by the American Society for Radiation Oncology. *Circulation* **121**:833–840

Loves S, Ruinemans-Koerts J, de Boer H (2008) Letrozole once a week normalizes serum testosterone in obesity-related male hypogonadism. *Eur J Endocrinol* **158**:741–747

MacDonald AA, Herbison GP, Showell M, Farquhar CM (2010) The impact of body mass index on semen parameters and reproductive hormones in human males: a systematic review with meta-analysis. *Hum Reprod Update* **16**:293–311

Maggio M, Lauretani F, Ceda GP, Bandinelli S, Basaria S, Ble A, Egan J, Paolisso G, Najjar S, Jeffrey Metter E, Valenti G, Guralnik JM, Ferrucci L (2006) Association between hormones and metabolic syndrome in older Italian men. *J Am Geriatr Soc* **54**:1832–1838

Malkin CJ, Pugh PJ, Jones RD, Kapoor D, Channer KS, Jones TH (2004) The effect of testosterone replacement on endogenous inflammatory cytokines and lipid profiles in hypogonadal men. *J Clin Endocrinol Metab* **89**:3313–3318

Marin P, Krotkiewski M, Bjorntorp P (1992a) Androgen treatment of middle-aged, obese men: effects on metabolism, muscle and adipose tissues. *Eur J Med* **1**:329–336

Marin P, Holmang S, Jonsson L, Sjostrom L, Kvist H, Holm G, Lindstedt G, Bjorntorp P (1992b) The effects of testosterone treatment on body composition and metabolism in middle-aged obese men. *Int J Obes Relat Metab Disord* **16**:991–997

Marin P, Holmang S, Gustafsson C, Jonsson L, Kvist H, Elander A, Eldh J, Sjostrom L, Holm G, Bjorntorp P (1993) Androgen treatment of abdominally obese men. *Obes Res* **1**:245–251

Muller M, Grobbee DE, den Tonkelaar I, Lamberts SW, van der Schouw YT (2005) Endogenous sex hormones and metabolic syndrome in aging men. *Clin Endocrinol Metab.* **90**:2618–2623

Nettleship JE, Jones TH, Channer KS, Jones RD (2007) Physiological testosterone replacement therapy attenuates fatty streak formation and improves high-density lipoprotein cholesterol in the Tfm mouse: an effect independent of the classic androgen receptor. *Circulation* **116**:2427–2434

Oh JY, Barrett-Connor E, Wedick NM, Wingard DL (2002) Endogenous sex hormones and the development of type 2 diabetes in older men and women. *Diabetes Care* **25**:55–60

Pasquali R, Casimirri F, Cantobelli S, Melchionda N, Morselli Labate AM, Fabbri R, Capelli M, Bortoluzzi L (1991) Effect of obesity and body fat distribution on sex hormones and insulin in men. *Metabolism* **40**:101–104

Pitteloud N, Hardin M, Dwyer AA, Valassi E, Yialamas M, Elahi D, Hayes FJ (2005a) Increasing insulin resistance is associated with a decrease in Leydig cell testosterone secretion in men. *J Clin Endocrinol Metab* **90**:2636–2641

Pitteloud N, Mootha VK, Dwyer AA, Hardin M, Lee H, Eriksson KF, Tripathy D, Yialamas M, Groop L, Elahi D, Hayes FJ (2005b) Relationship between testosterone levels, insulin sensitivity, and mitochondrial function in men. *Diabetes Care* **28**:1636–1642

Sato K, Iemitsu M, Aizawa K, Ajisaka R (2008) Testosterone and DHEA activate the glucose metabolism-related signalling pathway in skeletal muscle. *Am J Physiol Endocrinol Metab* **294**:E961–E968

Seidell JC, Bjorntorp P, Sjostrom L, Kvist H, Sannerstedt R (1990) Visceral fat accumulation in men is positively associated with insulin, glucose, and C-peptide levels, but negatively with testosterone levels. *Metabolism* **39**:897–901

Selvin E, Feinleib M, Zhang L, Rohrmann S, Rifai N, Nelson WG, Dobs A, Basaria S, Golden SH, Platz EA (2007) Androgens and diabetes in men. Results from the Third National Health and Nutrition Examination Survey (NHANES III). *Diabetes Care* **30**:234–238

Simon D, Preziosi P, Barrett-Connor E, Roger M, Saintpaul M, Nahoul K, Papoz L (1992) Interrelation between plasma testosterone and plasma-insulin in healthy adult men – the Telecom study. *Diabetologia* **35**:173–177

Simon D, Charles MA, Nahoul K, Orssaud G, Kremski J, Hully V,

Joubert E, Papoz L, Eschwege E (1997) Association between plasma total testosterone and cardiovascular risk factors in healthy adult men: the Telecom Study. *J Clin Endocrinol Metab* **82**:682–685

Singh R, Artaza JN, Taylor WE, Gonzalez-Cadavid NF, Bhasin S (2003) Androgens stimulate myogenic differentiation and inhibit adipogenesis in C3H 10T1/2 pluripotent cells through an androgen receptor-mediated pathway. *Endocrinology* **144**: 5081–5088

Smith JC, Bennett S, Evans LM, Kynaston HG, Parmar M, Mason MD, Cockcroft JR, Scanlon MF, Davies JS (2001) The effects of induced hypogonadism on arterial stiffness, body composition and metabolic parameters in males with prostate cancer. *J Clin Endocrinol Metab* **86**:4261–4267

Smith MR, Finkelstein JS, McGovern FJ, Zietman AL, Fallon MA, Shoenfeld DA, Kantoff PW (2002) Changes in body composition during androgen deprivation therapy for prostate cancer. *J Clin Endocrinol Metab* **87**: 599–603

Smith MR, Lee H, Nathan DM (2006) Insulin sensitivity during combined androgen blockade for prostate cancer. *J Clin Endocrinol Metab* **91**:1305–1308

Stanworth RD, Kapoor D, Channer KS, Jones TH (2008) Androgen receptor CAG repeat polymorphism is associated with serum testosterone levels, obesity and serum leptin in men with type 2 diabetes. *Eur J Endocrinol* **159**: 736–746

Stanworth RD, Kapoor D, Channer KS, Jones TH (2009) Statin therapy is associated with lower total but not bioavailable or free testosterone in men with type 2 diabetes. *Diabetes Care* **32**:541–546

Stanworth RD, Kapoor D, Channer KS, Jones TH (2011) Dyslipidaemia is

associated with testosterone, oestradiol and androgen receptor CAG repeat polymorphism in men with type 2 diabetes. *Clin Endocrinol (Oxf)* **74**:624–630

Stellato RK, Feldman HA, Hamdy O, Horton ES, McKinlay JB (2000) Testosterone, sex hormone binding globulin and the development of type 2 diabetes in middle aged men. *Diabetes Care* **23**:490–494

Strain GW, Zumoff B, Miller L, Rosner W, Levit C, Kalin M, Hershcopf RJ, Rosenfeld RS (1988) Effect of massive weight loss on hypothalamic-pituitary-gonadal function in obese men. *J Clin Endocrinol Metab* **66**:1019–1023

Straton IM, Adler AI, Neil AW, Matthews DR, Manley SE, Cull CA, Hadden D, Turner RC, Holman RR (2000) Association of glycaemia with macrovascular and microvascular complications of type 2 diabetes (UKPDS 35): prospective observational study. *BMJ* **321**:405–412

Svartberg J, von Muhlen D, Sundsfjord J, Jorde R (2004a) Waist circumference and testosterone levels in community dwelling men. The Tromso study. *Eur J Epidemiol* **19**:657–663

Svartberg J, von Muhlen D, Schirmer H, Barrett-Connor E, Sundsfjord J, Jorde R (2004b) Association of endogenous testosterone with blood pressure and left ventricular mass in men: the Tromso study. *Eur J Endocrinol* **159**:65–71

Tibblin G, Adlerberth A, Lindstedt G, Bjorntorp P (1996) The pituitary–gonadal axis and health in elderly men: a study of men born in 1913. *Diabetes* **45**:1605–1609

Tsai EC, Boyko EJ, Leonetti DL, Fujimoto WY (2000) Low serum testosterone level as a predictor of increased visceral fat in Japanese-American men. *Int J Obes Relat Metab Disord* **24**:485–491

Van Pottelbergh I, Braeckman L, De Bacquer D, De Backer G, Kaufman JM (2003) Differential contribution

of testosterone and estradiol in the determination of cholesterol and lipoprotein profile in healthy middle-aged men. *Atherosclerosis* **166**:95–102

Wang C, Swerdloff RS, Iranmanesh A, Dobs A, Snyder PJ, Cunningham G, Matsumoto AM, Weber T, Berman N; Testosterone Gel Study Group (2000) Transdermal testosterone gel improves sexual function, mood, muscle strength and body composition parameters in hypogonadal men. *J Clin Endocrinol Metab* **85**:2839–2853

Wang C, Nieschlag E, Swerdloff R, Behre HM, Hellstrom WJ, Gooren LJ, Kaufman JM, Legros JJ, Lunenfeld B, Morales A, Morley JE, Schulman C, Thompson IM, Weidner W, Wu FCW (2008) Investigation, treatment and monitoring of late-onset hypogonadism in males: ISA, ISSAM, EAU, EAA and ASA recommendations. *Eur J Endocrinol* **159**:507–514

Wang C, Jackson G, Jones TH, Matsumoto AM, Nehra A, Perelman MA, Swerdloff RS, Traish A, Zitzmann M, Cunningham G (2011) Low testosterone associated with obesity and the metabolic syndrome contributes to sexual dysfunction and cardiovascular disease risk in men with type 2 diabetes. *Diabetes Care* **34**:1669–1675

Xu T, Wang X, Hou S, Zhu J, Zhang X, Huang X (2002) Effect of surgical castration on risk factors for arteriosclerosis of patients with prostate cancer. *Chin Med J* **115**:1336–1340

Yialamas MA, Dwyer AA, Hanley E, Lee H, Pitteloud N, Hayes FJ (2007) Acute sex steroid withdrawal reduces insulin sensitivity in healthy men with idiopathic hypogonadotrophic hypogonadism. *J Clin Endocrinol Metab* **92**: 4254–4259

Zimmet P, Magliano D, Matsuzawa Y, Alberti G, Shaw J

(2005) The metabolic syndrome: a global public health problem and a new definition. *J Atheroscler Thromb* **12**:295–300

Zitzmann M (2009) The role of CAG repeat androgen receptor polymorphism in andrology. *Front Horm Res* **37**:52–61

Zmuda JM, Thompson PD, Dickenson R, Baussermann LL (1996) Testosterone decreases lipoprotein (a) in men. *Am J Cardiol* **77**:1244–1247

Zumoff B, Miller LK, Strain GW (2003) Reversal of the hypogonadotropic hypogonadism of obese men by the administration of the aromatase inhibitor testolactone. *Metabolism* **52**:1126–1128

Testosterone and erection

Mario Maggi and Hermann M. Behre

12.1   Introduction

Erectile dysfunction (ED) is a multifactorial disorder, and several emotional, physical and medical factors contribute to the degree of dysfunction that significantly impairs the patient and partner's quality of life, having a detrimental effect on sexual and reproductive activity. A recent analysis of all population-based studies conducted in the USA indicates that ED is indeed the most common endocrine disorder in men (Golden *et al.* 2009). A European survey shows that ED affects almost 30% of men in an age-dependent manner (Corona *et al.* 2010a). In 1993, the NIH Consensus Development Panel on Impotence defined ED as "the inability to attain and/or maintain penile erection sufficient for satisfactory sexual performance" (NIH Consensus Conference 1993).

Penile erection is a neurovascular event that can be seen as an integrated feed-forward interaction within a biological dimension (with its cardiovascular, neuronal and hormonal determinants), an intrapsychic dimension (the individual's sexual identity and sense of well-being), and a marital dimension (the context for a sexual relationship). In each ED patient, biological, psychological

and lifestyle factors are simultaneously present and mutually interacting (Petrone *et al.* 2003). In other words, ED is a frustrating symptom deriving from a continuous spectrum of clinical pictures including physical illness (organic component of ED), reaction to life stresses (intrapsychic component of ED) or an unhappy couple relationship (relational component of ED) (Petrone *et al.* 2003). We strongly believe that the male hormone, testosterone, plays a relevant role in determining perturbations in all three aforementioned dimensions of ED (organic, intrapsychic and relational).

The prevalence and the severity of ED increase with advancing age (Rosen *et al.* 2003; Corona *et al.* 2004; 2010a; Lindau *et al.* 2007). In the Massachusetts Male Aging Study (Feldman *et al.* 1994), the proportion of subjects with severe ED increased from 5% at the age of 40 years to 15% at the age of 70. Elderly patients are often affected by multiple organic diseases, which can interfere with sexual functioning. In particular, cardiovascular and metabolic diseases with increased prevalence in the elderly (including CAD, myocardial infarction, hypertension,

Testosterone: Action, Deficiency, Substitution, ed. Eberhard Nieschlag and Hermann M. Behre, Assoc. ed. Susan Nieschlag.
Published by Cambridge University Press. © Cambridge University Press 2012.

hyperlipidemia, diabetes mellitus and peripheral vascular disease) could play a crucial role in the pathogenesis of many cases of age-related sexual dysfunction (Feldman *et al.* 1994; Rosen *et al.* 2003; Corona *et al.* 2004; 2010a; Lindau *et al.* 2007). Also testosterone declines gradually as a function of aging; however, its relationship with ED is still debated. Data from the EMAS (European Male Aging Study), a population-based study involving more than 3000 subjects from 8 European centers, showed an unadjusted annual age decline for total testosterone of 0.04 nmol/l per year (Wu *et al.* 2008). In line with the EMAS results, a significant age-dependent decline also of total testosterone of 0.09 nmol/l·year was observed in subjects with ED (Corona *et al.* 2011a).

12.2 Physiology of erection

Erection can be regarded as a complex neurovascular process that can be initiated by recruitment of penile afferent signals (*reflexogenic erection*) and by visual, auditory, tactile, olfactory and imaginary stimuli (*psychogenic erection*). Several brain regions have been identified that are involved in the initiation of penile erection. The effect of testosterone on these central mechanisms is described in depth in Chapter 5.

At the penile level, erection occurs when the two sponge-like cavernous bodies (corpora cavernosa) become engorged with blood. Corpora cavernosa are essentially composed of large endothelium-lined vascular lacunae separated by fibrous trabeculae. The amount of blood flow to the corpora cavernosa is regulated by the activity of SMC lining the penile arteries and cavernous spaces in tight communication with the overlying endothelial cells. Penile erection is a vascular (hydraulic), three-step phenomenon (increased arterial inflow, sinusoidal smooth muscle relaxation and decreased venous drainage). In the flaccid penis, SMC of corpora cavernosa are contracted and penile blood inflow is low. During erection, relaxation of trabecular SMC results in increased blood flow and pressure in the corpora cavernosa and expansion of sinusoidal spaces. The expanded corpora cavernosa cause mechanical compression of the emissary veins, restricting the venous outflow from the cavernosal spaces and facilitating an entrapment of blood in the cavernosal sinusoids. This blood engorgement finally results in penile rigidity.

A series of biochemical and hemodynamic events that are associated with activation of the central nervous system control the switch between muscle contraction and relaxation (Berridge 2008). Sympathetic nerve activity is mainly responsible for maintaining SMC in a contractile state (see Fig. 12.1A). The release of noradrenalin (NA) from nerve endings allows its binding to cognate receptors, which activate two separate pathways within the cells, favoring increase in intracellular calcium and sensitization to it (see Fig. 12.1A). Smooth muscle cell relaxation is primarily driven by the activity of parasympathetic and non-adrenergic, non-cholinergic (NANC) nerve endings, which control nitric oxide (NO) formation through NO synthase (NOS), present in both endothelial cells (eNOS) and neurons (nNOS) (see Fig. 12.1B). Nitric oxide diffuses into SMC and increases the formation of cyclic GMP, an action actively counteracted by a series of phosphodiesterases (PDEs), the most important of which is PDE5. In human corpora cavernosa, PDE5 alone accounts for the breakdown of the majority (70%) of the formed cGMP (Morelli *et al.* 2004). Relaxation of cavernous SMC increases blood flow into cavernosal sinuses and venous occlusion, resulting in penile engorgement and rigidity.

12.3 Direct effects of testosterone on penile growth and erection

Penile development from the urogenital sinus and genital tubercle is a process which is not well understood, but two members of the Hedgehog (Hh) gene family, Sonic hedgehog (*Shh*) and Indian hedgehog (*Ihh*), expressed early during anogenital differentiation, are known to direct division of the cloaca into separate urogenital and anorectal sinuses. *Shh*−/− mice have complete agenesis of the external genitalia and persistence of the cloaca; in humans, mutations affecting Hedgehog signaling and its downstream targets underlie several syndromes characterized by anorectal malformation (Podlasek 2009). Androgens and a functioning AR are also necessary for normal development of the human penis. In humans, the penis grows in phases, initially during early gestation and then continuing until approximately the age of five. A latency period follows until puberty, when penile size responds to the increase of testosterone levels. Growth ceases at the completion of pubertal growth despite continued high levels of circulating testosterone. In a prospective, longitudinal population-based study of 728 Danish and 1234 Finnish infant boys it was found that endogenous testosterone was

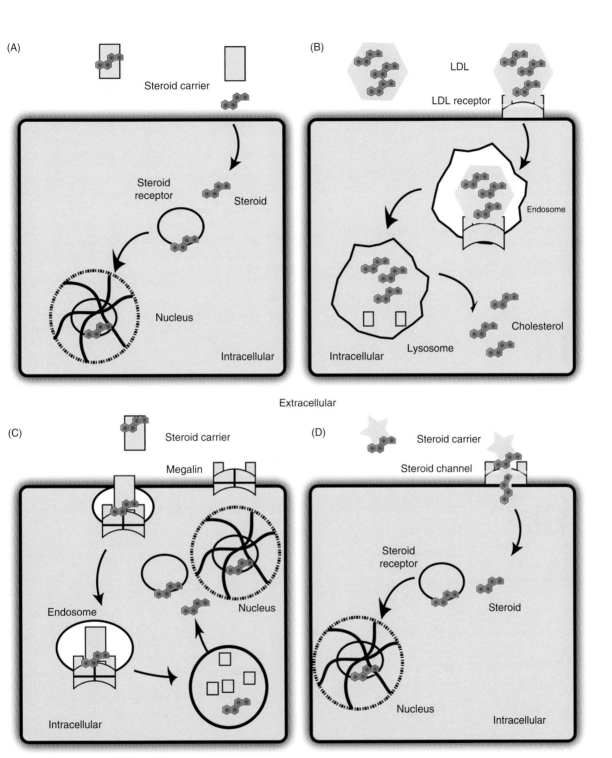

Fig. 2.5 Mechanisms by which steroidal hormones can enter cells. (A) The steroid hormone diffuses freely across the cell membrane, binds to an intracellular receptor and enters the nucleus to regulate gene expression. (B) Receptor-mediated endocytosis of steroid containing lipophilic molecules. The LDL binds its receptor and is taken up, degraded in lysosomes and the steroid cholesterol can enter different metabolic pathways. (C) Receptor-mediated endocytosis of steroids. The entire hormone carrier is endocytotically bound after binding to a carrier protein. Following the intracellular degradation of the carrier, the ligand hormone is released into the free cytoplasm. (D) Transport-mediated uptake of molecules through the membrane. The steroid carrier is recognized by a membrane receptor and the ligand is transported into the cell.

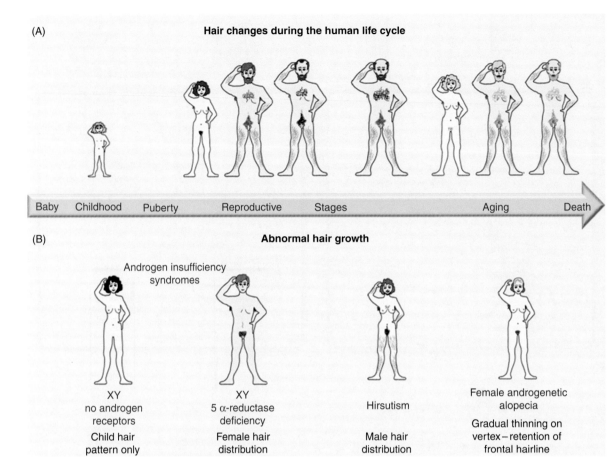

(A) **Hair changes during the human life cycle**

| Baby | Childhood | Puberty | Reproductive | Stages | Aging | Death |

(B) **Abnormal hair growth**

Androgen insufficiency syndromes

XY
no androgen receptors

Child hair pattern only

XY
5 α-reductase deficiency

Female hair distribution

Hirsutism

Male hair distribution

Female androgenetic alopecia

Gradual thinning on vertex – retention of frontal hairline

Fig. 7.1 Human hair varies with life stage and endocrine state. (A) Changes in hair distribution and color signal a person's age, state of maturity and sex. Visible (i.e. terminal) hair with protective functions normally develops in children on the scalp, eyelashes and eyebrows. Once puberty occurs, more terminal hair develops on the axilla and pubis in both sexes, and on the face, chest, limbs and often back in men. Androgens also stimulate hair loss from the scalp in men with the appropriate genes in a patterned manner, causing androgenetic alopecia. As age increases hair follicles lose their ability to make pigment, causing graying (canities). (B) People with various androgen insufficiency syndromes demonstrate that none of this occurs without functional androgen receptors and that only axillary and female pattern of lower pubic triangle hairs are formed in the absence of 5α-reductase type 2. Male pattern hair growth (hirsutism) occurs in women with abnormalities of plasma androgens or from idiopathic causes, and women may also develop a different form of hair loss, female androgenetic alopecia or female pattern hair loss (FPHL).

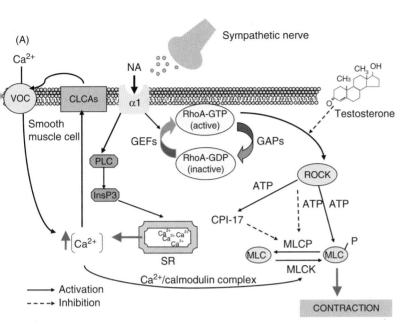

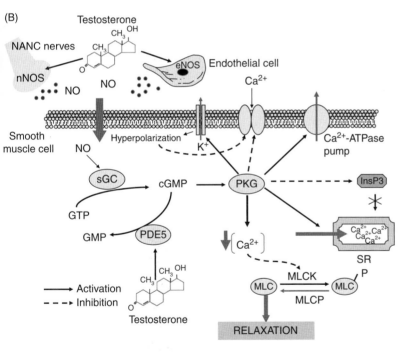

Fig. 12.1 Schematic representation of the biochemical events leading to penile flaccidity (A) or erection (B). The enzymatic steps for which a role for testosterone has been proposed are represented. See plate section for color version. (A) Noradrenalin (NA) binding generates inositol 1,4,5-trisphosphate (InsP3), which, by increasing intracellular calcium (Ca^{2+}) levels, activates Ca^{2+}-sensitive chloride channels (CLCAs), resulting in membrane depolarization with the diffusion of the stimulus to the neighboring cells and the opening of voltage-operated channels (VOC). The increased Ca^{2+} flow promotes, through calmodulin, activation of myosin light chain (MLC) kinase (MLCK) and cell contraction. Cell contraction is also obtained by altering the Ca^{2+} sensitivity through a NA-induced activation of a second pathway, RhoA/ROCK, which increases, through a series of kinase activation, the sensitivity of MLC to Ca^{2+}. Testosterone is supposed to negatively regulate the latter event. (B) Nitric oxide (NO) is generated by NO synthases in either non-adrenergic, non-cholinergic (NANC) neurons (nNOS) or endothelial cells (eNOS). Both steps are positively regulated by testosterone. Nitric oxide diffuses into SMC and activates a soluble guanylate cyclase (sGC), which in turn transforms GTP into cGMP. Cyclic GMP activates protein kinase G (PKG), which, through the indicated pathways, finally decreases intracellular Ca^{2+} levels, leading to relaxation. Phosphodiesterase type 5 (PDE5) metabolizes cGMP into GMP, thereby limiting its effects. The latter event is positively controlled by testosterone. Other abbreviations: cGMP, cyclic GMP; CPI-17, protein phosphatase 1 regulatory, subunit 14A; GAP, GTPase activating protein; GEF, guanine nucleotide exchange factor; MLCP, myosin light chain phosphatase; PLC, phospholipase C; rhoA, ras homolog gene family member A; ROCK, rho-associated, coiled-coil containing protein kinase; SR, sarcoplasmic reticulum.

significantly associated with penile size and growth rate (Boas *et al.* 2006). The exact mechanism of penile growth cessation remains unresolved, but is probably not only due to downregulation of ARs (Levy *et al.* 1996; Baskin *et al.* 1997). Although *Shh* expression is partially andro-gen dependent, in juvenile rats *Shh* signaling appears to be independent of testosterone (Bond *et al.* 2010).

Numerous studies in animal models have demon-strated a direct testosterone dependency of the erectile process. Experimental studies in animals and human cell cultures indicate that testosterone controls, dir-ectly or indirectly, the majority of mechanisms leading to erection and detumescence. First of all, it controls the commitment of penile cells towards a smooth muscle phenotype, favoring the functional and structural integrity that is necessary for penile erection (Traish *et al.* 2005; Morelli *et al.* 2007; Yassin and Saad 2008; Traish 2009; Corona and Maggi 2010). There is, in fact, general consensus on a trophic effect of testosterone on penile architecture in different animal species such as rabbit (Traish *et al.* 1999; 2003; Morelli *et al.* 2007), dog (Takahashi *et al.* 1991), mouse (Palese *et al.* 2003) and rat (Shabsigh *et al.* 1998; Zhang *et al.* 1999; Shen *et al.* 2003). In castrated animals, elastic and smooth muscle fibers are replaced by collagenous ones, which may result in fibrosis. It has also been shown that testosterone is involved in the maturation of penile tissue composition by promoting the commitment of pluripotent stem cells into the myogenic lineage, and inhibiting their differentiation towards adipogenic lineage. Androgen deficiency is associated with alterations in dorsal nerve structure and endothelial morphology, and accumulation of adipocytes in the subtunical region of the corpora cavernosa, which could impede blood outflow during sexual stimulation and contribute to venous leak (Traish *et al.* 2005; Morelli *et al.* 2007; Yassin and Saad 2008).

In addition, testosterone controls numerous enzymatic activities within the corpora cavernosa. A significant role of testosterone has been demonstrated for regulating NO formation (acting on eNOS and/or nNOS) in several animal models. Low testosterone conditions include senescence (Garban *et al.* 1995a; 1995b), diabetes mellitus type 1 and 2 (Vernet *et al.* 1995), metabolic syndrome (Filippi *et al.* 2009), adrenalectomy (Penson *et al.* 1997), hypophysectomy (Penson *et al.* 1996) and castration (Mills *et al.* 1992; Chamness *et al.* 1995; Lugg *et al.* 1995; 1996; Penson *et al.* 1997; Park *et al.* 1999). In castrated rats, both testosterone (Chamness *et al.* 1995; Lugg *et al.* 1995; Park *et al.* 1999) and DHT (Lugg *et al.* 1995; Park *et al.* 1999) replacement completely rescued NOS activity. It is still rather unclear which of the two major constitutive NOS isoforms, i.e. the neuronal (nNOS) or endothelial (eNOS) isoform, is mainly regulated by androgens in the rat penis. In the majority of studies androgens increased nNOS protein (Chamness *et al.* 1995; Park *et al.* 1999; Marin *et al.* 1999) or mRNA (Reilly *et al.* 1997; Schirar *et al.* 1997; Park *et al.* 1999); although positive effects on eNOS were also reported (Marin *et al.* 1999; Filippi *et al.* 2009). Other studies were negative on eNOS (Park *et al.* 1999) or nNOS in both rat (Lugg *et al.* 1996;

Penson *et al.* 1996; 1997) and rabbit (Traish *et al.* 1999) models of androgen ablation.

In addition, it has been demonstrated that testosterone also regulates the activity of the RhoA/ROCK pathway negatively, decreasing calcium sensitivity within penile SMC overall in both castration-induced (Wingard *et al.* 2003) and diabetes-induced hypogonadism (Vignozzi *et al.* 2007). RhoA is a member of the small monomeric GTPase family which plays a role not only in mediating smooth muscle contraction, through the activation of its downstream kinase (ROCK), but also in the regulation of several cellular processes, such as stress fiber formation and cell migration.

Under the same experimental conditions (surgical or chemical castration, diabetes/metabolic-syndrome-induced hypogonadism), it has been shown that testosterone also positively regulates the expression of PDE5 (Traish *et al.* 1999; Morelli *et al.* 2004; Zhang *et al.* 2005; 2006; Vignozzi *et al.* 2007; Filippi *et al.* 2009). Because testosterone positively controls both the enzymatic steps necessary for initiation (positive effect on NOS and negative on RhoA/ROCK) and the end (positive on PDE5) of the erectile process, its net effect on erection ends up as modest. Erections are indeed still possible in hypogonadal conditions where decreased cGMP formation, due to impaired NO production, is most probably counterbalanced by reduced PDE5 activity and cGMP hydrolysis.

However, it should be considered that, both in animals and men, testosterone acts mainly on sexual interest (Rochira *et al.* 2003; Vignozzi *et al.* 2005) and only partially on sexual potency. Accordingly, not all castrated men become impotent (Heim and Hursch 1979). Indeed, in prostatic cancer patients undergoing medical or surgical castration, sexual intercourse was preserved in 20–45% of subjects (Ellis and Grayhack 1963). Penile erections in response to powerful stimuli, such as erotic visual stimulation, have also been documented in hypo-androgenized individuals (Kwan *et al.* 1983; Bancroft and Wu 1983; Greenstein *et al.* 1995). According to Davidson (1986), in hypogonadal men "the decreased libido apparently leads to a secondary decrease in erectile performance during sexual situations, due probably to lack of interest or pleasure." Hence, erections are still possible without androgens, although less frequent because of low sexual interest. It has been reported since ancient times that eunuchs who were castrated after puberty were capable of maintaining erections. Accordingly, it was a custom in ancient Rome that women would use more potent eunuchs for pleasure without the risk of procreation (Dettenhofer 2009). Infants frequently have erections upon the slightest tactile stimulation, but, until puberty, boys do not engage in sexual activity outside the context of play. The paradox of a normal erection (upon adequate sexual stimulation) in hypo-androgenized individuals, in which NO formation is substantially hampered, finds an intriguing solution in the observation published almost three decades ago by Kwan et al. (1983). They found that the erectile response to explicit pornographic films in hypogonadal individuals was comparable to that of normal ones, while the time to penile detumescence was prolonged by a factor of two in the hypogonadal men as compared to eugonadal controls. The demonstration that cGMP breakdown through PDE5 is androgen dependent helps in understanding this apparent paradox, because, in a low-androgen milieu, cGMP catabolism is impaired (see Fig. 12.1; Morelli et al. 2004; Zhang et al. 2005).

Vasoactive intestinal peptide (VIP) is one of the first penile neurotransmitters characterized for facilitating erectile function. It signals though the G-protein-coupled receptor VPAC2 and, upon Gs α and adenylyl cyclase activation, it stimulates cAMP formation. Within the penis of hypogonadal rats, VIP signaling was substantially increased (Zhang et al. 2011), partially rescuing castration-induced ED. Testosterone supplementation to hypogonadal rats partially downregulated this pathway.

12.4 Association between androgen level and erectile activity in men with erectile dysfunction

The most widely used parameter to predict adequacy of penile circulation is cavernous peak systolic velocity (PSV, cm/s), measured 5–20 minutes after an intracavernous injection of a vasodilating agent (Corona et al. 2008). Fig. 12.2 shows an association between circulating testosterone and penile blood flow, as well as reported erectile activity, in a large series of subjects attending an andrological clinic for sexual dysfunction. As shown in Fig. 12.2A, penile blood flow, as detected by penile color Doppler ultrasound (PCDU) after PGE1 injection (10 μg), is positively related to testosterone plasma levels. The receiver operating characteristic (ROC) curve is a graphical plot of the sensitivity, or true positive rate, vs. false positive rate (1 − specificity or 1 − true negative rate), for a binary classifier system as its discrimination threshold is varied. The ROC curve analysis for severely impaired PSV (<25 cm/s) showed an overall accuracy of 65.3% in predicting low testosterone ($p < 0.0001$), with a specificity and sensitivity to detect abnormal testosterone (below 12 nmol/l) of 72.5% and 51.6%, respectively (see Fig. 12.2B).

Interestingly, in patients with ED, the evaluation of penile flow could be used not only to identify those deserving further investigation, but also to stratify future cardiovascular risk (Corona et al. 2011b). It has been shown that, in ED subjects, a dynamic PSV below 25 cm/s is associated with a relevant increase of cardiovascular risk (Corona et al. 2010b): the risk of major adverse cardiovascular events (MACE) increases by 5% for each 5 cm/s decrement of the dynamic PSV. In particular, male hypogonadism has been associated with increased mortality in patients affected by specific diseases, such as hypopituitarism, Klinefelter syndrome, mental retardation, and in specific populations, such as veterans and Japanese men, with at least one cardiovascular factor (Corona et al. 2011b). In line with these findings, it has been recently reported that, in ED subjects, low testosterone predicted MACE lethality (Corona et al. 2010c) and forthcoming MACE; the latter particularly in normal weight and overweight subjects (Corona et al. 2011c).

Penile nocturnal erections are a naturally occurring phenomenon during rapid eye movement (REM) sleep in all normal healthy males from infancy to old age, and they have no association with dream content (Montorsi and Oettel 2005). Although it is well accepted that sleep-related erections (SREs) deteriorate with ED, quite surprisingly the physiological role of sleep-related erections is still poorly understood. Testosterone seems to play a crucial role in the regulation of nocturnal erections. An androgenic control of SREs during REM sleep has been postulated for a long time. Karacan and Hirshkowitz (1991) noted that, in boys, SREs increase at the onset of puberty, suggesting a role of testosterone in such a process. In addition, testosterone levels peak near the transition from non-REM to REM sleep close to the onset of an SRE episode (Roffwarg et al. 1982). In the early 1980s Cunningham et al. (1982) reported that hyperprolactinemia-induced hypogonadism was associated with a reduction of SREs. These results were confirmed by

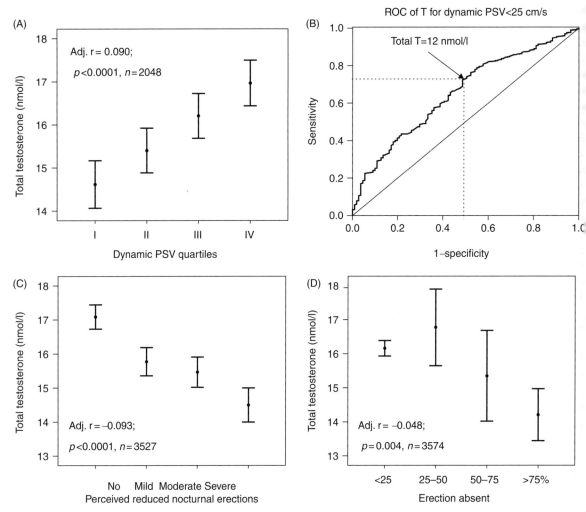

Fig. 12.2 Age-adjusted association (Adj. r) of reported erectile activity with blood levels of total testosterone (T) in the indicated number (n) of subjects with sexual dysfunction, studied at the University of Florence (Italy). (A) Association of maximal peak systolic velocity (PSV) at PCDU (after 10 μg PGE1), reported as quartiles, and total T. (B) ROC curve of PSV < 25 cm/s for total testosterone in the same population as in panel A. The arrow shows the sensitivity (ordinate) and 1 – specificity (abscissa) for total testosterone = 12 nmol/l. (C) Association between perceived reduced nocturnal/morning erections of increasing intensity (no, mild, moderate, severe) and total T. (D) Association between reported severe ED (erection absence, percentage of cases) and total T.

Kwan et al. (1983) around the same time and more recently by Carani et al. (1995). Testosterone levels correlate with the measured frequency of sleep erections (Cunningham et al. 1982; Roffwarg et al. 1982; Kwan et al. 1983; Karacan and Hirshkowitz 1991; Carani et al. 1995; Hirshkowitz and Schmidt 2005; Montorsi and Oettel 2005; Rochira et al. 2006), and TRT in hypogonadal men has been shown to increase the frequency, magnitude, duration and rigidity of SREs (Cunningham et al. 1982; O'Carroll et al. 1985; Hirshkowitz and Schmidt 2005; Montorsi and Oettel 2005; Rochira et al. 2006).

SREs can be easily measured non-invasively through the use of a nocturnal penile tumescence (NPT) test. Interestingly, the decreased frequency of SREs has been recognized recently as a possible predictive symptom of testosterone deficiency in community-dwelling men (Wu et al. 2010). It has been reported recently that investigation of SREs, through a validated (and costless) questionnaire (SIEDY item no. 13, Petrone et al. 2003), is able to predict NPT test results with an accuracy of about 70%. Using this questionnaire, it has been demonstrated that perceived reduced SREs were significantly associated with total (Fig. 12.2C), analog free, calculated free and calculated bioavailable testosterone, even after adjustment for age (Corona *et al.* 2011d).

In contrast to the clear-cut androgen dependence of both penile blood flow and spontaneous/nocturnal erections, reported sex-related erections were less clearly associated with testosterone blood levels. Only subjects reporting a severe ED show lower blood levels of testosterone (Corona and Maggi 2010). This indicates that penile erection is associated with the androgen milieu, even though other factors (i.e. intrapsychic, relational) might mitigate the patient's perception during sexual activity. Accordingly, Rhoden *et al.* (2002), in a large consecutive series of 1071 mainly eugonadal men aged from 40 to 90 years, found no significant association between serum testosterone levels and the prevalence or severity of ED as assessed by the questionnaire of the simplified International Index of Erectile Function (IIEF-5).

12.5   Effects of testosterone therapy on erection

Since the early beginnings of testosterone therapy of hypogonadal patients it has been known that testosterone restores normal male sexual behavior and erectile function (see Chapter 5). However, studies on the effect of TRT are surprisingly scanty, of short duration and often not placebo controlled. In order to emphasize the most important outcomes of TRT, meta-analysis was performed. In fact meta-analysis can pool trials with different results and offer clinicians and patients a single best estimate of the effect of TRT. Meta-analysis is particularly useful when there are a variety of reports with low statistical power; thus, pooling data can improve power and provide more robust results.

The first meta-analysis on TRT for ED in hypogonadal patients confirmed the significant improvement of erections after initiation of testosterone therapy (Jain *et al.* 2000). Pooled data on placebo-controlled studies showed an improvement of erectile function in 36 of 55 men treated with testosterone; whereas significantly fewer men responded to placebo treatment (9 out of 45) (Jain *et al.* 2000). A meta-analysis of 17 randomized placebo-controlled clinical trials (Isidori *et al.* 2005) indicated that, in comparison to placebo, a significant, but moderate, improvement of all aspects of sexual function was found in the studies of middle-age and elderly men with low

testosterone (testosterone concentration < 12 nmol/l or <346 ng/dl). Interestingly, meta-regression analysis demonstrated that the effect of TRT on erectile function was inversely related to the baseline testosterone concentration. Hence, the more severe the hypogonadism, the more significant or impressive are the results obtained with TRT. Conversely, no effect was observed for baseline testosterone levels higher than 12 nmol/l.

A subsequent meta-analysis (Boloña *et al.* 2007), including only trials devoted to men with sexual dysfunction at baseline, emphasized the possible role of aging as a moderator in evaluating the effect of TRT on sexual function. In particular, analyzing the studies according to men's age, they reported a sizable and significant effect of TRT on erectile function in the two trials including young patients, and a minimal and non-significant effect in those including older ones (mean age > 50 years). This last observation is not surprising. In fact, while hypogonadism can be the main cause of ED in younger patients, it is generally only one element of a multifactorial ED in older ones.

12.6   Combined therapy with testosterone and phosphodiesterase type 5 inhibitors in patients with erectile dysfunction

Oral therapy with inhibitors of the phosphodiesterase type 5 (PDE5i), e.g. sildenafil, vardenafil and tadalafil, is highly effective in treating ED (Tsertsvadze *et al.* 2009). However, in placebo-controlled phase III clinical trials and post-marketing evaluation, approximately 15 to 40% of patients do not respond to this medication (Tsertsvadze *et al.* 2009). Because PDE5 is androgen dependent (Morelli *et al.* 2004), it has been suggested that the combination of TRT and PDE5 inhibitors can be used to improve PDE5i outcomes in hypogonadal men. All observations emphasize that hypogonadism must be ruled out and, if present, adequately treated, before the prescription of any PDE5i. On the other hand, in an uncontrolled study Greenstein *et al.* (2005) reported that the combination of sildenafil was able to restore the 100% success rate in 48 mild hypogonadal ED patients, previously treated only with testosterone gel.

At present, various uncontrolled studies (Kalinchenko *et al.* 2003; Chatterjee *et al.* 2004; Foresta *et al.*

Table 12.1 Trials assessing the effect of combined therapy with testosterone (T) and sildenafil/tadalafil in men with erectile dysfunction unresponsive to testosterone (11), to PDE5i (1–3,6,10,12) or directly the combination of the two treatments (4,5,7,8, 9,13)

	References	n	Baseline testosterone levels (ng/dl)	Therapy	Overall efficacy (%)
1	Aversa et al. 2003[a]	20	<400	T patch/sildenafil 100 mg	80
2	Kalichenko et al. 2003	120	<340	Oral TU/sildenafil 100 mg	70
3	Shabsigh et al. 2004[a]	75	<400	T gel/sildenafil 100 mg	70
4	Chatterjee et al. 2004	12	<400 (75%)	T im/sildenafil 50–100 mg	100
5	Foresta et al. 2004	15	<200	T patch/sildenafil 50 mg	Normal NPT test par
6	Shamloul et al. 2005	40	<340	Oral TU/sildenafil 50–100 mg	Improvement
7	Greenstein et al. 2005	31	<400	T gel/sildenafil 100 mg	63
8	Tas et al. 2006	23	<400	T im/sildenafil 50–100 mg	34
9	Rochira et al. 2006[a]	24	< 200	T im/sildenafil 50 mg	Improved NPT test par
10	Hwang et al. 2006	32	<300	Oral TU/sildenafil 100 mg	57
11	Rosenthal et al. 2006	90	<350	T gel/sildenafil 100 mg	92
12	Yassin et al. 2006	69	<340	T gel/tadalafil 20 mg	65
13	Buvat et al. 2011[a]	73	<300	T gel/tadalafil 10 mg daily	51

Abbreviations: TU, testosterone undecanoate; NPT, nocturnal penile tumescence; Par, parameters.
[a] Placebo-controlled studies.

2004; Shamloul et al. 2005; Hwang et al. 2006; Rosenthal et al. 2006; Tas et al. 2006; Yassin et al. 2006) and four randomized, placebo-controlled studies (Aversa et al. 2003; Shabsigh et al. 2004; Rochira et al. 2006; Buvat et al. 2011) suggest that hypogonadism might hinder the effects of PDE5i on erectile function (Table 12.1). In particular, the combination of testosterone and PDE5i is able to improve the overall efficacy from 34 to 100% (see Table 12.1). In addition, one study suggested that the proportion of patients improved by the combination with testosterone increased with the duration of testosterone (65% after 10 weeks vs. 43% after only 4 weeks) (Aversa et al. 2003).

Three randomized, controlled studies support the concept of a positive interaction between TRT and PDE5i responsiveness. The first study included 20 patients with arteriogenic ED as diagnosed by dynamic color duplex ultrasound (PCDU). These men had normal sexual desire, serum levels of total and free testosterone in the lower quartile of the normal range, and had not responded to the highest dose of sildenafil (100 mg) on six consecutive attempts (Aversa et al. 2003). Patients were randomized to transdermal non-scrotal testosterone patches (5 mg/d; n = 10) or placebo patches (n = 10), and received 100 mg sildenafil tablets on demand. The PCDU revealed a significant increase of arterial inflow to cavernous arteries of the penis in the testosterone-treated men; whereas this parameter remained unchanged in the placebo group. Effects on erectile function were assessed by the International Index of

Erectile Function (IIEF) questionnaire (Rosen *et al.* 1997). Compared to placebo plus sildenafil, treatment with testosterone and sildenafil resulted in a significantly increased score of erectile function domain, the intercourse satisfaction domain, and the overall satisfaction domain of the IIEF. The scores of the sexual desire domain and orgasmic function domain remained unchanged, indicating that the treatment effect of testosterone was not only due to central effects on sexual desire. The Global Assessment Question (GAQ) "Has the treatment you received … improved your erections" was positively affirmed by 80% of men in the testosterone/sildenafil group compared to 10% in the placebo/sildenafil group at the end of treatment (Aversa *et al.* 2003).

This pilot study was followed by a randomized, double-blind, placebo-controlled, 12-week multicenter study in 70 men with low or low-normal serum testosterone (morning levels before 10 a.m. < 13.88 nmol/l) and non-responders to 100 mg of sildenafil during a 4-week run-in period (Shabsigh *et al.* 2004). Patients were randomly assigned to therapy with placebo gel and sildenafil (group I, *n* = 33) or 5 g/d of testosterone gel and sildenafil (group II, *n* = 37). While the severity of ED was similar in both groups at baseline, the erectile function domain, as well as the orgasmic function domain of the IIEF, improved significantly in group II at study week four, and scores remained at this level up to the end of the study. However, it should be noted that the difference between both groups lost significance following week four because of improvement of the total IIEF score and score of the erectile function domain in group I. In addition, no control group treated only with testosterone and oral placebo was included in this study.

Recently, results from a multicenter, multinational, double-blind, placebo-controlled study of 173 men, 45–80 years of age, non-responders to treatment with different PDE5 inhibitors, with baseline total testosterone levels ≤ 13.88 nmol/l or bioavailable testosterone ≤ 3.47 nmol/l were reported (Buvat *et al.* 2011). Men were first treated with tadalafil 10 mg once a day for 4 weeks; if not successful, they were randomized to receive placebo or 5 mg of testosterone gel, to be increased to 10 mg testosterone if results were clinically unsatisfactory. Erectile function improved progressively over a period of at least 12 weeks in both the placebo and testosterone treatment groups. In the overall population, with a mean baseline testosterone level of 11.7 ± 3.47 nmol/l, no

additional effect of testosterone administration to men optimally treated with PDE5i was encountered. However, the differences between the testosterone and placebo groups were significant for both Erectile Function Domain Score of the IIEF and Sexual Encounter Profile 3 in those men with baseline testosterone ≤ 10.4 nmol/l.

These three randomized, placebo-controlled studies provide evidence that patients with ED and low-normal or subnormal testosterone levels, who do not respond to PDE5i therapy, might benefit from a combined therapy. However, the real efficacy of this approach needs to be proven in larger placebo-controlled studies, because the meta-analysis by Tsertsvadze *et al.* (2009) did not support this view. It should be noted that the recent study by Buvat was not included in the Tsertsvadze meta-analysis.

Nevertheless, an international consultation, collaborating with major urological and sexual medicine societies convened in Paris, July 2009 (International Consultation of Sexual Medicine, ICSM-5), and recommended screening for testosterone deficiency in all patients with ED (Buvat *et al.* 2010).

12.7 Prevalence of testosterone deficiency in patients with erectile dysfunction

Recognition of hypogonadism in subjects with sexual dysfunction has been greatly helped by recent consensus among professional societies (Petak *et al.* 2002; Wang *et al.* 2009; Bhasin *et al.* 2010). It has been universally recognized that diagnosis of androgen deficiency should be made only in *symptomatic men* with unequivocally low serum testosterone levels, as neither criterion is consistently reliable when considered alone. All the guidelines recommend that total testosterone, the major parameter to be measured, should be sampled in the morning on at least two separate occasions before making a diagnosis. Testosterone substitution should be offered to symptomatic individuals when circulating total testosterone is below 8 nmol/l (231 ng/dl) (Wang *et al.* 2009). In addition, there is also general agreement that a total testosterone level above 12 nmol/l (346 ng/dl) does not require substitution. When total testosterone is between 8 and 12 nmol/l in the presence of typical hypogonadal symptoms, a testosterone treatment trial should be considered (Wang *et al.* 2009).

Among the different symptoms, sexual dysfunction represents the most specific symptom associated with low testosterone (Wu *et al.* 2010). Recent data from the EMAS recognized that a triad of sexual symptoms (low libido, and reduced spontaneous and sex-related erections) is the only syndromic association with decreased testosterone levels (Wu *et al.* 2010); whereas other proposed hypogonadal symptoms did not segregate with the androgen deficiency. In that large European survey, the simultaneous presence of the three sexual symptoms combined with a total testosterone level of less than 11 nmol/l and a free testosterone level of less than 220 pmol/l were therefore considered the minimal criteria for the diagnosis of hypogonadism (Wu *et al.* 2010). Conversely, in subjects with total testosterone below 8 nmol/l, the presence of sexual symptoms was unhelpful.

In epidemiological studies in ED subjects, serum testosterone below 10.4 nmol/l was found in 12% of 7000 men, compiled from nine large series (including 4% of 944 men less than 50 years old, and 14.7% of 4342 men more than 50 years old) (Buvat and Bou Jaoudé 2006). In one consecutive series of 1022 men with ED, Buvat and Lemaire (1997) detected serum concentrations of testosterone below 10.4 nmol/l in 8.0% of men. However, 40% of these patients had normal serum levels at repeated determination (Buvat and Lemaire 1997). Pituitary tumors were discovered in two men with low testosterone. Determination of testosterone only in cases of low sexual desire or abnormal physical examination would have overlooked 40% of men with low testosterone, and 37% of men subsequently improving during testosterone substitution therapy (Buvat and Lemaire 1997). A larger study involving 3547 men with ED revealed a prevalence of testosterone deficiency (serum concentration less than 9.7 nmol/l) of 18.7% (Bodie *et al.* 2003). In another consecutive series of 2794 men with ED aged 25–80 years, testosterone was <6.94 nmol/l in 7%, <10.4 nmol/l in 23%, <12 nmol/l in 33%, and <13.88 nmol/l in 47% of men (Köhler *et al.* 2008).

The difference in the prevalence of testosterone deficiency in patients with ED could be explained by different patient populations, different age of men with ED, differences in primary, secondary or tertiary care centers, different definitions of low testosterone levels, or single versus repeated testosterone determinations. It should be noted that none of these studies really fulfils the principles of evidence-based

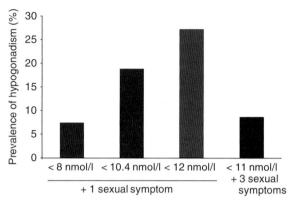

Fig. 12.3 Prevalence (%) of hypogonadism in subjects with sexual dysfunction (*n* = 3608), studied at the University of Florence (Italy), according to different biochemical thresholds for low testosterone. The proportion of hypogonadal subjects as derived from the new proposed criteria based on the EMAS (Wu *et al.* 2010) is also represented (three sexual symptoms and total testosterone below 11 nmol/l).

medicine, as no study included a control group of age-matched men without ED.

Fig. 12.3 shows the different prevalences of hypogonadism in 3608 subjects referred to an andrological clinic for sexual dysfunction (University of Florence). All subjects were, by definition, symptomatic, because they reported at least one symptom of sexual dysfunction. The data are essentially in keeping with results from Bodie *et al.* (2003) and Köhler *et al.* (2008), and show variable detection of male hypogonadism ranging from 7.4% (below 8 nmol/l) to 27.2% (below 12 nmol/l). However, when the strict criteria from the EMAS were applied (total testosterone below 11 nmol/l and at least three sexual symptoms), the resulting percentage of ED men with hypogonadism was lower (8.2%), but still higher than in the general population, according to the EMAS (2.1%).

12.8 Effects of sexual activity and treatment of erectile dysfunction on testosterone

Studies in rhesus macaques indicate that testosterone plasma levels are increased by exposure to a receptive female and copulation (Herndon *et al.* 1981). Hence, sexual activity and sex hormones appear to be intimately related. Accordingly, Fabbri *et al.* (1988) reported that, in non-organic impotent men, both bioactive LH and testosterone serum levels were significantly lower than in normal men. However, it is still unclear whether, in mating male individuals, testosterone is higher to allow better sexual and reproductive fitness (affecting libido/penile erections and/or spermatogenesis) or the reverse is true: sexual activity positively affects testosterone production. An often-cited, single observation, published in *Nature* almost 40 years ago, opted for the second scenario. An island resident observed an increase in beard growth on the day preceding, and during, his occasional visits to his mainland lover (Anonymous 1970).

During the following years only scanty reports substantiated this anecdotal account, demonstrating a time-related rise in testosterone level during sexual intercourse (Fox *et al.* 1972; Dabbs and Mohammed 1992) or exposure to erotic movies (LaFerla *et al.* 1978). Conversely, other reports addressing the question of a sexual-activity-induced rise in testosterone plasma levels were negative (Raboch and Starka 1973; Stearns *et al.* 1973; Lee *et al.* 1974; Kraemer *et al.* 1976). However, Stoleru *et al.* (1993), sampling male volunteers every 10 min for 12 h, found an increased pulsatile release of LH, with a concomitant increase in testosterone, occurring soon after exposure to erotic, but not neutral, movies. In normal healthy men and patients with ED, serum levels of testosterone increase significantly during the tumescence, as well as the rigidity phase of penile erection, and return to baseline in the detumescence phase (Becker *et al.* 2000; 2001).

In a consecutive series of 2302 male patients with ED (mean age 53.2 ± 12.5 years) an association was found between SIEDY Scale 2 score (which measures the relational component of ED: Petrone *et al.* 2003) and decreased intercourse frequency, severe ED, lower dynamic PSV at PCDU, and clinical and biochemical hypogonadism (Corona *et al.* 2009). Alternative models were explored using these different factors as dependent variables, in order to evaluate the specific relationship among the parameters. Multiple logistic regression analysis indicated that low penile blood flow and decreased intercourse frequency are bi-directionally coupled to poor relational domain, while the association with hypogonadism was mediated through sexual hypo-activity or inertia. In other words, this suggests that good sex is the prerequisite for a good couple relationship and a good couple relationship is the cornerstone for successful and happy couple sexual activity, which is accompanied by higher testosterone levels (Corona *et al.* 2009).

Accordingly, it was described that among subjects with sexual dysfunction, unfaithful men, reporting higher sexual intercourse frequency, have a lower prevalence of biochemical and clinical hypogonadism (Fisher *et al.* 2009). Similar results were previously reported by van Anders *et al.* (2007). In Corona's study, the sexual-frequency-dependent reduction of both total and free testosterone was not accompanied by a compensatory rise in LH levels, suggesting the presence of a central, hypothalamic-pituitary failure. Similar results were obtained in a rat experimental model (Vignozzi *et al.* 2009). Hypogonadotropic hypogonadism was observed occurring three months after bilateral denervation of the penis, obtained through resection of the rats' cavernous nerves (Vignozzi *et al.* 2009). It was speculated that sexual inactivity, induced by cavernous denervation, could lead to a state of overt hypogonadotropic hypogonadism (Vignozzi *et al.* 2009). This could also be the case in patients, considering that decreased penile blood flow and decreased sexual activity were associated with lower androgens and presence of hypogonadal symptoms, with inappropriately low LH levels (Corona *et al.* 2009).

Jannini *et al.* produced evidence that substantiated the hypothesis of an LH-mediated, sex-induced drive in testosterone production (Jannini *et al.* 1999; Carosa *et al.* 2002; 2004). In a controlled, non-randomized study they demonstrated that effective psychological, medical (prostaglandin E1, yohimbine) or mechanical (vascular surgery, penile prostheses, vacuum devices) therapy of ED leads to a sustained increase of serum testosterone levels (Jannini *et al.* 1999). The testosterone rise they found was independent of the kind of therapies employed, but strictly related to the successful outcome of therapeutic intervention. Hence, they speculated that sexual inertia resets the reproductive axis to lower activity, somehow inducing a secondary hypogonadism, characterized by reduced LH bioactivity (Carosa *et al.* 2002). Consequently, restoring sex normalizes sex hormones, including bioavailable LH and testosterone (Jannini *et al.* 1999; Carosa *et al.* 2004). However, RCTs are awaited to prove this interesting hypothesis.

12.9 Conclusion

There is clear evidence from experimental studies that testosterone influences erectile function not only indirectly by increased libido, but has direct effects on the penis. Whereas testosterone substitution therapy is effective for treatment of ED in hypogonadal patients, the effects of testosterone on erectile function in normal men seem to be marginal. Recent studies suggest that therapy combining testosterone and phosphodiesterase type 5 inhibitors could be useful in so-called "PDE5i non-responders" with low-normal or subnormal testosterone levels.

12.10 Key messages

- Positive effects of testosterone on erection are mediated by central stimulation of libido and sexual activity, but also by direct effects on the penis.
- Experimental studies suggest that the integrity of the smooth muscles of the penile arteries and the corpora cavernosa, as well as the biological activity of nitric oxide, the predominant cellular transmitter for normal erection, are androgen dependent.
- Impaired erectile function is a classical symptom of hypogonadism. Testosterone therapy of hypogonadal patients significantly improves erectile function. Testosterone not only enhances spontaneous sleep-related erections, but – to a lesser degree – also erectile response.
- In eugonadal men, variations of testosterone levels within the normal range or levels exceeding the upper limit of normal have no or very limited influence on erectile function.
- The true prevalence of testosterone deficiency as a cause for ED is not known, but seems to be less than 20%. Recent consensus statements recommend screening for testosterone deficiency in patients with ED.
- Randomized, placebo-controlled studies indicate that patients with ED and low-normal or subnormal testosterone levels benefit from therapy combining testosterone and phosphodiesterase type 5 inhibitors.
- Preliminary, non-randomized studies suggest that effective therapy of ED increases serum testosterone levels.

12.11 References

Anonymous (1970) Effects of sexual activity on beard growth in man. *Nature* 226:869–870

Aversa A, Isidori AM, Spera G, Lenzi A, Fabbri A (2003) Androgens improve cavernous vasodilation and response to sildenafil in patients with erectile dysfunction. *Clin Endocrinol (Oxf)* 58:632–638

Bancroft J, Wu FC (1983) Changes in erectile responsiveness during androgen replacement therapy. *Arch Sex Behav* 12:59–66

Baskin LS, Sutherland RS, DiSandro MJ, Hayward SW, Lipschutz J, Cunha GR (1997) The effect of testosterone on androgen receptors and human penile growth. *J Urol* 158:1113–1118

Becker AJ, Uckert S, Stief CG, Truss MC, Machtens S, Scheller F, Knapp WH, Hartmann U, Jonas U (2000) Cavernous and systemic testosterone levels in different phases of human penile erection. *Urology* 56:125–129

Becker AJ, Uckert S, Stief CG, Scheller F, Knapp WH, Hartmann U,

Jonas U (2001) Cavernous and systemic testosterone plasma levels during different penile conditions in healthy males and patients with erectile dysfunction. *Urology* 58:435–440

Berridge MJ (2008) Smooth muscle cell calcium activation mechanisms. *J Physiol* 586:5047–5061

Bhasin S, Cunningham GR, Hayes FJ, Matsumoto AM, Snyder PJ, Swerdloff RS, Montori VM; Task Force, Endocrine Society (2010) Testosterone therapy in men with androgen deficiency syndromes: an Endocrine Society clinical practice guideline. *J Clin Endocrinol Metab* 95:2536–2559

Boas M, Boisen KA, Virtanen HE, Kaleva M, Suomi AM, Schmidt IM, Damgaard IN, Kai CM, Chellakooty M, Skakkebaek NE, Toppari J, Main KM (2006) Postnatal penile length and growth rate correlate to serum testosterone levels: a longitudinal study of 1962 normal boys. *Eur J Endocrinol* 154:125–129

Bodie J, Lewis J, Schow D, Monga M (2003) Laboratory evaluations of erectile dysfunction: an evidence based approach. *J Urol* 169:2262–2264

Boloña ER, Uraga MV, Haddad RM, Tracz MJ, Sideras K, Kennedy CC, Caples SM, Erwin PJ, Montori VM (2007) Testosterone use in men with sexual dysfunction: a systematic review and meta-analysis of randomized placebo-controlled trials. *Mayo Clin Proc* 82:20–28

Bond CW, Angeloni NL, Podlasek CA (2010) Analysis of testosterone effects on sonic hedgehog signaling in juvenile, adolescent and adult sprague dawley rat penis. *J Sex Med* 7:1116–1125

Buvat J, Bou Jaoudé G (2006) Significance of hypogonadism in erectile dysfunction: *World J Urol* 24:657–667

Buvat J, Lemaire A (1997) Endocrine screening in 1,022 men with erectile dysfunction: clinical significance and cost-effective strategy. *J Urol* 158:1764–1767

Buvat J, Maggi M, Gooren L, Guay AT, Kaufman J, Morgentaler A, Schulman C, Tan HM, Torres LO, Yassin A, Zitzmann M (2010)

Endocrine aspects of male sexual dysfunctions. *J Sex Med* 7: 1627–1656

Buvat J, Montorsi F, Maggi M, Porst H, Kaipia A, Colson MH, Cuzin B, Moncada I, Martin-Morales A, Yassin A, Meuleman E, Eardley I, Dean JD, Shabsigh R (2011) Hypogonadal men nonresponders to the PDE5 inhibitor tadalafil benefit from normalization of testosterone levels with a 1% hydroalcoholic testosterone gel in the treatment of erectile dysfunction (TADTEST study). *J Sex Med* 8:284–293

Carani C, Granata ARM, Bancroft J, Marrama P (1995) The effects of testosterone replacement on nocturnal penile tumescence and rigidity and erectile response to visual erotic stimuli in hypogonadal men. *Psychoneuroendocrinology* 20:743–753

Carosa E, Benvenga S, Trimarchi F, Lenzi A, Pepe M, Simonelli C, Jannini EA (2002) Sexual inactivity results in reversible reduction of LH bioavailability. *Int J Impot Res* 14:93–99

Carosa E, Martini P, Brandetti F, Di Stasi SM, Lombardo F, Lenzi A, Jannini EA (2004) Type V phosphodiesterase inhibitor treatments for erectile dysfunction increase testosterone levels. *Clin Endocrinol (Oxf)* 61:382–386

Chamness SL, Ricker DD, Crone JK, Dembeck CL, Maguire MP, Burnett AL, Chang TS (1995) The effect of androgen on nitric oxide synthase in the male reproductive tract of the rat. *Fertil Steril* 63:1101–1107

Chatterjee R, Wood S, McGarrigle HH, Lees WR, Ralph DJ, Neild GH (2004) A novel therapy with testosterone and sildenafil for erectile dysfunction in patients on renal dialysis or after renal transplantation. *J Fam Plann Reprod Health Care* 30:88–90

Corona G, Maggi M (2010) The role of testosterone in erectile dysfunction. *Nat Rev Urol* 7:46–56

Corona G, Mannucci E, Mansani R, Petrone L, Giommi R, Mancini M, Bartolini M, Forti G, Maggi M (2004) Aging and pathogenesis of erectile dysfunction. *Int J Impot Res* 16:395–402

Corona G, Fagioli G, Mannucci E, Romeo A, Rossi M, Lotti F, Sforza A, Morittu S, Chiarini V, Casella G, Di Pasquale G, Bandini E, Forti G, Maggi M (2008) Penile Doppler ultrasound in patients with ED: role of peak systolic velocity measured in the flaccid state in predicting arteriogenic ED and silent coronary artery disease. *J Sex Med* 5: 2623–2634

Corona G, Mannucci E, Lotti F, Boddi V, Jannini EA, Fisher AD, Monami M, Sforza A, Forti G, Maggi M (2009) Impairment of couple relationship in male patients with sexual dysfunction is associated with overt hypogonadism. *J Sex Med* 6:2591–2600

Corona G, Lee DM, Forti G, O'Connor DB, Maggi M, O'Neill TW, Pendleton N, Bartfai G, Boonen S, Casanueva FF, Finn JD, Giwercman A, Han TS, Huhtaniemi IT, Kula K, Lean ME, Punab M, Silman AJ, Vanderschueren D, Wu FC; EMAS Study Group (2010a) Age related changes in general and sexual health in middle-aged and older men: results from the European Male Ageing Study (EMAS). *J Sex Med* 7:1362–1380

Corona G, Monami M, Boddi V, Cameron-Smith M, Lotti F, de Vita G, Melani C, Balzi D, Sforza A, Forti G, Mannucci E, Maggi M (2010b) Male sexuality and cardiovascular risk. A cohort study in patients with erectile dysfunction. *J Sex Med* 7:1918–1927

Corona G, Monami M, Boddi V, Cameron-Smith M, Fisher AD, de Vita G, Melani C, Balzi D, Sforza A, Forti G, Mannucci E, Maggi M (2010c) Low testosterone is associated with an increased risk of MACE lethality in subjects with erectile dysfunction. *J Sex Med* 7:1557–1564

Corona G, Rastrelli G, Ricca V, Maggi M (2011a) Testosterone deficiency in the aging male and its relationship with sexual dysfunction and cardiovascular diseases. *Horm Mol Biol Clin Investig* 4:509–520. DOI 10.1515/hmbci.2010.048

Corona G, Rastrelli G, Vignozzi L, Mannucci E, Maggi M (2011b) Testosterone, cardiovascular disease and the metabolic syndrome. *Best Pract Res Clin Endocrinol Metab* 25:337–353

Corona G, Rastrelli G, Monami M, Melani C, Balzi D, Sforza A, Forti G, Mannucci E, Maggi M (2011c) Body mass index regulates hypogonadism-associated CV risk: results from a cohort of subjects with erectile dysfunction. *J Sex Med* 8:2098–2105

Corona G, Rastrelli G, Balercia G, Sforza A, Forti G, Mannucci E, Maggi M (2011d) Perceived reduced sleep-related erections in subjects with erectile dysfunction: psychobiological correlates. *J Sex Med* 8:1780–1788

Cunningham GR, Kracan I, Ware JC, Lantz GD, Thornby JI (1982) The relationships between serum testosterone and prolactin levels and nocturnal penile tumescence (NPT) in impotent men. *J Androl* 3:241–247

Dabbs JM Jr, Mohammed S (1992) Male and female salivary testosterone concentrations before and after sexual activity. *Physiol Behav* 52:195–197

Davidson JM (1986) Androgen replacement therapy in a wider context: clinical and basic aspects. In: Dennerstein L, Fraser I (eds) *Hormones and Behavior*. Elsevier Science Publishers, New York, pp 433–441

Dettenhofer MH (2009) Women, eunuchs and imperial courts. In: Sheidel W (ed) *Rome and China: Comparative Perspectives on Ancient World Empires*. Oxford University Press, Oxford, pp 83–89

Ellis WJ, Grayhack JT (1963) Sexual function in aging males after orchidectomy and estrogen therapy. *J Urol* **89**:895–899

Fabbri A, Jannini EA, Ulisse S, Gnessi L, Moretti C, Frajese G, Isidori A (1988) Low serum bioactive luteinizing hormone in nonorganic male impotence: possible relationship with altered gonadotropin-releasing hormone pulsatility. *J Clin Endocrinol Metab* **67**:867–875

Feldman HA, Goldstein I, Hatzichristou DG, Krane RJ, McKinlay JB (1994) Impotence and its medical and psychosocial correlates: results of the Massachusetts Male Aging Study. *J Urol* **151**:54–61

Filippi S, Vignozzi L, Morelli A, Chavalmane AK, Sarchielli E, Fibbi B, Saad F, Sandner P, Ruggiano P, Vannelli GB, Mannucci E, Maggi M (2009) Testosterone partially ameliorates metabolic profile and erectile responsiveness to PDE5 inhibitors in an animal model of male metabolic syndrome. *J Sex Med* **6**:3274–3288

Fisher AD, Corona G, Bandini E, Mannucci E, Lotti F, Boddi V, Forti G, Maggi M (2009) Psychobiological correlates of extramarital affairs and differences between stable and occasional infidelity among men with sexual dysfunctions. *J Sex Med* **6**:866–875

Foresta C, Caretta N, Rossato M, Garolla A, Ferlin A (2004) Role of androgens in erectile function. *J Urol* **171**:2358–2362

Fox CA, Ismail AA, Love DN, Kirkham KE, Loraine JA (1972) Studies on the relationship between plasma testosterone levels and human sexual activity. *J Endocrinol* **52**:51–58

Garban H, Vernet D, Freedman A, Rajfer J, Gonzalez-Cadavid N (1995a) Effect of aging on nitric oxide-mediated penile erection in rats. *Am J Physiol* **268**:H467–H475

Garban H, Marquez D, Cai L, Rajfer J, Gonzalez-Cadavid NF (1995b) Restoration of normal adult penile erectile response in aged rats by long-term treatment with androgens. *Biol Reprod* **53**:1365–1372

Golden SH, Robinson KA, Saldanha I, Anton B, Ladenson PW (2009) Clinical review: prevalence and incidence of endocrine and metabolic disorders in the United States: a comprehensive review. *J Clin Endocrinol Metab* **94**:1853–1878

Greenstein A, Plymate SR, Katz PG (1995) Visually stimulated erection in castrated men. *J Urol* **153**:650–652

Greenstein A, Mabjeesh NJ, Sofer M, Kaver I, Matzkin H, Chen J (2005) Does sildenafil combined with testosterone gel improve erectile dysfunction in hypogonadal men in whom testosterone supplement therapy alone failed? *J Urol* **173**:530–532

Heim N, Hursch CJ (1979) Castration for sex offenders: treatment or punishment? A review and critique of recent European literature. *Arch Sex Behav* **8**:281–304

Herndon JG, Perachio AA, Turner JJ, Collins DC (1981) Fluctuations in testosterone levels of male rhesus monkeys during copulatory activity. *Physiol Behav* **26**:525–528

Hirshkowitz M, Schmidt MH (2005) Sleep-related erections: clinical perspectives and neural mechanisms. *Sleep Med Rev* **9**:311–329

Hwang TI, Chen HE, Tsai TF, Lin YC (2006) Combined use of androgen and sildenafil for hypogonadal patients unresponsive to sildenafil alone. *Int J Impot Res* **18**:400–404

Isidori AM, Giannetta E, Gianfrilli D, Greco EA, Bonifacio V, Aversa A (2005) Effects of testosterone on sexual function in men: results of a meta-analysis. *Clin Endocrinol (Oxf)* **63**:381–394

Jain P, Rademaker AW, McVary KT (2000) Testosterone supplementation for erectile dysfunction: results of a meta-analysis. *J Urol* **164**:371–375

Jannini EA, Screponi E, Carosa E, Pepe M, Lo Giudice F, Trimarchi F, Benvenga S (1999) Lack of sexual activity from erectile dysfunction is associated with a reversible reduction in serum testosterone. *Int J Androl* **22**:385–392

Kalinchenko SY, Kozlov GI, Gontcharov NP, Katsiya GV (2003) Oral testosterone undecanoate reverses erectile dysfunction associated with diabetes mellitus in patients failing on sildenafil citrate therapy alone. *Aging Male* **6**:94–99

Karacan I, Hirshkowitz K (1991) Aging and sleep apnea in impotent men with arterial risk factors. In: Smirne S, Franceschi M, Ferini-Strambi L (eds) *Sleep and Ageing*. Masson, Milan, pp 135–148

Köhler TS, Kim J, Feia K, Bodie J, Johnson N, Makhlouf A, Monga M (2008) Prevalence of androgen deficiency in men with erectile dysfunction. *Urology* **71**:693–697

Kraemer HC, Becker HB, Brodie HK, Doering CH, Moos RH, Hamburg DA (1976) Orgasmic frequency and plasma testosterone levels in normal human males. *Arch Sex Behav* **5**:125–132

Kwan M, Greenleaf WJ, Mann J, Crapo L, Davidson JM (1983) The nature of androgen action on male sexuality: a combined laboratory-self-report study on hypogonadal men. *Clin Endocrinol Metab* **57**:557–562

LaFerla JJ, Anderson DL, Schalch DS (1978) Psychoendocrine response to sexual arousal in human males. *Psychosom Med* **40**:166–172

Lee PA, Jaffe RB, Midgley AR Jr (1974) Lack of alteration of serum gonadotropins in men and women following sexual intercourse. *Am J Obstet Gynecol* **120**:985–987

Levy JB, Seay TM, Tindall DJ, Husmann DA (1996) The effects of androgen administration on phallic androgen receptor expression. *J Urol* **156**:775–779

Lindau ST, Schumm LP, Laumann EO, Levinson W, O'Muircheartaigh CA, Waite LJ (2007) A study of sexuality and health among older adults in the United States. *New Engl J Med* **357**:762–774

Lugg J, Ng C, Rajfer J, Gonzalez-Cadavid N (1996) Cavernosal nerve stimulation in the rat reverses castration-induced decrease in penile NOS activity. *Am J Physiol* **271**:E354–E361

Lugg JA, Rajfer J, Gonzalez-Cadavid NF (1995) Dihydrotestosterone is the active androgen in the maintenance of nitric oxide-mediated penile erection in the rat. *Endocrinology* **136**:1495–1501

Marin R, Escrig A, Abreu P, Mas M (1999) Androgen-dependent nitric oxide release in rat penis correlates with levels of constitutive nitric oxide synthase isoenzymes. *Biol Reprod* **61**:1012–1016

Mills TM, Wiedmeier VT, Stopper VS (1992) Androgen maintenance of erectile function in the rat penis. *Biol Reprod* **46**:342–348

Montorsi F, Oettel M (2005) Testosterone and sleep-related erections: an overview. *J Sex Med* **2**:771–784

Morelli A, Filippi S, Mancina R, Luconi M, Vignozzi L, Marini M, Orlando C, Vannelli GB, Aversa A, Natali A, Forti G, Giorgi M, Jannini EA, Ledda F, Maggi M (2004) Androgens regulate phosphodiesterase type 5 expression and functional activity in corpora cavernosa. *Endocrinology* **145**:2253–2263

Morelli A, Corona G, Filippi S, Ambrosini S, Forti G, Vignozzi L, Maggi M (2007) Which patients with sexual dysfunction are suitable for testosterone replacement therapy? *J Endocrinol Invest* **30**:880–888

NIH Consensus Conference (1993) Impotence. NIH Consensus Development Panel on Impotence. *JAMA* **270**:83–90

O'Carroll R, Shapiro C, Bancroft J (1985) Androgens, behaviour and nocturnal erection in hypogonadal men: the effects of varying the replacement dose. *Clin Endocrinol (Oxf)* **23**:527–538

Palese MA, Crone JK, Burnett AL (2003) A castrated mouse model of erectile dysfunction. *J Androl* **24**:699–703

Park KH, Kim SW, Kim KD, Paick JS (1999) Effects of androgens on the expression of nitric oxide synthase mRNAs in rat corpus cavernosum. *BJU Int* **83**:327–333

Penson DF, Ng C, Cai L, Rajfer J, Gonzalez-Cadavid NF (1996) Androgen and pituitary control of penile nitric oxide synthase and erectile function in the rat. *Biol Reprod* **55**:567–574

Penson DF, Ng C, Rajfer J, Gonzalez-Cadavid NF (1997) Adrenal control of erectile function and nitric oxide synthase in the rat penis. *Endocrinology* **138**: 3925–3932

Petak SM, Nankin HR, Spark RF, Swerdloff RS, Rodriguez-Rigau LJ; American Association of Clinical Endocrinologists (2002) American Association of Clinical Endocrinologists Medical Guidelines for clinical practice for the evaluation and treatment of hypogonadism in adult male patients – 2002 update. *Endocr Pract* **8**:440–456

Petrone L, Mannucci E, Corona G, Bartolini M, Forti G, Giommi R, Maggi M (2003) Structured interview on erectile dysfunction (SIEDY): a new, multidimensional instrument for quantification of pathogenetic issues on erectile dysfunction. *Int J Impot Res* **15**:210–220

Podlasek CA (2009) Sonic hedgehog, apoptosis, and the penis. *J Sex Med* **6** Suppl 3:334–339

Raboch J, Starka L (1973) Reported coital activity of men and levels of plasma testosterone. *Arch Sex Behav* **2**:309–315

Reilly CM, Zamorano P, Stopper VS, Mills TM (1997) Androgenic regulation of NO availability in rat penile erection. *J Androl* **18**:110–115

Rhoden EL, Telöken C, Sogari PR, Souto CA (2002) The relationship of serum testosterone to erectile function in normal aging men. *J Urol* **167**:1745–1748

Rochira V, Zirilli L, Madeo B, Balestrieri A, Granata AR, Carani C (2003) Sex steroids and sexual desire mechanism. *J Endocrinol Invest* **26**:29–36

Rochira V, Balestrieri A, Madeo B, Granata AR, Carani C (2006) Sildenafil improves sleep-related erections in hypogonadal men: evidence from a randomized, placebo-controlled, crossover study of a synergic role for both testosterone and sildenafil on penile erections. *J Androl* **27**:165–175

Roffwarg HP, Sachar EJ, Halpern F, Hellman L (1982) Plasma testosterone and sleep: relationship to sleep stage variables. *Psychosom Med* **44**:73–84

Rosen R, Altwein J, Boyle P, Kirby RS, Lukacs B, Meuleman E, O'Leary MP, Puppo P, Robertson C, Giuliano F (2003) Lower urinary tract symptoms and male sexual dysfunction: the multinational survey of the aging male (MSAM-7). *Eur Urol* **44**:637–649

Rosen RC, Riley A, Wagner G, Osterloh IH, Kirkpatrick J, Mishra A (1997) The international index of erectile function (IIEF): a multidimensional scale for assessment of erectile dysfunction. *Urology* **49**:822–830

Rosenthal BD, May NR, Metro MJ, Harkaway RC, Ginsberg PC (2006) Adjunctive use of AndroGel (testosterone gel) with sildenafil to treat erectile dysfunction in men with acquired androgen deficiency syndrome after failure using sildenafil alone. *Urology* **67**:571–574

Schirar A, Chang C, Rousseau JP (1997) Localization of androgen receptor in nitric oxide synthase- and vasoactive intestinal peptide-containing neurons of the major pelvic ganglion innervating the rat penis. *J Neuroendocrinol* **9**:141–150

Shabsigh R, Raymond JF, Olsson CA, O'Toole K, Buttyan R (1998) Androgen induction of DNA synthesis in the rat penis. *Urology* **52**:723–728

Shabsigh R, Kaufman JM, Steidle C, Padma-Nathan H (2004) Randomized study of testosterone gel as adjunctive therapy to sildenafil in hypogonadal men with erectile dysfunction who do not respond to sildenafil alone. *J Urol* **172**:658–663

Shamloul R, Ghanem H, Fahmy I, El-Meleigy A, Ashoor S, Elnashaar A, Kamel I (2005) Testosterone therapy can enhance erectile function response to sildenafil in patients with PADAM: a pilot study. *J Sex Med* **2**:559–564

Shen ZJ, Zhou XL, Lu YL, Chen ZD (2003) Effect of androgen deprivation on penile ultrastructure. *Asian J Androl* **5**:33–36

Stearns EL, Winter JS, Faiman C (1973) Effects of coitus on gonadotropin, prolactin and sex steroid levels in man. *J Clin Endocrinol Metab* **37**:687–691

Stoleru SG, Ennaji A, Cournot A, Spira A (1993) LH pulsatile secretion and testosterone blood levels are influenced by sexual arousal in human males. *Psychoneuroendocrinology* **18**:205–218

Takahashi Y, Hirata Y, Yokoyama S, Ishii N, Nunes L, Lue TF, Tanagho EA (1991) Loss of penile erectile response to intracavernous injection of acetylcholine in castrated dog. *Tohoku J Exp Med* **163**:85–91

Tas A, Ersoy A, Ersoy C, Gullulu M, Yurtkuran M (2006) Efficacy of sildenafil in male dialysis patients with erectile dysfunction unresponsive to erythropoietin and/ or testosterone treatments. *Int J Impot Res* **18**:61–68

Traish AM (2009) Androgens play a pivotal role in maintaining penile tissue architecture and erection: a review. *J Androl* **30**:363–369

Traish AM, Park K, Dhir V, Kim NN, Moreland RB, Goldstein I (1999) Effects of castration and androgen replacement on erectile function in a rabbit model. *Endocrinology* **140**:1861–1868

Traish AM, Munarriz R, O'Connell L, Choi S, Kim SW, Kim NN, Huang YH, Goldstein I (2003) Effects of medical or surgical castration on erectile function in an animal model. *J Androl* **24**:381–387

Traish AM, Toselli P, Jeong SJ, Kim NN (2005) Adipocyte accumulation in penile corpus cavernosum of the orchiectomized rabbit: a potential mechanism for veno-occlusive dysfunction in androgen deficiency. *J Androl* **26**:242–248

Tsertsvadze A, Fink HA, Yazdi F, MacDonald R, Bella AJ, Ansari MT, Garritty C, Soares-Weiser K, Daniel R, Sampson M, Fox S, Moher D, Wilt TJ (2009) Oral phosphodiesterase-5 inhibitors and hormonal treatments for erectile dysfunction: a systematic review and meta-analysis. *Ann Intern Med* **151**:650–661

van Anders SM, Hamilton LD, Watson NV (2007) Multiple partners are associated with higher testosterone in North American men and women. *Horm Behav* **51**:454–459

Vernet D, Cai L, Garban H, Babbitt ML, Murray FT, Rajfer J, Gonzalez-Cadavid NF (1995) Reduction of penile nitric oxide synthase in diabetic BB/WORdp (type I) and BBZ/WORdp (type II) rats with erectile dysfunction. *Endocrinology* **136**:5709–5717

Vignozzi L, Corona G, Petrone L, Filippi S, Morelli AM, Forti G, Maggi M (2005) Testosterone and sexual activity. *J Endocrinol Invest* **28**:39–44

Vignozzi L, Morelli A, Filippi S, Ambrosini S, Mancina R, Luconi M, Mungai S, Vannelli GB, Zhang XH, Forti G, Maggi M (2007) Testosterone regulates RhoA/Rho-kinase signaling in two distinct animal models of chemical diabetes. *J Sex Med* **4**:620–630

Vignozzi L, Filippi S, Morelli A, Marini M, Chavalmane A, Fibbi B, Silvestrini E, Mancina R, Carini M, Vannelli GB, Forti G, Maggi M (2009) Cavernous neurotomy in the rat is associated with the onset of an overt condition of hypogonadism. *J Sex Med* **6**:1270–1283

Wang C, Nieschlag E, Swerdloff R, Behre HM, Hellstrom WJ, Gooren LJ, Kaufman JM, Legros JJ, Lunenfeld B, Morales A, Morley JE, Schulman C, Thompson IM, Weidner W, Wu FC; International Society of Andrology; International Society for the Study of Aging Male; European Association of Urology; European Academy of Andrology; American Society of Andrology (2009) Investigation, treatment, and monitoring of late-onset hypogonadism in males: ISA, ISSAM, EAU, EAA, and ASA recommendations. *Eur Urol* **55**:121–130

Wingard CJ, Johnson JA, Holmes A, Prikosh A (2003) Improved erectile function after Rho-kinase inhibition in a rat castrate model of erectile dysfunction. *Am J Physiol Regul Integr Comp Physiol* **284**:R1572–R1579

Wu FC, Tajar A, Pye SR, Silman AJ, Finn JD, O'Neill TW, Bartfai G, Casanueva F, Forti G, Giwercman A, Huhtaniemi IT, Kula K, Punab M, Boonen S, Vanderschueren D; European Male Aging Study Group (2008) Hypothalamic-pituitary-testicular axis disruptions in older men are differentially linked to age and modifiable risk factors: the European Male Aging Study. *J Clin Endocrinol and Metab* **93**:2737–2745

Wu FC, Tajar A, Beynon JM, Pye SR, Silman AJ, Finn JD, O'Neill TW, Bartfai G, Casanueva FF, Forti G, Giwercman A, Han TS, Kula K, Lean ME, Pendleton N, Punab M, Boonen S, Vanderschueren D, Labrie F, Huhtaniemi IT; EMAS Group (2010) Identification of late-onset hypogonadism in middle-aged and elderly men. *N Engl J Med* **363**:123–135

Yassin AA, Saad F (2008) Testosterone and erectile dysfunction. *J Androl* **29**:593–604

Yassin AA, Saad F, Diede HE (2006) Testosterone and erectile function in hypogonadal men unresponsive to tadalafil: results from an open-label uncontrolled study. *Andrologia* **38**:61–68

Zhang MG, Shen ZJ, Zhang CM, Wu W, Gao PJ, Chen SW, Zhou WL (2011) Vasoactive intestinal polypeptide, an erectile neurotransmitter, improves erectile function more significantly in castrated rats than in normal rats. *BJU* **108**:440–446

Zhang XH, Hu LQ, Zheng XM, Li SW (1999) Apoptosis in rat erectile tissue induced by castration. *Asian J Androl* **1**:181–185

Zhang XH, Morelli A, Luconi M, Vignozzi L, Filippi S, Marini M, Vannelli GB, Mancina R, Forti G, Maggi M (2005) Testosterone regulates PDE5 expression and in vivo responsiveness to tadalafil in rat corpus cavernosum. *Eur Urol* **47**:409–416

Zhang XH, Filippi S, Morelli A, Vignozzi L, Luconi M, Donati S, Forti G, Maggi M (2006) Testosterone restores diabetes-induced erectile dysfunction and sildenafil responsiveness in two distinct animal models of chemical diabetes. *J Sex Med* **3**:253–264

Chapter 13

Testosterone and the prostate

John T. Isaacs and Samuel R. Denmeade

13.1 Introduction

During evolution, mammals developed accessory sex glands, which in males of the species are named either for their anatomical position in adult animals or for their assumed functions (Price and Williams-Ashman 1961). The only gland present in all orders of male mammals, even the egg-laying monotremes, is the prostate. The term "prostate" has an interesting but confusing history which has been extensively reviewed by Marx and Karenberg (2009). According to these authors, in ancient Greek the masculine term "*prostatēs*" literally meant "someone who stands before someone or something" and is the origin of the term "president" or "principal." This term, however, was never used in ancient Greece in a medical sense. It was not until the Renaissance that anatomists discovered the prostate, initially naming it the "glandulous body." In 1600 the French physician du Laurens introduced the metaphoric denomination

"*prostatae*." However, he and his contemporaries misinterpreted the history of the organ and the term, chose the wrong gender when translating it into Latin, and believed that it designated a double organ. Only in the 1800s was this anatomical error corrected, while the grammatical one lived on in the term "prostate."

Thus, the gland that in male mammals "stands before" the base of the bladder and produces and releases secretion into the male ejaculate is defined as the prostate. In most male mammals, there are additional glands that likewise release excretion into the ejaculate, and these glands are given a variety of names depending on the species. In humans, the male accessory sex tissues consist of the prostate including the periurethral glands (aka glands of Littre), seminal vesicles, and bulbourethral glands (Cowper's glands) (Fig. 13.1). Although it is believed that the prostate is important in protecting the lower urinary tract from

Testosterone: Action, Deficiency, Substitution, ed. Eberhard Nieschlag and Hermann M. Behre, Assoc. ed. Susan Nieschlag.
Published by Cambridge University Press. © Cambridge University Press 2012.

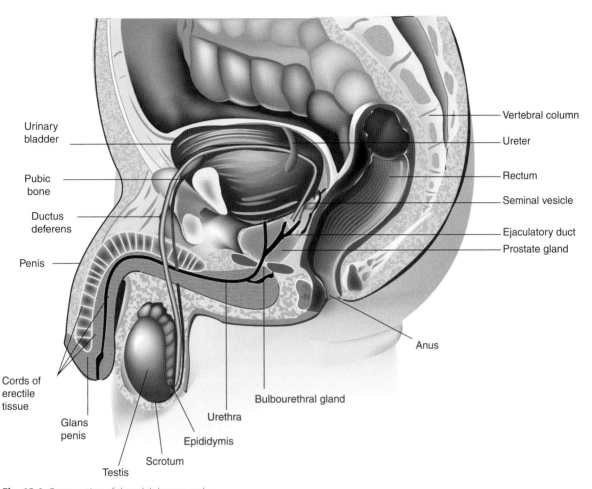

Urinary bladder

Pubic bone

Ductus deferens

Penis

Cords of erectile tissue

Glans penis

Testis

Scrotum

Epididymis

Urethra

Bulbourethral gland

Anus

Vertebral column

Ureter

Rectum

Seminal vesicle

Ejaculatory duct

Prostate gland

Fig. 13.1 Cross-section of the adult human male.

infection and for fertility, it is frequently the site of infection and inflammation, and sperm harvested from the epididymis without exposure to seminal or prostatic fluid can produce fertilization and successful birth (Silver *et al.* 1988). Thus, the prostate makes nothing that is absolutely required for male fertility.

The fact that the specific function of the prostate is not fully understood might not be so problematic if it were not the case that the prostate is the most common site of neoplastic transformation in men, with nearly one million men dying of prostate cancer globally each year (Jemal *et al.* 2011). Furthermore, the prostate is the most common site of benign neoplastic disease in males (Berry *et al.* 1984). More than 50% of all men above the age of 50 have benign prostatic hyperplasia (BPH), with 25% of men eventually requiring treatment for this condition (Berry *et al.* 1984). Thus, it is remarkable that, despite the high prevalence of

prostatic diseases, the etiologies of neither prostatic cancer nor BPH are known. A major reason why both the specific function of the prostate and etiology of the prostatic neoplasms have been difficult to elucidate is that the gross structure and histological appearance of this gland vary widely in the animal kingdom, and thus comparative animal studies have been problematic.

In fact, no organ system varies so widely among the animal species as the male sex accessory tissues (Price and Williams-Ashman 1961) (Fig. 13.2). In contrast to humans, rats and mice have a prostate that is composed of four anatomically and biochemically distinct prostatic lobes (i.e. the ventral, dorsal, lateral and anterior lobes: the last of these also called the coagulating gland). In addition, these species have seminal vesicles and preputial glands. Many species (e.g. primates (monkeys) and marsupials like opossum) have a segmented prostate and seminal vesicles (Fig. 13.2). Bulls have very small prostates and

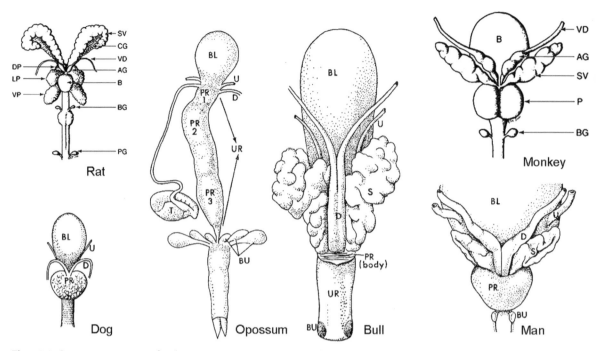

Fig. 13.2 Comparative anatomy of male accessory sex tissue in a series of mammals (rat, opossum, bull, dog, monkey and man). Abbreviations: BL or B, bladder; U or UR, urethra; P or PR or PG, prostate; S or SV, seminal vesicle; BU or BG, bulbourethral gland; D or AG, ampulla of ductus (vas) differens; T, testis; CG, coagulating gland (aka anterior prostate lobe); VP, ventral prostate lobe; LP, later prostate lobe; DP, dorsal prostate lobe; VD, vas deferens.

large seminal vesicles (Fig. 13.2). The normal human prostate is not composed of anatomically separate or segmented lobes as in many animals, but is instead divided into four zones (Fig. 13.3). The peripheral zone comprises 70 to 75% of the gland, the central zone 20 to 25%, and the transitional zone 5%, while the anterior surface consists of the fibromuscular stroma (McNeal *et al.* 1988). Most cancers develop in the peripheral zone. Benign prostatic hyperplasia develops in the transitional zone as a part of the aging process. In contrast, the dog has a well-developed prostate which has no zonal anatomy and completely lacks seminal vesicles (Fig. 13.2). Importantly, the dog is the only species other than man which spontaneously develops both BPH and prostatic cancer with aging (Isaacs 1984). Besides this anatomical variation, there is a large variation among the different species in the secretory products produced and released by the prostate into the ejaculate (Mann and Mann 1981).

For example, the human prostatic epithelial cells synthesize and secrete a series of unique proteins into the ejaculate (Coffey 1992). These include serine protease, PSA, human glandular kallikrein-2 (HK2) and prostatic-specific acid phosphatase. The essentially exclusive production of these proteins by normal and malignant prostatic cells has allowed the abnormal detection of these proteins in the serum of men to be useful as a means of (1) initially detecting prostatic cancer in asymptomatic men, (2) monitoring residual presence of systemic micrometastatic disease in men who have undergone radical prostatectomy for presumed localized disease, and (3) monitoring the response of clinically detected metastatic disease to systemic therapy. Although other animal species synthesize prostate-specific proteins (e.g. prostatein and probasin in the rat and the arginine esterase in the dog), there are no genes directly homologous to PSA or HK2, based on DNA sequence, in the dog or rat genome (Olsson *et al.* 2004). There is a homologous prostatic-specific acid phosphatase gene in the rat; however, the level of expression is nearly 1000-fold lower in rat versus human prostate epithelial cells (Coffey 1992).

13.2 Evolutionary selection of testosterone as master regulator of male reproduction

Based on such varied anatomy and biochemistry, it has been difficult to utilize animal models to define

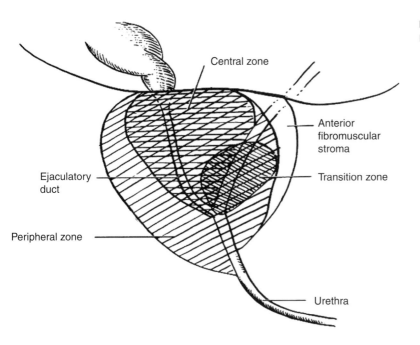

Fig. 13.3 Zonal anatomy of the human prostate.

the etiology of either BPH or prostatic cancer. It is known, however, that during mammalian evolution, testosterone was selected as the master regulator for the embryonic development and postnatal growth and maintenance of the prostate and the other male accessory sex tissues, as well as spermatogenesis, bone and muscle maturation and libido. Why testosterone was selected during mammalian evolution as the master regulator for male physiology and reproduction is not fully known. It is known that during evolution, all the members of the steroid receptors (i.e. estrogen (ERα and ERβ), mineralocorticoid (MR), glucocorticoid (GR), progesterone (PR), and androgen (AR)) descended from a single ancestral receptor which branched off from the rest of the nuclear receptor (NR) superfamily early in animal evolution (Eick and Thornton 2011). The similarity of all the invertebrate receptor sequences to the vertebrate ERs suggests that the ancestral steroid receptor protein was likely to have been ER-like in both sequence and in function, and that the other steroid receptors proliferated and diversified through a series of its gene duplications. Phylogenetic studies have documented that the enzymes of estrogen synthesis, which converts cholesterol to progesterone to testosterone to estrogen, co-evolved with the ER receptors and were present before the evolution of the steroid receptors sensitive to these latter two steroids (Eick and

Thornton 2011). In fact, the presence of testosterone may have been an important driving factor for the development of the AR, which is the last of the steroid receptors to have evolved (Eick and Thornton 2011).

Another driving factor involved in the selective pressure for testosterone becoming the master regulator of reproduction during evolution relates to the unique danger of reproduction in mammals. During mammalian evolution, breeding became episodically timed for optimal survival of both parents and offspring. Thus, as well as reduced sexual libido and sperm maturation, the male accessory sex glands are atrophic during the seasonal period when breeding is not optimal. When environmental conditions (i.e. food/temperature/light etc.) are appropriate, male mammals come into "breeding season." Such seasonal breeding has great reproductive advantage and was selected during evolution to restrict the energy requirements for maintaining male accessory sex glands, sperm maturation, and sexual libido, thus limiting the dangers associated with the maniacal focus upon procreation at the expense of self-survival (i.e. suppression of normal flight instinct in the presence of predators) to the minimal time frame of the breeding season. Since the breeding season for many mammals is short, evolutionary pressure drove development of a neuroendocrine (i.e. pineal gland-hypothalamic-pituitary) axis to restrict high

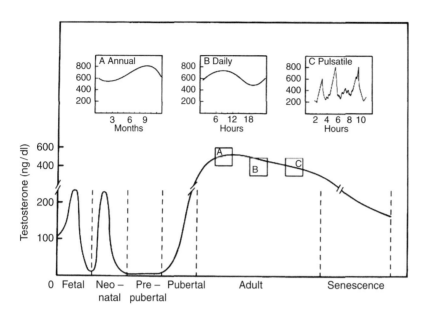

Fig. 13.4 Serum testosterone levels during various stages of development and aging in human males.

production and secretion of testosterone into the circulation by the testes to only the breeding season.

Coincident with the evolution of seasonal breeding, there was also selective pressure to develop a mechanism for the rise of testosterone to rapidly induce sexual libido, sperm maturation and full growth of the atrophic male accessory sex tissues needed for reproduction during the short breeding season. Thus during evolutionary selection of testosterone as the master regulator of seasonal male reproduction, there was co-selection of enzymes needed to regulate intracellular ligand and the AR needed to generate intracellular signaling induced by its ligand binding (Eick and Thornton 2011). In contrast with the other mammals, human males eventually evolved away from strict seasonal breeding and acquired the ability to sustain serum testosterone at a sufficiently high chronic level to maintain the male accessory sex glands, spermatogenesis and libido in a fully developed adult state so that fertility is constant. Such constant fertility is a definitive advantage for the highly mobile human species. This is because it enables reproduction to occur despite environment restrictions, allowing man to populate all of the biological niches throughout the world as opposed to "locking" the species to specific indigenous breeding ranges, like other mammals. Apparently, the price of such reproductive "freedom," however, is the acquisition of BPH and prostate cancer by the human male.

13.3 Role of testosterone in the development and maintenance of the human prostate

The urogenital sinus derived from the endoderm layer is the embryonic anlagen from which the prostate develops in utero. For the human prostate to develop normally, a critical level of androgenic stimulation is required at specific times during its development in utero (Wilson 1984). In the developing male, the fetal testis secretes testosterone into the fetal circulation at levels sufficient to stimulate the differentiation and growth of a portion of the urogenital sinus tissue, producing the definitive prostate gland. In humans, this begins during the first three months of fetal growth and remains high until the last months of pregnancy (Fig. 13.4). If sufficient serum testosterone is not present at this critical state of intrauterine development, the prostate does not develop (Wilson 1984).

During the first several months after birth, serum testosterone again rises before decreasing to a low baseline value (Fig. 13.4). This neonatal spike in serum testosterone is critical for "male imprinting" of the hypothalamic-pituitary-testicular axis begun during embryonic development (Gorski 2002; Grumbach 2002). After this neonatal period, serum testosterone remains low in humans until puberty when levels rise to the adult range (Frasier *et al.* 1969) (Fig. 13.4). Until puberty, the human prostate remains small (approximately <2 g; Isaacs 1984). During puberty, the human prostate grows to its adult size of approximately 20 g (Isaacs 1984). Between the age of 10 and 20 years, the rate of prostatic growth is exponential, with a prostatic weight-doubling time of ~3 years (Isaacs 1984). This period of exponential growth corresponds to the time period when the serum testosterone level is rising from initially low levels seen before the age of 10 to the high levels seen in an adult human male (Frasier *et al.* 1969; Fig. 13.4). If a boy is castrated before the age of 10, the serum testosterone levels do not rise to their normal adult level, and the proliferative growth of the human prostate between 10 and 20 years of life is completely blocked (Moore 1944; Huggins and Johnson 1947). These results demonstrate that a physiological level of testosterone is chronically required for the normal growth of the human prostate. This chronic requirement for testosterone derives from the necessity for androgens to regulate the total prostatic cell number by affecting both the rate of cell proliferation and of cell death. Androgen does this by stimulating the rate of cell proliferation (i.e. agonistic ability of androgen) while simultaneously inhibiting the rate of cell death (antagonistic ability of androgen) (Kyprianou and Isaacs 1988). Because of this dual agonist/antagonist effect of androgen on the prostate, the rate of cell proliferation is greater than the rate of cell death during the normal prostatic growth period occurring between 10 and 20 years of age. Having reached its maximum adult size by 20 years of age, the prostate normally ceases its continuous net growth (Isaacs 1984). This does not mean, however, that the cells of the adult prostate in men over 20 years of age do not continuously turn over with time, but that the rate of prostatic cell proliferation is balanced by an equal rate of prostatic cell death, such that neither involution nor overgrowth of the gland normally occurs with time. Thus the adult prostate in men over 20 is an example of a steady-state self-renewing tissue. If an adult male whose prostate is in this steady-state maintenance condition is castrated, serum testosterone levels rapidly decrease to low values comparable to those seen in males younger than 10 years of age. As a result, the prostate rapidly involutes (Peters and Walsh 1987). Such involution demonstrates that a physiological level of testosterone is chronically required, not only for initial development, but also for maintenance of the normal prostate. To define the molecular

mechanisms responsible for how testosterone stimulates such developmental and growth effects, an understanding of its metabolism and the role of the AR as an integrator of intracellular androgen signaling is required.

13.4 Testosterone metabolism in the prostate

The hypothalamic-pituitary-testicular axis regulates the serum level of testosterone via a series of feedback loops resulting in the testes secreting into the blood 6 mg of testosterone per day (Coffey 1992). In the serum, the total testosterone is ~ 20 nM, with 98% of the testosterone bound to a series of high-affinity (i.e. testosterone binding protein (TeBG)) or low-affinity (i.e. albumin) binding proteins. The 2% non-protein bound (i.e. "free testosterone") level is ~0.4 nM, and it is this "free testosterone" which is able to diffuse from the blood into the extracellular fluid of the prostatic stromal compartment into the prostate epithelial cells (Coffey 1992). Within these epithelial cells, testosterone is enzymatically converted to 5α-dihydrotestosterone (Bruchovsky and Wilson 1968). The enzymes responsible for the irreversible conversion of testosterone to DHT are the membrane-bound NADPH-dependent Δ4-3-ketosteroid 5α-oxidoreductases (i.e. SRD5A, aka 5α-reductases) (Fig. 13.5; Bruchovsky and Wilson 1968). Phylogenetic analysis of proteins with a steroid 5α-reductase domain from multiple species indicates that this SRD5A family can be separated in to three main groups consisting of: (1) the SRD5A1-SRD5A2 group; (2) the SRD5A3 group containing the human ortholog to the yeast DFG10 gene; and (3) the GPSN2-SRD5A2L2 group, supporting the idea that different classes of lipids can be substrates for these enzymes and suggesting that the substrate of the enzyme encoded by the common ancestral gene was potentially not a steroid (Cantagrel *et al.* 2010).

Within the prostate, SRD5A1–3 isoforms are expressed. Each of the isozymes has been cloned and the complete DNA-based sequence and amino acid composition are known (Andersson and Russell 1990; Jenkins *et al.* 1991; Labrie *et al.* 1992; Thigpen *et al.* 1992; Uemura *et al.* 2008). The genes encoding the proteins for all of the SRD5A isozymes have a similar structure containing five exons separated by four introns. The three genes share approximately 46% sequence homology and encode for a protein of 29 000 kDa molecular weight. The SRD5A1 isozyme is

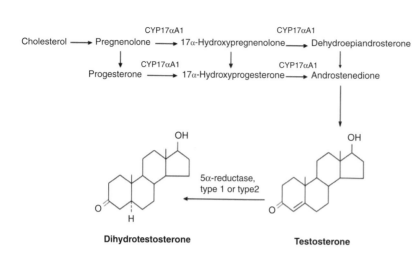

Fig. 13.5 Overview of the metabolic pathway for conversion of cholesterol to testosterone, indicating the role of CYP17A1 in this conversion and the 5α-reductase-catalyzed conversion to DHT.

encoded by a gene on human chromosome 5p15 (Jenkins *et al.* 1991). It has a neutral pH optimum, a requirement for high concentration of testosterone to saturate the enzyme (high K_m = 3 µM), and is rather insensitive to finasteride inhibition (K_i ~ 300 nM) (Andersson and Russell 1990; Jenkins *et al.* 1991). The type 1 isozyme is expressed at low levels by the prostate basal epithelial cells and is the predominant 5α-reductase isozyme in skin; it is also present in the liver (Jenkins *et al.* 1992; Normington and Russell 1992; Berman and Russell 1993).

The SRD5A2 isozyme is encoded by a gene on human chromosome 2p23 (Thigpen *et al.* 1992). It has an acidic (pH 5.0) optimum and has a lower K_m (0.5 µM) for testosterone. The SRD5A2 isozyme is the predominant 5α-reductase in androgen target tissue, including the prostate, where it is expressed in the stromal cells (Berman and Russell 1993; Bayne *et al.* 1998). Analysis of individuals with male pseudo-hermaphroditism caused by 5α-reductase deficiency has revealed no mutation in the type 1 isozyme gene (Jenkins *et al.* 1992). In contrast, molecular analysis demonstrated that mutation in the SRD5A2 gene accounts for this disorder (Thigpen *et al.* 1992). Based on these results, it has been suggested that the SRD5A1 isozyme functions in a catabolic manner in the metabolic removal of androgens by non-target tissue, whereas SRD5A2 isozyme functions in an anabolic role to amplify the androgenicity of testosterone by effectively converting it to DHT within androgen target tissue (Normington and Russell 1992). The SRD5A3 isoform is encoded by a gene on human chromosome 4q12 (Cantagrel *et al.* 2010) and is normally expressed in prostate basal, but not

secretory/luminal epithelial cells or prostate stromal cells (Godoy *et al.* 2011). While SRD5A3 can reduce testosterone to DHT, its major normal function appears to be in anabolic metabolism, where it reduces the isoprene unit of polyprenols to form dolichols, required for synthesis of dolichol-linked monosaccharides, and the oligosaccharide precursor used for N-glycosylation (Cantagrel *et al.* 2010).

Once formed via the 5-reductase, DHT can reversibly bind to the AR, which will be discussed in the next section, to regulate prostatic cellular proliferation and survival. Alternatively, DHT can be further reductively metabolized to 5x-androstane-3,17-diol (3α-diol) by the 3α-hydroxysteroid dehydrogenase type 3 isozyme (i.e. 3α-HSD type 3 enzyme, aka AKR1C2) (Rizner *et al.* 2003; Fig. 13.6). Once formed, 3α-diol can he re-oxidized back to DHT via an oxidative 3α-HSD enzyme not fully characterized in the normal prostate, or glucuronidated at position 3 and excreted by the prostate (Rizner *et al.* 2003). 3α-Diol can also be oxidized at its l7β-hydroxy position by 17β-HSD type 2 or type 6 isozymes to form 5α-androsterone, or can also be glucuronidated at position 3 and excreted (Biswas and Russell 1997; Rizner *et al.* 2003; Fig. 13.6). Dihydrotestosterone can also be either oxidatively metabolized at its l7β-hydroxy group by the 17β-HSD type 2 isozyme to form 5α-androstane-3,17-dione (Rizner *et al.* 2003), or reductively metabolized at its 3-keto group to produce 5α-androstane-3,17β-diol (3β-diol) by l7β-HSD type 7 isozyme (Torn *et al.* 2003; Fig. 13.6). Interestingly, it has been documented that the endogenous estrogen in the prostate is not l7β-estradiol but 3β-diol (Weihua *et al.* 2001). Also it has been documented

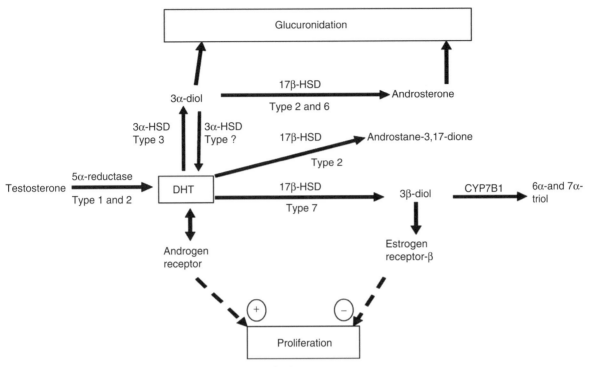

Fig. 13.6 Summary of enzymatic pathway of androgen within the human prostate.

that, within the normal prostate, both the isoforms of the estrogen receptor (i.e. ERα and ERβ) are expressed and both bind 3β-diol (Weihua *et al.* 2001). The ERα is expressed predominately in the prostatic stromal cells, while ERβ is expressed in the epithelial cells (Fixemer *et al.* 2003). The Gustafsson group which initially discovered ERβ has postulated that 3β-diol binding to the ERβ within prostatic epithelial cells results in antagonism of the AR signaling for epithelial cell proliferation (Weihua *et al.* 2002). The level of such an ER-dependent anti-proliferative effect is thus dependent upon the level of 3β-diol. This 3β-diol level is itself regulated by the activity of the CYP7B1 enzyme which hydroxylates 3β-diol to 5α-androstane-3β,6α,17β-triol (6α-triol) and 5α-androstane-3β,7α,17β-triol (7α-triol) (Isaacs *et al.* 1979; Weihua *et al.* 2002; Fig 13.6).

13.5 Androgen receptor as integrator of androgen signaling in the prostate

Androgen receptor is the integrator of androgen signaling in the prostate, as documented by the fact that germline truncation mutations early in the first exon of the gene preventing expression of AR result in complete androgen insensitivity syndrome and no prostate develops (Gottlieb *et al.* 1999). AR is a ligand-dependent zinc finger DNA-binding protein whose genomic binding coordinates formation of transcriptional complexes at the regulatory elements of targeted genes. The *AR* gene is located on the long arm of the X chromosome (*i.e.* Xq11.2) and encodes a protein with three critical domains: (1) an N-terminal domain involved in homotypic dimerization and binding with other transcriptional coactivator or co-repressor proteins; (2) a DNA-binding domain with two zinc finger binding motifs and hinge region; and (3) a C-terminal steroid LBD, which is also involved in homotypic dimerization and coactivation binding (Dehm and Tindall 2007; Fig. 13.7). This C-terminal LBD is also where 90 kDa heat shock protein (*i.e.* HSP90) dimers bind to stabilize the AR protein during its folding, subsequent to its synthesis. Specific interaction with androgenic ligands results in the conformational activation of AR. This allows the dissociation of the HSP90 dimer proteins and thus the binding and dimerization of the occupied AR to AREs present in the promoter and enhancer regions in AR-regulated genes (Fig. 13.8; Wang *et al.* 2005). This initial genomic AR binding allows further binding

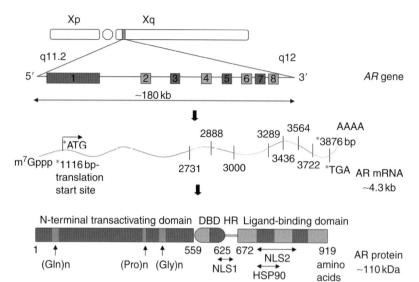

Fig. 13.7 Organization of the *AR* gene, mRNA and protein. AR is coded by a 180 kb gene located on the long arm of the X chromosome (i.e. 11q11.2) and, hence, is present as a single gene copy per cell. Upper panel indicates the position of the 8 exons of *AR* gene mRNA; middle panel indicates which exon encodes which base pairs (bp) in mRNA; and the lower panel aligns the individual exons with the encode portion of the AR protein.

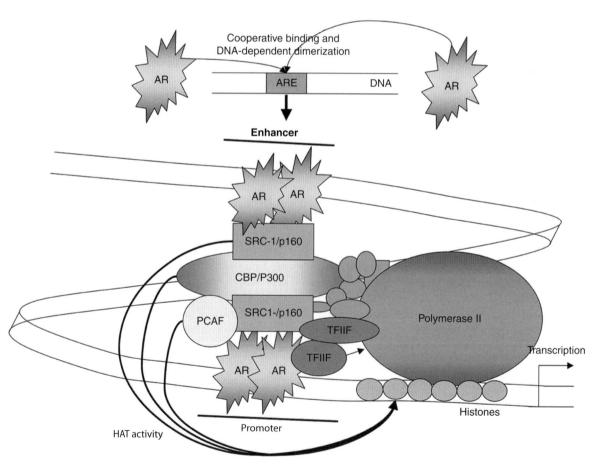

Fig. 13.8 Overview of transcriptional complex organized by AR at the ARE of the promoter/enhancer region of the PSA gene. The AR assembles a transcription initiation complex on the promoter/enhancer regions of androgen-regulated genes like PSA. Ligand-bound AR undergoes a DNA-dependent dimerization in the nucleus and recruits a number of transcription factors that acetylate histones, recruit additional transcription factors and DNA polymerase, and initiate transcription of the target gene.

to specific regions of the bound AR by additional nuclear proteins (i.e. transcriptional coactivator proteins like SRC-1, ARA 70, etc., and general transcription factors like TFII H and F) to produce transcriptional complexes that can activate or repress specific gene expression. For activation, formation of an active transcriptional complex is required, resulting in site-directed chromatin remodeling via histone acetylation and methylation that enhances target gene expression (Fig. 13.8). SRC-1 is a member of the p160 transcriptional coactivator gene family that includes *SRC-1, TIF2* (also termed *GRIP-1* and *SRC-2*), and *p/CIP* (also termed *RAC3, ACTR, AIBI* and *SRC-3*). Cell-free in-vitro transcription and in-vivo experiments have indicated that the SRC-1 family members enhance AR-dependent transactivation of nuclear genes; the mechanism for such enhancement involves binding of p160 proteins to the DNA-bound AR (Fig. 13.8). This allows the p160 to acetylate histones via its histone acetyltransferase (HAT) activity. Additional coactivators with histone acetyltransferase activity such as CBP, p300 or p/CAF also bind to the p160/AR complex. This results in chromatin remodeling and additional binding of general transcription factors such as TFIIH and TFIIF with the AR coactivation complexes (Litvinov *et al.* 2003; Dehm and Tindall 2007; Fig. 13.8).

Both testosterone and DHT can bind to AR; however, within the prostate, the metabolic pathways described in Fig. 13.6 are regulated so that DHT is present at a fivefold molar excess compared to testosterone (i.e. 10 nM for DHT vs. 2.0 nM for testosterone; Page *et al.* 2011). In addition, DHT has nearly a 10-fold higher AR binding affinity than testosterone (i.e. K_d of ~0.1 nM for DHT vs. ~1.0 nM for testosterone) (Litvinov *et al.* 2003). Thus, with regard to prostate physiology, testosterone is actually a "prohormone," with DHT being the active intracellular androgenic hormone. The extensive metabolic pathway for androgen within the prostate (Fig. 13.6) functions as a means for autoregulation, so that the prostatic level of DHT remains constant despite fluctuations in serum testosterone. This is significant since there are episodic and diurnal variations in both total and free serum testosterone levels in humans (Plymate *et al.* 1989; Fig. 13.3). Because growth versus regression (i.e. death) of the prostate epithelial cells is determined by the specific level of prostatic DHT (Kyprianou and Isaacs 1987), a constant prostatic DHT level is critically required for the dose-dependent ability of DHT to bind to

and regulate the function of the AR (Liao et *al.* 1972; Dehm and Tindall 2007).

13.6 Mechanism of androgen action in the prostate

To understand the mechanism for AR-dependent signaling in prostate, an understanding of the two phases of the development of the prostate is needed. The first ontogeny phase is initiated during embryonic life and continues into the early neonate period. During embryonic life, the prostate develops from the endodermal derived UGS anlagen in males under the stimulation of systemic androgen from the testes (Fig. 13.3). Such ontogeny requires reciprocal paracrine interactions between UGS stromal cells and UGS epithelial cells, driven by a critical level of circulating androgen (Fig. 13.9). Prostate ontogeny is initiated by an epithelial-to-stroma paracrine interaction permanently committing UGS mesenchymal stem cells denoted no. 1 (Fig. 13.9), to producing a subset of differentiated progeny denoted no. 2 (Fig. 13.9), which mature into smooth muscle cells (SMC) denoted no. 3 (Fig. 13.9), expressing both SRD5A2 enzyme and AR protein (Isaacs 2008).

The commitment of UGS stromal stem cells to produce SMC expressing both of these proteins is dependent upon paracrine factors (i.e. Sonic hedgehog, etc.) secreted by ectoderm UGS epithelial cells denoted no. 4 (Fig. 13.9) (Isaacs 2008). This induction is mandatory since genetically inherited defects in either SRD5A2 or AR prevent prostate development (Litvinov *et al.* 2003). This is because expression of SRD5A2 by these SMC allows them to irreversibly convert testosterone to DHT. Dihydrotestosterone is 10 times more potent than testosterone in its ability to stimulate AR-dependent transcription (Litvinov *et al.* 2003). Thus, this 5α-reductase activity amplifies the low levels of circulating androgen secreted by the embryonic testes to produce a sufficient level of DHT to bind and activate AR signaling in these SMC, denoted no. 5 (Fig. 13.9). This AR signaling stimulates synthesis and secretion of soluble paracrine and autocrine growth factors (GF) and survival factors (SF), termed andromedins (e.g. IGF-1, FGF-7 and-10, and VEGF) by these SMC, denoted no. 6 (Fig. 13.9). Once secreted by the SMC, andromedins diffuse and bind to their cognate receptors on specific cell types. Within the stromal compartment, such andromedin binding stimulates myogenesis, denoted

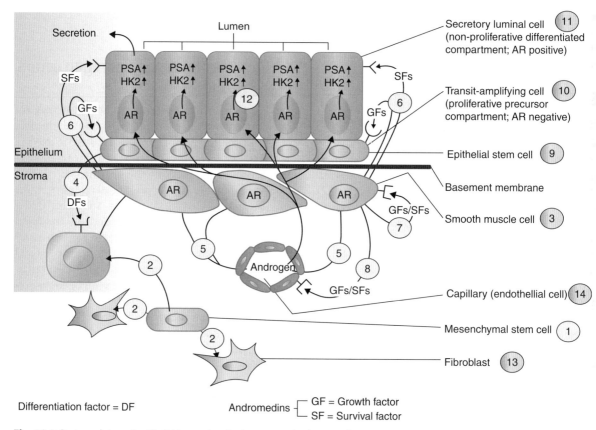

Fig. 13.9 Reciprocal stromal epithelial interactions in the prostate. In the normal prostate, growth and maintenance of prostatic epithelium depends on paracrine signaling of andromedins (growth and survival factors) produced by supporting stromal cells (smooth muscle and fibroblasts). Andromedins are secreted due to androgen signaling through AR, a nuclear hormone receptor expressed by prostate luminal epithelia but not by basal epithelia. Details for the specific numbers are provided in the text.

no. 7 (Fig. 13.9), and vasculogenesis, denoted no. 8 (Fig. 13.9). Within the epithelial compartment, andromedins stimulate epithelium to mature from medullary cords of undifferentiated epithelium which contain epithelial stem cells, denoted no. 9 (Fig. 13.9), with no canalization, into a simple, stratified, glandular epithelium composed of a basal layer of cuboidal cells denoted no. 10 (Fig. 13.9), upon which resides a second layer of columnar secretory luminal cells denoted no. 11(Fig. 13.9), adjacent to a patent lumen (Isaacs 2008).

During the embryonic and early postnatal period, the circulating level of testosterone is sufficient to allow the normal stroma to epithelial interaction for the initial ontogeny of the prostate. The circulating level of testosterone decreases within the first year of life, however, such that the prostate does not continue to grow (Fig. 13.3). A second phase of prostate growth is initiated during puberty, inducing the prostate to reach its normal adult size by 18–20 years of age. This second prostate growth phase is induced because, at puberty, circulating testosterone rises again to a sufficient level to re-stimulate adequate production of stromal andromedins (Fig. 13.3). Such positive paracrine stimulatory loops (Fig. 13.9) do not go unopposed, however, since the prostate does not normally continue to grow once it has reached its adult size, even though there is no decrease in andromedin levels. Instead, the prostate reaches its normal adult size and then net growth ceases even though circulating levels of androgen are maintained. After reaching its adult size, the prostate epithelial compartment enters a steady-state maintenance phase, in which the rate of epithelial proliferation balances the rate of death such that neither overgrowth nor regression of the gland normally occurs (Litvinov et al. 2003). The realization that both the stromal and epithelial compartments are organized into interactive stem cell units provides a mechanistic understanding of how the reciprocal positive feedback loops are regulated so that the steady-state size of the prostate is maintained without overgrowth in the young adult.

13.7 Organization of prostate epithelial and stromal stem cell units

Stem cells are defined by their capacity for self-renewal, multi-lineage differentiation and replicative quiescence. Pluripotent embryonic stem cells possess the most plasticity and can give rise to all tissues of an organism. During embryogenesis, there is a developmental process which results in the creation of tissue-restricted stem cells, termed adult stem cells, which lose their pluripotency, but retain ability to self-renew and undergo multi-lineage differentiation to maintain the tissue. Adult stem cells are generally quiescent and reside in a specialized cellular location known as a niche. The niche provides a microenvironment that maintains the balance between quiescence and self-renewal of the stem cell population. The concept of adult stem cells in the prostate first emerged to explain the profound capacity of this tissue for cyclic regeneration, using male rats as a model (Isaacs 1987).These results documented that, even after 30 rounds of cyclic androgen-ablation-induced prostate regression followed by androgen-replacement-induced restoration, which induced more than 60 additional epithelial cell population doublings, the prostate epithelial compartment is completely able to repopulate itself normally (Isaacs 1987). This remarkable prostatic regenerative capacity documents that the self-renewal of stem cells within the adult prostate is androgen independent.

Since these original studies 25 years ago, a large number of independent groups have added to the knowledge of how prostate epithelial stem cell units are organized. The results of these combined efforts are summarized in Fig. 13.10. Prostate epithelial stem cells, denoted no. 9 in Fig. 13.9, are present in niches within the basal layer of the epithelial compartment at a very low frequency (i.e. 0.5–1%). A defining characteristic of a prostate epithelial stem cell is that it does not express the AR or p63 proteins (Litvinov et al. 2009). This is consistent with the fact that embryonic UGS epithelial cells from either AR or p63 knock-out mice undergo prostatic ontogeny and glandular renewal when transplanted in combination with wild-type UGS mesenchymal cells (Isaacs 2008).

While an individual prostate stem cell possesses high self-renewal capacity, it proliferates infrequently to renew itself and simultaneously generate progeny for two distinct cell lineages (Fig. 13.10). The first and much less frequent lineage commitment is for terminal differentiation into a proliferation-quiescent neuroendocrine cell (NE in Fig. 13.10), which secretes a series of peptide growth factors. The second and much more common lineage commitment is for differentiation into a progenitor that undergoes a limited number of proliferative replications (i.e. amplifications), before transiting a maturation process of terminal differentiation (Isaacs 2008). This progenitor is termed a transit-amplifying (TA) cell, denoted no. 10 in Fig. 13.9. A transit-amplifying cell does not express AR protein and is dependent for proliferation, but not survival, on andromedins produced by stromal cells. One of the defining characteristics of a transit-amplifying cell is its obligatory expression of p63, as well as other basal markers such as cytokeratins 5 and 14, Jagged-1 and Notch-1 (Litvinov et al. 2006).

An individual transit-amplifying progenitor cell undergoes a limited number of amplifying cell divisions, expanding the cell population derived from a single stem cell, before maturing into an intermediate cell. This maturation involves downregulation of p63, Jagged-1, Notch-1 and basal cytokeratins 5 and 14 expression. A defining characteristic of an intermediate cell is its unique expression of PSCA. This cell is termed intermediate because it expresses both luminal lineage-specific cytokeratins 8 and 18, as well as the basal lineage-specific cytokeratins 5 and 15, and AR mRNA, but not AR protein (Litvinov et al. 2006). As an intermediate cell migrates upward from the basal layer to form the luminal layer, it stops expressing PSCA and now expresses AR protein. Engagement of the AR pathway within a luminal cell, denoted no. 12 in Fig. 13.9, induces its differentiation from a cuboidal into a columnar secretory luminal cell expressing prostate specific markers like PSA.

We have recently documented that an additional function of the ligand-occupied AR in prostatic secretory luminal cells is to suppress the ability of these secretory cells to proliferate even in the presence of continuously high andromedin levels (unpublished data: Vander Griend DJ, Litvinov IV, Chen S, Dalrymple SL, Antony L, Luo J, DeMarzo AM, Meeker AK, Isaacs JT. Oncogenic addiction of prostate cancer cells to androgen receptor involves loss of c-Myc suppression by

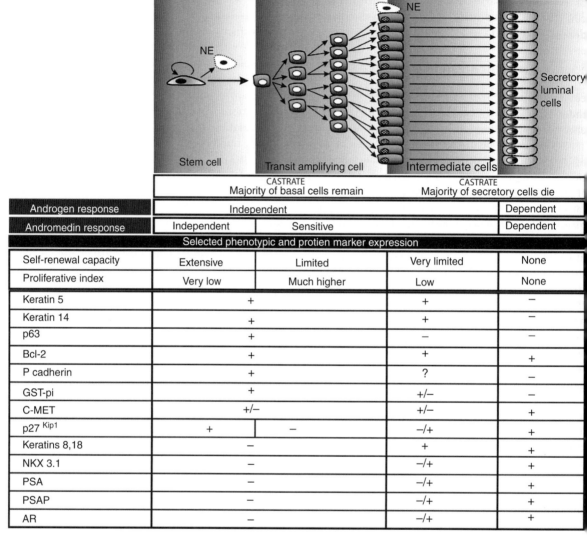

	Basal compartment		Luminal compartment	
		CASTRATE Majority of basal cells remain	CASTRATE Majority of secretory cells die	
Androgen response	Independent			Dependent
Andromedin response	Independent	Sensitive		Dependent
	Selected phenotypic and protien marker expression			
Self-renewal capacity	Extensive	Limited	Very limited	None
Proliferative index	Very low	Much higher	Low	None
Keratin 5	+		+	−
Keratin 14	+		+	−
p63	+		−	−
Bcl-2	+		+	+
P cadherin	+		?	−
GST-pi	+		+/−	−
C-MET	+/−		+/−	+
p27 Kip1	+	−	−/+	+
Keratins 8,18	−		+	+
NKX 3.1	−		−/+	+
PSA	−		−/+	+
PSAP	−		−/+	+
AR	−		−/+	+

Fig. 13.10 Stem cell model of prostatic epithelial cell compartmentalization. The prostate gland consists of a number of stem cell units that arise from one stem cell. Such a stem cell is located in the basal epithelial layer of the prostate and, upon division, gives rise to a population of transit-amplifying cells. The latter divide in the basal layer, and a fraction of them differentiate and move into the secretory luminal epithelial layer. As transit-amplifying cells differentiate and move into a secretory luminal layer from the basal layer, they acquire expression of a number of genetic markers, as indicated. Symbols: +/−, low-level retention of expression by a subset of transit-amplifying (i.e. intermediate) cells; +, expression of marker; −, lack of detectable expression of marker.

androgen receptor/β-Catenin/TCF-4 complexes). These studies document that proliferation of human prostate epithelial cells is dependent upon c-Myc expression induced by WNT-independent formation and binding of nuclear β-catenin/TCF-4 complexes to both the 5′ and the 3′ c-Myc enhancers, thus initiating transcription. When prostate epithelial cells expressing AR are exposed to androgen, c-Myc expression is suppressed and the cells arrest in G_0

and undergo terminal secretory luminal differentiation. The mechanism for such androgen-dependent AR-mediated G_0 growth arrest is independent of Rb, p21, p27, FoxP3, or downregulation of growth factors receptors. Instead, G_0 growth arrest involves the formation of AR/β-catenin/TCF-4 complexes which are unable to bind the 5′/3′ enhancers and initiate c-Myc transcription. Such binding to β-catenin/TCF-4 complexes does not occur when AR is mutated in its DNA-binding domain. The causal importance of this mechanism is confirmed by the ability of constitutive c-Myc expression to prevent androgen-dependent growth arrest of AR-expressing prostate epithelial cells. It is this ligand-occupied AR suppression of proliferation of the secretory luminal cells which prevents the androgen-stimulated stroma to epithelial positive feed-forward loop (Fig. 13.9) from inducing continuous net prostatic growth in the presence of a continuous supply of andromedins.

Since secretory luminal cells are the terminal stage of maturation of a hierarchical expanding population of cells comprising an individual stem cell unit (Fig. 13.10), these secretory luminal cells are quantitatively the major epithelial phenotype present in the gland even though they are proliferatively quiescent (i.e. terminally differentiated). Unlike their proliferating precursors, terminally differentiated secretory luminal cells, denoted no. 11 in Fig. 13.9, acquire a dependence on stromally derived andromedins for their survival. Hence, androgen deprivation induces apoptosis of these secretory luminal cells due to a decrease in andromedin levels. It is the death of these secretory luminal cells which predominately accounts for the regression of the prostate induced by androgen deprivation.

Besides prostate epithelial stem cells, there are also mesenchymal stem cells within prostate stroma. This conclusion is based upon the demonstration that there is a self-renewing subpopulation of prostate stromal cells from BPH tissue which express: (1) mesenchymal stem cell markers; (2) strong proliferative potential; and (3) ability to differentiate in to fibroblastic, myogenic, adipogenic and osteogenic lineages (Lin et al. 2007). Of these potential lineages, the most characteristic commitment of progeny from prostate mesenchymal stem cell is to differentiate into a fibroblast, denoted no. 13, or a smooth muscle cell, denoted no. 3 (Fig. 13.9). This latter commitment, as discussed earlier, is due to embryonic paracrine effects of prostate epithelial cells, denoted no. 4 in Fig. 13.9, which permanently commit the mesenchymal stem cells to give rise to a subset of progeny which can mature into AR-expressing SMC (Cunha et al. 1996). In the adult, the maturation of these SMC requires paracrine factors secreted by prostate epithelial cells, resulting in their expression of both 5α-reductase and AR proteins (Bayne et al. 1998). Once these SMC mature, androgen binding to AR induces their secretion of andromedins, denoted no. 6

(Fig. 13.9), including insulin-like growth factor 1 (IGF-1), FGF-7 and-10, and vascular endothelial growth factor (VEGF) (Isaacs 2008).

Insulin-like growth factor 1 is not only a paracrine factor for prostate epithelial cells but also a critical autocrine factor, denoted no. 7 in Fig. 13.9, for prostate stromal cells (Isaacs 2008). Another androgen-dependent paracrine factor produced by SMC, denoted no. 8 (Fig. 13.9), is VEGF. Vascular endothelial growth factor maintains the endothelial cells, denoted no. 14 (Fig. 13.9), and thus the blood supply in the prostate stromal compartment affecting both the stromal and epithelial cells (Joseph et al. 1997).

13.8 Androgen in benign prostatic hyperplasia and the clinical use of SRD5A inhibitors for its treatment

The realization that prostate is organized in to stem cell units provides a framework for understanding the mechanism for preventing either the regression or overgrowth of the normal adult gland. At about the age of 40, however, in the vast majority of men, this kinetic balance is disrupted and, with further aging, the gland enlarges and eventually produces BPH (Rhodes et al. 1999). In BPH, there is an increase in the cellular content of the transition zone of the prostate (Fig 13.3). This neoplastic growth involves: (1) an enhanced number of epithelial and stromal stem cell units; (2) an enhanced number of proliferations by transit-amplifying cells before these mature into non-proliferating luminal secretory cells; and/or (3) decreased ability of AR to limit the proliferation of luminal secretory cells. Benign prostatic hyperplasia characteristically is associated with an enhanced number of stromal cells. Since at least a subset of these stromal cells express AR and thus andromedins, androgen regulation within these stromal cells may be abnormal, leading to enhanced andromedin production. Theoretically, to inhibit such enhanced andromedin production, androgen ablation could be utilized to treat BPH. Unfortunately, such systemic androgen ablation has other unacceptable side-effects on bone density, muscle mass and libido. For these reasons, BPH is often treated medically with SRD5A inhibitors, since they decrease prostate tissues levels of DHT without lowering the systemic level of testosterone (Nasland and Miner 2007).

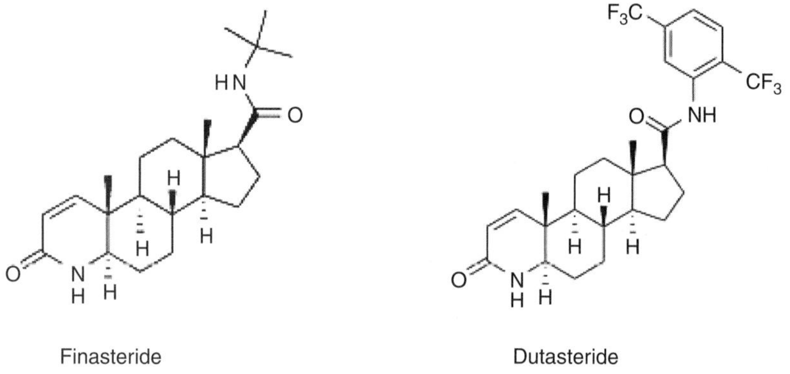

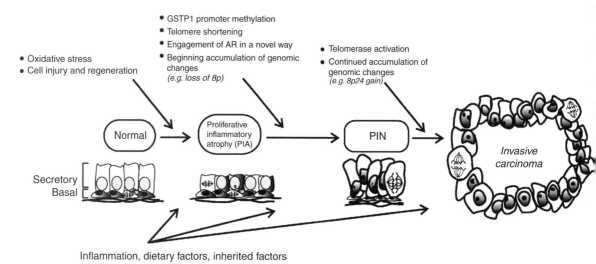

Finasteride

Dutasteride

Fig. 13.11 Chemical structure of the two clinically approved SRD5A inhibitors finasteride and dutasteride.

- Oxidative stress
- Cell injury and regeneration

- GSTP1 promoter methylation
- Telomere shortening
- Engagement of AR in a novel way
- Beginning accumulation of genomic changes *(e.g. loss of 8p)*

- Telomerase activation
- Continued accumulation of genomic changes *(e.g. 8p24 gain)*

Normal

Proliferative inflammatory atrophy (PIA)

PIN

Invasive carcinoma

Secretory
Basal

Inflammation, dietary factors, inherited factors

Fig. 13.12 Overview of prostatic carcinogenesis. PIN = prostatic intraepithelial neoplasia.

There are two clinically approved, orally active, small molecule SRD5A inhibitors: finasteride and dutasteride (Fig. 13.11). Finasteride is the older of the two approved drugs, and it is a competitive inhibitor of the human SRD5A1 isozyme with a $K_i = 360 \pm 40$ nM, and an irreversible inhibitor of the human SRD5A2 isozyme with a K_i of 69 ± 1 nM (Xu *et al.* 2006). Due to its rapid serum half-life, finasteride is a SRD5A2 selective drug (Xu *et al.* 2006). Like finasteride, dutasteride is also a competitive inhibitor of human SRD5A1 with a K_i of 6 ± 1 nM, and an irreversible inhibitor of the human SRD5A2 isozyme with a K_i of 7 ± 3 nM (Xu *et al.* 2006). Due to its extended serum half-life (i.e. >3 days), dutasteride is a dual SRD5A1 and 2 inhibitor (Xu *et al.* 2006). Chronic daily treatment with either of these SRD5A inhibitors lowers prostatic DHT, which decreases stromal andromedin production, thus reducing the size of

the BPH-enlarged prostate by 25%, without lowering serum testosterone and thus minimizing androgen-ablation side-effects (Foley and Kirby 2003).

13.9 Role of androgen in prostate carcinogenesis

Prostate carcinogenesis is the result of the accumulation of multiple genetic and epigenetic changes, whereby chronic and acute inflammation, in conjunction with dietary and other environmental factors, targets prostate epithelial cells for injury and destruction (De Marzo *et al.* 2007; Nelson *et al.* 2007; Fig. 13.12). The precursor for most peripheral zone prostatic carcinomas is thought to be high-grade prostatic intraepithelial neoplasia (HGPIN) (McNeal and Bostwick 1986). It is believed that HGPIN arises from low-grade PIN.

The cell type of origin for HGPIN is incompletely understood. A widely held view of carcinogenesis is that the common carcinomas generally arise in self-renewing tissues in which dividing cells acquire somatic genetic alterations in growth-regulatory genes. In normal human prostate epithelium, cell division takes place almost exclusively in the basal cell compartment where the tissue stem and presumably the transit-amplifying cells reside (Bonkhoff et al. 1994; Bonkhoff 1998). The secretory luminal cells do not normally proliferate and are the terminally differentiated cells that perform the androgen-regulated differentiated functions of the prostate, such as PSA production and secretion. Both prostate cancer and HGPIN cells possess many phenotypic and morphological features of secretory luminal cells (i.e. cytokeratin 8 and 18, PSA, HK, *PSMA* and AR expression); yet they also contain features of the basal transit-amplifying cell compartment such as c-MET expression, DNA replication and extensive self-renewal (Verhagen et al. 1992; De Marzo et al. 1998a; Meeker et al. 2002; van Leenders et al. 2002). Thus, in carcinoma these stem cell and transit-amplifying cell–like features have been shifted up from the basal into the secretory luminal compartment (De Marzo et al. 1998b; Meeker et al. 2002). Based upon these facts, it has been postulated that the cell of origin for prostate cancer is an intermediate, prostatic epithelial cell, presumably derived from the basal transit-amplifying population, which undergoes the initial malignant molecular changes allowing gene expression and morphological features of both basal and secretory luminal cells (Verhagen et al. 1992; De Marzo et al. 1998a; De Marzo et al. 1998b; Meeker et al. 2002; van Leenders et al. 2002; Vander Griend et al. 2008).

This conclusion is also supported by the demonstration that increased proliferation occurs as a regenerative response in cells with a transit-amplifying or intermediate phenotype (Meeker et al. 2002; van Leenders et al. 2002). The site of these phenotypically intermediate, initiated cells appears not to be random within the prostate. Instead, they are enriched in sites of focal glandular atrophy where the luminal epithelial cells, atrophic in appearance, are quite proliferative and often surrounded by inflammation within the gland. Therefore, these sites have been termed "proliferative inflammatory atrophy" (PIA) (De Marzo et al. 1999; Fig. 13.12). In this process, glutathione S-transferase pi 1 (GSTP1) expression is elevated in many of the cells in PIA as a genome-protective

measure. Although elevated in many of the cells in PIA, GSTP1 expression is eventually lost in some cells as the result of aberrant methylation of the CpG islands of the GSTP1 gene promoter (Lin et al. 2001). Indeed, such aberrant methylation of the GSTP1 promoter is one of the earliest molecular abnormalities characteristic of prostate cancer cells. This heritable epigenetic alteration places these cells at increased risk for the accumulation of additional genetic damage, with acceleration of the neoplastic process toward PIN (Lin et al. 2001). One of these additional genetic changes involves telomerase shortening by PIN cells. This appears to increase their genetic instability, driving further genetic damage and producing invasive cancers (Meeker et al. 2002; Fig. 13.12).

During the initiation of prostate carcinogenesis, there are distinct "hard wiring" changes in the AR signaling pathways. Normally the proliferating transit-amplifying cells in the basal epithelial layer do not express the androgen receptor, or express only low levels of AR. As discussed, during their maturation, these cells eventually express higher levels of AR. Once a critical AR level is reached, the occupancy of AR with ligand inhibits proliferation of these cells and induces their differentiation into secretory luminal cells. In contrast, the intermediate type of proliferating cells in PIA variably expresses higher levels of AR, and such AR expression is further enhanced in proliferating cells in HGPIN (De Marzo et al. 2001). Associated with this enhanced expression of the AR is the decreased expression of ERβ by HGPIN cells (Fixemer et al. 2003). These results document that "hard wiring" changes occur in the AR/ERβ signaling pathways even at this early stage of cancer development, since now AR-expressing/ERβ-negative cells are proliferating and not growth arrested.

These changes produce "gain of function" ability by AR so that it now engages the molecular signaling pathways directly, stimulating the proliferation and survival of these initiated prostatic cells (Vander Griend et al. 2010). Unlike the paracrine situation in the normal prostate, in which such growth regulation is initiated by AR binding to genomic sequences in the nuclei of stromal cells, during prostatic carcinogenesis genomic AR binding within the transformed cells itself activates this growth regulation. Due to these "hard wiring" changes, there is a conversion from paracrine to a cell-autonomous autocrine AR signaling pathway in invasive prostate cancer (Gao and

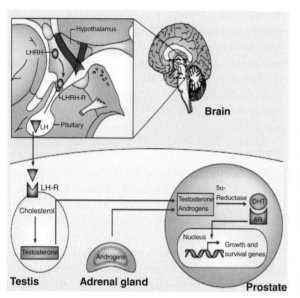

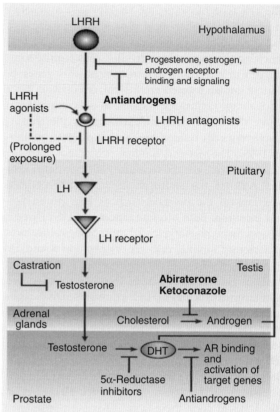

Fig. 13.13 Overview of the hypothalamic-pituitary-testicular axis and sites of therapeutic disruption by chemical agents.

Isaacs 1998; Gao *et al.* 2001; Vander Griend *et al.* 2010). These "gain of function" hard wiring changes pathologically allow androgen/AR complexes to bind to and enhance expression of survival and proliferation genes which physiologically are not affected by these complexes in either normal transit-amplifying or secretory luminal cells (Gao and Isaacs 1998; Gao *et al.* 2001; Vander Griend *et al.* 2010).

13.10 Androgen ablation as therapy for metastatic prostate cancer

Due to the fact that, during prostate carcinogenesis, AR is converted from a growth suppressor to an oncogene promoting cancer cell proliferation, patients with metastatic prostate cancer initially receive long-acting super-agonists of luteinizing hormone-releasing hormone (LHRH) which downregulate the cell surface expression of LHRH receptors on gonadotrophs in the anterior pituitary; thus preventing release of LH from these cells (Fig. 13.13). Downregulation of LH release

into the blood results in inhibition of testosterone production and secretion by the testes, producing a medical castration (Denmeade and Isaacs 2002; Fig. 13.13). These drugs rarely actually cure the cancer, however, because the initial response is almost always followed by a relapse to a castration-resistant stage.

The development of the castration-resistant state is not commonly associated with the loss of AR expression (Hobisch *et al.* 1996; Taplin *et al.* 1999; Linja *et al.* 2001; Shah *et al.* 2004). In fact, enhanced expression of AR is the most common phenotypic change characteristically associated with the development of castration-resistant prostate cancer (Chen *et al.* 2004; Taylor *et al.* 2010). While less than 10% of these cancers have undergone *AR* mutations (Taplin *et al.* 2003), approximately 30% of such castration-resistant prostatic cancers over-express AR due to amplification in the gene (Brown *et al.* 2002; Hyytinen *et al.* 2002; Taylor *et al.* 2010). A growing body of additional evidence points to the accumulation of molecular changes that reduce the threshold of

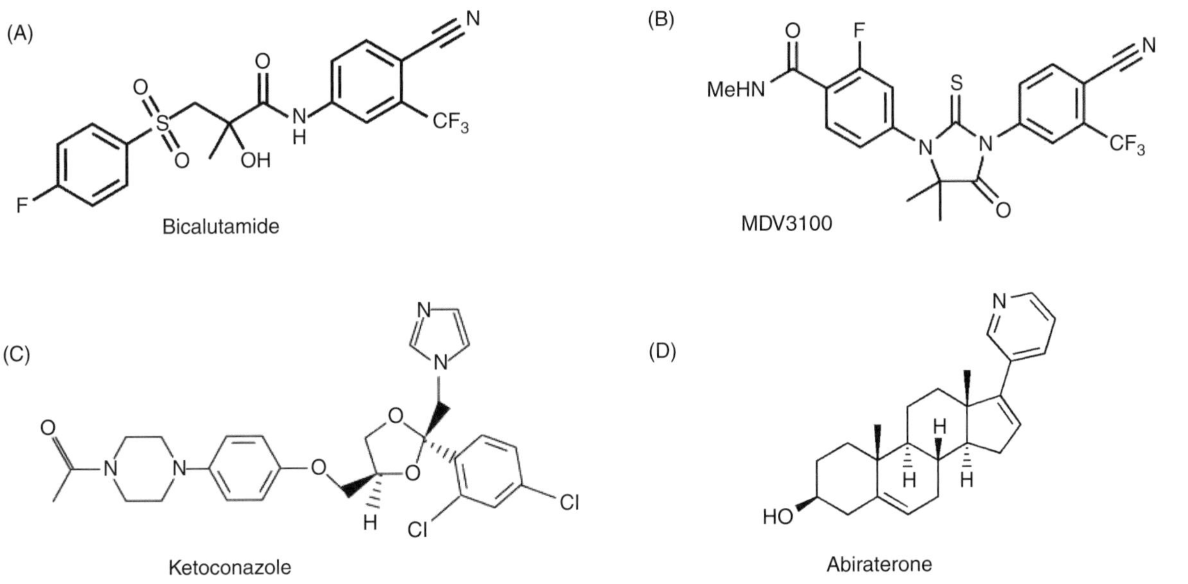

Fig. 13.14 Chemical structure of agents targeted at disrupting androgenic stimulation of prostate cancer cells. A=bicalutamide (Casodex); B=MDV3100; C=ketoconazole; and D=abiraterone.

AR ligand required for proliferation and survival (Isaacs and Isaacs 2004). Thus the AR is still a therapeutic target in castration-resistant prostate cancer.

In an attempt to block the residual AR signaling in the castration-resistant state, competitive AR antagonists (i.e. antiandrogens, like bicalutamide (Casodex; Fig. 13.14A) and, in more recent phase II clinical trials, the novel AR antagonist MDV3100 (Fig. 13.14B; Scher *et al.* 2010)) are often combined with LHRH super-agonists (Evans *et al.* 2011). Unfortunately, such additional androgen-ablation therapies are also usually not curative (Evans *et al.* 2011). To more fully suppress circulating androgen production, particularly that derived from both the adrenals as well as testes within such castrate-resistant metastatic patients, LHRH super-agonists have been combined with inhibitors of the cytochrome P450 steroid 17α-mono-oxygenase enzyme (i.e. CYP17A1 aka 17α-hydroxylase/17,20 lyase), which converts pregnenolone/progesterone into DHEA and androstenedione, since these intermediates must be formed for production of testosterone in both glands (Fig. 13.3). In clinical trials, either the non-selective inhibitor, ketoconazole (Fig. 13.14C; Keizman *et al.* 2012) or the more specific inhibitor, abiraterone (Fig. 13.14D; de Bono *et al.* 2011) have been used based upon the idea that castration-resistant prostate cancer (CRPC) remains hormone driven, with intratumoral steroid synthesis fueling tumor growth (Cai *et al.* 2011).

Despite encouraging clinical results with next generation drugs (e.g. MDV3100 and abiraterone) targeted at inhibiting the residual AR signaling in patients with CRPC, responses are variable and short-lived (Evans *et al.* 2011; de Bono *et al.* 2011).

13.11 SRD5A inhibitors for the prevention of prostate cancer

The realization that AR signaling is converted from a suppressor to an oncogenic stimulator of epithelial cell proliferation early in prostate carcinogenesis has raised the issue of whether prostate cancer development can be prevented by reducing AR signaling. Based upon their safe use in the treatment of BPH, two large RCTs, the Prostate Cancer Prevention Trial (PCPT) (Thompson *et al.* 2003) and the Reduction by Dutasteride of Prostate Cancer Events (REDUCE) trial (Andriole *et al.* 2010) evaluated daily use of finasteride 5 mg versus placebo for seven years and daily use of dutasteride 0.5 mg versus placebo for four years, respectively, for the reduction in the risk of prostate cancer in men at least 50 years of age. The trials demonstrated an overall 25% reduction in prostate cancer diagnoses with finasteride 5 mg and dutasteride treatment. This overall reduction was due to a decreased incidence of lower risk (i.e. Gleason Score 6) prostate cancers. However, both trials showed an increased incidence of high-grade (i.e. Gleason

Score >7) prostate cancer with finasteride and dutasteride treatment. Based upon an expert panel review of these results in June of 2011, the FDA informed healthcare professionals that the *Warnings and Precautions* section of the labels for the SRD5A inhibitor class of drugs had to be revised to include new safety information about the increased risk of being diagnosed with a more serious form of prostate cancer (high-grade prostate cancer). This risk appears to be low, but healthcare professionals should be aware of this safety information, and weigh the known benefits against the potential risks when deciding to start or continue treatment with SRD5A inhibitors in men.

13.12 New direction for treatment of castration-resistant prostate cancer: bipolar androgen therapy

Androgen ablation is highly effective palliative therapy for metastatic prostate cancer, but eventually all men relapse. The demonstration that AR expression continues in androgen-ablated patients has resulted in the classification "castration-resistant prostate cancer" (CRPC), and has led to the development of new second-line agents targeted at reducing residual AR signaling. Paradoxical to these second-line approaches is the observation that the growth of AR-expressing human CRPC can be inhibited by supraphysiological levels of androgens. This response appears to be due to high-dose androgen inhibiting re-licensing of DNA in CRPC cells expressing high levels of AR (Litvinov *et al.* 2006; Vander Griend *et al.* 2007; D'Antonio *et al.* 2009; Denmeade and Isaacs 2010). It may also be due to recently described effects of androgen in inducing double strand DNA breaks (Haffner *et al.* 2010). Based on available preclinical data demonstrating the effects of supraphysiological levels of testosterone on inhibition of growth of CRPC xenografts, we have initiated a clinical trial in men with CRPC testing the effect of monthly treatments with an im depot injection of testosterone. This im formulation achieves supraphysiological levels of testosterone that cannot be achieved with standard testosterone gel-based applications. The supraphysiological testosterone level is followed by a rapid drop to castrate levels of testosterone with each cycle of therapy (Denmeade and Isaacs 2010). This "bipolar androgen therapy" does not allow time for prostate cancer cells to adapt their AR expression in response

to environmental conditions. The goal is to determine if a clinical response can be achieved through this non-adaptive rapid cycling approach in men with CRPC.

13.13 Side-effects of androgen replacement/ablation in the aging male

Besides its effects upon normal and abnormal growth and physiology of the prostate, testosterone is also critical for maintenance of bone and muscle metabolism, as well as libido. For this reason, aging males who have an insufficient level of serum testosterone (i.e. hypogonadal males) suffer clinically from loss of bone and muscle mass as well as a decreased libido. Such aging hypogonadal males are candidates for exogenous testosterone replacement. Due to its growth-promoting effects on the prostate, however, such hormonal replacement therapy could enhance the development of BPH and/or prostate cancer. Thus, the decision to initiate such replacement hormonal therapy must be evaluated on risk vs. benefit analysis for each patient individually (see Chapter 16).

The side-effects observed in naturally developed hypogonadal males are also a problem in males either at high risk of developing prostate cancer that are treated with androgen-ablation therapy as a preventative modality, or in patients with clinically established prostate cancer who are being given androgen-ablation as therapy. In order to allow replacement hormonal therapy in hypogonadal patients and lessen side-effects of such testosterone-ablative therapies in patients with established prostate cancer, small molecule SARMs are being developed which retain the positive androgenic effects on bone, muscle and libido, but which have little or no growth-stimulatory effects on the prostate (Bhasin and Jasuja 2009). This approach is possible due to the increasing basic knowledge about the mechanism(s) of such androgenic effects at the molecular level (Litvinov *et al.* 2003). These molecular studies have documented that the binding of natural and synthetic SARMs induces a spectrum of conformational changes in the androgen receptor. This spectrum of conformations results in differential ability of the SARM-occupied AR to dimerize and bind to specific target genes and specific transcriptional cofactors, inducing either stimulation or repression of transcription. Thus, the development of such SARMs will usher in an exciting time during which clinical testing will determine whether modulating testosterone's effects will have an impact on the prevention and treatment of multiple diseases of the aging male.

13.14 Key messages

- The prostate is the most common site of neoplastic transformation in the human body.
- There are two types of prostatic neoplasms: one benign (i.e. BPH); the other malignant (i.e. prostate carcinoma).
- Testosterone is the major growth and functional regulator of both the normal and abnormal prostate.
- The prostate epithelium which gives rise to prostate cancer is organized functionally in stem cell units composed of stem cells, transit-amplifying cells, intermediate cells and secretory luminal cells.
- Testosterone is a prohormone in the prostate, where it is metabolized to both a more potent androgen (i.e. DHT) and to an estrogenic metabolite (i.e. 3β-diol).
- Dihydrotestosterone binds to the AR within prostatic stromal cells to induce the production and secretion of paracrine growth factors known as andromedins.
- Andromedins diffuse into the epithelial compartment where they stimulate the proliferation of transit-amplifying cells and the survival of transit-amplifying, intermediate and secretory luminal cells (i.e. paracrine androgen axis in normal prostate).
- Dihydrotestosterone binds to the AR in secretory luminal cells and directly induces the transcription of prostate differentiation markers, such as PSA, HK2 and prostatic-specific acid phosphatase, and induces their terminal

growth arrest by downregulating c-Myc expression.
- Prostate cancers are derived from epithelial cells. During prostatic carcinogenesis, molecular changes induce a conversion from a paracrine to an autocrine pathway so that the AR then directly stimulates the proliferation and survival of prostate cancer cells.
- Therapies which lower androgen levels or block AR signaling have both preventative and treatment effect on prostatic cancer and BPH.
- Besides its effects upon normal and abnormal growth and physiology of the prostate, testosterone is also a critical regulator of bone and muscle metabolism, as well as libido. Therefore, therapies which reduce testosterone's effects on the development and clinical progression of either BPH or prostate cancer have major side-effects upon quality of life.
- In addition, there are aging males who suffer from abnormally low serum testosterone levels with similar quality-of-life side-effects. These patients can be supplemented with exogenous testosterone, but they must be carefully monitored for development of BPH and prostate cancer.
- To allow replacement therapy in patients with low serum testosterone and lessen side-effects of testosterone, ablative therapies in patients with established prostate cancer, small molecule selective androgen response modifiers (SARMs) are being developed, which retain the positive androgenic effects on bone, muscle and libido, but which have little or no growth stimulatory effects on the prostate.

13.15 References

Andersson S, Russell DW (1990) Structural and biochemical properties of cloned and expressed human and rat steroid 5α-reductases. *Proc Natl Acad Sci USA* **87**:3640–3644

Andriole GL, Bostwick DG, Brawley OW, Gomella LG, Marberger M, Montorsi F, Pettaway CA, Tammela TL, Teloken C, Tindall DJ, Somerville MC, Wilson TH, Fowler IL, Rittmaster RS; REDUCE Study Group (2010) Effect of

dutasteride on the risk of prostate cancer. *N Engl J Med* **362**:1192–1202

Bayne CW, Donnelly F, Chapman K, Bollina P, Buck C, Habib F (1998) A novel coculture model for benign prostatic hyperplasia expressing both isoforms of 5alpha-reductase. *J Endocrinol Metab* **83**:206–213

Berman DM, Russell DW (1993) Cell-type-specific expression of rat 5 alpha-reductase isozymes. *Proc Natl Acad Sci USA* **90**:9359–9363

Berry SI, Coffey DS, Walsh PC, Ewing LL (1984) The development of human benign prostatic hyperplasia with age. *J Urol* **132**:474–479

Bhasin S, Jasuja R (2009) Selective androgen receptor modulators as function promoting therapies. *Curr Opin Clin Nutr Metab Care* **12**:232–240

Biswas MC, Russell DW (1997) Expression cloning and characterization of oxidative 17β- and 3α-hydroxysteroid dehyrogenases from rat and human prostate. *J Biol Chem* **272**:15959–15966

Bonkhoff H (1998) Neuroendocrine cells in benign and malignant prostate tissue: morphogenesis proliferation and androgen receptor status. *Prostate Suppl* **8**:18–22

Bonkhoff H, Stein U, Remberger K (1994) The proliferative function of basal cells in the normal and hyperplastic human prostate. *Prostate* **24**:114–118

Brown RS, Edwards J, Dogan A, Payne H, Harland SJ, Bartlett TM, Masters JR (2002) Amplification of the androgen receptor gene in bone metastases from hormone-refractory prostate cancer. *Pathol* **98**:237–244

Bruchovsky N, Wilson JD (1968) The conversion of testosterone in 5α-androstan-17β-ol-3one by the rat prostate in vivo and in vitro. *J Biol Chern* **243**:2012–2021

Cai C, Chen S, Ng P, Bubley GJ, Nelson PS, Mostaghel EA, Marck B, Matsumoto AM, Simon N, Wang H, Chen S, Balk SP (2011) Intratumoral de novo steroid synthesis activates androgen receptor in castration-resistant prostate cancer and is upregulated by treatment with CYP17A1 inhibitors. *Cancer Res* **71**:6503–6513

Cantagrel V, Lefeber DJ, Ng BG, Guan Z, Silhavy JL, Bielas SL, Lehle L, Hombauer H, Adamowicz M, Swiezewska E, DE Brouwer AP, Blumel P, Sykut-Cegielska J, Houliston S, Swistun D, Ali BR, Dobyns WB, Babovic-Vuksanovic D, van Bokhoven H, Wevers RA, Raetz CR, Freeze HH, Morava E, Al-Gazali L, Gleeson JG (2010) SRD5A3 is required for converting polyprenol to dolichol and is mutated in a congenital glycosylation disorder. *Cell* **142**:203–217

Chen CD, Welsbie DS, Tran C, Baek SH, Chen R, Vessella R, Rosenfeld M, Sawyers CL (2004) Molecular determinants of resistance to

antiandrogen therapy. *Nat Med* **10**:33–39

Coffey DS (1992) The molecular biology endocrinology and physiology of the prostate and seminal vesicles. In: Walsh PC, Retik AB, Stamey TA, Vaughan EL (eds) *Campbell's Textbook of Urology.* Saunders, Philadelphia, pp 221–266

Cunha GR, Hayward SW, Daihiya R, Foster BA (1996) Smooth muscle epithelial interactions in normal and neoplastic prostate development. *Acta Anat* **155**:63–72

D'Antonio JM, Vander Griend DJ, Isaacs JT (2009) DNA licensing as a novel androgen receptor mediated therapeutic target for prostate cancer. *Endocr Relat Cancer* **16**:325–332

de Bono JS, Logothetis CJ, Molina A, Fizazi K, North S, Chu L, Chi KN, Jones RJ, Goodman OB Jr, Saad F, Staffurth JN, Mainwaring P, Harland S, Flaig TW, Hutson TE, Cheng T, Patterson H, Hainsworth JD, Ryan CJ, Sternberg CN, Ellard SL, Fléchon A, Saleh M, Scholz M, Efstathiou E, Zivi A, Bianchini D, Loriot Y, Chieffo N, Kheoh T, Haqq CM, Scher HI; COU-AA-301 Investigators (2011) Abiraterone and increased survival in metastatic prostate cancer. *N Engl J Med* **364**:1995–2005

Dehm SM, Tindall DJ (2007) Androgen receptor structural and functional elements: role and regulation in prostate cancer. *Mol Endocrinol* **21**:2855–2863

De Marzo AM, Meeker AK, Epstein JI, Coffey DS (1998a) Prostate stem cell compartments: expression of the cell cycle inhibitor p27kip I in normal hyperplastic and neoplastic cells. *Am Pathol* **153**:911–919

De Marzo AM, Nelson WG, Meeker AK, Coffey DS (1998b) Stem cell features of benign and malignant prostate epithelial cells. *J Urol* **160**:2381–2392

De Marzo AM, Marchi VL, Epstein JI, Nelson WG (1999) Proliferative

inflammatory atrophy of the prostate: implications for prostatic carcinogenesis. *Am J Pathol* **155**:1985–1992

De Marzo AM, Putzi NIT, Nelson WG (2001) New concepts in the pathology of prostatic epithelial carcinogenesis *Urology* **57** (Suppl 1):103–114

De Marzo AM, Platz EA, Sutcliffe S, Xu J, Gronberg H, Drake CG, Nakai Y, Isaacs WB, Nelson WG (2007) Inflammation in prostate carcinogenesis. *Nat Rev Cancer* **7**:256–269

Denmeade SR, Isaacs JT (2002) A history of prostate cancer treatment *Nat Rev Cancer* **2**:389–396

Denmeade SR, Isaacs JT (2010) Bipolar androgen therapy: the rationale for rapid cycling of supraphysiologic androgen/ablation in men with castration resistant prostate cancer. *Prostate* **70**:1600–1607

Eick GN, Thornton JW (2011) Evolution of steroid receptors from an estrogen-sensitive ancestral receptor. *Mol Cell Endocr* **334**:31–38

Evans MJ, Smith-Jones PM, Wongvipat J, Navarro V, Kim S, Bander NH, Larson SM, Sawyers CL (2011) Noninvasive measurement of androgen receptor signaling with a positron-emitting radiopharmaceutical that targets prostate-specific membrane antigen. *Proc Natl Acad Sci USA* **108**:9578–9582

Fixemer F, Remberger K, Bonkhoff H (2003) Differential expression of the estrogen receptor beta (ERbeta) in human prostate tissue, premalignant changes, and in primary, metastatic, and recurrent prostatic adenocarcinoma. *Prostate* **54**:59–87

Foley CL, Kirby KS (2003) 5 alpha-reductase inhibitors: what's new? *Curr Opin Urol* **13**:31–37

Frasier SD, Gafford F, Horton RD (1969) Plasma androgens in childhood and adolescence. *J CLin Endocrinol Metab* **29**:1404–1408

Gao J, Isaacs JT (1998) Development of an androgen receptor null model for identifying the site of initiation for androgen stimulation of proliferation and suppression of programmed (apoptotic) death of PC-82 human prostate cancer cells. *Cancer Res* **58**:3299–3306

Gao J, Arnold JT, Isaacs JT (2001) Conversion from a paracrine to an autocrine mechanism of androgen-stimulated growth during malignant transformation of prostatic epithelial cells. *Cancer Res* **61**:5038–5044

Godoy A, Kawinski E, Li Y, Oka D, Alexiev B, Azzouni F, Titus MA, Mohler J (2011) 5α reductase type 3 expression in human benign and malignant tissues: a comparative analysis during prostate cancer progression. *Prostate* **71**:1033–1046

Gorski RA (2002) Hypothalamic imprinting by gonadal steroid hormones. *Adv Exp Med Biol* **11**:57–70

Gottlieb B, Vasiliou DM, Lumbroso R, Beitel LK, Pinsky L, Trifiro MA (1999) Analysis of exon 1 mutations in the androgen receptor gene. *Hum Mutat* **14**:527–539

Grumbach MM (2002) The neuroendocrinology of human puberty revisited. *Horm Res* **57** (Suppl 2):2–14

Haffner MC, Aryee MJ, Toubaji A, Esopi DM, Albadine R, Gurel B, Isaacs WB, Bova GS, Liu W, Xu J, Meeker AK, Netto G, De Marzo AM, Nelson WG, Yegnasubramanian S (2010) Androgen-induced TOP2B mediated double strand breaks and prostate cancer gene rearrangement. *Nat Genet* **42**:668–675

Hobisch A, Culig Z, Radnayr C, Bartsch C, Klocker H, Hittinair A (1996) Androgen receptor status of lymph node metastases from prostate cancer: *Prostate* **28**:129–135

Huggins C, Johnson MA (1947) Carcinoma of the bladder and prostate. *JAMA* **135**:1146–1152

Hyytinen ER, Haapala K, Thompson I, Lappalainen I, Roiha M, Rantala I, Helin HJ, Janne OA, Vihinen NI, Palvimo JJ, Koivisto PA (2002) Pattern of somatic androgen receptor gene mutations in patients with hormone-refractory prostate cancer. *Lab Invest* **82**:1391–1598

Isaacs JT (1984) Common characteristics of human and canine benign prostatic hyperplasia. In: Kimball FA (ed) *New Approaches to the Study of Benign Prostatic Hyperplasia*. AR Liss, New York, pp 217–234

Isaacs JT (1987) Control of cell proliferation and cell death in the normal and neoplastic prostate: a stem cell model. In: Rogers CH, Coffey DS, Cunha G, Grayhack J, Hinman F, Horton R (eds) *Benign Prostatic Hyperplasia*. Report No. INH 87–2881. Department of Health and Human Services, National Institutes of Health, Bethesda, MD, pp 85–94

Isaacs JT (2008) Prostate stem cells and benign prostatic hyperplasia. *Prostate* **68**:1025–1034

Isaacs JT, Isaacs WB (2004) Androgen receptor outwits prostate cancer drugs. *Nat Med* **10**:26–27

Isaacs JT, McDermott IR, Coffey DS (1979) The identification and characterization of a new $C^{19}O^3$ steroid metabolite in the rat ventral prostate: 5α-androstane-3β,6α,17β-triol. *Steroids* **33**:639–675

Jemal A, Bray F, Center MM, Ferlay ME, Ward E, Forman D (2011) Global cancer statistics. *CA Cancer J Clin* **61**:69–90

Jenkins EP, Hsieh C-L, Milatovich A, Norminton K, Berman DM, Franke U, Russel PW (1991) Characterization and chromosomal mapping of a human steroid 5α-reductase gene and pseudogene and mapping of the mouse homologue. *Genomics* **11**:1102–1112

Jenkins EP, Anderson S, Imperato-McGinley J, Wilson JD, Russell DW (1992) Genetic and pharmacologic evidence for more

than one human steroid 5α-reductase. *J Clin Invest* **89**:293–300

Joseph IB, Nelson JB, Denmeade SR, Isaacs JT (1997) Androgens regulate vascular endothelial growth factor content in normal and malignant prostatic tissue. *Clin Cancer Res* **3**:2507–2511

Keizman D, Huang P, Carducci MA, Eisenberger MA (2012) Contemporary experience with ketoconazole in patients with metastatic castration-resistant prostate cancer: clinical factors associated with PSA response and disease progression. *Prostate* **72**:461–467

Kyprianou N, Isaacs JT (1987) Quantal relationship between prostatic dihydrotestosterone and prostatic cell content: critical threshold concept. *Prostate* **11**:41–50

Kyprianou N, Isaacs JT (1988) Activation of programmed cell death in the rat ventral prostate after castration. *Endocrinology* **122**:552–562

Labrie F, Sugimoto Y, Luu-The V, Simard J, Lachance Y, Bachuarov D, Leblanc G, Durocher F, Paquet N (1992) Structure of human type II 5a-reductase gene. *Endocrinology* **131**:1571–1573

Liao S, Leong T, Tymocyko JL (1972) Structural recognition in interactions of androgens and receptor problems and in their association with nuclear components. *J Steroid Biochem* **3**:401–407

Lin VK, Wang SY, Vasquez DV, Xu CC, Zhang S, Tang L (2007) Prostatic stromal cells derived from benign prostatic hyperplasia specimens posses stem cell like property. *Prostate* **67**:1265–1276

Lin X, Tascilar M, Lee WH, Vles WJ, Lee BH, Veerawamy R, Asgari K, Freije D, van Rees B, Gage WR, Bova GS, Isaacs WB, Brooks JD, de Weese TL, De Marzo AM, Nelson WG (2001) GSTPI CpG island hypermethylation is responsible for the absence of GSTPI expression in human prostate cancer cells. *Am J Pathol* **159**:1815–1826

Linja MJ, Savinainen KJ, Sakamaki OR, Tammela TLJ, Vessella RL, Visakorpi T (2001) Amplification and overexpression of androgen receptor gene in hormone-refractory prostate cancer. *Cancer Res* **61**:3550–3555

Litvinov IV, De Marzo AM, Isaacs JT (2003) Is the Achilles' heel for prostate cancer therapy a gain of function in androgen receptor signaling? *J Clin Endorinol Metab* **88**:2972–2982

Litvinov IV, Vander Griend DJ, Antony L, Dalrymple S, De Marzo AM, Drake CG, Isaacs JT (2006) Androgen receptor as a licensing factor for DNA replication in androgen-sensitive prostate cancer cells. *Proc Natl Acad Sci USA* **103**:15085–15090

Litvinov IV, Vander Griend DJ, Xu Y, Antony L, Dalrymple SL, Isaacs JT (2009) Low-calcium serum-free medium selects for growth of normal prostate stem cells. *Cancer Res* **66**:8598–8607

Mann T, Mann CL (1981) *Male Reproductive Function and Semen.* Springer-Verlag, New York

Marx FJ, Karenberg A (2009) History of the term prostate. *Prostate* **69**:208–213

McNeal JE, Bostwick DG (1986) Intraductal dysplasia: a premalignant lesion of the prostate. *Hum Pathol* **17**:64–71

McNeal JE, Redwine EA, Freiha FS, Stamey TA (1988) Zonal distribution of prostatic adenocarcinoma. *Am J Surg Pathol* **12**:897

Meeker AK, Hicks JL, Platz EA, March GE, Bennett CJ, Delannoy MJ, De Marzo AM (2002) Telomere shortening is an early somatic DNA alteration in human prostate tumorigenesis. *Cancer Res* **62**:6406–6409

Moore RA (1944) Benign hypertrophy and carcinoma of the prostate:

occurrence and experimental production in animals. *Surgery* **16**:152–167

Nasland MJ, Miner M (2007) A review of the clinical efficacy and safety of 5alpha-reductase inhibitors for the enlarged prostate. *Clin Ther* **29**:17–25

Nelson WG, Yegnasubramanian S, Agoston AT, Bastian PJ, Lee BH, Nakayama M, De Marzo AM (2007) Abnormal DNA methylation, epigenetics, and prostate cancer. *Front Biosci* **12**:4254–4266

Normington K, Russell DW (1992) Tissue distribution and kinetic characteristics of rat steroid 5α-reductase isozymes. *J Biol Chem* **267**:19548–19554

Olsson AY, Valtonen-Andre C, Lilja H, Lundwall A (2004) The evolution of the glandular kallikrein locus: identification of orthologs and pseudogenes in the cotton-top tamarin. *Gene* **343**:347–355

Page ST, Lin DW, Mostaghel EA, Marck BT, Wright JL, Wu J, Amory JK, Nelson PS, Matsumoto AM (2011) Dihydrotestosterone administration does not increase intraprostatic androgen concentration or alter prostate androgen action in heathy men: a randomized-controlled trial. *J Clin Endrocrinol Metab* **96**:430–437

Peters CA, Walsh PC (1987) The effect of nafaralin acetate, a luteinizing hormone-releasing hormone agonist, on benign prostatic hyperplasia. *N Engl J Med* **317**:599–604

Plymate SR, Tenover JS, Brenner WJ (1989) Circadian variation in testosterone sex hormone-binding globulin and calculated non-sex hormone-binging globulin bound testosterone in healthy young and elderly man. *J Androl* **10**:366–371

Price D, Williams-Ashman GH (1961) The accessory reproductive glands of mammals. In: Young WC (ed) *Sex and Internal Secretions*, 3rd edn. Williams & Wilkins, Baltimore, MD, pp 366–488

Rhodes T, Girman CJ, Jacobsen SJ, Roberts RO, Guess HA, Lieber MM (1999) Longitudinal prostate growth rates during 5 years in randomly selected community men 40 to 79 years old. *J Urol* **161**:1174–1179

Rizner TL, Lin HK, Peehl DM, Steckelbroeck S, Bauman DR, Penning TM (2003) Human type 3 3α-hydroxysteroid dehydrogenase (also-keto reductase 1C2) and androgen metabolism in prostate cells. *Endocrinology* **144**:2922–2932

Scher HI, Beer TM, Higano CS, Anand A, Taplin ME, Efstathiou E, Rathkopf D, Shelkey J, Yu EY, Alumkal J, Hung D, Hirmand M, Seely L, Morris MJ, Danila DC, Humm J, Larson S, Fleisher M, Sawyers CL; Prostate Cancer Foundation/Department of Defense Prostate Cancer Clinical Trials Consortium (2010) Antitumour activity of MDV3100 in castration-resistant prostate cancer: a phase 1–2 study. *Lancet* **375**:1437–1446

Shah RB, Mehra R, Chinnaiyan AM, Shen R, Ghosh D, Zhou M, Macvicar GR, Varambally S, Harwood J, Bismar TA, Kim R, Rubin MA, Pienta KJ (2004) Androgen-independent prostate cancer is a heterogeneous group of diseases: lessons from a rapid autopsy program. *Cancer Res* **64**:9209–9216

Silver SJ, Balmacoda J, Borrero C (1988) Pregnancy with sperm aspiration from the proximal head of the epididymis: a new treatment for congenital absence of the vas deferens. *Fertil Steril* **50**:525–530

Taplin ME, Bubley GJ, Ko TJ, Small EJ, Upton M, Rajeshjuma B, Balk SP (1999) Selection for androgen receptor mutations in prostate cancers treated with androgen antagonist. *Cancer Res* **59**:2511–2515

Taplin ME, Rajeshkumar B, Halabi S, Werner CP, Woda BA, Picus J, Stadler W, Hayes DF, Kantoff PW, Vogelzang NJ, Small EJ; Cancer and Leukemia Group B Study 9663

(2003) Androgen receptor mutations in androgen-independent prostate cancer: cancer and Leukemia Group B Study 9663. *J Clin Oncol* **21**:2673–2678

Taylor BS, Schultz N, Hieronymus H, Gopalan A, Xiao Y, Carver BS, Arora VK, Kaushik P, Cerami E, Reva B, Antipin Y, Mitsiades N, Landers T, Dolgalev I, Major JE, Wilson M, Socci ND, Lash AE, Heguy A, Eastham JA, Scher HI, Reuter VE, Scardino PT, Sander C, Sawyers CL, Gerald WL (2010) Integrative genomic profiling of human prostate cancer. *Cancer Cell* **18**:11–22

Thigpen AE, Davis DL, Milatovich A, Mendonca BD, Imperato-McGinley J, Griggin J, Franke U, Wilson JD, Russel DW (1992) Molecular genetics of steroid 5α-reductase 2 deficiency. *J Clin Invest* **90**:799–809

Thompson IM, Goodman PJ, Tangen CM, Lucia MS, Miller GJ, Ford LG, Lieber MM, Cespedes RD, Atkins JN, Lippman SM, Carlin SM, Ryan A, Szczepanek CM, Crowley JJ, Coltman CA Jr (2003) The influence of finasteride on the development of prostate cancer. *N Engl J Med* **349**:215–224

Torn S, Nokelainen P, Kurlela R, Pulkka A, Menjivar M, Ghosh S, Coca-Prados M, Peltoketo H, Isomaa V, Vihko P (2003) Production purification and functional analysis of recombinant human and mouse 17β-hydroxysteroid dehydrogenase type 7. *Biochem Biophys Res Commun* **305**:37–45

Uemura M, Tamura K, Chung S, Honma S, Okuyama A, Nakamura Y, Nakagawa H (2008) Novel 5α-steroid reductase (SRD5A3, type-3) is overexpressed in hormone-refractory prostate cancer. *Cancer Sci* **99**:81–86

Vander Griend DJ, Litvinov IV, Isaacs JT (2007) Stabilizing androgen receptor in mitosis inhibits prostate cancer proliferation. *Cell Cycle* **6**:647–651

Vander Griend DJ, Karthaus WL, Dalrymple S, Meeker A, DeMarzo AM, Isaacs JT (2008) The role of CD133 in normal human prostate stem cells and malignant cancer-initiating cells. *Cancer Res* **68**:9703–9711

Vander Griend DJ, D'Antonio J, Gurel B, Antony L, DeMarzo AM, Isaacs JT (2010) Cell-autonomous intracellular androgen receptor signaling drives the growth of human prostate cancer initiating cells. *Prostate* **70**:90–99

van Leenders G, van Balken B, Aalders T, Hulsbergen-van de Kaa C, Ruiter D, Schalken J (2002) Intermediate cells in normal and malignant prostate epithelium express c-MET: implications for prostate cancer invasion. *Prostate* **51**:98–107

Verhagen AP, Ramaekers FC, Aalders TW, Schaafsma HE, Debruyne FM, Schalken JA (1992) Colocalization of basal and luminal cell-type cytokertins in human prostate cancer. *Cancer Res* **52**:6182–6187

Wang Q, Carroll JS, Brown M (2005) Spatial and temporal recruitment of androgen receptor and its coactivators involves chromosomal looping and polymerase tracking. *Mol Cell* **19**:631–642

Weihua Z, Makela S, Andersson LC, Salmi S, Saji S, Webster JI, Jenson EV, Nilsson S, Warner M, Gustafsson J-A (2001) A role for estrogen receptor beta in the regulation of growth of the ventral prostate. *Proc Natl Acad Sci USA* **98**:6330–6335

Weihua Z, Lathe R, Warner M, Gustafsson J-A (2002) An endocrine pathway in the prostate ERβ, AR, 5α-androstane-3β ,17β-diol, and CYP7B1, regulates prostate growth. *Proc Natl Acad Sci USA* **99**:13589–13594

Wilson JD (1984) The endocrine control of sexual differentiation. *Harvey Lect* **79**:145–172

Xu Y, Dalrymple SL, Becker RE, Denmeade SR, Isaacs JT (2006) Pharmacologic basis for the enhanced efficacy of dutasteride against prostatic cancers. *Clin Cancer Res* **12**:4072–4079

Clinical use of testosterone in hypogonadism and other conditions

Eberhard Nieschlag and Hermann M. Behre

14.1 Use of testosterone in male hypogonadism

The primary clinical use of testosterone is substitution therapy for male hypogonadism. Hypogonadism may be caused by lesions of the hypothalamo-pituitary system (secondary hypogonadism), the testes themselves (primary hypogonadism) or a mixture of both as in LOH. Lesions in the target organs may also cause hypogonadism (see Chapters 3 and 19). An overview of the various disease entities and syndromes is provided in Table 14.1, and for a detailed description the reader is referred to the textbook in andrology by Nieschlag *et al.* (2010). In recent years it became clear that there are strong interrelationships between hypogonadism on the one side and the metabolic syndrome as well as cardiovascular disorders on the other side; two special chapters (10 and 11) are therefore dedicated to these exciting developments.

The clinical signs and symptoms of all syndromes and disease entities are predominantly due to a lack of testosterone or its action. The most frequent disorders requiring testosterone substitution are Klinefelter syndrome (incidence 1 in 500 men), Kallmann syndrome, isolated hypogonadotropic hypogonadism (IHH), late-onset hypogonadism (LOH), anorchia and pituitary insufficiency. Some disorders such as varicocele, orchitis, maldescended testes and Sertoli-cell-only syndrome may not, or only eventually, require testosterone substitution. Although discrete endocrine alterations may be noted by laboratory tests in these patients, the endocrine capacity of the Leydig cells remains high enough to maintain serum testosterone in the lower physiological range.

Testosterone: Action, Deficiency, Substitution, ed. Eberhard Nieschlag and Hermann M. Behre, Assoc. ed. Susan Nieschlag. Published by Cambridge University Press. © Cambridge University Press 2012.

Table 14.1 Overview of disorders with male hypogonadism classified according to localization of cause

Hypothalamic-pituitary origin (hypogonadotropic syndromes = secondary hypogonadism)

Isolated hypogonadotropic hypogonadism (IHH) including Kallmann syndrome

Congenital adrenal hypoplasia

Prader–Labhart–Willi syndrome

Laurence–Moon–Biedl syndrome

Constitutional delay of puberty

Pituitary insufficiency/adenomas

Pasqualini syndrome

Isolated lack of FSH

Biological inactive LH or FSH

Hyperprolactinemia

Hemochromatosis

Testicular origin (hypergonadotropic syndromes = primary hypogonadism)

Congenital anorchia

Acquired anorchia

Maldescended testes

Klinefelter syndrome

XYY syndrome

XX male

Gonadal dysgenesis

Testicular tumors including Leydig cell tumors

Varicocele

Sertoli-cell-only syndrome

General disease e.g. renal failure, liver cirrhosis, metabolic syndrome, diabetes, myotonia dystrophica

Disorders of sexual differentiation due to enzyme defects in testosterone biosynthesis or LH-receptor defects (Leydig cell aplasia)

Exogenous factors

Mixed primary and secondary hypogonadism

Late-onset hypogonadism

Target organ resistance to sex steroids

Complete androgen insensitivity (CAIS) (testicular feminization)

Reifenstein syndrome (partial androgen insensitivity; PAIS)

Perineoscrotal hypospadias with pseudovagina

Aromatase deficiency

Estrogen resistance

Gynecomastia

In order to achieve fertility in patients with hypothalamic (IHH) or pituitary insufficiency, treatment with gonadotropins (hCG/hMG) or pulsatile GnRH is required temporarily (e.g. Büchter *et al.* 1998; Depenbusch *et al.* 2002; Warne *et al.* 2009). Once a pregnancy has been induced these patients will go back on testosterone substitution. Individuals with hypogonadism of testicular origin in whom infertility cannot be treated require testosterone substitution continuously. In all these patients testosterone substitution is a lifelong therapy.

There is general agreement that patients with "classical" disorders of primary or secondary hypogonadism should receive testosterone substitution therapy. However, there is a relatively large group of patients in whom hypogonadism develops as a corollary of other acute or chronic diseases. Although these patients lack testosterone and show symptoms of hypogonadism, testosterone is usually not administered to them. Just why substitution is withheld is not quite clear. Probably in many physicians' minds testosterone is still predominantly associated with sexual functions. However, the better the general effects of testosterone on well-being, mood, bones, muscles and red blood are understood, the more frequently testosterone substitution will be considered. Chapter 17 is dedicated to the possible use of testosterone in these non-gonadal diseases. Similarly, LOH occurring with increasing incidence in aging men, and representing a combined form of primary and secondary hypogonadism, is associated with symptoms of testosterone deficiency. But there is no general agreement on treatment strategies of this condition, and Chapter 16 deals with LOH and the controversies and unresolved problems surrounding this area. Chapter 18 analyses and compares the various guidelines for treatment of testosterone deficiency issued by different societies and organizations. As is stated there, most of the recommendations are not strictly evidence based, and clinical experience prevails as the major criterion. Therefore, for the time being, the principle may be followed that any type of hypogonadism documented by decreased serum testosterone concentrations deserves testosterone substitution, unless there is a clear contraindication, of which there are only a few.

14.1.1 Classification and symptoms of hypogonadism

The time of onset of testosterone deficiency is of greater importance for the clinical symptoms than localization of the cause. Lack of testosterone or testosterone action during weeks 8 to 14 of fetal life, the period of sexual differentiation, leads to the development of intersexual genitalia (see Chapter 3). Lack of testosterone at the end of fetal life results in maldescended testes and small penis size. In later life the onset of testosterone deficiency before or after completion of puberty determines clinical appearance (Table 14.2).

If testosterone is lacking from the time of normal onset of puberty onwards, eunuchoidal body proportions will develop; i.e. arm span exceeds the standing height, and lower length of body (from soles to symphysis) exceeds upper length (from symphysis to top of the cranium), and bone mass will not develop to its normal level. The distribution of fat will remain prepubertal and feminine; i.e. emphasis of hips, buttocks and lower belly. Voice mutation will not occur. The frontal hairline will remain straight without lateral recession; beard growth is absent or scanty; the pubic hairline remains straight. Hemoglobin and erythrocytes will be in the lower-normal to subnormal range. Early development of fine perioral and periorbital wrinkles is characteristic. Muscles remain underdeveloped. The skin is dry due to lack of sebum production, and free of acne. The penis remains small; the prostate is underdeveloped. Spermatogenesis will not be initiated, and the testes remain small. If an ejaculate can be produced it will have a very small volume. Libido and normal erectile function will not develop.

A lack of testosterone occurring in adulthood cannot change body proportions, but will result in decreased bone mass and osteoporosis, as well as in accumulation of abdominal fat. Early-on, lower backache and, at an advanced stage, vertebral fractures may occur.

Once mutation has taken place the voice will not change again. Lateral hair recession and baldness when present will persist, the secondary sexual hair will become scanty and, in advanced cases, a female hair pattern may again develop. Mild anemia may develop. Muscle mass and power decrease. The skin will become atrophied and wrinkled. Gynecomastia may develop. The prostate will decrease in volume while the penis will not, or only minimally, change its size, but will lose its function for coitus (Chapter 12). Spermatogenesis will decrease and, as a consequence, also the size of the testes, which will become softer. Libido and sexual arousability will decrease or disappear, while potency will be less affected.

14.1.2 Initiation of substitution therapy and choice of preparation

Testosterone substitution is started when the diagnosis is established and serum testosterone levels below

Table 14.2 Symptoms of hypogonadism relative to age of manifestation

Affected organ/function	Onset of lack of testosterone	
	Before	After
	completed puberty	
Larynx	No voice mutation	No change
Hair	Horizontal pubic hairline, straight frontal hairline, diminished beard growth	Diminishing secondary body hair, decreased beard growth
Skin	Absent sebum production, lack of acne, pallor, skin wrinkling	Decreased sebum production, lack of acne, pallor, skin wrinkling, hot flashes
Bones	Eunuchoid tall stature, arm span > height, osteoporosis	Arm span = height, osteoporosis
Bone marrow	Low degree anemia	Low degree anemia
Muscles	Underdeveloped	Atrophy
Prostate	Underdeveloped	Atrophy
Penis	Infantile	No change of size, loss of function
Testes	Small volume, often maldescended testes	Decrease of volume and consistency
Spermatogenesis	Not initiated	Arrest
Ejaculate	Not produced	Low volume
Libido	Not developed	Loss
Erectile function	Not developed	Erectile dysfunction

the normal range are found, taking into account the various influences on serum testosterone levels, including diurnal variations. In order to establish a diagnosis by documenting low serum testosterone levels, usually determination of testosterone in a serum sample taken between 07.00 and 11.00 in the morning is sufficient (Vermeulen and Verdonck 1992). Pooled sera will not improve diagnostic accuracy (see Chapter 4).

The symptoms of androgen deficiency can be prevented or reversed by testosterone treatment. It is important that a preparation with natural testosterone is selected for treatment so that all functions of testosterone and its active metabolites, DHT and estradiol, can be exerted (Fig. 14.1). Of all testosterone preparations and routes of application described in Chapter 15, im injection or oral ingestion of testosterone esters were formerly the most widely accepted and practiced modalities for the treatment of all forms of hypogonadism. Over the last two decades, transdermal testosterone preparations have become a valuable alternative, first transdermal patches and, more recently, transdermal gels. The transdermal preparations have the advantage that at least some mimic the normal physiological diurnal rhythm and thus represent the most physiological form of substitution.

For full im substitution, pharmacokinetic and clinical studies show that 200–250 mg testosterone enanthate or testosterone cypionate must be injected every two weeks (Nieschlag *et al.* 1976; Schulte-Beerbühl and Nieschlag 1980; Snyder and Lawrence 1980; Sokol *et al.* 1982; Cunningham *et al.* 1990). More recently, testosterone undecanoate dissolved in castor oil and injected intramuscularly has been shown to be effective in substitution therapy (Behre *et al.* 1999a; von Eckardstein and Nieschlag 2002; Zitzmann and Nieschlag 2007; Brabrand *et al.* 2011). Peak values remain within the normal range. In order to achieve a steady state at the beginning of substitution, the second 1000 mg injection is given 6 weeks after the first; further injections follow 10–14 weeks later. Individual intervals are determined according to serum testosterone levels which are measured immediately before the next injection. These determinations are then repeated in yearly intervals. Values

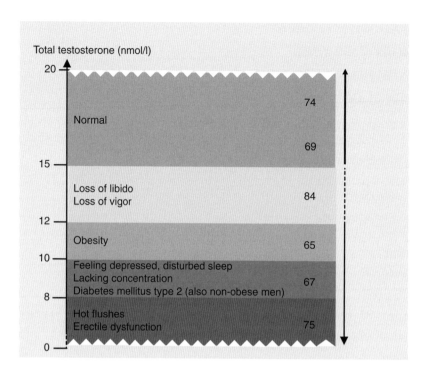

Total testosterone (nmol/l)

Normal	74
	69
Loss of libido Loss of vigor	84
Obesity	65
Feeling depressed, disturbed sleep Lacking concentration Diabetes mellitus type 2 (also non-obese men)	67
Hot flushes Erectile dysfunction	75

Fig. 14.1 Threshold levels of serum testosterone for various symptoms of late-onset hypogonadism (LOH) in 434 patients (Zitzmann *et al.* 2006). See plate section for color version.

that are too high lead to extension of injection intervals, and those that are too low to a shortening in injection intervals. Slow intergluteal injections are recommended. No adverse side-effects have been observed, even after many years of use (Zitzmann and Nieschlag 2007). If the dose of testosterone undecanoate injected is lowered, e.g. to 750 mg, the injection intervals need to be shortened to maintain normal serum levels (Wang *et al.* 2010).

Testosterone pellet implants were among the first modalities applied for TRT (see Chapter 1). If three to six implants are inserted, slowly declining serum testosterone levels in the normal range are achieved for four to six months. There is, however, an initial burst release, so that supraphysiological levels of about 50 nmol/l result. Commercially, pellets are only available in a few countries.

If oral substitution is preferred, 40 mg testosterone undecanoate capsules must be given two to four times daily. These doses have been shown to be effective in the majority of hypogonadal men in either open (Franchi *et al.* 1978; Morales *et al.* 1997) or double-blind controlled studies (Luisi and Franchi 1980; Skakkebaek *et al.* 1981) when libido and potency as well as physical and mental activity were taken as parameters. Although relatively high testosterone doses are consumed with this regimen, liver function

is not negatively affected, as was shown in 35 men taking 80–200 mg testosterone undecanoate over 10 years (Gooren 1994). The patients need to be instructed to ingest the capsules together with a meal in order to guarantee adequate absorption from the gut (Bagchus *et al.* 2003).

Transdermal testosterone preparations mimic physiological diurnal variations, and their kinetic profile is closest to the ideal substitution. They may be used as first choice and are especially well suited for patients who suffer from fluctuating symptoms caused by other preparations. In addition, upon removal, testosterone is immediately eliminated and they are therefore specifically suited for substitution in advanced age (Wang *et al.* 2008).

Scrotal patches consisting of a thin film containing 15 mg native testosterone were the first on the market. They were applied daily in the evening and led to sufficient serum testosterone levels for 22–24 hours. Adequate long-term substitution effect was achieved without serious side-effects under regular use, as has been observed in patients treated for up to 10 years with these patches (Behre *et al.* 1999b). Later developments superseded this initially useful preparation.

Non-scrotal transdermal systems also result in physiological serum levels with an appropriate number of systems, which have to be applied in the evening. As resorption of testosterone depends on the use of enhancers, in some cases considerable skin reactions limit the use of the systems. Although the patches mentioned above are hardly used today, recently a new testosterone patch was developed causing little skin irritation and which must be changed only every other day; however, two systems with either 1.8 or 2.4 mg resorbed per day must be used (Raynaud et al. 2009).

A further transdermal application is the use of testosterone gels, which are applied to large skin areas in order to allow sufficient amounts of the hormone to be resorbed. These gels are applied in the morning to the upper arm, shoulders and abdomen and are left to dry for five minutes. During this time contact with women or children, direct as well as through wash-rags and towels (de Ronde 2009), must be avoided, because of the danger of contamination. Thereafter the danger is negligible especially if the skin is washed after evaporation of the alcohol. Physiological levels result when the gel is applied in the morning. Long-term use over several years showed good results (Wang et al. 2004; McNicholas and Ong 2006). If a preparation with a higher testosterone concentration is used, less gel needs to be applied and good clinical results are obtained. If this gel is applied to the scrotum, only one fifth of the amount required when used on other skin areas is necessary for substitution (Kühnert et al. 2005). However, the scrotal application has not yet been licensed.

The choice of testosterone preparation and route of administration is ultimately up to the patient, who over time may gather experience with several preparations and develop his own preference. Younger patients will be more inclined to choose long-acting preparations, while the older patient (> 50 years) should be advised to use a short-acting preparation at least initially (Wang et al. 2008). If therapy has to be stopped due to developing contraindications (e.g. prostate disease), serum testosterone levels will immediately decline to endogenous levels.

If a patient has pronounced androgen deficiency, has never received testosterone and has passed the age of puberty, he is immediately treated with a full maintenance dose of testosterone. In cases of secondary hypogonadism when fertility is requested, testosterone therapy can be interrupted and GnRH or hCG/hMG therapy can be implemented until sperm counts increase and a pregnancy has been induced.

Testosterone therapy does not prevent the chance of initiating or reinitiating spermatogenesis with releasing or gonadotropic hormones. Once spermatogenesis has been induced it can be maintained for some time with hCG alone, keeping intratesticular testosterone concentrations high (Depenbusch et al. 2002).

Patients with residual testosterone production may not require a full maintenance dose, e.g. Klinefelter patients in an early phase of testosterone deficiency. In these cases injection intervals of testosterone esters may be extended; these cases may also be suited for low-dose testosterone undecanoate therapy (i.e. 40 mg once or twice daily) or intermittent transdermal treatment (e.g. every second or third day). This dose does not entirely suppress the residual endogenous testosterone production and supplements the lacking hormone.

Finally, the question needs to be addressed at which serum testosterone levels substitution therapy should be initiated. Based on clinical experience and many studies in normal and hypogonadal men, we considered 12–40 nmol/l as the normal range for many years (Nieschlag et al. 2010), i.e. starting treatment when – in the presence of relevant symptoms – testosterone levels dropped below 12 nmol/l. However, in other countries different levels were considered to be the limit to start substitution; e.g. 7.5 nmol/l in France, 7.5 to 8.0 nmol/l in the UK and 9.0 nmol/l in Spain (Nieschlag et al. 2004). This prompted a systematic investigation in patients suspected of LOH, and symptom-specific testosterone threshold levels resulted (Fig. 14.1). With regard to the different lower limits of normal, this implies that physicians consider different symptoms as an indication to start substitution, and the lower limit of 12 nmol/l could be raised rather than lowered. The 12 nmol/l threshold received further support from a recent study on reference ranges for normal men based on several cohorts and liquid chromatography–tandem mass spectrometry leading to 12.1 nmol/l (= 348 ng/dl) as the lower limit of normal (2.5th percentile (Bhasin et al. 2011)). In the same study, 243 pmol/l (= 70 pg/dl) was estimated to be the lower limit of free testosterone.

14.1.3 Surveillance of testosterone substitution therapy

The physiological effects of testosterone can be used for monitoring the efficacy of testosterone substitution therapy (Table 14.2). Since therapy aims at replacing the testosterone endogenously lacking, and since physiological serum concentrations are well known, serum testosterone levels also provide a good parameter for therapy surveillance. Guidelines for monitoring testosterone therapy in general were first issued by the World Health Organization (1992), followed by various societies and organizations as summarized in Chapter 18.

14.1.3.1   Behavior and mood

The patient's general well-being is a good parameter to monitor the effectiveness of replacement therapy. Under sufficient testosterone replacement the patient feels physically and mentally active, vigorous, alert and in good spirits; too low testosterone levels will be accompanied by lethargy, inactivity and depressed mood (Burris et al. 1992; Wang et al. 1996; Zitzmann and Nieschlag 2001) (see also Chapter 5).

14.1.3.2   Sexuality

The presence and frequency of sexual thoughts and fantasies correlate with appropriate testosterone substitution; while loss of libido and sexual desire are a sign of subnormal testosterone values. Spontaneous erections such as those during the morning phase of sleep will not occur if testosterone replacement is inadequate; however, erections due to tactile or visual erotic stimuli may be present even with low testosterone levels. The frequency of ejaculations and sexual intercourse correlate with serum testosterone levels in the normal to subnormal range. Therefore, detailed psychological exploration or a diary on sexual activity and interests are useful adjuncts in assessing testosterone substitution. For objective evaluation of psychosexual effects, weekly questionnaires on sexual thoughts and fantasies, sexual interest and desire, satisfaction with sexuality, frequency of erections and number of morning erections and ejaculations may be used (e.g. Lee et al. 2003; Rosen et al. 2011). These questionnaires are specifically suited for monitoring substitution therapy and less for diagnosing hypogonadism.

Priapism has been reported to occur in individual cases, mostly at the beginning of testosterone substitution in adult patients as well as in boys with delayed puberty (Endres et al. 1987; Zelissen and Stricker 1988; Ruch and Jenny 1989; Arrigo et al. 2005; Ichioka et al. 2006). This is an extremely rare effect and may have become even rarer since the new testosterone preparations avoid supraphysiological testosterone serum levels. Decreasing the testosterone dose is the rational consequence, but intervention by aspirating blood from the corpora cavernosa may be acutely necessary.

14.1.3.3   Phenotype

Muscles and physical strength grow under testosterone treatment, and the patient develops a more vigorous appearance (e.g. Wittert et al. 2003). The increase in lean body mass at the expense of body fat usually results in a decrease of body weight (Rolf et al. 2002). The distribution of subcutaneous fat that shows feminine characteristics in hypogonadism (hips, lower abdomen, nates) may change with increasing muscle mass. In particular, testosterone reduces abdominal fat.

The appearance and maintenance of a male sexual hair pattern is a good parameter for monitoring testosterone replacement (see Chapter 7). In particular, beard growth and frequency of shaving can easily be recorded. Hair growth in the upper pubic triangle is an important indicator of sufficient androgen substitution. While women, boys and untreated hypogonadal patients have a straight frontal hairline, androgenization is accompanied by temporal recession of the hairline and – if a predisposition exists – by the development of baldness. The *pattern* of male sexual hair is of greater importance than the *intensity* of hair growth. The AR polymorphism plays a role in male hair growth and pattern (see Chapter 3). A well-substituted patient may have to shave daily. However, if there is no genetic disposition for dense beard growth, additional testosterone will not increase facial hair.

Sebum production correlates with circulating testosterone levels, and hypogonadal men may suffer from dry skin. In an early phase of treatment patients may even complain about the necessity of shampooing more frequently; they have to be informed that this is a part of normal maleness. The occurrence of acne may be a sign of supraphysiological testosterone levels, and the dose should be reduced accordingly.

Gynecomastia may be caused by increased conversion to estradiol during testosterone therapy, especially under testosterone enanthate injections. After initiation of androgen therapy and consequent decrease of estradiol serum levels, gynecomastia usually disappears. If gynecomastia pre-exists due to an increased estradiol/testosterone ratio in hypogonadal men, it may decrease during adequate testosterone therapy. However, in severe cases mastectomy by an experienced plastic surgeon may be required.

Patients who have not undergone pubertal development will experience voice mutation soon after initiation of testosterone therapy (Akcam *et al.* 2004). During normal pubertal development the voice begins to break when serum testosterone levels reach about 10 nmol/l and SHBG drops (Pedersen *et al.* 1986). Mutation of the voice is very reassuring for the patient and helps him to adjust to his environment by closing the gap between his chronological and biological age. It is specifically important for the patient to be recognized as an adult male on the phone. Once the voice has mutated it is no longer a useful parameter for monitoring replacement therapy since the size of the larynx, the vocal chords and thus the voice achieved will be maintained without requiring further androgens.

In patients who have not gone through puberty, penis growth will be induced by testosterone treatment and normal erectile function will develop. Since penile androgen receptors diminish during puberty, growth will cease even under continued testosterone treatment (Shabsigh 1997; see Chapter 12).

Patients who did not undergo puberty before the onset of hypogonadism may also develop eunuchoidal body proportions because of retarded closure of the epiphyseal lines of the extremities. Testosterone treatment will briefly stimulate growth, but will then lead to closure of the epiphyses and will arrest growth. In these patients, an X-ray of the left hand and distal end of the lower arm should be made before treatment to determine bone age. The epiphyseal closure may be followed by further X-rays during the course of treatment. In addition, body height and arm span – as measured from the tip of the right to the tip of the left middle finger – should be measured until no further growth occurs. Continued growth, in particular of the arm span, indicates inadequate androgen substitution or extremely rare cases of estrogen resistance or aromatase deficiency (see Chapters 8 and 19).

14.1.3.4 Blood pressure and cardiac function

Overdosing androgens, as can be observed during misuse of testosterone and anabolic steroids, may increase blood pressure by increasing blood electrolytes and water retention, leading in extreme cases to edema (see Chapter 25). During effective testosterone substitution therapy in hypogonadal men

such side-effects are not observed (e.g. Whitworth *et al.* 1992). To the contrary, systolic and diastolic blood pressure decrease under regular testosterone substitution. Regular blood pressure measurement should be performed during testosterone therapy, especially during inception of treatment when the testosterone dosages have to be adjusted, and in men with additional problems of the heart and kidneys. In patients with severe cardiovascular problems testosterone must be administered very carefully and in low doses (Basaria *et al.* 2010; Aaronson *et al.* 2011; Chapter 11).

14.1.3.5 Serum testosterone

When serum testosterone levels are used to judge the quality of testosterone substitution it is necessary to be aware of the pharmacokinetic profiles of the different testosterone preparations (Chapter 15). Moreover, in longitudinal surveillance of testosterone therapy it is important to use assay systems that strictly undergo internal and external quality control (Chapter 4). Generally, testosterone serum levels should be measured just before the injection of the next dose of long-acting preparations or transdermal application. The time point of the last injection or administration of oral or transdermal testosterone must be recorded to interpret the serum levels measured.

Levels below the lower normal limit at the end of a three-week interval after testosterone enanthate injection should prompt shorter injection frequency of two-week intervals. Conversely, if the levels are in the high physiological range at the end of the injection interval, the dosing intervals may be extended.

When using the im depot preparation of testosterone undecanoate, peak values remain within the normal range. In order to achieve a steady state at the beginning of substitution the second 1000 mg injection is given 6 weeks after the first; further injections follow 10 to 14 weeks later. Individual intervals are determined according to serum testosterone levels, which are measured immediately before the next injection. These determinations are then repeated in yearly intervals. Values that are too high should lead to extension of injection intervals, those that are too low to a shortening of injection intervals (Zitzmann and Nieschlag 2007).

Low serum testosterone levels two to four hours after ingestion of oral testosterone undecanoate should prompt counseling of the patient so that the capsule is taken together with a meal and testosterone is better absorbed. However, it is difficult to base monitoring of treatment with oral testosterone undecanoate on serum testosterone levels, and other parameters are of more importance if this mode of therapy is chosen.

When transdermal preparations are applied, serum testosterone levels may be measured just before the next dose is administered. Initial measurements, however, are only meaningful after two or three weeks following initiation of therapy, since it takes time until the skin builds up a reservoir and steady state serum levels are reached.

After initiation of testosterone substitution, measuring serum testosterone under the conditions mentioned above is recommendable after 3 to 6 and 12 months, and thereafter annually.

In blood, testosterone is bound to SHBG and other proteins. Only about 2% of testosterone is not bound and is available for biological action of testosterone (free testosterone). Since total testosterone correlates well with free testosterone, separate determination of free testosterone is not necessary for routine monitoring (see also Chapter 4).

14.1.3.6 Serum dihydrotestosterone

Determination of DHT does not play a role in routine monitoring of TRT, but may be of importance in experimental use of testosterone preparations and monitoring biological effects of androgens. Due to the high 5α-reductase activity in skin, transdermal testosterone application is associated with increased serum DHT levels; this applies especially to scrotal application. The DHT adds to the overall androgenicity of the preparation, and a patient receiving transdermal treatment may be well substituted clinically although his serum testosterone does not reflect this. In these cases occasional measurement of serum DHT may be indicated (Kühnert et al. 2005; see also Chapter 4).

14.1.3.7 Serum estradiol

In sensitive patients, very high serum testosterone levels, as may occur under testosterone enanthate, may be converted to estrogens and cause gynecomastia. This is an indication to reduce the dose or switch to another testosterone preparation. In this case monitoring serum estradiol levels may explain the clinical findings.

14.1.3.8 Gonadotropins

The determination of LH and FSH plays a key role in establishing the diagnosis of hypogonadotropic (i.e. secondary) or hypergonadotropic (i.e. primary) hypogonadism. However, during surveillance of testosterone therapy they are of less importance. Negative-feedback regulation between hypothalamus, pituitary and testes causes negative correlation between serum testosterone and LH, as well as to some extent to FSH levels in normal men.

In cases with primary hypogonadism (e.g. intact hypothalamic and pituitary function), FSH and in particular LH increase with decreasing testosterone levels and may normalize under testosterone treatment. This is especially the case in patients with acquired anorchia (e.g. due to accidents or iatrogenic castration). However, in the most frequent form of primary hypogonadism, i.e. in patients with Klinefelter syndrome, LH and FSH often do not show significant suppression during testosterone substitution. Moreover, oral or transdermal testosterone may have only little effect on gonadotropins. Therefore LH is not a good indicator of sufficient TRT.

14.1.3.9 Erythropoiesis

Since erythropoiesis is androgen dependent, hypogonadal patients usually present with mild anemia (with values in the female normal range) which normalizes under testosterone treatment. Therefore, hemoglobin, red blood cell count and hematocrit are good parameters for surveillance of replacement therapy. If sufficient stimulation is lacking despite adequate testosterone therapy, lack of iron should be ruled out and treated if necessary. At the beginning of therapy red blood values should be assessed every three months, and later on annually. If too much testosterone is administered, supraphysiological levels of hemoglobin, erythrocytes and hematocrit as a sign of polycythemia can develop, indicating that the testosterone dose should be scaled down (Calof et al. 2005). In some cases phlebotomy may be required acutely. The erythropoietic response not only depends on the serum testosterone levels, but also on the age of the patient and androgen receptor polymorphism. Older patients and those with shorter CAG repeats react more sensitively to testosterone (Zitzmann and Nieschlag 2007).

Testosterone has been claimed to potentiate sleep apnea (see Chapter 17); however, only case reports about the incidence of sleep apnea during testosterone treatment have been published and, paradoxically, hypogonadism has also been cited as a cause of this condition (Luboshitzky *et al.* 2002; Attal and Chanson 2010). Increased hematocrit and increased mass of pharyngeal muscle bulk, as well as neuroendocrine effects of testosterone during therapy were discussed as possible reasons. The development of signs and symptoms of obstructive sleep apnea during testosterone therapy warrants a formal sleep study and treatment with continuous positive airway pressure (CPAP) if necessary. If the patient is unresponsive or cannot tolerate continuous positive airway pressure, the testosterone must be reduced or discontinued.

14.1.3.10   Liver function

The testosterone preparations proposed for testosterone replacement do not have negative side-effects on liver function. Nevertheless, many physicians believe that testosterone may disturb liver function. This impression derives from 17α-methyltestosterone and other 17α-alkylated anabolic steroids which are indeed liver toxic and which should no longer be used in the clinic (see Chapter 25).

Monitoring liver function is of special interest in hypogonadal patients with concomitant diseases that affect liver function, or in patients whose hypogonadism is induced by general diseases. In such cases additional medication is necessary that may influence liver function and thus influence testosterone metabolism, e.g. by increasing SHBG production.

14.1.3.11   Lipid metabolism

Lipid profiles may change under testosterone substitution. Presumed adverse effects such as decreasing high-density lipoprotein (HDL) levels and increasing low-density lipoprotein (LDL) levels have been reported when comparing different treatment modalities (Jockenhövel 1999). However, beneficial effects were also seen, especially in older hypogonadal men, as LDL levels decreased under testosterone substitution and HDL increased. The CAG repeat length of the androgen receptor has a modifying role in the effects on lipid parameters (Zitzmann *et al.* 2003), and pharmacogenetic considerations may in the future influence dose and route of testosterone administration. Currently, it appears sufficient to monitor lipids under testosterone therapy in those patients with grossly abnormal lipid profiles.

14.1.3.12   Prostate

Before initiating testosterone treatment a prostate carcinoma must be excluded. This is done by digital rectal examination (DRE) and PSA determination. Imaging techniques such as transrectal ultrasonography (TRUS) are not considered mandatory, but may add information.

Prostate volume as determined by transrectal ultrasonography is a sensitive end-organ parameter for surveillance. Testosterone substitution therapy increases prostate volume in hypogonadal men, but only to the extent seen in age-matched controls (Behre *et al.* 1994). Prostate volume growth also depends on the AR polymorphism (Zitzmann *et al.* 2003). Prostate-specific antigen increases slightly during therapy but remains within the normal range (Behre *et al.* 1999a; Zitzmann and Nieschlag 2007). Since testosterone therapy must be terminated if a prostate carcinoma occurs and prostate carcinoma is a disease of advanced age, patients above 45 years of age under testosterone treatment should be regularly investigated, first after 3–6 months and 12 months and then at yearly intervals (Wang *et al.* 2008). Measurement of PSA and palpation of the prostate, if possible supported by transrectal ultrasonography, should be performed. As a sign of adequate prostate and seminal vesicle stimulation, ejaculate volume will increase into the normal range.

14.1.3.13   Bone mass

Testosterone replacement therapy in hypogonadal men will increase the low bone mineralization, preventing or reversing osteoporosis and possibly bone fractures (Snyder 1999; Chapter 8). In particular, with respect to bones it is important to use testosterone preparations that can be converted into estrogens since this hormone plays a significant role in bone metabolism (Ohlsson and Vandenput 2009). Bone density should be measured in patients receiving testosterone substitution, prior to treatment and regularly every two years as long as treatment continues. Quantitative computer tomography (QCT) of the lumbar spine provides accurate information; other validated methods are dual photon absorptiometry and dual energy X-ray absorptiometry. Also sonographic measurement of bone density (for example, of the phalangi) provides a useful and inexpensive parameter for monitoring (Zitzmann *et al.* 2002).

14.2 Treatment of delayed puberty in boys

Androgen replacement therapy in male adolescents with constitutional delay of growth and puberty has been shown to be beneficial psychologically as well as physiologically, and should be initiated promptly on diagnosis (de Lange *et al.* 1979; Rosenfeld *et al.* 1982; Albanese and Stanhope 1995; Rogol 2005). Boys with delayed puberty are at risk for not obtaining adequate peak bone mass and for having deficiencies in developing social skills, an impaired body image and low self-esteem. Younger boys with short stature, delayed bone age (at least 10.5 years), and delayed pubertal development in the absence of other endocrinological abnormalities can be treated with 50–100 mg of testosterone enanthate or cypionate im, every four weeks for three months, whereas boys >14 years old may be treated with 250 mg (im, every four weeks for three months). After a three-month "wait and see" period, another course of treatment may be offered if pubertal development does not continue. An increase in testes size is the most important indicator of spontaneous pubertal development (testes volume >3 ml). Overtreatment with testosterone may result in premature closure of the epiphyses of long bones, resulting in reduced adult height. Therefore, treatment of patients who have not yet reached full adult height has to be undertaken carefully.

Low-dose oral testosterone undecanoate has been tested for the treatment of constitutional delay of puberty (Albanese *et al.* 1994; Brown *et al.* 1995). For example, treatment of 11–14-year-old prepubertal boys with 20 mg testosterone undecanoate per day for six months resulted in an increase in growth velocity without advancing bone age and pubertal development (Brown *et al.* 1995). Such "mild" treatment appears to be suited for an early phase when virilization is not yet requested. Transdermal testosterone should also be a useful method to induce puberty. However, experience in a larger series of patients has not yet been reported.

At the beginning of therapy it is often difficult to distinguish between boys with constitutional delay of growth and puberty, who require only temporary androgen replacement, and boys with idiopathic hypogonadotropic hypogonadism, who require lifelong androgen therapy to stimulate puberty and to maintain adult sexual function. However, boys with permanent hypogonadotropic hypogonadism will not have testicular growth induced by androgen therapy. Because pubertal growth is a product of the interaction of growth hormone (GH) and insulin-like growth factor 1 (IGF-1) and the hypothalamic-pituitary-gonadal axis, boys with concomitant GH deficiency will require the simultaneous administration of GH and androgens for the treatment of delayed puberty.

In boys with secondary causes of delayed puberty, development can also be induced by pulsatile GnRH or hCG/hMG respectively. This therapy has the advantage that testicular development is induced simultaneously. However, we prefer to induce initial virilization by testosterone and to stimulate spermatogenesis at a later stage with the more demanding GnRH or gonadotropin therapy.

14.3 Overall stature

The effect of testosterone on epiphyseal closure may be used to treat boys who are dissatisfied with their prospective final overall body height (for review see Drop *et al.* 1998). Treatment has to start before the age of 14. Doses of 500 mg testosterone enanthate have to be administered every two weeks for at least a year to produce effects (Bettendorf *et al.* 1997). This treatment should be reserved for special cases since tall stature is not a disease but rather a cosmetic and psychological problem. However, social and psychological conflicts caused by this condition should not be underestimated. It should also be remembered that testosterone is not registered for this treatment, which has therefore to be considered "experimental." Combining ethinyl estradiol with testosterone injections has no additional height-reducing effect (Decker *et al.* 2002).

An additional reservation comes from the possible effects of such high-dose testosterone treatment at this early age on fertility, the prostate, the cardiovascular system, on bones and other organs. Long-term follow-up of men treated on average 10 years earlier with high-dose testosterone for tall stature revealed no negative effects on sperm parameters and reproductive hormones in comparison to controls (de Waal *et al.* 1995; Lemcke *et al.* 1996; Hendriks *et al.* 2010). Prostate morphology as evaluated by ultrasonography did not show any abnormalities, and serum lipids were not different from the control group. Slightly lower sperm motility was attributable to a higher incidence of varicocele and maldescended testes in the treated men rather than to the treatment as such. Thus it appears that, as far as evaluated, high-dose reatment has no long-term negative side-effects n these adolescents.

14.4   Micropenis and microphallus

Enlargement of a micropenis or microphallus can be achieved in children by treatment with 25–50 mg of testosterone enanthate or cypionate (im, every three to four weeks for three months; Ishii *et al.* 2004) or with 1.25–5% testosterone cream, 5% DHT cream or 10% testosterone propionate cream (twice daily for three months). High-dose androgen therapy may be necessary to achieve some androgenization in male pseudohermaphroditism caused by 5α-reductase deficiency and certain AR defects.

14.5   Ineffective use of testosterone in male infertility

Since testosterone has been used so effectively in the treatment of endocrine insufficiency of the testes, its use has also been attempted in the treatment of idiopathic male infertility. Testosterone rebound was one of the earliest modalities in this regard. The published success rate in terms of pregnancies varied considerably from center to center, but remained low overall (Charny and Gordon 1978). All studies were uncontrolled trials without placebo and double-blinding, and therefore inconclusive. Testosterone rebound therapy cannot be recommended for treatment of infertility and is no longer practiced.

More recently, testosterone undecanoate has been tested for the treatment of idiopathic male infertility. However, a significant increase in pregnancy rates could not be demonstrated (Pusch 1989; Comhaire *et al.* 1995). When testosterone undecanoate was given combined with tamoxifen and/or hMG, an improvement of semen parameters was observed (Adamopoulos *et al.* 1995; 1997). However, in these studies no pregnancy rates were reported. The therapeutic goal of every infertility treatment should be an increase in pregnancy rates; therefore, studies in which only improved semen parameters are reported, without examining the pregnancy rates, must be considered as inconclusive in terms of infertility treatment. Similarly, after many years of clinical use, no significant effect of mesterolone on pregnancy rates could be demonstrated in an extensive WHO-sponsored multicenter trial (World Health Organization 1989).

Thus, to date testosterone and other androgens have no place in evidence-based treatment of idiopathic male infertility (Kamischke and Nieschlag 1999).

14.6   Contraindications to testosterone treatment

Effects and side-effects of testosterone therapy have been described in detail above. Here the major reasons for not initiating or for interrupting testosterone therapy are briefly summarized.

The major contraindication to testosterone therapy is a *prostate carcinoma*. A patient with an existing prostate carcinoma should not receive testosterone. A carcinoma has to be excluded before starting therapy, and the patient on testosterone should be checked regularly for prostate cancer (digital exploration, PSA, transrectal sonography and biopsy, if necessary). (See also Chapter 13.)

Breast cancer cells often are hormone sensitive, especially estrogen sensitive, and therefore, for reasons of safety, breast cancer is considered a contraindication to testosterone treatment. However, breast cancer is a relatively rare cancer in men and no cases of testosterone substitution and occurrence of breast cancer have been published, as an extended literature search revealed. Thus, this warning cannot be substantiated.

In some countries *sexual offenders* may be or have been treated by castration or antiandrogenic therapy. It would be a serious mistake to administer testosterone to such patients. Relapses and renewed crimes could be the consequence and the responsibility of the prescribing physician. The same holds true for pharmacological androgen deprivation therapy (ADT) using GnRH analogs or antiandrogens, which is currently the preferred therapy for sexual offenders.

Testosterone *suppresses spermatogenesis*: a phenomenon exploited for hormonal male contraception (see Chapter 23). In hypogonadal patients with reduced spermatogenetic function, testosterone administration will also decrease sperm production. Such patients who wish to father children, e.g. by techniques of artificial fertilization, should not receive testosterone substitution therapy, at least not for the time their sperm are necessary for fertilization of eggs. This is of increasing importance as not only residual sperm in patients with secondary hypogonadism but also with Klinefelter syndrome may be able to fertilize eggs via intracytoplasmatic sperm injection (ICSI) and induce pregnancies (e.g. Lanfranco *et al.* 2004).

14.7 Overall effect of testosterone

Testosterone has many biological functions and, as demonstrated in this chapter, testosterone is a safe medication. There are only very few reasons why testosterone should be withheld from a hypogonadal patient (see Section 14.6). Nevertheless, to date many hypogonadal men still do not receive the benefit of testosterone therapy because they are not properly diagnosed and the therapeutic consequences are not drawn (e.g. Bojesen *et al.* 2003). Some physicians even believe that the shorter life expectancy of men compared to women could be attributed to effects of testosterone. However, large epidemiological studies of healthy men or of patients have demonstrated that men with lower testosterone serum levels have a shorter life expectancy than those with higher testosterone levels (Shores *et al.* 2006; Laughlin *et al.* 2008; Haring *et al.* 2010; Bojesen *et al.* 2011). It remains currently unresolved whether testosterone levels are just an indicator of the general health status or whether there is a causal positive relationship between testosterone levels and longevity. By the same token it remains unresolved today whether testosterone treatment of hypogonadal men may extend or shorten their life expectancy. Without doubt, however, testosterone substitution significantly improves the quality of life of hypogonadal men.

14.8 Key messages

- The primary indications for testosterone therapy are the various forms of male hypogonadism. For substitution, testosterone preparations should be used that can be converted to 5α-dihydrotestosterone (DHT) as well as to estradiol, in order to develop the full spectrum of testosterone action.
- Injectable, oral and transdermal testosterone preparations are available for clinical use. The best preparation is the one that replaces testosterone serum levels at as close to physiological concentrations as possible. This objective is best reached by testosterone gels and by injectable testosterone undecanoate.
- In seven decades of clinical use testosterone has proven to be a very safe medication. No toxic effects are known. The only important contraindication is the presence of a prostate carcinoma which should be excluded before substitution is initiated.
- Testosterone therapy should be monitored by patients' well-being, alertness and sexual activity, by occasional measurement of serum testosterone levels, hemoglobin and hematocrit, by bone density measurements and prostate parameters (rectal examination, PSA and transrectal sonography).
- Testosterone can be used to initiate puberty in boys with constitutional delay of pubertal development. Careful dosing does not lead to premature closure of the epiphysis and reduced height.
- High-dose testosterone treatment in early puberty may prevent expected over-tall stature in boys. Negative long-term effects of this treatment have not become evident to date.
- Testosterone treatment is not indicated in idiopathic male infertility.

14.9 References

Aaronson AJ, Morrissey RP, Nguyen CT, Willix R, Schwarz ER (2011) Update on the safety of testosterone therapy in cardiac disease. *Expert Opin Drug Saf* 10:697–704

Adamopoulos DA, Nicopoulou S, Kapolla N, Vassipoulos P, Karamertzanis M, Kontogeorgos L (1995) Endocrine effects of testosterone undecanoate as a supplementary treatment to menopausal gonadotropins or tamoxifen citrate in idiopathic oligozoospermia. *Fertil Steril* 64:818–824

Adamopoulos DA, Nicopoulou St, Kapolla N, Karamertzanis M, Andreou E (1997) The combination of testosterone undecanoate with tamoxifen citrate enhances the effects of each agent given independently on seminal parameters in men with idiopathic oligozoospermia. *Fertil Steril* 67:756–762

Akcam T, Bolu E, Merati AL, Durmus C, Gerek M, Ozkaptan Y (2004) Voice changes after androgen therapy for hypogonadotrophic hypogonadism. *Laryngoscope* 114:1587–1591

Albanese A, Stanhope R (1995) Predictive factors in the determination of final height in boys with constitutional delay of growth and puberty. *J Pediatr* 126:545–550

Albanese A, Kewley GD, Long A, Pearl KN, Robins DG, Stanhope R

(1994) Oral treatment for constitutional delay of growth and puberty in boys: a randomized trial of an anabolic steroid or testosterone undecanoate. *Arch Dis Child* **71**:315–317

Arrigo T, Crisafulli G, Salzano G, Zirilli G, De Luca F (2005) High-flow priapism in testosterone-treated boys with constitutional delay of growth and puberty may occur even when very low doses are used. *J Endocrinol Invest* **28**:390–391

Attal P, Chanson P (2010) Endocrine aspects of obstructive sleep apnea. *J Clin Endocrinol Metab* **95**:483–495

Bagchus WM, Hust R, Maris F, Schnabel PG, Houwing NS (2003) Important effect of food on the bioavailability of oral testosterone undecanoate. *Pharmacotherapy* **23**:319–325

Basaria S, Coviello AD, Travison TG, Storer TW, Farwell WR, Jette AM, Eder R, Tennstedt S, Ulloor J, Zhang A, Choong K, Lakshman KM, Mazer NA, Miciek R, Krasnoff J, Elmi A, Knapp PE, Brooks B, Appleman E, Aggarwal S, Bhasin G, Hede-Brierley L, Bhatia A, Collins L, LeBrasseur N, Fiore LD, Bhasin S (2010) Adverse events associated with testosterone administration. *N Engl J Med* **363**:109–222

Behre HM, Bohmeyer J, Nieschlag E (1994) Prostate volume in testosterone-treated and untreated hypogonadal men in comparison to age-matched normal controls. *Clin Endocrinol* **40**:341–349

Behre HM, Abshagen K, Oettel M, Hübler D, Nieschlag E (1999a) Intramuscular injection of testosterone undecanoate for the treatment of male hypogonadism: phase I studies. *Eur J Endocrinol* **140**:414–419

Behre HM, von Eckardstein S, Kliesch S, Nieschlag E (1999b) Long-term substitution therapy of hypogonadal men with transscrotal testosterone over 7–10 years. *Clin Endocrinol* **50**:629–635

Bettendorf M, Heinrich UE, Schönberg DK, Grulich-Henn J (1997) Short-term, high dose testosterone treatment fails to reduce adult height in boys with constitutional tall stature. *Eur J Pediatr* **156**:911–915

Bhasin S, Pencina M, Jasuja GK, Travison TG, Coviello A, Orwoll E, Wang PY, Nielson C, Wu F, Tajar A, Labrie F, Vesper H, Zhang A, Ulloor J, Singh R, D'Agostino R, Vasan RS (2011) Reference ranges for testosterone in men generated using liquid chromatography tandem mass spectrometry in a community-based sample of healthy nonobese young men in the Framingham heart study and applied to three geographically distinct cohorts. *J Clin Endocrinol Metab* **96**: 2430–2439

Bojesen A, Juul S, Gravholt CH (2003) Prenatal and postnatal prevalence of Klinefelter syndrome: a national registry study. *J Clin Endocrinol Metab* **88**:622–626

Bojesen A, Stockholm K, Juul S, Gravholt CH (2011) Socioeconomic trajectories affect mortality in Klinefelter syndrome. *J Clin Endocrinol Metab* **96**:2098–2104

Brabrand S, Fosså SD, Cvancarova M, Lehne G (2011) Androgen substitution with testosterone undecanoate in survivors of bilateral testicular cancer requires individually-adjusted injection intervals. *BJU Int* **107**:1080–1087

Brown D, Butler CGE, Kelnar CJH, Wu FCW (1995) A double blind, placebo controlled study of the effects of low dose testosterone undecanoate on the growth of small for age, prepubertal boys. *Arch Dis Child* **73**:141–145

Büchter D, Behre HM, Kliesch S, Nieschlag E (1998) Pulsatile GnRH or human chorionic gonadotropin/ human menopausal gonadotropin as effective treatment for men with hypogonadotropic hypogonadism: a review of 42 cases. *Eur J Endocrinol* **149**:298–303

Burris AS, Banks SM, Carter CS, Davidson JM, Sherins RJ (1992) A long-term prospective study of the physiologic and behavioural effects of hormone replacement in untreated hypogondadal men. *J Androl* **14**:297–304

Calof OM, Singh AB, Lee ML, Kenny AM, Urban RJ, Tenover JL, Bhasin S (2005) Adverse events associated with testosterone replacement in middle-aged and older men: a meta-analysis of randomized, placebo-controlled trials. *J Gerontol A Biol Sci Med Sci* **60**:1451–1457

Charny CW, Gordon JA (1978) Testosterone rebound therapy: a neglected modality. *Fertil Steril* **29**:64–68

Comhaire F, Schoonjans F, Abelmassih R, Gordts S, Campo R, Dhont M, Milingos S, Gerris J (1995) Does treatment with testosterone undecanoate improve the in-vitro fertilizing capacity of spermatozoa in patients with idiopathic testicular failure? (Results of a double blind study). *Hum Reprod* **10**:2600–2602

Cunningham GR, Hirshkowitz M, Korenman SG, Karacan I (1990) Testosterone replacement therapy and sleep-related erections in hypogonadal men. *J Clin Endocrinol Metab* **70**:792–797

Decker R, Pratsch C-J, Sippell WG (2002) Combined treatment with testosterone (T) and ethinylestradiol (EE2) in constitutionally tall boys: is treatment with T plus EE2 more effective in reducing final height in tall boys than T alone? *J Clin Endocrinol Metab* **87**:1634–1639

de Lange WE, Snoep MC, Doorenbos H (1979) The effect of short-term testosterone treatment in boys with delayed puberty. *Acta Endocrinol* **91**:177–183

Depenbusch M, von Eckardstein S, Simoni M, Nieschlag E (2002) Maintenance of spermatogenesis in hypogonadotropic hypogonadal men with hCG alone. *Eur J Endocrinol* **147**:617–624 de Ronde W (2009) Hyperandrogenism after transfer of topical testosterone gel: case report and review of published and unpublished studies. *Hum Reprod* 24:425–428

de Waal WJ, Vreeburg JTM, Bekkering F, de Jong FH, de Muinck Keizer-Schrama SMPF, Drop SLS, Weber RFA (1995) High dose testosterone therapy for reduction of final height in constitutionally tall boys: does it influence testicular function in adulthood? *Clin Endocrinol* 43:87–95

Drop SLS, de Waal WJ, de Muinck Keizer-Schrama SMPF (1998) Sex steroid treatment of constitutionally tall stature. *Endocr Rev* 19:540–558

Endres W, Shin YS, Rieth M, Block T, Schmiedt E, Knorr D (1987) Priapism in Fabry's disease during testosterone treatment. *Klin Wschr* 65:925

Franchi F, Luisi M, Kicovic PM (1978) Long-term study of oral testosterone undecanoate in hypogonadal males. *Int J Androl* 1:270–278

Gooren LJG (1994) A ten year safety study of the oral androgen testosterone undecanoate. *J Androl* 15:212–215

Haring R, Völzke H, Steveling A, Krebs A, Felix SB, Schöfl C, Dörr M, Nauck M, Wallaschofski H (2010) Low serum testosterone levels are associated with increased risk of mortality in a population-based cohort of men aged 20–79. *Eur Heart J* 31:1494–1501

Hendriks AE, Boellaard WP, van Casteren NJ, Romijn JC, de Jong FH, Boot AM, Drop SL (2010) Fatherhood in tall men treated with high-dose sex steroids during adolescence. *J Clin Endocrinol Metab* 95:5233–5240

Ichioka K, Utsunomiya N, Kohei N, Ueda N, Inoue K, Terai A (2006) Testosterone-induced priapism in Klinefelter syndrome. *Urology* 67:622.e17–622.e18

Ishii T, Sasaki G, Hasegawa T, Sato S, Matsuo N, Ogata T (2004) Testosterone enanthate therapy is effective and independent of SRD5A2 and AR gene polymorphisms in boys with micropenis. *J Urol* 172:319–324

Jockenhövel F (1999) Influence of various modes of androgen substitution on serum lipids and lipoproteins in hypogonadal men. *Metabolism* 48:590–596

Kamischke A, Nieschlag E (1999) Analysis of medical treatment of male infertility. *Hum Reprod* 14:1–23

Kühnert B, Byrne M, Simoni M, Köpcke W, Gerss J, Lemmnitz G, Nieschlag E (2005) Testosterone substitution with a new transdermal, hydroalcoholic gel applied to scrotal or non-scrotal skin: a multicentre trial. *Eur J Endocrinol* 153:317–326

Lanfranco F, Kamischke A, Zitzmann M, Nieschlag E (2004) Klinefelter's syndrome. *Lancet* 364:273–283

Laughlin GA, Barrett-Connor E, Bergstrom J (2008) Low serum testosterone and mortality in older men. *J Clin Endocrinol Metab* 93:68–75

Lee KK, Berman N, Alexander GM, Hull L, Swerdloff RS, Wang C (2003) A simple self-report diary for assessing psychosexual function in hypogonadal men. *J Androl* 25:688–698

Lemcke B, Zentgraf J, Behre HM, Kliesch S, Bramswig JH, Nieschlag E (1996) Long-term effects on testicular function of high-dose testosterone treatment for excessively tall stature. *J Clin Endocrinol Metab* 81:296–301

Luboshitzky R, Aviv A, Hefetz A, Herer P, Shen-Orr Z, Lavie L, Lavie P (2002) Decreased pituitary-gonadal secretion in men with obstructive sleep apnea. *J Clin Endocrinol Metab* 87:3394–3398

Luisi M, Franchi F (1980) Double-blind group comparative study of testosterone undecanoate and mesterolone in hypogonadal male patients. *J Endocrinol Invest* 3:305–308

McNicholas T, Ong T (2006) Review of Testim gel. *Expert Opin Pharmacother* 7:477–484

Morales A, Johnston B, Heaton JPW, Lundie M (1997) Testosterone supplementation for hypogonadal impotence: assessment of biochemical measures and therapeutic outcomes. *J Urol* 157:849–854

Nieschlag E, Cüppers HJ, Wiegelmann W, Wickings EJ (1976) Bioavailability and LH suppressing effect of different testosterone preparations in normal and hypogonadal men. *Horm Res* 7:148

Nieschlag E, Behre HM, Bouchard P, Corrales JJ, Jones TH, Stalla GK, Webb SM, Wu FC (2004) Testosterone replacement therapy: current trends and future directions. *Hum Reprod Update* 10:409–419

Nieschlag E, Behre HM, Nieschlag S (eds) (2010) *Andrology. Male Reproductive Health and Dysfunction*, 3rd edn. Springer-Verlag, Berlin

Ohlsson C, Vandenput L (2009) The role of estrogens for male bone health. *Eur J Endocrinol* 160:883–889

Pedersen MF, Moller S, Krabbe S, Bennett P (1986) Fundamental voice frequency measured by electroglottography during continuous speech. A new exact secondary sex characteristic in boys in puberty. *Int J Ped Otohinol* 11:21–27

Pusch HH (1989) Oral treatment of oligozoospermia with testosterone-undecanoate: results of a double-blind-placebo-controlled trial. *Andrologia* 21:76–82

Raynaud JP, Augès M, Liorzou L, Turlier V, Lauze C (2009) Adhesiveness of a new testosterone-in adhesive matrix patch after extreme conditions. *Int J Pharmacol* **375**:28–32

Rogol AD (2005) New facets of androgen replacement therapy during childhood and adolescence. *Expert Opin Pharmacother* **6**:1319–1336

Rolf C, von Eckardstein S, Koken U, Nieschlag E (2002) Testosterone substitution of hypogonadal men prevents the age-dependent increases in body mass index, body fat and leptin seen in healthy ageing men: results of a cross-sectional study. *Eur J Endocrinol* **146**:505–511

Rosen RC, Araujo AB, Connor MK, Gerstenberger EP, Morgentaler A, Seftel AD, Miner MM, Shabsigh R (2011) The NERI Hypogonadism Screener: psychometric validation in male patients and controls. *Clin Endocrinol* **74**:248–256

Rosenfeld RG, Northcraft GB, Hintz RL (1982) A prospective, randomized study of testosterone treatment of constitutional delay of growth and development in male adolescents. *Pediatrics* **69**:681–687

Ruch W, Jenny P (1989) Priapism following testosterone administration for delayed male puberty. *Am J Med* **86**:256

Schulte-Beerbühl M, Nieschlag E (1980) Comparison of testosterone, dihydrotestosterone, luteinizing hormone, and follicle-stimulating hormone in serum after injection of testosterone enanthate or testosterone cypionate. *Fertil Steril* **33**:201–203

Shabsigh R (1997) The effects of testosterone on the cavernous tissue and erectile function. *World J Urol* **15**:21–26

Shores MM, Matsumoto AM, Sloan KL, Kivlajam DR (2006) Low serum testosterone and mortality in male veterans. *Arch Intern Med* **166**:1660–1665

Skakkebaek NE, Bancroft J, Davidson DW, Warner P (1981) Androgen replacement with oral testosterone undecanoate in hypogonadal men: a double blind controlled study. *Clin Endocrinol* **14**:49–61

Snyder PJ (1999) Effect of testosterone treatment on bone mineral density in men over 65 years of age. *J Clin Endocrinol Metab* **84**:1966–1972

Snyder PJ, Lawrence DA (1980) Treatment of male hypogonadism with testosterone enanthate. *J Clin Endocrinol Metab* **51**:1335–1339

Sokol RZ, Palacios A, Campfield LA, Saul C, Swerdloff RS (1982) Comparison of the kinetics of injectable testosterone in eugonadal and hypogonadal men. *Fertil Steril* **37**:425–430

Vermeulen A, Verdonck G (1992) Representatives of a single point plasma testosterone level for the long term hormonal milieu in men. *J Clin Endocrinol Metab* **74**:939–942

von Eckardstein S, Nieschlag E (2002) Treatment of male hypogonadism with testosterone undecanoate injection at extended intervals of 12 weeks: a phase II study. *J Androl* **23**:419–425

Wang C, Alexander G, Berman N, Salehian B, Davidson T, McDonald V, Steiner B, Hull H, Callegari C, Swerdloff R (1996) Testosterone replacement therapy improves mood in hypogonadal men – a clinical research center study. *J Clin Endocrinol Metab* **81**: 3578–3583

Wang C, Cunningham G, Dobs A (2004) Long-term testosterone gel (AndroGel) treatment maintains beneficial effects on sexual function and mood, lean and fat mass, and bone mineral density in hypogonadal men. *J Clin Endocrinol Metab* **89**:2085–2098

Wang C, Nieschlag E, Swerdloff R, Behre HM, Hellstrom WJ, Gooren LJ, Kaufman JM, Legros JJ, Lunenfeld B, Morales A, Morley JE, Schulman C, Thompson IM, Weidner W, Wu FC (2008) Investigation, treatment and monitoring of late onset hypogonadism in males. *Eur J Endocrinol* **159**:507–514

Wang C, Harnett M, Dobs AS, Swerdloff RS (2010) Pharmacokinetics and safety of long-acting testosterone undecanoate injections in hypogonadal men: an 84-week phase III clinical trial. *J Androl* **31**:457–465

Warne DW, Decosterd G, Okada H, Yano Y, Koide N, Howles CM (2009) A combined analysis of data to identify predictive factors for spermatogenesis in men with hypogonadotropic hypogonadism treated with recombinant human follicle-stimulating hormones and human chorionic gonadotropin. *Fertil Steril* **92**:594–604

Whitworth JA, Scoggins BA, Andrews J, Williamson PM, Brown MA (1992) Haemodynamic and metabolic effects of short term administration of synthetic sex steroids in humans. *Clin Exp Hypertens* **14**:905–922

Wittert GA, Chapman IM, Haren MT, Mackintosh S, Coates P, Morley JE (2003) Oral testosterone supplementation increases muscle and decreases fat mass in healthy elderly males with low-normal gonadal status. *J Gerontol A Biol Sci Med Sci* **58**:618–625

World Health Organization, Task Force on the Diagnosis and Treatment of Infertility (1989) Mesterolone and idiopathic male infertility: a double-blind study. *Int J Androl* **12**:254–264

World Health Organization, Nieschlag E, Wang C, Handelsman DJ, Swerdloff RS, Wu F, Einer-Jensen N, Waites G (1992) *Guidelines for the Use of Androgens*. WHO, Geneva

Zelissen PMJ, Stricker BHC (1988) Severe priapism as a complication of testosterone substitution therapy. *Am J Med* **85**:273

Zitzmann M, Nieschlag E (2001) Testosterone levels in healthy men and their relation to behavioural and physical characteristics: facts and constructs. *Eur J Endocrinol* **144**:183–197

Zitzmann M, Nieschlag E (2007) Androgen receptor gene CAG repeat length and body mass index modulate the safety of long-term intramuscular testosterone undecanoate therapy in hypogonadal men. *J Clin Endocrinol Metab* **92**:3844–3853

Zitzmann M, Rolf C, Brune M, Vieth V, Nieschlag E (2002) Monitoring bone density in hypogonadal men by quantitative phalangeal ultrasound. *Bone* **31**: 422–429

Zitzmann M, Depenbusch M, Gromoll J, Nieschlag E (2003) Prostate volume and growth in testosterone-substituted hypogonadal men are dependent on the CAG repeat polymorphism of the androgen receptor gene: a longitudinal pharmacogenetic study. *J Clin Endocrinol Metab* **88**: 2049–2054

Zitzmann M, Faber S, Nieschlag E (2006) Association of specific symptoms and metabolic risks with serum testosterone in older men. *J Clin Endocrinol Metab* **91**:4335–4343

Testosterone preparations for clinical use in males

Hermann M. Behre and Eberhard Nieschlag

15.1   Introduction

Although testosterone has been in clinical use for almost 70 years, it has only slowly attracted interest from clinical researchers. This is partly due to the fact that hypogonadal men requiring testosterone treatment constitute only a minority of all patients, and hypogonadism is not a life-threatening disease. Since development of new preparations is mainly a task of the pharmaceutical industry, and hypogonadal patients did not promise to contribute a substantial economic profit, development of testosterone preparations was slow. Only recently has the question of testosterone treatment of senescent men (see Chapter 16) and, to a certain extent, also the search for a hormonal male contraceptive (see Chapter 22) spurred interest in the pharmacology and application of testosterone.

Today oral, buccal, injectable, implantable and transdermal testosterone preparations are available for clinical use. There are only a few, especially few not-industry-sponsored, clinical studies available comparing the various preparations with the goal of identifying the optimal preparation for substitution purposes. While the older injectable testosterone preparations produce supraphysiological serum testosterone levels, newer preparations achieve levels closer to the physiological range. We are only beginning to understand which serum levels are required to achieve the various biological effects of testosterone and to avoid adverse side-effects. In particular, very little is known about long-term effects of testosterone therapy inherent to different preparations. Similarly, the role of the AR polymorphism in

Testosterone: Action, Deficiency, Substitution, ed. Eberhard Nieschlag and Hermann M. Behre, Assoc. ed. Susan Nieschlag.
Published by Cambridge University Press. © Cambridge University Press 2012.

modifying testosterone action individually is becoming understood only slowly, but may lead to a pharmacogenetic concept for the therapeutic application of testosterone (Zitzmann 2009; see also Chapter 3).

Under these circumstances it appears that the consensus reached by a Workshop Conference on Androgen Therapy organized jointly by the WHO, NIH and FDA in 1990 still provides the best therapeutic guidelines: "The consensus view was that the major goal of therapy is to replace testosterone levels at as close to physiological concentrations as is possible" (World Health Organization 1992). Until other evidence is provided, all testosterone preparations are best judged by this principle.

An important question is which androgen preparation should be used for clinical purposes. Numerous androgenic steroids have been synthesized and used clinically in the past. The synthetic androgens were produced with the aim of selectively enhancing certain aspects of testosterone activity, e.g. the anabolic effect on muscles or the hematopoietic effect. Some of these molecules proved to have toxic side-effects, in particular upon long-term use (as required for substitution of hypogonadism), or the desired efficacy and safety were inadequate in controlled clinical trials (as advocated by evidence-based medicine) (see Chapter 25). In addition, some of these steroids cannot be converted to 5α-DHT or estrogen, as is testosterone, and therefore cannot develop the full spectrum of activities of testosterone. The important biological significance of these conversions is described in Chapter 2. For these reasons, synthetic preparations have almost disappeared from the market, and testosterone as produced naturally is the prevailing androgen used in clinical medicine. In its various preparations testosterone has been available for over seven decades and, as one of the oldest "drugs" in clinical use, has demonstrated its high safety. However, new insights into the molecular mechanisms of androgen action may lead to the development of steroids suited for specific purposes (see Chapter 21). Whether such steroids may become useful and safe for clinical use remains to be seen.

As all other androgens, testosterone derives from the basic structure of androstane. This molecule consists of three cyclohexane and one cyclopentane ring (perhydrocyclopentanephenanthrene ring) and a methyl group each in position 10 and 13. Androstane itself is biologically inactive and gains activity through oxygroups in position 3 and 17. Testosterone, the quantitatively most important androgen synthesized in the organism, is characterized by an oxy group in position 3, a hydroxy group in position 17 and a double bond in position 4 (Fig. 15.1).

Three approaches have been used to make testosterone therapeutically effective: (1) various routes of administration; (2) esterification in position 17; and (3) chemical modification of the molecule. In addition, these approaches have been combined. Since it is of practical clinical relevance, the route of administration is used here for categorizing the various conventional and new testosterone preparations for clinical use in males (overview in Table 15.1).

15.2 Testosterone preparations for oral administration

15.2.1 Unmodified testosterone

Unmodified testosterone as physiologically secreted by the testes would appear to be the first choice when considering substitution therapy. When ingested orally in its unmodified form, testosterone is absorbed well from the gut but is effectively metabolized and inactivated in the liver before it reaches the target organs ("first-pass effect"). Only when a dose of 200 mg is ingested, which exceeds 30-fold the amount of testosterone produced daily by a normal man, is the metabolizing capacity of the liver overcome. With such doses an increase in peripheral testosterone blood levels becomes measurable and clinical effects can be observed (Johnsen *et al.* 1974; Nieschlag *et al.* 1975). The testosterone-metabolizing capacity of the liver, however, is age- and sex-dependent. An oral dose of 60 mg unmodified testosterone does not affect peripheral testosterone levels in normal adult men, but produces a significant rise in prepubertal boys and women (Nieschlag *et al.* 1977). This demonstrates that testosterone induces liver enzymes responsible for its own metabolism (Johnsen *et al.* 1976). When the liver is severely damaged its metabolizing capacity decreases. Thus, in patients with liver cirrhosis a dose of 60 mg testosterone (ineffective in normal men) produces high serum levels (Nieschlag *et al.* 1977).

In hypogonadal men with normal liver function, 400–600 mg testosterone must be administered daily if the patient is to be substituted by oral testosterone (Johnsen *et al.* 1974) – a dose exceeding the testosterone production of a normal man almost 100-fold. Aside from being uneconomical, the possibility of adverse effects of such huge testosterone doses cannot be excluded, especially when given over long periods of time as required for substitution therapy.

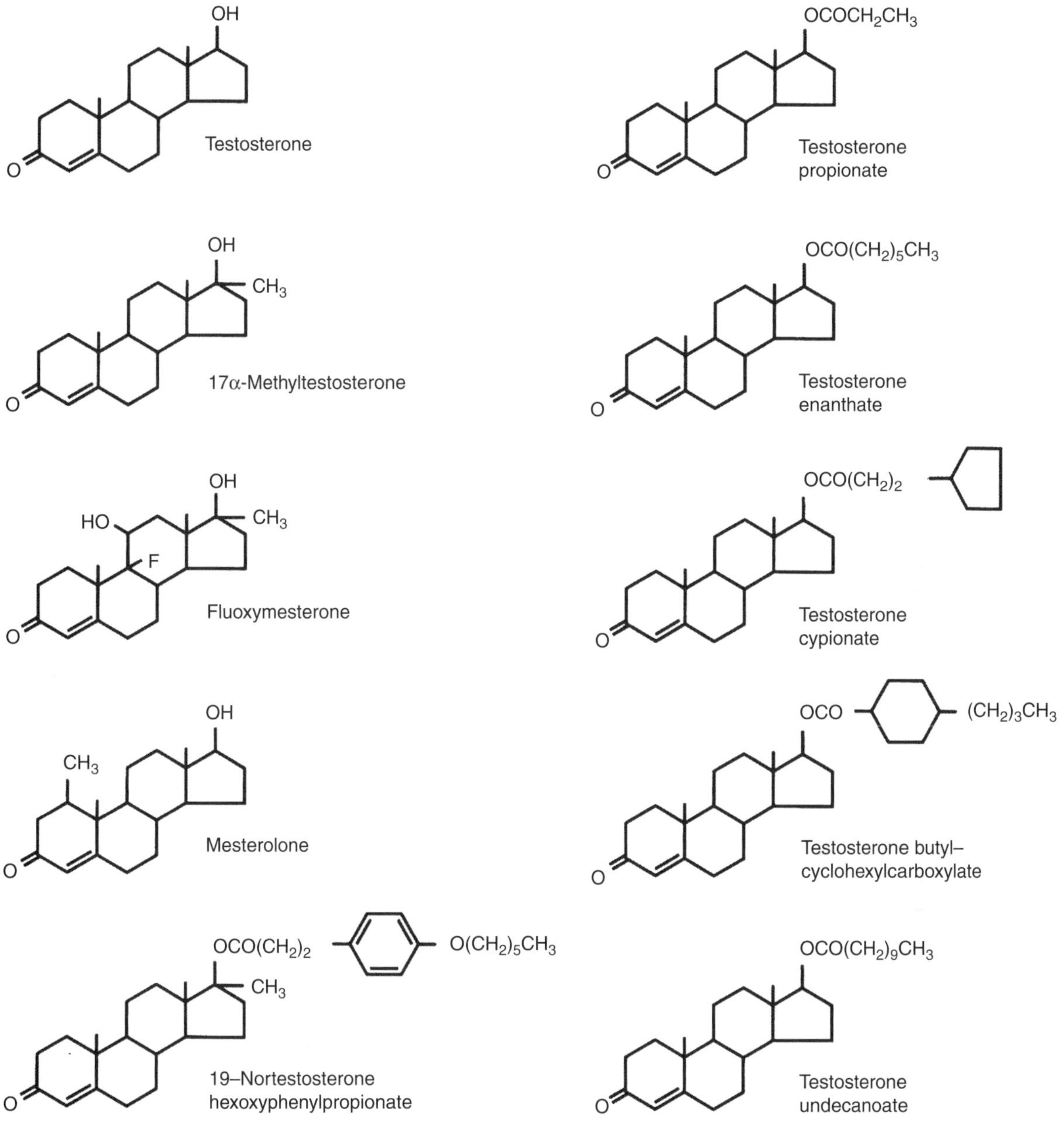

Fig. 15.1 Molecular structure of testosterone and clinically used testosterone esters and derivatives.

Recently, administration of high doses of testosterone has been re-examined with and without concomitant inhibition of 5α-reductase by dutasteride or finasteride (Snyder *et al.* 2010; Amory *et al.* 2011). Administration of 150–400 mg oral testosterone in various formulations twice daily or 300–600 mg daily with and without concomitant 5α-reductase inhibitors to hypogonadal men or men with experimental hypogonadism increased serum levels of testosterone to the normal or supraphysiological range. In addition, three-times 300 mg of oral testosterone per day was tested in normal men with suppressed endogenous testosterone by GnRH antagonist administration (Lee *et al.* 2011). Long-term studies with data on potential side-effects of these high-dose testosterone preparations and the clinical relevance of significantly decreased DHT levels are awaited to estimate the clinical perspective of this therapeutic approach.

Table 15.1 Mode of application and dosage of various testosterone preparations

Preparation	Route of application	Full substitution dose
In clinical use		
Testosterone undecanoate	Oral	2–4 capsules at 40 mg/day
Testosterone tablets	Buccal	30 mg twice daily
Testosterone enanthate	Intramuscular injection	200–250 mg every 2–3 weeks
Testosterone cypionate	Intramuscular injection	200 mg every 2 weeks
Testosterone undecanoate	Intramuscular injection	1000 mg every 10–14 weeks
Testosterone implants	Implantation under the abdominal skin	4 implants at 200 mg every 5–6 months
Transdermal testosterone patch	Non-scrotal skin	2 systems per day or every second day depending on preparation
Transdermal testosterone gel (1–2.5%)	Non-scrotal skin	Starting dose 40–62.5 mg/day depending on preparation
Testosterone solution (2%)	Axillary	Starting dose 60 mg/day
In advanced clinical development		
Testosterone undecanoate (self-emulsifying drug delivery system)	Oral	Not yet determined
Obsolete		
17α-Methyltestosterone	Oral	
Fluoxymesterone	Sublingual/oral	

15.2.2   17α-Methyltestosterone

Several attempts have been made to modify the testosterone molecule by chemical means in order to render it orally effective; i.e. to delay metabolism in the liver. In this regard, the longest-known testosterone derivative is 17α-methyltestosterone (Ruzicka *et al.* 1935), which is a fully effective oral androgen preparation. 17α-Methyltestosterone is quickly absorbed, and maximal blood levels are observed 90 to 120 minutes after ingestion. The half-life in blood amounts to approximately 150 minutes (Alkalay *et al.* 1973).

Ever since this steroid was introduced for clinical use, hepatotoxic side-effects such as an increase in serum liver enzymes (Carbone *et al.* 1959), cholestasis of the liver (Werner *et al.* 1950; de Lorimer *et al.* 1965) and peliosis of the liver (Westaby *et al.* 1977) have been reported repeatedly. It is of interest that humans are more susceptible to the hepatotoxic effects of methyltestosterone than rats (Heywood *et al.* 1977a) or dogs (Heywood *et al.* 1977b). Later, an association between long-term methyltestosterone treatment and liver tumors was found (e.g. Farrell *et al.* 1975; Boyd and Mark 1977; Goodman and Laden 1977; Paradinas *et al.* 1977; Falk *et al.* 1979).

The hepatotoxic side-effects are due to the alkyl group in the 17α position, and have also been reported for other steroids with this configuration (Krüskemper and Noell 1967). Because of the side-effects methyltestosterone should no longer be used therapeutically for hypogonadism, in particular since effective alternatives are available (Nieschlag 1981). The German Endocrine Society declared methyltestosterone obsolete in 1981, and the German Federal Health Authority ruled that methyltestosterone should be withdrawn from the market (Anonymous 1988). In other countries, however, methyltestosterone is still in use, a practice which should be terminated.

15.2.3   Fluoxymesterone

The androgenic activity of fluoxymesterone was enhanced over that of testosterone by the introduction of fluorine and the addition of a hydroxy group into the steroid skeleton of testosterone. This substance also contains a 17α-methyl group, and accordingly there is a risk of hepatotoxicity with long-term use. Therefore, this androgen has disappeared from the market.

15.2.4 Mesterolone

Mesterolone can be considered a derivative of the 5α-reduced testosterone metabolite 5α-dihydrotestosterone (DHT), which is protected from rapid metabolism in the liver by a methyl group in position 1 (Gerhards *et al.* 1966) and thus becomes orally active. It is free of liver toxicity. Unlike testosterone, mesterolone cannot be metabolized to estrogens (Breuer and Gütgemann 1966), and at a molecular level acts like DHT. Because of its limited effectiveness in suppressing pituitary gonadotropin secretion (Aakvaag and Stromme 1974; Gordon *et al.* 1975), it can only be considered an incomplete androgen. Altogether, mesterolone is not suited for the substitution of hypogonadism.

15.2.5 Testosterone undecanoate

When testosterone is esterified in the 17β-position with a long fatty acid side chain such as undecanoic acid, and given orally, its route of absorption from the gastrointestinal tract is slightly shifted from the vena portae to the lymph and reaches the circulation via the thoracic duct (Coert *et al.* 1975; Horst *et al.* 1976; Shackleford *et al.* 2003). Absorption is improved if the ester is taken in arachis oil (Nieschlag *et al.* 1975) and with a meal (Frey *et al.* 1979; Bagchus *et al.* 2003). After oral ingestion of a 40 mg capsule, of which 63%, i.e. 25 mg, is testosterone, maximum serum levels are reached two to six hours later (Nieschlag *et al.* 1975). Thus, with two to four capsules (80 to 160 mg) per day, testosterone substitution of hypogonadism can be achieved.

Pharmacokinetics of testosterone undecanoate after single-dose administration in oleic acid was tested in 8 hypogonadal patients and 12 normal men (Schürmeyer *et al.* 1983). On average, maximum levels of serum testosterone could be observed five hours after testosterone undecanoate administration. However, the serum testosterone profile showed high interindividual variability of the time when maximum concentrations were reached, as well as of the maximum levels themselves, which ranged from 17 to 96 nmol/l. When the individual serum concentration

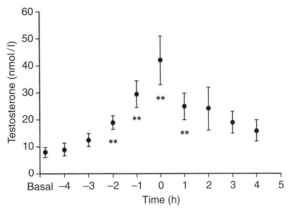

Fig. 15.2 Single-dose pharmacokinetics of testosterone undecanoate dissolved in oleic acid after oral administration of 120 mg of the ester to eight hypogonadal patients. Because of high interindividual variability of testosterone serum concentrations after administration of testosterone undecanoate, individual curves were all centralized about the time of maximal serum concentrations (time 0). Asterisks indicate significant higher testosterone serum concentrations compared to pretreatment values (basal) (mean ± standard error of mean (SEM)).

versus time curves were centralized about the time of maximal serum concentrations, serum concentrations significantly different from basal values were seen only two hours before and one hour after the time of maximal serum concentrations in hypogonadal patients (Fig. 15.2; Schürmeyer *et al.* 1983). Based on this observation it can be deduced that, even with administration of testosterone undecanoate in oleic acid three times daily, only short-lived testosterone peaks resulting in high fluctuations can be obtained.

The initial commercial preparation of oral testosterone undecanoate in oleic acid had to be refrigerated (2–8 °C) in the pharmacy for reasons of stability; whereas patients had to store it at room temperature to ensure optimal absorption. The shelf-life at room temperature was only three months. Therefore, a new, more stable pharmaceutical formulation of testosterone undecanoate was developed in which the oleic acid was replaced by castor oil. This new formulation can be stored at room temperature for three years. The lipid content in food influences absorption of this oral testosterone undecanoate preparation and could explain some of the intraindividual variability of testosterone levels. A low liquid meal with, at most, 5 g of lipid is not sufficient for adequate absorption of testosterone undecanoate. However, a "normal" meal containing approximately 19 g of lipid efficiently increases serum testosterone levels after oral administration of testosterone undecanoate capsules (Schnabel *et al.* 2007).

Recently, testosterone undecanoate was formulated into a new proprietary self-emulsifying drug delivery system (SEDDS) preparation for oral application. This SEDDS is intended to promote solubilization and the intestinal lymphatic absorption of lipophilic testosterone esters and thereby reduce first-pass hepatic metabolism. Pharmacokinetic studies in hypogonadal men up to 28 days showed that 200 mg testosterone twice daily given as testosterone undecanoate SEDDS (100 mg testosterone = 158.3 mg testosterone undecanoate) increased mean serum levels of testosterone to the normal range in most subjects, but not when taken in the fasting state (Yin *et al.* 2012; Fig. 15.3). Currently, this testosterone preparation is being tested in a large international phase III study.

15.3 Testosterone preparations for sublingual or buccal administration

17α-Methyltestosterone was found to be more effective when applied sublingually than when ingested orally (Escamilla 1949). This type of substitution should, however, not be practiced, because of the liver toxicity of methyltestosterone summarized above.

The solubility of the hydrophobic testosterone molecule can be enhanced by incorporation into hydroxypropyl-β-cyclodextrins (Pitha *et al.* 1986), which are macro-ring structures consisting of cyclic oligosaccharides. When testosterone incorporated into such cyclodextrins is administered sublingually, steep increases in serum testosterone occur, lasting for one or two hours (Stuenkel *et al.* 1991). Hypogonadal men treated with three-times-daily doses for 60 days showed improvement of their condition (Salehian *et al.* 1995; Wang *et al.* 1996). This is an interesting approach to testosterone substitution, but unless more constant serum levels can be achieved this therapy would require repeated daily applications and would have the same disadvantages as conventional oral testosterone undecanoate therapy.

Administration of testosterone via the buccal mucosa bypasses the liver and avoids first-pass clearance by delivering the drug directly into systemic circulation. Compared to sublingual administration, buccal mucosa is less permeable and potentially better suited for sustained delivery systems.

Whereas earlier buccal testosterone preparations were not very acceptable to the patients, a new

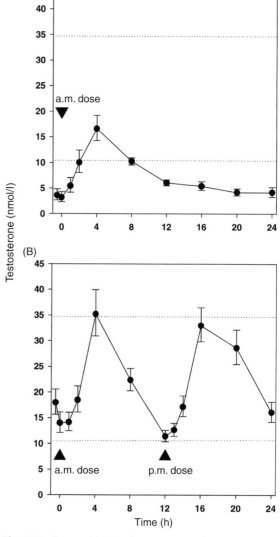

Fig. 15.3 Pharmacokinetics of testosterone undecanoate formulated into a proprietary self-emulsifying drug delivery system (SEDDS) (mean ± SEM) (adapted with permission from Yin *et al.* 2012). (A) Single dose pharmacokinetics after oral dosing of 200 mg testosterone in 12 hypogonadal men (100 mg testosterone = 158.3 mg testosterone undecanoate). (B) Multiple dose pharmacokinetics on day seven after 300 mg testosterone administered twice daily for seven days.

testosterone bioadhesive buccal system was designed to adhere rapidly to the buccal mucosa and gellify, for delivering testosterone steadily into the circulation. The pharmacokinetics were evaluated in 82 hypogonadal men (Wang *et al.* 2004). The tablet (30 mg testosterone) was applied twice daily to the upper gums for three months; 86.6% of the patients reached an average testosterone concentration over 24 hours within the physiological range. Local problems associated with tablet use were transient in most patients. Long-term acceptability and compliance of this mode of testosterone delivery to hypogonadal patients has still to be awaited. For example, in Germany this preparation was launched some years ago for treatment of hypogonadism but has disappeared from the market in the meantime.

15.4 Testosterone preparations for nasal administration

The first-pass effect of the liver can also be avoided by applying testosterone to the nasal mucosa (Danner and Frick 1980). However, unreliable absorption patterns and short-lived serum peaks prevented this form of application from further development to become a desirable option for long-term substitution therapy. Recently, this form of application has been re-examined: 7.6 mg of nasal testosterone was given either twice or three times a day in 21 severely hypogonadal men for 14 days (Mattern *et al.* 2008). In the group treated three times a day, serum levels of testosterone were maintained in most patients within the normal range. Further long-term studies will be necessary to fully evaluate the potential of this mode of testosterone application.

15.5 Testosterone preparations for rectal administration

In order to avoid the first-pass effect of the liver, testosterone can be applied rectally in suppositories (Hamburger 1958). Administration of a suppository containing 40 mg testosterone results in an immediate and steep rise of serum testosterone lasting for about four hours. Effective serum levels can be achieved by repeated applications (Nieschlag *et al.* 1976). This therapy, however, never gained much popularity probably because the patients find it unacceptable to use suppositories three times daily on a long-term routine basis.

15.6 Testosterone preparations for intramuscular administration

The most widely used testosterone substitution therapy is the im injection of testosterone esters. Unmodified testosterone has a half-life of only 10 minutes and would have to be injected very frequently. Esterification of the testosterone molecule at position 17, for example, with propionic or enanthic acid, prolongs the activity of testosterone in proportion to the length of the side chain when administered intramuscularly (Junkmann 1952; 1957). The deep im injection of testosterone esters in oily vehicle is generally safe and well tolerated, but can cause minor side-effects such as local pain (Mackey *et al.* 1995).

Studies applying GC-MS that allow discrimination between endogenous testosterone and exogenously administered deuterium-labeled testosterone propionate-19,19,19-d3 and its metabolite testosterone-19,19,19-d3 were able to show that after im administration, the testosterone ester is slowly absorbed into the general circulation and then rapidly converted to the active unesterified metabolite (Fujioka *et al.* 1986). The observation that the duration at the injection site is the major factor determining the residence time of the drug in the body agrees with pharmacokinetic studies in rats showing that the androgen ester 19-nortestosterone decanoate, when injected into the musculus gastrocnemius of the rat in vivo, is absorbed unchanged from the injection depot in the muscle into the general circulation according to first-order kinetics, with a long half-life of 130 h (van der Vies 1965). Comparisons of the absorption kinetics of different testosterone esters clearly show that the half-lives of the absorption of the esters increase when the esterified fatty acids have a longer chain (van der Vies 1985). In addition, pharmacokinetics are influenced by the oily vehicle, the injection site and the injection volume (Minto *et al.* 1997).

After absorption from the intramuscular depot, the testosterone ester is rapidly hydrolyzed in plasma, as was shown by in-vitro rat studies (van der Vies 1970) and in-vivo human studies (Fujioka *et al.* 1986). The rate of hydrolysis again depends on the structure of the acid chain, but this process is much faster than release from the injection depot (van der Vies 1985). The metabolism of the testosterone ester to the unesterified testosterone occurs rapidly, so that testosterone enanthate or testosterone have nearly identical intravenous pharmacokinetics (Sokol and Swerdloff 1986). Similarly, the duration of action of the orally effective ester testosterone undecanoate seems to be dependent on the duration of absorption of the uncleaved lipophilic testosterone undecanoate via the ductus thoracicus from the gut (Maisey *et al.* 1981; Schürmeyer *et al.* 1983).

In men treated with testosterone, the testosterone concentration measurable in the serum is the sum of endogenous testosterone and exogenous testosterone hydrolyzed from the injected ester. Hypogonadal patients are characterized by impaired or absent endogenous testosterone secretion; exogenous testosterone administration can further suppress endogenous testosterone secretion only to a limited degree, if at all. Accordingly, in hypogonadal patients the serum concentration versus time profile is mainly a reflection of the pharmacokinetics of exogenously administered testosterone ester alone. In this chapter the evaluation of pharmacokinetic parameters for different testosterone esters is based on the increases of testosterone serum concentrations over basal levels in hypogonadal patients.

15.6.1 Testosterone propionate

Single-dose pharmacokinetics of 50 mg testosterone propionate after im injection to seven hypogonadal patients, and the best-fit pharmacokinetic profile, are shown in Fig. 15.4 (Nieschlag *et al.* 1976). Maximal testosterone levels in the supraphysiological range were seen shortly after injection (40.2 nmol/l, t_{max} = 14 h). Testosterone levels below the normal range were observed following day two (57 h) after injection. The calculated values were 1843 nmol·h/l for area under the curve (AUC); 1.5 d for mean residence time (MRT); and 0.8 d for terminal half-life (Table 15.2).

Based on single-dose pharmacokinetic parameters, a multiple-dose pharmacokinetic simulation was performed. Expected testosterone serum concentrations after multiple dosing of 50 mg testosterone propionate, twice per week (e.g. injections Mondays and Thursdays, 8 a.m.), are shown in Fig. 15.5. Shortly after injection, high supraphysiological testosterone serum concentrations of up to 45 nmol/l are observed. At the end of the injection interval (three and four days, respectively), testosterone serum concentrations below the lower range of normal testosterone values are projected (7 nmol/l and 3 nmol/l, respectively).

Judged by the data from pharmacokinetic analysis and simulation, administration of testosterone propionate is not suitable for substitution therapy of male hypogonadism because of its short-term kinetics resulting in wide fluctuations of testosterone serum concentrations and maximal injection intervals of three days for the 50 mg dose.

Table 15.2 Comparative pharmacokinetics of different testosterone esters after intramuscular injection to hypogonadal patients

Testosterone ester	Terminal elimination half-life (d)
Testosterone propionate	0.8
Testosterone enanthate	4.5
Testosterone buciclate	29.5
Testosterone undecanoate	33.9

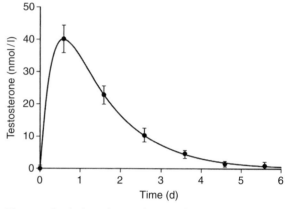

Fig. 15.4 Single-dose pharmacokinetics of testosterone propionate in seven hypogonadal patients. *Closed circles*, mean ± SEM of testosterone serum concentrations actually measured; *curve*, best-fit pharmacokinetic profile.

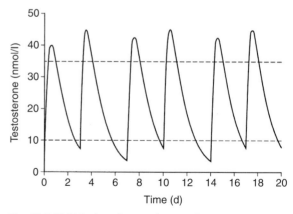

Fig. 15.5 Multiple-dose pharmacokinetics of testosterone propionate after injection of 50 mg testosterone propionate twice per week (e.g. Mondays and Thursdays). *Solid curve*, pharmacokinetic simulation; *broken lines*, range of normal testosterone values.

15.6.2 Testosterone enanthate

Single-dose pharmacokinetics of testosterone enanthate after im administration of 250 mg testosterone enanthate to seven hypogonadal patients and the best-fit pharmacokinetic profile are shown in Fig. 15.6 (Nieschlag *et al.* 1976). Maximal testosterone levels in the supraphysiological range were seen shortly after injection (39.4 nmol/l, $t_{max} = 10$ h). Testosterone levels below the normal range were observed following day 12 after injection. The calculated values were 9911 nmol·h/l for AUC, 8.5 d for MRT and 4.5 d for terminal half-life (Table 15.2).

Based on the pharmacokinetic parameters of single-dose pharmacokinetics, multiple-dose pharmacokinetic simulations for equal doses of 250 mg testosterone enanthate and injection intervals of one to four weeks were performed. With weekly injection intervals, supraphysiological maximal testosterone serum concentrations up to 78 nmol/l are observed at steady state shortly after injection, and supraphysiological

minimal testosterone serum concentrations up to 40 nmol/l just before the next injection (Fig. 15.7). Injecting 250 mg of testosterone enanthate every two weeks results in maximal supraphysiological

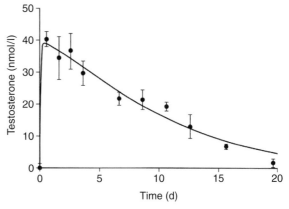

Fig. 15.6 Single-dose pharmacokinetics of testosterone enanthate in seven hypogonadal patients. *Closed circles*, mean ± SEM of testosterone serum concentrations actually measured; *curve*, best-fit pharmacokinetic profile.

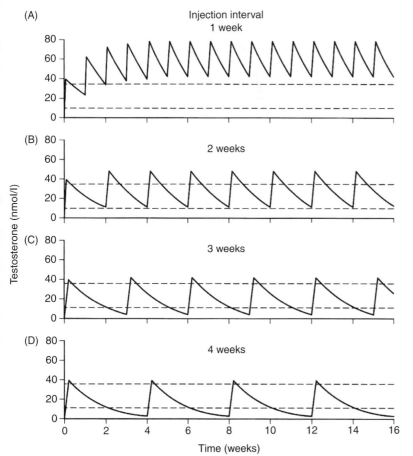

Fig. 15.7 Multiple-dose pharmacokinetics of testosterone enanthate after injection of 250 mg testosterone enanthate every week (A), every second week (B), every three weeks (C) and every four weeks (D). *Solid curves*, pharmacokinetic simulations; *broken lines*, range of normal testosterone values.

testosterone serum concentrations of up to 51 nmol/l shortly after injection and testosterone serum levels at the lower range for normal testosterone serum concentration shortly before the next injection. If the injection interval is extended to three weeks, testosterone serum concentrations below the normal range are observed 14 days after injection. With injection intervals of four weeks, testosterone serum concentrations are in the subnormal range at week three and four, and effective testosterone substitution is not guaranteed (Fig. 15.7).

The calculated testosterone serum concentrations at steady state obtained by computer simulation correspond well to the results of published studies describing multiple-dose testosterone enanthate pharmacokinetics. In a clinical trial for male contraception, 20 healthy men were injected with 200 mg/wk of testosterone enanthate for 12 weeks (Cunningham *et al.* 1978). Minimal serum concentrations of testosterone at steady state, i.e. the testosterone serum concentration just before the next injection, were measured at 31.2 to 39.5 nmol/l after weekly injection of 200 mg testosterone enanthate. Very similar data were obtained in further contraceptive studies when normal men received 200 mg/wk testosterone enanthate injections for 18 months (Anderson and Wu 1996; Wu *et al.* 1996). The data from these studies fit well with the computer-calculated minimal testosterone serum concentrations of 40 nmol/l and maximal testosterone levels of 78 nmol/l after multiple injections of testosterone enanthate at a dosage of 250 mg/wk.

Snyder and Lawrence (1980) administered 100 mg/wk (*n* = 12), 200 mg/2 wks (*n* = 10), 300 mg/3 wks (*n* = 9) and 400 mg/4 wks (*n* = 6) testosterone enanthate to hypogonadal patients during a study period of three months. Blood was drawn during the last injection period, when steady state had been reached, every day (100 mg/wk) up to every fourth day (400 mg/4 wks). Similar to the computer simulation described above for 250 mg testosterone enanthate and injection intervals of one to four weeks, initial supraphysiological testosterone serum levels were seen shortly after injection. In the 100 mg/wk treatment group, where daily blood sampling was performed, mean peak serum concentrations were seen 24 h after injection. Comparable to the results of the computer simulation, after injection of 200 mg/2 wks testosterone enanthate, following initial supraphysiological testosterone serum levels, values fell to progressively lower values before the next injection,

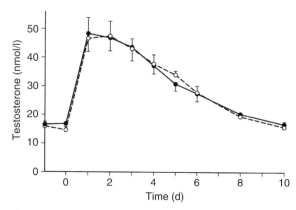

Fig. 15.8 Comparative pharmacokinetics of 194 mg of testosterone enanthate and 200 mg of testosterone cypionate after im injection to six normal volunteers. •, mean ± SEM of testosterone levels after testosterone enanthate injections; o, mean ± SEM of testosterone levels after testosterone cypionate injections.

eventually reaching the lower normal limit (Snyder and Lawrence 1980). Similar results were described after injection of 300 mg/3 wks or 400 mg/4 wks testosterone enanthate. The authors conclude that the testosterone enanthate doses of 200 mg have to be injected every two weeks or doses of 300 mg every three weeks to guarantee effective substitution therapy.

15.6.3 Testosterone cypionate and testosterone cyclohexanecarboxylate

Testosterone cypionate (cyclopentylpropionate) pharmacokinetics were compared with those of testosterone enanthate in a crossover study involving six healthy men aged 20–29 years. Three subjects received 194 mg of testosterone enanthate, followed seven weeks later by 200 mg of testosterone cypionate and vice versa (amount of unesterified testosterone 140 mg in both preparations). The serum testosterone profiles were identical after injection of both preparations in equivalent doses, both in terms of maximal concentrations and in terms of duration of elevation above basal levels (Fig. 15.8; Schulte-Beerbühl and Nieschlag 1980).

In a subsequent clinical study, the pharmacokinetics of testosterone cyclohexanecarboxylate were compared to the pharmacokinetics of testosterone enanthate in a single-blind, crossover study in seven healthy young men (Schürmeyer and Nieschlag 1984). After injection of either testosterone enanthate or testosterone cyclohexanecarboxylate, testosterone concentrations in serum increased sharply and reached maximum levels, four to five times above basal, 8–24 h after injection. During the following days a parallel decay of testosterone levels occurred after injection of either ester preparation, with testosterone serum concentrations slightly, but significantly lower after testosterone cyclohexanecarboxylate injection compared to testosterone enanthate injection two, three and seven days after administration. Basal serum levels were reached seven days after testosterone cyclohexanecarboxylate administration and nine days after injection of testosterone enanthate.

Because testosterone cypionate, testosterone cyclohexanecarboxylate and testosterone enanthate had comparable suppressing effects on LH and consequently on endogenous testosterone secretion, it can be concluded from these studies in normal volunteers that all three esters with similar molecular structure possess comparable pharmacokinetics of exogenous testosterone serum concentrations. Testosterone cypionate or testosterone cyclohexanecarboxylate do not provide a more advantageous pharmacokinetic profile than testosterone enanthate. This observation is in agreement with a clinical study of replacement therapy with single-dose administration of 200 mg of testosterone cypionate in 11 hypogonadal patients (Nankin 1987).

15.6.4 Testosterone ester combinations

Testosterone ester mixtures have been widely used for substitution therapy of male hypogonadism (e.g. Testoviron® Depot 50: 20 mg testosterone propionate and 55 mg testosterone enanthate; Testoviron® Depot 100: 25 mg testosterone propionate and 110 mg testosterone enanthate; Sustanon® 250: 30 mg testosterone propionate, 60 mg testosterone phenylpropionate, 60 mg testosterone isocaproate and 100 mg testosterone decanoate). These combinations are used following the postulate that the so-called short-acting testosterone ester (e.g. testosterone propionate) is the effective testosterone for substitution during the first days of treatment, and the so-called long-acting testosterone (e.g. testosterone enanthate) warrants effective substitution for the end of the injection interval. However, this assumption is not supported by the pharmacokinetic parameters of the individual testosterone esters. Both testosterone propionate and testosterone enanthate cause highest testosterone serum concentrations shortly after injection (Fig. 15.4 and Fig. 15.6). Accordingly, addition of testosterone propionate to testosterone enanthate only increases the initial undesired testosterone peak and worsens the pharmacokinetic profile that ideally should follow zero-order kinetics (Fig. 15.9). The computer simulation agrees well with the limited published single-dose testosterone values that have been measured in hypogonadal patients treated with the combination of testosterone propionate and testosterone enanthate. Maximal increases of approximately 40 nmol/l testosterone over basal values are described one day after im administration of a testosterone ester combination

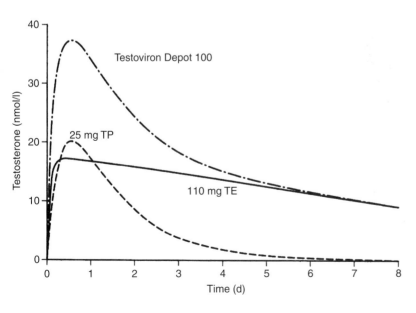

Fig. 15.9 Pharmacokinetic profile of Testoviron® Depot 100 (110 mg testosterone enanthate (TE) and 25 mg testosterone propionate (TP)) in comparison to the pharmacokinetics of the individual testosterone esters of the mixture. *Curves*, pharmacokinetic simulations.

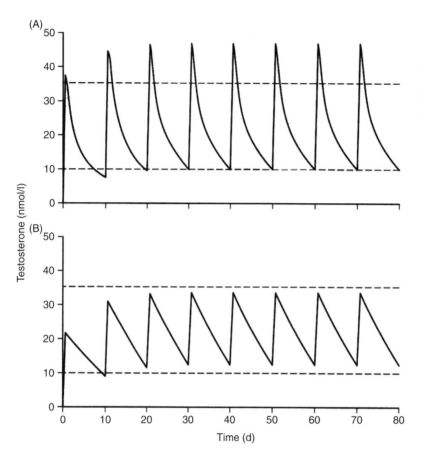

Fig. 15.10 Multiple-dose pharmacokinetics of (A) the testosterone ester mixture Testoviron® Depot 100 (110 mg testosterone enanthate and 25 mg testosterone propionate = 100 mg unesterified testosterone) every 10 d, in comparison with (B) 139 mg testosterone enanthate (= 100 mg unesterified testosterone) every 10 d. *Solid curves,* pharmacokinetic simulations; *broken lines,* range of normal testosterone values.

of 115.7 mg testosterone enanthate and 20 mg testosterone propionate to three hypogonadal patients (Fukutani *et al.* 1974).

A comparison of computer-simulated testosterone serum concentrations after multiple-dose injections of Testoviron® Depot 100 (110 mg testosterone enanthate and 25 mg testosterone propionate = 100 mg unesterified testosterone) every 10 d, and 139 mg testosterone enanthate (= 100 mg unesterified testosterone) every 10 d is shown in Fig. 15.10. As can be expected from the single-dose kinetics of the individual esters, injection of the testosterone ester mixture (Fig. 15.10A) produces a much wider fluctuation of testosterone serum concentrations relative to injection of testosterone enanthate alone (Fig. 15.10B). This simulation shows that injections of testosterone enanthate alone produce a more favorable pharmacokinetic profile in comparison to injections of testosterone propionate and testosterone enanthate ester mixtures in comparable doses. For treatment of male hypogonadism there is no advantage in combining the available short- and long-acting testosterone esters.

15.6.5 Testosterone buciclate

The disadvantage of all esters described so far is that they produce initially supraphysiological testosterone levels, which may exceed normal levels several-fold, and then slowly decline, so that before the next injection pathologically low levels may be reached. Some patients recognize these ups and downs of testosterone levels in parallel variations of general well-being, sexual activity and emotional stability. Despite these disadvantages, testosterone enanthate and cypionate are still the standard intramuscular therapy for male hypogonadism in various countries.

Because of these shortcomings of the available esters, the WHO initiated a steroid synthesis program (Crabbé *et al.* 1980), out of which a series of new testosterone esters was developed. When tested in laboratory rodents, a specific ester was identified that showed greatly prolonged activity, namely *testosterone-trans-4-n-butylcyclohexyl-carboxylate*, generic name *testosterone buciclate*. This preparation is injected intramuscularly in an aqueous solution, in

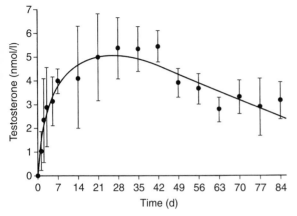

Fig. 15.11 Single-dose pharmacokinetics of testosterone buciclate after im injection of 600 mg of the ester to four hypogonadal patients. *Closed circles*, mean ± SEM of testosterone serum concentrations actually measured (increase over baseline); *curve*, best-fit pharmacokinetic profile.

injected dose of testosterone buciclate from 600 to 1000 mg prolongs the duration of action significantly, but does not lead to significantly higher maximal serum levels of testosterone.

The long duration of action of testosterone buciclate was also demonstrated in a contraceptive study with this new testosterone ester. After a single im injection of 1200 mg testosterone buciclate at a concentration of 400 mg/ml to eight normal men, serum levels of testosterone remained within the normal range, whereas gonadotropins and spermatogenesis were significantly suppressed for at least 18 weeks (Behre *et al.* 1995). These studies demonstrate that the long-acting testosterone buciclate is well suited for substitution therapy of male hypogonadism as well as for male contraception. However, this compound has not been developed into a marketable product and is currently not available.

contrast to the other testosterone esters which are dissolved in oily solution.

To assess the pharmacokinetics of testosterone buciclate in men, the first clinical study was performed in eight men with primary hypogonadism (Behre and Nieschlag 1992). The men were randomly assigned to two study groups and were given either 200 mg (group I) or 600 mg (group II) testosterone buciclate, intramuscularly. Whereas in group I serum androgen levels did not rise to normal values, in group II androgens increased significantly and were maintained in the normal range up to 12 weeks, with maximal serum levels (c_{max}) of 13.1 ± 0.9 nmol/l (mean $\pm$ SEM) in study week six (t_{max}). No initial burst release of testosterone was observed in either study group. Pharmacokinetic analysis revealed a terminal elimination half-life of 29.5 ± 3.9 days (Fig. 15.11; Table 15.2).

Because of the promising results of the first clinical study with testosterone buciclate, a follow-up study was initiated. After complete wash-out from previous therapy, all hypogonadal men received a single im injection of 1000 mg testosterone buciclate. As in the previous study with lower doses, no initial burst release of testosterone was observed. Maximal testosterone serum levels were observed nine weeks (t_{max}) after injection, with a mean value of 13.1 ± 1.8 nmol/l (c_{max}). Following peak concentrations, testosterone serum levels gradually declined and remained within the normal range up to week 16. This study demonstrated that an increase of the

15.6.6 Testosterone undecanoate

While testosterone undecanoate has been available for oral substitution for more than three decades, it was first demonstrated in China that im administration of testosterone undecanoate in tea seed oil (125 mg/ml) has a prolonged duration of action (Wang *et al.* 1991). In a clinical study in Asian hypogonadal men, eight patients received one im injection of 500 mg, and seven of the initial eight hypogonadal patients one injection of 1000 mg testosterone undecanoate (in 8 ml tea seed oil) in a crossover design (Zhang *et al.* 1998). Follow-up blood samples were obtained weekly up to week nine after injection. In both study groups, mean serum levels of testosterone were above the upper limit of normal during the first two weeks after injection. Thereafter, mean serum concentration remained in the normal range up to week seven after injection in the 500 mg dose group and at least up to week nine in the 1000 mg dose group. The terminal elimination half-lives were 18.3 ± 2.3 and 23.7 ± 2.7 days for the 500 mg dose and 1000 mg dose groups, respectively. Administration of 500 mg of this testosterone preparation every four weeks, after an initial loading dose of 1000 mg, for up to 12 months, to 308 healthy men for male contraception, maintained serum levels of testosterone in the normal range when measured directly before the next injection (Gu *et al.* 2003).

In the first study in Caucasian men, im injections of 250 mg or 1000 mg testosterone undecanoate in tea seed oil were given to 14 hypogonadal patients (Behre *et al.* 1999a). Follow-up examinations were performed 1, 2, 3, 5 and 7 days after injection and then weekly up to study week eight. Whereas no prolonged increase of testosterone was observed in the 250 mg group, serum levels of testosterone in the higher dose group increased from 4.8 ± 0.9 nmol/l (mean $\pm$ SEM) to maximum levels of 30.5 ± 4.3 nmol/l at day 7 (t_{max}). Testosterone levels remained within the normal range up to week seven (13.5 ± 1.2 nmol/l). Non-linear regression analysis revealed a terminal elimination half-life for intramuscular testosterone undecanoate of 20.9 ± 6.0 days (Fig. 15.12).

Similar to the preclinical study in monkeys, the clinical study in hypogonadal men demonstrated favorable pharmacokinetics of intramuscular testosterone undecanoate. Because of the relatively low concentration of 125 mg testosterone undecanoate per milliliter of tea seed oil, however, administration of the 1000 mg dose requires an injection volume of 8 ml, which renders im administration impracticable. Therefore, the preparation was reformulated and testosterone undecanoate dissolved in castor oil at a higher concentration of 250 mg/ml. Fourteen hypogonadal patients received one im injection of 1000 mg of the reformulated testosterone undecanoate preparation (Behre *et al.* 1999a). Maximal serum levels with the reformulated preparation were lower than with the Chinese preparation and remained within the mid-normal range (Fig. 15.12). Pharmacokinetic analysis revealed a long terminal elimination half-life of 33.9 ± 4.9 days (Table 15.2).

Due to these favorable pharmacokinetics, a first, prospective, open-label study with repeated im injection was initiated (Nieschlag *et al.* 1999). Thirteen hypogonadal men received four im injections of 1000 mg testosterone undecanoate in castor oil at

six-week intervals. Following the first injection, mean serum levels of testosterone were never found below the lower limit of normal (Fig. 15.13). However, peak and trough serum concentrations of testosterone increased during the six-month treatment, with testosterone levels above the upper normal limit after the third and fourth injection. Therefore, in 7 of the 14 hypogonadal men, injections were given at gradually increasing intervals between the 5th and 10th injection, and from then on every 12 weeks (von Eckardstein and Nieschlag 2002). During steady state, serum levels of testosterone remained in the normal range with maximal concentrations of 32.0 ± 11.7 nmol/l (mean $\pm$ SD) one week after injection, and nadir levels before the next injection of 12.6 ± 3.7 nmol/l (Fig. 15.14).

During the last decade, testosterone undecanoate dissolved in castor oil became one of the favorite intramuscular testosterone esters for treatment of hypogonadal men (see Chapter 14) and for clinical studies of

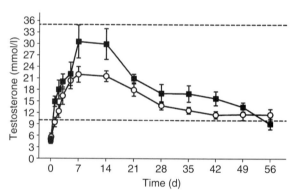

Fig. 15.12 Serum concentrations (mean $\pm$ SEM) of testosterone after single-dose im injections of 1000 mg testosterone undecanoate in tea seed oil in 7 hypogonadal men (■) or castor oil in 14 hypogonadal men (○). Broken lines indicate normal range of testosterone (from Behre *et al.* 1999a, adapted with permission of the European Journal of Endocrinology).

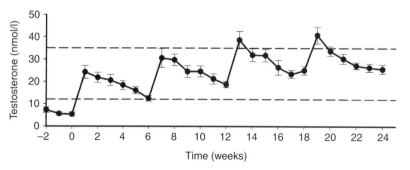

Fig. 15.13 Serum concentrations (mean $\pm$ SEM) of testosterone after multiple im injections of 1000 mg testosterone undecanoate in castor oil in 13 hypogonadal men. Broken lines indicate normal range of testosterone (adapted with permission from Nieschlag *et al.* 1999, copyright 1999, Blackwell Publishing).

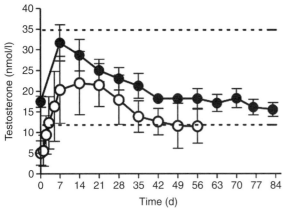

Fig. 15.14 Serum concentrations (mean ± SD) of testosterone after single injection of 1000 mg testosterone undecanoate in castor oil in hypogonadal men (o) and during multiple injections with the same dose every 12 weeks (●). Broken lines indicate normal range of testosterone (adapted with permission from von Eckardstein and Nieschlag 2002).

hormonal male contraception (see Chapter 22). Large-scale studies involving 1493 hypogonadal patients, comprising 6333 im injections and 1103 patient-years of treatment, demonstrated that this form of testosterone treatment is well tolerated, effective and safe (Zitzmann and Nieschlag 2007; Zitzmann *et al.* 2011).

15.6.7   Testosterone decanoate

Testosterone decanoate differs from testosterone undecanoate by one carbon atom in the ester side chain. It has been widely administered for many years as part of a mixture with shorter-action testosterone esters; however, it has not been available as a single preparation. To date there are no detailed studies published on the pharmacokinetics of administration of testosterone decanoate to hypogonadal men. However, im injections of 400 mg of testosterone decanoate were given four times at injection intervals of four weeks to normal men in a contraceptive study (Anderson *et al.* 2002). Endogenous testosterone was suppressed by concomitant administration of etonogestrel implants. Nadir testosterone levels before the next injection were in the lower normal range; whereas serum levels were at the upper normal limit one week after injection. From these limited data it can be concluded that testosterone decanoate seems to have an improved pharmacokinetic profile over testosterone enanthate, but does not allow similar prolonged injection intervals

of about 12 weeks, as demonstrated for testosterone undecanoate in hypogonadal men.

15.6.8   Testosterone microcapsules

Testosterone can be encapsuled in a biodegradable matrix composed of lactide/glycolide copolymer which is suitable for im injection. When microcapsule injections containing 315 mg of testosterone were given to eight hypogonadal men, serum testosterone levels slowly increased to peak levels at about 8 weeks and fell thereafter to reach pathological levels again by 11 weeks (Burris *et al.* 1988). In later studies the size-range and the testosterone loading of the microcapsules were adjusted so that, in hypogonadal men, im injections of 630 mg of testosterone in microcapsules (two im injections, 2.5 ml volume for each injection) resulted in serum levels of testosterone within the normal range for about 70 days (Bhasin *et al.* 1992). Similar results were obtained after subcutaneous injection of up to 534 mg of testosterone in microcapsules (total injection volume up to 5 ml) in hypogonadal men, albeit with a pronounced early peak and a relatively long period of low-normal serum total testosterone (Amory *et al.* 2002). These clinical studies demonstrated that the microspheres can be adapted to the required needs, but further long-term studies are needed to evaluate the clinical potential of this form of testosterone administration.

15.7   Testosterone pellets for subdermal administration

Subdermal testosterone pellet implantation was among the earliest effective modalities employed for clinical application of testosterone, which became an established form of androgen replacement therapy by 1940 (Deanesly and Parkes 1938; Vest and Howard 1939). With the advent of other modalities, e.g. intramuscular testosterone ester injections, it went out of general use. However, investigations in the 1990s redefined the favorable pharmacokinetic profiles and clinical pharmacology of testosterone implants (Handelsman *et al.* 1990; Jockenhövel *et al.* 1996).

The original testosterone implants were manufactured by high-pressure tableting of crystalline steroid with a cholesterol excipient. These proved brittle, hard to standardize or sterilize and exhibited surface unevenness and fragmentation during invivo absorption, to produce an uneven late release rate. These limitations were overcome in the 1950s by switching to high-temperature molding whereby molten testosterone was cast into cylindrical moulds to produce more robust implants. These have more uniform composition, resulting in a more steady and prolonged release and reduced tissue reaction. Sterilization is achieved by a combination of high-temperature exposure during manufacture together with surface sterilization or, more recently, gamma-irradiation. The testosterone implants are currently available in two sizes with a common diameter of 4.5 mm: 6 mm length for the 100 mg and 12 mm length for the 200 mg implant. Pellets are usually implanted under the skin of the lower abdominal wall under sterile conditions using a trochar and cannula.

The estimated half-life of absorption of testosterone from subdermal implants is 2.5 months. On average, approximately 1.3 mg of testosterone is released per day from the 200 mg pellet. Testosterone implants demonstrate a minor and transient accelerated initial "burst" release, which lasts for 1–2 days (Jockenhövel *et al.* 1996). The most comprehensive pharmacokinetic evaluation of testosterone implants was conducted in a random-sequence, crossover clinical study of 43 androgen-deficient men with primary or secondary hypogonadism (Handelsman *et al.* 1990). Patients were treated sequentially with three regimens – six 100 mg, three 200 mg or six 200 mg implants – at intervals of at least six months. Implantation of testosterone pellets resulted in a highly reproducible and dose-dependent time-course for circulation of total and free testosterone. Testosterone concentrations reached baseline by six months after either of the 600 mg dose regimens but remained significantly elevated after six months following the 1200 mg dose. The standard dose for hypogonadal men is 800 mg every six months, which can be titrated individually (Fig. 15.15).

Pellet implantation is generally well tolerated (Handelsman *et al.* 1997; Kaminetsky *et al.* 2011). Adverse events after implantations were extrusions (8.5–12% per procedure), bruising (2.3–8.8%) and infections (0.6–4%) (Handelsman *et al.* 1997; Kelleher *et al.* 1999). Due to the long-lasting effect and the inconvenience of removal, preferably pellets should be used by men in whom the beneficial effects and tolerance for androgen replacement therapy have already been established by treatment with shorter-acting testosterone preparations.

In a recent randomized, crossover clinical trial comparing subdermal testosterone pellets versus injectable testosterone undecanoate in 38 hypogonadal patients, no consistent differences were seen in a comprehensive range of pharmacodynamic measures reflecting androgen effects on biochemistry and hematology, muscle mass and strength, quality of life, mood and sexual function (Fennell *et al.* 2010). However, 91% of men preferred the injectable over the implantable form of testosterone therapy.

15.8 Testosterone preparations for transdermal administration

15.8.1 Testosterone patches

The skin easily absorbs steroids and other drugs, and transdermal drug delivery has become a widely used therapeutic modality. The scrotum shows the highest rate of steroid absorption, about 40-fold higher than the forearm (Feldmann and Maibach 1967). This difference in absorption rates has been exploited for the development of a transdermal therapeutic system (TTS) to deliver testosterone. Large 40 and 60 cm^2 polymeric membranes loaded with 10 or 15 mg testosterone, when attached to the scrotal skin deliver sufficient amounts of the steroid to provide hypogonadal men with serum levels in the physiological range (Bals-Pratsch *et al.* 1986; 1988; Findlay *et al.* 1987; Korenman *et al.* 1987). The application of the patch to scrotal skin requires hair clipping or shaving

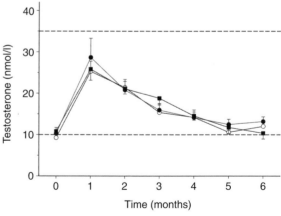

Fig. 15.15 Blood total testosterone (mean ± SEM) in 43 hypogonadal men receiving four 200 mg pellets (800 mg) implanted either under the skin of the lateral abdominal wall (in 4 tracks (●); n = 9, or in 2 tracks (○); n = 16) or in the hip region (■; n = 18). (Adapted with permission from Kelleher *et al.* 2001, copyright 2001, Blackwell Publishing.)

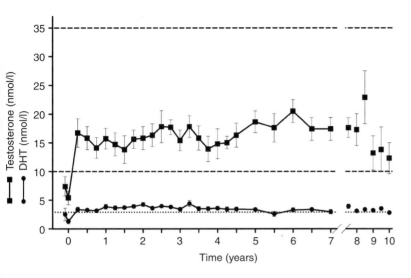

Fig. 15.16 Serum concentrations (mean ± SEM) of testosterone (■) and DHT (●) in 11 hypogonadal men before and during treatment with trans-scrotal testosterone patches. Broken lines indicate normal range of testosterone, dotted line upper normal limit of DHT (adapted with permission from Behre *et al.* 1999b, copyright 1999, Blackwell Publishing).

to optimize adherence. The membranes need to be renewed every day. When applied in the morning and worn until the next morning the resulting serum testosterone levels resemble the normal diurnal variations of serum testosterone in normal men without supraphysiological peaks (Bals-Pratsch *et al.* 1988). Long-term therapy up to 10 years with daily administration of the scrotal patch in 11 hypogonadal men produced steady-state serum levels of testosterone and estradiol in the normal range, and serum levels of DHT at or slightly above the higher limit of normal without significant adverse side-effects (Fig. 15.16; Behre *et al.* 1999b). However, with the introduction of testosterone gels for treatment of hypogonadism, scrotal testosterone patches lost popularity and the marketing has been discontinued.

While testosterone is readily absorbed by genital skin, transdermal systems for use on non-genital skin require enhancers to facilitate sufficient testosterone passage through the skin. The permeation-enhanced testosterone patch delivers 5 mg/day testosterone when applied to non-scrotal skin. If one or two such systems are worn for 24 hours physiological serum testosterone levels can be mimicked, as with scrotal patches (Fig. 15.17) (Brocks *et al.* 1996; Meikle *et al.* 1996). Due to the alcoholic enhancer used and the occlusive nature of the systems, the application is associated with skin irritation in up to 60% of the subjects, with most users discontinuing application because of the skin irritation (Jordan 1997; Parker and Armitage 1999). Preapplication of corticosteroid cream to the skin has been reported to decrease the

severity of skin irritation, although the effects on pharmacokinetics of testosterone are unclear.

Recently, a new thin, transparent and comfortable testosterone-in-adhesive matrix patch was launched that has to be applied only every second day. The adhesiveness seems to be quite good, even after physical exercise and after sauna (Raynaud *et al.* 2009). Depending on the size of the patch (30, 45 or 60 cm^2), the average daily release is 1.2, 1.8 or 2.4 mg of testosterone. The recommended initial dosing regimen is two 60 cm^2 patches every two days, which can be modified depending on the serum levels of testosterone achieved (Fig. 15.18). In a randomized, open label, multicenter, one-year study involving 224 hypogonadal patients, testosterone serum levels were above 3 ng/ml in 85% of patients after application of two patches of 60 cm^2 every 48 h, and remained stable over 12 months of testosterone therapy (Raynaud *et al.* 2008b).

15.8.2 Testosterone gels

In 2000, a 1% colorless hydroalcoholic gel containing 25 or 50 mg testosterone in 2.5 or 5 g gel was approved for clinical use in hypogonadism. The gel dries in less than 5 min without leaving a visible residue on the skin. About 9 to 14% of the testosterone in the gel is bioavailable. Application of the testosterone gel increased serum testosterone levels into the normal range within one hour after application (Wang *et al.* 2000). Steady-state serum levels are achieved 48–72 hours after initiation of therapy;

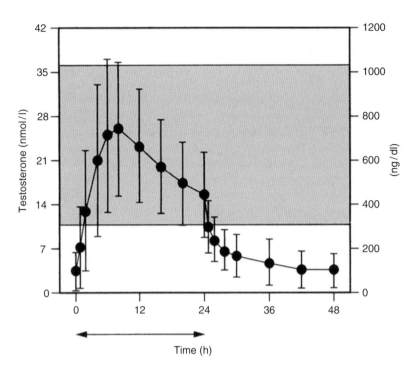

Fig. 15.17 Serum concentrations (mean ± SD) of testosterone during and after nighttime application of two non-scrotal testosterone systems to the backs of 34 hypogonadal men. Shaded area indicates normal range of testosterone (adapted with permission from Meikle *et al.* 1996, copyright 1996, The Endocrine Society).

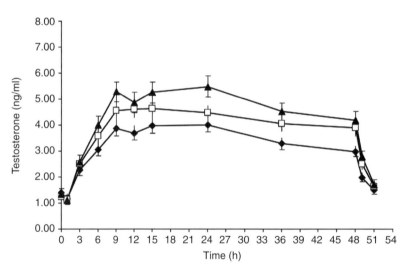

Fig. 15.18 Serum concentrations (mean ± SEM) of testosterone during single 48 h application of two matrix patches (♦, 30 cm^2; □, 45 cm^2; ▲, 60 cm^2) and 1–3 h after removal (adapted with permission from Raynaud *et al.* 2008a).

whereas pretreatment serum testosterone levels are seen four days after stopping application. The application of the testosterone gel at four sites (application skin areas approximately four times that of one site) resulted in an AUC of testosterone which was 23% higher compared to application of the same amount of gel on one site. However, this difference did not achieve statistical significance in the nine hypogonadal men tested (Wang *et al.* 2000).

Long-term pharmacokinetics of the transdermal testosterone gel were evaluated in 227 hypogonadal men (Swerdloff *et al.* 2000). Patients were randomly assigned to application of 5 or 10 g of the testosterone gel or two patches of a non-scrotal testosterone system. After 90 days of testosterone gel treatment, the dose was titrated up (5 to 7.5 g) or down (10 to 7.5 g) if the preapplication serum testosterone levels were outside the normal adult male range. During

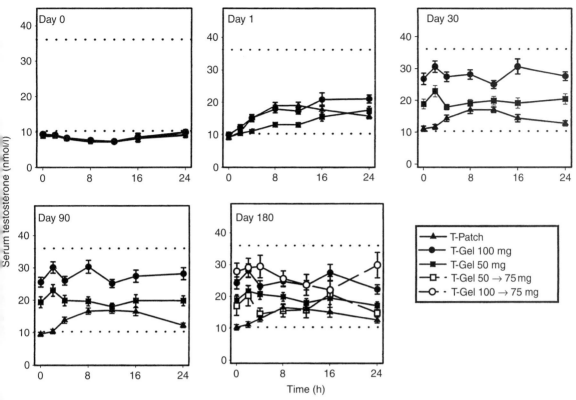

Fig. 15.19 Serum concentrations (mean ± SEM) of testosterone before (day 0) and after transdermal testosterone applications on days 1, 30, 90 and 180. Time 0 was 8 a.m., when blood sampling usually began. On day 90, the dose in the subjects applying testosterone gel (T gel) 50 or 100 mg was up- or down-titrated if their preapplicaton serum testosterone levels were below or above the normal adult male range, respectively. Dotted lines denote the adult normal range (adapted with permission from Swerdloff *et al.* 2000, copyright 2000, The Endocrine Society).

long-term treatment mean serum levels of testosterone were maintained in the mid-normal range with 5 g of gel and in the upper normal range with 10 g of gel (Fig. 15.19). Testosterone gel application resulted in dose-proportionate increases in serum DHT and estradiol as well as dose-proportionate decreases of gonadotropins.

The advantages of the testosterone gel over the early testosterone patches are a lower incidence of skin irritation, the ease of application, the invisibility of the dried gel, and the ability to deliver testosterone dose dependently to the low, mid- or upper normal range. A potential adverse side-effect of testosterone gel application is the transfer of testosterone to women or children upon close contact with the skin. Transfer of transdermal testosterone from the skin can be avoided by applying gel to skin covered by clothing, or showering after application. This preparation has gained a significant market share of androgen formulations in Europe and the United States.

Since then, a number of other testosterone gels have been under development. Two randomized, controlled studies demonstrated a dose-dependent increase of testosterone serum levels to the normal range in hypogonadal men after 90 days of application of 5 g/d or 10 g/d of another hydroalcoholic topical gel containing 1% testosterone compared to non-scrotal testosterone patches (*n* = 208; McNicholas *et al.* 2003) or compared to non-scrotal testosterone patches and placebo gel (*n* = 406; Steidle *et al.* 2003). Recent data from a registry study in 849 hypogonadal patients treated over 12 months demonstrated high compliance with this form of testosterone replacement (Khera *et al.* 2011).

A new testosterone gel at a concentration of 2% instead of the 1% of the earlier preparations was launched first in Sweden and Germany in 2005. This gel is provided in a metered-dose pump allowing adjusted dosing starting from 10 mg testosterone (0.5 g, 1 pump actuation) up to higher doses in 10-mg steps. The recommended starting dose is

40–60 mg of testosterone, e.g. 4–6 pump actuations or 2–3 g of the testosterone gel per day. In a recent large-scale, placebo-controlled study involving 220 hypogonadal men with diabetes mellitus and/or metabolic syndrome, good safety profile of this testosterone preparation was demonstrated, with no significant differences in the frequencies of adverse events or serious adverse events between patients treated with testosterone or placebo gel (Jones *et al.* 2011). Hypogonadal patients applied a starting dose of 3 g of the 2% testosterone gel (60 mg testosterone), and dose adjustments to 2 g (40 mg testosterone) or 4 g (80 mg testosterone) were made dependent on the serum levels of testosterone measured. In another recent study it was demonstrated that BMI has no significant

effect on normalization of testosterone concentration after application of this testosterone gel in hypogonadal men, and at least 75% of patients achieved serum levels in the normal range after three months of gel application (Dobs *et al.* 2011).

To date, the testosterone gel with the highest concentration of testosterone is a 2.5% topical gel. Recently, it has been launched in sachets containing 2.5 g gel (62.5 mg testosterone) or 5 g gel (125 mg testosterone). Application of 5 g/d of this 2.5% hydroalcoholic gel increased serum levels of testosterone to the normal range in 14 gonadotropin-suppressed normal men (Rolf *et al.* 2002a). Washing of the skin after 10 minutes did not influence the pharmacokinetic profile. No interpersonal testosterone transfer

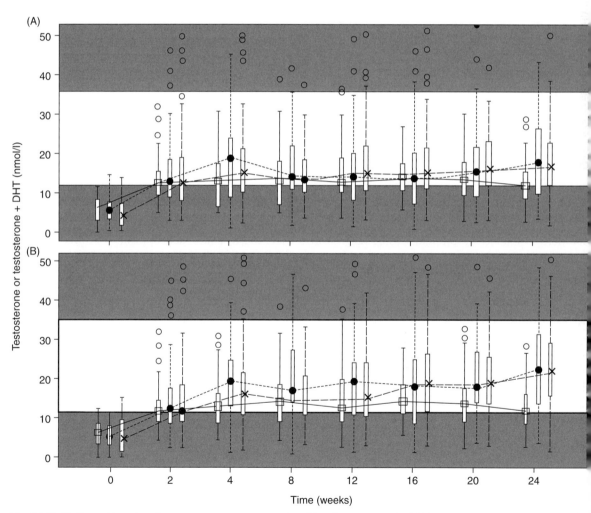

Fig. 15.20 Median and box plots of testosterone serum concentrations (A) and testosterone plus DHT serum concentrations (B), measured at 10 a.m., at weeks 0–24 in patients treated with the dermal 2.5% testosterone gel (–□–), scrotal 2.5% testosterone gel (–●–) and non-scrotal testosterone patch (–×–) (from Kühnert *et al.* 2005, adapted with permission of the European Journal of Endocrinology).

could be detected after evaporation of the alcohol vehicle of this testosterone gel (Rolf *et al.* 2002b). In a randomized, controlled, multicenter clinical trial, initial application of 5 g of the testosterone gel, with the possibility of dose adjustment down to 2.5 g or up to 10 g after four and eight weeks of treatment, resulted in significantly higher testosterone serum levels, well within the normal range, compared to a control group treated with non-scrotal testosterone patches (initially 2 patches, with individual adjustments to 1–3 patches per day) (Fig. 15.20; Kühnert *et al.* 2005). In the same study it could be demonstrated that scrotal application of only 1 g of the testosterone gel also normalized

serum levels of testosterone (with dose adjustments to 1 g of 1% testosterone gel to 2.5 g of 2.5% testosterone gel). Unfortunately, the scrotal application, despite being well tolerated by the patients, has not been approved by regulatory bodies.

Recently, the initial 1% hydroalcoholic testosterone gel has been reformulated to a 1.62% gel with increased viscosity and increased skin permeation, allowing delivery of testosterone also with a lower volume of gel. In a multicenter, randomized, placebo-controlled study, 2.5 g of this gel preparation was applied once daily for up to 182 days to either upper arms/shoulders or abdomen of hypogonadal patients (Kaufman *et al.* 2011; Fig. 15.21).

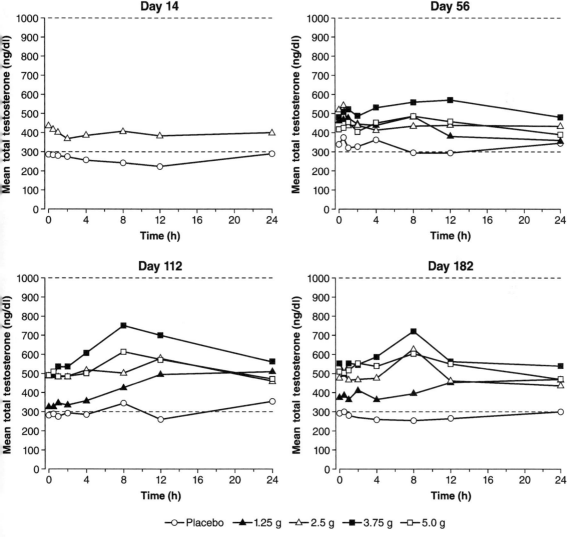

Fig. 15.21 Mean concentrations of serum testosterone on day 14, 56, 112 and 182 after daily application of 1.62% dermal testosterone gel. Dotted lines indicate normal testosterone range. On day 14, all patients in the testosterone group applied 2.5 g gel (adapted with permission from Kaufman *et al.* 2011).

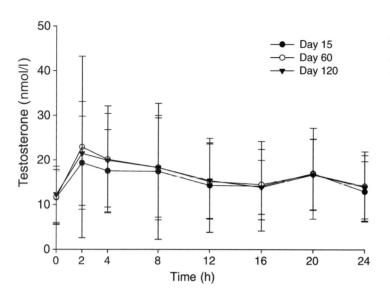

Fig. 15.22 Serum concentrations (mean ± SD) of testosterone at day 15, 60 and 120 in hypogonadal patients after daily application of testosterone topical solution to the axillae (adapted with permission from Wang *et al.* 2011).

Dose adjustments down to 1.25 g and up to 3.75 g or 5.0 g were made 14 d, 28 d or 42 d after initiation of treatment depending on serum testosterone levels. After titration, 7.3% of patients were treated with 1.25 g/d, 25.6% with 2.5 g/d, 28.2% with 3.75 g/d and 38.9% with 5 g/d. After 182 days of therapy, 82.2% of hypogonadal patients achieved average serum levels of testosterone within the normal eugonadal range.

15.8.3 Testosterone topical solution

A 2% formulation of a testosterone solution was approved by the FDA in November 2010. It is a non-occlusive topical formulation administered to the axilla, with an applicator instead of with the hands as for the testosterone gels. The safety, pharmacokinetics and efficacy of the topical solution were evaluated in an open-label, multicenter clinical trial (Wang *et al.* 2011). All hypogonadal patients started with a daily dose of 60 mg of the testosterone solution. Doses could be adjusted on days 45 and 90 to achieve serum levels of testosterone in the normal range. Most of the patients (97/135) stayed at the 60 mg dose after 120 days of therapy; 3/135 used the 30 mg dose; 25/135 the 90 mg dose; and 10/135 the 120 mg dose. After four months of therapy, 84.1% of hypogonadal patients had average serum levels of testosterone within the normal range (10.4–36.4 nmol/l) (Fig. 15.22). Application site erythema was noted in 5.2% of patients. This mode of testosterone application might reduce the undesired transfer of testosterone to other persons, as it is applied not by hand but by using an applicator, so it might be a favorable new option for testosterone replacement of hypogonadal men.

15.9 Key messages

- Oral, buccal, injectable, subdermal implantable and transdermal testosterone preparations are available for clinical use. The best preparation is the one that replaces testosterone serum levels at as close to physiological concentrations as possible.
- Oral administration of testosterone undecanoate in oleic acid or castor oil results in high interindividual and intraindividual variability of serum testosterone values. A new oral testosterone undecanoate preparation (proprietary self-emulsifying drug delivery system) shows an improved pharmacokinetic profile.
- Daily or twice-daily buccal administration of testosterone tablets increases serum testosterone to the normal range. Relatively low acceptability of this application form seems to be a disadvantage.
- The older testosterone esters for im injection (testosterone propionate, testosterone enanthate, testosterone cypionate, testosterone cyclohexanecarboxylate) are still widely used, but are suboptimal for the treatment of male hypogonadism. Doses and injection intervals most frequently used in the clinic lead to initial supraphysiological testosterone levels and subnormal values before the next injection. To obtain testosterone serum concentrations continuously in the normal range, unacceptably frequent small doses would have to be injected.

- Intramuscular injection of 1000 mg testosterone undecanoate to hypogonadal men maintains serum levels of testosterone within the normal range for three months. Injection intervals can be adjusted for individual patient needs.
- A single implantation procedure of testosterone pellets provides serum levels of testosterone in the normal range for up to six months. Pellet extrusion occurs in about 10% of the implantation procedures. Due to the long-lasting effect and the inconvenience of removal, preferably pellets should be used by men in whom the beneficial effects and tolerance for androgen replacement therapy have already been established.
- Transdermal application of testosterone by scrotal or non-scrotal patches increases serum levels of testosterone to the normal range and even mimics the physiological circadian testosterone rhythm.

- Daily administration of testosterone gel increases serum levels of testosterone in hypogonadal patients dose-dependently to the normal range. Whereas skin irritation is minimal, a potential adverse side-effect of testosterone gel application is the transfer of testosterone to women or children upon close contact with the skin. Various gel preparations have been launched with testosterone concentrations of 1–2.5%.
- If a 2.5% testosterone gel is applied to the scrotal skin, only about 20% of the amount of gel needed for non-genital application is required for substitution.
- Administration of a 2% formulation of a topical testosterone solution applied to the axilla using a special applicator normalizes serum testosterone levels in 84% of hypogonadal men after four months of treatment and has a good skin safety profile.

15.10　References

Aakvaag A, Stromme SB (1974) The effect of mesterolone administration to normal men on the pituitary-testicular function. *Acta Endocrinol* **77**:380–386

Alkalay D, Khemani L, Wagner WE, Bartlett MF (1973) Sublingual and oral administration of methyltestosterone. A comparison of drug bioavailability. *J Clin Pharmacol New Drugs* **13**:142–151

Amory JK, Anawalt BD, Blaskovich PD, Gilchriest J, Nuwayser ES, Matsumoto AM (2002) Testosterone release from a subcutaneous, biodegradable microcapsule formulation (Viatrel) in hypogonadal men. *J Androl* **23**:84–91

Amory JK, Bush MA, Zhi H, Caricofe RB, Matsumoto AM, Swerdloff RS, Wang C, Clark RV (2011) Oral testosterone with and without concomitant inhibition of 5α-reductase by dutasteride in hypogonadal men for 28 days. *J Urol* **185**:626–632

Anderson RA, Wu FC (1996) Comparison between testosterone enanthate-induced azoospermia and oligozoospermia in a male contraceptive study. II. Pharmacokinetics and pharmacodynamics of once weekly administration of testosterone enanthate. *J Clin Endocrinol Metab* **81**:896–901

Anderson RA, Zhu H, Cheng L, Baird DT (2002) Investigation of a novel preparation of testosterone decanoate in men: pharmacokinetics and spermatogenic suppression with etonogestrel implants. *Contraception* **66**:357–364

Anonymous (1988) Methyltestosteron-Monographie. *Bundesanzeiger* **40**:5140–5141

Bagchus WM, Hust R, Maris F, Schnabel PG, Houwing NS (2003) Important effect of food on the bioavailability of oral testosterone undecanoate. *Pharmacotherapy* **23**:319–325

Bals-Pratsch M, Knuth UA, Yoon YD, Nieschlag E (1986) Transdermal testosterone substitution therapy for male hypogonadism. *Lancet* **2**:943–946

Bals-Pratsch M, Langer K, Place VA, Nieschlag E (1988) Substitution therapy of hypogonadal men with transdermal testosterone over one year. *Acta Endocrinol (Copenh)* **118**:7–13

Behre HM, Nieschlag E (1992) Testosterone buciclate (20 Aet-1) in hypogonadal men: pharmacokinetics and pharmacodynamics of the new long-acting androgen ester. *J Clin Endocrinol Metab* **75**:1204–1210

Behre HM, Baus S, Kliesch S, Keck C, Simoni M, Nieschlag E (1995) Potential of testosterone buciclate for male contraception: endocrine differences between responders and nonresponders. *J Clin Endocrinol Metab* **80**:2394–2403

Behre HM, Abshagen K, Oettel M, Hubler D, Nieschlag E (1999a) Intramuscular injection of testosterone undecanoate for the treatment of male hypogonadism: phase I studies. *Eur J Endocrinol* **140**:414–419

Behre HM, von Eckardstein S, Kliesch S, Nieschlag E (1999b) Long-term substitution therapy of hypogonadal men with transscrotal testosterone over

7–10 years. *Clin Endocrinol (Oxf)* **50**:629–635

Bhasin S, Swerdloff RS, Steiner B, Peterson MA, Meridores T, Galmirini M, Pandian MR, Goldberg R, Berman N (1992) A biodegradable testosterone microcapsule formulation provides uniform eugonadal levels of testosterone for 10–11 weeks in hypogonadal men. *J Clin Endocrinol Metab* **74**:75–83

Boyd PR, Mark GJ (1977) Multiple hepatic adenomas and a heptatocellular carcinoma in a man on oral methyl testosterone for eleven years. *Cancer* **40**: 1765–1770

Breuer H, Gütgemann D (1966) Wirkung von 1alpha-Methyl-5alpha-androstan-17β-ol-3-on (Mesterolon) auf die Steroidausscheidung beim Menschen. *Arzneimittelforschung* **16**:759–762

Brocks DR, Meikle AW, Boike SC, Mazer NA, Zariffa N, Audet PR, Jorkasky DK (1996) Pharmacokinetics of testosterone in hypogonadal men after transdermal delivery: influence of dose. *J Clin Pharmacol* **36**:732–739

Burris AS, Ewing LL, Sherins RJ (1988) Initial trial of slow-release testosterone microspheres in hypogonadal men. *Fertil Steril* **50**:493–497

Carbone JV, Grodsky GM, Hjelte V (1959) Effect of hepatic dysfunction on circulating levels of sulphobromopthalein and its metabolites. *J Clin Invest* **38**:1989–1996

Coert A, Geelen J, de Visser J, van der Vies J (1975) The pharmacology and metabolism of testosterone undecanoate (TU), a new orally active androgen. *Acta Endocrinol* **79**:789–800

Crabbé P, Diczfalusy E, Djerassi C (1980) Injectable contraceptive synthesis: an example of international cooperation. *Science* **209**:992–994

Cunningham GR, Silverman VE, Kohler PO (1978) Clinical evaluation of testosterone enanthate for induction and maintenance of reversible azoospermia in man. In: Patanelli DJ (ed) *Hormonal Control of Male Fertility (Workshop Proceedings)*, NIH Publication No. 78-1097. US Department of Health, Education, and Welfare (NIH), Bethesda, MD, pp 71–87

Danner C, Frick G (1980) Androgen substitution with testosterone-containing nasal drops. *Int J Androl* **3**:429–431

Deanesly R, Parkes AS (1938) Further experiments on the administration of hormones by the subcutaneous implantation of tablets. *Lancet* **232**:606–608

de Lorimer AA, Gordan GS, Löwe RC, Carbone JV (1965) Methyltestosterone: related steroids and liver function. *Arch Intern Med* **116**:289–294

Dobs A, McGettigan J, Norwood P, Potts S, Gould E (2011) Baseline body mass index (BMI) has no effect upon normalization of testosterone concentrations with testosterone 2% gel [abstract]. *Endocr Rev* **32** (03_MeetingAbstracts):P1–353

Escamilla RF (1949) Treatment of preadolescent eunuchoidism with (methyl)testosterone linguets. *Amer Pract* **3**:425

Falk H, Thomas LB, Popper H, Ishak KG (1979) Hepatic angiosarcoma associated with androgenic-anabolic steroids. *Lancet* **2**:1120–1123

Farrell GC, Joshua DE, Uren RF, Baird PJ, Perkins KW, Kronenberg H (1975) Androgen-induced hepatoma. *Lancet* **1**:430–432

Feldmann RJ, Maibach HI (1967) Regional variation in percutaneous penetration of 14C cortisol in man. *J Invest Dermatol* **48**:181–183

Fennell C, Sartorius G, Ly LP, Turner L, Liu PY, Conway AJ, Handelsman DJ (2010) Randomized cross-over clinical trial of injectable vs. implantable depot testosterone for maintenance of testosterone replacement therapy in androgen deficient men. *Clin Endocrinol (Oxf)* **73**:102–109

Findlay JC, Place VA, Snyder PJ (1987) Transdermal delivery of testosterone. *J Clin Endocrinol Metab* **64**:266–268

Frey H, Aakvaag A, Saanum D, Falch J (1979) Bioavailability of oral testosterone in males. *Eur J Clin Pharmacol* **16**:345–349

Fujioka M, Shinohara Y, Baba S, Irie M, Inoue K (1986) Pharmacokinetic properties of testosterone propionate in normal men. *J Clin Endocrinol Metab* **63**:1361–1364

Fukutani K, Isurugi K, Takayasu H, Wakabayashi K, Tamaoki B-I (1974) Effects of depot testosterone therapy on serum levels of luteinizing hormone and follicle-stimulating hormone in patients with Klinefelter's syndrome and hypogonadotropic eunuchoidism. *J Clin Endocrinol Metab* **39**:856–864

Gerhards E, Gibian H, Kolb KH (1966) Zum Stoffwechsel von 1alpha-Methyl-5alpha androstan-17β-ol-3-on (Mesterolon) beim Menschen. *Arneimittelforschung* **16**:458–463

Goodman MA, Laden AMJ (1977) Hepatocellular carcinoma in association with androgen therapy. *Med J Aust* **1**:220–221

Gordon RD, Thomas MJ, Poyntin JM, Stocks AE (1975) Effect of mesterolone on plasma LH, FSH and testosterone. *Andrologia* **7**:287–296

Gu YQ, Wang XH, Xu D, Peng L, Cheng LF, Huang MK, Huang ZJ, Zhang GY (2003) A multicenter contraceptive efficacy study of injectable testosterone undecanoate in healthy Chinese men. *J Clin Endocrinol Metab* **88**:562–568

Hamburger C (1958) Testosterone treatment and 17-ketosteroid excretion. *Acta Endocrinol* **28**:529–536

Handelsman DJ, Conway AJ, Boylan LM (1990) Pharmacokinetics and pharmacodynamics of testosterone pellets in man. *J Clin Endocrinol Metab* **70**:216–222

Handelsman DJ, Mackey MA, Howe C, Turner L, Conway AJ (1997) Analysis of testosterone implants for androgen replacement therapy. *Clin Endocrinol* **47**:311–316

Heywood R, Hunter B, Green OP, Kennedy SJ (1977a) The toxicity of methyl testosterone in the rat. *Toxicol Lett* **1**:27–31

Heywood R, Chesterman H, Ball SA, Wadsworth PF (1977b) Toxicity of methyl testosterone in the beagle dog. *Toxicology* **7**:357–365

Horst HJ, Höltge WJ, Dennis M, Coert A, Geelen J, Voigt KD (1976) Lymphatic absorption and metabolism of orally administered testosterone undecanoate in man. *Klin Wschr* **54**:875–879

Jockenhövel F, Vogel E, Kreutzer E, Reinhard W, Lederbogen S, Reinwein D (1996) Pharmacokinetics and pharmacodynamics of subcutaneous testosterone implants in hypogonadal man. *Clin Endocrinol* **45**:61–71

Johnsen SG, Bennet EP, Jensen VG (1974) Therapeutic effectiveness of oral testosterone. *Lancet* **2**: 1473–1475

Johnsen SG, Kampmann JP, Bennet EP, Jörgensen F (1976) Enzyme induction by oral testosterone. *Clin Pharmacol Ther* **20**:233–237

Jones TH, Arver S, Behre HM, Buvat J, Meuleman E, Moncada I, Morales AM, Volterrani M, Yellowlees A, Howell JD, Channer KS; TIMES2 Investigators (2011) Testosterone replacement in hypogonadal men with type 2 diabetes and/or metabolic syndrome (the TIMES2 study). *Diabetes Care* **34**:828–837

Jordan WP (1997) Allergy and topical irritation associated with transdermal testosterone administration: a comparison of scrotal and nonscrotal transdermal systems. *Am J Contact Dermat* **8**:108–113

Junkmann K (1952) Über protrahiert wirksame Androgene. *Arch Path Pharmacol* **215**:85–92

Junkmann K (1957) Long-acting steroids in reproduction. *Recent Prog Horm Res* **13**:389–419

Kaminetsky JC, Moclair B, Hemani M, Sand M (2011) A phase IV prospective evaluation of the safety and efficacy of extended release testosterone pellets for the treatment of male hypogonadism. *J Sex Med* **8**:1186–1196

Kaufman JM, Miller MG, Garwin JL, Fitzpatrick S, McWhirter C, Brennan JJ (2011) Efficacy and safety study of 1.62% testosterone gel for the treatment of hypogonadal men. *J Sex Med* **8**:2079–2089

Kelleher S, Conway AJ, Handelsman DJ (1999) A randomized controlled clinical trial of antibiotic impregnation of testosterone pellet implants to reduce extrusion rate. *Eur J Endocrinol* **146**:513–518

Kelleher S, Conway AJ, Handelsman DJ (2001) Influence of implantation site and track geometry on the extrusion rate and pharmacology of testosterone implants. *Clin Endocrinol (Oxf)* **55**:531–536

Khera M, Bhattacharya RK, Blick G, Kushner H, Nguyen D, Miner MM (2011) Improved sexual function with testosterone replacement therapy in hypogonadal men: real-world data from the Testim Registry in the United States (TRiUS). *J Sex Med* **8**:3204–3213

Korenman SG, Viosca S, Garza D, Guralnik M, Place V, Campbell P, Davis SS (1987) Androgen therapy of hypogonadal men with transscrotal testosterone system. *Am J Med* **83**:471–478

Krüskemper HI, Noell G (1967) Steroidstruktur und Lebertoxizität. *Acta Endocrinol* **54**:73–80

Kühnert B, Byrne M, Simoni M, Köpcke W, Gerss J, Lemmnitz G, Nieschlag E (2005) Testosterone substitution with a new transdermal, hydroalcoholic gel applied to scrotal or non-scrotal skin: a multicentre trial. *Eur J Endocrinol* **153**:317–326

Lee A, Rubinow K, Clark RV, Caricofe RB, Bush MA, Zhi H, Roth MY, Page ST, Bremner WJ, Amory JK (2011) Pharmacokinetics of modified slow-release oral testosterone over nine days in normal men with experimental hypogonadism. *J Androl* Aug 25 [Epub ahead of print]

Mackey MA, Conway AJ, Handelsman DJ (1995) Tolerability of intramuscular injections of testosterone ester in oil vehicle. *Hum Reprod* **10**:862–865

Maisey NM, Bingham J, Marks V, English J, Chakraborty J (1981) Clinical efficacy of testosterone undecanoate in male hypogonadism. *Clin Endocrinol* **14**:625–629

Mattern C, Hoffmann C, Morley JE, Badiu C (2008) Testosterone supplementation for hypogonadal men by the nasal route. *Aging Male* **11**:171–178

McNicholas TA, Dean JD, Mulder H, Carnegie C, Jones NA (2003) A novel testosterone gel formulation normalizes androgen levels in hypogonadal men, with improvements in body composition and sexual function. *BJU Int* **91**:69–74

Meikle AW, Arver S, Dobs AS, Sanders SW, Rajaram L, Mazer N (1996) Pharmacokinetics and metabolism of a permeation-enhanced testosterone transdermal system in hypogonadal men: influence of application site – a clinical research center study. *J Clin Endocrinol Metab* **81**:1832–1840

Minto CF, Howe C, Wishart S, Conway AJ, Handelsman DJ (1997). Pharmacokinetics and pharmacodynamics of nandrolone esters in oil vehicle: effects of ester, injection site and injection volume. *J Pharmacol Exp Ther* **281**:93–102

Nankin HR (1987) Hormone kinetics after intramuscular testosterone cypionate. *Fertil Steril* **47**:1004–1009

Nieschlag E (1981) Ist die Anwendung von Methyltestosteron obsolet? *Dtsch med Wschr* **106**:1123–1125

Nieschlag E, Mauss J, Coert A, Kicovic P (1975) Plasma androgen levels in men after oral administration of testosterone or testosterone undecanoate. *Acta Endocrinol* **79**:366–374

Nieschlag E, Cüppers HJ, Wiegelmann W, Wickings EJ (1976) Bioavailability and LH-suppressing effect of different testosterone preparations in normal and hypogonadal men. *Horm Res* **7**:138–145

Nieschlag E, Cüppers EJ, Wickings EJ (1977) Influence of sex, testicular development and liver function on the bioavailability of oral testosterone. *Europ J Clin Invest* **7**:145–147

Nieschlag E, Büchter D, von Eckardstein S, Abshagen K, Simoni M, Behre HM (1999) Repeated intramuscular injections of testosterone undecanoate for substitution therapy in hypogonadal men. *Clin Endocrinol (Oxf)* **51**:757–763

Paradinas FJ, Bull TB, Westaby D, Murray-Lyon IM (1977) Hyperplasia and prolapse of hepatocytes into hepatic veins during longterm methyltestosterone therapy: possible relationships of these changes to the development of peliosis hepatis and liver tumours. *Histopathology* **1**:225–246

Parker S, Armitage M (1999) Experience with transdermal testosterone replacement therapy for hypogonadal men. *Clin Endocrinol (Oxf)* **50**:57–62

Pitha J, Harman SM, Michel ME (1986) Hydrophilic cyclodextrin derivatives enable effective oral administration of steroidal hormones. *J Pharm Sci* **75**:165–167

Raynaud JP, Aumonier C, Gualano V, Betea D, Beckers A (2008a) Pharmacokinetic study of a new testosterone-in-adhesive matrix patch applied every 2 days to hypogonadal men. *J Steroid Biochem Mol Biol* **109**:177–184

Raynaud JP, Legros JJ, Rollet J, Augès M, Bunouf P, Sournac M, Fiet J (2008b) Efficacy and safety of a new testosterone-in-adhesive matrix patch applied every 2 days for 1 year to hypogonadal men. *J Steroid Biochem Mol Biol* **109**:168–176

Raynaud JP, Augès M, Liorzou L, Turlier V, Lauze C (2009) Adhesiveness of a new testosterone-in-adhesive matrix patch after extreme conditions. *Int J Pharm* **375**:28–32

Rolf C, Kemper S, Lemmnitz G, Eickenberg U, Nieschlag E (2002a) Pharmacokinetics of a new transdermal testosterone gel in gonadotrophin-suppressed normal men. *Eur J Endocrinol* **146**:673–679

Rolf C, Knie U, Lemmnitz G, Nieschlag E (2002b) Interpersonal testosterone transfer after topical application of a newly developed testosterone gel preparation. *Clin Endocrinol (Oxf)* **56**:637–641

Ruzicka L, Goldberg MW, Rosenberg HR (1935) Herstellung des 17-Methyl-testosterons und anderer Androsten- und Androstanderivate. Zusammenhänge zwischen chemischer Konstitution und männlicher Hormonwirkung. *Helv Chim Acta* **18**:1487–1498

Salehian B, Wang C, Alexander G, Davidson T, McDonald V, Berman N, Dudley RE, Ziel F, Swerdloff RS (1995) Pharmacokinetics, bioefficacy, and safety of sublingual testosterone cyclodextrin in hypogonadal men: comparison to testosterone enanthate – a clinical research center study. *J Clin Endocrinol Metab* **80**:3567–3575

Schnabel PG, Bagchus W, Lass H, Thomsen T, Geurts TB (2007) The effect of food composition on serum testosterone levels after oral

administration of Andriol Testocaps. *Clin Endocrinol (Oxf)* **66**:579–585

Schulte-Beerbühl M, Nieschlag E (1980) Comparison of testosterone, dihydrotestosterone, luteinizing hormone, and follicle-stimulating hormone in serum after injection of testosterone enanthate or testosterone cypionate. *Fertil Steril* **33**:201–203

Schürmeyer T, Nieschlag E (1984) Comparative pharmacokinetics of testosterone enanthate and testosterone cyclohexanecarboxylate as assessed by serum and salivary testosterone levels in normal men. *Int J Androl* **7**:181–187

Schürmeyer T, Wickings EJ, Freischem CW, Nieschlag E (1983) Saliva and serum testosterone following oral testosterone undecanoate administration in normal and hypogonadal men. *Acta Endocrinol* **102**:456–462

Shackleford DM, Faassen WA, Houwing N, Lass H, Edwards GA, Porter CJ, Charman WN (2003) Contribution of lymphatically transported testosterone undecanoate to the systemic exposure of testosterone after oral administration of two Andriol formulations in conscious lymph duct-cannulated dogs. *J Pharmacol Exp Ther* **306**:925–933

Snyder CN, Clark RV, Caricofe RB, Bush MA, Roth MY, Page ST, Bremner WJ, Amory JK (2010) Pharmacokinetics of 2 novel formulations of modified-release oral testosterone alone and with finasteride in normal men with experimental hypogonadism. *J Androl* **31**:527–535

Snyder PJ, Lawrence DA (1980) Treatment of male hypogonadism with testosterone enanthate. *J Clin Endocrinol Metab* **51**:1335–1339

Sokol RZ, Swerdloff RS (1986) Practical considerations in the use of androgen therapy. In: Santen JR, Swerdloff RS (eds) *Male*

Reproductive Dysfunction. Marcel Dekker, New York, pp 211–225

Steidle C, Schwartz S, Jacoby K, Sebree T, Smith T, Bachand R; North American AA2500 T Gel Study Group (2003) AA2500 testosterone gel normalizes androgen levels in aging males with improvements in body composition and sexual function. *J Clin Endocrinol Metab* **88**:2673–2681

Stuenkel CA, Dudley RE, Yen SC (1991) Sublingual administration of testosterone hydroxypropyl-β-cyclodextrin inclusion complex simulates episodic androgen release in hypogonadal men. *J Clin Endocrinol Metab* **72**:1054–1059

Swerdloff RS, Wang C, Cunningham G, Dobs A, Iranmanesh A, Matsumoto AM, Snyder PJ, Weber T, Longstreth J, Berman N (2000) Long-term pharmacokinetics of transdermal testosterone gel in hypogonadal men. *J Clin Endocrinol Metab* **85**:4500–4510

van der Vies J (1965) On the mechanism of action of nandrolone phenylpropionate and nandrolone decanoate in rats. *Acta Endocrinol* **49**:271–282

van der Vies J (1970) Model studies in vitro with long-acting hormonal preparations. *Acta Endocrinol* **64**:656–669

van der Vies J (1985) Implications of basic pharmacology in the therapy with esters of nandrolone. *Acta Endocrinol Suppl (Copenh)* **271**:38–44

Vest SA, Howard JE (1939) Clinical experiments with androgens. IV: a method of implantation of crystalline testosterone. *J Am Med Assoc* **113**:1869–1872

von Eckardstein S, Nieschlag E (2002) Treatment of male hypogonadism with testosterone undecanoate injected at extended intervals of 12 weeks: a phase II study. *J Androl* **23**:419–425

Wang C, Eyre R, Clark D, Kleinberg C, Newman I, Iranmanesh A, Veldhuis R, Dudley RE, Berman N, Davidson T, Barstow TS, Sinow R, Alexander G, Swerdloff R (1996) Sublingual testosterone replacement improves muscle mass and strength, decreases bone resorption and increases bone formation markers in hypogonadal men – a clinical research center study. *J Clin Endocrinol Metab* **81**:3654–3662

Wang C, Berman N, Longstreth JA, Chuapoco B, Hull L, Steiner B, Faulkner S, Dudley RE, Swerdloff RS (2000) Pharmacokinetics of transdermal testosterone gel in hypogonadal men: application of gel at one site versus four sites: a general clinical research center study. *J Clin Endocrinol Metab* **85**:964–969

Wang C, Swerdloff R, Kipnes M, Matsumoto AM, Dobs AS, Cunningham G, Katznelson L, Weber TJ, Friedman TC, Snyder P, Levine HL (2004) New testosterone buccal system (Striant) delivers physiological testosterone levels: pharmacokinetics study in hypogonadal men. *J Clin Endocrinol Metab* **89**:3821–3829

Wang C, Ilani N, Arver S, McLachlan RI, Soulis T, Watkinson A (2011) Efficacy and safety of the 2% formulation of testosterone topical solution applied to the axillae in androgen-deficient men. *Clin Endocrinol (Oxf)* **75**:836–843

Wang L, Shi DC, Lu SY, Fang RY (1991) The therapeutic effect of domestically produced testosterone undecanoate in Klinefelter syndrome. *New Drugs Mark* **8**:28–32

Werner SC, Hamger FM, Kritzler RA (1950) Jaundice during methyltestosterone therapy. *Am J Med* **8**:325–331

Westaby D, Ogle SJ, Paradinas FJ, Randell JB, Murray-Lyon IM (1977) Liver damage from long-term methyltestosterone. *Lancet* **2**:261–263

World Health Organization, Nieschlag E, Wang C, Handelsman DJ, Swerdloff RS, Wu F, Einer-Jensen N, Waites G (1992) *Guidelines for the Use of Androgens.* WHO, Geneva

Wu FCW, Farley TMM, Peregoudov A, Waites GMH (1996) Effects of testosterone enanthate in normal men: experience from a multicenter contraceptive efficacy study. World Health Organization Task Force on Methods for the Regulation of Male Fertility. *Fertil Steril* **65**:626–636

Yin AY, Htun M, Swerdloff RS, Diaz-Arjonilla M, Dudley RE, Faulkner S, Bross R, Leung A, Baravarian S, Hull L, Longstreth JA, Kulback S, Flippo G, Wang C (2012) Re-examination of pharmacokinetics of oral testosterone undecanoate in hypogonadal men with a new self-emulsifying formulation. *J Androl* **33**:190–201

Zhang GY, Gu YQ, Wang XH, Cui YG, Bremner WJ (1998) A pharmacokinetic study of injectable testosterone undecanoate in hypogonadal men. *J Androl* **19**:761–768

Zitzmann M (2009) Pharmacogenetics of testosterone replacement therapy. *Pharmacogenomics* **10**:1341–1349

Zitzmann M, Nieschlag E (2007) Androgen receptor gene CAG repeat length and body mass index modulate the safety of long-term intramuscular testosterone undecanoate therapy in hypogonadal men. *J Clin Endocrinol Metab* **92**:3844–3853

Zitzmann M, Hanisch JU, Mattern A, Maggi M (2011) Testosterone replacement therapy in male hypogonadism: Final results from the largest international substitution trial involving 1493 patients [abstract]. *Endocr Rev* **32** (03_MeetingAbstracts):P1–347

Androgens in male senescence

Jean-Marc Kaufman, Guy T'Sjoen, and Alex Vermeulen

16.1 Introduction

"Andropause," defined as the male equivalent of the menopause, which in women signals the end of reproductive life and a near total cessation of sex steroid production by the gonads, does not exist. Indeed, aging in healthy men is normally not accompanied by abrupt or drastic alterations of gonadal function, and androgen production as well as fertility can be largely preserved until very old age.

The limited data available suggests that aging has limited influence on sperm quality and fertilizing capacity (Nieschlag et al. 1982; Rolf et al. 1996; Jung et al. 2002). Most consistently reported changes of population means for semen parameters are limited to a decrease of ejaculate volume and sperm motility, with a decrease in total sperm output and percentage spermatozoa with normal morphology reported in some studies (Rolf et al. 1996; Ng et al. 2004; Lazarou and Morgentaler 2008). Moreover, decreased ejaculatory frequency, as observed in elderly men (Rolf et al. 1996), might account for at least part of these age-related changes (Cooper et al. 1993). Serum inhibin B, a marker of Sertoli cell function and spermatogenesis, was shown to be relatively well maintained in healthy elderly men, albeit at the cost of clearly increased FSH stimulation that compensates for an age-related

Testosterone: Action, Deficiency, Substitution, ed. Eberhard Nieschlag and Hermann M. Behre, Assoc. ed. Susan Nieschlag. Published by Cambridge University Press. © Cambridge University Press 2012.

regression of Sertoli cell mass and function (Mahmoud *et al.* 2000).

Concerning hormonal testicular function, it is now well established that mean serum testosterone levels decrease progressively in generally healthy elderly men, even though there is a considerable interindividual variability in the extent of the changes (Kaufman and Vermeulen 2005). Well over 20% of otherwise apparently healthy men over 60 years of age present with decreased testosterone levels compared to serum levels in young adults. Moreover, this age-dependent decline in androgen production can be accentuated by co-morbidity, with transient or more permanent adverse effects on Leydig cell function (Kaufman and Vermeulen 2005; Travison *et al.* 2007). The relative contribution of aging versus subtle co-morbidities as cause of the declining mean serum testosterone levels in study populations of apparently healthy aging men inevitably remains an area of some controversy.

The extent to which a relative hypoandrogenism in the elderly contributes to clinical signs and symptoms of aging remains an issue not fully explored but deserving further attention, as many clinical features of aging in men are reminiscent of those of hypogonadism in younger subjects. Accumulating evidence indicates that clearly decreased serum testosterone levels in elderly men predict poorer health and survival. The indications for androgen supplementation to aging men, as well as its potential merits, remain a subject of debate.

16.2 Declining endocrine testicular function in senescence

16.2.1 Testosterone production and serum levels

Early reports of decreased spermatic vein testosterone blood concentrations (Hollander and Hollander 1958) and decreased testosterone blood production rates (Kent and Acone 1966) in elderly men compared to younger individuals were subsequently confirmed by several studies performed in the seventies (Vermeulen *et al.* 1972; Giusti *et al.* 1975; Baker *et al.* 1977). However, the observation of reduced testosterone blood production rate does not necessarily imply lower testosterone plasma levels. Indeed, the blood production rate is the product of the mean plasma levels and the metabolic clearance rate, whereby the latter is also reduced in elderly men (Kent and Acone 1966; Vermeulen *et al.* 1972; Coviello *et al.* 2006).

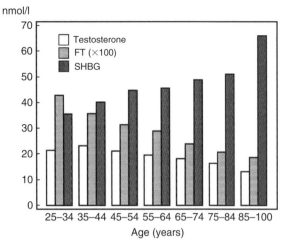

nmol/l

Fig. 16.1 Mean serum levels of testosterone, free testosterone (FT) and sex hormone-binding globulin (SHBG) according to age in a cross-sectional study of 300 healthy men (according to data in Vermeulen *et al.* 1996).

Whether aging in healthy men is also associated with decreased serum testosterone concentrations has long been a controversial issue. But a decline of serum levels from the fourth or fifth decade of life on, or even earlier according to some reports, has been demonstrated in a series of cross-sectional studies which included healthy ambulatory young and elderly men sampled in the morning (Vermeulen 1991; Kaufman and Vermeulen 2005; Mohr *et al.* 2005 for review). The observed mean serum testosterone values at age 75 years are about two-thirds of those at age 25 years (Fig. 16.1).

An age-related decrease of serum testosterone levels has also been documented in longitudinal studies (Morley *et al.* 1997; Zmuda *et al.* 1997; Harman *et al.* 2001; Feldman *et al.* 2002; Andersson *et al.* 2007; Travison *et al.* 2007; Liu *et al.* 2007a; Lapauw *et al.* 2008). In fact, the longitudinally assessed decline of serum testosterone tends to be even larger than apparent from cross-sectional analyses, which might be due to a bias towards healthier subjects in the latter, while during longitudinal follow-up more elderly subjects are likely to show deterioration than an improvement of their general health status relative to the baseline situation.

Whereas mean serum testosterone levels in the adult male population decrease with age, at all ages there is a large interindividual variability of serum testosterone levels, with some elderly men having frankly low serum testosterone levels while many

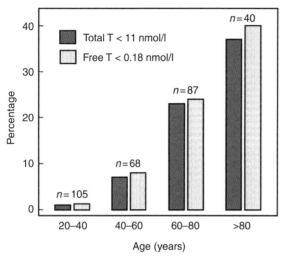

Fig. 16.2 Proportion of healthy men presenting with subnormal serum levels for total testosterone (Total T <11 nmol/l) or free testosterone (Free T <0.18 nmol/l) (from Kaufman and Vermeulen 1997).

others have perfectly preserved testosterone secretion, with serum levels well within the normal range for young adults. With advancing age, a progressively larger proportion of men present with subnormal values relative to those in young adults; in a group of 300 healthy men aged 20 to 100 years (Vermeulen *et al.* 1996), we observed a subnormal testosterone level in less than 1% of men below age 40 years but in more than 20% of men older than 60 years (Fig. 16.2). In an unselected, population-based sample of the Third National Health and Nutrition Examination Survey (NHANES III; USA), the prevalence of men with low serum testosterone defined as below 300 ng/dl (10.4 nmol/l) was 25% (Rohrmann *et al.* 2011). Also in an unselected, population-based sample, Araujo *et al.* (2007) observed a prevalence of over 20% of low total testosterone (<300 ng/dl) in men over 60 years of age, but in this study the prevalence was rather similar in younger men aged 40 to 60 years, which can be explained by the presence of co-morbidity and mainly a high prevalence (>30%) of obesity in this study population. A similar proportion of men over 65 years with serum testosterone below 300 ng/dl, without further age-related changes in this age-group, was reported for the large unselected population in the MrOS study (Orwoll *et al.* 2006a). In an unselected German population of primary care patients with mean age of 59 years, 20% presented with serum testosterone below 300 ng/dl (Schneider

et al. 2009). These findings illustrate that in unselected populations the age-related decrease of total serum testosterone seen in apparently healthy men tends to be masked by a higher prevalence of low testosterone in younger age groups.

16.2.2 Sex hormone-binding globulin and free testosterone serum levels

Whereas some authors may still argue that total testosterone concentrations are not reduced in perfectly healthy elderly men, there is virtually unanimity amongst authors that the free and non-specifically bound serum testosterone, which is generally considered to represent the serum testosterone fractions readily available for biological activity, does indeed decrease with age (Kaufman and Vermeulen 2005 for review). In healthy ambulatory men, mean serum levels of free testosterone and of non-SHBG-bound or so-called "bioavailable" testosterone (i.e. the sum of the free fraction and the fraction loosely bound to albumin) decrease by as much as 50% between the ages of 25 and 75 years (Vermeulen *et al.* 1996; Ferrini and Barrett-Connor 1998). The sharper decline of these fractions in comparison with total testosterone is explained by an age-associated increase of SHBG concentrations, and confirmed in longitudinal studies (Morley *et al.* 1997; Harman *et al.* 2001; Feldman *et al.* 2002; Andersson *et al.* 2007; Travison *et al.* 2007; Lapauw *et al.* 2008). In 300 healthy men aged 25–100 years we observed an approximately log linear decrease of free testosterone levels at a rate of 1.2% per year (Fig. 16.1); while total serum testosterone remained relatively stable up to the age of 55 years and declined thereafter at a rate of 0.85% per year (Vermeulen *et al.* 1996). The decline in serum testosterone persists in old age. In a group of apparently healthy older men ($n = 218$) with population-based recruitment, aged 71 to 86 years at baseline, the percentual yearly decline assessed longitudinally over four years amounted to 1.26%, 1.33% and 2.43% for total, free and non-SHBG-bound testosterone, respectively (Lapauw *et al.* 2008).

As is the case for total testosterone, there is a great between-subject variability in prevailing free (or bioavailable) testosterone levels in elderly men, ranging from markedly low levels to levels in the upper normal range for young adults (Fig. 16.3), the proportion of men with subnormal free testosterone levels increasing with age (Fig. 16.2). As a result of the more rapid

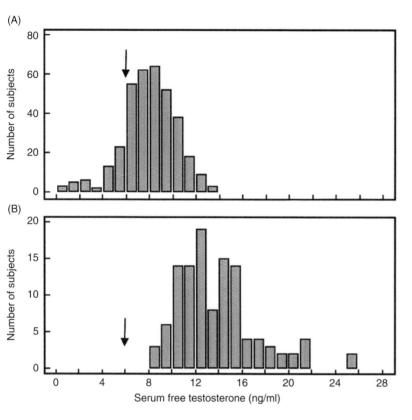

Fig. 16.3 Histogram for the distribution of serum free testosterone in (A) 353 community-dwelling elderly men without major health problems, aged 70 to 85 years and (B) in a younger control population of healthy men aged 23 to 58 years; the lower limit for the laboratory normal range is indicated by the arrows.

decline of free testosterone, the prevalence of elderly men with low free testosterone is greater than for low total testosterone (Kaufman and Vermeulen 2005; Rohrmann *et al.* 2011). However, as discussed below, limits of normality are somewhat arbitrary as the sensitivity threshold for androgen action may vary from tissue to tissue and according to age.

16.2.3 Tissue levels and metabolism of androgens

It is generally considered that free testosterone diffuses passively within the cell. It should be mentioned, however, that during transit through the capillaries, a large part of the albumin-bound testosterone dissociates and becomes bioavailable. Testosterone bound by SHBG is not directly available to the cells, but the physiopathology of SHBG is still incompletely understood. It has been shown that in some tissues (e.g. in the prostate and epididymis) cellular membranes carry SHBG receptors (Rosner *et al.* 1991; Porto *et al.* 1992), the activation of which stimulates intracellular cAMP production. Moreover, the SHBG–androgen complex might be internalized by several cell types.

Androgen receptors are present at highest concentrations in the accessory sex organs; whereas concentrations in other androgen-sensitive tissues such as the heart and bone are much lower. Tissue concentrations both of androgen receptors (Rajfer *et al.* 1989) and of androgens decrease with age (Deslypere and Vermeulen 1981; 1985).

Overall, the influence of the aging process on the metabolism of testosterone manifests itself essentially by a decrease of the metabolic clearance rate (Vermeulen *et al.* 1972; Coviello *et al.* 2006), which results from an age-associated decrease of cardiac output and of hepatic as well as tissue perfusion, and from increased binding of plasma testosterone to SHBG.

Of major physiological significance is the activating biotransformation in the tissues, with testosterone acting as a prohormone and being metabolized into the more potent androgen DHT by type 2 or type 1 5α-reductase, and to estrogens by the cytochrome P450 aromatase enzyme. Production of DHT occurs in, or in the close vicinity of the target cells, as does also its catabolic metabolism, with only a minor fraction escaping to the general circulation; whereas DHT produced in the liver is locally glucuronoconjugated and does not reach the general circulation. Blood production rate thus largely underestimates total DHT production in the organism. Aromatization of testosterone in (subcutaneous) fat and in striated muscle is the major contribution to circulating estradiol in men; both estradiol in the systemic circulation and estradiol locally produced in the target tissues can contribute to estrogen-mediated testosterone effects. The expression both of 5α-reductase activity and of the aromatase enzyme coded by the CYP19 gene can be differentially regulated in different target tissues (Russell and Wilson 1994; Kamat *et al.* 2002), local biotransformation to DHT and estrogens being potentially important regulatory components in the modulation of tissue effects of testosterone.

No data are available concerning the possible influence of aging on blood conversion rates of testosterone to DHT. Reports on age-related changes of DHT serum levels are not consistent, but do not suggest major changes, and in any case serum DHT is not a reliable parameter of tissue DHT formation (Labrie *et al.* 1995).

The conversion of testosterone to estradiol increases with age (Siiteri and MacDonald 1975; Lakshman *et al.* 2010), which appears to be the consequence of an increase of both aromatase tissue activity and of fat mass in the elderly (Vermeulen *et al.* 1996; Vermeulen and Kaufman 2002). This increasing global aromatase activity compensates for the decreased substrate availability, i.e. the declining testosterone and androstenedione plasma levels, so that the serum estradiol levels do not show much change or only slight decline during aging in men (Vermeulen *et al.* 1996; Ferrini and Barrett-Connor 1998; Vermeulen and Kaufman 2002; Orwoll *et al.* 2006a). However, there is a decrease with age of the serum testosterone-to-estradiol ratio and, as a consequence of the age-related increase in SHBG, also a moderate decrease of serum free and bioavailable estradiol (FE2 and Bio E2).

Serum levels of 5α-androstane-3α,17β-diol-glucuronide (ADG) decrease significantly with age (Deslypere *et al.* 1982), a consequence of the decreased serum concentrations of the precursors (70% testosterone and 30% DHEAS). A decrease of the ratio of 5α/5β metabolites in urine indicates an age-related decrease of type 2 5α-reductase activity (Vermeulen *et al.* 1972; Zumoff *et al.* 1976).

16.2.4 Factors affecting serum testosterone levels in elderly men

16.2.4.1 Influence of physiological factors and lifestyle

The physiological basis underlying the large interindividual variation in serum testosterone levels seen at any age is not yet fully elucidated, but several physiological variables and factors related to lifestyle have been identified that account for part of the wide range of normal values observed in healthy men. In any case, the apparent interindividual variability of testosterone levels is not merely artefactual as a result of a cross-sectional design of the clinical studies, as single-point plasma testosterone estimates reflect, fairly well, longer-term androgen status in healthy men (Vermeulen and Verdonck 1992).

The circadian variation of serum testosterone, with highest levels in the early morning and lowest levels in the late afternoon, should not play an important role in the wide range of normal testosterone levels if they are consequently evaluated in the morning (preferably before 10 a.m.), as should be the rule. However, recent reports suggest that serum testosterone is higher in fasting state (Sartorius *et al.* 2011). The ultradian pattern of episodic testosterone secretion undoubtedly contributes to the variability of testosterone levels (Veldhuis *et al.* 1987; Spratt *et al.* 1988). Therefore, although single time-point estimates are a valid approach for clinical studies, the existence of fluctuations in serum testosterone should be taken into account when assessing the androgen status of individual elderly subjects (Morley *et al.* 2002). The occurrence of circannual variations with amplitudes of up to 35% have been reported, with the highest testosterone levels measured between October and December for studies performed in the western hemisphere (Smals *et al.* 1976; Svartberg *et al.* 2003). However, other studies failed to find such variations or observed a maximum rather in spring or summer (Svartberg *et al.* 2003; Ruhayel *et al.* 2007; Brambilla *et al.* 2007).

Heredity appears to play an important role, as concluded from studies in twins and siblings (Meikle *et al.* 1986; 1988; Ring *et al.* 2005; Bogaert *et al.* 2008), with up to 60% of the variability of serum testosterone attributable to genetic factors. Nevertheless, nongenetic factors also have a substantial impact on testosterone serum levels.

The genetic basis for the heredity of serum (free) testosterone and SHBG is presently largely unknown. Reports of ethnic differences in serum testosterone levels have been inconsistent, with small differences tending to disappear if adjustments are made for differences in body composition, especially for abdominal adiposity (Winters *et al.* 2001; Gapstur *et al.* 2002; Heald *et al.* 2003; Rohrmann *et al.* 2007). Recently, regional and racial differences in sex steroids were reported for elderly men in the large MrOS study. Serum testosterone was 20% higher in Asian men living in Hong Kong or Japan, but not in the USA compared to the other groups. Again these differences tended to disappear, at least for total testosterone, when adjusted for BMI (Orwoll *et al.* 2010).

There has been considerable interest for the role of a polymorphic trinucleotide CAG-repeat contained in exon 1 of the *AR*, which encodes a functionally relevant polyglutamine tract of variable length. A CAG-repeat length exceeding the normal range of 15–31 results in diminished AR transactivation capacity. There is evidence that androgen activity is also affected by variations in *AR* gene CAG-repeat length within the normal range: shorter repeats being associated with increased AR transactivation capacity and clinical correlates of increased androgen activity (Zitzmann and Nieschlag 2003). Several studies have shown positive associations of serum total and free-testosterone levels with *AR* CAG-repeat length, which likely reflect the effect of the polymorphism on androgen sensitivity and consequently on the negative feedback set point for serum testosterone (Crabbe *et al.* 2007; Stanworth *et al.* 2008; Huhtaniemi *et al.* 2009; Lindström *et al.* 2010). The effect of this AR polymorphism on serum testosterone may be absent or reduced in the more elderly; possibly because of altered negative feedback regulation (Van Pottelbergh *et al.* 2003a; Harkonen *et al.* 2003). Other polymorphisms in the androgen receptor (Bogaert *et al.* 2009) and other genes involved in the pituitary-gonadal function (Eriksson *et al.* 2006; Vanbillemont *et al.* 2009; Huhtaniemi *et al.* 2010) have been reported to affect testosterone levels.

Several metabolic and hormonal factors influence SHBG serum levels. Insulin and insulin-like factor I (IGF-1) inhibit SHBG production and, in clinical studies, insulin was found to be inversely correlated with serum SHBG and testosterone levels (Haffner *et al.* 1988; Vermeulen *et al.* 1996).

In clinical studies, body composition and, in particular, adiposity emerges as an important determinant of SHBG levels. For the whole range of clinically encountered BMI values there is a highly significant negative correlation with SHBG and testosterone serum levels, which is explained at least in part by increased insulin levels (Khaw and Barrett-Connor 1992; Giagulli *et al.* 1994; Yeap *et al.* 2009a). In elderly men this inverse relationship between BMI and SHBG levels as well as total testosterone can be clearly demonstrated notwithstanding the background of an age-related rise of SHBG levels (Vermeulen *et al.* 1996; Mohr *et al.* 2006; Orwoll *et al.* 2006a; Wu *et al.* 2008). Similarly, a negative association of serum SHBG and total testosterone with leptin levels has been observed in elderly men (Haffner *et al.* 1997; Van Den Saffele *et al.* 1999). Negative associations with serum testosterone levels tend to be most pronounced for indices of abdominal adiposity (Khaw and Barrett-Connor 1992; Vermeulen *et al.* 1999a; Couillard *et al.* 2000; Kupelian *et al.* 2008; Hall *et al.* 2008; Grossmann 2011). Whereas in younger men moderate obesity mainly affects total serum testosterone by lowering SHBG binding capacity, with decreased free testosterone seen in morbid obesity (BMI > 35–40) as a result of neuroendocrine disturbances (Giagulli *et al.* 1994), elderly men might be even more sensitive to the negative effects of adiposity on free or bioavailable testosterone (Vermeulen *et al.* 1999a; Van Den Saffele *et al.* 1999; Couillard *et al.* 2000; Mohr *et al.* 2006). In this context it is interesting to note that Andersson *et al.* (2007) described a birth cohort effect with higher serum total testosterone, but not free testosterone, in older generations resulting from a decline of SHBG in more recent generations. This appears to be explained by a parallel increase of BMI in the latter generations. When discussing the effects of adiposity on serum androgens one should keep in mind the caveat that, as discussed later, the relation is bidirectional, with low serum testosterone favoring increased adiposity.

Overt alterations in thyroid hormone levels have marked effects on SHBG levels, with thyrotoxicosis resulting in a several-fold increase of SHBG levels and marked increase of total serum testosterone (Vermeulen *et al.* 1971). More subtle changes in thyroid hormone levels can also affect SHBG and testosterone levels, with significant increases of SHBG and testosterone levels seen in subclinical hyperthyroidism, with suppressed serum thyroid-stimulating hormone without clinical hyperthyroidism or elevation of thyroid hormone levels above normal (Faber *et al.* 1990; Giagulli and Vermeulen 1992).

Concerning lifestyle factors, reports on the effects of diet on serum testosterone levels have not always been concordant, but it seems possible to conclude that diet influences testosterone levels mainly indirectly through changes in SHBG levels, fiber-rich, vegetarian diets being associated with higher SHBG and testosterone levels than western-type diets with high fat content. Further, low protein intake is associated with decreased IGF-1, which in turn may result in increased SHBG and total testosterone (Kaufman and Vermeulen 2005 for review). In men aged 40 to 70 years in the Massachusetts Male Aging Study, fiber intake and protein intake, but not carbohydrate, fat or total caloric intake, were independent positive and negative determinants, respectively, of serum SHBG (Longcope *et al.* 2000).

Current smoking at all ages has generally been associated with 5 to 15% higher total and free serum testosterone levels than in non-smokers (Barrett-Connor and Khaw 1987; Dai *et al.* 1988; Field *et al.* 1994; Vermeulen *et al.* 1996). In the European Male Ageing Study (EMAS), including men 40 to 79 years without exclusion of co-morbidities, smoking was associated with increased serum levels of LH, SHBG and total, but not free, testosterone (Wu *et al.* 2008). Alcohol abuse, also in the absence of liver cirrhosis, may accentuate the age-associated decrease of testosterone levels, estradiol serum levels being increased (Cicero 1982; Irwin *et al.* 1988; Ida *et al.* 1992); moderate alcohol consumption has no adverse effect (Sparrow *et al.* 1980; Longcope *et al.* 2000).

Both physical and psychological stress and strenuous physical activity result in transient or more prolonged decreases of serum (free) testosterone (Kaufman and Vermeulen 2005 for review); although elderly men have been reported to be more resistant to stress such as the metabolic stress of fasting (Bergendahl *et al.* 1998).

Low serum (free) testosterone has also been associated with low income and with recent loss of spouse (Travison *et al.* 2007; Hall *et al.* 2008). Whether sexual activity influences serum testosterone levels remains a controversial issue as limited literature data are not consistent.

16.2.4.2 Testosterone serum levels in disease

There is considerable evidence that the aging process *per se* adversely affects testosterone production, but this will remain controversial as it may not be realistic to definitely exclude subtle co-morbidities in apparently healthy older men without selecting out a poorly representative group of "super-healthy elderly." In any case, diseases and/or their treatment can be associated with transient or more permanent decreases of testosterone production (Handelsman 1994; Turner and Wass 1997). Considering the high prevalence of diseases and use of medication that can adversely affect testosterone levels in the elderly, it is evident that in daily practice the age-associated decline in testosterone levels may often be accentuated by intercurrent disease (Mohr *et al.* 2005; Orwoll *et al.* 2006b; Travison *et al.* 2007; Schneider *et al.* 2009).

Acute critical illness, such as acute myocardial infarction or surgical trauma, is associated with temporary, but often profound and prolonged decrease of serum (free) testosterone (Wang *et al.* 1978; Woolf *et al.* 1985; Swartz and Young 1987; Spratt *et al.* 1993; Impallomeni *et al.* 1994; Vandenberghe *et al.* 2001).

A series of chronic diseases can induce more long-standing decreases in testosterone levels (Handelsman 1994; Turner and Wass 1997). Both testosterone and SHBG levels tend to be decreased in elderly men with insulin resistance, metabolic syndrome and type 2 diabetes (Andersson *et al.* 1994; Kupelian *et al.* 2008; Yeap *et al.* 2009a; Grossmann 2011).

Coronary atherosclerosis has been reported to be accompanied by lower or similar testosterone levels as compared to controls (Poggi *et al.* 1976; Lichtenstein *et al.* 1987; Swartz and Young 1987; Phillips *et al.* 1994; Alexandersen *et al.* 1996; Hak *et al.* 2002). Low serum testosterone has also been associated with carotid artery atherosclerosis, incident stroke and aneurisms of the aorta abdominalis (van den Beld *et al.* 2003; Yeap *et al.* 2009b; 2010). However, it is not clear whether decreased testosterone levels represented a consequence of atherosclerosis or rather a pre-existent risk factor for cardiovascular disease (see Wu and von Eckardstein 2003 for review).

In COPD and in patients with other hypoxic pulmonary diseases, serum testosterone levels are often decreased with inappropriately low gonadotropin levels, also in the absence of systemic glucocorticoid treatment (Semple *et al.* 1984; Kamischke *et al.* 1998). Sleep apnea syndrome is commonly accompanied by relative hypogonadotropic hypogonadism, potentially reversible by nasal continuous positive airways pressure therapy; massive obesity is often a contributing factor (Worstman *et al.* 1987; Grunstein *et al.* 1989; Luboshitzky *et al.* 2002).

Chronic renal failure is often accompanied by hypogonadism with complex pathophysiology, involving the different compartments of the hypothalamo-pituitary-gonadal axis (Handelsman and Dong 1993; Veldhuis *et al.* 1993). In chronic liver disease, decreased (free) testosterone levels are accompanied by increased SHBG, androstenedione and estrone levels (Baker *et al.* 1979; Elewaut *et al.* 1979). Hypogonadism in hemochromatosis is multifactorially determined, with a major contribution of pituitary insufficiency (Duranteau *et al.* 1993).

Moderate impairment of testicular function has been observed in active rheumatic diseases (Tapia-Serrano *et al.* 1991). In the elderly, as in the young, Leydig cell function may be adversely affected by endocrine diseases such as Cushing syndrome and pituitary tumors; in particular, prolactinomas. There is substantial overlap between symptoms of hypogonadism and hypothyroidism, which itself is a possible cause of hypogonadism (Brenta *et al.* 1999).

Finally, in the elderly there is a rather high prevalence of the use of medications, and concomitant use of several drugs is far from exceptional. This may further negatively affect gonadal function already impaired by underlying disease. Such a situation is typically encountered in COPD patients treated with glucocorticoids (Kamischke *et al.* 1998). Their chronic use may impair Leydig cell function, which induces a dose-dependent suppression of testosterone levels by combined actions at the testicular and at the hypothalamo-pituitary level, and by a decrease of SHBG serum levels (MacAdams *et al.* 1986; Kamischke *et al.* 1998). Opiates can induce hypogonadotropic hypogonadism (Daniell 2002; Rajagopal *et al.* 2004). Secretion of LH and Leydig cell function may be adversely affected by hyperprolactinemia during chronic use of neuroleptic drugs and related compounds (Bixler *et al.* 1977). Leydig cell function can be mildly affected by cytotoxic chemotherapy (Howell *et al.* 2001).

If only as a reminder, one has to mention hormonal treatment of prostate cancer, which is aimed at inducing profound hypogonadism by suppression of LH and testosterone secretion by use of a GnRH analog and/or by blockade of androgen effects with an antiandrogen. As to the use of 5α-reductase inhibitors in benign prostate hypertrophy, under treatment with finasteride testosterone levels are unchanged or modestly elevated (Vermeulen *et al.* 1989a), but treatment can result in mild symptoms of hypogonadism (Thompson *et al.* 2003) by mitigating androgen effects in those tissues where androgenic effects are largely mediated by DHT. Spironolactone can reduce testosterone production through an inhibitory action on the 17-hydroxylase-lyase activity (Stripp *et al.* 1975).

Several classes of antihypertensive drugs, including β-blockers, may adversely affect erectile function, and hypertensive patients under treatment may show mildly decreased serum testosterone levels (Turner and Wass 1997); considering the many confounding factors in these patients, an adverse effect of antihypertensive treatment on serum testosterone is not to be considered as established.

16.3 Physiopathology of declining testosterone levels in senescence

16.3.1 Primary testicular changes

Primary testicular factors undoubtedly play an important role in the age-associated decline of Leydig cell function, as indicated by a reduced absolute secretory response to stimulation with hCG (Longcope 1973; Nieschlag *et al.* 1973; 1982; Rubens *et al.* 1974; Harman and Tsitouras 1980; Nankin *et al.* 1981). Diminished testicular secretory capacity in the elderly has also been confirmed for the response to recombinant human LH following downregulation of endogenous LH with leuprorelin (Mulligan *et al.* 2001), and for the response to prolonged "physiologic" intermittent stimulation by endogenous LH during a two-week pulsatile GnRH infusion (Mulligan *et al.* 1999). This decrease in testicular reserve for testosterone secretion appears to result from a reduced number of Leydig cells (Sniffen 1950; Harbitz 1973; Neaves *et al.* 1984). There is, moreover, evidence for involvement of vascular changes (Sasano and Ichijo 1969; Suoranta 1971), the deficient oxygen supply inducing changes in testicular steroid metabolism (Pirke *et al.* 1980; Vermeulen and Deslypere 1986). In healthy community-dwelling elderly men 70 years or older, mean testicular volume is decreased by about 30% as compared to young men (Mahmoud *et al.* 2003).

In apparent agreement with the view of a primary testicular defect are observations of moderate increases of basal gonadotropin levels in elderly men as observed in several, but not all, studies on the age-related decline of testicular function (Vermeulen 1991; Tsitouras and Bulat 1995 for review). Although there have been some discordant findings (Urban *et al.* 1988; Mitchell *et al.* 1995), this increase is not limited to immunoreactive forms of the gonadotropins, as it is also demonstrated for levels measured by bioassay (Tenover *et al.* 1988; Kaufman *et al.* 1991; Matzkin *et al.* 1991). Part of the age-related increase of gonadotropin levels may result from reduced plasma clearance (Kaufman *et al.* 1991; Bergendahl *et al.* 1998). The increase of LH with age is usually of rather modest amplitude and inconsistent (Morley *et al.* 1997), but may be more prominent when considering populations with substantial prevalence of co-morbidity (Wu *et al.* 2008; Tajar *et al.* 2010). In a longitudinal assessment in community-dwelling men over age 70 years, both serum LH and FSH were independent predictors of serum (free) testosterone decrease (Lapauw *et al.* 2008).

16.3.2 Altered neuroendocrine regulation

Although the combined observations of a diminished testicular reserve for testosterone secretion with increased basal gonadotropin levels reveal involvement of a primary testicular factor in the age-related decline of Leydig cell function, other mechanisms must also be involved. Indeed, the responses to hCG challenges in elderly men indicate that the secretory reserve of the Leydig cells, albeit diminished, should still be sufficient to allow for a normalization of plasma testosterone levels, provided the endogenous drive by pituitary LH is adequate. The latter is indeed the case in some of the elderly, who present with well-maintained serum testosterone and elevated serum LH and are sometimes referred to as having "compensated hypogonadism" (Tajar *et al.* 2010). However, many elderly men with serum testosterone below the range for young men have normal or only slightly elevated serum LH. In the presence of a persistent status of relative hypoandrogenism, such LH levels should be regarded as inappropriately low and indicative of alterations in the neuroendocrine regulation of LH secretion. The relative inadequacy of the gonadotropin response to hypoandrogenism in elderly men has also been shown during experimental muting of endogenous testosterone suppression by administration of an antiandrogen (Veldhuis *et al.* 2001).

Assessment of the secretory capacity of the pituitary gonadotropes by in-vivo challenge with small,

"near physiologic" doses of synthetic GnRH has revealed a preserved or, in accordance with a status of relative hypoandrogenism, even moderately increased LH response in the elderly compared to the young (Kaufman *et al.* 1991; Mulligan *et al.* 1999). If the pituitary secretory capacity is maintained, hypothalamic mechanisms must be involved in the apparent failure of the feedback regulation to produce an adequate LH rise in response to hypoandrogenism (Vermeulen and Kaufman 1992).

Several changes in the neuroendocrine control of Leydig cell function likely situated at the hypothalamic level have been documented in elderly men. Circadian rhythm of LH and testosterone secretion is clearly blunted in elderly men (Bremner *et al.* 1983; Tenover *et al.* 1988; Plymate *et al.* 1989). Furthermore, the pulsatile pattern of LH secretion controlled by intermittent secretion of GnRH is altered, with increased irregularity of LH pulses (Pincus *et al.* 1997; Veldhuis *et al.* 2000). Whereas mean LH pulse frequency remains essentially unchanged in the elderly (Winters *et al.* 1984; Tenover *et al.* 1987; 1988; Urban *et al.* 1988; Vermeulen *et al.* 1989b), there is a diminished frequency of LH pulses with larger amplitude and resulting decrease of the mean LH pulse amplitude (Vermeulen *et al.* 1989b; Veldhuis *et al.* 1992), parameters of the stimulating effect on the Leydig cells. Considering the preserved pituitary LH secretory capacity, this decrease in LH pulse amplitude must by inference be attributed to decreased stimulation by endogenous GnRH, with reduced size of the bolus of the neuropeptide intermittently released into the pituitary portal circulation. This could in turn result either from a decreased number of GnRH-secreting neurons, from their less efficient intermittent recruitment and/or synchronization, and/or from downregulation of their activity by external local and/or systemic factors. This last possibility is supported by evidence for increased responsiveness to the negative feedback effects of testosterone in the elderly (Winters *et al.* 1984; 1997; Deslypere *et al.* 1987; Mulligan *et al.* 1999). The latter might also underlie the fact that LH pulse frequency, governed by the hypothalamic GnRH pulse generator and expected to increase in a state of hypoandrogenism, has been found by most authors to remain unchanged and thus inappropriately low; an increased LH pulse frequency in elderly men having been reported only by one group (Veldhuis *et al.* 1992; Mulligan *et al.* 1995).

The decreased hypothalamic drive of LH secretion in the elderly is not the consequence of an increased inhibitory tone by endogenous opioids, which on the contrary is rather reduced (Vermeulen *et al.* 1989b; Mikuma *et al.* 1994), does not result from increased inhibition by endogenous estrogens (T'Sjoen *et al.* 2005a), or from relative leptin deficiency (Van Den Saffele *et al.* 1999). The mechanisms underlying the apparent relative deficiency of GnRH secretion in elderly men remain to be fully elucidated. Moreover, the role in their presentation of additional risk factors, such as increased adiposity, apart from aging *per se*, remains a matter of debate (Wu *et al.* 2008; Sartorius *et al.* 2011).

16.3.3 Increase of serum sex hormone-binding globulin

The progressive increase of plasma SHBG binding capacity with age should be regarded as a third important aspect of the pathophysiological mechanisms responsible for the age-related changes in circulating testosterone levels. Indeed, against the background of a relative inability to respond optimally to hypoandrogenism by increased testosterone secretion in the elderly, due to the aforementioned testicular and neuroendocrine alterations, an independent progressive increase of SHBG binding capacity results in a steeper decline of the non-specifically bound testosterone fractions, i.e. free and bioavailable serum testosterone levels.

The substantial increase of SHBG concentrations in elderly men (Vermeulen *et al.* 1996; Orwoll *et al.* 2006a; Liu *et al.* 2007a; Wu *et al.* 2008) is remarkable as it occurs in the face of increased fat mass and insulin levels – factors that are known to be strong negative determinants of SHBG levels. But the cause of these increased SHBG levels remains unclear. It is unlikely that the decreased testosterone levels *per se* are responsible, as the increase in SHBG levels is observed at an earlier age than the decrease of testosterone levels, and the estradiol serum levels are rather similar in young and elderly men (Vermeulen *et al.* 1996). Serum SHBG and testosterone levels have been reported to be inversely correlated to 24-hour GH and IGF-1 levels (Erfurth *et al.* 1996; Pfeilschifter *et al.* 1996; Vermeulen *et al.* 1996), and it has been proposed that decreased activity of the somatotropic axis may play a role in the age-associated increase of SHBG levels and ensuing decrease of free testosterone levels (Vermeulen *et al.* 1996).

16.4 Clinical relevance of hypoandrogenism of senescence

16.4.1 General background

In contrast with the menopause, the decline of androgen levels in men is slowly progressive until the eighth decade, with a substantial proportion of men maintaining normal (free) testosterone levels. Frankly decreased testosterone levels in elderly men are thus by far not a generalized phenomenon and, as fertility is also usually well preserved until old age, there is no such phenomenon as an andropause or male climacterium. Subnormal serum testosterone with accompanying signs and symptoms of androgen deficiency in aging men is presently most commonly referred to as late-onset hypogonadism (LOH) (Wang *et al.* 2008). A key question is the clinical relevance of the apparent partial androgen deficiency occurring in some elderly men.

Many of the clinical features of aging in men are reminiscent of the clinical changes seen in hypogonadism in young men, with a decrease in general well-being, mood changes, a decrease of energy and virility, a decrease in sexual pilosity and skin thickness, a decrease in muscular mass and strength, an increase in upper and central body fat, a decrease in bone density and increased prevalence of osteoporotic fractures, insomnia, sweating and hot flushes, a decrease in libido and sexual drive, and markedly increased prevalence of ED. However, in the elderly this symptomatology develops slowly and progressively, with symptoms that are variable, subtle and not specific. Hence, the clinical picture at best suggests the possibility of a hypoandrogenic state in elderly men, and it is equally plausible that many observed clinical changes and the age-related decrease in serum testosterone levels are coincident and independent consequences of aging.

Much available information is still derived from cross-sectional studies, which revealed mostly only weak correlations between androgen status and clinical parameters. This is not surprising as clinical changes are often multifactorially determined, a complex clinical picture arising from concurrent effects of the aging process *per se*, a relative hypoandrogenism and intercurrent diseases. In elderly men there is a striking interindividual variability not only of the prevailing testosterone levels but also of the pace of "clinical aging." Furthermore, there is increasing evidence that androgen requirements may vary not only between individuals but within the same person, with different signs and symptoms of hypogonadism associated with different testosterone levels (Bhasin *et al.* 2005; Zitzmann *et al.* 2006; Wu *et al.* 2008). In any event, decreased androgen levels can at best be responsible for part of the clinical changes observed in aging men.

More recently an increasing amount of data became available from prospective studies assessing the relationship of sex steroid levels with various intermediary and clinical health outcomes, including frailty and mortality in aging men. The difficulty in interpretation of these studies often is deciding whether the hypoandrogenism is a specific and direct cause of the health problem or rather a more general marker of poorer health.

The studies examining the effects of androgen treatment in elderly men provide precious information, but should also be interpreted with caution, as the demonstration of beneficial effects of a pharmacological intervention does not necessarily imply that the corrected clinical sign or symptom was due to pre-existent androgen deficiency.

16.4.2 Hypoandrogenism of senescence and sexual activity

Aging in men is accompanied by a decrease in libido and sexual activity. Mean coital frequency was reported to be about four times a week at age 20–25 years and decreasing to less than twice a month between age 75 and 80 years (Masters 1986; Tsitouras and Bulat 1995).

Whereas normal libido requires adequate testosterone levels, as shown by the effect of testosterone withdrawal (Basaria *et al.* 2002) and that of replacement therapy in hypogonadal males (Hajjar *et al.* 1997; Snyder *et al.* 2000; Kunelius *et al.* 2002; Steidle *et al.* 2003; Isidori *et al.* 2005a), the correlation of libido with plasma testosterone levels is rather poor; the testosterone concentration required to sustain sexual activity and maintain libido appears to be rather low, probably at or below the lower end of the normal range in young men (Gooren 1987; Bhasin *et al.* 2001), and there is evidence indicating that healthy adults have substantially higher androgen levels than required for normal sexual behavior (Udry *et al.* 1985; Buena *et al.* 1993).

Nevertheless, in an experimental setting with graded testosterone replacement, there was a clear dose-response effect on libido and erectile function, but not on parameters of sexual activity, in the elderly, at variance with the absence of such a dose-response effect in young men (Bhasin *et al.* 2001; Gray *et al.* 2005). Several authors reported differences in parameters of sexual desire or activity according to endogenous serum testosterone levels in the elderly (Tsitouras *et al.* 1982; Davidson *et al.* 1983; Schiavi *et al.* 1990; Travison *et al.* 2006; Zitzmann *et al.* 2006; Araujo *et al.* 2007; Wu *et al.* 2010), but there is a broad overlap of serum testosterone levels in sexually less or more active elderly men in these studies. Moreover, other studies failed to find an association between androgen levels and the perception of sexual functioning (Perry *et al.* 2001; T'Sjoen *et al.* 2004).

Although potency and nocturnal penile tumescence (NPT) require adequate testosterone levels, and although several studies show that hormonal alterations might play some role in 6 to 45% of cases (Morley 1986), most frequently the cause of impotence in elderly males is non-hormonal. There exists, nevertheless, a correlation between bioavailable testosterone levels and the frequency of NPT (Morley 1986). Erections in response to visual stimuli, on the other hand, are largely testosterone independent in normal subjects (Kwan *et al.* 1983; Bancroft 1984); suggesting that whereas testosterone is required to sustain NPT, it is much less required to maintain response to external stimuli. Still, testosterone levels have been reported to correlate inversely with the latency of erection in response to visual stimuli (Rubin *et al.* 1979; Lange *et al.* 1980). Testosterone stimulates the activity of the nitric oxide synthase enzyme, which may explain reported synergistic effects between androgens and inhibitors of phosphodiesterase type 5 (Aversa *et al.* 2003).

Notwithstanding the rather mitigated picture of the role of testosterone in the regulation of erectile function, the manifest major contribution of non-hormonal factors in the pathogenesis of ED in the elderly, and failure to observe an association between serum testosterone and erectile function in several studies (Korenman *et al.* 1990; Feldman *et al.* 1994; Rhoden *et al.* 2002), more recent studies in elderly men reported increased prevalence of ED with decreased serum (free) testosterone (Zitzmann *et al.* 2006; Wu *et al.* 2010). A dose-response effect of testosterone on erectile function was demonstrated in elderly men (Gray *et al.* 2005), and, in a meta-analysis of testosterone replacement treatment, a positive effect on erectile function was shown; however, the treatment effects are rather modest, essentially restricted to men with initially low or low-normal serum testosterone, and seen mostly in studies of shorter duration (Isidori *et al.* 2005b).

The relative contribution of testosterone itself and of its metabolites DHT and estradiol in the maintenance of normal sexual function has not been extensively studied. At present there is no conclusive evidence for a major role of estradiol (Davidson *et al.* 1983), even though estradiol may contribute to some aspects of male sexual behavior (Carani *et al.* 1997). As to DHT, it can maintain sexual function (de Lignieres 1993; Kunelius *et al.* 2002), but 5α-reduction of testosterone to DHT is not an absolute requirement, as indicated by only limited occurrence of sexual dysfunction during treatment with the 5α-reductase inhibitor finasteride (Thompson *et al.* 2003).

16.4.3 Testosterone and cardiovascular risk profile

There is a gender gap for cardiovascular disease (CVD) and cardiovascular mortality, with men being at higher risk. Extensive reviews have failed to provide compelling evidence that this gender difference can be explained on the basis of distinctive patterns of endogenous sex hormone exposure in adulthood (Liu *et al.* 2003; Wu and von Eckardstein 2003).

Suppression of plasma testosterone levels in men with a GnRH analog increases HDL-C, an effect prevented by co-administration of testosterone (Goldberg *et al.* 1985; Moorjani *et al.* 1987; Bagatell *et al.* 1992), which seems in accordance with the generally held view that testosterone is responsible for a more atherogenic plasma lipid profile in postpubertal males as compared to women in their reproductive years. Experimental graded testosterone exposure in elderly men, resulting in hypogonadal to supraphysiological levels, dose-dependently decreased HDL-C (Bhasin *et al.* 2005). However, within a window situated around physiological serum testosterone levels in men, most authors have consistently observed a positive association between endogenous serum testosterone and HDL-C concentrations in healthy men (see Bagatell and Bremner 1995; Wu and von Eckardstein 2003 for review), which is the case not only for total but also for free testosterone (Haffner *et al.* 1993; Van Pottelbergh *et al.* 2003b). Furthermore, serum

testosterone has been shown to be inversely associated with serum triglycerides, total cholesterol, LDL cholesterol (LDL-C), fibrinogen and plasminogen activator type 1. In a multivariate analysis in an occupation-based cohort of 715 middle-aged men, free testosterone was most significantly positively associated with HDL-C and apolipoprotein B; while free estradiol was a stronger positive predictor of apolipoprotein E (Van Pottelbergh *et al.* 2003b). Obviously, body composition and insulin sensitivity are important confounders in the context of associations of serum sex steroid concentrations with cardiovascular risk factors (Wu and von Eckardstein 2003), and although in a number of studies associations between serum testosterone and HDL-C tend to persist after adjustments for these confounders, the statistical corrections may account only in part for their impact.

The metabolic syndrome and type 2 diabetes mellitus represent significant risk factors for CVD. A number of cross-sectional studies have described negative associations of serum (free) testosterone with prevalence of (components of) metabolic syndrome and type 2 diabetes (Grossmann 2011 for review). Moreover, prospective studies have shown that low serum testosterone predicts the development of metabolic syndrome and diabetes (Rodriguez *et al.* 2007; Kupelian *et al.* 2008; Grossmann 2011 for review), also in non-obese men (Kupelian *et al.* 2006).

A previous extensive literature review (Wu and von Eckardstein 2003), which included a large number of cross-sectional studies as well as a small number of then-available nested, case-control studies and prospective cohort studies, failed to establish a relationship between serum testosterone levels and CVD; similarly, observational studies also failed to establish a relationship between serum DHEA or its sulfate (DHEAS) with CVD. A recent meta-analysis of 19 prospective, population-based cohort and nested case-control studies showed a weak negative association of serum total testosterone with CVD: estimated summary relative risk (RR) was 0.89 for a change of 1 standard deviation in total testosterone level (95% CI 0.83 to 0.96). Age of study population and year of publication modified the relationship between serum testosterone and CVD. The estimated summary RR was 1.01 (0.95 to 1.08) for studies including middle-aged men, and 0.84 (0.76 to 0.92) for studies including men over 70 years of age; the latter studies showed a particularly pronounced association if published after 1 January 2007. From this meta-analysis it was concluded that, in elderly men, endogenous testosterone may weakly protect against CVD or that, alternatively, low testosterone may indicate poor general health (Ruige *et al.* 2011). In another recent meta-analysis of community-based studies, partially overlapping with the first one, the lower tertile of serum testosterone compared to the upper tertile was associated with 35% and 25% increased risk of all-cause mortality ($n = 11$ studies) and CVD mortality (7 studies), respectively. Age, baseline serum testosterone, length of follow-up and whether blood was sampled in the morning were factors contributing to substantial heterogeneity between studies (Araujo *et al.* 2011).

In conclusion, "high" testosterone levels within the physiological range do not cause an atherogenic lipid profile. On the contrary, moderately low serum testosterone levels are accompanied by lower HDL-C and higher LDL-C levels. Nevertheless, whereas higher endogenous testosterone may confer a limited protective effect against CVD in the elderly, low serum testosterone might rather represent a negative indicator of general health status.

The effects of exogenous testosterone on cardiovascular risk factors are mixed with possibly deleterious changes such as reductions in HDL-C and apolipoprotein A1, besides potentially favorable changes such as a decrease in serum fibrinogen, a reduction in abdominal fat mass, and augmented insulin sensitivity (Emmelot-Vonk 2008). According to a meta-analysis, testosterone treatment moderately reduces fat mass and total cholesterol, in particular in men with initially low serum testosterone (<10 nmol/l), has no effect on LDL-C, and reduces HDL-C, mainly in men with initially higher (>10 nmol/l) serum testosterone (Isidori *et al.* 2005a).

There has been considerable interest in possible beneficial direct vascular effects of androgens on coronary arteries in men with CAD, but this non-genomic action of testosterone may require rather high blood concentrations. Although the long-term effects of testosterone treatment on risk for CAD in elderly men are not established and the available evidence would certainly not allow for any claim of established favorable long-term effects, there appears to be no basis to suggest that androgen therapy aiming at near physiological serum levels should be withheld out of fear of adverse effects on cardiovascular risk (see Liu *et al.* 2003; Wu and von Eckardstein 2003; Kaufman and Vermeulen 2005). A recent report of increased incidence of cardiovascular-related adverse events during transdermal testosterone treatment in a rather small group of elderly men with limited mobility and high prevalence of chronic disease has raised concerns concerning the cardiovascular safety of serum testosterone in subjects at higher risk (Basaria *et al.* 2010).

16.4.4 Body composition and sarcopenia

Aging in men is associated with a decrease of lean body mass and an increase of fat mass, especially in the upper body and central body regions (Forbes and Reina 1970; Tenover 1994; Vermeulen *et al.* 1999a). Fat mass increases from around a mean of 20% of body weight in young men to 30% or more in the elderly; whereas muscle mass may decrease by as much as 35 to 40% from age 20 to 80 years (Bross *et al.* 1999). In a study in community-dwelling healthy men (Vermeulen *et al.* 1999a), we found a mean fat mass of 22.3% of body weight in 61 middle-aged men with mean age of 42 years, as compared to 29.4% in 271 men with mean age of 76 years, BMI being similar in both groups and lean body mass 30% lower in the elderly.

Fat mass, and in particular abdominal fat mass, is negatively associated with serum (free) testosterone levels (Vermeulen *et al.* 1999a; van den Beld *et al.* 2000). However, the direction of this association remains unclear, as low testosterone may be a positive determinant of adiposity; whereas, conversely, adiposity appears to be a negative determinant of serum testosterone. Moreover, altered activity of the somatotropic axis may also play an important role in age-related changes in body composition. In any case, a negative association of free testosterone with fat mass in elderly men persists after correction for serum IGF-1 levels, which are positively correlated to serum (free) testosterone and negatively to fat mass (Vermeulen *et al.* 1999a).

In a majority of controlled trials of several months duration with administration of androgens to elderly men with low or (low) normal serum (bioavailable) testosterone, treatment resulted in a modest decrease of total and/or abdominal fat mass (Gruenewald and Matsumoto 2003). In a meta-analysis, testosterone treatment was found to reduce fat mass by 1.6 kg (95% CI: 2.5 to 0.6), corresponding to 6.2% (9.2 to 3.3). Nevertheless, in this context GH may have a larger effect than testosterone (Münzer *et al.* 2001).

The age-associated loss of muscle mass is accompanied by decreased muscle strength, which occurs regardless of the level of physical activity (Rogers and Evans 1993). Muscle weakness is an important component of frailty in old age, contributing to functional limitation in activities of daily living and related problems such as an increased risk for falls (Rubenstein et al. 1994; Guralnik et al. 1995; Bhasin and Tenover 1997; Rolland et al. 2011). Information on the association of endogenous androgens and muscle mass is scarce. Van den Beld et al. (2000) and Vermeulen et al. (1999a) found no association of serum (free or non SHBG-bound) testosterone with lean body mass in sizable populations of ambulant elderly men. Similarly, Roy et al. (2002) found no association of lean mass with testosterone, independent of age, in men aged 20 to 90 years from the Baltimore Longitudinal Study of Aging. Several studies suggest a positive association of serum (free or bioavailable) testosterone levels with muscle function and strength (Abbasi et al. 1993; Häkkinen and Pakarinen 1994; van den Beld et al. 2000; Roy et al. 2002). Recent, large, cross-sectional and longitudinal observational studies have shown associations of low serum (free or bioavailable) testosterone with prevalent as well as worsening frailty in elderly men (Orwoll et al. 2006b; Cawthon et al. 2009; Hyde et al. 2010; Krasnoff et al. 2010; Travison et al. 2011), although this was not confirmed in all studies (Mohr et al. 2007; Schaap et al. 2008).

Experimental exposure of elderly men to testosterone levels varying from hypogonadal to supraphysiological serum levels resulted in dose-dependent increases of muscle mass and strength (Bhasin et al. 2005; Sattler et al. 2009). The response to testosterone in the elderly appears similar to that in young men (Bhasin et al. 2005). Several controlled studies of more than three months duration with androgen administration in elderly men with low or (low) normal serum testosterone (see Gruenewald and Matsumoto 2003; Isidori et al. 2005b for review) have shown increases of lean body mass (Snyder et al. 1999a; Kenny et al. 2001; Münzer et al. 2001; Ferrando et al. 2002; Steidle et al. 2003; Basaria et al. 2010). Findings on muscle force and various measures of functionality have been heterogeneous (Isidori et al. 2005b; Rolland et al. 2011 for review). Sih et al. (1997) observed a significant increase in grip strength in testosterone-treated men over the age of 50 years (mean age 68 years) with low bioavailable serum testosterone, in a prospective, randomized, placebo-controlled trial of 12 months duration; lower extremity muscle strength was not evaluated. Ferrando et al.

(2002) observed improved leg and arm muscle strength and an increase in muscle net protein balance in a small number of older men treated with testosterone for six months. Muscle strength measured by isokinetic peak torque was increased in flexion of the dominant knee, but not in knee extension or shoulder contraction during three months of transdermal administration of DHT in older men with low-normal serum testosterone (Ly et al. 2001). In this last study there was no effect of treatment on tests of gait, balance or mobility; no effect of treatment on muscle strength was observed in the studies by Kenny et al. (2001) and Snyder et al. (1999a). Crawford et al. (2003) reported increased muscle mass and strength during androgen treatment in men with mean age around 60 years under treatment with glucocorticoids. In intermediate-frail and frail elderly men, six months of testosterone treatment had beneficial effects on body composition, muscle strength, physical function and quality of life (Srinivas-Shankar 2010); beneficial effects were not maintained six months after end of treatment (O'Connell et al. 2011). In elderly men with limited mobility and high prevalence of chronic disease, transdermal testosterone treatment planned for six months improved muscle strength and stair climbing, but the trial was prematurely discontinued because of a high rate of adverse events (Basaria et al. 2010). In a study in older men with low-normal serum testosterone, Emmelot-Vonk et al. (2008) observed an increase of lean body mass, but no beneficial effect on functional status and mixed metabolic effects of six months testosterone therapy.

The data discussed in this section indicate that an age-associated partial hypoandrogenism might play a contributory role in the sarcopenia of older men, which is multifactorially determined, and that the elderly can respond to pharmacological treatment with testosterone, in particular if serum testosterone is initially low. However, whether androgen treatment plays a role in the management of sarcopenia and frailty in elderly men is not clear, as several issues need to be clarified, such as optimal treatment modalities, safety in frail elderly, and longer-term persistence of effects.

16.4.5 Senile osteoporosis

Aging of men is accompanied by continuous bone loss, which persists and may even accelerate in old age, and by exponential increase of vertebral and hip fracture incidence. Although age-specific fracture incidence in men is only about half that in women, one out of three to four fractures in the elderly occurs in men, and the consequences of fractures in men are more severe in terms of morbidity and mortality (see Orwoll and Klein 1995; Kaufman and Goemaere 2008; Khosla 2010 for review).

Profound hypogonadism in older men induces high bone turnover, accelerated bone loss and increased fracture risk, similar to the effects seen in younger men (Stoch et al. 2001; Mittan et al. 2002; Shahinian et al. 2005; Fink et al. 2006), and there are indications that TRT in men with acquired hypogonadism may result in partial recovery of bone density (Katznelson et al. 1996; Behre et al. 1997). Hypogonadism has also been reported to be a risk factor for hip fracture in elderly men (Stanley et al. 1991; Jackson et al. 1992; Boonen et al. 1997), but, besides low bone mass, other factors related to testosterone, such as muscle weakness, may be involved in the occurrence of hip fractures. In community-dwelling men over the age of 60 years from the Dubbo Osteoporosis Epidemiology Study, serum testosterone adjusted for serum SHBG and estradiol was associated with risk for osteoporotic factures (Meier et al. 2008).

There is strong evidence that aromatization of testosterone to estradiol is of major importance for preservation of the skeleton in elderly men. A preponderant role of estrogen in the regulation of bone metabolism in elderly men has been elegantly demonstrated in a short-term intervention study with selective manipulation of testosterone and estradiol levels (Falahati-Nini et al. 2000). This is further confirmed by bone loss observed in elderly men during treatment with an aromatase inhibitor that increased testosterone and decreased estradiol levels (Burnett-Bowie et al. 2009). In cross-sectional studies in elderly men, associations of bone mineral status or biochemical markers of bone turnover with sex steroid levels have been rather weak, although statistically significant. In several of the latter studies (free or bioavailable) estradiol was more strongly associated with BMD and/or bone turnover markers than (free or bioavailable) testosterone. Serum (free or bioavailable) estradiol, but not serum testosterone, is inversely associated with prospectively assessed bone loss in elderly men (Khosla et al. 2001; Van Pottelbergh et al. 2003a; Cauley et al. 2010). Moreover, changes in BMD, the personal clinical fracture history of the subjects and the fracture history in their first-degree relatives, were found to be associated with a polymorphism of the CYP19 gene that encodes for the aromatase enzyme, independently of serum estradiol levels, suggesting indirectly that local aromatization of testosterone in bone tissue might play a role (Van Pottelbergh et al. 2003a). Low estradiol levels have been associated with prevalent vertebral fractures in elderly men of the Rancho Bernardo Study (Barrett-Connor et al. 2000). In the MrOS Sweden cohort, low serum estradiol and high serum SHBG were associated with increased fracture risk (Mellström et al. 2008). There are indications for a serum (bioavailable) estradiol threshold effect for both bone loss and fracture risk (Mellström et al. 2008; Khosla 2010).

In community-dwelling men over age 70 years, we found no association of BMD or bone metabolism with a CAG-repeat polymorphism of the androgen receptor gene (Van Pottelbergh et al. 2001), while such an association has been reported for younger men (Zitzmann et al. 2001; Guadalupe-Grau et al. 2010).

Currently available, controlled data on the effects of testosterone treatment in elderly men are limited. Observed effects of androgen treatment in elderly men on biochemical indices of bone turnover have been rather heterogeneous (Orwoll and Oviatt 1992; Sih et al. 1997; Snyder et al. 1999b; Kenny et al. 2001), although in a meta-analysis treatment does appear to reduce levels of bone resorption markers (Isidori et al. 2005b).

In a randomized, double-blind trial of transdermal administration of testosterone by scrotal patch (6 mg/day) or placebo to men with normal or low serum testosterone (n = 108), Snyder et al. (1999b) found that, after three years of treatment, lumbar spine bone mineral density was increased in the placebo group as well as in the active treatment group, both receiving calcium and vitamin D supplements, without significant testosterone treatment effect; there was no change in BMD at the hip region in either treatment group. It is interesting to note that these negative findings for testosterone effects on bone were accompanied by significant treatment effects on fat mass and lean body mass. Kenny et al. (2001) reported prevention of bone loss at the hip during one year of treatment with transdermal testosterone (5 mg/day by body patch) as compared to placebo in healthy elderly men aged 65 to 87 years, but differences between placebo and active treatment were rather small. In a study of elderly men with initially moderately low serum testosterone, Amory *et al.* (2004) observed a significant increase of BMD at the spine and hip compared to placebo during 36 months of treatment with testosterone enanthate im 200 mg/wk, with or without associated treatment with the 5α-reductase inhibitor finasteride. In frail older men with low bioavailable serum testosterone, a history of fracture and/or low BMD, Kenny *et al.* (2010) observed an increase of spine BMD during transdermal testosterone treatment (5 mg/day), but interpretation is limited by a high drop-out rate. Crawford *et al.* (2003) found a beneficial effect of 12 months administration of testosterone, but not of the only minimally aromatizable androgen nandrolone, on BMD in men treated with glucocorticoids who had initially low or low-normal serum testosterone levels. In a meta-analysis and systematic review, testosterone treatment was found to favorably affect BMD at the spine, but not at the hip (Isidori *et al.* 2005b; Tracz *et al.* 2006).

Compared to findings of testosterone administration in younger hypogonadal men on bone effects, these are rather disappointing and may be explained by the fact that many men in these studies had either normal or near normal initial androgen levels; a further explanation might be the possible existence of a threshold effect with testosterone and derived estrogen requirements for near maximal bone effects lying at the lower end of the physiological range for sex steroid levels, which would be in line with the estradiol threshold for bone loss and fracture risk reported in several observational studies. A post-hoc analysis of the study by Snyder *et al.* (1999b), indicating that only those men with initially low serum total testosterone (< 300–350 ng/dl) increased their BMD during treatment supports this view, as do the positive results from the study by Amory *et al.* (2004) which included men with generally lower serum testosterone (i.e. baseline testosterone 283 ± 49 ng/dl).

In summary, the evidence suggests that declining sex steroid levels may adversely impact on the preservation of skeletal integrity in elderly men, and indicates that aromatization of testosterone to estradiol is a major component of the regulation of bone homeostasis in the elderly. The skeletal effects of testosterone deficiency are modulated by aromatase activity, which in turn is affected by factors such as adiposity and heredity. Testosterone treatment has mostly only modest beneficial effects on BMD in the elderly; mainly limited to men with initially low serum

testosterone and to effects on the lumbar spine. In view of the modest bone effects, of the lack of relevant studies with testosterone specifically in osteoporotic men, and of the availability of better validated specific osteoporosis medication such as bisphosphonates, osteoporosis as such is not an indication for testosterone therapy.

16.4.6 Additional clinical variables

Men have higher hemoglobin levels and red cell mass than women, and testosterone has a dose-dependent stimulatory effect on erythropoiesis that is more pronounced in elderly compared to young men (Coviello *et al.* 2008). Elderly men tend to have similar or only slightly lower hematocrit than young men. There is no documentation of association between endogenous androgen levels and parameters of erythropoiesis in elderly men.

Aging is associated with a deterioration of multiple aspects of cognitive performance. Hypogonadal men tend to show diminished spatial skills and, albeit findings have not been consistent, several observational studies in elderly men have reported positive associations of cognitive functions such as verbal memory and spatial skills with endogenous androgen levels (Kaufman and Vermeulen 2005 for review). In a long-term follow-up study, low serum testosterone was associated with increased risk of Alzheimer's disease (Moffat *et al.* 2004). In several, but not all intervention studies, androgen administration to elderly men resulted in improved spatial cognition and working memory, with decreased verbal fluency (see Muller *et al.* 2003; Gruenewald and Matsumoto 2003 for review). In a study in men 66 to 86 years of age with normal cognitive function, treatment with testosterone enanthate 200 mg every other week, a supraphysiological dose, resulted in a deterioration of cognitive functions (Maki *et al.* 2007).

Endogenous free and bioavailable testosterone levels were reported to be inversely associated with depressive mood and depressive symptoms in aging men (Barrett-Connor *et al.* 1999; Delhez *et al.* 2003), but other studies failed to confirm such associations (T'Sjoen *et al.* 2005b; Kaufman and Vermeulen 2005 for review), or reported the opposite association of less depressive symptoms in elderly men with lower serum testosterone (Perry *et al.* 2001). Similarly, the findings on association of low serum testosterone in the elderly with prevalence and incidence of depression have been inconsistent (Delhez *et al.* 2003; Joshi *et al.* 2010).

Aging evidently is often associated with a decrease of quality of life. The few available studies failed to establish a relation between endogenous androgen levels and quality of life (QoL), such as evaluated with the SF-36 questionnaire (Dunbar *et al.* 2001; T'Sjoen *et al.* 2004). Whereas testosterone therapy has been reported to improve some aspects of QoL in some studies (Snyder *et al.* 1999a; Crawford *et al.* 2003; Srinivas-Shankar *et al.* 2010), other studies failed to objectivate a beneficial effect of testosterone treatment on overall QoL or mood in elderly men (Ly *et al.* 2001; Kunelius *et al.* 2002; Gruenewald and Matsumoto 2003; Steidle *et al.* 2003; Kaufman and Vermeulen 2005 for review).

16.4.7   Conclusions

The extent of the clinical consequences of relative hypoandrogenism in elderly men remains difficult to pinpoint. Nevertheless, in many instances there is a significant, albeit usually weak, association between some aging-related clinical changes and serum levels of testosterone and/or its aromatized metabolite estradiol, which generally persists after adjustment for major confounders such as age and adiposity. In any case, it is also evident that the androgen status is at best only one of many factors that influence the pace and clinical expression of the aging process in men. Although associations between plasma androgen levels and the prevailing clinical status have been generally weak or even absent, this does not necessarily imply that the decline in testosterone levels in elderly men is not clinically relevant. Indeed, one may question whether a single time-point androgen measurement for estimation of the androgen status is sufficiently representative of this status in preceding years, during which clinical changes have accumulated to produce the present clinical picture in the investigated subject. Moreover, serum levels are at best imperfect parameters of testosterone action in the tissues. In this regard more recent prospective studies tend to reveal more robust associations between sex steroid levels and clinical parameters, including clinically relevant end-points such as frailty, fractures or mortality. A crucial question remains whether low androgen status and clinical outcome are causally and specifically related, or whether both

are rather more or less independent reflections of generally poorer health status.

16.5   Androgen therapy in elderly men

16.5.1   Who should be considered for treatment?

The age-associated decrease in serum testosterone levels raises the issue of the potential role of androgen substitution in elderly males. This implies a number of questions which, with the currently available evidence, can at best receive pragmatic interim answers: who should be treated, how and for how long?

As to the first question, in theory androgen administration to elderly men could be either "substitutive" to alleviate symptoms and prevent complications of partial or more complete androgen deficiency, or rather "pharmacological," to elderly men who are not necessarily androgen deficient, with specific treatment goals such as the prevention or treatment of osteoporosis, of frailty, or adjuvant treatment of ED. A few usually small-scaled studies pertaining to particular clinical situations with indications of potential treatment benefits and risks (Gruenewald and Matsumoto 2003; Kaufman and Vermeulen 2005; Fernandez-Balsells *et al.* 2010 for review) notwithstanding, for no single indication in elderly men is the present level of evidence sufficient to justify "pharmacological" androgen treatment in elderly men, thus leaving us with only the "substitutive" treatment to be considered at this time.

It is generally not a matter for debate that prolonged androgen deficiency in young men results in symptoms affecting QoL and carries a risk for longer-term complications, so that intervention to reestablish physiological androgen levels is required unless there is a specific contraindication for such an intervention. As to the elderly, there is no *a priori* medical or moral justification for withholding the benefits of "substitutive" treatment from symptomatic hypogonadal elderly men. Nevertheless a prudent, sufficiently conservative approach to such treatment seems advisable in view of limited data and clinical experience for this population, the low specificity of the symptoms of hypogonadism in the elderly, and the potential for greater susceptibility for adverse treatment effects.

This brings up the key issue of how to diagnose androgen deficiency in elderly men and thus the question of what the testosterone requirements are in elderly men (Vermeulen 2001). The question to be asked is whether elderly men are equally, less or more sensitive to testosterone action compared to the young. The answer to this question is limited on the one hand by lack of specificity of signs and symptoms of androgen deficiency, while on the other hand no useful direct biochemical measure of tissue activity of testosterone and its bioactive metabolites is available. Moreover, adding to the complexity, testosterone requirements for normal functioning may differ according to the tissue and physiological functions under consideration (Zitzmann *et al.* 2006), whereas the large between-subject variability of serum testosterone levels seen at all ages may be the expression of individual differences in androgen sensitivity (Crabbe *et al.* 2007; Huhtaniemi *et al.* 2009).

In view of the still unresolved issue of what should be considered "physiologic" or "optimal" androgen levels in elderly men, in many cases a margin of uncertainty will persist. Therefore diagnosis of hypogonadism in elderly men should be based on an appropriately conservative evaluation of clinical and hormonal findings (Kaufman and Vermeulen 2005; Wang *et al.* 2008; Bhasin *et al.* 2011).

As to the testosterone threshold levels compatible with a diagnosis of hypogonadism, in the absence of definitive evidence of altered sensitivity to androgens in the elderly, the least arbitrary attitude is probably to use the same lower normal limit as in young men, i.e. around 11 nmol/l (or 320 ng/dl) for total serum testosterone, around 0.225 nmol/l (or 6.5 ng/dl for serum free testosterone, and around 5 nmol/l (or 145 ng/dl) for bioavailable (i.e. non-specifically bound) testosterone. Although values for the lower end of the reference range for total testosterone in young men reported by various, experienced groups are usually not very different, there is some variation, with proposed lower normal values usually ranging between 280 and 350 ng/dl (9.7 and 12 nmol/l), and with differences explained by issues of methodology and standardization of testosterone assays and selection of the reference population (Rosner *et al.* 2007; Wang *et al.* 2008; Wheeler and Barnes 2008; Bhasin *et al.* 2011). Using liquid chromatography–tandem mass spectrometry (LC-MS/MS) to measure serum testosterone in a selected group of healthy non-obese young men, Bhasin *et al.* (2011) reported lower normal levels of 348 ng/dl and 7.0 ng/dl for total and free testosterone, defined as the 2.5th percentile.

We found that no more than 1% of healthy men aged 20–40 years old, but over 20% of men older than 65 years, present with a total serum testosterone below 11 nmol/l (Fig. 16.2): a prevalence of low testosterone in the same order of magnitude as reported by others for men over 65 years of age (Orwoll *et al.* 2006a; Araujo *et al.* 2007). Parameters of the biologically active fraction of serum testosterone, i.e. serum free testosterone and bioavailable testosterone, are in principle more appropriate for the evaluation of the androgen status. Their use will result in classification of an even larger proportion of elderly men as being hypoandrogenic, as the age-dependent decrease is steeper than for total testosterone. On the other hand, in a number of situations with low serum SHBG, such as in obesity and during treatment with glucocorticoids, these measurements may reveal a better preserved androgen status than indicated by serum total testosterone. In any case, taking into account the present lack of information on the long-term benefit–risk ratio for androgen treatment in elderly men, and the uncertainty about androgen requirements in the elderly, it seems advisable to apply the above cutoff values conservatively. In such a conservative approach to treatment of the elderly, intervention thresholds may differ from diagnostic criteria, considering for treatment only those men with frankly low testosterone, i.e. a (free) testosterone level clearly low relative to the proposed diagnostic thresholds for hypogonadism.

Available evidence does not support the alternative view that treatment might be justified in men with higher prevalent serum testosterone, i.e. within the lower normal range for young men, on the basis that elderly men would be less sensitive to androgen action. Indeed, whereas reports of decreased tissue concentration of androgen receptors in the elderly (Roehrborn *et al.* 1987) might suggest decreased sensitivity, data from functional studies indicate that in older men there is rather an increased sensitivity of LH secretion to the negative feedback action of testosterone (Winters *et al.* 1984; 1997; Deslypere *et al.* 1987). In elegant studies with suppression of endogenous testosterone secretion and subsequent exposure to graded doses of exogenous testosterone, Bhasin *et al.* (2005) showed that the elderly are as responsive as the young to the anabolic effects of testosterone, such as on fat mass, muscle mass and force, with indications of higher sensitivity to stimulation of erythropoiesis and decrease of HDL-C. Furthermore, the lower level of the serum testosterone range in young men appeared to be a valid threshold for occurrence of symptoms of hypogonadism also in the elderly (Wu *et al.* 2010; Bhasin *et al.* 2011). Moreover, as discussed above, whereas most studies on testosterone administration to elderly men have included a large proportion of men with serum testosterone within the lower normal range for young men, probably based on the rationale that these low-normal levels might in fact be suboptimal for many of these subjects, treatment effects were generally disappointing for those men without clearly low initial serum testosterone levels.

As to serum gonadotropin levels, although a markedly elevated serum LH certainly adds weight to the finding of a decreased serum testosterone, pointing towards a predominantly testicular factor in this particular patient (Tajar *et al.* 2010), elevated serum LH is not a prerequisite for the diagnosis of testosterone deficiency in older men, the age-associated decline of Leydig cell function being usually of mixed testicular and neuroendocrine origin, in particular whenever overweight and/or other co-morbidities contribute to the low testosterone of the subject.

As to objective signs of relative androgen deficiency, a decrease of muscle mass and strength and a concomitant increase in central body fat and osteoporosis can most easily be objectified, but are not specific signs. Decreased libido and sexual desire, loss of memory, difficulty in concentration, forgetfulness, insomnia, irritability and depressed mood, as well as decreased sense of well-being, are rather subjective feelings or impressions, less easily objectified and not easy to differentiate from hormone-independent aging. Of the latter indications, sexual symptoms have been reported to be most consistently related to low serum testosterone (Wu *et al.* 2010). Complaints of excessive sweating are not uncommon, whereas true hot flushes do occur in elderly men, although they are mainly prevalent in severe acquired hypogonadism such as under hormonal treatment for prostate cancer.

A number of questionnaires have been developed for use in clinical or epidemiological settings to help describe and semi-quantify symptoms in different areas of relevance to elderly men, such as questionnaires on self-perceived health status, on depressive mood, on urinary symptoms, on erectile function, or on coping with activities of daily living. There are also questionnaires that have been proposed as dedicated instruments to quantify symptoms of LOH and to screen for androgen deficiency in elderly men (Heinemann *et al.* 1999; Morley *et al.* 2000; Smith *et al.* 2000). These instruments lack specificity (Morley *et al.* 2000; Dunbar *et al.* 2001; Delhez *et al.* 2003; T'Sjoen *et al.* 2004), and their use for screening or diagnostic purposes should be discouraged (Wang *et al.* 2008; Bhasin *et al.* 2011). Indeed, considering the high prevalence in older men of non-specific symptoms loosely associated with hypoandrogenism, spontaneous active reporting of complaints may have the merit of higher specificity, whereas soliciting of complaints with screening questionnaires may lead to over-diagnosis and overtreatment.

In conclusion, according to the present state of the art, androgen supplementation should probably only be considered in the presence of androgen serum levels clearly below the lower normal limit for young men, together with unequivocal signs and symptoms of androgen deficiency, after having excluded reversible causes of low serum androgen and after careful screening for contraindications. The decision to treat will finally depend upon the balance between possible benefits and risks, integrating the most recent evidence available for androgen treatment as well as the evidence available for possible pharmacological and non-pharmacological alternatives. Indeed, the lack of reliable data on the long-term risk–benefit ratio imposes a critical and conservative attitude in accordance with a basic principle of clinical practice; i.e. *primum non nocere*.

From a practical point of view, serum testosterone should be assessed in the morning before 10 a.m., and low values obtained when sampling has been performed later during the day need to be verified by a morning sample. Low values should be confirmed by a second sample, ideally obtained with an interval of at least a couple of weeks. The reference range for serum testosterone should be validated for the type of assay used and preferably also for each laboratory; whereas for estimates of free or bioavailable testosterone one should use valid methods. As to the latter, it has been shown that free testosterone can be reliably calculated from serum total testosterone and SHBG using an equation derived from the mass action law, except when there are gross abnormalities in plasma proteins or when the subjects are treated with substances with high affinity for SHBG (e.g. DHT), the calculation being easily done with a simple algorithm on a personal or pocket computer. Neither the commercially available direct immunoassays for free testosterone, nor the simple ratio of total serum testosterone over serum SHBG should be regarded as reliable options in men (Vermeulen *et al.* 1999b).

16.5.2   Potential benefits

From the preceding sections of this chapter and from literature reviews (Gruenewald and Matsumoto 2003; Kaufman and Vermeulen 2005; Isidori *et al.* 2005a; 2005b; Ottenbacher *et al.* 2006; Bhasin *et al.* 2010), it emerges that testosterone administration to elderly men can induce potentially beneficial effects, but the results are often mitigated and without demonstrated impact on end-points that are directly relevant for the clinic. Several studies have shown improvement of lean body mass and sometimes also of muscle strength, but whether these changes are sufficient to make a meaningful difference in terms of functionality is still unclear. Positive effects on BMD are seen only in men with frankly low serum testosterone, and we have no information on the effect of treatment on fracture rates. Abdominal fat may decrease and insulin sensitivity may improve, whereas high-dose testosterone may have direct beneficial effects on heart and arteries, but we have no indication of gains in terms of hard cardiovascular end-points. There have been reports of favorable effects on mood, cognition and general well-being, but the findings are not always consistent and we have no data indicating that treatment may prevent or help treat depression, or have substantial longer-term effects on cognition and QoL. Androgen therapy has beneficial effects on sexual functioning in men with initially low serum testosterone levels, although the treatment effects may be small and usually significant for only some indices of sexual function.

A major limitation is the scarcity of controlled data. No more than a few hundred elderly men in total have been included in controlled trials, and among these only a minority in trials of at least one year's duration; less than half these men received active treatment with testosterone. Moreover, a substantial proportion of men included had initially (low) normal serum testosterone.

16.5.3   Potential risks

As to the risks of androgen replacement therapy in elderly men, we consider here only effects of "physiological" doses of testosterone and not those of massive "pharmacological" doses, as used by bodybuilders. Traditionally, it has been a matter of concern that prolonged treatment with androgen may increase the risk of cardiovascular disease. The complex relationship between endogenous and exogenous androgens and cardiovascular risk is discussed in Section 16.4.3. In-depth review of the literature (Liu *et al.* 2003; Wu and von Eckardstein 2003) suggests that exogenous androgen administration has both potentially favorable as well as possible adverse effects on cardiovascular risk. With the evidence currently available, improving cardiovascular risk can certainly not be considered an indication for androgen treatment, but there is also no suggestion that treatment with moderate, close to physiological doses carries an unacceptable risk that should prevent initiating otherwise indicated androgen treatment. A recent meta-analysis (Fernandez-Balsells *et al.* 2010) found no difference in the rates of death, myocardial infarction, revascularization procedures or cardiac arrhythmias between testosterone therapy and placebo/non-intervention in adult men. Testosterone treatment is associated with a decrease of HDL-C; the other lipid fractions, blood pressure and incidence of diabetes are not affected.

Androgen treatment results in a significant increase of hematocrit and blood hemoglobin level, and androgen treatment is associated with increased incidence of erythrocytosis (Calof *et al.* 2005; Fernandez-Balsells *et al.* 2010). Moreover, the stimulatory effects of testosterone administration on erythropoiesis have been shown to be increased in the elderly as compared to young men (Coviello *et al.* 2008). Polycythemia is not uncommon and may necessitate dose reduction, temporary interruption of treatment, or alternative measures such as phlebotomy. The occurrence of polycythemia appears to be more likely when the subjects are exposed to markedly supraphysiological androgen levels, as is often the case with treatment regimens consisting of im administration of depot preparations of testosterone esters at intervals of two to three weeks (Dobs *et al.* 1999). Nevertheless, significant increases of hematocrit and hemoglobin levels are also seen during transdermal administration of either testosterone (Snyder *et al.* 1999a; Steidle *et al.* 2003) or DHT (Ly *et al.* 2001; Kunelius *et al.* 2002), occasionally leading to erythrocytosis. Monitoring for occurrence of exaggerated elevations of hematocrit or hemoglobin concentrations during androgen treatment in elderly men is advisable, keeping in mind that some patients, in particular some with pulmonary disease, can have a high *a priori* risk of erythrocytosis.

The assertion that testosterone therapy may exacerbate obstructive sleep apnea (Sandblom *et al.* 1983) is essentially based on a few case reports. Whereas largely supraphysiological testosterone doses may indeed increase the risk of sleep apnea, this does not seem to be the case during treatment with more physiological dosages (Calof *et al.* 2005; Liu *et al.* 2007b). Nevertheless, clinical practice guidelines suggest that testosterone therapy should not be initiated in men with severe untreated sleep apnea (Bhasin *et al.* 2010).

Gynecomastia, related to the conversion of testosterone to estradiol in peripheral tissues, mainly fat tissue, which is relatively increased in elderly men, is a not uncommon but benign side-effect in elderly men, especially in the obese. This side-effect is probably less frequent when patients are not exposed to supraphysiological serum levels of testosterone. Although testosterone causes some sodium and water retention, this effect does usually not cause a problem, although this might be relevant in patients with congestive heart failure, hypertension or renal insufficiency. Hepatotoxicity is very rare when non-oral routes of administration of testosterone are used.

Of greater concern are the possible effects on the prostate, which is an androgen-dependent organ (Bhasin *et al.* 2003). In a meta-analysis by Calof *et al.* (2005), the combined rate of all prostate events was significantly greater in testosterone-treated compared to placebo-treated men (odds ratio 1.78; 95% CI: 1.07–2.95). Rates of prostate cancers, PSA greater than 4 ng/dl and prostate biopsies were numerically, but not significantly greater in testosterone-treated men. In a recent meta-analysis, Fernandez-Balsells *et al.* (2010) found no significant effect of testosterone therapy on outcomes such as prostate cancer incidence or need for prostate biopsy when compared to placebo/non-intervention.

Concerning benign prostatic hyperplasia (BPH), studies to date failed to observe important growth of the prostate (Wallace *et al.* 1993; Behre *et al.* 1994) and failed to find any relationship between plasma and BPH tissue levels of testosterone, DHT or estradiol. It appears that tissue levels are determined by enzyme activity in the tissue itself, rather than by surrounding plasma androgen levels. Treatment does not seem to result in increased voiding symptoms or postvoid residual volume (Gruenewald and

Matsumoto 2003), and only in cases of severe lower urinary tract obstructive symptoms is benign prostate disease considered a contraindication for androgen treatment (Bhasin *et al.* 2003; 2010; Wang *et al.* 2008). Prostate-specific antigen (PSA) levels, a parameter of androgen stimulation of prostate tissue, increase moderately during treatment but usually within the normal range, and after stopping treatment the values return to pretreatment levels (Behre *et al.* 1994, Hajjar *et al.* 1997). Small significant increases in PSA have also been observed under transdermal administration of testosterone to elderly men; only rarely is a more important rise in PSA seen (Snyder *et al.* 1999a; Kenny *et al.* 2001). Levels of PSA and prostate size were reported to remain unchanged (Ly *et al.* 2001; Kunelius *et al.* 2002) or even decreased (de Lignieres 1993) under transdermal DHT administration to older men, even though on close examination small PSA increases in comparison with placebo might occur (Ly *et al.* 2001). One could hypothesize that DHT treatment could have a relative prostate-sparing effect through a reduction of estradiol and/or DHT levels in prostate tissue as a result of suppression of concentrations in the systemic circulation of their precursor, i.e. testosterone.

Undoubtedly clinical prostate carcinoma is an androgen-sensitive tumor. Hence presence of a clinical prostate carcinoma is an absolute contraindication to testosterone supplementation. Subclinical carcinoma, only detectable on histology but undetectable by biochemical or clinical procedures, is found in a majority of men over 70 years old. Only a small minority of these subclinical carcinomas will further develop to a clinical carcinoma. It is not known whether testosterone treatment would stimulate the progression of subclinical carcinoma, and so far no available data indicate that testosterone substitution will activate subclinical carcinoma (Jackson *et al.* 1989; Schröder 1996). However, all studies so far concern only small numbers of carefully selected elderly males treated for short periods of time. In any case, before starting testosterone supplementation careful exclusion of a prostate carcinoma by rectal examination and serum PSA and, when required, supplemented by ultrasonography and biopsy, is mandatory. It is advised to perform controls of rectal examination, PSA and a symptom questionnaire for benign prostatic hyperplasia after 3 to 6 and 12 months in stable patients; thereafter yearly controls (Bhasin *et al.* 2003; 2010; Wang *et al.* 2008). Referral for urological work-up prior to therapy is required in case of palpable nodule or indurations on rectal examination, PSA level above 4 ng/ml or above 3 ng/ml in subjects at higher risk for prostate cancer. During therapy, a palpable nodule or indurations, an increase of PSA greater than 1.4 ng/dl or a PSA velocity of more than 0.4 ng/ml·yr using six-month PSA as reference, or an International Prostate Symptom Score (IPSS) greater than 19 should also prompt further urological evaluation (Bhasin *et al.* 2010).

16.5.4 Modalities of androgen substitution

In young healthy men, testosterone levels vary between 11 and 35 nmol/l and show a circadian variation with amplitude of $\pm$ 35%, highest levels being reached in the early morning and nadir values in the evening around 6–8 p.m. Therefore, when supplementing testosterone, the aim should be to alleviate symptoms related to the relative androgen deficiency, if possible by achieving plasma testosterone levels in the physiological range. As discussed in Section 16.5.1, in the absence of convincing evidence that androgen requirements change with age, physiological levels in young men should be aimed for. There is presently no evidence that it is clinically important to mimic the nycthemeral variations as found in young adults. Nevertheless, constant levels in the upper normal range will result in 24-hour mean levels that are supraphysiological as compared to the situation in young men subject to nycthemeral variations of serum testosterone.

Taken that the hypothalamic-pituitary-testicular axis is sensitive to negative feedback, and even more so in elderly males, the dose administered should increase testosterone levels up to the physiological range and not merely suppress LH secretion with only replacement of the deficient testosterone production by an inadequate dose of exogenous testosterone. In practical terms, full replacement doses are usually required.

Obviously, considering the fact that metabolization of testosterone to DHT and estradiol constitutes an important component for the regulation and full expression of testosterone effects, treatment with testosterone is the most physiological approach and the preferable option with the currently available evidence, but the debate is certainly not closed in view of interesting data obtained with alternative treatments such as transdermal DHT and in view of the intensive

ongoing research aimed at the development of "selective androgen receptor modulators" having tissue-specific properties. Moreover, other options such as stimulation of endogenous sex steroid production and a possible role for selective estrogen receptor modulators for particular indications in elderly men (e.g. osteoporosis) might also deserve to be further explored. With the currently available evidence there is no place for treatment with DHEA in elderly men.

For testosterone administration, new improved options have become available that avoid the large periodic oscillations between markedly supraphysiological testosterone levels and deficiently low concentrations, and some of these newer modes of administration allow individual tailoring of treatment. The pharmacology and practical aspects of testosterone replacement are discussed in detail in Chapter 13.

16.6 Key messages

- Mean total serum testosterone decreases progressively in healthy men over the age of 60 years (30% decrease between the ages of 25 and 75 years). Age-associated decrease of the bioavailable fractions of serum testosterone is steeper as a consequence of an age-related increase of serum SHBG (50% decrease of free or bioavailable testosterone between the ages of 25 and 75 years).
- There is great interindividual variability of prevailing androgen levels in the elderly, ranging from perfectly preserved to frankly hypogonadal. Part of the interindividual variability in serum testosterone levels is explained by heredity, physiological factors and lifestyle-related factors.
- The proportion of men with "subnormal" testosterone relative to levels in young men increases with age (>20% after age 60 years); whether androgen requirements change in aging men remains to be definitely established, but available evidence suggests that androgen requirements are not increased.
- The age-related decline in Leydig cell function can be accentuated transiently or more permanently by co-morbidity and medication.
- The contribution of lifestyle-related factors and/or subclinical co-morbidities in the age-related

decline of serum testosterone in apparently healthy men remains an area of debate.

- The age-related decline of testosterone production is the result of primary testicular changes as well as of failure of the hypothalamic regulatory mechanisms to respond adequately to the hypoandrogenic state.
- Many of the clinical features of aging in men are reminiscent of clinical changes seen in hypogonadism in younger men; relative hypoandrogenism may be involved in some, but certainly not all clinical changes.
- Although testosterone levels required for normal sexual activity may be rather low and the factors most commonly involved in sexual dysfunction in elderly men are not hormonal, serum testosterone levels below the range for young men are associated with sexual symptoms.
- Hypoandrogenism may be involved in the sarcopenia of elderly men.
- The role of hypoandrogenism in male senile osteoporosis remains to be confirmed; recent data indicate that aromatization of testosterone to estradiol plays an important role in the regulation of bone metabolism in elderly men.
- In the present state of the art, androgen supplementation should only be considered in the presence of androgen serum levels clearly below the lower normal limit for younger men, together with unequivocal signs and symptoms

of androgen deficiency, in the absence of other reversible causes of decreased androgen levels and after screening for contraindications.

- Available dedicated questionnaires assessing aging male symptomatology lack specificity, and their use for screening purposes should be discouraged.
- The longer-term risk–benefit ratio for androgen administration to elderly men is unknown.
- Possible benefits of the treatment include an improved sense of general well-being, of libido and of muscle strength, with increase of lean body mass and limited decrease of fat mass.
- So far, the limited data on safety of TRT in the elderly have been rather reassuring: larger-scale studies of longer duration are still needed to assess safety, in particular at the prostate level; development of erythrocytosis is one of the most troublesome side-effects, which may be less frequent if largely supraphysiological androgen levels are avoided.
- Androgen replacement therapy in the elderly requires careful monitoring by an experienced physician.

Acknowledgement

Part of this work was supported by the Fonds voor Wetenschappelijk Onderzoek Vlaanderen, Grants G.3062.92 and G.0058.97 and G.0331.02.

16.7   References

Abbasi AA, Drinka PJ, Mattson DE, Rudman D (1993) Low circulating levels of insulin-like growth factors and testosterone in chronically institutionalized elderly men. *J Am Geriatr Soc* **41**:975–982

Alexandersen P, Haarbo J, Christiansen C (1996) The relationship of natural androgens to coronary heart disease in males: a review. *Atherosclerosis* **125**:1–13

Amory JK, Watts NB, Easley KA, Sutton PR, Anawalt BD, Matsumoto AM, Bremner WJ, Tenover JL (2004) Exogenous testosterone or testosterone with finasteride increases bone mineral density in older men with low serum

testosterone. *J Clin Endocrinol Metab* **89**:503–510

Andersson AM, Jensen TK, Juul A, Petersen JH, Jørgensen, Skakkebaek NE (2007) Secular decline in male testosterone and sex hormone binding globulin serum levels in Danish population surveys. *J Clin Endocrinol Metab* **92**:4696–4705

Andersson B, Marin P, Lissner L, Vermeulen A, Björntorp P (1994) Testosterone concentration in women and men with NIDDM. *Diabetes Care* **17**:405–411

Araujo AB, Esche GR, Kupelian V, O'Donnell AB, Travison TG, Williams RE, Clark RV, McKinlay JB (2007) Prevalence of symptomatic androgen deficiency

in men. *J Clin Endocrinol Metab* **92**:4241–4247

Araujo AB, Dixon JM, Suarez EA, Murad MH, Guey LT, Wittert GA (2011) Clinical review: endogenous testosterone and mortality in men: a systematic review and meta-analysis. *J Clin Endocrinol Metab* **96**:3007–3019

Aversa A, Isidori AM, Spera G, Lenzi A, Fabbri A (2003) Androgens improve cavernous vasodilation and response to sildenafil in patients with erectile dysfunction. *Clin Endocrinol* **58**:632–638

Bagatell CJ, Bremner WJ (1995) Androgen and progestogen effects on plasma lipids. *Prog Cardiovasc Dis* **38**:255–271

Bagatell CJ, Knopp RH, Vale WW, Rivier JE, Bremner WJ (1992) Physiologic testosterone levels in normal men suppress high-density lipoprotein cholesterol levels. *Ann Int Med* **116**:967–973

Baker HWG, Burger HG, de Kretser D, Hudson B (1977) Endocrinology of aging: pituitary testicular axis. In: James VHT (ed) *Proceedings of the 5th International Congress of Endocrinology*. Excerpta Medica Foundation, Amsterdam, pp 479–183

Baker HWG, Burger HG, de Kretser DM, Dulmanis A, Hudson B, O'Connor S, Paulson CA, Purcell N, Rennie GC, Seah CS, Taft HP, Wang C (1979) A study of the endocrine manifestations of hepatic cirrhosis. *Q J Med* **177**:145–178

Bancroft J (1984) Androgens, sexuality and the aging male. In: Labrie F, Proulx L (eds) *Endocrinology*. Elsevier, Amsterdam, pp 913–916

Barrett-Connor E, Von Mühlen DG, Kritz-Silverstein D (1999) Bioavailable testosterone and depressed mood in older men: the Rancho Bernardo Study. *J Clin Endocrinol Metab* **84**:573–577

Barrett-Connor E, Mueller JE, Von Mühlen DG, Laughlin GA, Schneider DL, Sartoris DJ (2000) Low levels of estradiol are associated with vertebral fractures in older men: the Rancho Bernardo Study. *J Clin Endocrinol Metab* **85**:219–223

Barrett-Connor EL, Khaw KT (1987) Cigarette smoking and serum sex hormones in men. *Am J Epidemiol* **128**:796–805

Basaria S, Lieb II J, Tang AM, DeWeese T, Carducci M, Eisenberger M, Dobs AS (2002) Long-term effects of androgen deprivation therapy in prostate cancer patients. *Clin Endocrinol* **56**:779–786

Basaria S, Coviello AD, Travison TG, Storer TW, Farwell WR, Jette AM, Eder R, Tennstedt S, Ulloor J, Zhang A, Choong K, Lakshman KM, Mazer NA, Miciek R, Krasnoff J, Elmi A, Knapp PE, Brooks B,

Appleman E, Aggarwal S, Bhasin G, Hede-Brierley L, Bhatia A, Collins L, LeBrasseur N, Fiore LD, Bhasin S (2010) Adverse events associated with testosterone administration. *N Engl J Med* **363**:109–122

Behre HM, Bohmeyer J, Nieschlag E (1994) Prostate volume in testosterone-treated and untreated hypogonadal men in comparison to age-matched normal controls. *Clin Endocrinol* **40**:341–349

Behre HM, Kliesch S, Leifke E, Link TM, Nieschlag E (1997) Long term effect of testosterone therapy on bone mineral density in hypogonadal men. *J Clin Endocrinol Metab* **82**:2386–2390

Bergendahl M, Aloi JA, Iranmanesh A, Mulligan TM, Veldhuis JD (1998) Fasting suppresses pulsatile luteinizing hormone (LH) secretion and enhances order lines of LH release in young but not in older men. *J Clin Endocrinol Metab* **83**:1967–1975

Bhasin S, Tenover JS (1997) Age-associated sarcopenia – issues in the use of testosterone as an anabolic agent in older men. *J Clin Endocrinol Metab* **82**:1659–1660

Bhasin S, Woodhouse L, Casaburi R, Singh AB, Bhasin D, Berman N, Chen XH, Yarasheski KE, Magliano L, Dzekov C, Dzekov J, Bross R, Phillips J, Sinha-Hikim I, Shen RQ, Storer TW (2001) Testosterone dose-response relationships in healthy young men. *Am J Physiol Endocrinol Metab* **281**: E1172–E1181

Bhasin S, Singh AB, Mac RP, Carter B, Lee MI, Cunningham GR (2003) Managing the risk of prostate disease during testosterone replacement therapy in older men: recommendations for a standardized monitoring plan. *J Androl* **24**:299–311

Bhasin S, Woodhouse L, Casaburi R, Singh AB, Phong Mac R, Lee M, Yarasheski KE, Sinha-Hikim I,

Dzekov C, Dzeko v J, Magliano L, Storer TW (2005) Older men are as responsive as young men to the anabolic effects of graded doses of testosterone on the skeletal muscle. *J Clin Endocrinol Metab* **90**:678–688

Bhasin S, Cunningham GR, Hayes FJ, Matsumoto AM, Snyder PJ, Swerdloff RS, Montori VM (2010) Testosterone therapy in men with androgen deficiency syndromes: an Endocrine Society Clinical Practice Guideline. *J Clin Endocrinol Metab* **95**: 2536–2559

Bhasin S, Pencina M, Jasuja GK, Travison TG, Coviello A, Orwoll E, Wang PY, Nielson C, Wu F, Tajar A, Labrie F, Vesper H, Zhang A, Ulloor J, Singh R, D'Agostino R, Vasan RS (2011) Reference ranges for testosterone in men generated using liquid chromatography tandem mass spectrometry in a community-based sample of healthy nonobese young men in the Framingham Heart Study and applied to three geographically distinct cohorts. *J Clin Endocrinol Metab* **96**:2430–2439

Bixler EO, Santen RJ, Kales A (1977) Inverse effects of thioridazine (Melleril) on serum prolactin and testosterone concentrations in normal men. In: Troen P, Nankin HR (eds) *The Testis in Normal and Infertile Men*. Raven, New York, pp 405–409

Bogaert V, Taes Y, Konings P, Van Steen K, De Bacquer D, Goemaere S, Zmierczak H, Crabbe P, Kaufman JM (2008) Heritability of blood concentrations of sex-steroids in relation to body composition in young adult male siblings. *Clin Endocrinol* **69**:129–135

Bogaert V, Vanbillemont G, Taes Y, De Bacquer D, Deschepper E, Van Steen K, Kaufman JM (2009) Small effect of the androgen receptor gene GGN repeat polymorphism on serum testosterone levels in healthy men. *Eur J Endocrinol* **161**:171–177

Boonen S, Vanderschueren D, Xiao GC, Verbeke G, Dequeker J, Geusens P, Broos P, Bouillon R (1997) Age related (Type II) femoral neck osteoporosis in men: biochemical evidence for both hypovitaminosis D- and androgen deficiency-induced bone resorption. *J Bone Miner Res* 12:2119–2126

Brambilla DJ, O'Donnell AB, Matsumoto AM, McKinlay (2007) Lack of seasonal variation in serum sex hormone levels in middle-aged to older men in the Boston area. *J Clin Endocrinol Metab* **92**: 4224–4229

Bremner WJ, Vitiello MV, Prinz PN (1983) Loss of circadian rhythmicity in blood testosterone levels with aging in normal men. *J Clin Endocrinol Metab* 56:1278–1281

Brenta G, Schnitman M, Gurfinkiel M, Damilano S, Pierini A, Sinay I, Pisarev MA (1999) Variations of sex hormone-binding globulin in thyroid dysfunction. *Thyroid* 9:273–277

Bross R, Javanbakth M, Bhasin S (1999) Anabolic interventions for aging-associated sarcopenia. *J Clin Endocrinol Metab* 84:3420–3430

Buena F, Swerdloff RS, Steiner BS, Lutchmansingh P, Peterson MA, Pandian MR, Galmarini M, Bhasin S (1993) Sexual function does not change when serum testosterone levels are pharmacologically varied within the normal male range. *Fertil Steril* 59:1118–1123

Burnett-Bowie SA, McKay EA, Lee H, Leder BZ (2009) Effects of aromatase inhibition on bone mineral density and bone turnover in older men with low testosterone levels. *J Clin Endocrinol Metab* **94**:4785–4792

Calof OM, Singh AB, Lee ML, Kenny AM, Urban RJ, Tenover JL, Bhasin S (2005) Adverse events associated with testosterone supplementation of older men. *J Gerontol A Biol Sci Med Sci* 60:1451–1457

Carani C, Qin K, Simoni M, Faustini-Fustini M, Serpente S, Boyd J,

Korach KS, Simpson ER (1997) Effect of testosterone and estradiol in a man with aromatase deficiency. *N Engl J Med* 337:91–95

Cauley JA, Ewing SK, Taylor BC, Fink HA, Ensrud KE, Bauer DC, Barrett-Connor E, Marshall, Orwoll ES, for the Osteoporotic Fractures in Men Study (MrOS) Research Group (2010) Sex steroid hormones in older men: longitudinal associations with 4.5-year change in hip bone mineral density – the osteoporotic fractures in men study. *J Clin Endocrinol Metab* 95:4314–4323

Cawthon PM, Ensrud KE, Laughlin GA, Cauley JA, Dam TTL, Barrett-Connor E, Fink HA, Hoffman AR, Lau E, Lane NE, Stefanick ML, Cummings SR, Orwoll ES, for the Osteoporotic Fractures in Men (MrOS) Research Group (2009) Sex hormones and frailty in older men: the Osteoporotic Fractures in Men (MrOS) Study. *J Clin Endocrinol Metab* 94:3806–3815

Cicero TJ (1982) Alcohol induced defects in the hypothalamo-pituitary luteinizing hormone action in the male. *Alcoholism* 6:207–215

Cooper TG, Keck C, Oberdieck U, Nieschlag E (1993) Effects of multiple ejaculations after extended periods of sexual abstinence on total motile and normal sperm numbers as well as on accessory gland secretions from healthy normal and oligospermic men. *Hum Reprod* 8:1251–1258

Couillard C, Gagnon J, Bergeron J, Leon AS, Rao DC, Skinner JS, Wilmore JH, Desprès JP, Bouchard C (2000) Contribution of body fatness and adipose tissue distribution to the age variation in plasma steroid hormone concentration in men: the HERITAGE family study. *J Clin Endocrinol Metab* 1026–1031

Coviello AD, Lakshman K, Mazer NA, Bhasin S (2006) Differences in the apparent metabolic clearance rate of testosterone in young and older

men with gonadotropin suppression receiving graded doses of testosterone. *J Clin Endocrinol Metab* 91:4669–4672

Coviello AD, Kaplan B, Lakshman KM, Chen T, Singh AB, Bhasin S (2008) Effects of graded doses of testosterone on erythropoiesis in healthy young and older men. *J Clin Endocrinol Metab* 93:914–919

Crabbe P, Bogaert V, De Bacquer D, Goemaere S, Zmierczak H, Kaufman JM (2007) Part of the interindividual variation in serum testosterone levels in healthy men reflects differences in androgen sensitivity and feedback set point: contribution of the androgen receptor polyglutamine tract polymorphism. *J Clin Endocrinol* 92:3604–3610

Crawford BAL, Liu PY, Kean MT, Bleasel JF, Handelsman DJ (2003) Randomized placebo-controlled trial of androgen effects on muscle and bone in men requiring long-term systemic glucocorticoid treatment. *J Clin Endocrinol Metab* 88:3167–3176

Dai WS, Gutai JP, Kuller LH, Cauley JA (1988) Cigarette smoking and serum sex hormones in men. *Am J Epidemiol* **128**: 796–805

Daniell HW (2002) Hypogonadism in men consuming sustained-action oral opioids. *J Pain* 3:377–384

Davidson JM, Chen JJ, Crapo L, Gray GD, Greenleaf WJ, Catania JA (1983) Hormonal changes and sexual function in aging men. *J Clin Endocrinol Metab* 57:71–77

Delhez M, Hansenne M, Legros J-J (2003) Andropause and psychopathology: minor symptoms rather than pathological ones. *Psychoneuroendocrinology* **28**: 863–874

de Lignieres B (1993) Transdermal dihydrotestosterone treatment of 'andropause'. *Ann Med* **25**:235–241

Deslypere JP, Vermeulen A (1981) Aging and tissue androgens. *J Clin Endocrinol Metab* 53:430–434

Deslypere JP, Vermeulen A (1985) Influence of age on steroid concentration in skin and striated muscle in women and in cardiac muscle and lung tissue in men. *J Clin Endocrinol Metab* **60**:648–653

Deslypere JP, Sayed A, Punjabi U, Verdonck L, Vermeulen A (1982) Plasma 5α androstane-3α,17-diol and urinary 5α-androstane, 3α17-diol glucuronide, parameters of peripheral androgen action: a comparative study. *J Clin Endocrinol Metab* **54**:386–391

Deslypere JP, Kaufman JM, Vermeulen T, Vogelaers D, Vandalem JL, Vermeulen A (1987) Influence of age on pulsatile luteinizing hormone release and responsiveness of the gonadotrophs to sex hormone feedback in men. *J Clin Endocrinol Metab* **64**:68–73

Dobs AS, Meikle AW, Arver S, Sanders SW, Caramelli KE, Mazer NA (1999) Pharmacokonetics, efficacy, and safety of a permeation-enhanced testosterone transdermal system in comparison with biweekly injections of testosterone enanthate for treatment of hypogonadal men. *J Clin Endocrinol Metab* **84**:3469–3478

Dunbar N, Gruman C, Reisine S, Kenny A (2001) Comparison of two health status measures and their associations with testosterone levels in older men. *Aging Male* **4**:1–7

Duranteau L, Chanson P, Blumberg-Tick J, Thomas G, Brailly S, Lubetzki J, Schaison G, Bouchard P (1993) Non-responsiveness of serum gonadotropins and testosterone to pulsatile GnRH in hemochromatosis suggesting a pituitary defect. *Acta Endocrinol (Copenh)* **128**:351–354

Elewaut A, Barbier F, Vermeulen A (1979) Testosterone metabolism in normal males and male cirrhotics. *Z Gastroenterol* **17**:402–405

Emmelot-Vonk M, Verhaar HJJ, Hakhai Pour HR, Aleman A, Lock TMTW, Bosch JLH Ruud, Grobbee DE, van der Schouw YT (2008) Effect of testosterone supplementation on functional mobility, cognition, and other parameters in older men. *JAMA* **299**:39–52

Erfurth EM, Hagmar LE, Sääf M, Hall K (1996) Serum levels of insulin-like growth factor I and insulin-like growth factor binding protein 1 correlate with serum free testosterone and sex hormone binding globulin in healthy young and middle-aged men. *Clin Endocrinol* **44**:659–664

Eriksson AL, Lorentzon M, Mellström D, Vandenput L, Swanson C, Andersson N, Hammond GL, Jakobsson J, Rane A, Orwoll ES, Ljunggren O, Johnell O, Labrie F, Windahl SH, Ohlsson C (2006) SHBG gene promoter polymorphisms in men are associated with serum sex hormone-binding globulin, androgen and androgen metabolite levels, and hip bone mineral density. *J Clin Endocrinol Metab* **91**:5029–5037

Faber J, Perrild H, Johansen JS (1990) Bone Gla protein and sex hormone-binding globulin in nontoxic goiter: parameters for metabolic status at the tissue levels. *J Clin Endocrinol Metabol* **70**:49–55

Falahati-Nini A, Riggs BL, Atkinson EJ, O'Fallon WM, Eastell R, Khosla S (2000) Relative contributions of testosterone and estrogen in regulating bone resorption and formation in normal elderly men. *J Clin Invest* **106**:1533–1560

Feldman HA, Goldstein I, Hatzichristou DG, Krane RJ, Mckinlay JB (1994) Impotence and its medical and psychosocial correlates: results of the Massachusetts Male Aging Study. *J Urol* **151**:54–61

Feldman HA, Longcope C, Derby CA, Johannes CB, Araujo AB, Coviello AD, Bremner WJ, McKinlay JB (2002) Age trends in the level of serum testosterone and other hormones in middle aged men: longitudinal results from the Massachusetts Male Aging Study. *J Clin Endocrinol Metab* **87**:589–598

Fernandez-Balsells MM, Murad MH, Lane M, Lampropulos JF, Albuquerque F, Mullan RJ, Agrwal N, Elamin MB, Gallegos-Orozco JF, Wang AT, Erwin PJ, Bhasin S, Montori VM (2010) Adverse effects of testosterone therapy in adult men: a systematic review and meta-analysis. *J Clin Endocrinol Metab* **95**:2560–2575

Ferrando AA, Sheffield-Moore M, Yeckel CW, Gilkison C, Jiang J, Achacosa A, Lieberman SA, Tipton K, Wolfe RR, Urban RJ (2002) Testosterone administration to older men improves muscle function: molecular and physiological mechanisms. *Am J Physiol Metab* **282**:E601–E607

Ferrini LC, Barrett-Connor E (1998) Sex hormones and age: a cross-sectional study of testosterone and estradiol and their bioavailable fractions in community-dwelling men. *Am J Epidemiol* **147**:750–754

Field AE, Colditz GA, Willett WC, Longcope C, McKinlay JB (1994) The relation of smoking, age, relative weight and dietary intake to serum adrenal steroids, sex hormones and sex hormone binding globulin in middle age men. *J Clin Endocrinol Metab* **79**:1310–1316

Fink HA, Ewing SK, Ensrud KE, Barrett-Connor E, Taylor BC, Cauley JA, Orwoll ES for the Osteoporotic Fractures in Men Study Group (2006) Association of testosterone and estradiol deficiency with osteoporosis and rapid bone loss in older men. *J Clin Endocrinol Metab* **91**:2908–3915

Forbes GB, Reina JC (1970) Adult lean body mass declines with age: some longitudinal observations. *Metabolism* **19**:653–663

Gapstur SM, Gann PH, Kopp P, Colangelo L, Longcope C, Liu K (2002) Serum androgen concentrations in young men: a longitudinal analysis of associations with age, obesity and race. The CARDIA male hormone study. *Canc Epidemiol Biom Prev* **11**:1041–1047

Giagulli VA, Vermeulen A (1992) Increased plasma 5α-androstane-3α, 17β-diol glucuronide concentration in clinically euthyroid women with suppressed plasma thyrotropin levels: further evidence for generalized tissue overexposure to thyroid hormones in these subjects. *J Clin Endocrinol Metab* **74**:1465–1467

Giagulli VA, Kaufman JM, Vermeulen A (1994) Pathogenesis of decreased androgen levels in obese men. *J Clin Endocrinol Metab* **79**:997–1000

Giusti G, Gonnelli P, Borreli D, Fiorelli G, Forti G, Pazzagli M, Serio M (1975) Age related secretion of androstenedione, testosterone and dihydrotestosterone by the human testes. *Exp Gerontol* **10**:241–245

Goldberg RB, Rabin AN, Alexander AN, Coelle GC, Getz GE (1985) Suppression of plasma testosterone leads to an increase in serum total and high density lipoprotein cholesterol and apoproteins A-1 and B. *J Clin Endocrinol Metab* **60**:203–207

Gooren LJG (1987) Androgen levels and sex functions in testosterone treated hypogonadal men. *Arch Sex Beh* **16**:463–476

Gray PB, Singh AB, Woodhouse LJ, Storer TW, Casaburi R, Dzekov J, Dzekov C, Sinha-Hikim I, Bhasin S (2005) Dose-dependent effects of testosterone on sexual function, mood, and visuospatial cognition in older men. *J Clin Endocrinol Metab* **90**:3838–3846

Grossmann M (2011) Low testosterone in men with type 2 diabetes: significance and treatment. *J Clin Endocrinol Metab* **96**: 2341–2353

Gruenewald DA, Matsumoto AM (2003) Testosterone supplementation therapy for older men: potential benefits and risks *J Am Geriatr Soc* **51**:101–115

Grunstein RR, Handelsman DJ, Lawrence SJ, Blackwell C, Caterson ID, Sullivan CE (1989) Neuroendocrine dysfunction in sleep apnea: reversal by nasal continuous positive airway pressure. *J Clin Endocrinol Metab* **68**:352–358

Guadalupe-Grau A, Rodriguez-Gonzalez FG, Ponce-Gonzalez JG, Dorado C, Olmedillas H, Fuentes T, Perez-Gomez J, Sanchis-moysi J, Diaz-Chico BN, Calbet JAL (2010) Bone mass and the CAG and GGN androgen receptor polymorphisms in young men. *Plos One* **5**:e11529

Guralnik JM, Ferrucci L, Simonsick EM, Salive ME, Wallace RB (1995) Lower-extremity function in persons over 70 years as a predictor of subsequent disability. *N Engl J Med* **322**:556–561

Haffner SM, Katz MS, Stern MP, Dunn JF (1988) The relationship of sex hormones to hyperinsulinemia and hyperglycemia. *Metabolism* **37**:683–688

Haffner SM, Mykkänen L, Valdez RA, Stern MP, Katz MS (1993) Relationship of sex hormones to lipids and lipoproteins in non-diabetic men. *J Clin Endocrinol Metab* **77**:1610–1615

Haffner SM, Miettinen H, Karhapaa L, Laakso M (1997) Leptin concentrations, sex hormones and cortisol in non diabetic men. *J Clin Endocrinol Metab* **82**:1807–1809

Hajjar RR, Kaiser FE, Morley JE (1997) Outcomes of long-term testosterone replacement in older hypogonadal males: a retrospective analysis. *J Clin Endocrinol Metab* **82**:3793–3796

Hak AE, Witteman JC, de Jong FH, Geerlings MI, Hofman A, Pols HA (2002) Low levels of endogenous androgens increase the risk of atherosclerosis in elderly men: the Rotterdam study. *J Clin Endocrinol Metab* **87**:3632–3639

Häkkinen K, Pakarinen A (1994) Serum hormones and strength development during strength training in middle-aged and elderly

males and females. *Acta Physiol Scand* **150**:211–219

Hall SA, Esche GR, Araujo AB, Travison TG, Clark RV, Williams RE, McKinlay JB (2008) Correlates of low testosterone and symptomatic androgen deficiency in a population-based sample. *J Clin Endocrinol Metab* **93**: 3870–3877

Handelsman DJ (1994) Testicular dysfunction in systemic disease. *Endocr Metab Clin* **23**:839–852

Handelsman DJ, Dong Q (1993) Hypothalamo-pituitary-gonadal axis in chronic renal failure. *Endocr Metab Clin* **22**:145–161

Harbitz TB (1973) Morphometric studies of Leydig cells in elderly men, with special reference to the histology of the prostate. *Acta Pathol Microbiol Scand* **81**:301–314

Harkonen K, Huhtaniemi I, Makinen J, Hubler D, Irjala K, Koskenvuo M, Oettel M, Raitakari O, Saad F, Pollanen P (2003) The polymorphic androgen receptor gene CAG repeat, pituitary-testicular function and andropausal symptoms in ageing men. *Int J Androl* **26**:187–194

Harman SM, Tsitouras PD (1980) Reproductive hormones in aging men I. Measurment of sex steroids, basal luteinizing hormone and Leydig cell response to human chorionic gonadotropin. *J Clin Endocrinol Metab* **51**:35–40

Harman SM, Metter EJ, Tobin JD, Pearson J, Blackman MR (2001) Longitudinal effects of aging on serum total and free testosterone levels in healthy men. *J Clin Endocrinol Metab* **86**:724–730

Heald AH, Ivison F, Anderson SG, Cruickshank K, Laing I, Gibson JM (2003) Significant ethnic variation in total and free testosterone concentration. *Clin Endocrinol* **58**:262–266

Heinemann L, Zimmermann T, Vermeulen A, Thiel C, Hummel W (1999) A new 'aging males' symptoms' rating scale. *Aging Male* **2**:105–114

Hollander N, Hollander VP (1958) The microdetermination of testosterone in human spermatic vein blood. *J Clin Endocrinol Metab* **18**:966–970

Howell SJ, Radford JA, Adams JE, Smets EM, Warburton R, Shalet SM (2001) Randomized placebo-controlled trial of testosterone replacement in men with mild Leydig cell insufficiency following cytotoxic chemotherapy. *Clin Endocrinol (Oxf)* **55**:315–324

Huhtaniemi IT, Pye SR, Limer KL, Thomson W, O'Neill TW, Platt H, Payne D, John SL, Jiang M, Boonen S, Borghs H, Vanderschueren D, Adams JE, Ward KA, Bartfai G, Casanueva F, Finn JD, Forti G, Giwercman A, Han TS, Kula K, Lean MEJ, Pendleton N, Punab M, Silman AJ, Wu FCW; EMAS Study Group (2009) Increased estrogen rather than decreased androgen action is associated with longer androgen receptor CAG repeats. *J Clin Endocrinol Metab* **94**:277–284

Huhtaniemi IT, Pye SR, Holliday KL, Thomson W, O'Neill TW, Platt H, Payne D, John SL, Jiang M, Bartfai G, Boonen S, Casanueva FF, Finn JD, Forti G, Giwercman A, Han TS, Kula K, Lean MEJ, Pendleton N, Punab M, Silman AJ, Vanderschueren D, Labrie F, Wu FCW; European Male Aging Study Group (2010) Effect of polymorphisms in selected genes involved in pituitary-testicular function on reproductive hormones and phenotype in aging men. *J Clin Endocrinol Metab* **95**:1898–1908

Hyde Z, Flicker L, Almeida OP, Hankey GJ, McCaul KA, Chubb SAP, Yeap BB (2010) Low free testosterone predicts frailty in older men: the health in men study. *J Clin Endocrinol Metab* **95**:3165–3172

Ida Y, Tsyjimaru S, Nakamura K, Shirao I, Mukasa H, Egarni H, Nakazawa H (1992) Effect of acute and repeated alcohol ingestion on hypothalamic-pituitary-gonadal and hypothalamic-pituitary-adrenal functioning in normal males. *Drug Alcohol Dep* **31**:57–64

Impallomeni M, Kaufman BM, Palmer AJ (1994) Do acute diseases transiently impair anterior pituitary function in patients over the age of 75? A longitudinal study of the TRH test and basal gonadotrophin levels. *Postgrad Med J* **70**:86–91

Irwin M, Dreyfus E, Baird DS, Smith T, Schuckit M (1988) Testosterone in chronic alcoholic men. *Br J Addict* **83**:949–953

Isidori AM, Giannetta E, Gianfrilli D, Greco EA, Bonifacio V, Aversa A, Isidori A, Fabbri A, Lenzi A (2005a) Effects of testosterone on sexual function in men: results of a meta-analysis. *Clin Endocrinol* **63**:381–394

Isidori AM, Giannetta E, Greco EA, Gianfrilli D, Bonifacio V, Isidori A, Lenzi A, Fabbri A (2005b) Effects of testosterone on body composition, bone metabolism and serum lipid profile in middle-aged men: a meta-analysis. *Clin Endocrinol* **63**:280–293

Jackson JA, Waxman J, Spiekerman M (1989) Prostatic implications of testosterone replacement therapy. *Arch Intern Med* **149**:2364–2366

Jackson JA, Riggs MW, Spiekerman M (1992) Testosterone deficiency as a risk factor for hip fracture in men: a case control study. *Am J Med Sci* **304**:4–8

Joshi D, van Schoor NM, de Ronde W, Schaap LA, Comijs HC, Beekman ATF, Lips P (2010) Low free testosterone levels are associated with prevalence and incidence of depressive symptoms in older men. *Clin Endocrinol* **72**:232–240

Jung A, Schuppe HC, Schill WB (2002) Comparison of semen quality in older and younger men attending an andrology clinic. *Andrologia* **34**:116–122

Kamat A, Hinshelwood MM, Murry BA, Mendelson CR (2002) Mechanisms in tissue-specific regulation of estrogen biosynthesis in humans. *Trends Endocrinol Metab* **13**:122–128

Kamischke A, Kemper DE, Castel MA, Luthke M, Rolf C, Behre HM, Magnussen H, Nieschlag E (1998) Testosterone levels in men with chronic obstructive pulmonary disease with or without glucocorticoid therapy. *Eur Respir J* **11**:41–45

Katznelson L, Finkelstein JS, Schoenfeld DA, Rosenthal DI, Anderson EJ, Klibanski A (1996) Increase in bone density and lean body mass during testosterone administration in men with acquired hypogonadism. *J Clin Endocrinol Metab* **81**:4358–4365

Kaufman JM, Goemaere S (2008) Osteoporosis in men. *Best Pract Res Clin Endocrinol Metab* **22**:787–812

Kaufman JM, Vermeulen A (1997) Declining gonadal function in elderly men. *Baillière's Endocrinol Metab* **11**:289–309

Kaufman JM, Vermeulen A (2005) The decline of androgen levels in elderly men and its clinical and therapeutic implications. *Endocrine Rev* **26**:833–876

Kaufman JM, Giri M, Deslypere JP, Thomas G, Vermeulen A (1991) Influence of age on the responsiveness of the gonadotrophs to luteinizing hormone-releasing hormone in males. *J Clin Endocrinol Metab* **72**:1255–1260

Kenny A, Kleppinger A, Annis K, Rathier M, Browner B, Judge JO, McGee D (2010) Effects of transdermal testosterone on bone and muscle in older men with low bioavailable testosterone levels, low bone mass, and physical frailty. *JAGS* **58**:1134–1143

Kenny AM, Prestwood KM, Gruman CA, Marcello KM, Raisz LG (2001) Effects of transdermal testosterone on bone and muscle in older men with low bioavailable testosterone levels. *J Gerontol A Biol Sci Med Sci* **56**:M266–M272

Kent JZ, Acone AB (1966) Plasma androgens and aging. In: Vermeulen A, Exley D (eds) *Androgens in Normal and Pathological Conditions*. Excerpta Medica Foundation, Amsterdam, pp 31–35

Khaw KT, Barrett-Connor E (1992) Lower endogenous androgens predict central obesity in men. *Ann Epidemiol* 2:675–682

Khosla S (2010) Update in male osteoporosis. *J Clin Endocrinol Metab* 95:3–10

Khosla S, Melton LJ III, Atkinson EJ, O'Fallon WM (2001) Relationship of serum sex steroid levels to longitudinal changes in bone density in young versus elderly men. *J Clin Endocrinol Metab* 86: 3555–3561

Korenman SG, Morley JE, Mooradian AD, Davis SS, Kaiser FE, Silver AJ, Viosca SP, Garza D (1990) Secondary hypogonadism in older men: its relation to impotence. *J Clin Endocrinol Metab* 71:963–969

Krasnoff JB, Basaria S, Pencina MJ, Jasuja GK, Vasan RS, Ulloor J, Zhang A, Coviello A, Kelly-Hayes M, D'Agostino RB, Wolf PA, Bhasin S, Murabito JM (2010) Free testosterone levels are associated with mobility limitation and physical performance in community-dwelling men: the Framingham Offspring Study. *J Clin Endocrinol Metab* 95:2790–2799

Kunelius P, Lukkarinen O, Hannuksela ML, Itkonen O, Tapanainen JS (2002) The effects of transdermal dihydrotestosterone in the aging male: a prospective, randomized, double blind study. *J Clin Endocrinol Metab* 87:1467–1472

Kupelian V, Page ST, Araujo AB, Travison TG, Bremner WJ, McKinlay JB (2006) Low sex hormone-binding globulin, total testosterone, and symptomatic androgen deficiency are associated with development of the metabolic syndrome in nonobese men. *J Clin Endocrinol Metab* 91:843–850

Kupelian V, Hayes FJ, Link CL, Rosen R, McKinlay JB (2008) Inverse association of testosterone and the metabolic syndrome in men is consistent across race and ethnic groups. *J Clin Endocrinol Metab* 93:3403–3410

Kwan M, Greenleaf WJ, Mann J, Crapo L, Davidson J (1983) The nature of androgen action on male sexuality: a combined laboratory/self report study on hypogonadal men. *J Clin Endocrinol Metab* 57:557–562

Labrie F, Bélanger A, Simard J, Van Luu-The, Labrie C (1995) DHEA and peripheral androgen and estrogen formation: intracrinology. *Ann N Y Acad Sci* 774:16–28

Lakshman KM, Kaplan B, Travison TG, Basaria S, Knapp PE, Singh AB, La Valley MP, Mazer NA, Bhasin S (2010) The effects of injected testosterone dose and age on the conversion of testosterone to estradiol and dihydrotestosterone in young and older men. *J Clin Endocrinol Metab* 95: 3955–3964

Lange JD, Brown WA, Wincze J, Zwick W (1980) Serum testosterone concentration and penile tumescence changes in men. *Horm Behav* 14:267–270

Lapauw B, Goemaere S, Zmierczak H, Van Pottelbergh I, Mahmoud A, Taes Y, De Bacquer D, Vansteelandt S, Kaufman JM (2008) The decline of serum testosterone levels in community-dwelling men over 70 years of age: descriptive data and predictors of longitudinal changes. *Eur J Endocrinol* 159:459–468

Lazarou S, Morgentaler A (2008) The effect of aging on spermatogenesis and pregnancy outcomes. *Urol Clin N Am* 35:331–339

Lichtenstein MJ, Yarnell JWG, Elwood PC, Beswick AD, Sweetnam PM, Marks V, Teale D, Riad-Fahmy D (1987) Sex hormones, insulin, lipid and prevalent ischemic heart disease. *Am J Epidemiol* 126:647–657

Lindström S, Ma J, Altshuler D, Giovannucci E, Riboli E, Albanes D, Allen NE, Berndt SI, Boeing H, Bueno-de-Mesquita HB, Chanock SJ, Dunning AM, Feigelson HS, Gaziano JM, Haiman CA, Hayes RB, Henderson BE, Hunter DJ, Kaaks R, Kolonel LN, Le Marchand L, Martinez C, Overvad K, Siddiq A, Stampfer M, Stattin P, Stram DO, Thun MJ, Trichopoulos D, Tumino R, Virtamo J, Weinstein SJ, Yeager M, Kraft P, Freedman ML (2010) A large study of androgen receptor germline variants and their relation to sex hormone levels and prostate cancer risk. Results from the National Cancer Institute Breast and Prostate Cancer Cohort Consortium. *J Clin Endocrinol Metab* 95:E121–E127

Liu PY, Death AK, Handelsman DJ (2003) Androgens and cardiovascular disease. *Endocr Rev* 24:313–340

Liu PY, Beilin J, Meier C, Nguyen TV, Center JR, Leedman PJ, Seibel MJ, Eisman JA, Handelsman DJ (2007a) Age-related changes in serum testosterone and sex hormone binding globulin in Australian men: longitudinal analyses of two geographically separate regional cohorts. *J Clin Endocrinol Metab* 92:3599–3603

Liu PY, Caterson ID, Grunstein RR, Handelsman DJ (2007b) Androgens, obesity, and sleep-disordered breathing in men. *Endocrinol Metab Clin N Am* 36:349–363

Longcope C (1973) The effect of human chorionic gonadotropin on plasma steroid levels in young and old men. *Steroids* 21:583–592

Longcope C, Feldman HA, McKinlay JB, Araujo AB (2000) Diet and sex hormone-binding globulin. *J Clin Endocrinol Metab* 85:293–296

Luboshitzky R, Aviv A, Hefetz A, Herer P, Shen-Orr Z, Lavie L, Lavie P (2002) Decreased pituitary-gonadal secretion in men with obstructive sleep apnea. *J Clin Endocrinol Metab* **87**:3394–3398

Ly LP, Jimenez M, Zhuang TN, Celermajer DS, Conway AJ, Handelsman DJ (2001) A double-blind, placebo-controlled, randomized clinical trial of transdermal dihydrotestosterone gel on muscular strength, mobility, and quality of life in older men with partial androgen deficiency. *J Clin Endocrinol Metab* **86**:4078–4088

MacAdams MR, White RH, Chipps BE (1986) Reduction of serum testosterone levels during chronic glucocorticoid therapy. *Ann Intern Med* **104**:648–651

Mahmoud AM, Goemaere S, De Bacquer D, Comhaire FH, Kaufman JM (2000) Serum inhibin B levels in community-dwelling elderly men. *Clin Endocrinol* **53**:141–147

Mahmoud AM, Goemaere S, El-Garem Y, Van Pottelbergh I, Comhaire FH, Kaufman JM (2003) Testicular volume in relation to hormonal indices of gonadal function in community-dwelling elderly men. *J Clin Endocrinol Metab* **88**:179–184

Maki PM, Ernst M, London ED, Mordecai KL, Perschler P, Durso SC, Brandt J, Dobs A, Resnick SM (2007) Intramuscular testosterone treatment in elderly men: evidence of memory decline and altered brain function. *J Clin Endocrinol Metab* **92**:4107–4114

Masters WH (1986) Sex and aging – expectations and reality. *Hosp Pract* **15**:175–198

Matzkin H, Braf Z, Nava D (1991) Does age influence the bioactivity of follicle-stimulating hormone in men. *Age Ageing* **20**:199–205

Meier C, Nguyen TV, Handelsman DJ, Schindler C, Kushnir MM, Rockwood AL, Meikle AW, Center JR, Eisman JA, Seibel MJ (2008) Endogenous sex hormones and incident fracture risk in older men. *Arch Intern Med* **168**:47–54

Meikle AW, Bishop DT, Stringham JD, West DW (1986) Quantitating

genetic and non genetic factors to determine plasma sex steroid variation in normal male twins. *Metabolism* **35**:1090–1095

Meikle AW, Stringham JD, Bishop T, West DW (1988) Quantitation of genetic and nongenetic factors influencing androgen productions and clearance rates in men? *J Clin Endocrinol Metab* **67**: 104–109

Mellström D, Vandenput L, Mallmin H, Holmberg A, Lorentzon M, Oden A, Johansson H, Orwoll ES, Labrie F, Karlsson MK, Ljunggren O, Ohlsson C (2008) Older men with low serum estradiol and high serum SHBG have an increased risk of fractures. *J Bone Miner Res* **23**:1552–1560

Mikuma N, Kumamoto Y, Maruta H, Nitta T (1994) Role of the hypothalamic opioidergic system in the control of gonadotropin secretion in elderly men. *Andrologia* **26**:39–45

Mitchell R, Hollis S, Rothwell C, Robertsons WR (1995) Age related changes in the pituitary testicular axis in normal men; lower serum testosterone results from decreased bioactive LH drive. *Clin Endocrinol* **42**:501–507

Mittan D, LEE S, Miller E, Perez RC, Basler JW, Bruder JM (2002) Bone loss following hypogonadism in men with prostate cancer treated with GnRH analogs. *J Clin Endocrinol Metab* **87**:3656–3661

Moffat SD, Zonderman AB, Metter EJ, Kawas C, Blackman MR, Harman SM, Resnick SM (2004) Free testosterone and risk for Alzheimer disease in older men. *Neurology* **62**:188–193

Mohr BA, Guay AT, O'Donnell AB, McKinlay JB (2005) Normal, bound and nonbound testosterone levels in normally ageing men: results from the Massachusetts Male Ageing Study. *Clin Endocrinol* **62**:64–73

Mohr BA, Bhasin S, Link CL, O'Donnell AB, Mckinlay JB (2006) The effect of changes in adiposity

on testosterone levels in older men: longitudinal results from the Massachusetts male ageing study. *Eur J Endocrinol* **155**:443–452

Mohr BA, Bhasin S, Kupelian V, Araujo AB, O'Donnell AB, McKinlay JB (2007) Testosterone, sex hormone-binding globulin, and frailty in older men. *J Am Geriatr Soc* **55**:548–555

Moorjani S, Dupont A, Labrie F, Lupien PJ, Brun D, Gagné C, Giguère M, Bélanger A (1987) Increase in plasma high density lipoprotein concentration following complete androgen blockade in men with prostatic carcinoma. *Metabolism* **36**:244–250

Morley JE (1986) Impotence. *Am J Med* **80**:897–906

Morley JE, Kaiser FE, Perry HM III, Patrick P, Morley PM, Stauber PM, Vellas B, Baumgartner RN, Garry PJ (1997) Longitudinal changes in testosterone, luteinizing hormone and follicle stimulating hormone in healthy older men. *Metabolism* **46**:410–413

Morley JE, Charlton E, Patrick P, Kaiser FE, Cadeau P, McCready D, Perry HM III (2000) Validation of a screening questionnaire for androgen deficiency in aging males. *Metabolism* **49**:1239–1242

Morley JE, Patrick P, Perry HM III (2002) Evaluation of assays available to measure free testosterone. *Metabolism* **51**:554–559

Muller M, Grobbee DE, Thijssen JHH, van den Beld AW, van der Schouw YT (2003) Sex hormones and male health: effects on components of the frailty syndrome. *Trends Endocrinol Metab* **14**:289–296

Mulligan T, Iranmanesh A, Gheorghiu S, Godschalk M, Veldhuis JD (1995) Amplified nocturnal luteinizing hormone (LH) secretory burst frequency with selective attenuation of pulsatile (but not basal) testosterone secretion in healthy aging men: possible Leydig cell desensitization to endogenous LH signaling-a clinical research center study. *J Clin Endocrinol Metab* **80**:3025–3031

Mulligan T, Iranmanesh A, Kerzner R, Demers LW, Veldhuis JD (1999) Two-week pulsatile gonadotropin releasing hormone infusion unmasks dual (hypothalamic and Leydig cell) defects in the healthy aging male gonadotropic axis. *Europ J Endocrinol* **141**:257–266

Mulligan T, Iranmanesh A, Veldhuis JD (2001) Pulsatile iv infusion of recombinant human LH in leuprolide-suppressed men unmasks impoverished Leydig-cell secretory responsiveness to midphysiological LH drive in the aging male. *J Clin Endocrinol Metab* **86**:5547–5553

Münzer T, Haeman MS, Hees P, Shapiro E, Christmas C, Bellantoni MF, Stevens TE, O'Connor KG, Pabst KM, Clair C Sr, Sorkin JD, Blackman MR (2001) Effects of GH and/or sex steroid administration on abdominal subcutaneous and visceral fat in healthy aged women and men. *J Clin Endocrinol Metab* **86**:3604–3610

Nankin HR, Lin T, Murono EP, Osterman J (1981) The aging Leydig cell III. Gonadotropin stimulation in men. *J Androl* **2**:181–189

Neaves WB, Johnson L, Porter JC, Parker CR, Petty CS (1984) Leydig cell numbers, daily sperm production and gonadotropin levels in aging men. *J Clin Endocrinol Metab* **59**:756–763

Ng KK, Donat R, Chan L, Lalak A, Di Pierro I, Handelsman DJ (2004) Sperm output of older men. *Hum Reprod* **19**:1811–1815

Nieschlag E, Kley KH, Wiegelmann W, Solback HG, Krüskemper HL (1973) Lebensalter und endokrine Funktion der Testes des erwachsenen Mannes. *Deut Med Wschr* **98**:1281–1284

Nieschlag E, Lammers U, Freischem CW, Langer K, Wickings EJ (1982) Reproductive functions in young fathers and grandfathers. *J Clin Endocrinol Metab* **55**:676–681

O'Connell MDL, Roberts SA, Srinivas-Shankar U, Tajar A, Connolly MJ, Adams JE, Oldham JA, Wu FCW (2011) Do the effects of testosterone on muscle strength, physical function, body composition, and quality of life persist six months after treatment in intermediate-frail and frail elderly men? *J Clin Endocrinol Metab* **96**:454–458

Orwoll E, Lambert LC, Marshall LM, Phipps K, Blank J, Barrett-Connor E, Cauley J, Ensrud K, Cummings S, for the Osteoporotic Fractures in Men Study Group (2006a) Testosterone and estradiol among older men. *J Clin Endocrinol Metab* **91**:1336–1344

Orwoll E, Lambert LC, Marshall LM, Blank J, Barrett-Connor E, Cauley J, Ensrud K, Cummings SR, for the Osteoporotic Fractures in Men Study Group (2006b) Endogenous testosterone levels, physical performance, and fall risk in older men. *Arch Intern Med* **166**:2124–2131

Orwoll ES, Klein RF (1995) Osteoporosis in men. *Endocr Rev* **16**:87–115

Orwoll ES, Oviatt S (1992) Transdermal testosterone supplementation in normal older men. In: Program of the 74th Annual Meeting of the Endocrine Society. The Endocrine Society, Bethesda; Abstract 1071

Orwoll ES, Nielson CM, Labrie F, Barrett-Connor E, Cauley JA, Cummings SR, Ensrud K, Karlsson M, Lau E, Leung PC, Lunggren O, Mellström D, Patrick A, Stefanick ML, Nakamura K, Yoshimura N, Zmuda J, Vandenput L, Ohlsson C and for the Osteoporotic Fractures in Men (MrOS) Research Group (2010) Evidence for geographical and racial variation in serum sex steroid levels in older men. *J Clin Endocrinol Metab* **95**: E151–E160

Ottenbacher KJ, Ottenbacher ME, Ottenbacher AJ, Acha AA, Ostir GV (2006) Androgen treatment and muscle strength in elderly men: a meta-analysis. *J Am Geriatr Soc* **54**:1666–1673

Perry PJ, Lund BC, Arndt S, Holman T, Bever-Stille KA, Paulsen J, Demers LM (2001) Bioavailable testosterone as a correlate of cognition, psychological status, quality of life, and sexual function in aging males: implications for testosterone replacement therapy. *Ann Clin Psychiatry* **13**:75–80

Pfeilschifter J, Scheidt-Nave C, Leidig-Bruckner G, Woitge HW, Blum WF, Wüster C, Haack D, Ziegler R (1996) Relationship between circulating insulin-like growth factor components and sex hormones in a population based sample of 50–80 year old men and women. *J Clin Endocrinol Metab* **81**:2534–2540

Phillips GB, Pinkernell BJ, Jing TY (1994) The association of hypotestosteronemia with coronary heart disease. *Arterioscler Thromb* **14**:701–706

Pincus SM, Veldhuis JD, Mulligan T, Iranmanesh A, Evans WS (1997) Effects of age on the irregularity of LH and FSH serum concentrations in women and men. *Am J Physiol* **273**:E989–E995

Pirke KM, Sintermann R, Vogt HJ (1980) Testosterone and testosterone precursors in the spermatic vein and in the testicular tissue of old men. *Gerontology* **26**:221–230

Plymate SR, Tenover JS, Bremner WJ (1989) Circadian variation in testosterone, sex hormone-binding globulin, and calculated non sex hormone-binding globulin bound testosterone in healthy young and elderly men. *J Androl* **10**:366–371

Poggi UI, Arguelles AE, Rosner J, de Laborde NP, Cassini JH, Volmer MC (1976) Plasma testosterone and serum lipids in male survivors of myocardial infarction. *J Steroid Biochem* **7**:229–231

Porto CS, Abreu LC, Gunsalus GL, Bardin CW (1992) Binding of sex hormone binding globulin (SHBG) to testicular membranes and solubilized receptor. *Mol Cell Endocrinol* **89**:33–38

Rajagopal A, Vassilopoulou-Sellin R, Palmer JL, Kaur G, Bruera E (2004) Symptomatic hypogonadism in male survivors of cancer with chronic exposure to opioids. *Cancer* **100**:851–858

Rajfer JK, Namkun PC, Petra Ph (1989) Identification, partial characterization and age associated changes of a cytoplasmatic androgen receptor in the rat penis. *J Steroid Biochem* **33**: 1489–1492

Rhoden EL, Teloken C, Mafessoni R, Souto CA (2002) Is there any relation between serum levels of total testosterone and the severity of erectile dysfunction? *Int J Impot Res* **14**:167–171

Ring HZ, Lessov CN, Reed T, Marcux R, Holloway L, Swan GE, Carmelli D (2005) Heritability of plasma sex hormones and hormone binding globulin in adult male twins. *J Clin Endocrinol Metab* **90**:3653–3658

Rodriguez A, Muller DC, Metter EJ, Maggio M, Harman SM, Blackman MR, Andres R(2007) Aging, androgens, and the metabolic syndrome in a longitudinal study of aging. *J Clin Endocrinol Metab* **92**:3568–3572

Roehrborn CG, Lange JL, George FW, Wilson JD (1987) Changes in amount and intracellular distribution of androgen receptor in human foreskin as a function of age. *J Clin Invest* **79**:44–47

Rogers MA, Evans WJ (1993) Changes in skeletal muscle with aging: effects of exercise training. *Exercise Sports Sci Rev* **21**:65–102

Rohrmann S, Nelson WG, Rifai N, Brown TR, Dobs A, Kanarek N, Yager JD, Platz EA (2007) Serum estrogen, but not testosterone, levels differ between black and white men in a nationally representative sample of Americans. *J Clin Endocrinol Metab* **92**:2519–2525

Rohrmann S, Platz EA, Selvin E, Shielst MS, Joshut CE, Menket A, Feinleibt M, Basaria S, Rifai N, Dobs AS, Kanarek N, Nelson WG (2011) The prevalence of low sex steroid hormone concentrations in men in the Third National Health and Nutrition Examination Survey (NHANES III). *Clin Endocrinol* **75**:232–239

Rolf C, Behre M, Nieschlag E (1996) Reproductive parameters of older compared to younger men of infertile couples. *Int J Androl* **19**:135–142

Rolland Y, Dupuy C, Abellan van Kan G, Gillette S, Vellas B (2011) Treatment strategies for sarcopenia and frailty. *Med Clin N Am* **95**:427–438

Rosner W, Hryb DJ, Kahn MS, Nakhla HM, Romas NA (1991) Sex hormone binding globulin: anatomy and physiology of a new regulating system. *J Steroid Biochem Mol Biol* **40**:813–820

Rosner W, Auchus RJ, Azziz R, Sluss PM, Raff H (2007) Position statement: utility, limitations, and pitfalls in measuring testosterone: an Endocrine Society position statement. *J Clin Endocrinol Metab* **92**:405–413

Roy TA, Blackman MR, Harman SM, Tobin JD, Schrager M, Metter EJ (2002) Interrelationships of serum testosterone and free testosterone index with FFM and strength in aging men. *Am J Physiol Endocrinol Metab* **283**:E284–E294

Rubens R, Dhont M, Vermeulen A (1974) Further studies on Leydig cell function in old age. *J Clin Endocrinol Metab* **39**:40–45

Rubenstein LZ, Josephson KR, Robbins AS (1994) Falls in the nursing home. *Ann Intern Med* **121**: 442–451

Rubin HB, Henson DE, Falvo RE, High RW (1979) The relationship between men's endogenous levels of testosterone and their penile response to erotic stimuli. *Behav Res Ther* **17**:305–312

Ruhayel Y, Malm G, Haugen TB, Henrichsen T, Bjøsvikt C, Grotmol T, Saethert T, Malm J, Figenschau Y, Rylander L, Levine RJ, Giwercman A (2007) Seasonal variation in serum concentrations of reproductive hormones and urinary excretion of 6-sulfatoxymelatonin in men living north and south of the Arctic Circle: a longitudinal study. *Clin Endocrinol* **67**:85–92

Ruige JB, Mahmoud AM, De Bacquer D, Kaufman JM (2011) Endogenous testosterone and cardiovascular disease in healthy men: a meta-analysis. *Heart* **97**:870–875

Russell DW, Wilson JD (1994) Steroid 5α-reductase: two genes/two enzymes. *Annu Rev Biochem* **63**:25–61

Sandblom RE, Matsumoto AM, Scoene RB, Lee KA, Giblin EC, Bremner WJ, Pierson DJ (1983) Obstructive sleep apnea induced by testosterone administration *N Engl J Med* **308**:508–510

Sartorius G, Spasevska S, Idan A, Turner L, Allan L, Ly LP, Conway AJ, McLachlan RI, Handelsman DJ (2011) Older men reporting excellent asymptomatic health exhibit no decline in serum testosterone, dihydrotestosterone or estradiol with age: the healthy man study. *Endocr Rev* **32**:OR35–1 (abstract)

Sasano N, Ichijo S (1969) Vascular patterns of the human testes with special reference to its senile changes. *Tohoku J Exp Med* **99**:269–280

Sattler FR, Castaneda-Sceppa C, Binder EF, Schroeder ET, Wang Y, Bhasin S, Kawakubo M, Stewart Y, Yarasheski KE, Ulloor J, Colletti P, Roubenoff R, Azen SP (2009) Testosterone and growth hormone improve body composition and muscle performance in older men. *J Clin Endocrinol Metab* **94**:1991–2001

Schaap LA, Pluijm SMF, Deeg DJH, Penninx BW, Nicklas BJ, Lips P,

Harris TB, Newman AB, Kritchevsky SB, Cauley JA, Goodpaster BH, Tylavsky FA, Yaffe K, Visser M (2008) Low testosterone levels and decline in physical performance and muscle strength in older men: findings from two prospective cohort studies. *Clin Endocrinol* **68**:42–50

Schiavi RC, Schreiner-Engel P, Mandeli J, Schanzer H, Cohen E (1990) Healthy aging and male sexual function. *Am J Psychiatry* **147**:776–771

Schneider HJ, Sievers C, Klotsche J, Böhler S, Pittrow D, Lehnert H, Wittchen HU, Stalla GK (2009) Prevalence of low male testosterone levels in primary care in Germany: cross-sectional results from the DETECT study. *Clin Endocrinol* **70**:446–454

Schröder FH (1996) The prostate and androgens: the risk of supplementation. In: Oddens B, Vermeulen A (eds) *Androgens and the Aging Male.* Parthenon Publishing Group, New York, pp 223–226

Semple PD, Beastall GH, Brown TM, Stirling KW, Mills RJ, Watson WS (1984) Sex-hormone suppression and sexual impotence in hypoxic pulmonary fibrosis. *Thorax* **39**:46–51

Shahinian VB, Kuo Y, Freeman JL, Goodwin JS (2005) Risk of fracture after androgen deprivation for prostate cancer. *New Engl J Med* **352**:154–164

Sih R, Morley JE, Kaiser FE, Perry HM III, Patrick P, Ross C (1997) Testosterone replacement in older hypogonadal men: a 12 month randomized controlled trial. *J Clin Endocrinol Metab* **82**:1661–1667

Siiteri PK, MacDonald PC (1975) Role of extraglandular estrogen in human endocrinology. In: Greep RD, Astwood B (eds) *Handbook of Physiology*, Vol. II. American Physiological Society, Washington, DC, pp 491–508

Smals AGH, Kloppenburg PWC, Benraad TJ (1976) Circannual cycle in plasma testosterone levels in man. *J Clin Endocrinol Metab* **42**:979–982

Smith KW, Gruman C, Reisine S, Kenny A (2000) Construction and field validation of a self-administered screener for testosterone deficiency (hypogonadism) in aging men. *Clin Endocrinol (Oxf)* **53**:703–711

Sniffen RC (1950) The testes. I. The normal testis. *Arch Pathol* **50**:259–284

Snyder PJ, Peachey H, Berlin JA, Hannoush P, Berlin JA, Loh L, Lendrow DA, Holmes JH, Dlewati A, Santanna J, Rosen CJ, Strom BL (1999a) Effect of testosterone treatment on body composition and muscle strength in men over 65 years of age. *J Clin Endocrinol Metab* **84**:2647–2653

Snyder PJ, Peachey H, Berlin JA, Hannoush P, Berlin JA, Loh L, Holmes JH, Dlewati A, Staley J, Santanna J, Kapoor SC, Attie MF, Haddad JG Jr, Strom BL (1999b) Effect of testosterone treatment on bone mineral density in men over 65 years of age. *J Clin Endocrinol Metab* **84**:1966–1972

Snyder PJ, Peachey H, Berlin JA, Hannoush P, Haddad G, Dlewati A, Santanna J, Loh L, Lenrow DA, Holmes JH, Kapoor SC, Atkinson LE, Strom BL (2000) Effects of testosterone replacement in hypogonadal men. *J Clin Endocrinol Metab* **85**:2670–2677

Sparrow D, Silbert JE, Rowe JW (1980) The influence of age, alcohol consumption, and body build on gonadal function in men. *J Clin Endocrinol Metab* **51**:508–512

Spratt DI, O'Dea L, Schoenfeld D, Butler J, Narashimha H, Rao P, Crowley WF (1988) Neuroendocrine-gonadal axis in men: frequent sampling of LH, FSH and testosterone. *Am J Physiol* **254**: E658–E666

Spratt DI, Cox P, Orav J, Moloney J, Bigos T (1993) Reproductive axis suppression in acute illness is related to disease severity. *J Clin Endocrinol Metab* **76**:1548–1554

Srinivas-Shankar U, Roberts SA, Connolly MJ, O'Connell MDL, Adams JE, Oldham JA, Wu FCW (2010) Effects of testosterone on muscle strength, physical function, body composition, and quality of life in intermediate-frail and frail elderly men: a randomized, double-blind, placebo-controlled study. *J Clin Endocrinol Metab* **95**:639–650

Stanley HL, Schmitt BP, Poses RM, Deiss WP (1991) Does hypogonadism contribute to the occurrence of a minimal trauma hip fracture in elderly men? *JAGS* **39**:766–771

Stanworth RD, Kapoor D, Channer KS, Jones TH (2008) Androgen receptor CAG repeat polymorphism is associated with serum testosterone levels, obesity and serum leptin in men with type 2 diabetes. *Eur J Endocrinol* **159**:739–746

Steidle C, Schwartz S, Jacoby K, Sebree T, Smith T, Bachand R (2003) AA2500 testosterone gel normalizes androgen levels in aging males with improvements in body composition and sexual function. *J Clin Endocrinol Metab* **88**:2673–2681

Stoch AS, Parker RA, Chen L, Bubley G, Ko Y-J, Vincelette A, Greenspan SL (2001) Bone loss in men with prostate cancer treated with gonadotropin-releasing hormone agonists. *J Clin Endocrinol Metab* **86**:2787–2791

Stripp B, Taylor AA, Bartter FC, Gillette JR, Loriaux DL, Easley R, Menard RH (1975) Effect of spironolactone on sex hormones in man. *J Clin Endocrinol Metab* **41**:777–781

Suoranta H (1971) Changes in small vessels of the adult testes in relation to age and some pathological conditions. *Virchows Arch A Pathol Pathol Anat* **352**:765–781

Svartberg J, Jorde R, Sundsfjord J, Bønaa KH, Barrett-Connor E (2003) Seasonal variation of testosterone and waist to hip ratio in men: the

Tromsø Study. *J Clin Endocrinol Metab* **88**:3099–3104

Swartz CM, Young MA (1987) Low serum testosterone and myocardial infarction in geriatric male patients. *J Am Geriatr Soc* **35**:39–44

Tajar A, Forti G, O'Neill TW, Lee DM, Silman AJ, Finn JD, Bartfai G, Boonen S, Casanueva FF, Giwercman A, Han TS, Kula K, Labrie F, Lean MEJ, Pendleton N, Punab M, Vanderschueren D, Huhtaniemi IT, Wu FCW; EMAS Group (2010) Characteristics of secondary, primary, and compensated hypogonadism in aging men: evidence from the European Male Ageing Study. *J Clin Endocrinol Metab* **95**:1810–1818

Tapia-Serrano R, Jimenez-Baldera FJ, Murrieta S, Bravo-Gatica C, Guerra R, Mintz G (1991) Testicular function in active ankylosing spondylitis – therapeutic response to human chorionic gonadotrophin. *J Rheumatol* **18**:841–848

Tenover JS (1994) Androgen administration to aging men. *Endocrinol Metab Clin N Am* **23**:877–889

Tenover JS, Matsumoto AM, Plymate SR, Bremner WJ (1987) The effects of aging in normal men on bioavailable testosterone and luteinizing hormone secretion: response to clomiphene citrate. *J Clin Endocrinol Metab* **65**:1118–1126

Tenover JS, Matsumoto AM, Clifton DK, Bremmer WJ (1988) Age related alterations in the circadian rhythms of pulsatile luteinizing hormone and testosterone secretion in healthy men. *J Gerontol* **43**: M163–M169

Thompson IM, Goodman PJ, Tangen CM, Lucia MS, Miller GJ, Ford LG, Lieber MM, Cespedes RD, Atkins JN, Lippman SM, Carlin SM, Ryan A, Szczepanek CM, Crowley JJ, Coltman CA Jr (2003) The influence of finasteride on the development of prostate cancer. *N Engl J Med* **349**:215–224

Tracz MJ, Sideras K, Bolona ER, Haddad RM, Kennedy CC, Uraga MV, Caples SM, Erwin PJ, Montori VM (2006) Testosterone use in men and its effects on bone health. A systematic review and meta-analysis of randomized placebo-controlled trials. *J Clin Endocrinol Metab* **91**:2011–2016

Travison TG, Morley JE, Araujo AB, O'Donnell AB, McKinlay JB (2006) The relationship between libido and testosterone levels in aging men. *J Clin Endocrinol Metab* **91**:2509–2513

Travison TG, Araujo AB, Kupelian V, O'Donnell AB, McKinlay JB (2007) The relative contributions of aging, health, and lifestyle factors to serum testosterone decline in men. *J Clin Endocrinol Metab* **92**:549–555

Travison TG, Nguyen AH, Naganathan V, Stanaway FF, Blyth FM, Cumming RG, Le Couteur DG, Sambrook PN, Handelsman DJ (2011) Changes in reproductive hormone concentrations predict the prevalence and progression of the frailty syndrome in older men: the concord health and ageing in men project. *J Clin Endocrinol Metab* **96**:2464–2474

Tsitouras PD, Bulat T (1995) The aging male reproductive system. *Endocrinol Metab Clin* **24**:297–315

Tsitouras PD, Martin CE, Harman SM (1982) Relation of serum testosterone to sexual activity in healthy elderly men. *J Gerontol* **37**:288–293

T'Sjoen G, Goemaere S, De Meyere M, Kaufman JM (2004) Perception of males' aging symptoms, health and well-being in elderly community-dwelling men is not related to circulating androgen levels. *Psychoneuroendocrinology* **29**:201–214

T'Sjoen GG, Giagulli VA, Delva H, Crabbe P, De Bacquer D, Kaufman JM (2005a) Comparative assessment in young and elderly men of the gonadotropin response to aromatase inhibition. *J Clin Endocrinol Metab* **90**:5717–5722

T'Sjoen GG, De Vos S, Goemaere S, Van Pottelbergh I, Dierick M, Van Heeringen C, Kaufman JM (2005b) Sex steroid level, androgen receptor polymorphism, and depressive symptoms in healthy elderly men. *J Am Geriatr Soc* **53**:636–642

Turner HE, Wass JAH (1997) Gonadal function in men with chronic illness. *Clin Endocrinol* **47**:379–403

Udry JR, Billy JO, Morris NM, Groff TR, Raj MH (1985) Serum androgenic hormones motivate normal behavior in adolescent boys. *Fertil Steril* **43**:90–94

Urban RJ, Veldhuis JD, Blizzard R, Dufau ML (1988) Attenuated release of biologically active luteinizing hormone in healthy aging men. *J Clin Invest* **81**: 1020–1029

Vanbillemont G, Bogaert V, De Bacquer D, Lapauw B, Goemaere S, Toye K, Van Steen K, Taes Y, Kaufman JM (2009) Polymorphisms of the SHBG gene contribute to the interindividual variation of sex steroid hormone blood levels in young, middle-aged and elderly men. *Clin Endocrinol* **70**:303–310

van den Beld AW, de Jong FH, Grobbee DE, Pols HAP, Laberts SWJ (2000) Measures of bioavailable serum testosterone and estradiol and their relationships with muscle strength, bone density, and body composition in elderly men. *J Clin Endocrinol Metab* **85**:3276–3282

van den Beld AW, Bots ML, Janssen JA, Pols HA, Lamberts SW, Grobbee DE (2003) Endogenous hormones and carotid atherosclerosis in elderly men. *Am J Epidemiol* **157**:25–31

Vandenberghe G, Weekers F, Baxter RC, Wouters P, Iranmanesh A, Bouillon R, Veldhuis JD (2001) Five-day pulsatile gonadotropin releasing hormone administration unveils combined hypothalamic-pituitary-gonadal defects underlying profound hypoandrogenism in men with prolonged critical illness. *J Clin Endocrinol Metab* **86**:3217–3226

Van Den Saffele JK, Goemaere S, De Bacquer D, Kaufman JM (1999) Serum leptin levels in healthy ageing men: are decreased serum testosterone and increased adiposity in elderly men the consequence of leptin deficiency? *Clin Endocrinol* **51**:81–88

Van Pottelbergh I, Lumbroso S, Goemaere S, Sultan C, Kaufman JM (2001) Lack of influence of the androgen receptor gene, CAG repeat polymorphism on sex steroid status and bone metabolism in elderly men. *Clin Endocrinol* **55**:659–666

Van Pottelbergh I, Goemaere S, Kaufman JM (2003a) Bioavailable estradiol and an aromatase gene polymorphism are determinants of bone mineral density changes in men over 70 years of age. *J Clin Endocrinol Metab* **88**:3075–3081

Van Pottelbergh I, Braeckman L, De Bacquer D, De Backer G, Kaufman JM (2003b) Differential contribution of testosterone and estradiol in the determination of cholesterol and lipoprotein profile in healthy middle-aged men. *Atherosclerosis* **166**:95–102

Veldhuis JD, King JC, Urban RJ, Rogol AD, Evans WS, Kolp LA, Johnson ML (1987) Operating characteristics of the male hypothalamo-pituitary-gonadal axis. Pulsatile release of testosterone and follicle stimulating hormone and their temporal coupling with luteinizing hormone. *J Clin Endocrinol Metab* **65**:929–941

Veldhuis JD, Urban RJ, Lizarralde G, Johnson ML, Iranmanesh A (1992) Attenuation of luteinizing hormone secretory burst amplitude as a proximate basis for the hypoandrogenism of healthy aging men. *J Clin Endocrinol Metab* **75**:707–713

Veldhuis JD, Wilkowski MJ, Zwart AD, Urban RJ, Lizarralde G,

Iranmanesh A, Bolton WK (1993) Evidence for attenuation of hypothalamic gonadotropin-releasing hormone (GnRH) impulse strength with preservation of GnRH pulse frequency in men with chronic renal failure. *J Clin Endocrinol Metab* **76**:648–654

Veldhuis JD, Iranmanesh A, Godschalk M, Mulligan T (2000) Older men manifest multifold synchrony disruption of reproductive neurohormone outflow. *J Clin Endocrinol Metab* **85**:1477–1486

Veldhuis JD, Zwart A, Mulligan T, Iranmanesh A (2001) Muting of androgen negative feedback unveils impoverished gonadotropin-releasing hormone/luteinizing hormone secretory reactivity in healthy older men. *J Clin Endocrinol Metab* **86**:529–535

Vermeulen A (1991) Clinical Review 24: Androgens in the aging male. *J Clin Endocrinol Metab* **73**:221–224

Vermeulen A (2001) Androgen replacement therapy in the aging male – a critical evaluation. *J Clin Endocrinol Metab* **86**:2380–2390

Vermeulen A, Deslypere JP (1986) Intratesticular unconjugated steroids in elderly men. *J Steroid Biochem* **24**:1079–1083

Vermeulen A, Kaufman JM (1992) Role of the hypothalamo-pituitary function in the hypoandrogenism of healthy aging. *J Clin Endocrinol Metab* **74**:1226A–1226C

Vermeulen A, Kaufman JM (2002) Diagnosis of hypogonadism in the aging male. *Aging Male* **5**:170–176

Vermeulen A, Verdonck G (1992) Representativeness of a single point plasma testosterone level for the long term hormonal milieu in men. *J Clin Endocrinol Metab* **74**:939–942

Vermeulen A, Stoica T, Verdonck L (1971) The apparent free testosterone concentration, an index of androgenicity. *J Clin Endocrinol Metab* **33**:759–767

Vermeulen A, Rubens R, Verdonck L (1972) Testosterone secretion and

Metabolism in male senescence. *J Clin Endocrinol Metab* **34**:730–735

Vermeulen A, Giagulli VA, De Schepper P, Buntinx A, Stoner E (1989a) Hormonal effects of an orally active 4-azasteroid inhibitor of 5 alpha-reductase in humans. *Prostate* **14**:45–53

Vermeulen A, Deslypere JP, Kaufman JM (1989b) Influence of antiopioids on luteinizing hormone pulsatility in aging men. *J Clin Endocrinol Metab* **68**:68–72

Vermeulen A, Kaufman JM, Giagulli VA (1996) Influence of some biological indices on sex hormone binding globulin and androgen levels in aging and obese males. *J Clin Endocrinol Metab* **81**:1821–1827

Vermeulen A, Goemaere S, Kaufman JM (1999a) Sex hormones, body composition and aging. *Aging Male* **2**:8–16

Vermeulen A, Verdonck L, Kaufman JM (1999b) A critical evaluation of simple methods for the estimation of free testosterone in serum. *J Clin Endocrinol Metab* **84**:3666–3672

Wallace EM, Pye SD, Wild ST, Wu FCW (1993) Prostate specific antigen and prostate gland size in men receiving exogenous testosterone for male contraception. *Int J Androl* **16**:35–40

Wang C, Chan V, Yeung RTT (1978) Effect of surgical stress on pituitary testicular function. *Clin Endocrinol* **9**:255–266

Wang C, Nieschlag E, Swerdloff R, Behre HM, Hellstrom WJ, Gooren LJ, Kaufman JM, Legros JJ, Lunenfeld B, Morales A, Morley JE, Schulman C, Thompson IM, Weidner W, Wu FCW (2008) Investigation, treatment and monitoring of late-onset hypogonadism in males. *Eur J Endocrinol* **159**:507–514

Wheeler MJ, Barnes SC (2008) measurement of testosterone in the diagnosis of hypogonadism in the ageing male. *Clin Endocrinol* **69**:515–525

Winters SJ, Sherins RJ, Troen P (1984) The gonadotropin suppressive activity of androgen is increased in elderly men. *Metabolism* **33**:1052–1059

Winters SJ, Atkinson L for the Testoderm Study Group (1997) Serum LH concentrations in hypogonadal men during transdermal testosterone replacement through scrotal skin: further evidence that ageing enhances testosterone negative feedback. *Clin Endocrinol* **47**: 317–322

Winters SJ, Brufsky A, Weissfeld J, Trump DL, Dyky MA, Hadeed V (2001) Testosterone, sex hormone binding globulin and body composition in young adult African, American and Caucasian men. *Metabolism* **50**:1242–1247

Woolf PD, Hamill RW, McDonald JV, Lee LA, Kelly M (1985) Transient hypogonadotropic hypogonadism caused by critical illness. *J Clin Endocrinol Metab* **60**: 444–450

Worstman J, Eagleton LE, Rosner W, Dufau ML (1987) Mechanism for the hypotestosteronemia of the sleep apnea syndrome. *Am J Med Sci* **293**:221–225

Wu FC, von Eckardstein A (2003) Androgens and coronary artery disease. *Endocr Rev* **24**: 183–217

Wu FC, Tajar A, Pye SR, Silman AJ, Finn JD, O'Neill TW, Bartfai G, Casanueva F, Forti G, Giwercman A, Huhtaniemi IT, Kula K, Punab M, Boonen S, Vanderschueren D; The European Male Aging Study Group (2008) Hypothalamic-pituitary-testicular axis disruptions in older men are differentially linked to age and modifiable risk factor: the European male aging study. *J Clin Endocrinol Metab* **93**:2737–2745

Wu FCW, Tajar A, Beynon JM, Pye SR, Silman AJ, Finn JD, O'Neill TW, Bartfai G, Casanueva FF, Forti G, Giwercman A, Han TS, Kula K, Lean MEJ, Pendleton N, Punab M, Boonen S, Vanderschueren D, Labrie F, Huhtaniemi IT, for the EMAS Group (2010) Identification of late-onset hypogonadism in middle-aged and elderly men. *N Engl J Med* **363**: 123–135

Yeap BB, Chubb SAP, Hyde Z, Jamrozik K, Hankey GJ, Flicker L, Norman PE (2009a) Lower serum testosterone is independently associated with insulin resistance in non-diabetic older men: the health in men study. *Eur J Endocrinol* **161**:591–598

Yeap BB, Hyde Z, Almeida OP, Norman PE, Chubb P, Hamrozik K, Flicker L, Hankey GJ (2009b) Lower testosterone levels predict incident stroke and transient ischemic attack in older men. *J Clin Endocrinol Metab* **94**: 2353–2359

Yeap BB, Hyde Z, Norman PE, Chubb SAP, Golledge J (2010) Associations of total testosterone, sex hormone-binding globulin, calculated free testosterone, and luteinizing hormone with prevalence of abdominal aortic aneurysm in older men. *J Clin Endocrinol Metab* **95**:1123–1130

Zitzmann M, Nieschlag E (2003) The CAG repeat polymorphism within the androgen receptor gene and maleness. *Int J Androl* **26**:76–83

Zitzmann M, Brune M, Kornmann B, Gromoll J, Junker R, Nieschlag E (2001) The CAG repeat polymorphism in the AR gene affects bone density and bone metabolism in healthy males. *Clin Endocrinol* **55**:649–657

Zitzmann M, Faber S, Nieschlag E (2006) Association of specific symptoms and metabolic risks with serum testosterone in older men. *J Clin Endocrinol Metab* **91**:4335–4343

Zmuda JM, Cauley JA, Kriska A, Glynn NW, Gutai JP, Kuller LH (1997) Longitudinal relation between endogenous testosterone and cardiovascular disease risk factors in middle-aged men: a 13-year follow-up of former Multiple Risk Factor Intervention Trial Participants. *Am J Epidemiol* **146**:609–617

Zumoff B, Bradlow L, Finkelstein J, Boyar RM, Hellman L (1976) The influence of age and sex on the metabolism of testosterone. *J Clin Endocrinol Metab* **42**:703–706

17.1 Introduction

Male reproductive function is markedly influenced by non-gonadal disease, with mild androgen deficiency almost a universal consequence of chronic disease. While this centrally mediated hormonal-axis response to chronic illness is inherently reversible, in theory, with sufficiently severe or prolonged underlying illness, this secondary androgen deficiency might contribute to the disease pathophysiology and clinical manifestations. Furthermore, androgens are therapeutic drugs with potent effects on androgen-sensitive tissues, such as muscle, bone, brain, liver or adipose

Testosterone: Action, Deficiency, Substitution, ed. Eberhard Nieschlag and Hermann M. Behre, Assoc. ed. Susan Nieschlag.
Published by Cambridge University Press. © Cambridge University Press 2012.

tissue, which may be exploited pharmacologically for therapeutic benefit, subject to comparable efficacy, safety and cost-effectiveness criteria as applicable to other xenobiotic drugs.

As an adjunct to standard medical care, androgen therapy may be considered as either physiological androgen replacement or, more usually, as pharmacological androgen therapy. Androgen replacement therapy aims to replicate endogenous androgen exposure, thereby limiting it to the use of testosterone in doses intended to produce physiological blood testosterone concentrations. To the degree it replicates endogenous androgen exposure, the expectation for safety may reasonably be compared with the benchmark of life-long health experience of eugonadal men.

By contrast, pharmacological androgen therapy is no different from pharmacotherapy with any xenobiotic drug used to achieve a therapeutic goal. It utilizes any androgen, without restriction to testosterone or reference to replacement doses, to optimal effect as judged by the standards of efficacy, safety and cost-effectiveness applicable to other drugs. Pharmacological androgen therapy has usually involved synthetic, orally active androgens rather than testosterone, because of industry preference for oral medications. Nearly all orally active androgens are from the 17α-alkylated class of synthetic androgens which is now obsolete for androgen replacement therapy due to its class-specific risk of hepatotoxicity and the availability of suitable alternative testosterone products. The development of non-steroidal androgens, marketed as "selective androgen receptor modulators" (SARMs), offers new possibilities for adjuvant pharmacological androgen therapy. In contrast to the full spectrum of androgen effects of testosterone, such SARMs would be pure androgens not subject to tissue-specific activation by aromatization to a corresponding estrogen or to amplification of androgenic potency by 5a-reduction. In this context the endogenous pure androgens nandrolone and DHT can be considered prototype SARMs. SARMs are not the modern embodiment of so-called "anabolic steroids," an outdated term referring to hypothetical but non-existent non-virilizing androgens targeted exclusively to muscle, a failed concept lacking biological proof of principle (Handelsman 2011).

The goals of androgen therapy for non-gonadal disease must be considered in relation to the natural history of the underlying disease. Mild androgen deficiency, evident in altered blood hormonal levels but without distinctive clinical features, is a universal, non-specific biochemical consequence of systemic disease, which is reversible upon alleviation of the underlying disorder. If the androgen deficiency is unusually severe or prolonged, it might contribute to morbidity from the underlying disease but is unlikely to change the mortality (Liu et al. 2003a). The latter follows from recognizing that even severe, lifelong androgen deficiency has minimal influence on life expectancy, as seen in congenital genetic androgen insensitivity (Quigley et al. 1995), castration before puberty (Nieschlag et al. 1993; Jenkins 1998) or Klinefelter syndrome (Bojesen et al. 2004); by contrast, castration of institutionalized adults has been reported to prolong (Hamilton and Mestler 1969) or shorten (Eyben et al. 2005) life expectancy, although the latter studies are severely confounded by the reasons prompting castration (Eyman et al. 1990). Hence pharmacological androgen therapy in systemic disease can realistically aim to palliate symptoms and improve QoL without expecting to improve mortality unless it ameliorates the natural mortality history of the underlying disease. Furthermore, the potential short-term benefits of pharmacological androgen therapy on QoL must be balanced against potentially detrimental long-term effects of androgen therapy.

Recognizing the few well-established indications for pharmacological androgen therapy, placebo controls remain the hallmark of high-quality clinical studies. In addition, desirable clinical-trial design features include reliable, realistic diagnostic criteria, adequate power and duration, with valid, objective clinical end-points (rather than surrogates). Unfortunately, few studies fulfill such stringent criteria, and the available body of knowledge therefore provides little reliable guidance for practical therapeutics. Therefore this chapter focuses on better controlled clinical studies rather than covering the plethora of papers reported over more than seven decades since testosterone was first used clinically (Hamilton 1937). A comprehensive account of early, mostly poorly or uncontrolled, studies of androgen therapy up to the mid-1970s is contained in classical comprehensive textbooks (Krüskemper 1968; Kochakian 1976).

Effects of androgen replacement therapy (Chapter 14), as well as androgen effects on bone (Chapter 8), cardiovascular disease (Chapter 10) and related metabolic disorders (Chapter 11), prostate diseases (Chapter 13) and male aging (Chapter 16), as well as in women (Chapter 23), are covered in detail elsewhere in this book. Observational studies of systemic disease effects on male reproductive health are reviewed elsewhere (Handelsman 2010a).

17.2   Liver disease

17.2.1   Cirrhosis

In studies dating back to the 1960s, pharmacological androgen therapy does not alter the natural history of alcoholic cirrhosis (Rambaldi and Gluud 2006). The earliest controlled studies of androgen therapy to ameliorate the natural history of alcoholic cirrhosis claimed a survival benefit (Wells 1960), whereas another failed to confirm these findings (Fenster 1966); however, neither was large nor long enough to be definitive. The best evidence derived from the Copenhagen Study Group for Liver Disease, which enrolled 221 men with alcoholic cirrhosis in a three-year prospective, double-blinded, randomized, placebo-controlled study, testing oral micronized testosterone (600 mg daily) (Copenhagen Study Group for Liver Diseases 1986). This study showed convincingly no benefit in mortality, hepatic histology, liver hemodynamics and biochemical function or in sexual dysfunction. The negative outcome with sufficient power to exclude a 35% decrease in mortality was at variance with previous poorly controlled reports (Kopera 1976). The observation of portal vein thrombosis in three men treated with testosterone may be related to the distinctive testosterone pharmacokinetics in chronic liver disease (Nieschlag *et al.* 1977; Gluud et *al.* 1981), demonstrating markedly supraphysiological peripheral blood testosterone concentrations at standard clinical doses, presumably due to the high blood SHBG levels in chronic liver disease, and reflecting even more extreme portal blood testosterone concentrations(Gluud *et al.* 1987; 1988).

17.2.2   Hepatitis

Short-term controlled studies of androgen therapy in men with alcoholic hepatitis provide no convincing evidence of any clinical benefit (Rambaldi and Gluud 2006). A prospective, randomized, multicenter Veterans Administration study claimed a mortality benefit after 30 days of oxandrolone treatment (80 mg daily), compared with placebo in 263 men presenting with alcoholic hepatitis (Mendenhall *et al.* 1984). The imprecise entry criteria and end-points (Maddrey 1986) and short-term benefits of that study were not confirmed in a further study of 271 poorly nourished men with alcoholic hepatitis randomized to treatment with oxandrolone plus high calorie food supplements compared with a group receiving placebo without dietary supplementation (Mendenhall *et al.* 1993). This study showed no overall survival benefit on primary intention-to-treat analysis; however, post-hoc subgroup analysis claiming a significant short-term survival benefit remained unconvincing due to the study design and analysis methodology. Another small randomized, controlled study of 19 men and 20 women with alcoholic hepatitis treated with 80 mg oxandrolone, parenteral nutrition, both or neither for 21 days demonstrated modest improvement in hepatic biochemical function but did not report other clinical end-points (Bonkovsky *et al.* 1991).

17.2.3   Androgen-induced liver disorders

A consistent adverse feature of pharmacological androgen therapy, regardless of indication, is the risk of 17α-alkylated androgen-induced liver disorders (Ishak and Zimmerman 1987). These involve biochemical effects on hepatic function, hepatotoxicity (hepatitic or cholestatic) and liver tumor development (benign or malignant), and peliosis hepatis, reflecting the full range of class-specific adverse effects of oral 17α-alkylated androgens. No reliable estimates of the incidence or prevalence of such alkylated androgen-induced hepatotoxicity are available, although claims based on post-marketing surveillance suggest a low prevalence with low doses used in women in some (Phillips *et al.* 2003; Orr and Fiatarone Singh 2004) but not all reviews (Velazquez and Alter 2004). The East German national sports doping program using oral 17α-alkylated androgens resulted in deaths from liver failure and chronic liver disease (Franke and Berendonk 1997). Every marketed 17α-alkylated androgen is associated with hepatotoxicity; whereas other androgens (1-methyl androgens, nandrolone, testosterone, DHT) have minimal risk (Ishak and Zimmerman 1987; Velazquez and Alter 2004). Biochemical hepatic function is consistently impaired by oral 17α-alkylated androgens, most frequently manifest clinically as cholestasis. Androgen-induced hepatitis, peliosis and tumors are less frequent but unpredictable. Blood SHBG concentrations are significantly reduced by any oral androgen as well as supraphysiological circulating testosterone concentrations in peripheral or portal blood (Conway *et al.* 1988). This indicates that SHBG can serve as a useful, sensitive index of hepatic androgen over-dosage.

17.3 Hematological disorders

17.3.1 Erythropoiesis and polycythemia

Androgen therapy has long been used clinically to stimulate erythropoiesis (Shahidi 1973), since the original observational study of 68 women with breast cancer demonstrating significant, sometimes dramatic, increases in hemoglobin after administering 100 mg testosterone or dihydrotestosterone propionate injections three times weekly (Kennedy and Gilbertsen 1957). In addition, androgen therapy has smaller and less consistent effects on other bone marrow cell lineages that produce neutrophils and platelets. Androgen therapy increases hemoglobin in healthy men (Palacios et al. 1983; Wu et al. 1996) as well as augmenting the hemoglobin responses to recombinant human erythropoietin (EPO) in renal anemia (Ballal et al. 1991) and iron supplementation in iron deficiency anemia (Victor et al. 1967). The molecular mechanism of androgen-induced stimulation of erythrogenesis remains poorly understood. Stimulation of erythropoietin secretion, augmentation of erythropoietin action and reduction in circulating levels of hepcidin, an iron transport protein (Bachman et al. 2010), have been proposed as non-exclusive mechanisms of action. The hemoglobin response to standard testosterone doses is usually modest in magnitude (typically ~10 g/l), with overt polycythemia occurring in a small proportion (~1%) of normal (Palacios et al. 1983; Wu et al. 1996) or hypogonadal (Krauss et al. 1991; Drinka et al. 1995) men; whereas high androgen doses produce higher rates (~8%) of polycythemia (Idan et al. 2010). This risk of androgen-induced polycythemia is increased in men with higher baseline hemoglobin (Idan et al. 2010), on higher androgen dose (Idan et al. 2010; Ip et al. 2010) or using injectable testosterone esters (Jockenhövel et al. 1997; Siddique et al. 2004) rather than more stable, steady-state testosterone delivery transdermally (Lakshman and Basaria 2009) or by depot implants (Handelsman et al. 1997); while the suspected contributions of high-altitude residence and hypoxia (Gore et al. 2007) and underlying chronic respiratory failure (Kent et al. 2011) or sleep apnea (Choi et al. 2006) remain to be confirmed. Androgen-induced polycythemia may be asymptomatic or produce significant clinical effects due to hyperviscosity and/or ischemia. It is usually reversible following interruption of androgen treatment, but occasionally acute clinical circumstances (e.g. unstable angina or transient ischemic attack) may warrant venesection. Following recovery from testosterone-induced polycythemia, its dose dependency allows for resuming testosterone treatment with careful monitoring, using a steady-state preparation gel or long-acting depot.

17.3.2 Anemia due to marrow failure

In severe aplastic anemia, a major study of 110 patients compared HLA-identical marrow transplantation with oral, im or no androgen therapy (Camitta et al. 1979). This showed a major survival advantage (70% vs. 35% six-month survival) for 47 patients having HLA-identical bone marrow transplantation compared with 63 patients in whom no donor was available who were randomized to oral (oxymetholone 3–5 mg/kg·day), intramuscular (nandrolone decanoate 3–5 mg/kg·wk) or no androgen therapy (Camitta et al. 1979). The latter three groups did not differ in survival; a finding consistent with another small randomized study that showed no survival benefit due to androgen therapy (50–100 mg nandrolone phenylpropionate weekly) compared with placebo vehicle injections (Branda et al. 1977).

In standard non-transplantation treatment for aplastic anemia, a randomized crossover study of 44 patients concluded that anti-thymocyte globulin (ATG) was superior to androgen therapy (nandrolone decanoate 5 mg/kg·wk). This conclusion was, however, flawed, as half the patients had failed prior androgen therapy, thus constituting an entry bias against androgen therapy (Young et al. 1988). Coupled with ATG, androgen therapy appears to offer morbidity but not mortality benefit in aplastic anemia. A randomized, controlled multicenter study of the European Bone Marrow Transplantation in Severe Aplastic Anaemia Study Group of 134 patients with newly diagnosed severe aplastic anemia receiving standard therapy (including ATG and methylprednisolone) demonstrated an improvement in transfusion independence due to treatment with oxymetholone (2 mg/kg·day) compared with placebo (Bacigalupo et al. 1993). However, there was no overall benefit in survival that was determined principally by the severity of disease based on leukocyte count. These findings confirmed the benefit of androgen therapy on transfusion independence but not survival from two smaller randomized, placebo-controlled studies involving 61 patients using oral metenolone acetate

(2–3 mg/kg·day) (Li Bock *et al.* 1976; Kaltwasser *et al.* 1988), but contradict another randomized, placebo-controlled study which found no benefit from androgen therapy (fluoxymesterone 25 mg/m^2·day or oxymetholone 4 mg/kg·day) over placebo in 53 patients (Champlin *et al.* 1985). None of these studies reported survival benefits or formally evaluated QoL, and all frequently observed female virilization.

An important pair of studies attempted to define the optimal dosage and type of androgen therapy for aplastic anemia (French Cooperative Group for the Study of Aplastic and Refractory Anaemias 1986). In the first study, 110 patients were randomized into four groups according to androgen (norethandrolone, fluoxymesterone) and dose (high, 1 mg/kg·day; low, 0.2 mg/kg·day). Survival was mainly influenced by disease severity, but, in less severe cases, high-dose androgen therapy significantly improved survival over low-dose androgen therapy. Despite randomization, there were imbalances between treatment groups with respect to disease severity and age that undermine the interpretability of the findings. In the second study, 125 patients were randomized to four different androgens – norethandrolone, stanozolol, fluoxymesterone (all at 1 mg/kg·day) or testosterone undecanoate (1.7 mg/kg·day). The fluoxymesterone treatment group had the best and stanozolol the worst survival; with norethandrolone and testosterone undecanoate being equivalent and intermediate in efficacy. Once again, however, the treatment groups were unbalanced with respect to disease severity and age. Hence the reported benefit limited to the less severe and older (>30 year) cases remains dubious. The superiority of any specific androgen remains to be unequivocally demonstrated, with particular difficulty in comparing effective doses of different androgens.

The French Cooperative Study Group also reported a series of cohort studies examining the efficacy of androgen therapy in patients with aplastic anemia. Their initial cohort randomized 352 men and women to treatment with metandienone (1 mg/kg·day), oxymetholone (2.5 mg/kg·day), metenolone acetate (2.5 mg/kg·day) or norethandrolone (1 mg/kg·day). The metandienone group had the best, whereas oxymetholone and metenolone groups exhibited equally the worst two-year survival from randomization (Cooperative Group for the Study of Aplastic and Refractory Anaemias 1979). However, treatment groups were unbalanced for disease severity, the principal determinant of survival. Despite post-hoc stratified

analyses, it remains ultimately difficult to conclude whether underlying disease prognosis or drug effects explained the differences in group survival. In a follow-up study from the same cohort who survived at least two years from initial randomization, 137 patients were re-randomized to rapid (3 month) or slow (20 month) withdrawal of their original androgen therapy. The slow withdrawal group had a higher rate of maintained remission consistent with androgen therapy, having maintained a clinical benefit, presumably via maintenance of hemoglobin levels, but no survival data were reported (Najean and Joint Group for the Study of Aplastic and Refractory Anaemias 1981). More recent findings continue to support an effective role for androgen therapy as part of immunosuppressive (non-transplant) therapy for aplastic anemia (Leleu *et al.* 2006).

Overall, androgen therapy does not improve survival in aplastic anemia but provides a morbidity benefit by maintaining hemoglobin and transfusion independence, although the improved quality of life has not been quantified. In severe aplastic anemia, bone marrow transplantation from an HLA-identical sibling (if feasible) is the preferred treatment and superior to androgen therapy. Androgen therapy may be useful in less severe aplastic anemia for which bone marrow transplantation is not available or justified (Marwaha *et al.* 2004; Jaime-Perez *et al.* 2011), or where the primary disease is refractory or relapses after primary marrow transplantation (Füreder and Valent 2011). However, the relative merits of androgen therapy compared with HLA-non-identical bone marrow transplantation or in the presence of failing or failed bone marrow transplantation have not been clearly defined. Although it is prudent to avoid injectable androgens in a population that may be thrombocytopenic, the preponderant use of oral 17α-alkylated androgens in aplastic anemia appears unjustified when non-hepatotoxic oral androgens such as 1-methyl androgens (metenolone, mesterolone) and testosterone undecanoate appear to be equally effective.

17.3.3 Myeloproliferative disorders

The use of androgen therapy in other causes of bone marrow failure has been less extensively studied. One controlled study of 29 patients with myeloproliferative disorders randomized patients to treatment with fluoxymesterone (30 mg daily) compared with transfusions alone, but was terminated prematurely due to slow recruitment and poor hemoglobin response, with only 4/14 achieving an increase of >10 g/l (Brubaker *et al.* 1982). These findings are supported by another randomized study of 56 patients with myelodysplasia which found oral metenolone acetate (2.5 mg/kg·day) no better than intravenous cytarabine or symptomatic maintenance therapy (Najean and Pecking 1979). Androgens remain part of standard supportive care for myeloproliferative disorders (Reilly 2006).

17.3.4 Thrombocytopenia

Experimental evidence suggests a role for endogenous (Whitnall *et al.* 2000) or synthetic androgens (Hosseinimehr *et al.* 2006) to reduce irradiation-induced marrow failure of platelets or leukocytes. A beneficial effect of androgen therapy in thrombocytopenia due to marrow failure has been suggested by a study in myelodysplasia associated with thrombocytopenia, in which 20 patients were randomized to receive either danazol (600 mg daily) or fluoxymesterone (1 mg/kg·day). Although both groups had an impressive response in termination of clinical bleeding (6/6) and increasing platelet count (11/20), the lack of a placebo group means that the contribution of natural remission could not be evaluated (Wattel *et al.* 1994).

The role of androgen therapy in immune thrombocytopenic purpura (ITP) remains poorly defined in the absence of controlled clinical trials. Two short-term observational studies have reported that danazol increases platelet counts in ITP as well as decreasing prednisone requirement (Ambriz *et al.* 1986) and reducing platelet-reactive immunoglobulin G (Ahn *et al.* 1983). Reports of long-term usage indicate sustained remission in over half the patients but with significant adverse hepatic and virilization effects (Maloisel *et al.* 2004; Rice 2004).

17.4 Renal disease

Men with chronic renal failure exhibit many non-specific features consistent with androgen deficiency including gynecomastia, impotence, testicular atrophy, impaired spermatogenesis and infertility, as well as somatic disorders of bone, muscle and other androgen-responsive tissues (Handelsman 1985; Handelsman and Dong 1993; Handelsman and Liu 1998). Such consequences of uremia are partially rectified during dialysis but reversed only by renal transplantation. There is little information on androgen replacement therapy in patients with end-stage renal disease, during dialysis or after renal transplantation. Only a single randomized, controlled study has examined androgen replacement therapy in uremic men (van Coevorden *et al.* 1986). Nineteen regularly hemodialyzed men were randomized to receive either oral testosterone undecanoate (240 mg daily) or placebo for 12 weeks. Although libido and sexual activity increased, hemoglobin was unchanged and no other androgen effects on bone, muscle, cognition and well-being were reported. Although transdermal testosterone has similar pharmacokinetics in uremic as in hypogonadal men (Singh *et al.* 2001), a phase IV single-center study showed that daily administration of 100 mg transdermal 1% gel failed to consistently increase serum testosterone or DHT in 40 uremic men with reduced blood testosterone levels (Brockenbrough *et al.* 2006). Consequently the failure to modify EPO requirement or clinical features (hemoglobin, bone density, body composition, lipids, sexual function or mood) remain inconclusive, and further studies achieving an increase in blood testosterone are required. A Cochrane review of therapeutic options for improving sexual function in chronic kidney disease failed to evaluate the effects of androgens (Vecchio *et al.* 2010).

Pharmacological androgen therapy has been evaluated in a randomized, placebo-controlled trial of nandrolone decanoate in dialyzed patients (Johansen *et al.* 1999). Twenty-nine patients were randomized by sequential allocation to 100 mg nandrolone decanoate intramuscularly each week (*n* = 14) or saline placebo (*n* = 15) for six months. Lean body mass (measured by DXA), timed walking and stair-climbing speed were all increased; self-reported fatigue fell but there was no change in handgrip strength. Peak oxygen consumption was also increased at three months, but not significantly so by the end of the sixth month. Larger placebo-controlled clinical studies of longer duration are needed to determine whether the impressive short-term benefits are sustainable and/or improve survival. A well-controlled, randomized phase II dose-finding study of 54 patients on optimized EPO therapy showed that 24 weeks of treatment with doses of 50, 100 or 200 mg nandrolone decanoate weekly (halved in women), for 24 weeks increased appendicular lean mass in a dose-dependent manner (Macdonald *et al.* 2007). This occurred without increasing fluid overload or any consistent improvement in physical functioning, but virilization of women was intolerable at doses higher than 50 mg weekly. It was concluded that body composition is enhanced by doses of 200 mg for men (50 mg for women) weekly, but improving physical functioning may require additional exercise interventions.

17.4.1 Effect of androgens on renal function

Based on the renotrophic effects of androgens (Mooradian *et al.* 1987), it has long been speculated that androgen therapy in patients with chronic renal failure or nephrotic syndrome might improve or slow the deterioration in underlying renal function. However, clinical evidence for renotrophic effects of androgen therapy has remained ambiguous due to the lack of adequately powered, placebo-controlled studies (Krüskemper 1968; Kopera 1976). The best clinical evidence is derived from a placebo-controlled study of elderly patients without renal disease (Dontas *et al.* 1967) and another evaluating uremic patients but without a control group (Wilkey *et al.* 1960). In the first study (Dontas *et al.* 1967), indices of both glomerular and tubular function improved with nandrolone phenylpropionate (25 mg injections weekly) after ~40 weeks. In the other (Wilkey *et al.* 1960), well-being and biochemical tests of renal function improved, but no detailed findings or analysis were presented for the 88 uremic patients treated with various doses of injectable testosterone propionate (50 mg daily) or cypionate (100 mg daily to monthly) and oral fluoxymesterone (5 mg daily) (Wilkey *et al.* 1960). Despite the biological basis for renotrophic effects, the lack of adequate clinical evidence precludes an established role for androgen therapy in the management of chronic renal failure.

More recently, the possibility that androgen therapy may be detrimental to the function of kidney transplants was suggested based on rodent experiments in which androgen therapy hastened, and androgen blockade delayed, chronic allograft nephropathy (Muller *et al.* 1999; Antus *et al.* 2001). These effects did not require aromatization of testosterone, nor were they gender specific (Antus *et al.* 2002). Although no systematic clinical data have been reported, case reports raised concerns about use of androgens in patients with kidney and other transplants (Schofield *et al.* 2002) and warrant further evaluation. Analogous but wider concerns have been raised about androgen therapy, based on experimental findings in animal models that androgen may produce deleterious effects on the kidneys, such as raising blood pressure and reducing renal function. Hence the potential amelioration due to the age-related decline in circulating androgen levels may represent an unrecognized benefit (Reckelhoff *et al.* 2005).

17.4.2 Anemia of end-stage renal failure

The anemia of end-stage renal failure has multiple contributory factors including EPO deficiency, toxic inhibitors of EPO action, androgen deficiency, micronutrient deficiency (iron, folate, pyridoxine), blood loss and hemolysis (Neff *et al.* 1985). The effect of androgen therapy on hemoglobin involves both increased circulating EPO concentration (Buchwald *et al.* 1977), and augmentation of EPO action (Balla *et al.* 1991). Erythropoietin deficiency is a major factor (Winearls 1995), and androgen therapy probably acts mainly by increasing EPO, since androgen therapy has no effect on hemoglobin after bilateral nephrectomy (von Hartitzsch and Kerr 1976), when the major source of endogenous EPO is removed. Androgen therapy has consistent effects on EPO secretion and hemoglobin concentrations (Navarro and Mora 2001), although circulating EPO is not consistently related to resultant increases in hemoglobin (Teruel *et al.* 1995). Endogenous testosterone is an important physiological determinant of red cell mass in men, since blockade of androgen action lowers hemoglobin levels (Weber *et al.* 1991; Teruel *et al.* 1997). Furthermore, post-transplant erythrocytosis may depend on EPO and possibly also endogenous testosterone (Chan *et al.* 1992). These findings suggest that androgens also have important actions in augmenting EPO effects. The intertwined roles of androgen and EPO deficiency and sensitivity in chronic renal failure remain difficult to disentangle (Silverberg *et al.* 2004; Daniell 2006; Diskin 2007).

Two randomized, placebo-controlled studies have shown that nandrolone treatment increases hemoglobin in patients with end-stage renal failure. One randomized 21 men to nandrolone (100 mg weekly) or placebo vehicle injections for five months in a crossover design (Hendler *et al.* 1974); while another randomized 18 patients to nandrolone decanoate (200 mg weekly) for three months (Williams *et al.* 1974). Both found significant increases in mean hemoglobin (15 g/l and 10 g/l, respectively), and one reported a clinically significant decreased transfusion requirement (Hendler *et al.* 1974). A further study confirmed the beneficial effects of nandrolone decanoate

(200 mg weekly) compared with placebo vehicle injections for four months (Buchwald *et al.* 1977); whereas three smaller and less well-conducted studies failed to show an increase in hemoglobin (Li Bock *et al.* 1976; Naik *et al.* 1978; van Coevorden *et al.* 1986). A further randomized, controlled clinical study compared four androgen regimens in dialyzed patients, finding that testosterone enanthate (4 mg/kg·wk) and nandrolone decanoate (3 mg/kg·wk) were more effective in increasing hematocrit than oxymetholone (1 mg/kg·day) and fluoxymesterone (0.4 mg/kg·day). However, whether these differences reflected different effective androgen doses, the androgen class (17α-alkylated or not) or route of administration (including pharmacokinetics) remains unclear (Neff *et al.* 1981). Future studies examining androgen replacement therapy using transdermal testosterone will be of interest, and preliminary studies indicate similar pharmacokinetic profile in uremic as in hypogonadal men (Singh *et al.* 2001).

There is accumulating evidence that androgen or EPO therapies are equally effective in maintaining hemoglobin in patients with chronic renal disease. A retrospective analysis of 84 patients receiving androgen therapy (nandrolone decanoate 200 mg weekly) for six months reported that men over 55 years of age had the best hemoglobin responses, and that this response was comparable with those treated with EPO (Teruel *et al.* 1996a). This was subsequently confirmed in two controlled, prospective studies which both treated with nandrolone decanoate 200 mg/wk or EPO (6000 U/wk) for six months. The first prospective study found very similar hemoglobin responses and safety profiles for 18 men over 50 years of age treated with androgen (nandrolone decanoate 200 mg/wk) compared with 6 men under 50 years and 16 women receiving EPO (6000 U/wk); however, the lack of randomization and non-comparability of groups by age and gender limits the interpretation of these findings (Teruel *et al.* 1996b). The second study (Gascon *et al.* 1999) randomized 33 patients over the age of 65 to receive im nandrolone decanoate 200 mg/wk ($n = 14$) or to continue EPO (mean dose of 6000 units/week; $n = 19$) for six months, and found comparable hematological parameters by the end of the study. However, it appears that all seven women were allocated, rather than randomized, to EPO since no woman received nandrolone. Recently, a randomized, controlled study in 27 men aged over 50 years reported that nandrolone decanoate (200 mg weekly

for six months) was equivalent to EPO (initial dose 50 units/kg·week, titrated to maintain hemoglobin between 11 and 13 g/dl) in maintaining hemoglobin (Navarro *et al.* 2002). These studies together suggest that im nandrolone decanoate (200 mg/week) in dialyzed men over 50 years of age is as effective as EPO in maintaining hemoglobin. However, the relative safety of these treatments requires further clarification.

Androgen therapy may also have an adjunctive role to EPO, perhaps as an EPO-sparing agent. This has been examined in two randomized (Berns *et al.* 1992; Gaughan *et al.* 1997) and one non-randomized (Ballal *et al.* 1991) EPO-controlled studies. In the most powerful study (Gaughan *et al.* 1997), 19 dialyzed patients were randomized to receive nandrolone (100 mg weekly) plus EPO (4500 U/wk) or EPO alone for 26 weeks. The addition of nandrolone to low-dose EPO (approximately equal to 60 U/kg·wk) resulted in a significantly greater rise in hematocrit. Similar significant additional increases in hemoglobin were reported in a small non-randomized study of eight men choosing to receive nandrolone decanoate (100 mg weekly) plus intermediate dose EPO (6000 U/wk) compared with EPO alone (Ballal *et al.* 1991) for 12 weeks. To the contrary, another small but randomized study employing a higher dose of EPO (120 U/kg·wk) was unable to detect any benefit of nandrolone decanoate (2 mg/kg·wk) for 16 weeks plus EPO compared with the same dose of EPO alone in 12 dialyzed patients (Berns *et al.* 1992). Whether these discrepancies are due to study design, age or EPO dose remains to be clarified; although it is possible that androgens have greatest synergism with submaximal EPO dosage, and that the higher EPO dose obviates any additional androgen-induced increase in hemoglobin. Randomized prospective studies to examine the use of low-dose subcutaneous EPO with adjunctive androgen therapy are needed (Horl 1999), particularly in older men.

A caveat on androgen therapy is the risk of polycythemia, which occurs as a rare idiosyncratic reaction among men with normal renal function receiving exogenous testosterone (Drinka *et al.* 1995). Testosterone-induced polycythemia may be more common among older men receiving im testosterone injections (Hajjar *et al.* 1997) and less common with more steady-state depot testosterone delivery, but has been observed with all forms of exogenous androgen (Jockenhövel *et al.* 1997).

17.4.3   Growth of boys on hemodialysis

One small, double-blind, placebo-controlled crossover study examined the effects of testosterone on short-term growth in boys with short stature on hemodialysis (Kassmann *et al.* 1992). After an eight-week run-in, eight boys (mean 3.9 SD below mean height for age) on regular hemodialysis were randomized to start on one of two four-week treatment periods separated by a six-week wash-out period before crossing over to the other treatment. Treatment consisted of 2 g/m²·day of a transdermal gel, corresponding to a topical daily dose of 50 mg/m²·day testosterone or placebo. Although a significant increase in short-term growth velocity (using knemometry) was reported overall, gain of final height was not reported and cannot be predicted from growth velocity. Furthermore, the small sample size and unbalanced randomization were limitations. Further larger and longer studies would be needed before even low-dose androgen therapy could be considered effective or safe.

17.4.4   Enuresis

Following suggestions from the 1940s that androgen therapy might improve childhood enuresis, a recent controlled clinical trial involving 30 boys aged 6–10 years has claimed a benefit for oral mesterolone treatment compared with placebo (El-Sadr *et al.* 1990). This study may have been flawed as the method of randomization leading to 20 being treated with mesterolone (20 mg daily for two weeks) compared with 10 on placebo (vitamin C) was not explained. The statistically significant increase in cystometric bladder capacity in the mesterolone-treated group was attributable to 6 boys who had dramatic increases; whereas the remainder did not differ from the 10 placebo-treated boys. Although no adverse effects were reported, the well-known potential hazards of androgen therapy in prepubertal children, including premature closure of epiphyses and short stature, precocious sexual maturation and psychological sequelae, would require detailed safety evaluation before androgen therapy could be considered acceptable for a benign functional disorder with favorable natural history in otherwise healthy children.

17.5   Muscular disorders
17.5.1   Frailty

Frailty is a clinical syndrome with features derived from the natural history of declining physical and mental function of aging people; notably the increased vulnerability to further deterioration, together with reduced recuperative power responding to adverse effects which have relatively minor detrimental impact at younger age. Although progressive declines in multiple organ systems all contribute to frailty, this syndrome is most evident in muscular function. The increased risk of fall, fractures and related adverse effects among the aging are ascribed to frailty. Consequently, frailty has steadily evolved into a framework for considering hormonal treatment for aging (Villareal and Morley 1994) including the use of testosterone (the andropause hypothesis). Currently, however, there is no evidence that frailty is improved by androgen administration to older men (Sullivan *et al.* 2005; Muller *et al.* 2006; Srinivas-Shankar *et al.* 2010; Kenny *et al.* 2010; Atkinson *et al.* 2010). This may reflect the fact that, although testosterone administration to older men consistently improves muscle mass and strength, such treatment effects may be insufficient to provide clinically meaningful improvement in physical performance or resilience of older men (O'Connell *et al.* 2011).

17.5.2   Muscular dystrophies

The effects of androgen therapy on neuromuscular disorders have been best studied by Griggs *et al.*, in a series of careful studies of myotonic dystrophy, a genetic myopathy due to a trinucleotide (CTG) repeat mutation in the myotonin (protein kinase) gene. Myotonic dystrophy is associated with testicular atrophy and biochemical androgen deficiency compared with age-matched healthy men or men with other neuromuscular wasting diseases (Griggs *et al.* 1985), although serum testosterone does not correlate with extent of muscle wasting. Since life expectancy in myotonic dystrophy is determined by respiratory muscular weakness leading to terminal pneumonia, androgen therapy aiming to improve muscular strength might prolong life. To test this hypothesis, a randomized, placebo-controlled study was undertaken in 40 men with myotonic dystrophy who were treated with either testosterone enanthate (3 mg/kg) or placebo injections each week for 12 months (Griggs *et al.* 1989). In a well-designed two-site study, muscle mass was increased as indicated by creatinine excretion and total body potassium, but there was no difference in quantitative measures of manual or respiratory muscle strength. Crucially, the lack of improved pulmonary function implies that mortality benefits would be unlikely. Androgen therapy may simply increase the mass of dysfunctional muscle.

The same investigators also examined the effect of androgen therapy in boys with Duchenne muscular dystrophy in a randomized, placebo-controlled study (Fenichel *et al.* 2001), following encouraging results from an uncontrolled pilot study of 10 boys treated for three months (Fenichel *et al.* 1997). Boys 5–10 years of age with Duchenne muscular dystrophy ($n = 51$) were randomly assigned to receive oxandrolone (0.1 mg/kg·day) or placebo for six months. Although the primary end-point (semi-quantitative average muscle strength score) and timed functional tests of gait were not significantly improved, oxandrolone produced a significant increase in some post-hoc comparisons such as quantitative myometry and in upper limb muscle strength score. Despite marginal efficacy, oxandrolone was granted FDA orphan drug status for treatment of Duchenne muscular dystrophy in 1997. While it may produce better growth and fewer side-effects than high-dose glucocorticoids, which are more effective but at the cost of more adverse effects including growth retardation and weight gain, the relative merits or oxandrolone (or other safer androgens) compared with intermittent, low-dose prednisone (Dubowitz *et al.* 2002) warrant direct evaluation. Similarly, the discrepancy between these findings is puzzling and the precise role of pharmacological androgen therapy in other forms of neurogenetic or degenerative neuromuscular disorders also deserves evaluation.

17.6 Rheumatological diseases

17.6.1 Hereditary angioedema

The efficacy of oral 17α-alkylated androgens in hereditary angioedema was established by a small, double-blind, placebo-controlled randomized crossover study (Spaulding 1960) in which six members of a single family received multiple periods of treatment or placebo. This study clearly demonstrated the efficacy of oral methyltestosterone in reducing the frequency of attacks well before the disease pathogenesis was understood. Subsequent studies confirmed these observations showing that androgen therapy increases C1-esterase inhibitor concentration, partially rectifying the underlying biochemical deficiency responsible for the disorder (Sheffer *et al.* 1977). Although other 17α-alkylated oral androgens such as fluoxymesterone, oxymetholone and stanozolol have

been used, danazol has become standard prophylactic therapy. This followed a randomized, double-blind, crossover study which showed increased blood C1-esterase inhibitor concentration together with a dramatic decrease (94% vs. 2%) in attack-free 28-day periods using 600 mg danazol daily compared with placebo in 93 courses among nine patients (Gelfand *et al.* 1976). Danazol doses are tapered to minimal levels that maintain adequate control of attack, and this dose minimization may explain the anecdotal impression that such danazol therapy has minimal effects on male fertility, although quantitative studies have not been reported. Recent studies suggest that stanozolol (1–2 mg daily) is about as effective as danazol (50–200 mg daily), but, despite their efficacy, hepatotoxicity and female virilization remain problems (Hosea *et al.* 1980; Cicardi *et al.* 1997). While it is assumed that the beneficial effects of androgen therapy in reducing frequency and severity of angioedema attacks are only exhibited by 17α-alkylated androgens, only very limited studies of non-17α-alkylated androgens such as nandrolone, 1-methyl androgens or testosterone (Spaulding 1960) have been reported. Since angioedema requires lifelong prophylaxis, further studies of non-hepatotoxic androgens should be undertaken. Noting that androgen effects are not fast enough for acute treatment, it is possible the oral route of administration may constitute a form of liver targeting (via first-pass exposure) for high hepatic androgen doses, which might not be feasible or safe for parenteral administration.

Long-term experience among allergy specialists continue to show androgens exhibiting reasonable cost-effectiveness in reducing frequency and severity of attacks balanced against adverse effects including hepatotoxicity and virilization (Sloane *et al.* 2007; Bork *et al.* 2008; Banerji *et al.* 2008; Craig 2008; Fust *et al.* 2011), and androgens remain the most widely used prophylaxis (Riedl *et al.* 2011).

17.6.2 Rheumatoid arthritis

The rationale for androgen therapy in rheumatoid arthritis is that (1) the lower prevalence in men suggests a protective role for androgens; (2) active disease is associated with reduction in endogenous testosterone production; (3) androgen effects on muscle and bone may improve morbidity in rheumatoid arthritis; and (4) androgen effects (e.g. fibrinolysis) may reduce disease activity.

The best designed and conducted study of androgen therapy involved 107 women with active rheumatoid arthritis according to American College of Rheumatology (ACR) criteria on stable standard (steroid, NSAID) treatment for at least three months who were randomized to treatment with fortnightly injections of either androgen therapy (testosterone propionate 50 mg plus progesterone 2.5 mg) or placebo for one year (Booij *et al.* 1996). The inclusion of a very low dose of progesterone, which the authors claim was biologically ineffective, was based on an old clinical practice aiming to reduce virilization from testosterone. Evaluated on a double-blinded, intention-to-treat basis, this study demonstrated significant improvement in the erythrocyte sedimentation rate (ESR), pain and disability scores and ACR improvement criteria, but not in the numbers of tender or swollen joint or joints requiring intra-articular steroid injections. There was a high dropout rate (39/107), mostly (28/39) due to inefficacy defined as any mid-study increase in anti-rheumatic medication; however, these were evenly distributed between treatment groups. As expected, virilization was the major adverse effect reported, but there were few other side-effects, and tolerability was good, as most androgen-treated patients (67% vs. 37% on placebo) wished to continue their allocated medication at the end of the study. The significant benefits of androgen therapy over placebo were predominantly in subjective measures rather than objective signs of disease activity. This raises the possibility that androgen therapy may preferentially improve mood or tolerance of disability rather than actually modifying disease impact or natural history. This well-designed study is a model for investigation of pharmacological androgen therapy in systemic disease.

Other studies of androgen therapy in rheumatoid arthritis are small, poorly designed and inconclusive. One uncontrolled study of seven men with rheumatoid arthritis treated with six months of androgen therapy (oral testosterone undecanoate 120 mg daily) observed a decline in disease activity (reduced numbers of tender joints and analgesic usage) together with minor immunological changes that were not correlated with disease activity. The lack of a placebo group in a disease with a remitting natural history renders such observations unconvincing (Cutolo *et al.* 1991). A larger study of 35 men with definite rheumatoid arthritis randomized them to injections of testosterone enanthate (250 mg monthly)

or placebo for nine months (Hall *et al.* 1996). This study noted that overall disease activity (defined by biochemical variables and clinical scales) was not improved by androgen therapy, and, indeed, significantly more men on testosterone therapy experienced disease "flare" during the study. The inclusion of men with inactive rheumatoid arthritis and initial use of an inadequate testosterone dose were limitations of this study. An older double-blind study randomized 40 patients with definite rheumatoid arthritis on stable NSAID to treatment with stanozolol 10 mg daily or placebo for six months on the basis that androgen therapy might increase fibrinolysis (Belch *et al.* 1986). This study found a significant improvement in the composite Mallaya disease activity index combining objective (ESR, hemoglobin, articular scores) and subjective (pain, morning stiffness) dimensions, despite the failure to influence measurable fibrinolysis. Adverse effects such as hepatotoxicity or virilization in females were not reported. Whether androgen therapy in men with rheumatoid arthritis can modify the natural history or whether it only improves mood and toleration of pain and disease remains to be clarified.

17.6.3 Other rheumatological disorders (systemic lupus erythematosus, Raynaud's, systemic sclerosis and Sjögren's disease, chronic urticaria)

Few well-controlled studies of androgen therapy have been reported in other rheumatological disorders. This includes male-preponderant rheumatological diseases (ankylosing spondylitis, gout) as well as the majority of female-preponderant autoimmune diseases.

In systemic lupus erythematosus (SLE), only two, small, uncontrolled studies (including together 5 men among 17 patients) using androgen therapy (nandrolone decanoate) have been reported (Hazelton *et al.* 1983; Lahita *et al.* 1992). This information is so limited that no conclusions can be drawn without larger and better-designed studies. Another double-blind study randomized 28 women with mild to moderate SLE to treatment with DHEA (200 mg daily) or placebo for three months. Treatment with this weak androgen precursor did not improve SLE disease activity index, number of flares, prednisone usage or physician overall assessment, although there was an improvement in the patients' overall assessment of well-being (Van Vollenhoven *et al.* 1995). These findings are reinforced by a well-controlled study of 60 women with quiescent SLE randomized to 200 mg DHEA or placebo for 12 months, where effects of placebo and expectation but not of DHEA were observed (Hartkamp *et al.* 2010). By contrast, another study of 41 women with glucocorticoid-treated SLE reported that the addition of low-dose DHEA (20–30 mg) for six months was superior to placebo for improving QoL (Nordmark *et al.* 2005). It is not clear whether this discrepancy reflects differences in underlying SLE activity or the effects of glucocorticoid suppression of adrenal function. A study using low (female) doses of transdermal testosterone (150 µg daily) for 12 weeks produced no benefit in 34 women with SLE (Gordon *et al.* 2008).

One study has examined the effects of treatment with stanozolol (10 mg daily) or placebo for 24 weeks in primary Raynaud's phenomenon and systemic sclerosis (Jayson *et al.* 1991). Although 43 patients (19 Raynaud's, 24 systemic sclerosis; including only 4 men) entered, only 28 patients (11 Raynaud's, 17 systemic sclerosis) completed the study. Compared with placebo, stanozolol significantly improved ultrasonic Doppler index as well as finger pulp and nail bed temperatures, but there was no difference in reported frequency or severity of vasospastic attacks, scleroderma skin score or grip strength. The clinical significance of the changes in digital small vessel function recorded in the absence of vasospasm and without reduction in attack rates is unclear.

A double-blind study randomized 20 women with primary Sjögren's syndrome to treatment with androgen (nandrolone decanoate 100 mg fortnightly) or placebo for six months (Drosos *et al.* 1988). Androgen therapy did not produce any significant improvement over placebo in objective validated measures of xerostomia (stimulated parotid flow rate measurements, labial salivary gland histology), xerophthalmia (Schirmer's I test, slit lamp eye examination after rose Bengal staining) or systemic disease (ESR), although the subjective assessment of xerostomia by patients and physicians as well as overall patient's well-being assessment were significantly better on nandrolone. Virilization was reported in nearly all nandrolone-treated women with this relatively high androgen dose, but none discontinued for this reason. Again these studies reinforce the observations that androgen therapy may significantly improve feelings of well-being regardless of the underlying disease activity. This is reinforced by well-controlled studies of 60 women with Sjögren's syndrome randomized to 200 mg DHEA or placebo for 12 months, where there was a striking placebo effect with expectation but not DHEA having clear apparent benefits (Hartkamp *et al.* 2008).

A recent randomized, double-blind study examined the role of stanozolol as an adjunct to standard antihistamine therapy for chronic urticaria. Patients (20 men, 30 women) were randomized to treatment with stanozolol 4 mg daily or placebo in addition to antihistamine (cetirizine 10 mg daily) for 12 weeks (Parsad *et al.* 2001). Over 70% improvement in physician and patient-scored urticaria was observed in 17/26 patients who received stanozolol, but in only 7/24 patients who received cetirizine alone. This highly statistically significant benefit was observed four weeks after starting treatment and continued throughout the study. Whether the benefits of stanozolol are gender specific, or whether other androgens are also effective, has not been established.

17.7 Bone disease

The role of androgens in bone development and disorders is discussed in Chapter 8. Androgen therapy to treat osteoporosis has the advantage for fracture prevention of not only increasing bone mass but possessing potentially synergistic beneficial effects on muscular strength and mental function to prevent falls due to frailty: an independent contributor to osteoporotic fractures. The evidence supporting androgen therapy, however, is limited. For treatment of idiopathic osteoporosis, the largest randomized, placebo-controlled study, involving 327 patients treated for nine months with one year of follow-up, had inadequate power to detect effects of androgen therapy (metandienone 2.5 mg daily) on fracture rates (Inkovaara *et al.* 1983). The only other controlled study randomized 21 men to receive either weekly injections of nandrolone decanoate 50 mg or no treatment for 12 months (Hamdy *et al.* 1998). It remains unclear whether the inconsistent and transient increase in bone density observed was due to the low dose, the minimally aromatized androgen or small sample size. Additionally, an uncontrolled study has claimed striking increase in lumbar (but not hip) bone density in non-androgen deficient men treated with testosterone ester injections 250 mg fortnightly for six months (Anderson *et al.* 1997).

An important area for androgen therapy to prevent or ameliorate bone loss and fractures may be steroid-induced osteoporosis. High-dose glucocorticoid therapy is commonly used for its immunosuppressive or anti-inflammatory effects in autoimmune and chronic inflammatory diseases and in transplantation medicine. Two controlled studies have examined androgen therapy in men taking regular high-dose glucocorticoid treatment. The first reported that testosterone may reverse the bone loss due to high-dose glucocorticoid therapy in 15 men with severe asthma (Reid *et al.* 1996). The subjects were randomly allocated to monthly testosterone injections (250 mg mixed testosterone esters) or no treatment for 12 months, with the control group crossing over to testosterone treatment for the second 12-month period. After 12 months of testosterone treatment, lumber spine BMD increased by 5% compared with no change on placebo. However, no benefit was noted in bone density overall or in three other sites. The limitations of this study (unblinded, sub-replacement testosterone dose) are addressed in a larger study randomizing 51 men to fortnightly injections of testosterone esters 200 mg, nandrolone decanoate 200 mg or matching oil vehicle placebo for 12 months (Crawford *et al.* 2003). This study observed improved muscular strength with both androgens but improved lumbar bone density and bone-specific QoL only in men treated with testosterone. This highlights the importance of aromatization in androgen therapy for bone but not muscle. Larger studies examining fracture outcome as well as earlier studies aimed to prevent the rapid initial bone loss would be most valuable.

17.8 Critical illness, trauma and surgery

Critical illness, trauma, burns, surgery and malnutrition all result in a catabolic state characterized by acute muscle breakdown which is reversed during recovery. These catabolic states are characteristically accompanied by functional hypogonadotropic androgen deficiency. This is due to functional partial GnRH deficiency as pulsatile GnRH administration can rescue LH pulsatility and hypoandrogenemia (Aloi *et al.* 1997; van den Berghe *et al.* 2001). This has long led to the hypothesis that androgen therapy might improve mortality or morbidity by pharmacologically enhancing nutritional supplementation and muscle,

bone and skin recovery where sustained androgen deficiency is sufficient to contribute significantly to the overall catabolic state. However, the endocrine responses to catabolic states such as critical illness are highly complex, involving widespread dysregulation of all pituitary hormonal axes, so that, if restoration of any anabolic hormones is effective, it may require multiple rather than individual replacement (or pharmacological doses) to be effective (Langouche and van den Berghe 2006). The success of intensive insulin therapy to regulate hyperglycemia (van den Berghe *et al.* 2001) has been disputed (Finfer *et al.* 2009), leaving uncertainty over targets and outcomes in clinical practice (Kavanagh and McCowen 2010), highlighting the caution that, whatever the promise of combination pituitary hormonal approaches, rigorous experimental evaluation is required before adoption (Langouche and van den Berghe 2006). Key surrogate outcome variables for evaluating the efficacy of androgen therapy in such catabolic states include (1) muscle mass, strength and function; (2) bone turnover and wound healing (particularly after burns); as well as (3) health service utilization variables such as duration of in-hospital stay and rate and extent of rehabilitation.

17.8.1 Muscle wasting

A number of studies have examined the effects of androgen therapy as an adjunct to elective surgery using improved nitrogen balance as a surrogate for muscle mass for their end-point. The best designed study randomized 60 patients after colorectal cancer surgery to receive either a single injection of stanozolol (50 mg) or no extra treatment. Participants were also randomized among three types of post-operative, peripheral-vein nutrition (standard dextrose-saline, amino acid supplementation or glucose-amino acid-fat mixture) and stratified by gender (Hansell *et al.* 1989). The primary end-point was cumulative nitrogen balance for the first four post-operative days, and this was consistently and significantly influenced only by nutritional supplementation. Stanozolol augmented nitrogen balance only on the third post-operative day in the group receiving amino acid supplements. This was largely attributable to its effects in women and gave no improvement over standard post-operative care on other post-operative days, with other nutritional supplements, nor had any influence on a wide range of other metabolic variables. Importantly, neither convalescence nor complication rates were influenced by androgen or nutritional therapy.

Other studies have largely confirmed these findings. The first randomized 44 men with tuberculosis requiring pulmonary resection to treatment with either high-dose norethandrolone (50 mg daily) or no extra treatment within strata of different intensity of post-operative hyperalimentation (Webb *et al.* 1960). This showed a modest, transient effect of androgen therapy on positive nitrogen balance restricted to the first-three post-operative days which was absent during the second-three post-operative days. The second study randomized 36 patients to one injection of stanozolol (50 mg) or placebo one day before surgery, with similar outcomes (Blamey *et al.* 1984). A third study randomized 30 men after gastric surgery for duodenal ulcer (vagotomy/pyloroplasty) to a single post-operative injection of nandrolone decanoate (50 or 100 mg), parenteral nutrition, both, or to standard treatment (Tweedle *et al.* 1973). This study reported that the eight-day post-operative nitrogen balance was best with the combination of nandrolone plus parenteral nutrition, and that each alone was superior to standard treatment, but no clinical outcome measures were reported. The fourth study randomized 20 patients recovering from multiple trauma to receive either nandrolone decanoate injections (50 mg on day three plus 25 mg on day six) or no extra treatment. It found that nandrolone plus standard enteral or parenteral nutrition was superior to no extra treatment in nitrogen balance, urinary 3-methyl histidine excretion and amino acid retention for the first 10 days of hospitalization (Hausmann *et al.* 1990). The only clinical outcome measure, however, was six-month survival, which did not differ according to androgen therapy. Finally, more recent studies have shown benefits in burned children randomized to oxandrolone or placebo. One study showed enhanced deposition of leg muscle, but not whole body protein, when evaluated in 26 children at six months after admission (Eyben *et al.* 2005). In another study, 35 burned children demonstrated increased synthesis of constitutive circulating proteins and reduced acute phase reactants as well as a reduced requirement for albumin supplementation (Thomas *et al.* 2004). However, neither study demonstrated improved clinical outcomes.

Other studies, however, have been unable to detect any clinical benefits. One well-designed study randomized 48 patients requiring hyperalimentation to supplemental treatment with either nandrolone decanoate (50 mg) or placebo injections biweekly, aiming to determine whether nitrogen balance could be improved within the first 21 days post-operatively (Lewis *et al.* 1981). No benefit was observed in nitrogen balance, weight gain, creatinine output, and serum albumin or immune function. These negative findings were supported by another study that examined a higher nandrolone dose. This study randomized 24 patients requiring intravenous alimentation to nandrolone decanoate (100 mg before starting and repeated one week later) or no extra treatment, and found increased fluid but not nitrogen balance, and did not find any clinical benefits (Young *et al.* 1983). Another study has examined the use of oral oxandrolone, randomizing 60 patients (including 5 women) requiring enteral nutrition to oxandrolone 20 mg each day or placebo for no more than 28 days, and reported no differences in nitrogen balance or clinically relevant outcomes such as infection rate or length of stay (Gervasio *et al.* 2000).

17.8.2 Skin healing

One group of investigators has performed two studies examining whether oxandrolone (20 mg/day) can promote skin healing after severe burn injury. The double-blind study randomized 20 patients with severe burns to receive oxandrolone or matching placebo for at least three weeks commencing two to three days after the injury (Demling and Orgill 2000). Oxandrolone therapy promoted skin healing in the standardized donor site, improved nitrogen balance and reduced weight loss, but did not alter length of hospital stay. Similar results were reported in an earlier non-blinded study of 36 patients randomized to receive GH ($n = 20$) or oxandrolone ($n = 16$) (Demling 1999). However, the non-randomly selected and non-equivalent control group ($n = 16$, with less severe burns) and the lack of blinding limit the interpretation of this study. Whether improved skin healing at the donor site will lead to improved overall recovery and specifically promote the healing of severely burned skin remains unproven. These indefinite findings need to be considered in the light of experimental evidence suggesting that androgens may retard skin wound healing (Gilliver *et al.* 2008; 2009).

Various studies have also examined whether androgens may improve recovery from burns injury in the context that numerous new pharmacological approaches are undergoing evaluation (Gauglitz *et al.* 2011). Burns injury is a salient test for the application of pharmacological androgen therapy where the intent – to modify the underlying natural history of the disorder – is particularly plausible. Recovery from burns depends primarily on the extent and severity of the burns injury but also on the impact of the injury on vital organ systems either directly (lungs) or indirectly (kidneys) during recovery. The gravity of the underlying disorder may be sufficient to justify the overriding relative contraindications of hepatotoxicity (alkylated androgens) and inappropriate virilization (use for women and children). The hypercatabolic state present during recovery provides the opportunity for exogenous androgens to ameliorate the clinical course and enhance rehabilitation from the burns injury. Four placebo-controlled studies have shown consistent clinical and biochemical benefits of oxandrolone relative to placebo in burned adults (Wolf *et al.* 2006; Przkora *et al.* 2007) and children (Murphy *et al.* 2004; Jeschke *et al.* 2007), despite the expected hepatotoxicity of oxandrolone. Large-scale, randomized, well-controlled trials are required to evaluate the definitive risks and benefits (Miller and Btaiche 2009); whether the same benefits could be obtained with non-hepatotoxic androgens also remains to be determined.

17.8.3 Rehabilitation

Two studies have examined whether short-term pharmacological androgen therapy can improve rehabilitation in older men. The first randomized 25 men scheduled for knee replacement to receive weekly doses of 300 mg testosterone enanthate or matched placebo during three weeks before surgery (Amory *et al.* 2002). The second randomized 15 men admitted to hospital for general physical rehabilitation to receive weekly injections of 100 mg testosterone enanthate or placebo for two months (Bakhshi *et al.* 2000). Small improvements in Functional Independence Measure (FIM) score and strength (hand-grip dynamometry) were reported only in the latter study which, however, suffered from the limitations of small sample size, non-matching saline placebo and unbalanced groups despite randomization (Honkanen and Lesser 2001). Further well-controlled studies focusing on rehabilitation following elective surgery in older men would be of interest; however, adverse outcomes of androgen therapy (on ventilator-dependent surgical patients) have also been reported (Bulger *et al.* 2004).

17.9 Immune disease

Androgen therapy for HIV/AIDS has been investigated mainly for its effects on disease-associated morbidity (weight loss, weakness, QoL) rather than to influence the underlying disease natural history. Indeed, randomized, placebo-controlled studies have consistently reported no androgen effect on CD4 count or viral load (Coodley and Coodley 1997; Grinspoon *et al.* 1998; Bhasin *et al.* 1998; Strawford *et al.* 1999; Sattler *et al.* 1999; Rabkin *et al.* 1999; Dobs *et al.* 1999; Bhasin *et al.* 2001), with two exceptions (Berger *et al.* 1996; Grinspoon *et al.* 2000), neither of which showed a consistent decrease in both CD4 count and viral load. One rationale for androgen therapy stems from the observation that body weight loss is an important terminal determinant of survival in AIDS and other fatal diseases (Grunfeld and Feingold 1992). It has been estimated that death occurs when lean body mass reaches 66% of ideal (Kotler *et al.* 1989), leading to the proposition that, if androgens (or other agents including megestrol or GH) increased appetite and/or body weight, death may be delayed. Given this hypothesis, the effect of androgen therapy may differ between men with AIDS wasting, and those without weight loss.

17.9.1 AIDS/HIV wasting

A number of randomized, placebo-controlled studies of androgen therapy in HIV-positive men with AIDS wasting have reported increased lean mass, but minimal effects on total body weight, possibly due to concomitantly reduced fat mass. In the most comprehensive study (Grinspoon *et al.* 1998; 2000), 51 men selected for both weight loss and low serum testosterone concentration were randomized to receive testosterone enanthate 300 mg or oil-based placebo intramuscularly every three weeks for six months. Although total weight, fat mass (DXA), total body water content (bioimpedance) and physical function were not changed by testosterone therapy, fat-free mass (DXA), lean mass (total body potassium) and muscle mass (urinary creatinine excretion) were all increased (Grinspoon *et al.* 1998). The increased lean body mass was sustained during the open-label, six month extension (Grinspoon *et al.* 1999). In contrast, the other four studies have examined body compositional changes less comprehensively (Dobs *et al.* 1999; Batterham and Garsia 2001) or not at all (Berger *et al.* 1996; Coodley and Coodley 1997). The first randomized 63 HIV seropositive men suffering from wasting and weakness to receive either 15 mg or 5 mg oxandrolone daily or placebo for 16 weeks (Berger *et al.* 1996). Both oxandrolone (but not control) groups demonstrated transient weight gain within the first month, peaking at the first week. Subsequently, while the high-dose group maintained mean weight gain and the other groups less so, the within-group variance increased, suggesting major within-group heterogeneity in time-course. There was also no clear dose-response relationship. A second placebo-controlled crossover study randomized 39 men with HIV-associated weight loss to receive injections of either testosterone cypionate 200 mg or placebo (of unstated type) every fortnight for three months before crossing over to the other treatment (Coodley and Coodley 1997). Although testosterone improved one of five aspects of QoL (overall well-being), there were no changes in the other components or in weight. However, the null effect could have been due to the lack of washout between treatments. A third study selected men with HIV-associated weight loss with serum testosterone concentrations in the low-normal range (Dobs *et al.* 1999). This multicenter, placebo-controlled study randomized 133 men to receive trans-scrotal testosterone patch (delivering nominal 6 mg testosterone per day) or matching placebo daily for 12 weeks. Testosterone treatment did not alter weight or lean mass (bioimpedance); however, inconsistent improvements in QoL were observed. These findings are supported by a study that randomized 15 men to receive nandrolone decanoate (100 mg/fortnight), megestrol acetate (400 mg/day) or dietary advice alone and reported that nandrolone did not increase weight or lean mass (bioimpedance) (Batterham and Garsia 2001). Confirmatory findings were also reported in a well-designed, multi-center study of 38 HIV-positive women with AIDS wasting (Mulligan *et al.* 2007). A further study of oxandrolone administration confirms the benefits of an androgen (Stenner *et al.* 1998), although there is little justification for using a hepatotoxic androgen when safer non-alkylated androgens are equally effective.

Studies in men with AIDS wasting have confirmed the additive effect of exercise. Two studies examined the effect of im testosterone therapy with or without exercise. In both, men were selected on the basis of HIV-associated weight loss and exposed to exercise consisting of a progressive resistance program three times each week throughout the study. In one study (Bhasin *et al.* 1998), 61 men were randomized to receive testosterone enanthate 100 mg/wk and/or resistance exercise for 16 weeks. Among the 49 evaluable men, testosterone or resistance exercise increased body weight, thigh muscle volume (MRI), muscle strength and lean body mass (deuterium oxide dilution and DXA) compared with the control (placebo, no exercise) group, but the combination did not promote further gains. Quality of life was not altered. In the other study (Grinspoon *et al.* 2000; Fairfield *et al.* 2001), 50 men were randomized to receive testosterone enanthate 200 mg/wk and/or resistance exercise for 12 weeks. Among the 43 evaluable men, testosterone or resistance exercise increased body weight, lean mass (DXA) and some components of strength, and reduced fat mass (DXA) (Grinspoon *et al.* 2000). The effect of the combination over testosterone therapy or exercise alone was not reported. Another study of 24 men with HIV-associated weight loss treated all with progressive resistance exercise and testosterone enanthate 100 mg each week "to suppress endogenous testosterone production" and then randomized half to additionally receive oxandrolone 20 mg each day or placebo tablets for eight weeks (Strawford *et al.* 1999). The addition of oxandrolone was reported to increase lean tissue accrual and strength; however, the lack of a no-treatment control and the concurrent use of two androgens makes interpretation difficult.

Further studies have used a three-arm study design to examine the influence of aromatization on beneficial androgen effects (Crawford *et al.* 2003) by contrasting the effects of the non-aromatizable pure androgen nandrolone with the aromatizable androgen testosterone and placebo (Gold *et al.* 2006; Sardar *et al.* 2010), with both demonstrating superior efficacy of nandrolone. Although consistent with the proposition that aromatization is unimportant for such androgen effects, this conclusion hinges on the difficulty of proving dose equivalence of the two androgen regimens.

17.9.2   HIV without wasting

In HIV-positive men without wasting, androgen-induced changes in body composition are more modest. One study of 41 HIV-positive men selected participants for low-normal serum testosterone concentrations (but not weight loss) and randomized them to 12 months of daily transdermal treatment with testosterone (delivering 5 mg testosterone daily) or placebo patch (Bhasin *et al.* 1998). Testosterone produced a greater reduction in fat mass (DXA) but no difference in lean mass, physical function (strength) or QoL. The additive effect of testosterone with exercise has also been examined in HIV-positive men without weight loss. In this study, all 30 men with stable weight were treated with supraphysiological weekly doses of im nandrolone decanoate (200 mg for the first dose, 400 mg for the second dose and 600 mg for all subsequent doses) and randomized, half to additionally receive progressive resistance exercise three times each week, or not, for 12 weeks (Sattler *et al.* 1999). Although resistance exercise augmented gains in muscular strength and lean body mass (DXA and bioimpedance), there was no additional effect on body weight. The lack of a no-treatment control and the unblinded exercise intervention limit the interpretation of this study. In this population of men with relatively stable HIV infection, another study examined the acceptability of testosterone route of delivery among 30 HIV-positive men treated for eight weeks with im injections every one to two weeks, then switched to eight weeks of daily application of a transdermal gel (Scott *et al.* 2007). The transdermal route demonstrated more stable blood testosterone levels and was preferred, although the one-way switch design was a limitation.

A well-designed study, examining 75 HIV-positive, non-wasted men with abdominal obesity treated with 10 g transdermal testosterone gel daily for 24 weeks, observed reduction in total body and subcutaneous fat depots but lesser effects on visceral fat mass (Bhasin *et al.* 2007).

17.10   Malignant disease

Androgen therapy could influence mortality from malignant disease via direct antitumor effects, or improve morbidity by maintaining weight, hemoglobin, neutrophil count, muscle mass and bone mass through its known actions. Reduced morbidity may also augment treatment by creating greater tolerance for more aggressive cytotoxic therapy. Despite encouraging results from animal models and uncontrolled clinical reports, human studies are unconvincing. Although older studies demonstrate a consistent but modest effect of androgen therapy in reducing the magnitude, duration and/or complications from chemotherapy-induced neutropenia, few well-controlled

clinical studies have shown unequivocal benefits of androgen therapy. The recent availability of recombinant human G-CSF/GM-CSF, with its greater efficacy and better tolerability reduces the benefits from androgen-induced prevention of neutropenia to cost-effective, second-line status.

Androgen therapy appears to have morbidity benefits in some but not all studies. One open, controlled study randomized 33 patients with lung or other non-hormone responsive solid cancers to standard chemotherapy plus nandrolone decanoate (200 mg weekly) or no additional treatment. In this study androgen therapy produced better maintenance of body weight, hemoglobin and less transfusion requirement, but no improved survival or physical performance (Spiers *et al.* 1981). Similarly, a cohort of 23 patients with inoperable lung cancer requiring palliative chest radiotherapy were randomized to receive or not to receive additional treatment with nandrolone phenylpropionate (loading dose 100 mg followed by 50 mg weekly during hospitalization). During radiotherapy (4500 cGy), androgen therapy maintained higher hemoglobin and lower transfusion requirements (Evans and Elias 1972). In contrast, two other studies have failed to demonstrate a definite benefit of androgen therapy. In one study of 40 adults (including 9 women) who had undergone esophageal resection for carcinoma, subjects were randomized to receive im injections of nandrolone decanoate 50 mg or oil-based placebo every three weeks for three months commencing one month after resection (Darnton *et al.* 1999). No treatment effect in weight, appetite or mid-arm circumference was detected, although appetite improved in both groups with time. In the other study, 37 patients with unresectable non-small cell lung cancer requiring standard combination chemotherapy were randomized to receive, or not, additional treatment with nandrolone decanoate (200 mg weekly for four weeks). Androgen therapy was associated with only a non-significant statistical trend towards improved survival (median 8.2 vs. 5.5 months) and less weight loss, but no improvement in marrow function (Chlebowski *et al.* 1986). The subtherapeutic dose employed by the first study (Darnton *et al.* 1999) and the greater myelosuppression resulting from aggressive modern combination chemotherapy in the second study (Chlebowski *et al.* 1986) may have negated any morbidity benefits.

Another study has examined the effect of androgen, progestin or corticosteroid treatment for an indefinite period of time on appetite and weight in 475 men and women with weight loss due to advanced incurable cancer (Loprinzi *et al.* 1999). Subjects were stratified by cancer type, prognosis and degree of weight loss before being randomized to receive fluoxymesterone 20 mg/day or megestrol acetate 800 mg/day or dexamethasone 3 mg/day in a double-blind fashion for a median duration of two months. Although survival or QoL was equivalent between groups, fluoxymesterone at the dose administered was significantly inferior for appetite stimulation and tended to result in less weight gain. Furthermore, hirsutism and virilization were major problems occurring in about 10% of all women. The role of fluoxymesterone to stimulate appetite is doubtful given the clear superiority of other agents and the dubious QoL consequences of this indication.

A study of 35 men with hematological malignancies in complete remission following treatment with cytotoxic chemotherapy evaluated the role of androgen therapy for compensated Leydig cell failure. Men with low-normal circulating testosterone and raised LH concentrations were randomized (single blind) to receive, for 12 months, transdermal placebo or testosterone patches (2.5–5 mg/day), dose titrated to maintain a serum testosterone concentration of >20 nM (Howell *et al.* 2001). Testosterone treatment did not alter bone turnover markers, hip, spine or forearm BMD (quantitative computed tomography and DXA), lean mass or fat mass (DXA), mood (hospital anxiety and depression scale) or sexual function. However, two out of five components of the multidimensional fatigue inventory were improved (activity was increased and physical fatigue was reduced). These inconsistent and minor effects were supported by a case control study showing minimal differences based on lower serum testosterone concentrations in similar men (Howell *et al.* 2000), suggesting that androgen replacement therapy offers little objective benefit for men with compensated Leydig cell failure post-cytotoxic therapy.

Pharmacological androgen therapy has also been evaluated for maintenance therapy for acute non-lymphocytic leukemia (ANLL), on the basis that enhanced proliferation of residual normal hematopoietic precursors would competitively suppress the growth of the leukemic clones. Among 114 / 212 patients with newly diagnosed ANLL who obtained complete remission after standard induction chemotherapy, 82 agreed to be randomized to undergo standard maintenance chemotherapy alone or in combination with BCG vaccination, stanozolol (0.1 mg/kg·d) or BCG vaccination plus stanozolol. After three years of follow-up, all four arms had similar rates of remission and adverse events (Mandelli *et al.* 1981).

Androgen therapy continues to have an established role in late-stage advanced breast cancer, usually as a late option after failure of other hormonal therapies and when the virilizing side-effects may be more acceptable. Few recent studies have focused on androgen therapy, so that clinically it now occupies a residual but diminishing role relative to modern hormonal and cytotoxic chemotherapy for breast cancer. The frequency and prognostic significance of AR expression in breast cancer (Gucalp and Traina 2010), together with recent experimental advances in understanding the role of androgen action in female reproductive physiology (Walters *et al.* 2010), may lead to re-examining the role of androgens in female hormone-dependent cancers.

17.11   Respiratory disease

17.11.1   Chronic obstructive lung disease

Advanced chronic airflow limitation is associated with weight loss and muscle depletion, possibly due to the increased energy required for breathing, or reduced serum testosterone concentrations (Kamischke *et al.* 1998). Interventions aimed at improving muscle bulk such as nutrition, exercise or androgens may therefore have an impact on the morbidity and/or mortality of the underlying respiratory disease. A few well-controlled studies examining the effects of androgens have been reviewed (Svartberg 2010). Six placebo-controlled, parallel-group studies (Schols *et al.* 1995; Ferreira *et al.* 1998; Creutzberg *et al.* 2003; Svartberg *et al.* 2004; Casaburi *et al.* 2004; Sharma *et al.* 2008) have been conducted involving 395 patients treated for 8–27 weeks with injectable nandrolone decanoate (3, 50 mg every fortnight), testosterone enanthate (2, 250 or 400 mg per month) or oral stanozolol (1, 12 mg daily). None showed any improvement in objective lung function, although five of six showed improvement in muscle. As in other medical conditions, it is possible that the effects of androgen may be due to mood elevation and improved coping mentality and behaviors rather than any direct impact on the natural history of the underlying disease.

389

The largest well-conducted prospective study demonstrated that short-term, low-dose androgen therapy (nandrolone decanoate) augmented the effects of nutritional supplementation in patients with moderate to severe chronic airways disease (Schols et al. 1995). From 233 consecutive patients with stable, moderate to severe and bronchodilator-unresponsive pulmonary disease admitted to an intensive pulmonary rehabilitation program, 217 were randomized into three groups. These were to receive eight weeks of treatment with (1) placebo injections; (2) a nutritional supplement (one high-fat, high-calorie drink daily) plus placebo injections; or (3) a nutritional supplement plus androgen injections (nandrolone decanoate (50 mg men, 25 mg women)) with im injections given fortnightly. Participants were also stratified according to the degree of baseline muscle depletion (body weight < 90% and/or lean mass < 67% ideal, or not) at entry. During the study all patients underwent a standardized exercise program. Both nutrition and androgen therapy increased body weight over placebo, with androgen therapy having more prominent effects on lean body mass and respiratory muscle strength, although there was no measurable improvement in submaximal exercise tolerance nor any major adverse effects. The lack of an androgen-alone arm and blinding with respect to nutritional supplementation made it difficult to evaluate the impact of androgen therapy relative to improved nutrition. After four years, follow-up of 203 of these men revealed no treatment effect on survival (Schols et al. 1998); however in a post-hoc analysis, those with larger increases in weight (including 24% of the initial placebo group) had a significantly decreased mortality risk.

Improvement in underlying pulmonary disease itself may ameliorate the gonadal dysfunction of systemic disease. In one study of men with chronic obstructive pulmonary disease with severe hypoxia and impotence, long-term oxygen therapy improved total and free testosterone and lowered SHBG (without changes in LH or FSH) in five men who had improved sexual function. The remaining seven who had unimproved sexual function had no changes in circulating hormone concentrations (Aasebo et al. 1993).

17.11.2 Obstructive sleep apnea

Obstructive sleep apnea is associated with reduced blood testosterone (Liu et al. 2007); a feature that is rectified by mechanical splinting of the upper airways using positive air pressure to maintain patency (Grunstein et al. 1989). A case report has indicated that sleep apnea may be precipitated in an obese man by testosterone administration (Sandblom et al. 1983), and high-dose testosterone can adversely affect sleep patterns in older men (Liu et al. 2003b). These considerations indicate caution is required when considering pharmacological androgen therapy, especially in obese men who are at higher risk of undiagnosed obstructive sleep apnea. Nevertheless, the actual risk of precipitating sleep apnea by testosterone administration to unselected older men remains low. Enquiring about heavy snoring and irregular sleep breathing and daytime somnolence are usually suitable screening tests.

Androgen therapy has been reported to increase sleep arousals from disordered breathing in a randomized crossover study of 11 hypogonadal men receiving testosterone enanthate (200–400 mg per fortnight) or no therapy. This study compared somnography during androgen therapy (3–7 days after a testosterone injection) with a no-treatment group consisting of patients after withdrawal (mean 53 days post-injection) of androgen therapy (Schneider et al. 1986). Anatomical and functional evaluation of the upper-airway patency in four patients showed no treatment-related difference, but this finding is inconclusive due to the small sample size. Another retrospective study examined the prevalence of obstructive sleep apnea in hemodialyzed men and the potential role of testosterone ester injections in its causation (Millman et al. 1985). Obstructive sleep apnea symptoms were common (12 / 29, 41%), particularly in those receiving regular testosterone enanthate injections (250 mg weekly) to stimulate erythropoiesis (9/12, 75%) compared with those not receiving testosterone (6/17, 35%). Withdrawal of testosterone, however, did not alter the signs or symptoms of sleep apnea in the five men studied both during and two months after cessation of testosterone treatment. This suggests that testosterone ester injections may not be a regular precipitant of obstructive sleep apnea. This is corroborated by further surveillance showing that sleep apnea is common among patients with chronic renal failure even before commencement of dialysis or testosterone treatment (Kimmel et al. 1989).

The effect of androgen therapy on sleep and breathing has been examined in only three randomized, placebo-controlled studies. In the largest study, among 108 older men (Snyder et al. 1999) randomized to receive a dose-titrated testosterone patch (approximately 6 mg/day) or matching placebo for three years, sleep breathing did not deteriorate, although the tracking device may lack sensitivity (Portier *et al.* 2000), and sleep architecture was not examined. In a small, randomized, placebo-controlled study, 10 men rendered acutely hypogonadal with leuprorelin (Leibenluft *et al.* 1997) were randomized to receive testosterone enanthate 200 mg every fortnight or oil placebo for four weeks. Testosterone did not alter overnight plethysmography-determined sleep parameters (except that time slept in stage 4 sleep was lengthened), but the effects on breathing were not reported. Whether the frequent overnight blood sampling may have influenced sleep is not clear. In the only randomized, placebo-controlled study to examine both sleep and breathing, 17 community-dwelling healthy men over the age of 60 were randomized to receive three injections of im testosterone esters at weekly intervals (500 mg, 250 mg and 250 mg) or matching oil-based placebo, and then crossed over to the other treatment after eight weeks washout (Liu *et al.* 2003b). Testosterone treatment shortened sleep (~1 hour), worsened sleep apnea (by ~7 events/hour) and increased the duration of hypoxemia (~5 min/night), but did not worsen function (driving ability and psychomotor performance). Together these studies suggest that high-dose administration of testosterone esters may have adverse effects on sleep and breathing in the short-term; however, the effects of longer-term use of lower, more physiological testosterone doses remains unknown.

A low frequency of obstructive sleep apnea complicating androgen therapy as an idiosyncratic effect cannot be excluded. Whether this idiosyncratic reaction is related to the pharmacokinetics of the testosterone formulation used, such as the extreme peak serum testosterone following im injections, has yet to be determined. Whether similar effects would occur with more physiological testosterone formulations remains to be established in properly controlled clinical trials, although the low frequency of such reactions would require very large studies.

17.11.3   Asthma

Few studies have examined androgen effects in asthma. One uncontrolled study of asthmatic women administered testosterone reported improved clinical status, but the lack of control group or fixed regimen are major limitations (Wulfsohn *et al.* 1964). A small, double-blind study of 15 steroid-dependent asthmatic boys randomized to ethylestrenol (0.1 mg/kg·d) or placebo for 12 months reported a significant improvement in peak expiratory flow rate in the androgen group compared with the placebo group (Kerrebijn and Delver 1969). Despite the claim of no acceleration of bone maturation (according to the ratio of bone-age/height velocity) in this older study, the safety of such androgen therapy in boys prior to completion of puberty is very doubtful, and androgen therapy has no place in the modern treatment of adolescent asthma.

17.12   Neurological disease
17.12.1   Cognitive function

Studies over the last decade provided promising evidence for beneficial effects of testosterone on cognitive function, with potential to ameliorate its decline with aging (Cherrier *et al.* 2001; 2003; 2004; 2005a). Furthermore, two pilot studies have been performed: one in 15 men with Alzheimer's disease and 17 with mild cognitive impairment (Cherrier *et al.* 2005b), and another in 16 men with Alzheimer's disease and 22 healthy controls (Lu *et al.* 2006), both showing modest, selective improvement in some but not all cognitive domains. However, subsequent studies in otherwise healthy older men have failed to replicate the Cherrier studies (Kenny *et al.* 2004; Haren *et al.* 2005; Gray *et al.* 2005; Vaughan *et al.* 2007), with one study showing detrimental effects of testosterone (Maki *et al.* 2007) on cognitive function. One limitation of the original positive studies was their lack of proper masking for oil-based injectable testosterone by using a saline placebo, which is a serious limitation for studies with subjective, psychological or effort-dependent end-points (Handelsman 2010b). Moreover, large observational (LeBlanc *et al.* 2010) and interventional (Young *et al.* 2010) studies found no corroborative effect of sex steroids on cognitive function at any age. Testosterone may have socio-behavioral effects (Zak *et al.* 2009), and it remains possible that non-specific mood or other psychological consequences of androgen deprivation may disrupt cognitive function. More powerful and specifically designed studies may be informative (Warren *et al.* 2008; Cherrier 2009).

17.12.2 Headache

The role of androgen withdrawal and therapy in men with cluster headache, an almost exclusively male disorder, has been examined in two controlled studies. In one, 60 men with chronic cluster headache were randomized single-blind to treatment with a single dose of a GnRH analog (3.75 mg leuprorelin depot) or vehicle injection (Nicolodi *et al.* 1993a). Self-reported frequency, intensity and duration of headache as well as sexual activity declined progressively during three successive 10-day periods after injection, compared with pre-injection baseline in those treated with leuprorelin; whereas there was no change in placebo-treated men. The therapeutic response was delayed in onset, corresponding temporally to the onset of castrate testosterone concentrations, and the benefit persisted in most men for the one-month post-treatment follow-up period, while no changes were noted at any stage in the placebo group. As headache is a remitting illness with subjective study end-points, the unmasking of active drug by the regular occurrence of sexual dysfunction in the treated group undermines the validity of the placebo-control group. The surprising absence of a placebo effect in the intended control group reinforces the possibility of an observer bias. Subsequently, another study was conducted in which 12 men with chronic cluster headache and 12 non-headache controls underwent treatment with very high-dose androgen therapy (testosterone propionate 100 mg daily) for 14 days (Nicolodi *et al.* 1993b). Remarkably, this produced a dramatic increase in self-reported sexual activity in the cluster headache group, but not the control group. These curious findings warrant more rigorous study with a double-blind study design utilizing more objective end-points.

17.12.3 Depression

Testosterone has long been considered effective for treatment of depression (Altschule and Tillotson 1948). Oral mesterolone was the first androgen studied for antidepressive effects. Laboratory evidence that a single dose of mesterolone (1–25 mg) mimics the effects of tricyclic antidepressants on the electroencephalogram led to a patent predicting that androgens might have beneficial effects on clinical depression (Itil *et al.* 1974). However, this was not confirmed in a double-blind clinical trial which randomized 52 depressed men to treatment with mesterolone (150–450 mg daily) or

placebo for six weeks (Itil *et al.* 1984). Both groups improved equally in scores for global clinical impression, physician's checklist for depression, self-rating and Hamilton depression rating, and there were no differences in objective measures (EEG, plasma monoamine oxidase levels).

A systematic review and meta-analysis has evaluated 23 studies using an androgen for depression (Zarrouf *et al.* 2009). In addition to 18 studies using testosterone, other studies utilized mesterolone (2), methyltestosterone (1), and the androgen precursor DHEA (2). After excluding 16 studies not meeting study-design quality criteria, 7 studies underwent formal meta-analysis to show a significant benefit of testosterone relative to placebo. Subgroup analysis showed that significant benefit was confined to the hypogonadal (vs. eugonadal) subgroup. However, this meta-analysis was significantly flawed by including the largest clinical trial which used DHEA, a very weak androgen in women but ineffective in men, as well as including women and men (Rabkin *et al.* 2006), whereas the other 6 studies included only men and used effective doses of testosterone. Due to the meta-analysis weighting by study size, this study had strongly disproportionate influence (44.5% weighting vs. others 5.1–18.1%), and the meta-analysis conclusions may not be robust to excluding the DHEA study. Some additional studies reported since the meta-analysis included one study of 23 men with mild depression using injectable testosterone (200 mg per 10 days) for six weeks (Seidman *et al.* 2009); however, some significant improvement attributed to testosterone cannot exclude the effects of expectation due to the use of inadequate masking (saline placebo for oil-based testosterone injections) (Handelsman 2010b). More conclusively, the largest study so far reported randomizing 100 depressed men who had responded poorly to conventional antidepressant therapy to adjunctive treatment with testosterone or matching placebo gel for six weeks. This study observed no significant difference in mood or measures of depression (Pope *et al.* 2010), although there was significant improvement in male sexual function (Amiaz *et al.* 2011). Whether subgroups of depressed men or specific features of their depression (e.g. sexual function) may respond more effectively remains to be better defined by further well-controlled clinical trials. The relatively non-specific mood-elevating effects of testosterone may be the basis for findings such as a significant improvement relative to placebo in immediate post-operative symptoms following open prostatectomy (Pourmand *et al.* 2008).

17.12.4   Other neurological disease

Observational studies of men with epilepsy, usually on anticonvulsant treatment, demonstrate impairment of male reproductive function including lowered blood testosterone levels and reduced sexual function and fertility (Isojarvi 2008), although the effects on other systemic androgen-dependent functions are not well reported and the role of testosterone is debatable (Talbot *et al.* 2008; Duncan *et al.* 2009). The principal common effect of enzyme-inducing anticonvulsants appears to be manifest as increasing blood SHBG levels creating a form of acquired partial androgen resistance. However, there have been few studies of testosterone effects in anticonvulsant-treated men with epilepsy (Herzog *et al.* 1998; 2010). The single controlled study examined 40 men with epilepsy and reduced sexual function and testosterone levels, who all received testosterone (im testosterone cypionate 300 mg fortnightly) for 12 weeks and were then randomized to receive an added aromatase inhibitor (anastrozole) or matching placebo tablet (Herzog *et al.* 2010). All participants demonstrated significant improvements in mood and QoL measures as well as in reduced seizure frequency. However, the lack of a no-testosterone control group provides little basis for valid interpretation of the before–after comparisons as indicative of testosterone effects. Despite some trends, there were no significant effects of aromatase inhibition on any end-point, although the study may have been underpowered for this analysis. Further placebo-controlled studies of testosterone would be of considerable interest to determine whether anticonvulsant treatment does represent an acquired androgen-resistant state.

The potential use of testosterone as adjunct therapy for men with schizophrenia has been evaluated by a preliminary study (Ko *et al.* 2008). This treated 30 men with schizophrenia with either transdermal testosterone or placebo gel daily for four weeks and showed improvement in negative schizophrenic symptoms. An inconclusive Cochrane analysis entitled "Testosterone for Schizophrenia" only included three studies using DHEA, an ineffective androgen precursor, and none with testosterone (Elias and Kumar 2007). Confusing DHEA with the potent androgen testosterone distorts discussion of

androgen effects (Pae 2009). On the contrary, a pilot study proposed the adjunctive use of estrogen therapy for men with schizophrenia (Kulkarni *et al.* 2011) based on the claim that estradiol treatment has shown promise in treatment of women with schizophrenia (Kulkarni *et al.* 2008). Such pharmacological estrogen therapy, creating an androgen-deficient state, causes increased adverse cardiovascular effects which necessitated premature termination of studies involving estrogen administration to men (VACURG 1967; Coronary Drug Project Research Group 1973) and which are also reported with modern medical castration for prostate cancer (Saylor and Smith 2010). Larger and longer duration placebo-controlled studies of testosterone administration would be of considerable interest.

Promising preliminary findings from placebo-controlled pilot studies have been reported for the use of testosterone in multiple sclerosis (Sicotte *et al.* 2007) and in Parkinson's disease (Okun *et al.* 2006). Further studies would be of great interest.

17.13   Vascular disease

The effect of androgen therapy in coronary artery (Wu and von Eckardstein 2003) and cardiovascular (Liu *et al.* 2003a) disease are reviewed in Chapter 10. This section will review studies of androgen therapy for peripheral vascular venous disease.

The use of androgen therapy in acute or chronic venous disease arises from their fibrinolytic effect, which may reduce venous fibrin plugging. One study of chronic venous insufficiency, aiming to test whether androgen therapy would reduce the rate of venous ulceration, involved 60 patients with venous skin changes but no ulceration being treated with below-knee compression stockings as standard therapy (McMullin *et al.* 1991). They were randomized to receive either stanozolol (10 mg daily) or placebo tablets for six months, and androgen therapy produced a significant but modest reduction in the area of venous skin changes but no change in prospective rate of new ulcers or skin oxygenation. The side-effects comprised mostly virilization, presumably due to stanozolol treatment of women.

Another prospective, two-center study examined the role of androgen therapy in prevention of post-operative deep venous thrombosis (DVT). In this study 200 patients scheduled for elective major abdominal surgery were randomized into three groups (Zawilska *et al.* 1990). The first received inhaled heparin (800 units/kg) one day prior to surgery alone; a second group received the same dose of inhaled heparin plus a single injection of nandrolone phenylpropionate (50 mg); and the third group received standard heparin prophylaxis (5000 units twice daily, subcutaneously). Treatments were from the day before surgery until the fifth post-operative day. Using daily ^{125}I-fibrinogen scanning to detect DVT in 183 evaluable patients, there was no significant difference in post-operative DVT or clinically significant bleeding episodes among the three groups. Unfortunately the study had major between-center differences and used a suboptimal detection method. It was also underpowered to reliably evaluate the claim that addition of nandrolone to nebulized heparin was as effective as standard heparin but with much lower bleeding risk. Larger and better-designed studies of the effects of androgen therapy on venous disease in men seem warranted.

17.14 Body weight

17.14.1 Wasting

Many older studies examined the role of androgen therapy to augment body weight in patients with wasting or cachexia from a variety of underlying medical diseases, as well as for cosmetic reasons in otherwise healthy people. For example, one double-blind study treated 28 healthy men and women and 26 male patients with wasting associated with chronic diseases (e.g. tuberculosis, chronic degenerative disorders) with placebo or one of two doses (25 mg or 50 mg daily) of norethandrolone for 12 weeks (Watson *et al.* 1959). The placebo group subsequently also crossed over to active treatment for another 12 weeks. Compared with placebo, both androgen groups had significantly improved body weight gain and reported improved appetite and well-being, but there was no dose-response relationship. Most patients had abnormal bromosulfophthalein retention, and nearly all women experienced some virilization. Very few other studies, however, were well-controlled, and the end-point of weight gain has little validity in isolation outside the context of the overall objectives of medical management for specific illnesses (see HIV/AIDS).

17.14.2 Obesity

The effects of testosterone on obesity and its associated metabolic syndrome and type 2 diabetes are reviewed in Chapter 11. Studies of testosterone administration in the metabolic syndrome (Corona *et al.* 2011a) and type 2 diabetes (Corona *et al.* 2011b) have been subjected to meta-analysis summaries. However, although massive obesity is associated with lowering of total testosterone, there are few well-designed, placebo-controlled clinical trials evaluating androgen therapy in men with uncomplicated obesity.

A series of studies by Marin *et al.* has raised interesting questions about the role of pharmacological androgen therapy in obesity. A pilot study reported reduced waist/hip circumference and improved insulin sensitivity following three months' transdermal treatment with testosterone (250 mg in 10 g gel daily) in eight men, but not with DHT (250 mg in 10 g gel daily) in nine men (Marin *et al.* 1992). The study design, lacking placebo controls or any dose finding, did not allow any conclusion as to whether this difference arose from differences in skin bioavailability or androgen type (aromatizable or not) or potency. The same investigators then reported a double-blind study in which 27 middle-aged men with abdominal obesity were randomized to placebo, testosterone or DHT treatment by daily topical application of a transdermal gel (125 mg in 5 g gel daily) for nine months (Marin *et al.* 1995). Testosterone treatment inhibited lipid uptake into adipose tissue triglycerides, decreased lipoprotein lipase activity, reduced visceral fat stores (CT scan) and increased euglycemic clamp insulin sensitivity compared with DHT and placebo groups (Marin 1995). The results of Marin *et al.* were not confirmed by another study which randomized 30 obese middle-aged men into three groups to receive oral oxandrolone (10 mg/day), testosterone enanthate (150 mg) injections fortnightly or placebo treatments for nine months using a double-dummy, double-blinded design (Lovejoy *et al.* 1995). Due to lowering of HDL-C by oral oxandrolone, a monitoring committee required the oxandrolone arm to be switched to injections of nandrolone decanoate (30 mg) fortnightly. None of the androgens (oxandrolone, nandrolone, testosterone) had any consistent overall effect on muscle or fat mass, but the interim change in study design reduced its power. The discrepancies between these studies require clarification with large sample size, longer duration and more clinically meaningful end-points.

Human chorionic gonadotropin has been widely used since the 1960s in ad-hoc and unproven low-dose regimens in combination with a low calorie diet to reduce obesity in middle-aged men (Young *et al.* 1976; Lijesen *et al.* 1995). A meta-analysis of controlled studies (Lijesen *et al.* 1995) concurs with the largest available single study (Young *et al.* 1976) that such low-dose hCG therapy is ineffective and has no valid role in the treatment of obesity.

17.15 Key messages

- Androgen replacement therapy aims to replicate but not exceed tissue androgen exposure of eugonadal men and hence is limited to testosterone in physiological doses. Although chronic diseases may cause mild androgen deficiency as a non-specific consequence of systemic illness, androgen replacement therapy may influence morbidity but is unlikely to improve mortality.

- Pharmacological androgen therapy utilizes androgens to maximal efficacy within adequate safety limits without regard to androgen class or dose. Such treatment is judged by the efficacy, safety and cost-effectiveness standards of other drugs. Very few studies of pharmacological androgen therapy fulfill the requirements of adequate study design (randomization, placebo control, objective end-points, adequate power and duration).

- Pharmacological androgen therapy has not reduced mortality or altered the natural history of any non-gonadal disease.

- Since 17α-alkylated androgens are hepatotoxic, other safer oral and parenteral androgens should be preferred where possible.

- Androgen therapy does not improve mortality or morbidity from acute or chronic alcoholic liver disease. The effects in non-alcoholic liver disease have not been studied.

- Androgen therapy does not improve survival in aplastic anemia but improves morbidity by maintaining hemoglobin and reducing transfusion dependence.

- In anemia of end-stage renal failure, androgen therapy is cheaper than, and augments the effects of, EPO, but whether it is equally or less effective remains controversial. Restricting the use of androgen therapy to older men has the most favorable risk–benefit.

- Androgen therapy prevents acute episodes of hereditary angioedema and probably chronic urticaria.

- Many important questions and opportunities remain for androgen therapy in non-gonadal disease, but careful clinical trials are essential for proper evaluation.

- Traditional indications for androgen therapy (e.g. osteoporosis, anemia, advanced breast cancer) persist until more specific and effective treatments become available. Nevertheless newer indications, lower cost and/or equivalent efficacy may still favor androgen therapy in some circumstances.

- The mood-elevating properties of androgen therapy may explain or augment adjuvant effects of androgen therapy on non-gonadal diseases.

- The best opportunities for future evaluation of adjuvant use of androgen therapy in men with non-gonadal disease include steroid-induced osteoporosis, wasting due to AIDS and cancer, and chronic respiratory, rheumatological and neurological diseases. In addition, the role of androgen therapy in recovery and/or rehabilitation after severe catabolic illness such as burns, critical illness or major surgery is promising but requires more detailed evaluation.

- Future studies of adjuvant androgen therapy require high-quality clinical data involving randomization and placebo controls as well as optimal dose-finding and real, rather than surrogate, end-points.

17.16   References

Aasebo U, Gyltnes A, Bremnes RM, Aakvaag A, Slordal L (1993) Reversal of sexual impotence in male patients with chronic obstructive pulmonary disease and hypoxemia with long term oxygen therapy. *J Steroid Biochem Mol Biol* **46**:799–803

Ahn YS, Harrington WJ, Simon SR, Mylvaganam R, Pall LM, So AG (1983) Danazol for the treatment of idiopathic thrombocytopenic purpura. *N Engl J Med* **308**:1396–1399

Aloi JA, Bergendahl M, Iranmanesh A, Veldhuis JD (1997) Pulsatile intravenous gonadotropin-releasing hormone administration averts fasting-induced hypogonadotropism and hypoandrogenemia in healthy, normal weight men. *J Clin Endocrinol Metab* **82**:1543–1548

Altschule MD, Tillotson KJ (1948) The use of testosterone in the treatment of depressions. *N Engl J Med* **239**:1036–1038

Ambriz R, Pizzuto J, Morales M, Chavez G, Guillen C, Aviles A (1986) Therapeutic effect of danazol on metrorrhagia in patients with idiopathic thrombocyotpenic purpura (ITP). *Nouv Rev Fr Hematol* **28**:275–279

Amiaz R, Pope HG, Mahne T, Kelly JF, Brennan BP, Kanayama G, Weiser M, Hudson JI, Seidman SN (2011) Testosterone gel replacement improves sexual function in depressed men taking serotonergic antidepressants: a randomized, placebo-controlled clinical trial. *J Sex Marital Ther* **37**:243–254

Amory JK, Chansky HA, Chansky KL, Camuso MR, Hoey CT, Anawalt BD, Matsumoto AM, Bremner WJ (2002) Preoperative supraphysiological testosterone in older men undergoing knee replacement surgery. *J Am Geriatr Soc* **50**:1698–1701

Anderson FH, Francis RM, Peaston RT, Wastell HJ (1997) Androgen supplementation in eugonadal men with osteoporosis: effects of six months treatment on bone formation and resorption. *J Bone Miner Res* **12**:472–478

Antus B, Yao Y, Liu S, Song E, Lutz J, Heemann U (2001) Contribution of androgens to chronic allograft nephropathy is mediated by dihydrotestosterone. *Kidney Int* **60**:1955–1963

Antus B, Yao Y, Song E, Liu S, Lutz J, Heemann U (2002) Opposite effects of testosterone and estrogens on chronic allograft nephropathy. *Transpl Int* **15**:494–501

Atkinson RA, Srinivas-Shankar U, Roberts SA, Connolly MJ, Adams JE, Oldham JA, Wu FC, Seynnes OR, Stewart CE, Maganaris CN, Narici MV (2010) Effects of testosterone on skeletal muscle architecture in intermediate-frail and frail elderly men. *J Gerontol A Biol Sci Med Sci* **65**:1215–1219

Bachman E, Feng R, Travison T, Li M, Olbina G, Ostland V, Ulloor J, Zhang A, Basaria S, Ganz T, Westerman M, Bhasin S (2010) Testosterone suppresses hepcidin in men: a potential mechanism for

testosterone-induced erythrocytosis. *J Clin Endocrinol Metab* **95**:4743–4747

Bacigalupo A, Chaple M, Hows J, Van Lint MT, McCann S, Milligan D, Chessells J, Goldstone AH, Ottolander J, van't Veer ET, Comotti B, Coser P, Broccia G, Bosi A, Locasciulli A, Catalano L, Battista R, Arcese W, Carotenuto M, Marmont AM, Gordon Smith EC (1993) Treatment of aplastic anaemia (AA) with antilymphocyte globulin (ALG) and methylprednisolone (MPred) with or without androgens: a randomized trial from the EBMT SAA working party. *Br J Haematol* **83**:145–151

Bakhshi V, Elliott M, Gentili A, Godschalk M, Mulligan T (2000) Testosterone improves rehabilitation outcomes in ill older men. *J Am Geriatr Soc* **48**:550–553

Ballal SH, Domoto DT, Polack DC, Marciulonis P, Martin KJ (1991) Androgens potentiate the effects of erythropoietin in the treatment of anemia of end-stage renal disease. *Am J Kidney Dis* **17**:29–33

Banerji A, Sloane DE, Sheffer AL (2008) Hereditary angioedema: a current state-of-the-art review, V: attenuated androgens for the treatment of hereditary angioedema. *Ann Allergy Asthma Immunol* **100** (1 Suppl 2): S19–S22

Batterham MJ, Garsia R (2001) A comparison of megestrol acetate, nandrolone decanoate and dietary counselling for HIV associated weight loss. *Int J Androl* **24**:232–240

Belch JJ, Madhok R, McArdle B, McLaughlin K, Kluft C, Forbes CD, Sturrock R (1986) The effect of increasing fibrinolysis in patients with rheumatoid arthritis: a double blind study of stanozolol. *Q J Med* **58**:19–27

Berger JR, Pall L, Hall CD, Simpson DM (1996) Oxandrolone in AIDS-wasting myopathy. *AIDS* **10**:1657–1662

Berns JS, Rudnick MR, Cohen RM (1992) A controlled trial of recombinant human erythropoietin and nandrolone decanoate in the treatment of anemia in patients on chronic hemodialysis. *Clin Nephrol* **37**:264–267

Bhasin S, Storer TW, Asbel-Sethi N, Kilbourne A, Hays R, Sinha-Hikim I, Shen R, Arver S, Beall G (1998) Effects of testosterone replacement with a nongenital, transdermal system, Androderm, in human immunodeficiency virus-infected men with low testosterone levels. *J Clin Endocrinol Metab* **83**:3155–3162

Bhasin S, Woodhouse L, Casaburi R, Singh AB, Bhasin D, Berman N, Chen X, Yarasheski KE, Magliano L, Dzekov C, Dzekov J, Bross R, Phillips J, Sinha-Hikim I, Shen R, Storer TW (2001) Testosterone dose-response relationships in healthy young men. *Am J Physiol Endocrinol Metab* **281**: E1172–E1181

Bhasin S, Parker RA, Sattler F, Haubrich R, Alston B, Umbleja T, Shikuma CM (2007) Effects of testosterone supplementation on whole body and regional fat mass and distribution in human immunodeficiency virus-infected men with abdominal obesity. *J Clin Endocrinol Metab* **92**:1049–1057

Blamey SL, Garden OJ, Shenkin A, Carter DC (1984) Modification of postoperative nitrogen balance with preoperative anabolic steroid. *Clin Nutr* **2**:187–192

Bojesen A, Juul S, Birkebaek N, Gravholt CH (2004) Increased mortality in Klinefelter syndrome. *J Clin Endocrinol Metab* **89**:3830–3834

Bonkovsky HL, Fiellin DA, Smith GS, Slaker DP, Simon D, Galambos JT (1991) A randomized, controlled trial of treatment of alcoholic hepatitis with parenteral nutrition and oxandrolone. I. Short-term effects on liver function. *Am J Gastroenterol* **86**:1200–1208

Booij A, Biewenga-Booij CM, Huber-Bruning O, Cornelis C, Jacobs JW, Bijlsma JW (1996) Androgens as adjuvant treatment in postmenopausal female patients with rheumatoid arthritis. *Ann Rheum Dis* **55**:811–815

Bork K, Bygum A, Hardt J (2008) Benefits and risks of danazol in hereditary angioedema: a long-term survey of 118 patients. *Ann Allergy Asthma Immunol* **100**:153–161

Branda RF, Amsden TW, Jacob HS (1977) Randomized study of nandrolone therapy for anemia due to bone marrow failure. *Arch Intern Med* **137**:65–69

Brockenbrough AT, Dittrich MO, Page ST, Smith T, Stivelman JC, Bremner WJ (2006) Transdermal androgen therapy to augment EPO in the treatment of anemia of chronic renal disease. *Am J Kidney Dis* **47**:251–262

Brubaker LH, Briere J, Laszlo J, Kraut E, Landaw SA, Peterson P, Goldberg J, Donovan P (1982) Treatment of anemia in myeloproliferative disorders: a randomized study of fluoxymesterone v transfusions only. *Arch Intern Med* **142**:1533–1537

Buchwald D, Argyres S, Easterling RE, Oelshlegel FJ Jr, Brewer GJ, Schoomaker EB, Abbrecht PH, Williams GW, Weller JM (1977) Effect of nandrolone decanoate on the anemia of chronic hemodialysis patients. *Nephron* **18**:232–238

Bulger EM, Jurkovich GJ, Farver CL, Klotz P, Maier RV (2004) Oxandrolone does not improve outcome of ventilator dependent surgical patients. *Ann Surg* **240**:472–478; discussion:478–480

Camitta BM, Thomas ED, Nathan DG, Gale RP, Kopecky KJ, Rappeport JM, Santos G, Gordon-Smith EC, Storb R (1979) A prospective study of androgens and bone marrow transplantation for treatment of severe aplastic anemia. *Blood* **53**:504–514

Casaburi R, Bhasin S, Cosentino L, Porszasz J, Somfay A, Lewis MI, Fournier M, Storer TW (2004) Effects of testosterone and resistance training in men with chronic obstructive pulmonary disease. *Am J Respir Crit Care Med* **170**:870–878

Champlin RE, Ho WG, Feig SA, Winston DJ, Lenarsky C, Gale RP (1985) Do androgens enhance the response to antithymocyte globulin in patients with aplastic anemia? A prospective randomized trial. *Blood* **66**:184–188

Chan PCK, Wei DCC, Tam SCF, Chan FL, Yeung WC, Cheng IKP (1992) Post-transplant erythrocytosis: role of erythropoietin and male sex hormones. *Nephrol Dial Transpl* **7**:137–142

Cherrier MM (2009) Testosterone effects on cognition in health and disease. *Front Horm Res* **37**:150–162

Cherrier MM, Asthana S, Plymate S, Baker L, Matsumoto AM, Peskind E, Raskind MA, Brodkin K, Bremner W, Petrova A, LaTendresse S, Craft S (2001) Testosterone supplementation improves spatial and verbal memory in healthy older men. *Neurology* **57**:80–88

Cherrier MM, Craft S, Matsumoto AH (2003) Cognitive changes associated with supplementation of testosterone or dihydrotestosterone in mildly hypogonadal men: a preliminary report. *J Androl* **24**:568–576

Cherrier MM, Plymate S, Mohan S, Asthana S, Matsumoto AM, Bremner W, Peskind E, Raskind M, Latendresse S, Haley AP, Craft S (2004) Relationship between testosterone supplementation and insulin-like growth factor-I levels and cognition in healthy older men. *Psychoneuroendocrinology* **29**:65–82

Cherrier MM, Matsumoto AM, Amory JK, Ahmed S, Bremner W, Peskind ER, Raskind MA, Johnson M, Craft S (2005a) The role of aromatization in testosterone supplementation: effects on cognition in older men. *Neurology* **64**:290–296

Cherrier MM, Matsumoto AM, Amory JK, Asthana S, Bremner W, Peskind ER, Raskind MA, Craft S (2005b) Testosterone improves spatial memory in men with Alzheimer disease and mild cognitive impairment. *Neurology* **64**:2063–2068

Chlebowski RT, Herrold J, Ali I, Oktay E, Chlebowski JS, Ponce AT, Heber D, Block JB (1986) Influence of nandrolone decanoate on weight loss in advanced non-small cell lung cancer. *Cancer* **58**:183–186

Choi JB, Loredo JS, Norman D, Mills PJ, Ancoli-Israel S, Ziegler MG, Dimsdale JE (2006) Does obstructive sleep apnea increase hematocrit? *Sleep Breath* **10**:155–160

Cicardi M, Castelli R, Zingale LC, Agostoni A (1997) Side effects of long-term prophylaxis with attenuated androgens in hereditary angioedema: comparison of treated and untreated patients. *J Allergy Clin Immunol* **99**:194–196

Conway AJ, Boylan LM, Howe C, Ross G, Handelsman DJ (1988) A randomised clinical trial of testosterone replacement therapy in hypogonadal men. *Int J Androl* **11**:247–264

Coodley GO, Coodley MK (1997) A trial of testosterone therapy for HIV-associated weight loss. *AIDS* **11**:1347–1352

Cooperative Group for the Study of Aplastic and Refractory Anaemias (1979) Androgen therapy of aplastic anaemia: a prospective study of 352 cases. *Scand J Haematol* **22**:343–356

Copenhagen Study Group for Liver Diseases (1986) Testosterone treatment of men with alcoholic cirrhosis: a double-blind study. *Hepatology* **6**:807–813

Corona G, Monami M, Rastrelli G, Aversa A, Tishova Y, Saad F, Lenzi A, Forti G, Mannucci E, Maggi M (2011a) Testosterone and metabolic syndrome: a meta-analysis study. *J Sex Med* **8**:272–283

Corona G, Monami M, Rastrelli G, Aversa A, Sforza A, Lenzi A, Forti G, Mannucci E, Maggi M (2011b) Type 2 diabetes mellitus and testosterone: a meta-analysis study. *Int J Androl* **34**:528–540

Coronary Drug Project Research Group (1973) The Coronary Drug Project. Findings leading to discontinuation of the 2.5-mg day estrogen group. *JAMA* **226**:652–657

Craig TJ (2008) Appraisal of danazol prophylaxis for hereditary angioedema. *Allergy Asthma Proc* **29**:225–231

Crawford BA, Liu PY, Kean M, Bleasel J, Handelsman DJ (2003) Randomised, placebo-controlled trial of androgen effects on bone and muscle in men requiring long-term systemic glucocorticoid therapy. *J Clin Endocrinol Metab* **88**:3167–3176

Creutzberg EC, Wouters EF, Mostert R, Pluymers RJ, Schols AM (2003) A role for anabolic steroids in the rehabilitation of patients with COPD? A double-blind, placebo-controlled, randomized trial. *Chest* **124**:1733–1742

Cutolo M, Balleari E, Giusti M, Intra E, Accardo S (1991) Androgen replacement therapy in male patients with rheumatoid arthritis. *Arthritis Rheum* **34**:1–5

Daniell HW (2006) Erythropoietin resistance during androgen deficiency. *Arch Intern Med* **166**:1923; author reply:1923–1924

Darnton SJ, Zgainski B, Grenier I, Allister K, Hiller L, McManus KG, Steyn RS (1999) The use of an anabolic steroid (nandrolone decanoate) to improve nutritional status after esophageal resection for carcinoma. *Dis Esophagus* **12**:283–288

Demling RH (1999) Comparison of the anabolic effects and complications of human growth hormone and the testosterone analog,

oxandrolone, after severe burn injury. *Burns* **25**:215–221

Demling RH, Orgill DP (2000) The anticatabolic and wound healing effects of the testosterone analog oxandrolone after severe burn injury. *J Crit Care* **15**:12–17

Diskin CJ (2007) Erythropoietin levels and androgens use: what is their relationship in the correction of anemia? *Arch Intern Med* **167**:309

Dobs AS, Cofrancesco J, Nolten WE, Danoff A, Anderson R, Hamilton CD, Feinberg J, Seekins D, Yangco B, Rhame F (1999) The use of a transscrotal testosterone delivery system in the treatment of patients with weight loss related to human immunodeficiency virus infection. *Am J Med* **107**:126–132

Dontas AS, Papanicolaou NT, Papanayiotou P, Malamos BK (1967) Long-term effects of anabolic steroids on renal functions in the aged subject. *J Gerontol* **22**:268–273

Drinka PJ, Jochen AL, Cuisinier M, Bloom R, Rudman I, Rudman D (1995) Polycythemia as a complication of testosterone replacement therapy in nursing home men with low testosterone levels. *J Am Geriatr Soc* **43**:899–901

Drosos AA, van Vliet-Dascalopoulos E, Andonopoulos AP, Galanopoulou V, Skopouli FN, Moutsopoulos HM (1988) Nandrolone decanoate (deca-durabolin) in primary Sjogren's syndrome: a double blind study. *Clin Exp Rheumatol* **6**:53–57

Dubowitz V, Kinali M, Main M, Mercuri E, Muntoni F (2002) Remission of clinical signs in early Duchenne muscular dystrophy on intermittent low-dosage prednisolone therapy. *Eur J Paediatr Neurol* **6**:153–159

Duncan S, Talbot A, Sheldrick R, Caswell H (2009) Erectile function, sexual desire, and psychological well-being in men with epilepsy *Epilepsy Behav* **15**:351–357

Elias A, Kumar A (2007) Testosterone for schizophrenia. *Cochrane Database Syst Rev* **3**:CD006197

El-Sadr A, Sabry AA, Abdel-Rahman M, El-Barnachawy R, Koraitim M (1990) Treatment of primary nocturnal enuresis by oral androgen mesterolone. A clinical and cystometric study. *Urology* **36**:331–335

Evans JT, Elias EG (1972) The erythropoietic response to anabolic therapy in patients receiving radiotherapy. *J Clin Pharmacol New Drugs* **12**:101–104

Eyben FE, Graugaard C, Vaeth M (2005) All-cause mortality and mortality of myocardial infarction for 989 legally castrated men. *Eur J Epidemiol* **20**:863–869

Eyman RK, Grossman HJ, Chaney RH, Call TL (1990) The life expectancy of profoundly handicapped people with mental retardation. *N Engl J Med* **323**:584–589

Fairfield WP, Treat M, Rosenthal DI, Frontera W, Stanley T, Corcoran C, Costello M, Parlman K, Schoenfeld D, Klibanski A, Grinspoon S (2001) Effects of testosterone and exercise on muscle leanness in eugonadal men with AIDS wasting. *J Appl Physiol* **90**:2166–2171

Fenichel G, Pestronk A, Florence J, Robison V, Hemelt VM (1997) A beneficial effect of oxandrolone in the treatment of Duchenne muscular dystrophy: a pilot study. *Neurology* **48**:1225–1226

Fenichel GM, Griggs RC, Kissel J, Kramer TI, Mendell JR, Moxley RT, Pestronk A, Sheng K, Florence J, King WM, Pandya S, Robison VD, Wang H (2001) A randomized efficacy and safety trial of oxandrolone in the treatment of Duchenne dystrophy. *Neurology* **56**:1075–1079

Fenster LF (1966) The nonefficacy of short-term anabolic steroid therapy in alcoholic liver disease. *Ann Intern Med* **65**:738–744

Ferreira IM, Verreschi IT, Nery LE, Goldstein RS, Zamel N, Brooks D,

Jardim JR (1998) The influence of 6 months of oral anabolic steroids on body mass and respiratory muscles in undernourished COPD patients. *Chest* **114**:19–28

Finfer S, Chittock DR, Su SY, Blair D, Foster D, Dhingra V, Bellomo R, Cook D, Dodek P, Henderson WR, Hebert PC, Heritier S, Heyland DK, McArthur C, McDonald E, Mitchell I, Myburgh JA, Norton R, Potter J, Robinson BG, Ronco JJ (2009) Intensive versus conventional glucose control in critically ill patients. *N Engl J Med* **360**:1283–1297

Franke WW, Berendonk B (1997) Hormonal doping and androgenization of athletes: a secret program of the German Democratic Republic government. *Clin Chem* **43**:1262–1279

French Cooperative Group for the Study of Aplastic and Refractory Anaemias (1986) Androgen therapy in aplastic anaemia: a comparative study of high and low-doses and of 4 different androgens. *Scand J Haematol* **36**:346–352

Füreder W, Valent P (2011) Treatment of refractory or relapsed acquired aplastic anemia: review of established and experimental approaches. *Leuk Lymphoma* **52**:1435–1445

Fust G, Farkas H, Csuka D, Varga L, Bork K (2011) Long-term efficacy of danazol treatment in hereditary angioedema. *Eur J Clin Invest* **41**:256–262

Gascon A, Belvis JJ, Berisa F, Iglesias E, Estopinan V, Teruel JL (1999) Nandrolone decanoate is a good alternative for the treatment of anemia in elderly male patients on hemodialysis. *Geriatr Nephrol Urol* **9**:67–72

Gaughan WJ, Liss KA, Dunn SR, Mangold AM, Buhsmer JP, Michael B, Burke JF (1997) A 6-month study of low-dose recombinant human erythropoietin alone and in combination with androgens for the treatment of anemia in chronic hemodialysis patients. *Am J Kidney Dis* **30**:495–500

Gauglitz GG, Williams FN, Herndon DN, Jeschke MG (2011) Burns: where are we standing with propranolol, oxandrolone, recombinant human growth hormone, and the new incretin analogs? *Curr Opin Clin Nutr Metab Care* **14**:176–181

Gelfand JA, Sherins RJ, Alling DW, Frank MM (1976) Treatment of hereditary angioedema with danazol: reversal of clinical and biochemical abnormalities. *N Engl J Med* **295**:1444–1448

Gervasio JM, Dickerson RN, Swearingen J, Yates ME, Yuen C, Fabian TC, Croce MA, Brown RO (2000) Oxandrolone in trauma patients. *Pharmacotherapy* **20**:1328–1334

Gilliver SC, Ruckshanthi JP, Hardman MJ, Nakayama T, Ashcroft GS (2008) Sex dimorphism in wound healing: the roles of sex steroids and macrophage migration inhibitory factor. *Endocrinology* **149**:5747–5757

Gilliver SC, Ruckshanthi JP, Hardman MJ, Zeef LA, Ashcroft GS (2009) 5alpha-dihydrotestosterone (DHT) retards wound closure by inhibiting re-epithelialization. *J Pathol* **217**:73–82

Gluud C, Bennett P, Dietrichson O, Johnsen SG, Ranek L, Svendsen LB, Juhl E (1981) Short-term parenteral and peroral testosterone administration in men with alcoholic cirrhosis. *Scand J Gastroenterol* **16**:749–755

Gluud C, Dejgard A, Bennett P, Svenstrup B (1987) Androgens and oestrogens before and following oral testosterone administration in male patients with and without alcoholic cirrhosis. *Acta Endocrinol (Copenh)* **115**:385–391

Gluud C, Bennett P, Svenstrup B, Micic S, Copenhagen Study Group for Liver Diseases (1988) Effect of oral testosterone treatment on serum concentrations of sex steroids, gonadotrophins and prolactin in alcoholic cirrhotic men. *Aliment Pharmacol Ther* **2**:119–128

Gold J, Batterham MJ, Rekers H, Harms MK, Geurts TB, Helmyr PM, Silva de Mendonca J, Falleiros Carvalho LH, Panos G, Pinchera A, Aiuti F, Lee C, Horban A, Gatell J, Phanuphak P, Prasithsirikul W, Gazzard B, Bloch M, Danner SA (2006) Effects of nandrolone decanoate compared with placebo or testosterone on HIV-associated wasting. *HIV Med* **7**:146–155

Gordon C, Wallace DJ, Shinada S, Kalunian KC, Forbess L, Braunstein GD, Weisman MH (2008) Testosterone patches in the management of patients with mild/moderate systemic lupus erythematosus. *Rheumatology (Oxford)* **47**:334–338

Gore CJ, Clark SA, Saunders PU (2007) Nonhematological mechanisms of improved sea-level performance after hypoxic exposure. *Med Sci Sports Exerc* **39**:1600–1609

Gray PB, Singh AB, Woodhouse LJ, Storer TW, Casaburi R, Dzekov J, Dzekov C, Sinha-Hikim I, Bhasin S (2005) Dose-dependent effects of testosterone on sexual function, mood and visuospatial cognition in older men. *J Clin Endocrinol Metab* **90**:3838–3846

Griggs RC, Kingston W, Herr BE, Forbes G, Moxley RT (1985) Lack of relationship of hypogonadism to muscle wasting in myotonic dystrophy. *Arch Neurol* **42**:881–885

Griggs RC, Pandya S, Florence JM, Brooke MH, Kingston W, Miller JP, Chutkow J, Herr BE, Moxley RT (1989) Randomized controlled trial of testosterone in myotonic dystrophy. *Neurology* **39**:219–222

Grinspoon S, Corcoran C, Askari H, Schoenfeld D, Wolf L, Burrows B, Walsh M, Hayden D, Parlman K, Anderson E, Basgoz N, Klibanski A (1998) Effects of androgen administration in men with the AIDS wasting syndrome. A randomized, double-blind, placebo-controlled trial. *Ann Intern Med* **129**:18–26

Grinspoon S, Corcoran C, Anderson E, Hubbard J, Stanley T, Basgoz N, Klibanski A (1999) Sustained anabolic effects of long-term androgen administration in men with AIDS wasting. *Clin Infect Dis* **28**:634–636

Grinspoon S, Corcoran C, Parlman K, Costello M, Rosenthal D, Anderson E, Stanley T, Schoenfeld D, Burrows B, Hayden D, Basgoz N, Klibanski A (2000) Effects of testosterone and progressive resistance training in eugonadal men with AIDS wasting. A randomized, controlled trial. *Ann Intern Med* **133**:348–355

Grunfeld C, Feingold KR (1992) Metabolic disturbances and wasting in the acquired immunodeficiency syndrome. *N Engl J Med* **327**:329–337

Grunstein RR, Handelsman DJ, Lawrence SJ, Blackwell C, Caterson ID, Sullivan CE (1989) Hypothalamic dysfunction in sleep apnea: reversal by nasal continuous positive airways pressure. *J Clin Endocrinol Metab* **68**:352–358

Gucalp A, Traina TA (2010) Triple-negative breast cancer: role of the androgen receptor. *Cancer J* **16**:62–65

Hajjar RR, Kaiser FE, Morley JE (1997) Outcomes of long-term testosterone replacement in older hypogonadal males: a retrospective analysis. *J Clin EndocrinolMetab* **82**:3793–3796

Hall GM, Larbre JP, Spector TD, Perry LA, Silva JAD (1996) A randomized trial of testosterone therapy in males with rheumatoid arthritis. *Br J Rheumatol* **35**:568–573

Hamdy RC, Moore SW, Whalen KE, Landy C (1998) Nandrolone decanoate for men with osteoporosis. *Am J Ther* **5**:89–95

Hamilton JB (1937) Treatment of sexual underdevelopment with synthetic male hormone substance. *Endocrinology* **21**:649–654

Hamilton JB, Mestler GE (1969) Mortality and survival: comparison of eunuchs with intact men and women in a mentally retarded population. *J Gerontol* **24**:395–411

Handelsman DJ (1985) Hypothalamic-pituitary gonadal dysfunction in chronic renal failure, dialysis, and renal transplantation. *Endocr Rev* **6**:151–182

Handelsman DJ (2010a) Testicular dysfunction in systemic diseases. In: Nieschlag E, Behre HM, Nieschlag S (eds) *Andrology. Male Reproductive Health and Dysfunction*, 3rd edn. Springer-Verlag, Berlin, pp 339–364

Handelsman DJ (2010b) Inadequate masking of testosterone. *J Am Coll Cardiol* **55**:2290; author reply:2290–2291

Handelsman DJ (2011) Commentary: androgens and "anabolic steroids": the one-headed Janus. *Endocrinology* **152**:1752–1754

Handelsman DJ, Dong Q (1993) Hypothalamo-pituitary gonadal axis in chronic renal failure. *Endocrinol Metab Clin North Am* **22**:145–161

Handelsman DJ, Liu PY (1998) Androgen therapy in chronic renal failure. *Baillieres Clin Endocrinol Metab* **12**:485–500

Handelsman DJ, Mackey MA, Howe C, Turner L, Conway AJ (1997) Analysis of testosterone implants for androgen replacement therapy. *Clin Endocrinol (Oxf)* **47**:311–316

Hansell DT, Davies JW, Shenkin A, Garden OJ, Burns HJ, Carter DC (1989) The effects of an anabolic steroid and peripherally administered intravenous nutrition in the early postoperative period. *J Parenter Enter* **13**:349–358

Haren MT, Wittert GA, Chapman IM, Coates P, Morley JE (2005) Effect of oral testosterone undecanoate on visuospatial cognition, mood and quality of life in elderly men with low-normal gonadal status. *Maturitas* **50**:124–133

Hartkamp A, Geenen R, Godaert GL, Bootsma H, Kruize AA, Bijlsma JW,

Derksen RH (2008) Effect of dehydroepiandrosterone administration on fatigue, well-being, and functioning in women with primary Sjogren syndrome: a randomised controlled trial. *Ann Rheum Dis* **67**:91–97

Hartkamp A, Geenen R, Godaert GL, Bijl M, Bijlsma JW, Derksen RH (2010) Effects of dehydroepiandrosterone on fatigue and well-being in women with quiescent systemic lupus erythematosus: a randomised controlled trial. *Ann Rheum Dis* **69**:1144–1147

Hausmann DF, Nutz V, Rommelsheim K, Caspari R, Mosebach KO (1990) Anabolic steroids in polytrauma patients. Influence on renal nitrogen and amino acid losses: a double-blind study. *J Parenter Enter* **14**:111–114

Hazelton RA, McCruden AB, Sturrock RD, Stimson WH (1983) Hormonal manipulation of the immune response in systemic lupus erythematosus: a drug trial of an anabolic steroid, 19-nortestosterone. *Ann Rheum Dis* **42**:155–157

Hendler ED, Goffinet JA, Ross S, Longnecker RE, Bakovic V (1974) Controlled study of androgen therapy in anemia of patients on maintenance hemodialysis. *N Engl J Med* **291**:1046–1051

Herzog AG, Klein P, Jacobs AR (1998) Testosterone versus testosterone and testolactone in treating reproductive and sexual dysfunction in men with epilepsy and hypogonadism. *Neurology* **50**:782–784

Herzog AG, Farina EL, Drislane FW, Schomer DL, Smithson SD, Fowler KM, Dworetzky BA, Bromfield EB (2010) A comparison of anastrozole and testosterone versus placebo and testosterone for treatment of sexual dysfunction in men with epilepsy and hypogonadism. *Epilepsy Behav* **7**:264–271

Honkanen L, Lesser GT (2001) Testosterone use for rehabilitation of older men. *J Am Geriatr Soc* **49**:339–340

Horl WH (1999) Is there a role for adjuvant therapy in patients being treated with epoetin? *Nephrol Dial Transpl* **14**:50–60

Hosea SW, Santaella ML, Brown EJ, Berger M, Katusha K, Frank MM (1980) Long-term therapy of hereditary angioedema with danazol. *Ann Intern Med* **93**:809–812

Hosseinimehr SJ, Zakaryaee V, Froughizadeh M (2006) Oral oxymetholone reduces mortality induced by gamma irradiation in mice through stimulation of hematopoietic cells. *Mol Cell Biochem* **287**:193–199

Howell SJ, Radford JA, Smets EM, Shalet SM (2000) Fatigue, sexual function and mood following treatment for haematological malignancy: the impact of mild Leydig cell dysfunction. *Br J Cancer* **82**:789–793

Howell SJ, Radford JA, Adams JE, Smets EM, Warburton R, Shalet SM (2001) Randomized placebo-controlled trial of testosterone replacement in men with mild Leydig cell insufficiency following cytotoxic chemotherapy. *Clin Endocrinol (Oxf)* **55**:315–324

Idan A, Griffiths KA, Harwood DT, Seibel MJ, Turner L, Conway AJ, Handelsman DJ (2010) Long-term effects of dihydrotestosterone treatment on prostate growth in healthy, middle-aged men without prostate disease: a randomized, placebo-controlled trial. *Ann Intern Med* **153**:621–632

Inkovaara J, Gothoni G, Halttula R, Heikinheimo R, Tokola O (1983) Calcium, vitamin D and anabolic steroid in treatment of aged bones: double-blind placebo-controlled long-term clinical trial. *Age Ageing* **12**:124–130

Ip FF, di Pierro I, Brown R, Cunningham I, Handelsman DJ, Liu PY (2010) Trough serum testosterone predicts the

development of polycythemia in hypogonadal men treated for up to 21 years with subcutaneous testosterone pellets. *Eur J Endocrinol* **162**:385–390

Ishak KG, Zimmerman HJ (1987) Hepatotoxic effects of the anabolic-androgenic steroids. *Semin Liver Dis* **7**:230–236

Isojarvi J (2008) Disorders of reproduction in patients with epilepsy: antiepileptic drug related mechanisms. *Seizure* **17**:111–119

Itil TM, Cora R, Akpinar S, Herrmann WM, Patterson CJ (1974) "Psychotropic" action of sex hormones: computerized EEG in establishing the immediate CNS effects of steroid hormones. *Curr Thera Res* **16**:1147–1170

Itil TM, Michael ST, Shapiro DM, Itil KZ (1984) The effects of mesterolone, a male sex hormone in depressed patients (a double blind controlled study. *Methods Find Exp Clin Pharmacol* **6**:331–337

Jaime-Perez JC, Colunga-Pedraza PR, Gomez-Ramirez CD, Gutierrez-Aguirre CH, Cantu-Rodriguez OG, Tarin-Arzaga LC, Gomez-Almaguer D (2011) Danazol as first-line therapy for aplastic anemia. *Ann Hematol* **90**:523–527

Jayson MI, Holland CD, Keegan A, Illingworth K, Taylor L (1991) A controlled study of stanozolol in primary Raynaud's phenomenon and systemic sclerosis. *Ann Rheum Dis* **50**:41–47

Jenkins JS (1998) The voice of the castrato. *Lancet* **351**:1877–1880

Jeschke MG, Finnerty CC, Suman OE, Kulp G, Mlcak RP, Herndon DN (2007) The effect of oxandrolone on the endocrinologic, inflammatory, and hypermetabolic responses during the acute phase postburn. *Ann Surg* **246**:351–360; discussion:360–362

Jockenhövel F, Vogel E, Reinhardt W, Reinwein D (1997) Effects of various modes of androgen substitution therapy on

erythropoiesis. *Eur J Med Res* **2**:293–298

Johansen KL, Mulligan K, Schambelan M (1999) Anabolic effects of nandrolone decanoate in patients receiving dialysis: a randomized controlled trial. *JAMA* **281**:1275–1281

Kaltwasser JP, Dix U, Schalk KP, Vogt H (1988) Effect of androgens on the response to antithymocyte globulin in patients with aplastic anaemia. *Eur J Haematol* **40**:111–118

Kamischke A, Kemper DE, Castel MA, Luthke M, Rolf C, Behre HM, Magnussen H, Nieschlag E (1998) Testosterone levels in men with chronic obstructive pulmonary disease with or without glucocorticoid therapy. *Eur Respir J* **11**:41–45

Kassmann K, Rappaport R, Broyer M (1992) The short-term effect of testosterone on growth in boys on hemodialysis. *Clin Nephrol* **37**:148–154

Kavanagh BP, McCowen KC (2010) Clinical practice. Glycemic control in the ICU. *N Engl J Med* **363**:2540–2546

Kennedy BJ, Gilbertsen AS (1957) Increased erythropoiesis induced by androgenic hormone therapy. *N Engl J Med* **256**:719–726

Kenny AM, Fabregas G, Song C, Biskup B, Bellantonio S (2004) Effects of testosterone on behavior, depression, and cognitive function in older men with mild cognitive loss. *J Gerontol A Biol Sci Med Sci* **59**:75–78

Kenny AM, Kleppinger A, Annis K, Rathier M, Browner B, Judge JO, McGee D (2010) Effects of transdermal testosterone on bone and muscle in older men with low bioavailable testosterone levels, low bone mass, and physical frailty. *J Am Geriatr Soc* **58**:1134–1143

Kent BD, Mitchell PD, McNicholas WT (2011) Hypoxemia in patients with COPD: cause, effects, and disease progression. *Int J Chron Obstruct Pulmon Dis* **6**:199–208

Kerrebijn KF, Delver A (1969) Ethylestrenol (Orgabolin): effects on asthmatic children during corticosteroid treatment. *Scand J Respir Dis* **68**:70–77

Kimmel PL, Miller G, Mendelson WB (1989) Sleep apnea syndrome in chronic renal disease. *Am J Med* **86**:308–314

Ko YH, Lew YM, Jung SW, Joe SH, Lee CH, Jung HG, Lee MS (2008) Short-term testosterone augmentation in male schizophrenics: a randomized, double-blind, placebo-controlled trial. *J Clin Psychopharmacol* **28**:375–383

Kochakian CD (ed) (1976) *Anabolic-Androgenic Steroids*. Springer-Verlag, Berlin

Kopera H (1976) Miscellaneous uses of anabolic steroids. In: Kochakian CD (ed) *Anabolic-Androgenic Steroids*. Springer-Verlag, Berlin, pp 535–625

Kotler DP, Tierney AR, Wang J, Pierson RN (1989) Magnitude of body-cell-mass depletion and the timing of death from wasting in AIDS. *Am J Clin Nutr* **50**:444–447

Krauss DJ, Taub HA, Lantinga LJ, Dunsky MH, Kelly CM (1991) Risks of blood volume changes in hypogonadal men treated with testosterone enanthate for erectile impotence. *J Urol* **146**:1566–1570

Krüskemper HL (1968) *Anabolic Steroids*. Academic Press, New York

Kulkarni J, de Castella A, Fitzgerald PB, Gurvich CT, Bailey M, Bartholomeusz C, Burger H (2008) Estrogen in severe mental illness: a potential new treatment approach. *Arch Gen Psychiatry* **65**:955–960

Kulkarni J, de Castella A, Headey B, Marston N, Sinclair K, Lee S, Gurvich C, Fitzgerald PB, Burger H (2011) Estrogens and men with schizophrenia: is there a case for adjunctive therapy? *Schizophr Res* **125**:278–283

Lahita RG, Cheng CY, Monder C, Bardin CW (1992) Experience with 19-nortestosterone in the therapy of systemic lupus erythematosus: worsened disease after treatment with 19-nortestosterone in men and lack of improvement in women. *J Rheumatol* **19**:547–555

Lakshman KM, Basaria S (2009) Safety and efficacy of testosterone gel in the treatment of male hypogonadism. *Clin Interv Aging* **4**:397–412

Langouche L, van den Berghe G (2006) The dynamic neuroendocrine response to critical illness. *Endocrinol Metab Clin North Am* **35**:777–791, ix

LeBlanc ES, Wang PY, Janowsky JS, Neiss MB, Fink HA, Yaffe K, Marshall LM, Lapidus JA, Stefanick ML, Orwoll ES (2010) Association between sex steroids and cognition in elderly men. *Clin Endocrinol (Oxf)* **72**:393–403

Leibenluft E, Schmidt PJ, Turner EH, Danaceau MA, Ashman SB, Wehr TA, Rubinow DR (1997) Effects of leuprolide-induced hypogonadism and testosterone replacement on sleep, melatonin, and prolactin secretion in men. *J Clin Endocrinol Metab* **82**:3203–3207

Leleu X, Terriou L, Duhamel A, Moreau AS, Andrieux J, Dupire S, Coiteux V, Berthon C, Micol JB, Guieze R, Facon T, Bauters F (2006) Long-term outcome in acquired aplastic anemia treated with an intensified dose schedule of horse antilymphocyte globulin in combination with androgens. *Ann Hematol* **85**:711–716

Lewis L, Dahn M, Kirkpatrick JR (1981) Anabolic steroid administration during nutritional support: a therapeutic controversy. *J Parent Ent Nutr* **5**:64–66

Li Bock E, Fulle HH, Heimpel H, Pribilla W (1976) Die Wirkung von Mesterolon bei Panmyelopathien und renalen Anaemien. *Med Klin* **71**:539–547

Lijesen GK, Theeuwen I, Assendelft WJ, Van Der Wal G (1995) The effect of human chorionic gonadotropin (HCG) in the treatment of obesity by means of the Simeons therapy: a criteria-based meta-analysis. *Br J Clin Pharmacol* **40**:237–243

Liu PY, Death AK, Handelsman DJ (2003a) Androgens and cardiovascular disease. *Endocr Rev* **24**:313–340

Liu PY, Yee BJ, Wishart SM, Jimenez M, Jung DG, Grunstein RR, Handelsman DJ (2003b) The short-term effects of high dose testosterone on sleep, breathing and function in older men. *J Clin Endocrinol Metab* **88**:3605–3613

Liu PY, Caterson ID, Grunstein RR, Handelsman DJ (2007) Androgens, obesity, and sleep-disordered breathing in men. *Endocrinol Metab Clin North Am* **36**:349–363

Loprinzi CL, Kugler JW, Sloan JA, Mailliard JA, Krook JE, Wilwerding MB, Rowland KM Jr, Camoriano JK, Novotny PJ, Christensen BJ (1999) Randomized comparison of megestrol acetate versus dexamethasone versus fluoxymesterone for the treatment of cancer anorexia/cachexia. *J Clin Oncol* **17**:3299–3306

Lovejoy JC, Bray GA, Greeson CS, Klemperer M, Morris J, Partington C, Tulley R (1995) Oral anabolic steroid treatment, but not parenteral androgen treatment, decreases abdominal fat in obese, older men. *Int J Obes* **19**:614–624

Lu PH, Masterman DA, Mulnard R, Cotman C, Miller B, Yaffe K, Reback E, Porter V, Swerdloff R, Cummings JL (2006) Effects of testosterone on cognition and mood in male patients with mild Alzheimer disease and healthy elderly men. *Arch Neurol* **63**:177–185

Macdonald JH, Marcora SM, Jibani MM, Kumwenda MJ, Ahmed W, Lemmey AB (2007) Nandrolone decanoate as anabolic therapy in chronic kidney disease: a randomized phase II dose-finding study. *Nephron Clin Pract* **106**:c125–c135

Maddrey WC (1986) Is therapy with testosterone or anabolic-androgenic steroids useful in the treatment of alcoholic liver disease? *Hepatology* **6**:1033–1035

Maki PM, Ernst M, London ED, Mordecai KL, Perschler P, Durso SC, Brandt J, Dobs A, Resnick SM (2007) Intramuscular testosterone treatment in elderly men: evidence of memory decline and altered brain function. *J Clin Endocrinol Metab* **92**:4107–4114

Maloisel F, Andres E, Zimmer J, Noel E, Zamfir A, Koumarianou A, Dufour P (2004) Danazol therapy in patients with chronic idiopathic thrombocytopenic purpura: long-term results. *Am J Med* **116**:590–594

Mandelli F, Amadori S, Dini E, Grignani F, Leoni P, Liso V, Martelli M, Neri A, Petti MC, Ferrini PR (1981) Randomized clinical trial of immunotherapy and androgenotherapy for remission maintenance in acute non-lymphocytic leukemia. *Leuk Res* **5**:447–452

Marin P (1995) Testosterone and regional fat distribution. *Obes Res* **3** Suppl 4:609S–612S

Marin P, Holmang S, Jonsson L, Sjostrom L, Kvist H, Holm G, Lindstedt G, Bjorntorp P (1992) The effects of testosterone treatment on body composition and metabolism in middle-aged obese men. *Int J Obes* **16**:991–997

Marin P, Oden B, Bjorntorp P (1995) Assimilation and mobilization of triglycerides in subcutaneous abdominal and femoral adipose tissue in vivo in men: effects of androgens. *J Clin Endocrinol Metab* **80**:239–243

Marwaha RK, Bansal D, Trehan A, Varma N (2004) Androgens in childhood acquired aplastic anaemia in Chandigarh, India. *Trop Doct* **34**:149–152

McMullin GM, Watkin GT, Coleridge Smith PD, Scurr JH (1991) Efficacy of fibrinolytic enhancement with

stanozolol in the treatment of venous insufficiency. *Austr N Zealand Surgery* **61**:306–309

Mendenhall CL, Anderson S, Garcia-Pont P, Goldberg S, Kiernan T, Seeff LB, Sorrell M, Tamburro C, Weesner R, Zetterman R, Chedid A, Chen T, Rabin L; Veterans Administration Cooperative Study on Alcoholic Hepatitis (1984) Short-term and long-term survival in patients with alcoholic hepatitis treated with oxandrolone and prenisolone. *N Engl J Med* **311**:1464–1470

Mendenhall CL, Moritz TE, Roselle GA, Morgan TR, Nemchausky BA, Tamburro CH, Schiff ER, McClain CJ, Marsano LS, Allen JI (1993) A study of oral nutritional support with oxandrolone in malnourished patients with alcoholic hepatitis. *Hepatology* **17**:564–576

Miller JT, Btaiche IF (2009) Oxandrolone treatment in adults with severe thermal injury. *Pharmacotherapy* **29**:213–226

Millman RP, Kimmel PL, Shore ET, Wasserstein AG (1985) Sleep apnea in hemodialysis patients: the lack of testosterone effect on its pathogenesis. *Nephron* **40**:407–410

Mooradian AD, Morley JE, Korenman SG (1987) Biological actions of androgens. *Endocr Rev* **8**:1–28

Muller M, van den Beld AW, van der Schouw YT, Grobbee DE, Lamberts SW (2006) Effects of dehydroepiandrosterone and atamestane supplementation on frailty in elderly men. *J Clin Endocrinol Metab* **91**:3988–3991

Muller V, Szabo A, Viklicky O, Gaul I, Portl S, Philipp T, Heemann UW (1999) Sex hormones and gender-related differences: their influence on chronic renal allograft rejection. *Kidney Int* **55**:2011–2020

Mulligan K, Zackin R, Von Roenn JH, Chesney MA, Egorin MJ, Sattler FR, Benson CA, Liu T, Umbleja T, Shriver S, Auchus RJ, Schambelan M (2007) Testosterone supplementation of megestrol

therapy does not enhance lean tissue accrual in men with human immunodeficiency virus-associated weight loss: a randomized, double-blind, placebo-controlled, multicenter trial. *J Clin Endocrinol Metab* **92**:563–570

Murphy KD, Thomas S, Mlcak RP, Chinkes DL, Klein GL, Herndon DN (2004) Effects of long-term oxandrolone administration in severely burned children. *Surgery* **136**:219–224

Naik RB, Gibbons AR, Gyde OH, Harris BR, Robinson BH (1978) Androgen trial in renal anaemia. *Proc Eur Dial Transplant Assoc* **15**:136–143

Najean Y, Pecking A (1979) Refractory anemia with excess of blast cells: prognostic factors and effect of treatment with androgens or cytosine arabinoside. Results of a prospective trial in 58 patients. Cooperative Group for the Study of Aplastic and Refractory Anemias. *Cancer* **44**:1976–1982

Najean Y; Joint Group for the Study of Aplastic and Refractory Anaemias (1981) Long-term follow-up in patients with aplastic anemia. A study of 137 androgen-treated patients surviving more than two years. *Am J Med* **71**:543–551

Navarro JF, Mora C (2001) In-depth review effect of androgens on anemia and malnutrition in renal failure: implications for patients on peritoneal dialysis. *Perit Dial Int* **21**:14–24

Navarro JF, Mora C, Macia M, Garcia J (2002) Randomized prospective comparison between erythropoietin and androgens in CAPD patients. *Kidney Int* **61**:1537–1544

Neff MS, Goldberg J, Slifkin RF, Eiser AR, Calamia V, Kaplan M, Baez A, Gupta S, Mattoo N (1981) A comparison of androgens for anemia in patients on hemodialysis. *N Engl J Med* **304**:871–875

Neff MS, Goldberg J, Slifkin RF, Eiser AR, Calamia V, Kaplan M, Baez A, Gupta S, Mattoo N (1985)

Anemia in chronic renal failure. *Acta Endocrinol Suppl* **271**:80–86

Nicolodi M, Sicuteri F, Poggioni M (1993a) Hypothalamic modulation of nociception and reproduction in cluster headache. I. Therapeutic trials of leuprolide. *Cephalgia* **13**:253–257

Nicolodi M, Sicuteri F, Poggioni M (1993b) Hypothalamic modulation of nociception and reproduction in cluster headache. II. Testosterone-induced increase of sexual activity in males with cluster headache. *Cephalgia* **13**:258–260

Nieschlag E, Cuppers HJ, Wickings EJ (1977) Influence of sex, testicular development and liver function on the bioavailability of oral testosterone. *Eur J Clin Invest* **7**:145–147

Nieschlag E, Nieschlag S, Behre HM (1993) Lifespan and testosterone. *Nature* **366**:215

Nordmark G, Bengtsson C, Larsson A, Karlsson FA, Sturfelt G, Ronnblom L (2005) Effects of dehydroepiandrosterone supplement on health-related quality of life in glucocorticoid treated female patients with systemic lupus erythematosus. *Autoimmunity* **38**:531–540

O'Connell MD, Tajar A, Roberts SA, Wu FC (2011) Do androgens play any role in the physical frailty of ageing men? *Int J Androl* **34**:195–211

Okun MS, Fernandez HH, Rodriguez RL, Romrell J, Suelter M, Munson S, Louis ED, Mulligan T, Foster PS, Shenal BV, Armaghani SJ, Jacobson C, Wu S, Crucian G (2006) Testosterone therapy in men with Parkinson disease: results of the TEST-PD Study. *Arch Neurol* **63**:729–735

Orr R, Fiatarone Singh M (2004) The anabolic androgenic steroid oxandrolone in the treatment of wasting and catabolic disorders: review of efficacy and safety. *Drugs* **64**:725–750

Pae CU (2009) Comments on "Short-term testosterone augmentation in male schizophrenics: a randomized, double-blind, placebo-controlled trial" by Dr Ko and colleagues. *J Clin Psychopharmacol* **29**:194–195; author reply:196–197

Palacios A, Campfield LA, McClure RD, Steiner B, Swerdloff RS (1983) Effect of testosterone enanthate on hematopoesis in normal men. *Fertil Steril* **40**:100–104

Parsad D, Pandhi R, Juneja A (2001) Stanozolol in chronic urticaria: a double blind, placebo controlled trial. *J Dermatol* **28**:299–302

Phillips EH, Ryan S, Ferrari R, Green C (2003) Estratest and Estratest HS (esterified estrogens and methyltestosterone) therapy: a summary of safety surveillance data, January 1989 to August 2002. *Clin Ther* **25**:3027–3043

Pope HG Jr, Amiaz R, Brennan BP, Orr G, Weiser M, Kelly JF, Kanayama G, Siegel A, Hudson JI, Seidman SN (2010) Parallel-group placebo-controlled trial of testosterone gel in men with major depressive disorder displaying an incomplete response to standard antidepressant treatment. *J Clin Psychopharmacol* **30**:126–134

Portier F, Portmann A, Czernichow P, Vascaut L, Devin E, Benhamou D, Cuvelier A, Muir JF (2000) Evaluation of home versus laboratory polysomnography in the diagnosis of sleep apnea syndrome. *Am J Respir Crit Care Med* **162**:814–818

Pourmand G, Salem S, Karami A, Baradaran N, Mehrsai A (2008) Anabolic-androgenic steroid effects on early morbid symptoms after open prostatectomy: a pilot study. *Aging Male* **11**:123–127

Przkora R, Herndon DN, Suman OE (2007) The effects of oxandrolone and exercise on muscle mass and function in children with severe burns. *Pediatrics* **119**:e109–e116

Quigley CA, DeBellis A, Marschke KB, El-Awady MK, Wilson EM, French FF (1995) Androgen receptor defects: historical, clinical and molecular perspectives. *Endocr Rev* **16**:271–321

Rabkin JG, Wagner GJ, Rabkin R (1999) Testosterone therapy for human immunodeficiency virus-positive men with and without hypogonadism. *J Clin Psychopharmacol* **19**:19–27

Rabkin JG, McElhiney MC, Rabkin R, McGrath PJ, Ferrando SJ (2006) Placebo-controlled trial of dehydroepiandrosterone (DHEA) for treatment of nonmajor depression in patients with HIV/AIDS. *Am J Psychiatry* **163**:59–66

Rambaldi A, Gluud C (2006) Anabolic-androgenic steroids for alcoholic liver disease. *Cochrane Database Syst Rev* **4**:CD003045

Reckelhoff JF, Yanes LL, Iliescu R, Fortepiani LA, Granger JP (2005) Testosterone supplementation in aging men and women: possible impact on cardiovascular-renal disease. *Am J Physiol Renal Physiol* **289**:F941–F948

Reid IR, Wattie DJ, Evans MC, Stapleton JP (1996) Testosterone therapy in glucocorticoid-treated men. *Arch Intern Med* **156**:1173–1177

Reilly JT (2006) Idiopathic myelofibrosis: pathogenesis to treatment. *Hematol Oncol* **24**:56–63

Rice L (2004) Danazol, idiopathic thrombocytopenic purpura, and thrombopoietin. *Am J Med* **117**:972–973; author reply:973

Riedl M, Gower RG, Chrvala CA (2011) Current medical management of hereditary angioedema: results from a large survey of US physicians. *Ann Allergy Asthma Immunol* **106**:316–322.e4

Sandblom RE, Matsumoto AM, Scoene RB, Lee KA, Giblin EC, Bremner WJ, Pierson DJ (1983) Obstructive sleep apnea induced by testosterone administration. *N Engl J Med* **308**:508–510

Sardar P, Jha A, Roy D, Majumdar U, Guha P, Roy S, Banerjee R, Banerjee AK, Bandyopadhyay D (2010) Therapeutic effects of nandrolone and testosterone in adult male HIV patients with AIDS wasting syndrome (AWS): a randomized, double-blind, placebo-controlled trial. *HIV Clin Trials* **11**:220–229

Sattler FR, Jaque SV, Schroeder ET, Olson C, Dube MP, Martinez C, Briggs W, Horton R, Azen S (1999) Effects of pharmacological doses of nandrolone decanoate and progressive resistance training in immunodeficient patients infected with human immunodeficiency virus. *J Clin Endocrinol Metab* **84**:1268–1276

Saylor PJ, Smith MR (2010) Adverse effects of androgen deprivation therapy: defining the problem and promoting health among men with prostate cancer. *J Natl Compr Canc Netw* **8**:211–223

Schneider BK, Pickett CK, Zwillich CW, Weil JV, McDermott MT, Santen RJ, Varano LA, White DP (1986) Influence of testosterone on breathing during sleep. *J Appl Physiol* **61**:618–623

Schofield RS, Hill JA, McGinn CJ, Aranda JM (2002) Hormone therapy in men and risk of cardiac allograft rejection. *J Heart Lung Transplant* **21**:493–495

Schols AM, Soeters PB, Mostert R, Pluymers RJ, Wouters EF (1995) Physiologic effects of nutritional support and anabolic steroids in patients with chronic obstructive pulmonary disease. A placebo-controlled randomized trial. *Am J Respir Crit Care Med* **152**:1268–1274

Schols AM, Slangen J, Volovics L, Wouters EF (1998) Weight loss is a reversible factor in the prognosis of chronic obstructive pulmonary disease. *Am J Respir Crit Care Med* **157**:1791–1797

Scott JD, Wolfe PR, Anderson P, Cohan GR, Scarsella A (2007) Prospective study of topical testosterone gel (AndroGel) versus intramuscular testosterone in testosterone-deficient HIV-infected men. *HIV Clin Trials* **8**:412–420

Seidman SN, Orr G, Raviv G, Levi R, Roose SP, Kravitz E, Amiaz R, Weiser M (2009) Effects of testosterone replacement in middle-aged men with dysthymia: a randomized, placebo-controlled clinical trial *J Clin Psychopharmacol* **29**:216–221

Shahidi NT (1973) Androgens and erythropoiesis. *N Engl J Med* **289**:72–80

Sharma S, Arneja A, McLean L, Duerksen D, Leslie W, Sciberras D, Lertzman M (2008) Anabolic steroids in COPD: a review and preliminary results of a randomized trial. *Chron Respir Dis* **5**:169–176

Sheffer AL, Fearon DT, Austen KF (1977) Methyltestosterone therapy in hereditary angioedema. *Ann Intern Med* **86**:306–308

Sicotte NL, Giesser BS, Tandon V, Klutch R, Steiner B, Drain AE, Shattuck DW, Hull L, Wang HJ, Elashoff RM, Swerdloff RS, Voskuhl RR (2007) Testosterone treatment in multiple sclerosis: a pilot study. *Arch Neurol* **64**:683–688

Siddique H, Smith JC, Corrall RJ (2004) Reversal of polycythaemia induced by intramuscular androgen replacement using transdermal testosterone therapy. *Clin Endocrinol (Oxf)* **60**:143–145

Silverberg D, Wexler D, Blum M, Schwartz D, Iaina A (2004) The use of androgens in anaemia resistant to erythropoietin and i.v. iron in patients with heart and renal failure. *Nephrol Dial Transplant* **19**:1021

Singh AB, Norris K, Modi N, Sinha-Hikim I, Shen R, Davidson T, Bhasin S (2001) Pharmacokinetics of a transdermal testosterone system in men with end stage renal disease receiving maintenance hemodialysis and healthy hypogonadal men. *J Clin Endocrinol Metab* **86**:2437–2445

Sloane DE, Lee CW, Sheffer AL (2007) Hereditary angioedema: safety of long-term stanozolol therapy. *J Allergy Clin Immunol* **120**:654–658

Snyder PJ, Peachey H, Hannoush P, Berlin JA, Loh L, Lenrow DA, Holmes JH, Dlewati A, Santanna J, Rosen CJ, Strom BL (1999) Effect of testosterone treatment on body composition and muscle strength in men over 65 years of age. *J Clin Endocrinol Metab* **84**:2647–2653

Spaulding WB (1960) Methyltestosterone therapy for hereditary episodic edema (hereditary angioneurotic edema). *Ann Intern Med* **53**:739–745

Spiers ASD, DeVita SF, Allar MJ, Richards S, Sedranak N (1981) Beneficial effects of an anabolic steroid during cytotoxic chemotherapy for metatstatic cancer. *J Med* **12**:433–446

Srinivas-Shankar U, Roberts SA, Connolly MJ, O'Connell MD, Adams JE, Oldham JA, Wu FC (2010) Effects of testosterone on muscle strength, physical function, body composition, and quality of life in intermediate-frail and frail elderly men: a randomized, double-blind, placebo-controlled study. *J Clin Endocrinol Metab* **95**:639–650

Stenner J, Holthaus K, Mackenzie SH, Crawford ED (1998) The effect of ejaculation on prostate-specific antigen in a prostate cancer-screening population. *Urology* **51**:455–459

Strawford A, Barbieri T, Van Loan M, Parks E, Catlin D, Barton N, Neese R, Christiansen M, King J, Hellerstein MK (1999) Resistance exercise and supraphysiologic androgen therapy in eugonadal men with HIV-related weight loss: a randomized controlled trial. *JAMA* **281**:1282–1290

Sullivan DH, Roberson PK, Johnson LE, Bishara O, Evans WJ, Smith ES, Price JA (2005) Effects of muscle strength training and testosterone in frail elderly males. *Med Sci Sports Exerc* **37**:1664–1672

Svartberg J (2010) Androgens and chronic obstructive pulmonary disease. *Curr Opin Endocrinol Diabetes Obes* 17:257–261

Svartberg J, Aasebo U, Hjalmarsen A, Sundsfjord J, Jorde R (2004) Testosterone treatment improves body composition and sexual function in men with COPD, in a 6-month randomized controlled trial. *Respir Med* 98:906–913

Talbot JA, Sheldrick R, Caswell H, Duncan S (2008) Sexual function in men with epilepsy: how important is testosterone? *Neurology* 70:1346–1352

Teruel JL, Marcen R, Navarro JF, Villafruela JJ, Fernandez-Lucas M, Liano F, Ortuno J (1995) Evolution of serum erythropoietin after androgen administration to hemodialysis patients: a prospective study. *Nephron* 70:282–286

Teruel JL, Aguilera A, Marcen R, Antolin JN, Otero GG, Ortuno J (1996a) Androgen therapy for anaemia of chronic renal failure. *Scand J Urol Nephr* 30:403–408

Teruel JL, Marcen R, Navarro-Antolin J, Aguilera A, Fernandez-Juarez G, Ortuno J (1996b) Androgen versus erythropoietin for the treatment of anemia in hemodialyzed patients: a prospective study. *J Am Soc Nephrol* 7:140–144

Teruel JL, Cano T, Marcen R, Villafruela JJ, Rivera M, Fernandez-Juarez G, Ortuno J (1997) Decrease in the haemoglobin level in haemodialysis patients undergoing antiandrogen therapy. *Nephro Dial Transplant* 12:1262–1263

Thomas S, Wolf SE, Murphy KD, Chinkes DL, Herndon DN (2004) The long-term effect of oxandrolone on hepatic acute phase proteins in severely burned children. *J Trauma* 56:37–44

Tweedle D, Walton C, Johnston IDA (1973) The effect of an anabolic steroid on postoperative nitrogen balance. *Br J Clin Pract* 27:130–132

VACURG (Veterans Administration Cooperative Urological Research Group) (1967) Carcinoma of the prostate: treatment comparisons. *J Urol* 98:516–522

van Coevorden A, Stolear JC, Dhaene M, van Herweghem JL, Mockel J (1986) Effect of chronic oral testosterone undecanoate administration on the pituitary-testicular axes of hemodialyzed male patients. *Clin Nephrol* 26:48–54

van den Berghe G, Wouters P, Weekers F, Verwaest C, Bruyninckx F, Schetz M, Vlasselaers D, Ferdinande P, Lauwers P, Bouillon R (2001) Intensive insulin therapy in the surgical intensive care unit. *N Engl J Med* 345:1359–1367

Van Vollenhoven RF, Engleman EG, McGuire JL (1995) Dehydroepiandrosterone in systemic lupus erythematosus. *Arthritis Rheum* 38:1826–1831

Vaughan C, Goldstein FC, Tenover JL (2007) Exogenous testosterone alone or with finasteride does not improve measurements of cognition in healthy older men with low serum testosterone. *J Androl* 28:875–882

Vecchio M, Navaneethan SD, Johnson DW, Lucisano G, Graziano G, Saglimbene V, Ruospo M, Querques M, Jannini EA, Strippoli GF (2010) Interventions for treating sexual dysfunction in patients with chronic kidney disease. *Cochrane Database Syst Rev* 12:CD007747

Velazquez I, Alter BP (2004) Androgens and liver tumors: Fanconi's anemia and non-Fanconi's conditions. *Am J Hematol* 77:257–267

Victor G, Shanmugasundaram K, Krishnamurthi CA, Rex PM, Nagarajan D (1967) Haemoglobin response to anabolic steroid in iron-deficiency anaemia. *J Assoc Physicians India* 15:177–183

Villareal DT, Morley JE (1994) Trophic factors in aging. Should older people receive hormonal replacement therapy? *Drugs Aging* 4:492–509

von Hartitzsch B, Kerr DNS (1976) Response to parenteral iron with and without androgen therapy in patients undergoing regular haemodialysis. *Nephron* 17:430–438

Walters KA, Simanainen U, Handelsman DJ (2010) Molecular insights into androgen actions in male and female reproductive function from androgen receptor knockout models. *Hum Reprod Update* 16:543–558

Warren MF, Serby MJ, Roane DM (2008) The effects of testosterone on cognition in elderly men: a review. *CNS Spectr* 13:887–897

Watson RN, Bradley MH, Callahan R, Peters BJ, Kory RC (1959) A six-month evaluation of an anabolic drug, norethandrolone, in underweight persons. *Am J Med* 26:238–248

Wattel E, Cambier N, Caulier MT, Sautiere D, Bauters F, Fenaux P (1994) Androgen therapy in myelodysplastic syndromes with thrombocytopenia: a report on 20 cases. *Br J Haematol* 87:205–208

Webb WR, Doyle RS, Howard HS (1960) Relative metabolic effects of calories, protein, and an anabolic steroid (19-nortestosterone) in early postoperative period. *Metabolism* 9:1047–1057

Weber JP, Walsh PC, Peters CA, Spivak JL (1991) Effect of reversible androgen deprivation on hemoglobin and serum erythropoietin in men. *Am J Hematol* 36:190–194

Wells R (1960) Prednisolone and testosterone propionate in cirrhosis of the liver: a controlled trial. *Lancet* 2:1416–1419

Whitnall MH, Elliott TB, Harding RA, Inal CE, Landauer MR, Wilhelmsen CL, McKinney L, Miner VL, Jackson WE 3rd, Loria RM, Ledney GD, Seed TM (2000) Androstenediol stimulates myelopoiesis and enhances resistance to infection in gamma-irradiated mice. *Int J Immunopharmacol* 22:1–14

Wilkey JL, Barson LJ, Kest L, Bragagni A (1960) The effect of testosterone on the azotemic patient: an intermediary report. *J Urol* **83**:25–29

Williams JS, Stein JH, Ferris TF (1974) Nandrolone decanoate therapy for patients receiving hemodialysis. A controlled study. *Arch Intern Med* **134**:289–292

Winearls CG (1995) Historical review of the use of recombinant human erythropoietin in chronic renal failure. *Nephrol Dial Transplant* **10** (Suppl 2):3–9

Wolf SE, Edelman LS, Kemalyan N, Donison L, Cross J, Underwood M, Spence RJ, Noppenberger D, Palmieri TL, Greenhalgh DG, Lawless M, Voigt D, Edwards P, Warner P, Kagan R, Hatfield S, Jeng J, Crean D, Hunt J, Purdue G, Burris A, Cairns B, Kessler M, Klein RL, Baker R, Yowler C, Tutulo W, Foster K, Caruso D, Hildebrand B, Benjamin W, Villarreal C, Sanford AP, Saffle J (2006) Effects of oxandrolone on outcome measures in the severely burned: a multicenter prospective randomized double-blind trial. *J Burn Care Res* **27**:131–139; discussion:140–141

Wu FC, von Eckardstein A (2003) Androgens and coronary artery disease. *Endocr Rev* **24**:183–217

Wu FCW, Farley TMM, Peregoudov A, Waites GMH; WHO Task Force on Methods for the Regulation of Male Fertility (1996) Effects of testosterone enanthate in normal men: experience from a multicenter contraceptive efficacy study. *Fertil Steril* **65**:626–636

Wulfsohn NL, Politzer WM, Henrico JS (1964) Testosterone therapy in bronchial asthma. *S Afr Med J* **38**:170–172

Young GA, Yule AG, Hill GL (1983) Effects of an anabolic steroid on plasma amino acids, proteins, and body composition in patients receiving intravenous hyperalimentation. *J Parent Ent Nutr* **7**:221–225

Young LA, Neiss MB, Samuels MH, Roselli CE, Janowsky JS (2010) Cognition is not modified by large but temporary changes in sex hormones in men. *J Clin Endocrinol Metab* **95**:280–288

Young N, Griffith P, Brittain E, Elfenbein G, Gardner F, Huang A,

Harmon D, Hewlett J, Fay J, Mangan K (1988) A multicenter trial of antithymocyte globulin in aplastic anemia and related diseases. *Blood* **72**:1861–1869

Young RL, Fuchs RJ, Woltjen MJ (1976) Chorionic gonadotropin in weight control. A double-blind crossover study. *JAMA* **236**:2495–2497

Zak PJ, Kurzban R, Ahmadi S, Swerdloff RS, Park J, Efremidze L, Redwine K, Morgan K, Matzner W (2009) Testosterone administration decreases generosity in the ultimatum game. *PLoS One* **4**:e8330

Zarrouf FA, Artz S, Griffith J, Sirbu C, Kommor M (2009) Testosterone and depression: systematic review and meta-analysis. *J Psychiatr Pract* **15**:289–305

Zawilska K, Tokarz A, Misiak A, Psuja P, Wislawski S, Szymczak P, Meissner J, Karon J, Lewandowski K, Lopaciuk S, Ziemski JM, Sowler J (1990) Nebulised heparin and anabolic steroid in the prevention of postoperative deep venous thrombosis following elective abdominal surgery. *Folia Haematologica* **117**:699–707

Review of guidelines on diagnosis and treatment of testosterone deficiency

Ronald S. Swerdloff and Christina C. L. Wang

18.1 Introduction

This is an effort to review and compare the guidelines on diagnosis, treatment options, outcomes and monitoring of men with low serum testosterone. The principal published guidelines are listed in Table 18.1.

18.2 What is a guideline?

18.2.1 Definition of guideline

A *guideline* is a statement by which to determine a course of action. A guideline aims to streamline particular processes according to a set routine or sound practice. By definition, following a guideline is never mandatory. Guidelines are thus not binding and should not be enforced. Medical guidelines are often created by medical professional societies to help physicians and other health professionals provide community-level standard of practice, and are sometimes used to reward practitioners for "desired behavior."

Testosterone: Action, Deficiency, Substitution, ed. Eberhard Nieschlag and Hermann M. Behre, Assoc. ed. Susan Nieschlag. Published by Cambridge University Press. © Cambridge University Press 2012.

Table 18.1 Comparison of recent guidelines on management of male hypogonadism

Organization / *Title* / Date of newest guideline	Applicable age	Diagnosis: symptoms, hormone tests and threshold	Screening	Treatment options listed	Serum testosterone goals	Exclusions	Monitoring requirements for testosterone treatment
American Association of Clinical Endocrinologists (Petak et al. 2002) *Medical guidelines for clinical practice for the evaluation and treatment of hypogonadism in adult male patients* 2002 Not evidence based	All ages; discusses LOH	Symptoms: desirable Hormones: TT: multiple <200–318 ng/dl (<6.9 to 11 nmol/l) Repeat TT required: not stated SHBG: can be used to calculate FT FT, BT, cFT: optional; no thresholds provided	Not stated	Many	Mid-normal		Symptoms: every 3–4 months in yr 1 serum T: recommended but frequency not stated DRE and prostate symptoms: every 6–12 months; PSA annually HCT: every 6 months for 18 months, and annually; T treatment adjusted if HCT>50% Lipids: initial; 6–12 months and annually
Swedish specialists (Abrahamsson et al. 2010) *Testosterone deficiency management program and treatment recommendations* Unpublished Not evidence based	All ages	Symptoms: required Hormones: TT: <8 nmol/l (230 ng/dl) probable deficiency; >12 nmol/l (346 nmol/l) probably normal; 8–12 nmol/l gray area Repeat TT required: not stated SHBG: yes FT, BT, cFT: no	No	Yes	Not stated	DRE abnormal; PSA > 3 ng/l; breast CA; HCT > 53% (relative); OSA (relative); heart failure (untreated)	T, PSA, hemoglobin, HCT: every 3 months for 1 yr then every 12 months DRE: every 12 months BMD: every 24 months Lipids: not stated
Canadian Physicians (Morales et al. 2010)	Older age group > age 40	Symptoms: required Hormones: TT: no threshold	Only "high risk men"; challenges specificity of	Yes	Not stated	Breast or prostate CA; abnormal PSA and DRE refer to urologist; IPSS > 21 relative	Serum T: every 3–6 months in year 1 and yearly thereafter

Table 18.1 (cont.)

Organization Title Date of newest guideline	Applicable age	Diagnosis: symptoms, hormone tests and threshold	Screening	Treatment options listed	Serum testosterone goals	Exclusions	Monitoring requirements for testosterone treatment
Practical guide to diagnosis, management and treatment of testosterone deficiency for Canadian physicians 2010		Repeat TT required: yes SHBG: only as part of cFT and cBT; no threshold levels given FT, BT, cFT: BT "gold standard"; cBT and cFT acceptable alternative; no threshold levels given	ADAM questionnaire			contraindication to T treatment; erythrocytosis; untreated OSA; severe CHF; men wishing biological fatherhood	PSA and DRE: every 3–6 months in year 1 and at yearly intervals Hemoglobin and HCT: every 3–6 months in year 1 and yearly thereafter Lipids: not stated
Endocrine Society (Bhasin et al. 2010) *Testosterone therapy in men with androgen deficiency syndromes: an Endocrine Society clinical practice guideline* 2010 Evidence based	Young and middle age men; older men equivocal	Symptoms: required Hormones: TT: for young and middle-aged men, below reference range for healthy young men established in individual laboratory. For older men, panel disagreed on threshold TT: <280 ng/dl (9.7 nmol/l) with symptoms or <200 ng/dl (6.9 nmol/l) Repeat TT required: yes SHBG: no, unless cFT or BT are used.	No, except in certain high-risk populations (e.g. HIV and glucocorticoid-receiving men)	Yes	Mid-normal (young and middle-aged men); older men unclear	Prostate CA; breast CA; PSA >4.0 ng/ml and/ or abnormal DRE (>3.0 PSA in high-risk e.g. African and first-degree relatives with prostate CA: refer to urologist; suggest prostate CA risk calculator be used. HCT >50%; IPSS >19; hyper-viscosity, untreated OSA; class III-IV CHF	Serum T: 3–6 months after starting T Rx PSA/DRE: no for age < 40; >40 – baseline DRE and PSA, 3–6 months after T Rx, then guidelines for age and race; increase in PSA > 1.4 ng/ml within any 12-month period or PSA velocity > 0.4 ng/ml per yr using PSA level after 6 months of T Rx as reference and PSA data available for >2years; IPSS > 19 HCT: baseline 3–6 months and annual

			FT, BT, cFT: no, except when TT is in gray zone or altered SHBG suspected					>54%: stop therapy and adjust dose Lipids: not stated
ISA, ISSAM, EAU, EAA, ASA (Wang et al. 2009) *Investigation, treatment and monitoring of late-onset hypogonadism in males* 2010 Evidence based	> age 60	Symptoms: not stated, improvement in signs and symptoms of T deficiency should be sought by 3–6 months of treatment Hormones: TT: <8 nmol/l (230 ng/dl); >12 nmol/l (350 ng/dl) not hypogonadal; 8–12 nmol/l (230–350 ng/dl) requires calculated FT or FT by equilibrium dialysis Repeat TT required: not stated, monitor improvement in signs and symptoms of T deficiency by 3–6 months of treatment SHBG: required for calculated FT FT, BT, cFT: FT <225 pmol/l (65 pg/ml) provides supportive evidence for T treatment; threshold values for BT are not generally available; salivary T not recommended for general use	No	Yes	Mid- to lower young adult male serum T levels	Prostate and breast CA; erythrocytosis; (HCT > 52%) untreated; OSA untreated; severe CHF; IPSS > 21 relative contraindication to T treatment	Serum T: not stated DRE and PSA: baseline, at 3–6 months, 12 months and annually after Rx; suspicious DRE/increased PSA or calculated risk leads to ultrasound-guided biopsy; men successfully treated for prostate CA with symptomatic hypogonadism are potential candidates for T Rx after a prudent interval if there is no clinical or laboratory evidence of residual CA HCT/hemoglobin: before Rx, 3–4 months and 12 months of Rx then annually; dose adjustment or periodic phlebotomy to keep hematocrit below 55% Lipids: not stated	

Table 18.1 (cont.)

Organization / *Title* / Date of newest guideline	Applicable age	Diagnosis: symptoms, hormone tests and threshold	Screening	Treatment options listed	Serum testosterone goals	Exclusions	Monitoring requirements for testosterone treatment
Practice Committee for the American Society for Reproductive Medicine (American Society for Reproductive Medicine 2006) *Treatment of androgen deficiency in the aging male* 2006 Not evidence based	> age 50	Symptoms: required Hormones: TT: < 200 ng/dl (<6.9 nmol/l) = hypogonadism; >400 (13.8 nmol/l) not deficient; 200–400 treatment could be beneficial Repeat TT required: not stated SHBG: yes for cFT or cBT FT, BT, cFT: FT or BT or cFT may be useful for "might benefit" group; values for BT that are <normal range for adult men supports the diagnosis of T deficiency	No	Yes	Not stated	Clinical prostate CA; breast CA; elevated HCT > 55%; and sensitivity to treatment; relative contraindications are: severe OSA; HCT> 52%; severe LUTS; and CHF	Serum T: levels over pretreatment but not >reference range for young adult males PSA: PSA >1.0 ng/ml within 3–6 months of Rx; PSA obtained 3 and 6 months after treatment and annually thereafter HCT, hemoglobin: at 3 and 6 months after Rx and annually Lipids: not stated
Andrology Australia (www. andrologyaustralia. org) *Testosterone deficiency fact sheet* 2005 Patient information sheet	All ages	Symptoms: required? Hormones: TT: <8 nmol/l (230 ng/ dl) Repeat TT required: not stated SHBG: no, unless as alternative if cFT or BT are used FT, BT, cFT: not stated	Not stated	Yes	Not stated	prostate and breast CA; relative exclusion men with OSA and CHF	Not stated

Abbreviations: T, testosterone; TT, total testosterone; FT, free testosterone; BT, bioavailable testosterone; cFT, calculated FT; cBT, calculated BT; DRE, digital rectal examination; PSA, prostate-specific antigen; LUTS, lower urinary tract symptoms; HCT, hematocrit; OSA, obstructive sleep apnea; CHF, chronic heart failure; IPSS, International Prostate Symptom Score; Rx, treatment; CA, cancer; ISA, International Society of Andrology; ISSAM, International Society for the Study of the Aging Male; EAU, European Association cf Urology; EAA, European Acadamy of Andrology; ASA, American Society of Andrology.

18.2.2   Selection of guideline committee members

Guideline committee members are usually selected by a professional organization because they are experienced and respected in the particular area of interest. In some cases guidelines can be written by special-interest groups with predetermined agendas.

18.2.3   Evidence-based versus expert-opinion criteria for guidelines

Guidelines can be based on expert opinion or on published evidence at defined levels of quality (evidence based). The highest quality for interventional studies is appropriately powered, double-blinded and placebo-controlled clinical trials. Unfortunately, many guidelines lack adequate high levels of evidence, and thus such guidelines are to a great extent expert-opinion formulated. This is the case for male hypogonadism.

In this review, the authors have surveyed a number of guidelines on androgen deficiency, and present the major consensus views as well as areas where there are significant differences in opinions. The guidelines are listed in Table 18.1. It will be noted that some guidelines focus on all age ranges and are independent of the etiologies of hypogonadism, while others focus on specific age groups (i.e. old age), etiologies (i.e. HIV, obesity), targeted symptoms (i.e. libido, osteoporosis) and outcomes. Some focus on different interventional approaches (testosterone treatment).

Evidence-based: the International Societies (Wang *et al.* 2009) and The Endocrine Society (Bhasin *et al.* 2010) guidelines rated the quality of the evidence and thus can be considered evidence based, although both acknowledged that much of the evidence is weak and the conclusions are thus to some extent "expert opinion." The authors of this chapter have participated on several of the guidelines committees referenced in this review, and can attest to the fact that there may be differences in the views of guideline committee members on specific areas; recommendations may represent a negotiated consensus view.

Expert opinion: a number of the reviewed guidelines provided opinions that were not rated by the quality of evidence. All guidelines provided literature support for what could be considered expert opinions. The guidelines on hypogonadism from the Canadian Physicians (Morales *et al.* 2010),

American Association of Clinical Endocrinologists (Petak *et al.* 2002), Swedish Specialists (Abrahamsson *et al.* 2010), the Endocrine Society of Australia (Conway *et al.* 2000) and American Society of Reproductive Medicine (American Society for Reproductive Medicine 2006) fall into this category.

Organization-based or other: many guidelines are identified as an official position of a medical or scientific society, while others appear to be an independent select group of "experts." Some guidelines seem to be sponsored by a pharmaceutical company. In this last situation it may not be clear if the recommendations were fully independent.

18.3   Definition of hypogonadism

Hypogonadism in the literal sense refers to a decreased function of the hormone secretory compartments of the testes (e.g. testosterone secretion by Leydig cells) and decreased sperm production by the germinal compartment. However, most often clinicians think of hypogonadism as androgen deficiency and its clinical manifestations. This review of hypogonadism guidelines will focus on testosterone deficiency.

18.3.1   Diagnosis of hypogonadism

The diagnosis of testosterone deficiency may be based only on the blood hormone level (serum testosterone) or require both a low serum testosterone and symptoms compatible with, or specific for, a low serum testosterone. Unfortunately, many symptoms lack sufficient specificity to be diagnostic for a low serum testosterone. Furthermore, blood levels of testosterone can be assayed as total testosterone, free testosterone or biologically active testosterone. Each type of measurement uses different methodologies which may vary in accuracy and specificity.

18.3.2   Age-group selective?

Testosterone deficiency in males differs in diagnostic approaches and clinical presentations in infants, children, pubertal, young and middle-aged adults and in old age. This review focuses on adults. Most guidelines are broad in reference to age group, but some have specifically dealt with androgen deficiency in the elderly, referred to in some guidelines as late onset hypogonadism (LOH) (Wang *et al.* 2009).

18.3.3 Hormone threshold

This is one of the most difficult aspects of defining hypogonadism. The standard approach is to take a reference range for a normal population (mean $\pm$ 2 SD) and define hypogonadism as below this population-based standard. This approach has several problems: (1) What population? (Age, race, exclusions for co-morbidities.) (2) What reference range? Unfortunately we lack a universally agreed-upon reference range (published reference ranges vary considerably depending on the laboratory methodology and population studied). (3) What testosterone assays used? For example, total testosterone, biologically active testosterone, and free testosterone. Free testosterone can be measured by analog displacement assays, calculated based on formulae of mass action or empirical formulae (Sartorius *et al.* 2009; Ly *et al.* 2010), assessed knowing SHBG and total testosterone levels, or determined by equilibrium dialysis (Vermeulen *et al.* 1999). (See Chapter 4.)

18.3.4 What level of testosterone is clinically relevant for the diagnosis?

There have been efforts to relate symptoms and signs of hypogonadism to serum testosterone levels using defined methodology. This is best exemplified by the data from the European Male Aging Study (Wu *et al.* 2010). These data suggest that different symptom components of hypogonadism seem to present at different serum testosterone concentrations in a population. Thus, decreased libido is evident at a higher serum testosterone level than other symptoms. Different guidelines create a threshold from anywhere below a defined reference range to levels below 200 ng/dl. In some guidelines, expert opinions were acknowledged to differ considerably (Wang *et al.* 2009). The problem is further complicated by the concept that there are individual patient differences in sensitivity to serum testosterone. This concept is inherent in the range of values that make up the bell-shaped curve of a reference population. Thus a "normal" man, A, may have a mean serum testosterone of 600 ng/dl, while equally "normal" man, B, may appear phenotypically indistinguishable in terms of signs and symptoms of androgen effect from a man with a mean serum testosterone of 400 ng/dl.

18.3.5 Symptoms required for the diagnosis of hypogonadism

Some guidelines refer only to objective evidence of a low serum testosterone to define hypogonadism,

while others insist on both a chemical deficiency and clinical signs or symptoms to merit the diagnosis of hypogonadism (Table 18.1).

18.4 Screening for androgen deficiency syndrome

Very few guidelines support the use of either population-based hormonal screening or questionnaires to find more cases of "hypogonadism" (Table 18.1; Wang *et al.* 2009; Bhasin *et al.* 2010). Guideline authors seem to be inhibited by the lack of clear hormone thresholds (see above) and limited evidence-based data to prove benefit for treatment of the full spectrum of symptoms, to support the use of population-based testosterone measurement screening. The case-finding questionnaires such as Androgen Deficiency in Aging Male (ADAM) (Morley *et al.* 2000), Aging Male Symptoms Rating Scale (AMS) (Heinemann *et al.* 2004) and the Massachusetts Male Aging Study Questionnaire (Smith *et al.* 2000) proposed for identification of hypogonadism are limited in practical use by the lack of specificity (despite great sensitivity). There is a new questionnaire for hypogonadal men that has not yet been validated in different populations (Rosen *et al.* 2011). Thus, essentially none of the guidelines have advocated population-based screening, although some have advocated use of hormone screening in high-risk groups. For example, the Endocrine Society supports measuring serum testosterone in patients receiving opioids and glucocorticoids and men with known HIV disease, and low trauma fractures, regardless of symptoms of low testosterone; while they recommend measurement of serum testosterone in men with type 2 diabetes mellitus, chronic renal disease and chronic obstructive pulmonary disease only when they have symptoms suggestive of low serum testosterone. A similar recommendation was stated for type 2 diabetes by the International Societies guidelines; the American Association of Clinical Endocrinologists (AACE) guidelines were silent on this topic.

18.5 Clinical manifestations of hypogonadism

18.5.1 Libido

Impaired libido is the classic symptom of low testosterone and is a focal point of the symptom complex in the discussion of most guidelines. The EMAS defined the serum testosterone level that is associated with low testosterone syndrome in middle-aged and elderly men (Wu *et al.* 2010). Impaired libido is also noted in LOH in several guidelines (Wang *et al.* 2009; Bhasin *et al.* 2010; Morales *et al.* 2010). The AACE guidelines of 2002 stated that most studies support the benefits of testosterone therapy for impaired sexual behavior in men with low testosterone (Petak *et al.* 2002). The ISA guidelines recommend that men with ED and/or decreased libido and documented low testosterone are candidates for testosterone therapy (Wang *et al.* 2009). The Canadian Physicians' guidelines are positive about the benefits of testosterone therapy for men with decreased sexual desire (Morales *et al.* 2010). The Endocrine Society guidelines recommend that "clinicians offer testosterone therapy to men with low serum testosterone levels and low libido and men with ED after evaluating for other causes of ED and consideration of other therapies for ED." They go on to state that the evidence that testosterone is beneficial for improving decreased libido is overall supportive but not always consistent across controlled studies reported in the literature (Bhasin *et al.* 2010).

18.5.2   Erectile function

Erectile dysfunction is also a classic symptom of men with low testosterone; unless the testosterone deficiency is very severe, it is often secondary to a co-morbid condition that responds better to phosphodiesterase 5 (PDE5) inhibitors than testosterone replacement. The ISA guideline on LOH discusses the possibility that testosterone treatment may be useful as a complementary treatment when older hypogonadal patients fail to respond to PDE5 inhibitors (Wang *et al.* 2009). The Canadian Physicians' guideline states that men with profound hypogonadism show significant improvement in ED when on TRT (Morales *et al.* 2010). For ED, the use of PDE5 inhibitors remains the principal treatment. In men with low testosterone and ED, the majority of experts seem to prefer initial treatment with PDE5 inhibitors and adding testosterone for decreased libido or other signs and symptoms of low testosterone. A properly powered study is needed to compare the benefits of PDE5 inhibitors and testosterone, alone and together, in men with ED and low testosterone.

18.5.3   Muscle strength and function

A number of guidelines list decreased muscle mass and strength as one of the symptom complexes seen in men with low testosterone (American Society for Reproductive Medicine 2006; Wang *et al.* 2009; Bhasin *et al.* 2010; Morales *et al.* 2010). Most but not all guidelines discuss improved muscle mass with testosterone treatment and emphasize variability of improvement in function. Meta-analyses of randomized trials in middle-aged men and placebo-controlled studies in older men have demonstrated that TRT is associated with greater improvement in grip strength and lean body mass and reduction in body fat mass than placebo (Isidori *et al.* 2005; Page *et al.* 2005; Srinivas-Shankar *et al.* 2010). In contrast, changes in performance-based measures of physical function in testosterone trials that recruited healthy older men selectively have been inconsistent across trials (Bhasin *et al.* 2010). It is hoped that the ongoing, larger sized, well-controlled testosterone interventional trials on improvement in physical function in older men with physical disabilities will provide more clarity to the important question of reduction in frailty after testosterone replacement.

18.5.4   Bone mineral loss and osteoporosis

Most trials have recognized that low testosterone is a risk factor for decreased BMD and fractures (especially in hypogonadal older men). Most experts agree that the prevalence of osteoporosis is greater in men with low, compared to normal, serum testosterone levels (Amin *et al.* 2000; Meier *et al.* 2008). Testosterone replacement therapy was found to increase bone density in hypogonadal men (Behre *et al.* 1997; Svartberg *et al.* 2008). While a few studies have not shown a clear benefit in bone density, many studies with exogenous testosterone have noted increases in BMD in hypogonadal aging males (Merza *et al.* 2006). Some studies have reported improvements in lumbar bone density (Snyder *et al.* 1999; Amory *et al.* 2004; Wang *et al.* 2004; Basurto *et al.* 2008; Svartberg *et al.* 2008). This has also been noted in two meta-analyses (Isidori *et al.* 2005; Tracz *et al.* 2006). Some studies (Amory *et al.* 2004; Wang *et al.* 2004; Nair *et al.* 2006) suggested improvements in hip bone mineral density; while meta-analysis studies (Isidori *et al.* 2005; Tracz *et al.* 2006) found femoral neck improvements to be inconclusive. The Endocrine Society guidelines state that the available data rule out a moderate to large testosterone effect on BMD; yet some studies have shown impressive increases in BMD in older men (Amory *et al.* 2004).

The Canadian Physicians guidelines say that "bone mineral density is increased by testosterone therapy in men with low testosterone levels" (Morales *et al.* 2010). American Association of Clinical Endocrinologists guidelines state that BMD should be assessed before and at one to two years; treatment options to maintain bone mass may include testosterone, implying that it is prescribed for other manifestations of hypogonadism (Petak *et al.* 2002). The ISA guidelines argue that bone density increases with testosterone treatment in hypogonadal men of all ages, but recognizes that the lack of data on reduction of fractures makes conclusions on the benefit of testosterone to treatment of hypogonadal men with low BMD difficult (Wang *et al.* 2009). It is clear from the review of guidelines that prevention of fractures has not been adequately assessed, and assessment of the long-term benefits of testosterone on bone strength and density requires larger-sized, well-controlled studies.

18.5.5   Cognition

There are very limited data on the effects of testosterone therapy in hypogonadal men; the Endocrine Society guidelines state that there were three placebo-controlled studies, but the results were imprecise on several dimensions of cognition and were insignificant after pooling (Bhasin *et al.* 2010).

18.5.6   Mood and well-being

Mild depressive states are reported in many hypogonadal men. The Canadian Physician guideline states that testosterone therapy may benefit emotional well-being (Morales *et al.* 2010). The Endocrine Society guidelines reviewed the interventional data and found that results of controlled studies on depression and QoL were imprecise and inconsistent (Bhasin *et al.* 2010).

18.5.7   Diabetes and metabolic syndrome

There are many studies suggesting that low serum testosterone may be a predictor of future metabolic syndrome and diabetes mellitus (Brand *et al.* 2010; Wang *et al.* 2011). Evidence that interventional replacement testosterone treatment will prevent or correct either metabolic syndrome or type 2 diabetes mellitus is limited. The Swedish Specialists (Abrahamsson *et al.* 2010) state, however, that hypothesis-generating studies show that, by normalizing testosterone

levels in cases of metabolic syndrome or type 2 diabetes, insulin resistance is reduced and this appears to improve both blood glucose control and dyslipidemia.

18.6   Potential risks of testosterone treatment

18.6.1   Prostate cancer

All guidelines and regulatory-agency-directed medicine instructions list non-cured prostate cancer as a contraindication for testosterone treatment. Paradoxically, most guidelines indicate that there was insufficient data to determine if long-term testosterone is a risk factor for developing prostate cancer in the future. The Endocrine Society guideline recommends against testosterone therapy without further urological evaluation in men with a palpable prostate nodule or induration. They made the same cautious statement in men with PSA > 4 ng/ml or > 3 ng/ml in men with high family risk or African racial derivation (Bhasin *et al.* 2010).

18.6.2   Severe lower urinary tract obstructive symptoms (LUTS) and benign prostate hyperplasia

This widely used symptom list is often given in guidelines as a relative or absolute contraindication for testosterone treatment (Wang *et al.* 2009; Bhasin *et al.* 2010); yet there is little evidence that symptoms are worsened with treatment. Despite this, some guidelines give contraindication thresholds for the International Prostate Symptom Score questionnaire (IPSS) >19 or 21, as examples.

18.6.3   Cardiovascular disease

Cardiovascular risk is discussed in many guidelines. The principal position is that low testosterone is associated with greater cardiovascular morbidity and mortality, but there is inadequate interventional data to say whether testosterone treatment of men with low testosterone will benefit cardiovascular status, worsen or not affect cardiovascular outcomes. The Swedish Specialists' guidelines (Abrahamsson *et al.* 2010) are more adamant that there is no increased risk from testosterone treatment on coronary disease. They do, however, say that fluid retention induced by testosterone may worsen CHF. This is also stated in other guidelines. A recent report of increased cardio-vascular risk of testosterone treatment of hypogonadal debilitated men (Basaria *et al.* 2010; see Chapter 10) represents a potential cautionary sign, but the finding requires confirmation as it differs from other investigators who report cardiovascular benefits from testosterone treatment (see Chapter 10).

18.6.4 Erythrocytosis

It was noted in most guidelines that testosterone will increase red blood cell mass, hemoglobin and hematocrit. The Endocrine Society guidelines recommend against treating men with low testosterone if their hematocrit is greater than 50% (Bhasin *et al.* 2010). The ISA guidelines place the threshold for entry into treatment at hematocrit of >52% (Wang *et al.* 2009), and the Swedish Specialists' guidelines (Abrahamsson *et al.* 2010) recommend hematocrit >53% as a relative contraindication The Canadian Physicians' (Morales *et al.* 2010) and AACE (Petak *et al.* 2002) guidelines do not define erythrocytosis, but list it as a contra-indication to treatment with testosterone.

18.6.5 Untreated sleep apnea

This is listed as a contraindication or relative contra-indication in most guidelines. The evidence for physiological doses of testosterone aggravating or causing obstructive sleep apnea is very weak but is usually listed in regulatory inserts as a risk.

18.7 Treatment options

Most guidelines reviewed available testosterone formulations, with some providing details on pharmacokinetics and drug-specific adverse effects. The ISA guidelines express concern about use of long-acting testosterone injectables for older men with LOH because of the protracted half-life that would delay withdrawal from drug in case of adverse effect (Wang *et al.* 2009). The formulation list is provided in many guideline documents, but, since it is the most recent, we refer readers to Table 6 in The Endocrine Society 2010 guidelines (Bhasin *et al.* 2010) and to Chapter 15.

18.8 Monitoring patients on testosterone treatment

Most guidelines recommend monitoring patients for improvements in symptoms, blood testosterone levels

and adverse effects. It is unclear what testosterone level should be a goal, for lack of benefit/risk data based on serum testosterone level attained. In general, normal range levels are recommended. Safety blood testing includes PSA, hematocrit or hemoglobin; physical examination includes digital rectal exam for prostate induration and nodules; history includes lower urinary tract symptoms (LUTS) and obstructive sleep apnea. The recommendation for frequency of testing is not consistent among guidelines but, in general, recommended at baseline, three to six months and annually thereafter. Some guidelines provide detailed PSA and hematocrit levels (Wang *et al.* 2009; Bhasin *et al.* 2010) for stopping treatment, evaluation with specialist or intervention (e.g. veni-section for erythrocytosis).

18.9 Conclusions

This chapter reviews a number of guidelines prepared by experts in a number of countries in North America and Europe for the clinical diagnosis and treatment of young adult, middle-aged and elderly hypogonadal men. These guideline committees reviewed the literature on the topic to provide evidence-based and/or expert opinion, with two guidelines attempting to provide an assessment of quality of the evidence: the Endocrine Society (Bhasin *et al.* 2010) and International Societies (Wang *et al.* 2009). These two guidelines concluded that the evidence to support many of the recommendations was either weak or reverted to expert opinion. McLachlan, in an editorial opinion on the 2010 Endocrine Society guidelines, stated "The evidence basis for informing clinical practice has developed only marginally; among the 45 new references cited from 2006, there are 7 small to moderate sized randomized controlled trials and several controlled studies of responses in young vs. older men; the remainder are commentaries, meta-analyses, or epidemiological studies. With their intimate understanding of the knowledge gaps and as required for writing summary guidelines, the authors [of this guideline] have filled in the blanks with considered commentary." His editorial also commented on the common use of vague terms that reflect the lack of hard data and the shifting sands of opinion (McLachlan 2010).

A second editorial on the Endocrine Society 2010 guidelines update was provided by Bradley Anawalt. He reiterated that "As with the original 2006 guidelines, the evidence for the 2010 guidelines is weak. On a rating scale of very low, low, moderate and high quality, all the recommendations were based on evidence judged to be very low or low and the majority of the recommendations were based on very low quality evidence" (Anawalt 2010). He pointed out many controversial areas in the Endocrine Society guidelines (most addressed by the guideline's authors themselves), including concern about the limited value of digital rectal exams as a monitoring safety tool to detect prostate cancer, the lack of consensus of the value of the prostate calculator as a tool to integrate the data on prostate risk, and the "conservative" recommendation of using a testosterone increase in PSA of >1.5 pg/ml·year as signal for a (urological) assessment (Wolf *et al.* 2010). There are some inconsistencies in his argument as it follows references (Andriole *et al.* 2009; Schroder *et al.* 2009) as to the limited value in reducing mortality rates by screening for prostate cancer in the general population. Anawalt argues for large-scale efficacy and safety studies to answer important questions about benefit/risk of TRT for symptomatic men with low testosterone.

The authors of this chapter are aware of an ongoing study ("T trial") in 800 hypogonadal men, age ≥ 65 years, using a carefully crafted, multiple end-point, placebo-controlled, double-blinded study design. The study will provide insights into the efficacy of reversal of symptoms by replacement testosterone treatment, but it is under-powered for judging cardiovascular disease and prostate safety issues. An interventional arm of the European Male Aging Study (EMAS) will provide valuable additional data as the age groups are wider and the populations differ.

It is also obvious to the present authors that the lack of specificity of the signs and symptoms of low serum testosterone, the uncertainty in the appropriate tests to identify hypogonadism, the lack of a clear threshold of serum testosterone levels for clinical phenotype, and the great impact of co-morbid conditions on the prevalence rate of androgen deficiency has led to uncertainty whether low serum testosterone is a cause of a disorder or a manifestation associated with many disorders. This is particularly true in androgen deficiency in older men.

Furthermore, the recommendations on serum testosterone goals for treatment and the type and frequency of monitoring are also mainly common sense opinions based on clinical experience rather than evidence based. There is a fairly strong opinion in most guidelines against population screening to detect the "syndromic" disorder of testosterone deficiency, as the rationale for treatment is not strongly science based.

The careful review of the available guidelines also demonstrates the bias of the various committees' members. There are the enthusiasts and naysayers in the identification of potentially treatable patients. It is our opinion that the divergences of opinion are resolvable as we gather more hard data from carefully powered, well-controlled, large-scale, interventional studies in men of all ages with low-testosterone disorder. Our bias is a cautious positive view that we will better define who should and who should not be treated and, for the former category, determine if the benefits of replacement therapy outweigh the risks.

18.10   Key messages

- Guidelines are guides designed to improve patient care and not enforceable rules.
- Guidelines can be evidence based, represent expert opinion, or a combination of evidence and opinion.
- Evidence-based guidelines are valued more than those based on expert opinion.
- Two groups (ISA and Endocrine Society) have attempted evidence-based guidelines, but both depend significantly on expert opinion.
- Highest quality, evidence-based guidelines require appropriately powered, well-controlled (ideally double-blinded, placebo-controlled) data that has been validated by confirmatory studies.
- Evidence-based guidelines for hypogonadism are considered to be of low quality.
- Guidelines based on expert opinion depend on the selection of the expert panel and are subject to uncertain validity.
- Guidelines on hypogonadism share some common conclusions but differ in diagnostic criteria, treatment indications and monitoring strategies.
- Guidelines are living documents and require revision as new data of improved quality become available.

18.11   References

Abrahamsson U, Arver S, Damber JE, Ekstrom U, Giwercman A, Lehtihet M, Link K, Nilsson J, Peeker R, Pousette A, Rosen T, Stroberg P, Willenheimer R (2010) [*Testosterone Deficiency Management Programme and Treatment Recommendations.*] Svensk Andrologisk Förening, Stockholm. Available at: www.svenskandrologi.se/res/Default/vardprogram.pdf (accessed Feb 22, 2012)

American Society for Reproductive Medicine (2006) Treatment of androgen deficiency in the aging male. *Fertil Steril* **86**:S236–S240

Amin S, Zhang Y, Sawin CT, Evans SR, Hannan MT, Kiel DP, Wilson PW, Felson DT (2000) Association of hypogonadism and estradiol levels with bone mineral density in elderly men from the Framingham study. *Ann Intern Med* **133**:951–963

Amory JK, Watts NB, Easley KA, Sutton PR, Anawalt BD, Matsumoto AM, Bremner WJ, Tenover JL (2004) Exogenous testosterone or testosterone with finasteride increases bone mineral density in older men with low serum testosterone. *J Clin Endocrinol Metab* **89**:503–510

Anawalt BD (2010) Guidelines for testosterone therapy for men: how to avoid a mad (t)ea party by getting personal. *J Clin Endocrinol Metab* **95**:2614–2617

Andriole GL, Crawford ED, Grubb RL 3rd, Buys SS, Chia D, Church TR, Fouad MN, Gelmann EP, Kvale PA, Reding DJ, Weissfeld JL, Yokochi LA, O'Brien B, Clapp JD, Rathmell JM, Riley TL, Hayes RB, Kramer BS, Izmirlian G, Miller AB, Pinsky PF, Prorok PC, Gohagan JK, Berg CD (2009) Mortality results from a randomized prostate-cancer screening trial. *N Engl J Med* **360**:1310–1319

Basaria S, Coviello AD, Travison TG, Storer TW, Farwell WR, Jette AM, Eder R, Tennstedt S, Ulloor J,

Zhang A, Choong K, Lakshman KM, Mazer NA, Miciek R, Krasnoff J, Elmi A, Knapp PE, Brooks B, Appleman E, Aggarwal S, Bhasin G, Hede-Brierley L, Bhatia A, Collins L, LeBrasseur N, Fiore LD, Bhasin S (2010) Adverse events associated with testosterone administration. *N Engl J Med* **363**:109–122

Basurto L, Zarate A, Gomez R, Vargas C, Saucedo R, Galvan R (2008) Effect of testosterone therapy on lumbar spine and hip mineral density in elderly men. *Aging Male* **11**:140–145

Behre HM, Kliesch S, Leifke E, Link TM, Nieschlag E (1997) Long-term effect of testosterone therapy on bone mineral density in hypogonadal men. *J Clin Endocrinol Metab* **82**:2386–2390

Bhasin S, Cunningham GR, Hayes FJ, Matsumoto AM, Snyder PJ, Swerdloff RS, Montori VM (2010) Testosterone therapy in men with androgen deficiency syndromes: an Endocrine Society clinical practice guideline. *J Clin Endocrinol Metab* **95**:2536–2559

Brand JS, van der Tweel I, Grobbee DE, Emmelot-Vonk MH, van der Schouw YT (2010) Testosterone, sex hormone-binding globulin and the metabolic syndrome: a systematic review and meta-analysis of observational studies. *Int J Epidemiol* **40**:189–207

Conway AJ, Handelsman DJ, Lording DW, Stuckey B, Zajac JD (2000) Use, misuse and abuse of androgens. The Endocrine Society of Australia consensus guidelines for androgen prescribing. *Med J Aust* **172**:220–224

Heinemann LA, Saad F, Heinemann K, Thai DM (2004) Can results of the Aging Males' Symptoms (AMS) scale predict those of screening scales for androgen deficiency? *Aging Male* **7**:211–218

Isidori AM, Giannetta E, Greco EA, Gianfrilli D, Bonifacio V, Isidori A, Lenzi A, Fabbri A (2005) Effects of testosterone on body composition,

bone metabolism and serum lipid profile in middle-aged men: a meta-analysis. *Clin Endocrinol (Oxf)* **63**:280–293

Ly LP, Sartorius G, Hull L, Leung A, Swerdloff RS, Wang C, Handelsman DJ (2010) Accuracy of calculated free testosterone formulae in men. *Clin Endocrinol (Oxf)* **73**:382–388

McLachlan RI (2010) Certainly more guidelines than rules. *J Clin Endocrinol Metab* **95**:2610–2613

Meier CT, Nguyen V, Handelsman DJ, Schindler C, Kushnir MM, Rockwood AL, Meikle AW, Center JR, Eisman JA, Seibel MJ (2008) Endogenous sex hormones and incident fracture risk in older men: the Dubbo Osteoporosis Epidemiology Study. *Arch Intern Med* **168**:47–54

Merza Z, Blumsohn A, Mah PM, Meads DM, McKenna SP, Wylie K, Eastell R, Wu F, Ross RJ (2006) Double-blind placebo-controlled study of testosterone patch therapy on bone turnover in men with borderline hypogonadism. *Int J Androl* **29**:381–391

Morales A, Bella AJ, Chun S, Lee J, Assimakopoulos P, Bebb R, Gottesman I, Alarie P, Dugre H, Elliott S (2010) A practical guide to diagnosis, management, and treatment of testosterone deficiency for Canadian Physicians. *Can Urol Assoc J* **4**:269–275

Morley JE, Charlton E, Patrick P, Kaiser FE, Cadeau P, McCready D, Perry HM III (2000) Validation of a screening questionnaire for androgen deficiency in aging males. *Metabolism* **49**:1239–1242

Nair KS, Rizza RA, O'Brien P, Dhatariya K, Short KR, Nehra A, Vittone JL, Klee GG, Basu A, Basu R, Cobelli C, Toffolo G, Dalla Man C, Tindall DJ, Melton LJ 3rd, Smith GE, Khosla S, Jensen MD (2006) DHEA in elderly women and DHEA or testosterone in elderly men. *N Engl J Med* **355**:1647–1659

Page ST, Amory JK, Bowman FD, Anawalt BD, Matsumoto AM,

Bremner WJ, Tenover JL (2005) Exogenous testosterone (T) alone or with finasteride increases physical performance, grip strength, and lean body mass in older men with low serum T. *J Clin Endocrinol Metab* **90**:1502–1510

Petak SM, Nankin HR, Spark RF, Swerdloff RS, Rodriguez-Rigau LJ (2002) American Association of Clinical Endocrinologists Medical Guidelines for clinical practice for the evaluation and treatment of hypogonadism in adult male patients – 2002 update. *Endocr Pract* **8**:440–456

Rosen RC, Araujo AB, Connor MK, Gerstenberger EP, Morgentaler A, Seftel AD, Miner MM, Shabsigh R (2011) The NERI Hypogonadism Screener: psychometric validation in male patients and controls. *Clin Endocrinol* **74**:248–256

Sartorius G, Ly LP, Sikaris K, McLachlan R, Handelsman DJ (2009) Predictive accuracy and sources of variability in calculated free testosterone estimates. *Ann Clin Biochem* **46**:137–143

Schroder FH, Hugosson J, Roobol MJ, Tammela TL, Ciatto S, Nelen V, Kwiatkowski M, Lujan M, Lilja H, Zappa M, Denis LJ, Recker F, Berenguer A, Maattanen L, Bangma CH, Aus G, Villers A, Rebillard X, van der Kwast T, Blijenberg BG, Moss SM, de Koning HJ, Auvinen A (2009) Screening and prostate-cancer mortality in a randomized European study. *N Engl J Med* **360**:1320–1328

Smith KW, Feldman HA, McKinlay JB (2000) Construction and field validation of a self-administered screener for testosterone deficiency (hypogonadism) in ageing men. *Clin Endocrinol* **53**:703–711

Snyder PJ, Peachey H, Hannoush P, Berlin JA, Loh L, Holmes JH, Dlewati A, Staley J, Santanna J, Kapoor SC, Attie MF, Haddad JG Jr, Strom BL (1999) Effect of testosterone treatment on bone mineral density in men over 65 years of age. *J Clin Endocrinol Metab* **84**:1966–1972

Srinivas-Shankar U, Roberts SA, Connolly MJ, O'Connell MD, Adams JE, Oldham JA, Wu FC (2010) Effects of testosterone on muscle strength, physical function, body composition, and quality of life in intermediate-frail and frail elderly men: a randomized, double-blind, placebo-controlled study. *J Clin Endocrinol Metab* **95**:639–650

Svartberg J, Agledahl I, Figenschau Y, Sildnes T, Waterloo K, Jorde R (2008) Testosterone treatment in elderly men with subnormal testosterone levels improves body composition and BMD in the hip. *Int J Impot Res* **20**:378–387

Tracz MJ, Sideras K, Bolona ER, Haddad RM, Kennedy CC, Uraga MV, Caples SM, Erwin PJ, Montori VM (2006) Testosterone use in men and its effects on bone health. A systematic review and meta-analysis of randomized placebo-controlled trials. *J Clin Endocrinol Metab* **91**:2011–2016

Vermeulen A, Verdonck L, Kaufman JM (1999) A critical evaluation of simple methods for the estimation of free testosterone in serum. *J Clin Endocrinol Metab* **84**:3666–3672

Wang C, Cunningham G, Dobs A, Iranmanesh A, Matsumoto AM, Snyder PJ, Weber T, Berman N, Hull L, Swerdloff RS (2004) Long-term testosterone gel (AndroGel) treatment maintains beneficial effects on sexual function and mood, lean and fat mass, and bone mineral density in hypogonadal men. *J Clin Endocrinol Metab* **89**:2085–2098

Wang C, Nieschlag E, Swerdloff RS, Behre HM, Hellstrom WJ, Gooren LJ, Kaufman JM, Legros JJ, Lunenfeld B, Morales A, Morley JE, Schulman C, Thompson IM, Weidner W, Wu FC (2009) Investigation, treatment, and monitoring of late-onset hypogonadism in males: ISA, ISSAM, EAU, EAA, and ASA recommendations. *J Androl* **30**:1–9

Wang C, Jackson G, Jones TH, Matsumoto AM, Nehra A, Perelman MA, Swerdloff RS, Traish A, Zitzmann M, Cunningham G (2011) Low testosterone associated with obesity and the metabolic syndrome contributes to sexual dysfunction and cardiovascular disease risk in men with type 2 diabetes. *Diabetes Care* **34**:1669–1675

Wolf AM, Wender RC, Etzioni RB, Thompson IM, D'Amico AV, Volk RJ, Brooks DD, Dash C, Guessous I, Andrews K, DeSantis C, Smith RA; American Cancer Society Prostate Cancer Advisory Committee (2010) American Cancer Society guideline for the early detection of prostate cancer: update 2010. *CA Cancer J Clin* **60**:70–98

Wu FC, Tajar A, Beynon JM, Pye SR, Silman AJ, Finn JD, O'Neill TW, Bartfai G, Casanueva FF, Forti G, Giwercman A, Han TS, Kula K, Lean ME, Pendleton N, Punab M, Boonen S, Vanderschueren D, Labrie F, Huhtaniemi IT (2010) Identification of late-onset hypogonadism in middle-aged and elderly men. *N Engl J Med* **363**:123–135

Chapter 19

Pathophysiology of estrogen action in men

Vincenzo Rochira, Daniele Santi, and Cesare Carani

19.1 Estrogens in men: historical development

Adult male sexual and reproductive functions were traditionally considered to be under the control of both gonadotropins and androgens. Hence, testosterone has long been considered the male hormone (Funk *et al.* 1930), and the concept of estrogen involvement on male physiology is new. In 1934 Zondek, however, first documented estrogen production in the male by demonstrating the intratesticular conversion of androgens into estrogens in male stallions (Zondek 1934). This mechanism was assumed to operate in men as well, but the real demonstration of estrogen production in the human male was provided only some years later in 1979 (MacDonald *et al.* 1979). Subsequent observations and studies, such as the characterization of the biochemical pathways (Heard *et al.* 1955; MacDonald *et al.* 1979) and the immunohistochemical demonstration of the estrogen

ligands in male tissues, including the reproductive system (Greco *et al.* 1992; Brodie and Inkster 1993), together with the advancements in testicular paracrinology (Saez 1994), all contributed to expand the comprehension of estrogen's role in men. Although the concept of testosterone as a prohormone for estrogen in men was old (Zondek 1934), the role of estrogens in men continued to be uncertain until the beginning of the nineties, and estrogens were left in the background for a long time in male physiology.

The idea that estrogens regulate several functions in men, also including human male reproduction, is a recent acquisition (Faustini-Fustini *et al.* 1999; Rochira *et al.* 2005), that has emerged only in the last 20 years (for review see Rochira *et al.* 2005), when the development of molecular biology allowed detailed characterization of estrogen receptors and their function (Couse *et al.* 1997), as well as the genes involved in the synthesis of estrogens (Simpson *et al.* 1994).

Testosterone: Action, Deficiency, Substitution, ed. Eberhard Nieschlag and Hermann M. Behre, Assoc. ed. Susan Nieschlag. Published by Cambridge University Press. © Cambridge University Press 2012.

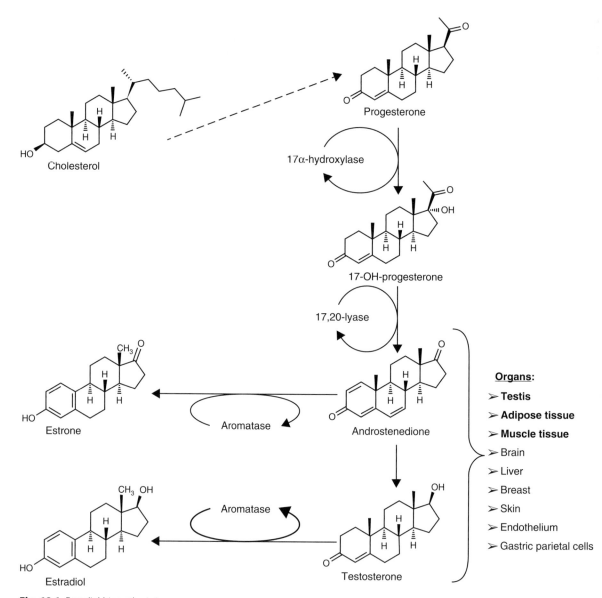

Fig. 19.1 Estradiol biosynthesis in men.

A further step was taken when animal models for congenital estrogen deficiency were generated (Korach 1994; Couse and Korach 1999). All the studies mentioned above, together with the discovery of mutations in the estrogen receptor alpha (ERα) (Smith *et al.* 1994), and/or in the aromatase enzyme in humans (Morishima *et al.* 1995; Carani *et al.* 1997) definitively changed some classical standpoints in endocrinology, providing evidence that estrogens also exert a wide range of biological effects in men and not only in women (Deroo and Korach 2006).

In males, estrogens derive from circulating androgens and are mainly produced by the testes, adipose and muscle tissue (Fig. 19.1). The key step for estrogen biosynthesis is the aromatization of C19 androgens, which are responsible for testosterone and androstenedione conversion into estradiol and estrone, respectively (Fig. 19.1). This conversion is regulated by the aromatase enzyme, a protein that belongs to the family of P450 mono-oxygenase enzyme complex (Simpson *et al.* 1994; Fig. 19.1). This enzyme is responsible for three consecutive hydroxylation reactions, the final result of which is

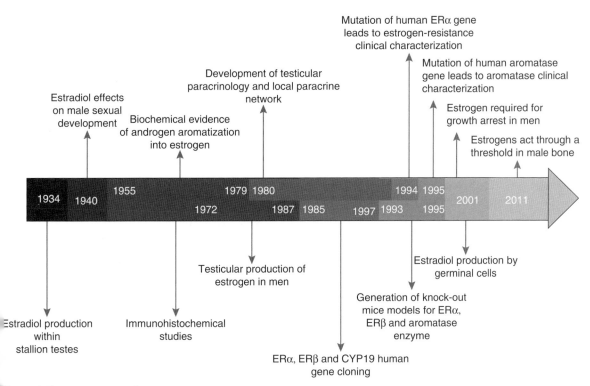

Fig. 19.2 Estrogens in men: milestones.

the aromatization of the A-ring of androgens (Simpson *et al.* 1994; Gruber *et al.* 2002; Fig. 19.1).

Circulating estrogens are reversibly bound, mainly to SHBG and, to a lesser degree, to albumin. Estrogen actions are mediated by binding to specific nuclear estrogen receptors (ERs), which are ligand-inducible transcription factors regulating the expression of target genes (Gruber *et al.* 2002; Deroo and Korach 2006). Two subtypes of nuclear ERs have been described (Gruber *et al.* 2002): ERα and the more recently discovered ERβ.

Other than the classical pathways based on transcriptional mechanisms, a non-genomic action enrolling cell-surface receptors of estrogens has been recently documented (Gruber *et al.* 2002).

Milestones of knowledge referring to estrogen physiology in men (for review see Rochira *et al.* 2005) are summarized in Fig. 19.2.

19.2 Estrogen action on the hypothalamic-pituitary unit: regulation of gonadotropin feedback

Animal and human models of congenital estrogen deficiency provide evidence that aromatization of

testosterone is required for normal functioning of the hypothalamic-pituitary testicular axis (Faustini-Fustini *et al.* 1999; Simoni *et al.* 1999). Accordingly, serum gonadotropins are high in all adult patients with aromatase deficiency, in the presence of normal to increased serum testosterone (Rochira and Carani 2009; Table 19.1 and Table 19.2), thus implying that estrogens are important for regulating the amount of circulating gonadotropins in men. A detailed study of the effects of different doses of transdermal estradiol on pituitary function in a man with congenital aromatase deficiency demonstrated that estrogens might control not only basal secretion of gonadotropins, but also their responsiveness to GnRH administration. In this study, estrogen administration to a male patient with aromatase deficiency decreased basal and GnRH-stimulated secretion of LH, FSH and α-subunit, in a dose-dependent manner (Rochira *et al.* 2002a). Furthermore, in men without congenital defects of estrogen function, the pharmacological inhibition of estrogen also results in a significant increase of both LH and FSH (Taxel *et al.* 2001; De Ronde and de Jong 2011; Saylam *et al.* 2011). All these data support an inhibitory effect of estrogens

Table 19.1 Phenotype of animal models of estrogen resistance and aromatase deficiency

	αERKO	βERKO mice	Estrogen resistance in men (ERα)	ArKO mice	Aromatase deficiency in men
Testis	Germ cells loss; enlarged seminiferous tubule	Normal	Normal volume (20–25 ml)	Normal at 14 wk	Normal or increased
Germ cells	Normal development of germ cells when transplanted in the wild type	Not described	Not described	Disruption of spermatogenesis at 1 year of age	Germ cell arrest at spermatocyte level Or Complete germ cell depletion
Sperm characteristics	Reduced number; motility and fertilizing capacity	Normal sperm count	Normal sperm count (25 × 10^6/ml) Reduced viability (18%)	Reduced sperm count and decreased viability at 8 months of age	From oligoasthenozoospermia to severe asthenospermia
Fertility	Infertile	Fertile	Fertile?	Infertile at 1 year	Infertile
Hormonal Pattern	LH ↑ FSH → T ↑ E$_2$↑	LH → FSH → T → E$_2$ →	LH ↑ FSH ↑ T → E$_2$ ↑	LH ↑ FSH → T ↑ E$_2$ Undetectable	LH → ↑ FSH ↑ T → ↑ E$_2$ Undetectable

Abbreviations: T, testosterone; E$_2$, estradiol.
Symbols: ↑ increase; → unchanged.

on gonadotropin secretion at the pituitary level (Faustini-Fustini *et al.* 1999; Simoni *et al.* 1999; Fig. 19.3) that operates from early to mid-puberty (Mauras *et al.* 2000; Wickman and Dunkel 2001) and that persists even during adulthood and advanced age (Taxel *et al.* 2001). The hypothalamic-pituitary gonadal axis, however, also responds to androgens, since the administration of DHT is able to decrease LH and FSH partially with a concomitant reduction in serum testosterone and estradiol (Idan *et al.* 2010).

More recently, estrogen action at hypothalamic level has also been documented (Raven *et al.* 2006; Rochira *et al.* 2006a), and the main influence is exerted by circulating estrogens, rather than by those locally produced (Raven *et al.* 2006; Rochira *et al.* 2006a; Fig. 19.3). The administration of anastrozole, a potent aromatase inhibitor, to men with IHH resulted, in fact, in a decrease of GnRH pulse frequency at the hypothalamic level and in a blunted pituitary responsiveness to GnRH (Hayes *et al.* 2000). Furthermore, estradiol administration lowers LH pulse frequency in normal subjects with pharmacologically induced estrogen

deficiency (Pitteloud *et al.* 2008a), as well as in aromatase-deficient men (Rochira *et al.* 2006a).

Estrogens are also able to modulate FSH secretion in men (Rochira *et al.* 2001; 2005). In normal men with pharmacologically induced sex steroid deprivation, estradiol, but not testosterone, is able to restore normal FSH serum levels (Pitteloud *et al.* 2008b). Due to the concomitant impairment of the patients' spermatogenesis, complete normalization of serum FSH was not achieved in all aromatase-deficient men during estradiol treatment, even in the presence of physiological levels of circulating estradiol (Rochira and Carani 2009); only supraphysiological levels of estrogens being necessary to obtain FSH normalization (Carani *et al.* 1997; Rochira *et al.* 2000).

Other than the gonadal axis, even growth hormone, prolactin and thyroid-stimulating hormone are partially modulated by estrogens in men, as documented by their abnormal secretion in men with aromatase deficiency (Rochira *et al.* 2002a; Rochira and Carani 2009).

Table 19.2 Summary of both well-established and supposed estrogen actions on male reproductive system

Function		Animals	Humans
Spermatogenesis	Well-established	Fluid reabsorption in the efferent ductules (ERα) Sperm concentration (ERα) Abnormal development of male reproductive structures after exposure to estrogen excess	Abnormal development of male reproductive structures after exposure to estrogen excess
	Supposed	Growth control of germ cells' proliferation during fetal life (ERβ) Germ cell differentiation Inhibition of germ cell apoptosis (ERβ) Control of cell adhesion (particularly on Sertoli cells)	Control of spermatogenesis and sperm maturation
Gonadotropin secretion	Well-established	Inhibition of gonadotropin secretion at pituitary level	Inhibition of gonadotropin secretion at both pituitary and hypothalamic level
	Supposed	Inhibition of gonadotropin secretion at hypothalamic level	—
Sexual behavior	Well-established	Promotion of mating copulative behavior	No effects on gender identity and sexual orientation
	Supposed	Determinant for partner preference	Possible positive role on male sexual behavior
Bone physiology	Well-established	Bone mineral density maintenance	Epiphyseal closure and growth arrest Acquisition of normal skeletal proportions Acquisition of peak bone mass Maintenance of bone mass
	Supposed	—	Anabolic effect on cortical bone Action on bone by means of a threshold (between 12 and 20 pg/ml of serum estradiol)
Glucose and lipid metabolism	Well-established	Modulation of insulin sensitivity and glucose tolerance Modulation of fat storage and adiposity	Control of insulin sensitivity Control of HDL-C production
	Supposed	Regulation of lipid metabolism	Control of glucose tolerance Regulation of total and LDL cholesterol Regulation of fat distribution

In conclusion, the control of gonadotropin feedback exerted by sex steroids is mainly related to estrogens, particularly to the amount circulating (Fig. 19.3).

19.3 Estrogens and male reproduction

In rodents and in men, immunocytochemical studies have revealed that ERs and the aromatase enzyme are expressed and functionally active throughout the male reproductive tract (Couse and Korach 1999; O'Donnell et al. 2001). Thus, it is now clear that the presence of estrogens and ERs in the male reproductive system ensures a physiological function of estrogens on male reproduction, and that both estrogen deficiency and excessive estrogen exposure may have deleterious reproductive effects in men (Sharpe 1998; Rochira et al. 2001; 2005; Rochira and Carani 2009).

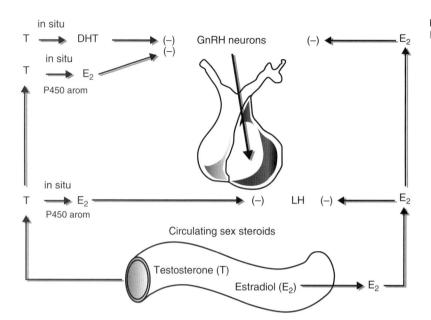

Fig. 19.3 Estrogen's role at hypothalamic and pituitary level.

19.3.1 Estrogen effects on male reproduction in rodents

The site of ERs and aromatase expression varies widely during development in rodents, and they are expressed at a very early stage (Rochira *et al.* 2005; 2009). ERα is abundant in efferent ductules from fetal life to adulthood, implying a crucial role in male reproduction (Hess *et al.* 2011); while ERβ is mainly expressed during fetal life, suggesting a major role in the development of male reproductive structures until birth (O'Donnell *et al.* 2001; Rochira *et al.* 2009). Accordingly, ERβ is probably the main target accounting for the effects of supraphysiological estrogen levels on abnormal development of reproductive structures during fetal life (Toppari and Skakkebaek 1998; O'Donnell *et al.* 2001; Rochira *et al.* 2009). In the adult male reproductive system of rodents, ERα is mainly expressed in the proximal (rete testis, efferent ductules, proximal epididymis), rather than in the distal (corpus and cauda of the epididymis, vas deferens) reproductive ducts (O'Donnell *et al.* 2001; Rochira *et al.* 2009). This peculiar distribution accounts for several important estrogen actions in the proximal ducts; especially the efferent ductules (Hess *et al.* 2011).

Estradiol may serve as a survival factor for round spermatids and to maintain spermatogenesis and promote normal sperm maturation (Carreau and Hess 2010). The lack of estradiol may promote apoptosis, with a resulting failure in elongated spermatid differentiation (Pentakainen *et al.* 2000).

Estrogen-deficient knock-out mice are useful models to investigate estrogen action in rodents (Couse and Korach 1999; O'Donnell *et al.* 2001). At present, four different lines of estrogen-deficient knock-out mice have been generated (Table 19.1): (1) ERα knock-out (αERKO) mice with disrupted *ERα* gene; (2) the βERKO mice, with an inactivated *ERβ*; and (3) the αβERKO mice with non-functioning *ERα* and *ERβ* (Couse and Korach 1999). The αERKO, βERKO and αβERKO mice provide helpful information on the loss of ER function (estrogen resistance). The knock-out of aromatase gene leads to aromatase knock-out (ArKO) mice, an experimental animal model useful for investigating the congenital lack of both circulating and locally produced estrogens since birth (Korach 1994; Couse and Korach 1999; O'Donnell *et al.* 2001). Estrogen-resistant knock-out mice have high levels of circulating estrogens with also the non-genomic pathway still functioning, while aromatase-deficient mice have no circulating estrogens and no active estrogen pathway (O'Donnell *et al.* 2001). The reproductive phenotype of estrogen-deficient knock-out mice is summarized in Table 19.1.

19.3.2 Knock-out models of estrogen deficiency

Male αERKO mice are infertile since the seminiferous epithelium is atrophic and degenerated, and both tubules and rete testis are dilated (Hess *et al.* 2011). The lack of estrogen-dependent fluid reabsorption leads to increased fluid back-pressure, resulting in a retroactive progressive swelling of the seminiferous tubules caused by the marked dilation of the tubules (Couse and Korach 1999; Hess *et al.* 2011; Table 19.1). In αERKO mice, serum LH is increased, inducing Leydig cell hyperplasia and increased serum testosterone while FSH is normal (Korach 1994; Couse and Korach 1999; Table 19.1).

Unlike αERKO mice, male ArKO mice are initially fully fertile, but fertility decreases with advancing age due to complete arrest of spermatogenesis at the level of early spermatids (Couse and Korach 1999). The early arrest of spermatogenesis suggests a failure in germ cell differentiation, as a consequence of estrogen lack in the testicular environment (Luconi *et al.* 2002), leading to a less severe degree of infertility than in αERKO mice (Couse and Korach 1999). Conversely, βERKO mice are fully fertile, also in adulthood (Couse and Korach 1999; Table 19.1). Gonadotropins are increased in ArKO mice due to the lack of an estrogen-inhibitory effect at the central level (see above) (Table 19.1).

In conclusion, a functional ERα, but not ERβ, is needed for the development and maintenance of normal fertility in male mice (Rochira *et al.* 2009).

19.3.3 Estrogen effects on male reproduction in men

Aromatase enzyme, ERα and ERβ are widely expressed throughout the male reproductive system, even in men, and they are also found in human sperm (Rochira *et al.* 2005; 2009; Carreau and Hess 2010). Accordingly, ERs are present in the human sperm membrane (Luconi *et al.* 1999), where they modulate a rapid non-genomic action. Thus, human ejaculated spermatozoa are responsive to estrogens throughout their run from the testes to the urethra, since they also express ERα and ERβ, and it seems that estrogens modulate sperm maturation (Luconi *et al.* 1999; Carreau and Hess 2010).

In the human testis both somatic and germ cells express aromatase, not only in immature germ cells,

but also in mature human spermatozoa (Pentakainen *et al.* 2000; Aquila *et al.* 2004). Thus, human spermatozoa are a site of estrogen biosynthesis and they should be considered a mobile endocrine unit producing and responding to estrogens (Rochira *et al.* 2009; Carreau and Hess 2010).

Data from human subjects with congenital estrogen deficiency document that all the eight affected men had an impairment of spermatogenesis, ranging from severe oligozoospermia and oligoasthenospermia to asthenospermia (Rochira *et al.* 2005; Zirilli *et al.* 2008; Rochira and Carani 2009). The variable degree of fertility impairment in men with congenital deficiency of estrogen action or synthesis does not allow any conclusions to be drawn, and whether these reproductive features are the consequence of a congenital lack of estrogen or they are only epiphenomena remains unsolved. Outside the context of estrogen deficiency, however, administration of aromatase inhibitors to infertile men with impaired testosterone-to-estradiol ratio resulted in an improvement of their fertility rate (Raman and Schlegel 2002; Saylam *et al.* 2011), suggesting the importance of estrogens in male reproduction. Finally, the role of estrogen in controlling sperm production and quality has been recently confirmed by the association of polymorphisms of estrogen-related genes with both sperm concentration and motility, but not with sperm morphology (Lee *et al.* 2011).

19.3.4 Inappropriate estrogen exposure

Many studies in animals suggest that inappropriate exposure to estrogens in utero and during the neonatal period impairs testicular descent, the hypothalamic-pituitary-gonadal axis and testicular function; in particular prenatal exposure to diethylstilbestrol (DES) results in abnormal development of male reproductive structures (Sharpe 1998; Toppari and Skakkebaek 1998).

In men, increased estrogen exposure has been supposed to impair fertility (Sharpe 1998; Toppari and Skakkebaek 1998), on the basis of the progressive decline in sperm count and the corresponding increase of environmental estrogens in some western countries. In the past, the inappropriate clinical use of DES in pregnant women was associated with a rise in the incidence of genital malformations at birth such as: epididymal cysts, meatal stenosis, hypospadias, cryptorchidism and microphallus. In addition, semen quality of men exposed to DES in utero resulted in greater impairment than in unexposed controls, but without clear indication of subfertility or clinical infertility (Wilcox *et al.* 1995).

In conclusion, animal studies strongly support the idea that exposure to estrogen excess affects the development and function of reproductive male organs, but the real impact of estrogen overexposure on human male fertility remains to be established.

However, the exact mode and site of action of estrogens in the male reproductive system remain only partially known, and further research is required to improve knowledge of this issue.

19.4 Estrogens and human male sexuality

19.4.1 Gender identity and sexual orientation

Sex steroids, mainly testosterone, modulate adult male sexual behavior in mammals (Robbins 1996). In men, sexual behavior is the result of the sum of the effects of cognitive processes, cultural environment, hormonal and genetic prerequisites (Rochira *et al.* 2003). The role of estrogen in male sexual behavior has been poorly investigated, and knowledge derives mainly from studies performed on animals or from rare models of human estrogen deficiency.

Testosterone aromatization to estradiol in the brain was considered the key step in the establishment of a male brain and in determining sexual dimorphism of the central nervous system in non-primate mammals (Gorski 1991; Pilgrim and Reisert 1992; Garcia-Falgueras and Swaab 2010). According to Dörner's hypothesis (Dörner 1988), prenatal and perinatal brain exposure to estrogens may be responsible for the establishment of a male brain (Roselli *et al.* 2009); an event occurring only in the male brain, and not in the female one. Accordingly, ovaries release very small amounts of estrogen that are also soon inactivated in rodents (Rochira *et al.* 2005; Roselli *et al.* 2009), while males produce a greater amount of androgens that are converted into estrogen. Thus, circulating estrogens are greater in males than in females during fetal life, which accounts for the sexual dimorphism of hypothalamic structures in rodents (Roselli *et al.* 2009; 2011).

The same mechanism also seems to be involved for the establishment of differences in hypothalamic structures between men and women (Dörner 1988; LeVay 1991). Prenatal hormonal exposure is classically considered to be involved in determining sexual orientation on the basis of some differences in hypothalamic structures found between heterosexual and homosexual men (LeVay 1991; Garcia-Falgueras and Swaab 2010). This hypothesis is supported by the concept that sexual differentiation of the brain takes place in parallel with the peak of testosterone secretion from the testis and the corresponding increase in serum estradiol during fetal life (Gorski 1991; Roselli *et al.* 2009; Garcia-Falgueras and Swaab 2010). According to this hypothesis, the intrinsic pattern of mammalian brain development is female, and estrogen is required for the development of a male brain (Dörner 1988; Garcia-Falgueras and Swaab 2010); thus emphasizing the role of estrogen aromatization locally in the brain (Roselli *et al.* 2009). Permanent changes in the organization of certain neural circuits, a prerequisite for sex-specific regulation of reproductive and sexual behavior, probably also occur under the effects of estrogen (Pilgrim and Reisert 1992; Roselli *et al.* 2009; Garcia-Falgueras and Swaab 2010). By considering all the factors mentioned above, the lack of estrogen action on the developing brain in males was believed to be strictly related to both dimorphism of hypothalamic structures, and the future development of sexual orientation (Gorski 1991; LeVay 1991; Roselli *et al.* 2009; Garcia-Falgueras and Swaab 2010), even though most of the data came from studies performed in rodents (Pilgrim and Reisert 1992; Roselli *et al.* 2009; Garcia-Falgueras and Swaab 2010). Recently, the role for local hypothalamic aromatase activity and expression in partner preference has been confirmed in rams (Roselli *et al.* 2004). In this study, the preferences of sexual partner were associated with both the volume of the ovine sexually dimorphic nucleus and different patterns of aromatase expression, providing the first demonstration that differences in aromatase expression within the brain are related to partner preferences and are involved in the determination of adult sexual behavior (Roselli *et al.* 2004).

Aromatase deficiency in men is an interesting model to study the role of estradiol in human male sexual behavior by considering the lack of aromatase activity from fetal life through adulthood (Rochira *et al.* 2005; 2009; Rochira and Carani 2009). All men with aromatase deficiency had a male gender identity and heterosexual orientation (Morishima *et al.* 1995;

Carani *et al.* 1999; 2005; Herrmann *et al.* 2002; Rochira *et al.* 2005; 2009; Maffei *et al.* 2007; Lanfranco *et al.* 2008; Rochira and Carani 2009). The fact that congenital aromatase deficiency does not affect psychosexual orientation and gender identity in humans allows the hypothesis that, in contrast to animals, psychological and social factors may be the most relevant determinants of gender role behavior in men, with hormones probably having a minor role (Rochira *et al.* 2005; Rochira and Carani 2009; Roselli *et al.* 2011).

In conclusion, aromatase has a key role in the control of male reproductive behavior, especially in animals (rodents and rams), where it induces organizational effects on the developing brain during fetal life (Wright *et al.* 2010). Local estrogen production within the brain and exposure to circulating estrogens are responsible for testosterone effects on sexual differentiation. Differences exist among species, however, and explain the essential role of aromatization in rodents (Roselli *et al.* 2011; Wright *et al.* 2010) and its poor effect in humans (Carani *et al.* 1999; 2005; Rochira *et al.* 2005; Rochira and Carani 2009).

19.4.2   Sexual behavior

In men, adult male sexual behavior is partially dependent on testosterone, the main hormone involved in male sexuality (Funk *et al.* 1930; Granata *et al.* 1997; Rochira *et al.* 2003; see also Chapter 5). Accordingly, testosterone deficiency frequently produces loss of libido and ED (Granata *et al.* 1997; Rochira *et al.* 2003). At the same time, TRT increases sexual interest and improves sexual behavior (Robbins 1996; Rochira *et al.* 2003).

In experimental animals, the knock-out of estrogen pathways or a condition of pharmacologically induced estrogen deficiency results in severe impairment of sexual behavior (Rochira *et al.* 2005; 2009). Accordingly, ArKO mice (Honda *et al.* 1998), αβERKO male mice and αERKO mice (Couse and Korach 1999) all exhibit a significant reduction in mounting frequency and a significant prolonged latency to mount when compared with wild-type animals (Couse and Korach 1999; O'Donnell *et al.* 2001). To the contrary, βERKO mice did not show any defect in any components of sexual behavior, including ejaculation (Couse and Korach 1999). These findings suggest that ERα is required for mounting behavior in male mice and that androgen receptor activation alone is not sufficient for fully normal sexual behavior in rodents (Rochira *et al.* 2005; 2009).

Much less is known about the role of estrogens in sexual behavior in the human male, since the proportion of testosterone effects on male sexual behavior that may be ascribed to its conversion into estradiol is still not known. A detailed sexual investigation of aromatase-deficient men documented an increase of all the parameters of sexual activity during estrogen treatment (Carani *et al.* 1999; 2005), but the best outcome in terms of sexual behavior was obtained only when a concomitant normalization of both serum testosterone and estradiol was reached (Carani *et al.* 2005), supporting the concept that both androgens and estrogens are required for normal sexual behavior in men. Outside the context of congenital lack of estrogens, it is difficult to obtain conclusive information on the role of estrogen on male sexual behavior because of inadequacy of studies and conflicting results in the literature.

Finally, estrogen receptors and the aromatase enzyme have been identified in the penile tissue of a large number of species, including humans (Crescioli *et al.* 2003; Dietrich *et al.* 2004; Goyal *et al.* 2007), suggesting direct estrogenic activity within the penis. At present, what we know about estrogen action within the penis derives from the observation that exposure of male offspring to estrogen-like endocrine disruptors in utero induces micropenis and hypospadias (Toppari *et al.* 1996) and that, in animals, penile development and function is estrogen dependent (Mowa *et al.* 2006). Estrogens seem to be involved in penile post-orgasm flaccidity (Vignozzi *et al.* 2004), in penile growth and in erection (Crescioli *et al.* 2003; Greco *et al.* 2006).

19.5   Estrogens and the male bone

Sex steroids, both estrogens and androgens, act on bone tissue and influence bone maturation and maintenance. The old concept that estrogens are implicated in the regulation of bone metabolism in women while androgens regulate the homeostasis of the skeleton in men is outdated.

The important role of estrogen in bone metabolism in men has been characterized in the last 15 years by means of the description of rare case reports of estrogen-deficient men and by several epidemiological studies (Rochira *et al.* 2006b; Khosla 2010).

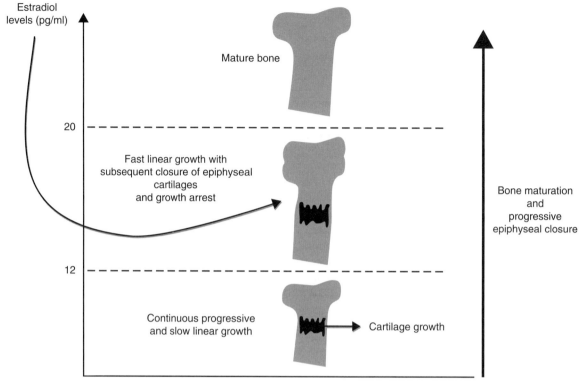

Fig. 19.4 Serum estradiol threshold for epiphyseal closure.

The relative contribution of androgens versus estrogens in the regulation of the male skeleton, however, is complex and partially unclear, but some estrogen actions on male bone, such as the acceleration of growth arrest are now well defined (see also Chapter 8).

19.5.1   Bone maturation

Pubertal growth in humans was traditionally considered as an androgen-dependent process since it progresses in parallel with the rise in serum testosterone. However, several studies have recently shown that part of the actions of androgens at puberty (induction of the growth spurt, bone maturation and ossification of the epiphyseal cartilages) is clearly mediated by estrogens in the human male (Zirilli *et al.* 2008). Accordingly, current evidence indicates that estrogens stimulate skeletal maturation in males as well as in females during many steps of skeletal development (Rochira *et al.* 2002b; Zirilli *et al.* 2008).

Estrogen serum levels increase simultaneously with testosterone levels throughout puberty, and correlate directly with chronological age, skeletal age, weight, height and pubertal stage (Klein *et al.* 1996). Besides, estrogens have a biphasic effect on growth plates since low doses of estradiol stimulate ulnar growth in boys, while higher doses lead to an inhibition of this process (Cutler 1997).

Nowadays, we know from aromatase-deficient men that estrogens are necessary in men for the completion of bone maturation, since they control epiphyseal closure and growth arrest (Carani *et al.* 1997; Herrmann *et al.* 2002; Maffei *et al.* 2004). Conversely, androgens alone are not sufficient to promote normal skeletal development during puberty (Faustini-Fustini *et al.* 1999; Rochira *et al.* 2002b; Zirilli *et al.* 2008). By considering the eight aromatase-deficient men described to date (Rochira and Carani 2009), a serum estradiol threshold exists above which bone maturation occurs, and comprises between 12 pg/ml and 20 pg/ml (Lanfranco *et al.* 2008; Fig. 19.4). Furthermore, the human model of male aromatase deficiency provides evidence on the pivotal role of estrogens in establishing normal skeletal proportions. Accordingly, the coexistence of continuing linear growth of long bones and eunuchoid body habitus in men affected by aromatase deficiency highlights the concept that estrogens, rather than androgens, are needed for harmonic skeletal growth (Zirilli *et al.* 2008; Rochira and Carani 2009). As a consequence, in hypogonadal men the disproportional growth of long bones is mainly due to relative estrogen deficiency (Faustini-Fustini *et al.* 1999; Maffei *et al.* 2004; Zirilli *et al.* 2008; Rochira and Carani 2009), as also confirmed by normal skeleton proportions in subjects affected by CAIS (Zachmann *et al.* 1986).

19.5.2 Bone mineral density

It is now generally accepted that estradiol is the main sex steroid required for bone homeostasis in men (Rochira *et al.* 2006b). The lack of DHT efficacy in increasing BMD in patients with benign prostate hyperplasia confirms the minor role of androgen on bone (Idan *et al.* 2010). The reduction of lumbar BMD by 1.5% in these patients was the result of the net compensation between the poor anabolic effects of high circulating DHT and the prevalent negative effect on BMD due to the reduction of testosterone and estradiol levels; the latter caused by the negative feedback of DHT on gonadotropin secretion (Idan *et al.* 2010). In a recent work, Khosla *et al.* (2011) stressed the concept that declining bioavailable estrogen levels also made a substantial contribution to age-related bone loss in men, but remarked that cortical bone and trabecular bone may respond differently to estrogen and to estrogen deficiency.

The relevance of estradiol to bone health derives mostly from the evidence that aromatase-deficient men have a less mineralized skeleton (Zirilli *et al.* 2008), and from several studies showing that serum estradiol levels directly correlate with BMD in men (Khosla 2010). Furthermore, estradiol treatment is effective in increasing BMD in men with aromatase deficiency, working in a dose-dependent fashion (Rochira *et al.* 2000; Zirilli *et al.* 2008; Rochira and Carani 2009). Estradiol seems to be protective for bone, but only when serum levels are above a threshold (Mellström *et al.* 2008); the precise threshold value, however, remains to be settled. In cohort studies this threshold has been set at around 12–20 pg/ml (Vandenput and Ohlsson 2010), and by studying the effects of estrogen treatment in aromatase-deficient men (Lanfranco *et al.* 2008), this threshold has been more precisely determined as being around 16 pg/ml (Fig. 19.4). This value has also been confirmed by

studies on fracture risk in older men (Mellström *et al.* 2008; Fig. 19.4), and recently Khosla *et al.* stated that a serum estradiol level above 25 pg/ml is certainly protective for bone in men (Khosla *et al.* 2011; Fig. 19.4).

In general, however, the estrogen regulation of bone remodeling is due to: (1) inhibition of activation of bone remodeling and of initiation of new basic multicellular units; (2) inhibition of the differentiation and promoting the apoptosis of osteoclasts, reducing bone resorption; (3) promotion of the commitment and differentiation of osteoblasts, and prevention of their apoptosis, maintaining bone formation at the cellular level (Khosla *et al.* 2011). For all these reasons, bone loss in man is mainly related to relative estrogen deficiency (Rochira *et al.* 2006b; Khosla 2010; Khosla *et al.* 2011).

Even though BMD is strongly estrogen dependent, direct action on bone is also exerted in men by androgens, particularly at puberty, probably accounting for sexual dimorphism of the bone mass (Rochira *et al.* 2006b; Vandenput and Ohlsson 2010). A mild to severe reduction of circulating testosterone in men, due to hypogonadism and/or aging, could be responsible for bone loss directly or indirectly through a concomitant decrease of circulating estradiol. This, with individual differences, may be a determinant for the severity of bone clinical manifestations (Rochira *et al.* 2006b).

In conclusion, estrogens seem to be the most important sex steroid involved in the final phases of skeletal maturation and mineralization, even if the exact mode and site of action of estrogens in bone and in epiphyseal cartilages are not yet completely known (Zirilli *et al.* 2008).

19.6 Estrogens and metabolism
19.6.1 Glucose metabolism

The role of estrogen in glucose and insulin metabolism in men is difficult to establish since separating the actions in-vivo of androgen *per se* from those of estrogen *per se* remains challenging. In estrogen-deficient men, insulin resistance and fasting glucose are increased and improve during estrogen treatment (Rochira *et al.* 2002b; 2007; Maffei *et al.* 2004). The same metabolic pattern is present in knock-out mice models of estrogen deficiency (Couse and Korach 1999). Severe impairment of the estrogen-to-testosterone ratio (increased androgens and decreased estrogens) seems to represent a condition for the development of insulin resistance in men (Maffei *et al.* 2004; Rochira *et al.* 2007), not only in men with congenital estrogen deficiency (Mauvais-Jarvis 2011).

19.6.2 Lipid metabolism

Congenital estrogen deficiency is associated with an altered lipid profile (Faustini-Fustini *et al.* 1999; Rochira *et al.* 2002b), mainly characterized by higher total cholesterol and triglyceride serum levels, higher LDL-C and very low HDL-C (Zirilli *et al.* 2008; Rochira and Carani 2009). It is noteworthy that HDL-C is inversely linked to serum testosterone; in fact, supraphysiological doses of testosterone decreased HDL-C in aromatase-deficient men (Maffei *et al.* 2004; Rochira *et al.* 2007). Conversely, estradiol treatment determined a moderate increase of HDL-C together with a small reduction of triglycerides, total cholesterol and LDL-C in aromatase-deficient subjects (Carani *et al.* 1997; Herrmann *et al.* 2002; Rochira *et al.* 2002b; Maffei *et al.* 2004). Overall, the effects of estrogen on lipid metabolism resemble those exerted in females (Deroo and Korach 2006).

19.7 Clinical and therapeutic implications

The knowledge of estrogen pathophysiology in men is of crucial importance for the understanding and clinical management of all conditions of congenital or acquired estrogen deficiency in men.

Clinical conditions of congenital estrogen deficiency in men are very rare and include estrogen resistance; aromatase deficiency; 17α-hydroxylase-17,20-lyase deficiency; 17,20-lyase deficiency and cytochrome P450 oxido-reductase deficiency (PORD) (Fukami *et al.* 2009; Rochira and Carani 2009); and congenital severe hypogonadism. Acquired estrogen deficiency is more common in clinical practice and includes transient estrogen deficiency in boys with delayed puberty, and all the conditions of acquired severe hypogonadism (Rochira *et al.* 2006b).

In all these clinical conditions, targeting circulating estrogens is of great importance, even in the case of testosterone replacement treatment, in order to ensure adequate effectiveness, such as in the case of bone health. Furthermore, estrogen may be useful as a marker of adequate testosterone treatment, especially when it is important to avoid overtreatment, as in the case of testosterone treatment during puberty. Accordingly, the amount of circulating estrogen is crucial for the closure of bone epiphyses, the achievement of final stature and for obtaining both adequate peak bone mass and skeletal proportions. Thus, serum estradiol could be a good surrogate for monitoring testosterone treatment, especially at puberty.

Estrogen replacement treatment in aromatase-deficient men should be started as soon as the diagnosis has been reached, taking into account that high doses of estrogen in adult men with aromatase deficiency leads to a rapid completion of skeletal maturation within six to nine months, through rapid bone elongation and an increase in height followed by quick epiphyseal closure and growth arrest (Rochira *et al.* 2009). Once epiphyseal closure has been achieved, estrogen treatment should be continued lifelong, with the main goal of preventing bone loss and to reduce risk of cardiovascular disease by reducing the dose of estradiol in order to maintain serum estradiol within the normal range for adult men (Rochira and Carani 2009).

It remains to be established if estrogen in men is a good target for improving or modulating male fertility, since conflicting results are available in the area of aromatase inhibitors used for the treatment of male infertility (Raman and Schlegel 2002; Rochira *et al.* 2009; Carreau and Hess 2010; Saylam *et al.* 2011). The real efficacy of antiestrogens is far from being elucidated, and it is a matter of debate whether the increase of sperm density induced by antiestrogens is actually related to a real improvement of both sperm fertility and pregnancy rates (Rochira *et al.* 2009; Carreau and Hess 2010).

19.8 Conclusions

Several lines of evidence support the view that estrogens are required for, and in part mediate, androgen actions on several tissues and organs in men. The progress made in the last 20 years in fields of estrogen pathophysiology in men has clarified the importance of estrogen in men but leaves some issues still unresolved. In particular, estrogen action on bone and gonadotropin secretion is now well characterized (Table 19.2), and part of the estrogen action on spermatogenesis is now known but needs further evidence. Conversely, the effect of estrogen on glucose and lipid metabolism is still controversial (Table 19.2).

A major area of uncertainty is the possible role of estrogen in boys before puberty. It is known that low levels of circulating estradiol are detected in infancy when using ultrasensitive assays (Bay *et al.* 2004), but their significance is not known.

19.9 Key messages

- Circulating estrogens inhibit gonadotropins by acting at both the hypothalamic and the pituitary level.
- Estrogens probably contribute to modulating sperm concentration and motility.
- Estrogens do not influence gender identity and sexual orientation in men.
- Estrogens are needed for bone maturation and growth arrest in men.
- Estrogens ensure normal skeletal proportions.
- Estrogens are necessary for the achievement of peak bone mass and subsequent maintenance of bone mineralization.
- Estrogens exert positive effects on insulin sensitivity and on levels of HDL cholesterol.
- Congenital estrogen deficiency is characterized by the absence of bone maturation, by continuing linear growth, and remains often not diagnosed until adulthood in men.
- Estrogen replacement treatment is effective on bone maturation and mineralization, on the normal functioning of the hypothalamic-pituitary-gonadal axis and on insulin sensitivity in aromatase-deficient men, but not in estrogen-resistant men.

19.10 References

Aquila S, Sisci D, Gentile M, Middea E, Catalano S, Carpino A, Rago V, Andò S (2004) Estrogen receptor (ER) alpha and ER beta are both expressed in human ejaculated spermatozoa: evidence of their direct interaction with phospatidylinositol-3-OH kinase/akt pathway. *J Clin Endocrinol Metab* **89**:1443–1451

Bay K, Andersson AM, Skakkebaek NE (2004) Estradiol levels in prepubertal boys and girls – analytical challenges. *Int J Androl* **27**:266–273

Brodie A, Inkster S (1993) Aromatase in the human testis. *J Steroid Biochem Molec Biol* **44**:549–555

Carani C, Qin K, Simoni M, Faustini-Fustini M, Serpente S, Boyd J (1997) Effect of testosterone and estradiol in a man with aromatase deficiency. *N Engl J Med* **337**:91–95

Carani C, Rochira V, Faustini-Fustini M, Balestrieri A, Granata ARM (1999) Role of estrogen in male sexual behaviour: insights from the natural model of aromatase deficiency. *Clin Endocrinol (Oxf)* **51**:517–525

Carani C, Granata AR, Rochira V, Caffagni G, Aranda C, Antunez P, Maffei LE (2005) Sex steroid and sexual desire in a man with a novel mutation of aromatase gene and hypogonadism. *Psychoneuroendocrinol* **30**:413–417

Carreau S, Hess RA (2010) Oestrogens and spermatogenesis. *Philos Trans R Soc Lond B Biol Sci* **365**:1517–1535

Couse JF, Korach KS (1999) Estrogen receptor null mice: what have we learned and where will they lead us? *Endocrine Rev* **20**:358–417

Couse JF, Lindzey J, Grandien K, Gustafsson JA, Korach KS (1997) Tissue distribution and quantitative analysis of estrogen receptor-α (ERα) and estrogen receptor-β (ERβ) messenger ribonucleic acid in the wild-type and ERα-knock-out mouse. *Endocrinology* **138**:4613–4621

Crescioli C, Maggi M, Vannelli GB, Ferruzzi P, Granchi S, Mancina R, Muratori M, Forti G, Serio M, Luconi M (2003) Expression of functional estrogen receptors in human fetal male external genitalia. *Clin Endocrinol Metab* **88**:1815–1824

Cutler GB Jr (1997) The role of estrogen in bone growth and maturation during childhood and adolescence, *J Steroid Biochem Mol Biol* **61**:141–144

De Ronde W, de Jong FH (2011) Aromatase inhibitors in men: effects and therapeutic options. *Reprod Biol Endocrinol* **9**:93

Deroo BJ, Korach KS (2006) Estrogen receptors and human disease. *J Clin Invest* **116**:561–570

Dietrich W, Haitel A, Huber JC, Reiter WJ (2004) Expression of estrogen receptors in human corpus cavernosum and male urethra. *J Histochem Cytochem* **52**:355–360

Dörner G (1988) Neuroendocrine response to estrogen and brain differentiation in heterosexuals, homosexuals, and transsexuals. *Arch Sex Behav* **17**:57–75

Faustini-Fustini M, Rochira V, Carani C (1999) Oestrogen deficiency in men: where are we today? *Eur J Endocrinol* **140**:111–129

Fukami M, Nishimura G, Homma K, Nagai T, Hanaki K, Uematsu A, Ishii T, Numakura C, Sawada H, Nakacho M, Kowase T, Motomura K, Haruna H, Nakamura M, Ohishi A, Adachi M, Tajima T, Hasegawa Y, Hasegawa T, Horikawa R, Fujieda K, Ogata T (2009) Cytochrome P450 oxidoreductase deficiency: identification and characterization of biallelic mutations and genotype-phenotype correlations in

35 Japanese patients. *J Clin Endocrinol Metab* **94**:1723–1731

Funk C, Harrow B, Lejwa A (1930) The male hormone. *Am J Physiol* **92**:440–449

Garcia-Falgueras A, Swaab DF (2010) Sexual hormones and the brain: an essential alliance for sexual identity and sexual orientation. *Endocr Dev* **17**:22–35

Gorski RA (1991) Sexual differentiation of the endocrine brain and its control. In: Motta M (ed) *Brain Endocrinology*, 2nd edn. Raven Press, New York, pp 71–104

Goyal HO, Braden TD, Williams CS, Williams J (2007) Role of estrogen in induction of penile dysmorphogenesis: a review. *Reproduction* **134**:199–208

Granata ARM, Rochira V, Lerchl A, Marrama P, Carani C (1997) Relationship between sleep-related erections and testosterone levels in men. *J Androl* **18**:522–527

Greco EA, Pili M, Bruzziches R, Corona G, Spera G, Aversa A (2006) Testosterone:estradiol ratio changes associated with long-term taladafil administration: a pilot study. *J Sex Med* **3**:716–722

Greco TL, Furlow JD, Duello TM, Gorski J (1992) Immunodetection of estrogen receptors in fetal and neonatal male mouse reproductive tracts. *Endocrinology* **130**:421–429

Gruber CJ, Tschugguel W, Schneeberger C, Huber J (2002) Production and actions of estrogens. *N Engl J Med* **346**:340–352

Hayes FJ, Seminara SB, Decruz S, Boepple PA, Crowley WF Jr (2000) Aromatase inhibition in the human male reveals a hypothalamic site of estrogen feedback. *J Clin Endocrinol Metab* **85**:3027–3035

Heard RD, Jellinck PH, O'Donnelll VJ (1955) Biogenesis of the estrogens: the conversion of testosterone-4-C14 to estrone in pregnant mare. *Endocrinology* **57**:200–204

Herrmann BL, Saller B, Janssen OE, Gocke P, Bockish A, Sperling H, Mann K, Broecker M (2002) Impact of estrogen replacement therapy in a male with congenital aromatase deficiency caused by a novel mutation in the CYP19 gene. *J Clin Endocrinol Metab* **87**:5476–5484

Hess RA, Fernandes SA, Gomes GR, Oliveira CA, Lazari MF, Porto CS (2011) Estrogen and its receptors in efferent ductules and epidydimis. *J Androl* **32**:600–613

Honda S, Harada N, Ito S, Takagi Y, Maeda S (1998) Disruption of sexual behavior in male aromatase-deficient mice lacking exons 1 and 2 of the *Cyp19* gene. *Biochem Biophys Res Comm* **252**:445–449

Idan A, Griffiths KA, Harwood DT, Seibel MJ, Turner L, Conway AJ, Handelsman DJ (2010) Long-term effects of dihydrotestosterone treatment on prostate growth in healthy, middle-aged men without prostate disease: a randomized, placebo-controlled trial. *Ann Intern Med* **153**:621–632

Khosla S (2010) Update on estrogens and the skeleton. *J Clin Endocrinol Metab* **95**:3569–3577

Khosla S, Melton LJ 3rd, Riggs BL (2011) The unitary model for estrogen deficiency and the pathogenesis of osteoporosis: is a revision needed? *J Bone Miner Res* **26**:441–451

Klein KO, Martha PO Jr, Blizzard RM, Herbst T, Rogol AD (1996) A longitudinal assessment of hormonal and physical alterations during normal puberty in boys. II. Estrogen levels as determined by an ultrasensitive bioassay. *J Clin Endocrinol Metab* **81**:3203–3207

Korach KS (1994) Insights from the study of animals lacking functional estrogen receptor. *Science* **266**:1524–1527

Lanfranco F, Zirilli L, Baldi M, Pignatti E, Corneli G, Ghigo E, Aimaretti G, Carani C, Rochira V (2008) A novel mutation in the human aromatase gene: insights on

the relationship among serum estradiol, longitudinal growth and bone mineral density in an adult man under estrogen replacement treatment. *Bone* **43**:212–218

Lee IW, Kuo PH, Su MT, Kuan LC, Hsu CC, Kuo PL (2011) Quantitative trait analysis suggests polymorphisms of estrogen-related genes regulate human sperm concentrations and motility. *Hum Reprod* **26**:1585–1596

LeVay S (1991) A difference in hypothalamic structure between heterosexual and homosexual men. *Science* **253**:1034–1037

Luconi M, Muratori M, Forti G, Baldi E (1999) Identification and characterization of a novel functional estrogen receptor on human sperm membrane which interferes with progesterone effects. *J Clin Endocr Metab* **84**:1670–1678

Luconi M, Forti G, Baldi E (2002) Genomic and nongenomic effects of estrogens: molecular mechanisms of action and clinical implications for male reproduction. *J Steroid Bioch Mol Biol* **80**:369–381

MacDonald PC, Madden JD, Brenner PF, Wilson JD, Siiteri PK (1979) Origin of estrogen in normal men and in women with testicular feminization. *J Clin Endocrinol Metab* **49**:905–916

Maffei L, Murata Y, Rochira V, Tubert G, Aranda C, Vasquez M, Clyne CD, Davis S, Simpson ER, Carani C (2004) Dysmetabolic syndrome in a man with a novel mutation of the aromatase gene: effects of testosterone, alendronate, and estradiol treatment. *J Clin Endocrinol Metab* **89**:61–70

Maffei L, Rochira V, Zirilli L, Antunez P, Aranda C, Fabre B, Simone ML, Pignatti E, Simpson ER, Houssami S, Clyne CD, Carani C (2007) A novel compound heterozygous mutation of the aromatase gene in an adult man: a reinforced evidence on the relationships among congenital estrogen deficiency, adiposity and the metabolic syndrome. *Clin Endocrinol* 67:218–224

Mauras N, O'Brien KO, Klein KO, Hayes V (2000) Estrogen suppression in males: metabolic effects. *J Clin Endocrinol Metab* 85:2370–2377

Mauvais-Jarvis F (2011) Estrogen and androgen receptors: regulators of fuel homeostasis and emerging targets for diabetes and obesity. *Trends Endocrinol Metab* 22:24–33

Mellström D, Vandenput L, Mallmin H, Holmberg AH, Lorentzon M, Odén A, Johansson H, Orwoll ES, Labrie F, Karlsson MK, Ljunggren O, Ohlsson C (2008) Older men with low serum estradiol and high serum SHBG have an increased risk of fractures. *J Bone Miner Res* 23:1552–1560

Morishima A, Grumbach MM, Simpson ER, Fisher C, Qin K (1995) Aromatase deficiency in male and female sibling caused by a novel mutation and the physiological role of estrogens. *J Clin Endocrinol Metab* 80:3689–3699

Mowa CN, Jesmin S, Miyauchi T (2006) The penis: a new target and source of estrogen in male reproduction. *Histol Histopathol* 21:53–67

O'Donnelll L, Robertson KM, Jones ME, Simpson ER (2001) Estrogen and spermatogenesis. *Endocr Rev* 22:289–318

Pentakainen V, Erkkila K, Suomaleinen L, Parvinen M, Dunkel L (2000) Estradiol acts as a germ cell survival factor in the human testis. *J Clin Endocrinol Metab* 85:2057–2067

Pilgrim C, Reisert J (1992) Differences between male and female brains – developmental mechanisms and implications. *Horm Metab Res* 24:353–359

Pitteloud N, Dwyer AA, DeCruz S, Lee H, Boepple PA, Crowley WF Jr, Hayes FJ (2008a) Inhibition of luteinizing hormone secretion by testosterone in men requires aromatization for its pituitary but

not its hypothalamic effects: evidence from the tandem study of normal and gonadotropin-releasing hormone-deficient men. *J Clin Endocrinol Metab* 93:784–791

Pitteloud N, Dwyer AA, DeCruz S, Lee H, Boepple PA, Crowley WF Jr, Hayes FJ (2008b) The relative role of gonadal sex steroids and gonadotropin-releasing hormone pulse frequency in the regulation of follicle-stimulating hormone secretion in men. *J Clin Endocrinol Metabol* 93:2686–2692

Raman JD, Schlegel PN (2002) Aromatase inhibitor for male infertility. *J Urol* 167:624–629

Raven G, de Jong FH, Kaufman JM, de Ronde W (2006) In men, peripheral estradiol levels directly reflect the action of estrogens at the hypothalamopituitary level to inhibit gonadotropin secretion. *J Clin Endocrinol Metab* 91:3324–3328

Robbins A (1996) Androgens and male sexual behavior. *Trends Endocrinol Metab* 7:345–350

Rochira V, Carani C (2009) Aromatase deficiency in men: a clinical perspective. *Nature Reviews* 5:559–568

Rochira V, Faustini-Fustini M, Balestrieri A, Carani C (2000) Estrogen replacement therapy in a man with congenital aromatase deficiency: effects of different doses of transdermal estradiol on bone mineral density and hormonal parameters. *J Clin Endocrinol Metab* 85:1841–1845

Rochira V, Balestrieri A, Madeo B, Baraldi E, Faustini-Fustini M, Granata AR, Carani C (2001) Congenital estrogen deficiency: in search of the estrogen role in human male reproduction. *Mol Cell Endocrinol* 178:107–115

Rochira V, Balestrieri A, Faustini-Fustini M, Borgato S, Beck-Peccoz P, Carani C (2002a) Pituitary function in a man with congenital aromatase deficiency: effect of different doses of

transdermal estradiol on basal and stimulated pituitary hormones. *J Clin Endocrinol Metab* 87:2857–2862

Rochira V, Balestrieri A, Madeo B, Spaggiari A, Carani C (2002b) Congenital estrogen deficiency in men: a new syndrome with different phenotypes; clinical and therapeutic implications in men. *Mol Cell Endocrinol* 193:19–28

Rochira V, Zirilli L, Madeo B, Balestrieri A, Granata AR, Carani C (2003) Sex steroids and sexual desire mechanism. *J Endocrinol Invest* 26:29–36

Rochira V, Granata ARM, Madeo B, Zirilli L, Rossi G, Carani C (2005) Estrogens in males: what have we learned in the last 10 years? *Asian J Androl* 7:3–20

Rochira V, Zirilli L, Genazzani AD, Balestrieri A, Aranda C, Fabre B, Antunez P, Diazzi C, Carani C, Maffei L (2006a) Hypothalamic-pituitary-gonadal axis in two men with aromatase deficiency: evidence that circulating estrogens are required at the hypothalamic level for the integrity of gonadotropin negative feedback. *Eur J Endocrinol* 155:513–522

Rochira V, Balestrieri A, Madeo B, Zirilli L, Granata ARM, Carani C (2006b) Osteoporosis and male age-related hypogonadism: role of sex steroids on bone patho (physiology). *Eur J Endocrinol* 154:175–185

Rochira V, Madeo B, Zirilli L, Caffagni G, Maffei L, Carani C (2007) Oestradiol replacement treatment and glucose homeostasis in two men with congenital aromatase deficiency: evidence for a role of oestradiol and sex steroids imbalance on insuline sensitivity in men. *Diabet Med* 24:1491–1495

Rochira V, Madeo B, Zirilli L, Carani C (2009) Estrogens and male reproduction. In: de Groot L, McLachlan RI (eds) *Endocrinology of Male Reproduction*. www.endotext.org/male/male17/maleframe17.htm (MDText.com,

Inc), South Dartmouth, MA, Chapter 17

Roselli CE, Larkin K, Resko JA, Stellflug JN, Stormshak F (2004) The volume of a sexually dimorphic nucleus in the ovine medial preoptic area/anterior hypothalamus varies with sexual partner preference. *Endocrinology* **145**:478–483

Roselli CE, Liu M, Hurn PD (2009) Brain aromatization: classic roles and new perspectives. *Semin Reprod Med* **27**:207–217

Roselli CE, Estill CT, Stadelman HL, Meaker M, Stormshak F (2011) Separate critical periods exist for testosterone-induced differentiation of the brain and genitals in sheep. *Endocrinology* **152**:2409–2415

Saez JM (1994) Leydig cells: endocrine, paracrine, and autocrine regulation. *Endocr Rev* **15**:574–626

Saylam B, Efesoy O, Cayan S (2011) The effect of aromatase inhibitor letrozole on body mass index, serum hormones, and sperm parameters in infertile men. *Fertil Steril* **95**:809–811

Sharpe RM (1998) The roles of oestrogen in the male. *Trends Endocrinol Metab* **9**:371–377

Simoni M, Rochira V, Faustini-Fustini M, Carani C (1999) Estrogen resistance and aromatase deficiency. In: Beck-Peccoz P (ed) *Regulation of Pituitary Hormone Secretion*, HypoCCS Series, Vol. 3. BioScientifica Ltd, Bristol, pp 85–95

Simpson ER, Mahendroo MS, Means GD, Kilgore MW, Hinshelwood MM, Graham-Lorence S, Amarneh B, Ito Y, Fisher CR, Michael MD (1994) Aromatase cytochrome P450, the enzyme responsible for estrogen biosynthesis. *Endocr Rev* **15**:342–355

Smith EP, Boyd J, Frank GR, Takahashi H, Cohen RM, Specker B, Williams TC, Lubahn DB, Korach KS (1994) Estrogen resistance caused by a mutation in the estrogen-receptor gene in a man. *N Engl J Med* **331**: 1056–1061

Taxel P, Kennedy DG, Fall PM, Willard AK, Clive JM, Raisz LG (2001) The effect of aromatase inhibition on sex steroids, gonadotropins, and markers of bone turnover in older men. *J Clin Endocrinol Metab* **86**:2869–2874

Toppari J, Skakkebaek NE (1998) Sexual differentiation and environmental endocrine disruptors. *Baillières Clin Endocrinol Metab* **12**:143–155

Toppari J, Larsen JC, Christiansen P, Giwercman A, Grandjean P, Guillette LJ Jr, Jégou B, Jensen TK, Jouannet P, Keiding N (1996) Male reproductive health and environmental xenoestrogens. *Environ Health Persp* **104**:741–803

Vandenput L, Ohlsson C (2010) Sex steroid metabolism in the regulation of bone health in men. *J Steroid Biochem Mol Biol* **121**:582–588

Vignozzi L, Filippi S, Luconi M, Morelli A, Mancina R, Marini M,

Vennelli GB, Granchi S, Orlando C, Gelmini S, Ledda F, Forti G, Maggi M (2004) Oxytocin receptor is expressed in the penis and mediates an estrogen-dependent smooth muscle contractility. *Endocrinology* **145**:1823–1834

Wickman S, Dunkel L (2001) Inhibition of P450 aromatase enhances gonadotropin secretion in early and midpubertal boys: evidence for a pituitary site of action of endogenous E. *J Clin Endocrinol Metab* **86**:4887–4894

Wilcox AJ, Baird DD, Weinberg CR, Hornsby PP, Herbst AL (1995) Fertility in men exposed prenatally to diethylstilbestrol. *N Engl J Med* **332**:1411–1416

Wright CL, Schwarz JS, Dean SL, McCarthy MM (2010) Cellular mechanisms of estradiol-mediated sexual differentiation of the brain. *Trends Endocrinol Metab* **21**:553–561

Zachmann M, Prader A, Sabel AH, Crigler JF, Ritzen MF, Atares M, Ferrandez AF (1986) Pubertal growth in patients with androgen insensitivity: indirect evidence for the importance of estrogens in pubertal growth of girls. *J Pediatr* **108**:694–697

Zirilli L, Rochira V, Diazzi C, Caffagni G, Carani C (2008) Human models of aromatase deficiency. *J Steroid Biochem Molec Biol* **109**:212–218

Zondek B (1934) Mass excretion of oestrogenic hormone in the urine of the stallion. *Nature* **33**:209–210

Chapter 20

Dehydroepiandrosterone and androstenedione

Bruno Allolio, Wiebke Arlt, and Stefanie Hahner

20.1   Introduction

Man, together with higher primates, has adrenals secreting large amounts of dehydroepiandrosterone (DHEA) and its sulfate ester, DHEAS. The physiological role of these steroid hormones is still not fully understood. However, in recent years a growing number of careful investigations have helped to better appreciate the function of DHEA(S).

Dehydroepiandrosterone is distinct from the two other major adrenocortical steroids – cortisol and aldosterone – in declining with advancing age. Moreover, administration of DHEA to experimental animals has demonstrated a multitude of beneficial effects on the prevention of cancer, heart disease, diabetes and obesity (Svec and Porter 1998). This has led to the assumption that the age-related decline of DHEA may play a role in

the degenerative changes observed in human aging and that administration of DHEA may reverse some of these changes. Moreover, the still ongoing availability of DHEA as a food supplement in the USA and its marketing as an anti-aging drug resulted in large scale self-administration without medical supervision.

However, in rodents circulating levels of DHEA and DHEAS are several orders of magnitude lower than in humans and no age-related decline in DHEA concentrations has been documented. This indicates that experimental studies in laboratory animals receiving high doses of DHEA have little bearing for human physiology.

This chapter, therefore, will focus mainly on data generated in humans. Dehydroepiandrosterone (sulfate), or DHEA(S), will refer to both DHEA and DHEAS. In addition, clinical studies concerning

Testosterone: Action, Deficiency, Substitution, ed. Eberhard Nieschlag and Hermann M. Behre, Assoc. ed. Susan Nieschlag. Published by Cambridge University Press. © Cambridge University Press 2012.

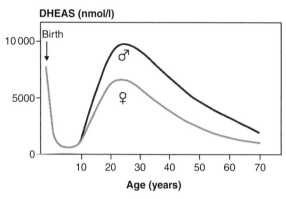

Fig. 20.1 Serum DHEAS concentrations during the human life cycle.

androstenedione, another less widely used steroid hormone precursor, will also be covered.

20.2 Dehydroepiandrosterone secretion and age

In humans and in some non-human primates, the secretion of DHEA(S) shows a characteristic pattern throughout the life cycle (Orentreich *et al.* 1984; Fig. 20.1). Dehydroepiandrosterone (sulfate) is secreted in high quantities by the fetal zone of the adrenal cortex, leading to high circulating DHEAS levels at birth. As the fetal zone involutes, a sharp fall in serum DHEA(S) concentrations is observed post-partum to almost undetectable levels after the first months of life. Levels remain low until they gradually increase between the 6th and 10th years of age; a phenomenon termed adrenarche (Sklar *et al.* 1980; Auchus and Rainey 2004). Recently it has been suggested that a rise in intra-adrenal cortisol during childhood adrenal growth may lead to inhibition of 3β-hydroxysteroid dehydrogenase type 2 and thereby contribute to the initiation of adrenarche (Topor *et al.* 2011). Dehydroepiandrosterone (sulfate) concentrations peak during the third decade, followed by a steady decline with advancing age, so that levels during the eighth and ninth decade are only 10–20% of those in young adults (Orentreich *et al.* 1992). This decline has been termed "adrenopause" in spite of unchanged or even increased cortisol secretion during aging (Laughlin and Barrett-Connor 2000). The age-related decline in DHEA(S) levels shows high interindividual variability (Spencer *et al.* 2007), and is associated with a reduction in size of the zona reticularis (Parker *et al.* 1997). Dehydroepiandrosterone secretion follows a diurnal rhythm similar to that

of cortisol, while DHEAS does not vary throughout the day. There is a clear gender difference in DHEA(S) concentrations, with lower DHEAS concentrations in adult women compared to men (Orentreich *et al.* 1984). The physiological basis for this gender difference is not fully clear. Some of the circulating DHEA in males may be contributed by the testes (Nieschlag *et al.* 1973). Roth *et al.* (2011) demonstrated that both DHEA and androstenedione are highly concentrated (27-fold and 175-fold, respectively) in the human testes, and respond to hCG. However, substantial changes in intratesticular DHEA or androstenedione were not reflected by the circulating concentrations of these steroids. No contribution from the ovaries has been reported, although they may indirectly affect DHEA(S) levels (Cumming *et al.* 1982).

There is also a clear genetic component to circulating DHEA(S) levels, which show high interindividual variability and vary significantly in populations of different ethnic origins (Spencer *et al.* 2007).

20.3 Epidemiology

There is some gender effect of high DHEAS levels in epidemiological studies: an inverse correlation between DHEAS levels and death from any cause was reported for men (>50 years of age) but not for women (Barrett-Connor and Goodman-Gruen 1995). In a prospective cohort study in 622 subjects of 65 years and older, mortality at two and four years was associated with low serum DHEAS at baseline in men but not in women (Berr *et al.* 1996). Similarly in a report including men (*n* = 963) and women (*n* = 1171) >65 years of age, all cause and cardiovascular disease mortality were highest in the lowest DHEAS quartile for men. Again no significant association of circulating DHEAS and mortality was found for women (Trivedi and Khaw 2001). In addition, Mazat *et al.* (2001) found no association between mortality and DHEAS levels in women; whereas in men the relative risk of death was 1.9 (*p* < 0.01) for those with the lowest concentrations of DHEAS. However, in a more recent study in 270 postmenopausal women undergoing coronary angiography for suspected CAD, lower DHEAS concentrations were predictive of higher cardiovascular and all-cause mortality (Shufelt *et al.* 2010). As DHEAS was related to severity of CAD, it was suggested that low DHEAS was mechanistically linked to atherosclerosis. Furthermore, in 302 postmenopausal women hospitalized for stroke, DHEAS

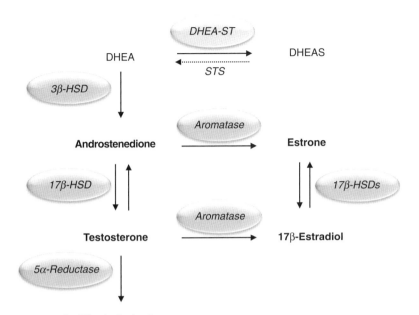

Fig. 20.2 Bioconversion of DHEA and androstenedione to sex steroids. Abbreviations: 3β-HSD, 3β-hydroxysteroid dehydrogenase activity; 17β-HSD, 17β-hydroxysteroid dehydrogenase activity; STS, steroid sulfatase activity; DHEA-ST, DHEA sulfotransferase activity (mainly mediated by SULT2A1).

was inversely related to stroke severity; whereas the outcome (handicap, death) was directly associated with DHEAS and androstenedione levels. The sex difference observed in many (but not all) studies may be related, in part, to sex-specific differences in bioconversion of DHEA(S) (Arlt *et al.* 1998; 1999a; see below).

In addition, low DHEAS levels may be a non-specific marker of poor health status and thereby associated with an increased risk of severe illness and death. Low DHEA(S) concentrations have been found in SLE, dementia, breast cancer and rheumatoid arthritis, and there is an inverse relationship between serum DHEAS levels and severity of disease (Deighton *et al.* 1992). Thus, low DHEAS levels may indicate the presence of a not yet apparent disease, which determines a future risk of morbidity or even mortality.

20.4 Mechanisms of action

20.4.1 Dehydroepiandrosterone

Three mechanisms of action have been described for DHEA: as a precursor for active sex steroids, as a neurosteroid interacting with receptors in the central nervous system, and as a ligand for a specific DHEA receptor.

As the human steroidogenic enzyme P450c17 converts almost no 17α-hydroxyprogesterone to androstenedione, the biosynthesis of virtually all sex steroids begins with the conversion of 17-hydroxypregnenolone to DHEA. Thus, only DHEA is converted to

androstenedione by the activity of 3β-hydroxysteroid dehydrogenase (3β-HSD) and then further converted to testosterone and estradiol by isoenzymes of 17β-hydroxysteroid dehydrogenase (17β-HSD) and P450 aromatase, respectively (Fig. 20.2). Only lipophilic DHEA can be converted intracellularly to androgens and estrogens. Thus the local availability and activity of DHEA sulfotransferase (SULT2A1) and steroid sulfatase determines the ratio of DHEA activation (via conversion to sex steroids) to inactivation (via secretion as DHEAS back into the circulation). It has consistently been shown that oral DHEA is readily converted to both DHEAS and downstream steroids (e.g. androstenedione) (Arlt *et al.* 1998; 1999a). Accordingly, a genome-wide association study in 14 846 subjects found an association of serum DHEAS with polymorphisms in the *SULT2A1* gene (Zhai *et al.* 2011). It has also long been assumed that DHEAS undergoes continuous conversion to DHEA; thereby serving as a large circulating pool for DHEA generation (Allolio and Arlt 2002). However, this concept has been challenged by the results of intravenous administration of DHEAS in healthy men (Hammer *et al.* 2005). While DHEAS is generated from circulating DHEA via hepatic SULT2A1 activity in relevant amounts, only minute amounts of circulating DHEA arise from DHEAS, indicating that hepatic steroid sulfatase hardly contributes to circulating DHEA. This observation has profound implications, as it is now clear that changes in circulating DHEAS may not always reflect changes in DHEA availability. This has been convincingly demonstrated in patients with septic shock who have low circulating DHEAS in the presence of high DHEA concentrations (Arlt *et al.* 2006). Moreover, inactivating mutations in the cofactor enzyme PAPS synthase 2, that provides the sulfate donor PAPS to human DHEA sulfotransferase, have been shown to result in non-detectable DHEAS but high levels of DHEA and downstream androgens (Noordam *et al.* 2009). This finding has provided definitive evidence for a crucial role of DHEA sulfation in regulating the production of active androgens. The situation is different in pregnancy, as here DHEAS can be converted to DHEA due to abundant placental expression of steroid sulfatase (Reed *et al.* 2005). Furthermore, the situation may also be different in various target tissues (e.g. breast, prostate) where substantial steroid sulfatase activity may lead to the local generation of relevant amounts of DHEA and consecutively downstream sex steroids not reflected in the circulation (Stanway *et al.* 2007).

The widespread presence of 3β-HSD, 17β-HSD, 5α-reductase and P450 aromatase results in almost ubiquitous peripheral generation of sex steroids from DHEA. Tissues involved include liver, skin, prostate, bone, breast and brain. It has been estimated that 40% of the androgen pool in elderly men and 50–100% of estrogen synthesis in pre- and postmenopausal women results from adrenal steroids converted in peripheral tissues (Labrie 2010).

The concept of peripheral synthesis, action and metabolism of steroid hormones from inactive precursors within the same target cell has been coined "intracrinology." Such intracrine processes are difficult to study, as serum parameters may only partially reflect target cell physiology. Nonetheless there is evidence that the bioconversion of DHEA(S) follows a sexually dimorphic pattern, with preferential increases in androgenic activity in women and increases in circulating estrogens in men (Arlt *et al.* 1998; 1999a). However, in men with combined adrenal insufficiency and hypogonadism due to hypopituitarism, oral DHEA administration induces significant increases in both estrogens and androgens (Young *et al.* 1997). Moreover, after oral administration of DHEA to men a pronounced increase in circulating 5α-androstane-3α,17β-diol-glucuronide (ADG) is found, indicating increased peripheral androgen synthesis not reflected by changes in circulating

testosterone levels (Arlt *et al.* 1999a). As ADG is the major metabolite of DHT (Giagulli *et al.* 1989), it reflects increased DHT generation in peripheral androgen target tissues. Furthermore, DHEA can also be converted to hydroxylated metabolites like androst-5-ene-3β,7β,17β-triol (βAET), which has anti-inflammatory and cholesterol-lowering activity (Stickney *et al.* 2011). The potential clinical role of this and other steroids derived from the prohormone DHEA awaits further studies.

In addition, DHEA is considered a neurosteroid. There is compelling evidence for DHEA synthesis and action in the central nervous system. Several studies have demonstrated the synthesis of P450c17 and other key steroidogenic enzymes in the brain (Zwain and Yen 1999), thereby providing the tools to generate DHEA in the absence of adrenal and gonadal function. Dehydroepiandrosterone influences neuronal activity via interaction with various receptors (N-methyl-D-aspartate (NMDA) receptor, sigma receptor, γ-aminobutyric acid (GABA$_A$) receptor (Perez-Neri *et al.* 2008)). Dehydroepiandrosterone may also influence brain function by direct binding to dendritic brain microtubule-associated protein MAP2C (Laurine *et al.* 2003). Animal and in-vitro studies have shown that DHEA(S) affects neuronal growth and development and improves glial survival, learning and memory (Compagnone and Mellon 1998; Svec and Porter 1998). An intriguing observation is the direct interaction of DHEA with nerve growth factor (NGF) receptors. This binding of DHEA to NGF receptors is functional, mediating anti-apoptotic effects and providing a mechanism of its neuroprotective action (Lazaridis *et al.* 2011).

Third, there is growing evidence for DHEA action outside the brain via specific receptors, although such a specific DHEA receptor has not yet been fully characterized or even cloned. High-affinity binding sites for DHEA have been described in murine and human T-cells (Meikle *et al.* 1992; Okabe *et al.* 1995), but their specificity for DHEA remained questionable. High-affinity binding sites for DHEA were identified in bovine endothelial cells (Liu and Dillon 2002). In these cells DHEA activates eNOS via a G-protein-coupled plasma membrane receptor. Similarly, DHEA affects extracellular-signal-regulated kinase 1 (ERK-1) phosphorylation in human vascular smooth muscle cells, independently of androgen and estrogen receptors (Williams *et al.* 2002). Dehydroepiandrosterone also causes vascular endothelial proliferation

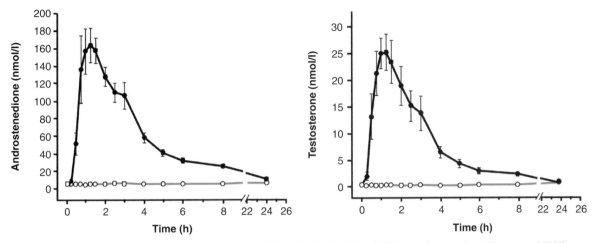

Fig. 20.3 Increase of testosterone in healthy young women after oral administration of 100 mg androstenedione (Kicman *et al.* 2003).

in a MAP-kinase dependent manner (Liu *et al.* 2008). It was shown in human and bovine vascular endothelial cells that DHEA leads to a significant production of H_2O_2 at physiological concentrations via specific membrane receptors. Furthermore, DHEA-induced endothelial cell proliferation was blocked by catalase, suggesting that H_2O_2 is a key molecule mediating the proliferative response to DHEA (Iruthayanathan *et al.* 2011). In vascular smooth muscle cells, DHEA affects phosphorylation and translocation of the transcription factor FoxO1, possibly by indirectly modifying mineralocorticoid receptor activity (Lindschau *et al.* 2011). Interaction with sigma receptors may also play a role outside the brain, as DHEA was shown to upregulate and stimulate sigma-1 receptors in the aorta and the kidney in experimental animals, inducing eNOS activity (Bhuiyan and Fukunaga 2010; Bhuiyan *et al.* 2011). These observations strengthen the concept of direct and specific hormonal activity of DHEA independent of its bioconversion to other steroids. Of note, a recent study has provided evidence for a distinct action of DHEAS in human neutrophils: DHEAS, but not unconjugated DHEA, was found to increase human neutrophil superoxide generation, a crucial mechanism underpinning neutrophil function, by direct interaction of DHEAS with protein kinase C (PKC) β (Radford *et al.* 2010). Of note, human neutrophils were shown to be capable of active and specific transmembrane import of hydrophilic DHEAS via the organic anion transporter polypeptide D (OATP-D) that appears as selectively expressed in neutrophils but no other human blood cell (Radford *et al.* 2010).

Taken together, there is clear evidence that DHEA has a complex and specific activity profile, which in part is gender specific due to its sex-related differential pattern of downstream bioconversion to potent sex steroids. While an interaction with several known receptors has been convincingly shown, a specific DHEA receptor remains to be characterized.

20.4.2 Androstenedione

Androstenedione is not only a product of DHEA metabolism, but may be regarded as a prohormone itself. It can be converted to testosterone by 17β-HSDs or to estrone by the aromatase enzyme complex (Leder *et al.* 2000). Accordingly, administration of androstenedione may alter circulating steroid hormone concentrations. In women, pronounced increases not only in circulating androstenedione but also in testosterone, DHT and free androgen index have been described following administration of 100 mg androstenedione (Kicman *et al.* 2003; Bassindale *et al.* 2004; Fig. 20.3). In contrast, in men the effects of oral androstenedione have been variable: in some trials serum total testosterone concentrations were not affected by 100 mg androstenedione (King *et al.* 1999; Brown *et al.* 2000). However, 300 mg androstenedione induced increases in testosterone levels (Leder *et al.* 2000). Importantly, clear increases in estrogens were observed after oral ingestion of androstenedione in young and elderly men (King *et al.* 1999; Brown *et al.* 2000; Leder *et al.* 2000) and less pronounced also in women (Brown *et al.* 2004), an effect quite similar to oral DHEA administration.

However, in postmenopausal women only an increase in testosterone and estrone, but not in estradiol was reported (Leder *et al.* 2002). The intracrine activation of androstenedione – similar to DHEA – was highlighted by a detailed analysis of the metabolism of orally administered androstenedione in young men (Leder *et al.* 2001), observing increases in the excretion rates of conjugated testosterone, androsterone, etiocholanolone and dihydrotestosterone. It was concluded that orally administered androstenedione is largely metabolized to androgen metabolites before release into the general circulation. Thus again the biological activity of androstenedione is incompletely reflected by circulating active sex steroids. Similar hormone profiles were obtained using sublingual androstenediol in young men (Brown *et al.* 2002). Clear increases in serum testosterone were found by bypassing first-pass hepatic metabolism using this sublingual administration. Intriguingly, longer-term administration of 200 mg/day androstenedione in elderly men led to an unexpected increase in circulating DHEAS (upstream of androstenedione) and a reduced increase to an acute challenge with androstenedione, suggesting enhanced androstenedione metabolism (Beckham and Earnest 2003).

At present there is no evidence that androstenedione has biological activity independent of its downstream conversion to sex steroids.

20.5 Treatment with DHEA: clinical studies

20.5.1 Patients with adrenal insufficiency

The classical approach to study the physiological role of a hormone in humans is to analyze the effect on a hormonal deficit and the changes induced by replacement of the missing hormone. Thus, adrenal insufficiency is the most useful model disease to understand the clinical activity of DHEA. In adrenal insufficiency, not only cortisol and (in primary adrenal insufficiency) aldosterone is lacking, but also DHEA, and one might speculate that replacement of cortisol and aldosterone alone is not sufficient to fully restore well-being in adrenal insufficiency. Intriguingly, it has recently been clearly demonstrated that, despite established replacement of glucocorticoids and mineralocorticoids, patients suffer from impaired well-being with increased fatigue, depression, loss of libido and impaired vitality (Jakobi *et al.* 2001;

Hahner *et al.* 2007; Erichsen *et al.* 2009). Jakobi *et al.* have provided some more insight into the mechanism of increased fatigue in conventionally treated patients with adrenal insufficiency. Muscle function (twitch tension, central activation) was reduced and patients self-terminated a submaximal fatigue protocol significantly earlier than controls (5 ± 1 vs. 10 ± 1 min, $p = 0.006$; Jakobi *et al.* 2001). Recent data furthermore demonstrate increased mortality in adrenal insufficiency patients, specifically from respiratory infections (Tomlinson *et al.* 2001; Bergthorsdottir *et al.* 2006; Bensing *et al.* 2008; Erichsen *et al.* 2009).

For replacement of DHEA(S) in adrenal insufficiency, an oral dose of 25–50 mg DHEA per day has consistently been found to restore circulating DHEA(S) into the normal range of young adults (Arlt *et al.* 1999b; Hunt *et al.* 2000). Due to the downstream bioconversion, lasting increases in circulating androgens have been demonstrated in women (Arlt *et al.* 1998; 1999b; Fig. 20.4).

So far, several trials have investigated the effect of DHEA replacement on well-being and on metabolic parameters in both primary and secondary adrenal insufficiency (Arlt *et al.* 1999b; Hunt *et al.* 2000; Callies *et al.* 2001; Johannsson *et al.* 2002; Lovas *et al.* 2003; Libe *et al.* 2004; Bilger *et al.* 2005; van Thiel *et al.* 2005; Brooke *et al.* 2006; Dhatariya *et al.* 2008; Gurnell *et al.* 2008). Dehydroepiandrosterone has shown beneficial effects on subjective health status, mood and sexuality. These effects could also be demonstrated in men who do not suffer from androgen deficiency owing to the preserved androgen production by their testes, suggesting that these effects are in part mediated by neurosteroidal activity (see also Chapter 17).

In the first double-blind study (Arlt *et al.* 1999b), treatment with DHEA in women with adrenal insufficiency raised the initially low concentrations of DHEA(S), androstenedione and testosterone into the normal range. Serum concentrations of SHBG, total cholesterol and HDL-C decreased significantly. Dehydroepiandrosterone improved well-being and sexuality: compared to placebo DHEA resulted in a significant decrease in the scores for depression and anxiety, as well as for a global severity index of the SCL-90-R questionnaire. Beneficial effects of DHEA treatment on anxiety and depression were also observed for the Hospital Anxiety and Depression Scale (HADS). A reduction in fatigue was evident from the Giessen Complaint List. Treatment with

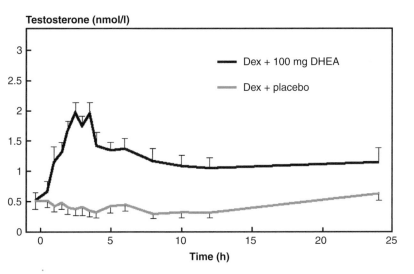

Fig. 20.4 Lasting increases of serum testosterone in healthy dexamethasone (Dex)-suppressed women after oral administration of 100 mg DHEA versus placebo (Arlt *et al.* 1998).

DHEA resulted in significant increases in the initially low scores of all four visual-analog scales for sexuality. Dehydroepiandrosterone did not affect fasting serum glucose, insulin and parameters of body composition (Callies *et al.* 2001). Using an incremental cycling test, maximum workload was 95.8 ± 20.4 W after DHEA, compared to 91.7 ± 24.1 W after placebo ($p = 0.057$).

Androgenic skin effects of DHEA treatment were reported in 19 out of the 24 women but were mostly mild and transient (Arlt *et al.* 1999b).

Improvement in mood and fatigue was also observed after DHEA replacement in Addison's disease in the trial reported by Hunt *et al.* (2000). The hormonal changes induced by DHEA in females were virtually identical to those reported by Arlt *et al.* (1999b), with increases in serum DHEA(S), androstenedione and testosterone into normal range for women. In males, serum testosterone and SHBG did not change. Hunt *et al.* (2000) found a significant increase in self-esteem after DHEA substitution. Using a Profile of Mood State Questionnaire it was demonstrated that evening mood and evening fatigue was improved by DHEA. No changes in BMD, BMI, serum cholesterol or insulin sensitivity were observed after DHEA treatment. As the beneficial effects in this study were also observed in male patients who exhibited no change in testosterone, it was concluded that DHEA acts directly at the central nervous system rather than via peripheral conversion to androgens (Hunt *et al.* 2000). The same group followed up on these results and performed the largest study so far in patients with primary adrenal insufficiency ($n = 106$), who received 12 months of DHEA replacement (50 mg/day) or placebo in a parallel-group study design (Gurnell *et al.* 2008). Results of this phase III trial demonstrated significant improvement of SF-36 role emotional function scores and some slight improvement also in further QoL scores during DHEA replacement. No significant benefit of DHEA treatment on fatigue or cognitive or sexual function could be demonstrated. In addition they found a reversal of loss of BMD at the femoral neck by DHEA replacement as assessed by DXA. Body composition analysis by DXA also revealed a significant increase in lean body mass, while fat mass remained unchanged (Gurnell *et al.* 2008).

In 38 women with secondary adrenal insufficiency due to hypopituitarism, DHEA (20–30 mg/day) was used (Johannsson *et al.* 2002). Dehydroepiandrosterone or placebo was given for six months in a randomized, placebo-controlled, double-blind study, followed by a six-month open treatment period. The percentage of partners of the patients who reported improved alertness, stamina and initiative in their spouses were 70%, 64% and 55%, respectively, in the DHEA group, and 11%, 6% and 11%, respectively, in the placebo group ($p < 0.05$). Sexual relations tended to improve ($p = 0.06$). An increase in or the reappearance of axillary and/or pubic hair was seen in all women given 30 mg DHEA and in 69% of women receiving 20 mg DHEA, but was not found in women receiving placebo. Glucose metabolism and lipoproteins remained unaffected by DHEA, with the exception of transient decrease in HDL-C. These values had significantly increased at 12 months ($p < 0.05$). Bone markers and BMD remained unchanged. Androgenic skin effects were more often seen during DHEA treatment.

The role of DHEA replacement in adolescent and young women was investigated by Bilger *et al.* (2005). Five young females with hypopituitarism, aged between 15 and 23 years, received DHEA 50 mg/day in a 12-month, double-blind, placebo-controlled crossover trial. A better life satisfaction was shown under DHEA replacement in the Life Situation Survey compared to placebo (110 vs. 102, $p = 0.05$). In addition, an improvement of maximal oxygen uptake (VO_2), and decreased percentage body fat was observed which did not reach significance in the small group investigated. Similarly, Binder and colleagues demonstrated, in a cohort of 23 young girls and women (13–25 years), that 12 months of DHEA treatment vs. placebo resulted in significant improvement of pubic hair Tanner stage and improved mood and well-being, specifically of depression and anxiety and the global severity index as assessed by the SCL-90-R (Binder *et al.* 2009).

Two studies have investigated the additive effect of DHEA to GH replacement in secondary adrenal insufficiency. Van Thiel *et al.* studied the effects of DHEA (50 mg/d) for 16 weeks versus placebo in GH- and ACTH-deficient men ($n = 15$), and postmenopausal women ($n = 16$), in a double-blind, placebo-controlled crossover study (van Thiel *et al.* 2005). A significant improvement by DHEA in SF-36 vitality scores in both men and women and in the HADS depression score in women was detected. However, no differences in fatigue scores, QoL assessment in GH deficiency in adults (QOL-AGHDA) or in the sexual functioning questionnaires could be demonstrated. Interestingly, IGF-1 levels increased in women during DHEA replacement by about 18%. No change in IGF-1 levels was observed in men, suggesting that the effect may be related to androgenic effects following normalization of androgen levels in women. This observation was also made by Brooke *et al.*, resulting in a decrease of GH replacement doses (Brooke *et al.* 2006). In this double-blind, placebo-controlled trial, 30 females and 21 males with hypopituitarism received DHEA 50 mg over six months, followed by an open phase of six months of DHEA treatment. Females showed improvement in QOL-AGHDA score, in SF-36 (Short Form 36) social functioning and general health perception after six months of DHEA; whereas men showed improvement in self esteem and depression

domains of the General Health Questionnaire after six months of DHEA.

Besides the results of these randomized trials, evidence from case reports (Kim and Brody 2001; Wit *et al.* 2001) in adrenal insufficiency is available. Kim and Brody (2001) have described a 24-year-old female with Addison's disease and the complaint of neither axillary nor pubic hair growth. Dehydroepiandrosterone was added to the conventional replacement therapy. Pubic hair growth changed from Tanner stage I to Tanner stage III within two years of receiving DHEA at a final dose of 25 mg daily. Similarly, Wit *et al.* (2001) used oral DHEAS (15 mg/m^2) for atrichia pubis in four female adolescents with panhypopituitarism ($n = 2$) or 17-hydroxylase deficiency ($n = 2$). They found DHEAS an efficacious treatment, leading from atrichia pubis to Tanner stage 4–5 pubic hair.

However, other studies could not find any beneficial effect of DHEA replacement (Lovas *et al.* 2003; Libe *et al.* 2004), and a more recent meta-analysis of RCTs of the effect of DHEA in adrenal insufficiency revealed only moderate beneficial effects on health-related QoL and depression (Alkatib *et al.* 2009). Effects on anxiety and sexual well-being were also small and did not reach statistical significance, which led to the conclusion that larger clinical trials are needed before the routine use of DHEA in adrenal insufficiency can be recommended.

20.5.2   Elderly subjects

The age-related decline in circulating DHEA(S) has led to a number of randomized trials to assess the effect of oral DHEA in otherwise healthy elderly subjects. In a first double-blind, placebo-controlled trial using a crossover design, 13 men and 17 women aged 40–70 years received either 50 mg DHEA or placebo for three months (and vice versa) (Morales *et al.* 1994). The subjects reported an improvement in well-being using a non-validated questionnaire for self-assessment of well-being. No change in insulin sensitivity and body composition was found (see also Sections 20.7.2 and 20.7.3). Bioavailable IGF-1 increased slightly during DHEA treatment, whereas HDL-C decreased in women. Short-term (two weeks) randomized, double-blind studies by Wolf *et al.* (1997; 1998) failed to demonstrate any benefit of DHEA on well-being, mood and cognition. Similarly, in a double-blind, placebo-controlled crossover trial, Arlt *et al.* (2001) found no effect of DHEA

(50 mg/day) on mood, well-being and sexuality in 20 men aged 50–69 years after four months of therapy. In another placebo-controlled, randomized crossover trial by van Niekerk et al., no effect of 50 mg/day DHEA for 13 weeks on well-being and cognition was found using a wide range of validated self-assessment questionnaires and standardized test batteries, respectively (van Niekerk et al. 2001). No effect of DHEA on activities of daily living was found after three months of 100 mg/d DHEA in 39 men aged 60–84 years in another placebo-controlled crossover trial (Flynn et al. 1999).

In the DHEAge study, Baulieu et al. (2000) investigated the effects of 50 mg/d DHEA vs. placebo in a double-blind, randomized, parallel study including 140 men and 140 women aged 60–79 years. In general the results were disappointing. Neither well-being nor cognition was improved by DHEA using a wide range of validated tools. In women > 70 years, gains in BMD were detected and libido was increased, but no significant changes were observed in men. Furthermore, no influence on well-being or cognition could be demonstrated after 12 months of DHEA treatment.

So far the longest trial by Nair et al. investigated the effect of DHEA and testosterone on QoL, body composition, physical performance and metabolism in elderly subjects (Nair et al. 2006). The authors found no significant effects of DHEA in these healthy elderly individuals with low baseline DHEA levels on QoL, body composition, physical performance or insulin sensitivity.

Several studies have investigated the role of DHEA for treatment of symptoms related to postmenopausal hormone deficiency (Davis et al. 2011). Dehydroepiandrosterone treatment has been shown to enhance parameters of sexual function in postmenopausal women after single-dose treatment with 300 mg (Hackbert and Heiman 2002) or longer term administration of an oral dose or vaginal cream (Schmidt et al. 2005; Labrie et al. 2009). Most of these studies, however, administered supraphysiological DHEA doses. Recent longer term studies with larger sample sizes using 50 mg/d DHEA showed no improvement in sexual function by DHEA and no change in general well-being (Nair et al. 2006; Kritz-Silverstein et al. 2008; Panjari et al. 2009).

Taking all studies on DHEA supplementation in elderly subjects together, the results show only very limited effects of DHEA compared to placebo. An important explanation for this lack of efficacy may be related to a selection bias. In almost all studies, only healthy subjects with excellent performance status at baseline were included, thereby leaving limited space for further improvement. However, from these studies it can be concluded that age-related low DHEA concentrations do not necessarily lead to impaired well-being, cognition and sexuality *per se* (Allolio and Arlt 2002).

20.5.3 Patients with impaired mood and well-being

Consistent with the effects of DHEA on mood and well-being in patients with adrenal insufficiency, beneficial effects were also observed in randomized, double-blind studies in patients with major depression (Wolkowitz et al. 1999) and midlife dysthymia (Bloch et al. 1999). Dehydroepiandrosterone also improved scores on an activities of daily living scale in patients with myotonic dystrophy (Sugino et al. 1998). Reiter et al. have reported an improvement in erectile function, sexual satisfaction and orgasmic function in 40–60-year-old men suffering from ED and receiving 50 mg/d DHEA for six months in a randomized, double-blind fashion (Reiter et al. 1999). To compare the efficacy of DHEA vs. placebo in Alzheimer's disease, 58 patients were randomized to six months of treatment with DHEA (100 mg/d) or placebo. A transient effect on cognitive performance narrowly missed significance (Wolkowitz et al. 2003), possibly because of the small patient sample. Strous et al. have studied the efficacy of DHEA (100 mg/d) in schizophrenic patients with prominent negative symptoms (Strous et al. 2003). In a double-blind trial, a significant improvement in negative symptoms ($p < 0.001$), as well as in depressive ($p < 0.05$) and anxiety ($p < 0.001$) symptoms was seen in individuals receiving DHEA.

It seems noteworthy that the pattern of improvement observed in these trials closely resembled the changes observed in patients with adrenal insufficiency.

20.5.4 Patients with immunological disorders

In a number of studies, DHEA supplementation has been used to modify immune functions and alter the course of immunopathies. Most studies have been performed in patients with SLE, a chronic auto-immune inflammatory disease of unknown etiology (van Vollenhoven *et al.* 1994; Chang *et al.* 2002). The concept of using DHEA in the treatment of SLE was based on the observation that women are more often affected and that androgens and DHEA concentrations are low in patients with SLE (Lahita *et al.* 1987). Moreover, androgen treatment can modify the disease progression in an animal model of SLE (Melez *et al.* 1980). After preliminary evidence of a glucocorticoid-sparing effect of DHEA in patients with mild SLE (van Vollenhoven *et al.* 1994), a randomized, double-blind, placebo-controlled trial was performed (van Vollenhoven *et al.* 1999). It demonstrated beneficial effects of DHEA on patient and physician overall assessment, SLE disease activity index (SLEDAI) and glucocorticoid requirements. This was confirmed in recent double-blind, randomized, placebo-controlled trials demonstrating that DHEA (200 mg/d) was well tolerated, reduced the number of SLE flares, reduced disease activity and allowed reduction of the dosage of glucocorticoids (Chang *et al.* 2002; Hartkamp *et al.* 2010). It is important to note that most of these studies included women only, and that it remains unclear whether similar results can be obtained in men. In a phase II uncontrolled pilot trial, DHEA (200 mg/d) was effective and safe in patients with refractory Crohn's disease and ulcerative colitis (Andus *et al.* 2003). However, to date no placebo-controlled trials have been performed in inflammatory bowel disease. In all these trials, side-effects were mild, with acne being the most frequently seen adverse event despite the use of undoubtedly supraphysiological DHEA doses (200 mg/d).

DHEA supplementation has also been used to enhance the antibody response to tetanus and influenza vaccines (Danenberg *et al.* 1997). However, in these randomized, placebo-controlled trials, no consistent effect of DHEA on protective antibody titers was found.

20.5.5 Dehydroepiandrosterone supplementation in diminished ovarian reserve

Dehydroepiandrosterone supplementation for diminished ovarian reserve (DOR) in patients undergoing artificial reproductive treatment has first been suggested by (Casson *et al.* 2000) to compensate for adrenocortical changes in aging women and to take advantage of the IGF-1 increase induced by DHEA. Furthermore, animal data have shown that androgen action in granulosa cells plays a crucial role for follicular development and function by promoting preantral growth (Sen and Hammes 2010). In women with DOR, DHEA administration was associated with increasing oocyte and embryo counts (Gleicher *et al.* 2010). Cohort studies in 89 DOR patients supplemented with DHEA and 101 controls indicated shorter time to pregnancy and higher pregnancy rates (28.1 vs. 10.9%; Barad *et al.* 2007). The same group reported that DHEA supplementation reduced embryo aneuploidy in a case control study of 22 consecutive patients (Gleicher *et al.* 2010). In a first randomized, open trial in 33 women with DOR, DHEA (75 mg/d) was associated with a significantly higher birth rate (23.1 vs. 4%, $p < 0.05$; Wiser *et al.* 2010). However, this sample size is rather small and the statistical evaluation of this trial has been heavily criticized (Kolibianakis *et al.* 2011). Despite the still weak overall evidence due to the current lack of rigorous randomized trials of sufficient size (Sunkara and Coomarasamy 2011; Yakin and Urman 2011), it is estimated that about one-third of all IVF centers today use DHEA supplementation in women with DOR (Gleicher and Barad 2011). Reported side-effects were generally mild and included oily skin, acne and hair loss.

20.6 Androstenedione administration in clinical studies

Effects of oral androstenedione have not been studied in women and have been largely disappointing in men. Short-term (five days) androstenedione (100 mg/d) administration had no anabolic effect on muscle protein metabolism in eugonadal young men (Rasmussen *et al.* 2000). In 30–56-year-old men, androstenedione (3×100 mg/d) for 28 days slightly reduced HDL-C without affecting PSA, suggesting some androgenic activity (Brown *et al.* 2000). Serum HDL-C was also reduced in an eight-week randomized trial in 20 young men receiving oral androstenedione (300 mg/d) (King *et al.* 1999). Androstenedione failed to enhance muscle adaptation to resistance training in this population (King *et al.* 1999).

At present, both treatment duration and sample sizes have been too limited to draw any firm conclusions on the clinical efficacy and the ergogenic activity of androstenedione. However, the profound increases in circulating testosterone observed in women after oral androstenedione deserve attention and should preclude its use as a food supplement (Kicman *et al.* 2003; Bassindale *et al.* 2004). Even more so as androstenedione currently belongs to the popular supplements in young athletes (Calfee and Fadale 2006) and its abuse is not easily detectable (Brown *et al.* 2004).

20.7 The emerging therapeutic profile of DHEA

20.7.1 Effects on the central nervous system

Improvement in mood and well-being have consistently been observed in patients with adrenal insufficiency (Arlt *et al.* 1999b; Hunt *et al.* 2000; Johannsson *et al.* 2002) and in patients with depressive disorders (Bloch *et al.* 1999; Wolkowitz *et al.* 1999) and schizophrenia (Strous *et al.* 2003); particularly improving symptoms of anxiety and depression and their physical correlates. It is important to note that improvements have only been observed in subjects with impaired mood and well-being at baseline, and that DHEA-induced improvements led to scores in the range of normal healthy subjects. This indicates that DHEA may normalize impaired well-being but will not lead to "supranormal" well-being in otherwise healthy subjects (irrespective of the presence of low endogenous DHEAS concentrations).

Several cases of mania have been reported with DHEA treatment (Kline and Jaggers 1999; Markowitz *et al.* 1999), and we also have observed a similar case in a woman with adrenal insufficiency receiving a daily dose of 25 mg DHEA; although a direct causal role for DHEA is difficult to establish.

The basis for the anxiolytic and antidrepressive activity of DHEA remains to be elucidated but may be related to both androgenic effects and neurosteroidal actions of DHEA.

In contrast, there is little evidence that DHEA affects memory or cognition. Negative results have been found not only in healthy elderly subjects (Baulieu *et al.* 2000) but also in adrenal insufficiency (Arlt *et al.* 2000). Moreover, in Addison's disease cognition is not impaired despite severe endogenous DHEA deficiency (Arlt *et al.* 2000). Thus it is unlikely that cognition is a major target of DHEA action.

Libido and sexual satisfaction are influenced by DHEA in women with adrenal insufficiency (Arlt *et al.* 1999b) and in elderly women with age-related low DHEAS (Baulieu *et al.* 2000). Also in men, only impaired sexuality benefits from DHEA administration (Reiter *et al.* 1999), while normal baseline performance cannot be enhanced (Arlt *et al.* 2001). The effect of DHEA on libido and sexuality is most likely a consequence of increased androgenic activity derived from DHEA by peripheral bioconversion. In recent years it has become increasingly clear that androgens play a key role for female sexuality (Shifren *et al.* 2000; Arlt 2003). In fact, the adrenals are a major source of female androgens (Labrie *et al.* 2003), and their fundamental role for female sexuality (Waxenberg *et al.* 1959) has been rediscovered by studies on the therapeutic potential of DHEA. The available evidence and the superior pharmacokinetic properties make DHEA a highly attractive tool for treatment of impaired sexuality in women. However, firm conclusions must await the results of further trials.

20.7.2 Metabolism and body composition

The effects of DHEA on metabolic parameters (e.g. lipids, insulin sensitivity) and body composition are mostly not consistent and largely unimpressive.

However, consistently observed in response to DHEA treatment in both hypoadrenal patients and elderly subjects is an increase in IGF-1 levels (Morales *et al.* 1998; Villareal *et al.* 2000; van Thiel *et al.* 2005; Brooke *et al.* 2006; Jankowski *et al.* 2006; von Muhlen *et al.* 2008; Weiss *et al.* 2009). Effects on lipids also appear to be relatively robust. The first study in patients with adrenal insufficiency already demonstrated a significant decrease of total cholesterol and HDL-C. Similarly, in the study by Dhatariya *et al.* (2005) or Srinivasan *et al.* (2010), DHEA additionally reduced total cholesterol, LDL-C and triglycerides and also HDL-C in hypoadrenal patients. The overall DHEA effect on the lipid profile is modest, mainly consisting of a HDL-C-lowering effect (Barnhart *et al.* 1999; Dayal *et al.* 2005; Nair *et al.* 2006; Srinivasan *et al.* 2010).The mechanisms for the reduction in HDL and total cholesterol are most likely mediated by the effects of androgens on increasing hepatic lipase activity, thus impairing hepatic cholesterol formation.

The majority of studies assessing the effect of oral DHEA on insulin sensitivity document no effect on insulin sensitivity in healthy elderlies receiving replacement doses of DHEA (Morales *et al.* 1994; Casson *et al.* 1995; Yen *et al.* 1995; Morales *et al.* 1998; Nair *et al.* 2006; Basu *et al.* 2007; Igwebuike *et al.* 2008; Panjari *et al.* 2009). Villareal *et al.* investigated 28 women and 28 men aged 65–78 years with age-related decrease in DHEA levels. The insulin area under the curve during the oral glucose tolerance test was significantly reduced after six months of DHEA therapy compared with placebo, and a significant increase in the insulin sensitivity index in response to DHEA was observed (Villareal and Holloszy 2004).

In a study in 28 hypoadrenal women receiving 50 mg oral DHEA over 12 weeks, Dhatariya *et al.* also observed lower fasting insulin and glucagon levels with DHEA. Insulin sensitivity, assessed by using a hyperinsulinemic-euglycemic clamp, was increased during DHEA administration (Dhatariya *et al.* 2005). However, no effects of DHEA on fasting glucose, insulin, or glucose–insulin ratio were observed in other studies in patients with adrenal insufficiency (Callies *et al.* 2001; Libe *et al.* 2004).

Body composition remains mostly unaffected by DHEA. Morales *et al.* reported an increase in muscle strength in men but not in women, aged 50–60 years, after six months of treatment with 100 mg/d DHEA (Morales *et al.* 1998). Application of a 10% DHEA cream to the skin daily over 12 months resulted in an increase in femoral muscle area in 15 women aged 60–70 years (Diamond *et al.* 1996). A decrease in fat mass and an increase in fat-free mass assessed by DXA measurement were furthermore observed by Villareal *et al.* (2000). However, no effect on body composition could be observed in several other large trials (Arlt *et al.* 2001; Percheron *et al.* 2003; Jankowski *et al.* 2006; Nair *et al.* 2006; von Muhlen *et al.* 2008).

The possibility of potentiating the response to exercise training has been investigated. Villareal *et al.* analyzed the effects of 10 months of DHEA 50 mg/d in combination with weightlifting exercise training during the last four months of the study (DHEA exercise group, $n = 29$; placebo exercise group, $n = 27$) in 28 women and 28 men aged 65–78 years. Dehydroepiandrosterone alone for six months did not significantly increase strength or thigh muscle volume. However, DHEA supplementation potentiated the effect of four months of weightlifting training on muscle strength, and on thigh muscle volume, measured by MRI (Villareal and Holloszy 2006). This potentiation was, however, not seen in

another study in 31 postmenopausal women receiving 12 weeks of DHEA 50 mg/d in addition to endurance and resistance exercise training; whereas exercising *per se* significantly increased insulin sensitivity and improved body composition (Igwebuike *et al.* 2008). Thus, at present a significant effect of DHEA on muscular function and body composition remains uncertain.

20.7.3 Skeletal system

Dehydroepiandrosterone replacement has been reported to increase BMD in elderly subjects. However, small sample size and short duration of treatment precluded clear conclusions in many trials. Jankowski *et al.* investigated 70 women and 70 men aged 60–88 years (Jankowski *et al.* 2006). They observed an increase in hip BMD in both sexes and, in women, also an increase in lumbar spine BMD after one year's treatment with 50 mg/d DHEA (Jankowski *et al.* 2006). Changes in BMD were associated with estradiol levels and free estrogen index at 12 months, suggesting that the effects were primarily mediated by increases in serum estradiol (Jankowski *et al.* 2008). Nair *et al.* performed a two-year, placebo-controlled, randomized, double-blind study involving 87 elderly men and 57 elderly women with low levels of sulfated DHEA (Nair *et al.* 2006). Men receiving DHEA 75 mg/d had an increase in BMD at the femoral neck. Women who received DHEA 50 mg/d had an increase in BMD at the ultradistal radius. Several other RCTs reported similar observations, with slight increases in BMD and changes in markers of bone turnover, mainly in women (Labrie *et al.* 1997; Baulieu *et al.* 2000; Villareal *et al.* 2000; von Muhlen *et al.* 2008).

In patients with adrenal insufficiency, DHEA reversed ongoing loss of BMD at the femoral neck but not at other sites in women receiving DHEA replacement (Gurnell *et al.* 2008). However, other studies could not detect relevant effects on bone mass (Hunt *et al.* 2000; Johannsson *et al.* 2002).

Dehydroepiandrosterone effects on bone markers were missing in men (Baulieu *et al.* 2000; Arlt *et al.* 2001; Kahn *et al.* 2002) and were variable in women with either increases, decreases or no change in bone resorption markers (Baulieu *et al.* 2000; Villareal *et al.* 2000; Callies *et al.* 2001) and increases or no change in osteocalcin (Baulieu *et al.* 2000; Callies *et al.* 2001).

At present it seems likely that beneficial effects of DHEA on BMD are small compared to other treatment options and restricted to women, possibly due to androgenic and estrogenic biotransformation of DHEA. Again, only large, prospective, controlled trials will settle this issue.

20.7.4 Skin

Skin is an important target of DHEA action: DHEA increases sebum secretion and skin hydration (Labrie *et al.* 1997; Baulieu *et al.* 2000), and has been reported to reduce facial skin pigmentation (yellowness) in elderlies (Baulieu *et al.* 2000). Androgenic changes such as acne and hirsutism, including facial hair growth, have been reported as possible side-effects in numerous controlled trials (Arlt *et al.* 1999b; Hunt *et al.* 2000; Lovas *et al.* 2003; Brooke *et al.* 2006; Gurnell *et al.* 2008).

20.7.5 Immune system

Based on data from animal experiments (Svec and Porter 1998) and from in-vitro studies (Meikle *et al.* 1992; Okabe *et al.* 1995), DHEA has been suggested as a steroid with immune-regulatory activity. This view is supported by the clinical studies in patients with SLE, demonstrating glucocorticoid-sparing activity of DHEA and clinical improvement (Chang *et al.* 2002). However, in these studies DHEA was given at a clearly supraphysiological dose (200 mg/d), and physiological replacement doses (50 mg/d) given to healthy elderlies in the DHEAge study did not have any effect on B- and T-cell populations, cytokine production or natural killer (NK) cell cytotoxicity (unpublished observations). In-vitro studies with human cells also show DHEA-induced increases in IL-2 secretion (Suzuki *et al.* 1991) and NK cell activity (Solerte *et al.* 1999) and inhibition of IL-6 release (Gordon *et al.* 2001). Secretion of IL-2 in SLE correlates with circulating DHEAS, and in-vitro DHEA restores IL-2 secretion from T-lymphocytes of SLE patients (Suzuki *et al.* 1995). No consistent in-vivo data on immune effects of DHEA in humans are reported. Again it is likely that beneficial effects of DHEA are more easily detectable in patients with immunopathies and an altered immune system at baseline (Hazeldine *et al.* 2010).

20.8 Practical approach to the patient with DHEA deficiency

At present there is still no established indication and no generally accepted pharmacological preparation of DHEA for treatment. However, there is growing evidence (Achermann and Silverman 2001; Allolio *et al.* 2007; Alkatib *et al.* 2009) that DHEA replacement in patients with adrenal insufficiency is beneficial in a significant percentage of cases. In these patients impaired well-being including depression, reduced vitality and increased fatigue (Hahner *et al.* 2007) has been documented: symptoms that are likely to respond to DHEA replacement (25–50 mg/day). Treatment usually starts with 25 mg/day. Serum DHEAS concentrations can easily be monitored and should be in the respective sex- and age-adjusted reference range (Orentreich *et al.* 1984). It is important to know that significant improvement may occur only after two to four months of treatment.

Treatment of elderlies with age-related physiologically low endogenous DHEA(S) is not justified. All available evidence indicates that the age-related decline in DHEA(S) concentration is not necessarily associated with impairment in well-being and mood or with increased fatigue. Accordingly, DHEA supplementation offers no apparent benefit for such a population. This is a situation very similar to postmenopausal hormone replacement: despite very low estradiol concentrations, estrogen replacement may be more often detrimental than beneficial. This does not exclude the possibility that certain subgroups of elderly subjects (e.g. patients with frailty) may benefit from DHEA supplementation, but these subgroups need to be defined. In particular, there is no evidence that DHEA supplementation reverses relevant aspects of aging.

Reports on beneficial effects of DHEA on a diminished ovarian reserve in IVF patients are intriguing but still inconclusive. Thus, despite the widespread use of pharmacological doses of DHEA (75 mg/day) in this setting, its use should be regarded as clearly experimental pending larger-scale, randomized studies that clearly demonstrate effectiveness.

20.9 Future perspectives

Important progress has been made in the field of DHEA research. The therapeutic potential of DHEA is more clearly visible (see Table 20.1), and DHEA has

Table 20.1 Action profile of DHEA

Central nervous system:

- Mood → (↑), well-being ↑ (→), anxiety ↓ (→), depression ↓, fatigue → (↓), cognitive function →
- Libido → (↑ in women), sexual satisfaction → (↑)

Metabolism:

- Insulin sensitivity →, fasting glucose →
- HDL cholesterol ↓ (→), total cholesterol →
- IGF-1 ↑ (→)

Muscle:

- Strength → (↑), muscle area →
- Lean body mass → (↑)

Bone:

- Bone mineral density → (↑ in women)
- Bone maker → (↑↓)

Skin:

- Sebum production ↑
- Skin hydration ↑
- Acne ↑

Immune system:

- Glucocorticoid demand in immunopathies (↓)
- Immune cell distribution → (B-cells, T-cells, NK cells)

Symbols: ↑ increase; → unchanged; ↓ reduced; () changes only found in some of the published studies.

become part of routine replacement in many patients with adrenal insufficiency and impaired well-being. However, large phase III trials are still necessary to firmly establish its role in the treatment of adrenal failure and to further define the spectrum of DHEA actions. In particular, it is difficult to separate androgenic from DHEA-specific effects. In this regard studies in male patients with adrenal insufficiency will be highly informative, as in this population DHEA-induced androgenic actions are expected to play virtually no role on the background of high endogenous testosterone concentrations.

Recent larger trials have again demonstrated that hopes of using DHEA as an anti-aging remedy were not justified. However, DHEA may have therapeutic potential for patients with psychiatric illnesses (depression, schizophrenia, dysthymia) or immunopathies and women with androgen deficiency-related complaints (e. g. loss of libido).

In these patient groups administration of DHEA must not be regarded as substitution therapy but rather as pharmacotherapy. Accordingly, only large, prospective, randomized, double-blind trials will allow definition of the benefits and also the risks of such DHEA pharmacotherapy. Much work remains to be done in this area.

An important contribution to the development of treatment strategies with DHEA will come from a better understanding of the mechanisms of action of DHEA. It is predicted that future DHEA research will be successful in identifying more specific direct actions of DHEA; e.g. the identification and characterization of the putative membrane-bound G-protein-coupled DHEA receptor. Of particular interest will be the investigation of specific DHEA actions on the immune and central nervous systems.

In conclusion, DHEA has emerged as a fascinating adrenal steroid, but its physiology and therapeutic potential are still waiting to be fully revealed.

20.10 Key messages

- DHEA(S) secretion shows a characteristic pattern during the human life cycle, with a prepubertal rise (adrenarche) and a continuous decline (adrenopause) after a peak in early adulthood. There is high interindividual variability and a sex difference in circulating DHEA(S) levels with higher concentrations in males.
- Low DHEA(S) concentrations predict imminent mortality in both men and women. Low DHEAS levels may be a non-specific marker of poor health and rather an epiphenomenon but not a cause of disease.
- Dehydroepiandrosterone exerts its biological activity via its downstream conversion to potent sex steroids, as a neurosteroid interacting with various receptors in the central nervous system, and also via a membrane-bound specific G-protein-coupled DHEA receptor, particularly in the vascular system.
- Like DHEA, androstenedione acts as a prohormone and is converted predominantly into androgens and to a minor extent into estrogens after oral administration.
- Treatment of patients with adrenal insufficiency (25–50 mg/day DHEA) improves QoL, depression and fatigue and may also improve sexuality in female patients. By

contrast, in healthy elderly subjects with age-related low endogenous DHEA(S), beneficial effects of DHEA supplementation remain doubtful.

- Dehydroepiandrosterone administration has been found to improve anxiety and depression in midlife dysthymia, patients with depression and schizophrenia. In systemic lupus erythematous, DHEA reduces disease activity and flares, and allows reduction of the glucocorticoid dose.

- In short-term studies, androstenedione and DHEA did not improve muscle function or muscle strength, although these steroids are prohibited as ergogenic drugs by the World Anti Doping Agency (WADA).

- The available clinical evidence suggests that the main target tissues for DHEA are the central nervous system, the skin and possibly the immune system. Beneficial effects on muscle function, bone and ovarian folliculogenesis remain to be fully established.

20.11   References

Achermann JC, Silverman BL (2001) Dehydroepiandrosterone replacement for patients with adrenal insufficiency. *Lancet* **357**:1381–1382

Alkatib AA, Cosma M, Elamin MB, Erickson D, Swiglo BA, Erwin PJ, Montori VM (2009) A systematic review and meta-analysis of randomized placebo-controlled trials of DHEA treatment effects on quality of life in women with adrenal insufficiency. *J Clin Endocrinol Metab* **94**:3676–3681

Allolio B, Arlt W (2002) DHEA treatment: myth or reality? *Trends Endocrinol Metab* **13**:288–294

Allolio B, Arlt W, Hahner S (2007) DHEA: why, when, and how much – DHEA replacement in adrenal insufficiency. *Ann Endocrinol (Paris)* **68**:268–273

Andus T, Klebl F, Rogler G, Bregenzer N, Scholmerich J, Straub RH (2003) Patients with refractory Crohn's disease or ulcerative colitis respond to dehydroepiandrosterone: a pilot study. *Aliment Pharmacol Ther* **17**:409–414

Arlt W (2003) Management of the androgen-deficient woman. *Growth Horm IGF Res* **13** (Suppl A): S85–S89

Arlt W, Justl HG, Callies F, Reincke M, Hubler D, Oettel M, Ernst M, Schulte HM, Allolio B (1998) Oral dehydroepiandrosterone for adrenal androgen replacement: pharmacokinetics and peripheral conversion to androgens and estrogens in young healthy females after dexamethasone suppression. *J Clin Endocrinol Metab* **83**:1928–1934

Arlt W, Haas J, Callies F, Reincke M, Hubler D, Oettel M, Ernst M, Schulte HM, Allolio B (1999a) Biotransformation of oral dehydroepiandrosterone in elderly men: significant increase in circulating estrogens. *J Clin Endocrinol Metab* **84**:2170–2176

Arlt W, Callies F, van Vlijmen JC, Koehler I, Reincke M, Bidlingmaier M, Huebler D, Oettel M, Ernst M, Schulte HM, Allolio B (1999b) Dehydroepiandrosterone replacement in women with adrenal insufficiency. *N Engl J Med* **341**:1013–1020

Arlt W, Callies F, Allolio B (2000) DHEA replacement in women with adrenal insufficiency – pharmacokinetics, bioconversion and clinical effects on well-being, sexuality and cognition. *Endocr Res* **26**:505–511

Arlt W, Callies F, Koehler I, van Vlijmen JC, Fassnacht M, Strasburger CJ, Seibel MJ, Huebler D, Ernst M, Oettel M, Reincke M, Schulte HM, Allolio B (2001) Dehydroepiandrosterone supplementation in healthy men with an age-related decline of dehydroepiandrosterone secretion. *J Clin Endocrinol Metab* **86**:4686–4692

Arlt W, Hammer F, Sanning P, Butcher SK, Lord JM, Allolio B, Annane D, Stewart PM (2006) Dissociation of serum dehydroepiandrosterone and dehydroepiandrosterone sulfate in septic shock. *J Clin Endocrinol Metab* **91**:2548–2554

Auchus RJ, Rainey WE (2004) Adrenarche – physiology, biochemistry and human disease. *Clin Endocrinol (Oxf)* **60**:288–296

Barad D, Brill H, Gleicher N (2007) Update on the use of dehydroepiandrosterone supplementation among women with diminished ovarian function. *J Assist Reprod Genet* **24**:629–634

Barnhart KT, Freeman E, Grisso JA, Rader DJ, Sammel M, Kapoor S, Nestler JE (1999) The effect of dehydroepiandrosterone supplementation to symptomatic perimenopausal women on serum endocrine profiles, lipid parameters, and health-related quality of life. *J Clin Endocrinol Metab* **84**:3896–3902

Barrett-Connor E, Goodman-Gruen D (1995) Dehydroepiandrosterone sulfate does not predict cardiovascular death in postmenopausal women. The Rancho Bernardo Study. *Circulation* **91**:1757–1760

Bassindale T, Cowan DA, Dale S, Hutt AJ, Leeds AR, Wheeler MJ, Kicman AT (2004) Effects of oral administration of androstenedione on plasma androgens in young women using hormonal contraception. *J Clin Endocrinol Metab* **89**:6030–6038

Basu R, Dalla Man C, Campioni M, Basu A, Nair KS, Jensen MD, Khosla S, Klee G, Toffolo G, Cobelli C, Rizza RA (2007) Two years of treatment with dehydroepiandrosterone does not improve insulin secretion, insulin action, or postprandial glucose turnover in elderly men or women. *Diabetes* **56**:753–766

Baulieu EE, Thomas G, Legrain S, Lahlou N, Roger M, Debuire B, Faucounau V, Girard L, Hervy MP, Latour F, Leaud MC, Mokrane A, Pitti-Ferrandi H, Trivalle C, de Lacharriere O, Nouveau S, Rakoto-Arison B, Souberbielle JC, Raison J, Le Bouc Y, Raynaud A, Girerd X, Forette F (2000)

Dehydroepiandrosterone (DHEA), DHEA sulfate, and aging: contribution of the DHEAge study to a sociobiomedical issue. *Proc Natl Acad Sci USA* **97**:4279–4284

Beckham SG, Earnest CP (2003) Four weeks of androstenedione supplementation diminishes the treatment response in middle aged men. *Br J Sports Med* **37**:212–218

Bensing S, Brandt L, Tabaroj F, Sjoberg O, Nilsson B, Ekbom A, Blomqvist P, Kampe O (2008) Increased death risk and altered cancer incidence pattern in patients with isolated or combined autoimmune primary adrenocortical insufficiency. *Clin Endocrinol (Oxf)* **69**:697–704

Bergthorsdottir R, Leonsson-Zachrisson M, Oden A, Johannsson G (2006) Premature mortality in patients with Addison's disease: a population-based study. *J Clin Endocrinol Metab* **91**:4849–4853

Berr C, Lafont S, Debuire B, Dartigues JF, Baulieu EE (1996) Relationships of dehydroepiandrosterone sulfate in the elderly with functional, psychological, and mental status, and short-term mortality: a French community-based study. *Proc Natl Acad Sci USA* **93**:13410–13415

Bhuiyan MS, Tagashira H, Fukunaga K (2011) Dehydroepiandrosterone-mediated stimulation of sigma-1 receptor activates Akt-eNOS signaling in the thoracic aorta of ovariectomized rats with abdominal aortic banding. *Cardiovasc Ther* **29**:219–230

Bhuiyan S, Fukunaga K (2010) Stimulation of Sigma-1 receptor by dehydroepiandrosterone ameliorates hypertension-induced kidney hypertrophy in ovariectomized rats. *Exp Biol Med (Maywood)* **235**:356–364

Bilger M, Speraw S, LaFranchi SH, Hanna CE (2005) Androgen replacement in adolescents and young women with

hypopituitarism. *J Pediatr Endocrinol Metab* **18**:355–362

Binder G, Weber S, Ehrismann M, Zaiser N, Meisner C, Ranke MB, Maier L, Wudy SA, Hartmann MF, Heinrich U, Bettendorf M, Doerr HG, Pfaeffle RW, Keller E (2009) Effects of dehydroepiandrosterone therapy on pubic hair growth and psychological well-being in adolescent girls and young women with central adrenal insufficiency: a double-blind, randomized, placebo-controlled phase III trial. *J Clin Endocrinol Metab* **94**:1182–1190

Bloch M, Schmidt PJ, Danaceau MA, Adams LF, Rubinow DR (1999) Dehydroepiandrosterone treatment of midlife dysthymia. *Biol Psychiatry* **45**:1533–1541

Brooke AM, Kalingag LA, Miraki-Moud F, Camacho-Hubner C, Maher KT, Walker DM, Hinson JP, Monson JP (2006) Dehydroepiandrosterone improves psychological well-being in male and female hypopituitary patients on maintenance growth hormone replacement. *J Clin Endocrinol Metab* **91**:3773–3779

Brown GA, Vukovich MD, Martini ER, Kohut ML, Franke WD, Jackson DA, King DS (2000) Endocrine responses to chronic androstenedione intake in 30- to 56-year-old men. *J Clin Endocrinol Metab* **85**:4074–4080

Brown GA, Martini ER, Roberts BS, Vukovich MD, King DS (2002) Acute hormonal response to sublingual androstenediol intake in young men. *J Appl Physiol* **92**:142–146

Brown GA, Dewey JC, Brunkhorst JA, Vukovich MD, King DS (2004) Changes in serum testosterone and estradiol concentrations following acute androstenedione ingestion in young women. *Horm Metab Res* **36**:62–66

Calfee R, Fadale P (2006) Popular ergogenic drugs and supplements in young athletes. *Pediatrics* **117**:e577–e589

Callies F, Fassnacht M, van Vlijmen JC, Koehler I, Huebler D, Seibel MJ, Arlt W, Allolio B (2001) Dehydroepiandrosterone replacement in women with adrenal insufficiency: effects on body composition, serum leptin, bone turnover, and exercise capacity. *J Clin Endocrinol Metab* **86**:1968–1972

Casson PR, Faquin LC, Stentz FB, Straughn AB, Andersen RN, Abraham GE, Buster JE (1995) Replacement of dehydroepiandrosterone enhances T-lymphocyte insulin binding in postmenopausal women. *Fertil Steril* **63**:1027–1031

Casson PR, Lindsay MS, Pisarska MD, Carson SA, Buster JE (2000) Dehydroepiandrosterone supplementation augments ovarian stimulation in poor responders: a case series. *Hum Reprod* **15**:2129–2132

Chang DM, Lan JL, Lin HY, Luo SF (2002) Dehydroepiandrosterone treatment of women with mild-to-moderate systemic lupus erythematosus: a multicenter randomized, double-blind, placebo-controlled trial. *Arthritis Rheum* **46**:2924–2927

Compagnone NA, Mellon SH (1998) Dehydroepiandrosterone: a potential signalling molecule for neocortical organization during development. *Proc Natl Acad Sci USA* **95**:4678–4683

Cumming DC, Rebar RW, Hopper BR, Yen SS (1982) Evidence for an influence of the ovary on circulating dehydroepiandrosterone sulfate levels. *J Clin Endocrinol Metab* **54**:1069–1071

Danenberg HD, Ben-Yehuda A, Zakay-Rones Z, Gross DJ, Friedman G (1997) Dehydroepiandrosterone treatment is not beneficial to the immune response to influenza in elderly subjects. *J Clin Endocrinol Metab* **82**:2911–2914

Davis SR, Panjari M, Stanczyk FZ (2011) Clinical review: DHEA replacement for postmenopausal women. *J Clin Endocrinol Metab* **96**:1642–1653

Dayal M, Sammel MD, Zhao J, Hummel AC, Vandenbourne K, Barnhart KT (2005) Supplementation with DHEA: effect on muscle size, strength, quality of life, and lipids. *J Womens Health (Larchmt)* **14**:391–400

Deighton CM, Watson MJ, Walker DJ (1992) Sex hormones in postmenopausal HLA-identical rheumatoid arthritis discordant sibling pairs. *J Rheumatol* **19**:1663–1667

Dhatariya K, Bigelow ML, Nair KS (2005) Effect of dehydroepiandrosterone replacement on insulin sensitivity and lipids in hypoadrenal women. *Diabetes* **54**:765–769

Dhatariya KK, Greenlund LJ, Bigelow ML, Thapa P, Oberg AL, Ford GC, Schimke JM, Nair KS (2008) Dehydroepiandrosterone replacement therapy in hypoadrenal women: protein anabolism and skeletal muscle function. *Mayo Clin Proc* **83**:1218–1225

Diamond P, Cusan L, Gomez JL, Belanger A, Labrie F (1996) Metabolic effects of 12-month percutaneous dehydroepiandrosterone replacement therapy in postmenopausal women. *J Endocrinol* **150** Suppl: S43–S50

Erichsen MM, Lovas K, Skinningsrud B, Wolff AB, Undlien DE, Svartberg J, Fougner KJ, Berg TJ, Bollerslev J, Mella B, Carlson JA, Erlich H, Husebye ES (2009) Clinical, immunological, and genetic features of autoimmune primary adrenal insufficiency: observations from a Norwegian registry. *J Clin Endocrinol Metab* **94**:4882–4890

Flynn MA, Weaver-Osterholtz D, Sharpe-Timms KL, Allen S, Krause G (1999) Dehydroepiandrosterone replacement in aging humans. *J Clin Endocrinol Metab* **84**:1527–1533

Giagulli VA, Verdonck L, Giorgino R, Vermeulen A (1989) Precursors of plasma androstanediol- and androgen-glucuronides in women. *J Steroid Biochem* **33**:935–940

Gleicher N, Barad DH (2011) Dehydroepiandrosterone (DHEA) supplementation in diminished ovarian reserve (DOR). *Reprod Biol Endocrinol* **9**: 67

Gleicher N, Weghofer A, Barad DH (2010) Dehydroepiandrosterone (DHEA) reduces embryo aneuploidy: direct evidence from preimplantation genetic screening (PGS). *Reprod Biol Endocrinol* **8**:140

Gordon CM, LeBoff MS, Glowacki J (2001) Adrenal and gonadal steroids inhibit IL-6 secretion by human marrow cells. *Cytokine* **16**:178–186

Gurnell EM, Hunt PJ, Curran SE, Conway CL, Pullenayegum EM, Huppert FA, Compston JE, Herbert J, Chatterjee VK (2008) Long-term DHEA replacement in primary adrenal insufficiency: a randomized, controlled trial. *J Clin Endocrinol Metab* **93**:400–409

Hackbert L, Heiman JR (2002) Acute dehydroepiandrosterone (DHEA) effects on sexual arousal in postmenopausal women. *J Womens Health Gend Based Med* **11**:155–162

Hahner S, Loeffler M, Fassnacht M, Weismann D, Koschker AC, Quinkler M, Decker O, Arlt W, Allolio B (2007) Impaired subjective health status in 256 patients with adrenal insufficiency on standard therapy based on cross-sectional analysis. *J Clin Endocrinol Metab* **92**:3912–3922

Hammer F, Subtil S, Lux P, Maser-Gluth C, Stewart PM, Allolio B, Arlt W (2005) No evidence for hepatic conversion of dehydroepiandrosterone (DHEA) sulfate to DHEA: in vivo and in vitro studies. *J Clin Endocrinol Metab* **90**:3600–3605

Hartkamp A, Geenen R, Godaert GL, Bijl M, Bijlsma JW, Derksen RH (2010) Effects of dehydroepiandrosterone on fatigue and well-being in women with quiescent systemic lupus erythematosus: a randomised controlled trial. *Ann Rheum Dis* **69**:1144–1147

Hazeldine J, Arlt W, Lord JM (2010) Dehydroepiandrosterone as a regulator of immune cell function. *J Steroid Biochem Mol Biol* **120**:127–136

Hunt PJ, Gurnell EM, Huppert FA, Richards C, Prevost AT, Wass JA, Herbert J, Chatterjee VK (2000) Improvement in mood and fatigue after dehydroepiandrosterone replacement in Addison's disease in a randomized, double blind trial. *J Clin Endocrinol Metab* **85**:4650–4656

Igwebuike A, Irving BA, Bigelow ML, Short KR, McConnell JP, Nair KS (2008) Lack of dehydroepiandrosterone effect on a combined endurance and resistance exercise program in postmenopausal women. *J Clin Endocrinol Metab* **93**:534–538

Iruthayanathan M, O'Leary B, Paul G, Dillon JS (2011) Hydrogen peroxide signaling mediates DHEA-induced vascular endothelial cell proliferation. *Steroids* **76**:1483–1490

Jakobi JM, Killinger DW, Wolfe BM, Mahon JL, Rice CL (2001) Quadriceps muscle function and fatigue in women with Addison's disease. *Muscle Nerve* **24**:1040–1049

Jankowski CM, Gozansky WS, Schwartz RS, Dahl DJ, Kittelson JM, Scott SM, Van Pelt RE, Kohrt WM (2006) Effects of dehydroepiandrosterone replacement therapy on bone mineral density in older adults: a randomized, controlled trial. *J Clin Endocrinol Metab* **91**:2986–2993

Jankowski CM, Gozansky WS, Kittelson JM, Van Pelt RE, Schwartz RS, Kohrt WM (2008) Increases in bone mineral density in response to oral dehydroepiandrosterone replacement in older adults appear to be mediated by serum estrogens.

J Clin Endocrinol Metab **93**:4767–4773

Johannsson G, Burman P, Wiren L, Engstrom BE, Nilsson AG, Ottosson M, Jonsson B, Bengtsson BA, Karlsson FA (2002) Low dose dehydroepiandrosterone affects behavior in hypopituitary androgen-deficient women: a placebo-controlled trial. *J Clin Endocrinol Metab* **87**:2046–2052

Kahn AJ, Halloran B, Wolkowitz O, Brizendine L (2002) Dehydroepiandrosterone supplementation and bone turnover in middle-aged to elderly men. *J Clin Endocrinol Metab* **87**:1544–1549

Kicman AT, Bassindale T, Cowan DA, Dale S, Hutt AJ, Leeds AR (2003) Effect of androstenedione ingestion on plasma testosterone in young women; a dietary supplement with potential health risks. *Clin Chem* **49**:167–169

Kim SS, Brody KH (2001) Dehydroepiandrosterone replacement in Addison's disease. *Eur J Obstet Gynecol Reprod Biol* **97**:96–97

King DS, Sharp RL, Vukovich MD, Brown GA, Reifenrath TA, Uhl NL, Parsons KA (1999) Effect of oral androstenedione on serum testosterone and adaptations to resistance training in young men: a randomized controlled trial. *JAMA* **281**:2020–2028

Kline MD, Jaggers ED (1999) Mania onset while using dehydroepiandrosterone. *Am J Psychiatry* **156**: 971

Kolibianakis EM, Venetis CA, Tarlatzis BC (2011) DHEA administration in poor responders. *Hum Reprod* **26**:730–731; author reply:731

Kritz-Silverstein D, von Muhlen D, Laughlin GA, Bettencourt R (2008) Effects of dehydroepiandrosterone supplementation on cognitive function and quality of life: the DHEA and Well-Ness (DAWN) Trial. *J Am Geriatr Soc* **56**:1292–1298

Labrie F (2010) DHEA, important source of sex steroids in men and even more in women. *Prog Brain Res* **182**:97–148

Labrie F, Diamond P, Cusan L, Gomez JL, Belanger A, Candas B (1997) Effect of 12-month dehydroepiandrosterone replacement therapy on bone, vagina, and endometrium in postmenopausal women. *J Clin Endocrinol Metab* **82**:3498–3505

Labrie F, Luu-The V, Labrie C, Belanger A, Simard J, Lin SX, Pelletier G (2003) Endocrine and intracrine sources of androgens in women: inhibition of breast cancer and other roles of androgens and their precursor dehydroepiandrosterone. *Endocr Rev* **24**:152–182

Labrie F, Archer D, Bouchard C, Fortier M, Cusan L, Gomez JL, Girard G, Baron M, Ayotte N, Moreau M, Dube R, Cote I, Labrie C, Lavoie L, Berger L, Gilbert L, Martel C, Balser J (2009) Effect of intravaginal dehydroepiandrosterone (Prasterone) on libido and sexual dysfunction in postmenopausal women. *Menopause* **16**:923–931

Lahita RG, Bradlow HL, Ginzler E, Pang S, New M (1987) Low plasma androgens in women with systemic lupus erythematosus. *Arthritis Rheum* **30**:241–248

Laughlin GA, Barrett-Connor E (2000) Sexual dimorphism in the influence of advanced aging on adrenal hormone levels: the Rancho Bernardo Study. *J Clin Endocrinol Metab* **85**:3561–3568

Laurine E, Lafitte D, Gregoire C, Seree E, Loret E, Douillard S, Michel B, Briand C, Verdier JM (2003) Specific binding of dehydroepiandrosterone to the N terminus of the microtubule-associated protein MAP2. *J Biol Chem* **278**:29979–29986

Lazaridis I, Charalampopoulos I, Alexaki VI, Avlonitis N,

Pediaditakis I, Efstathopoulos P, Calogeropoulou T, Castanas E, Gravanis A (2011) Neurosteroid dehydroepiandrosterone interacts with nerve growth factor (NGF) receptors, preventing neuronal apoptosis. *PLoS Biol* 9: e1001051

Leder BZ, Longcope C, Catlin DH, Ahrens B, Schoenfeld DA, Finkelstein JS (2000) Oral androstenedione administration and serum testosterone concentrations in young men. *JAMA* 283:779–782

Leder BZ, Catlin DH, Longcope C, Ahrens B, Schoenfeld DA, Finkelstein JS (2001) Metabolism of orally administered androstenedione in young men. *J Clin Endocrinol Metab* 86:3654–3658

Leder BZ, Leblanc KM, Longcope C, Lee H, Catlin DH, Finkelstein JS (2002) Effects of oral androstenedione administration on serum testosterone and estradiol levels in postmenopausal women. *J Clin Endocrinol Metab* 87:5449–5454

Libe R, Barbetta L, Dall'Asta C, Salvaggio F, Gala C, Beck-Peccoz P, Ambrosi B (2004) Effects of dehydroepiandrosterone (DHEA) supplementation on hormonal, metabolic and behavioral status in patients with hypoadrenalism. *J Endocrinol Invest* 27: 736–741

Lindschau C, Kirsch T, Klinge U, Kolkhof P, Peters I, Fiebeler A (2011) Dehydroepiandrosterone-induced phosphorylation and translocation of FoxO1 depend on the mineralocorticoid receptor. *Hypertension* 58:471–478

Liu D, Dillon JS (2002) Dehydroepiandrosterone activates endothelial cell nitric-oxide synthase by a specific plasma membrane receptor coupled to Galpha(i2,3). *J Biol Chem* 277:21379–21388

Liu D, Iruthayanathan M, Homan LL, Wang Y, Yang L, Dillon JS (2008)

Dehydroepiandrosterone stimulates endothelial proliferation and angiogenesis through extracellular signal-regulated kinase 1/2-mediated mechanisms. *Endocrinology* 149:889–898

Lovas K, Gebre-Medhin G, Trovik TS, Fougner KJ, Uhlving S, Nedrebo BG, Myking OL, Kampe O, Husebye ES (2003) Replacement of dehydroepiandrosterone in adrenal failure: no benefit for subjective health status and sexuality in a 9-month, randomized, parallel group clinical trial. *J Clin Endocrinol Metab* 88:1112–1118

Markowitz JS, Carson WH, Jackson CW (1999) Possible dihydroepiandrosterone-induced mania. *Biol Psychiatry* 45:241–242

Mazat L, Lafont S, Berr C, Debuire B, Tessier JF, Dartigues JF, Baulieu EE (2001) Prospective measurements of dehydroepiandrosterone sulfate in a cohort of elderly subjects: relationship to gender, subjective health, smoking habits, and 10-year mortality. *Proc Natl Acad Sci USA* 98:8145–8150

Meikle AW, Dorchuck RW, Araneo BA, Stringham JD, Evans TG, Spruance SL, Daynes RA (1992) The presence of a dehydroepiandrosterone-specific receptor binding complex in murine T cells. *J Steroid Biochem Mol Biol* 42:293–304

Melez KA, Boegel WA, Steinberg AD (1980) Therapeutic studies in New Zealand mice. VII. Successful androgen treatment of NZB/NZW F1 females of different ages. *Arthritis Rheum* 23:41–47

Morales AJ, Nolan JJ, Nelson JC, Yen SS (1994) Effects of replacement dose of dehydroepiandrosterone in men and women of advancing age. *J Clin Endocrinol Metab* 78:1360–1367

Morales AJ, Haubrich RH, Hwang JY, Asakura H, Yen SS (1998) The effect of six months treatment with a 100 mg daily dose of

dehydroepiandrosterone (DHEA) on circulating sex steroids, body composition and muscle strength in age-advanced men and women. *Clin Endocrinol (Oxf)* 49:421–432

Nair KS, Rizza RA, O'Brien P, Dhatariya K, Short KR, Nehra A, Vittone JL, Klee GG, Basu A, Basu R, Cobelli C, Toffolo G, Dalla Man C, Tindall DJ, Melton LJ 3rd, Smith GE, Khosla S, Jensen MD (2006) DHEA in elderly women and DHEA or testosterone in elderly men. *N Engl J Med* 355:1647–1659

Nieschlag E, Loriaux DL, Ruder HJ, Zucker IR, Kirschner MA, Lipsett MB (1973) The secretion of dehydroepiandrosterone and dehydroepiandrosterone sulphate in man. *J Endocrinol* 57:123–134

Noordam C, Dhir V, McNelis JC, Schlereth F, Hanley NA, Krone N, Smeitink JA, Smeets R, Sweep FC, Claahsen-van der Grinten HL, Arlt W (2009) Inactivating PAPSS2 mutations in a patient with premature pubarche. *N Engl J Med* 360:2310–2318

Okabe T, Haji M, Takayanagi R, Adachi M, Imasaki K, Kurimoto F, Watanabe T, Nawata H (1995) Up-regulation of high-affinity dehydroepiandrosterone binding activity by dehydroepiandrosterone in activated human T lymphocytes. *J Clin Endocrinol Metab* 80:2993–2996

Orentreich N, Brind JL, Rizer RL, Vogelman JH (1984) Age changes and sex differences in serum dehydroepiandrosterone sulfate concentrations throughout adulthood. *J Clin Endocrinol Metab* 59:551–555

Orentreich N, Brind JL, Vogelman JH, Andres R, Baldwin H (1992) Long-term longitudinal measurements of plasma dehydroepiandrosterone sulfate in normal men. *J Clin Endocrinol Metab* 75:1002–1004

Panjari M, Bell RJ, Jane F, Wolfe R, Adams J, Morrow C, Davis SR (2009) A randomized trial of oral

DHEA treatment for sexual function, well-being, and menopausal symptoms in postmenopausal women with low libido. *J Sex Med* 6:2579–2590

Parker CR Jr, Mixon RL, Brissie RM, Grizzle WE (1997) Aging alters zonation in the adrenal cortex of men. *J Clin Endocrinol Metab* 82:3898–3901

Percheron G, Hogrel JY, Denot-Ledunois S, Fayet G, Forette F, Baulieu EE, Fardeau M, Marini JF (2003) Effect of 1-year oral administration of dehydroepiandrosterone to 60- to 80-year-old individuals on muscle function and cross-sectional area: a double-blind placebo-controlled trial. *Arch Intern Med* 163:720–727

Perez-Neri I, Montes S, Ojeda-Lopez C, Ramirez-Bermudez J, Rios C (2008) Modulation of neurotransmitter systems by dehydroepiandrosterone and dehydroepiandrosterone sulfate: mechanism of action and relevance to psychiatric disorders. *Prog Neuropsychopharmacol Biol Psychiatry* 32:1118–1130

Radford DJ, Wang K, McNelis JC, Taylor AE, Hechenberger G, Hofmann J, Chahal H, Arlt W, Lord JM (2010) Dehdyroepiandrosterone sulfate directly activates protein kinase C-beta to increase human neutrophil superoxide generation. *Mol Endocrinol* 24:813–821

Rasmussen BB, Volpi E, Gore DC, Wolfe RR (2000) Androstenedione does not stimulate muscle protein anabolism in young healthy men. *J Clin Endocrinol Metab* 85:55–59

Reed MJ, Purohit A, Woo LW, Newman SP, Potter BV (2005) Steroid sulfatase: molecular biology, regulation, and inhibition. *Endocr Rev* 26:171–202

Reiter WJ, Pycha A, Schatzl G, Pokorny A, Gruber DM, Huber JC, Marberger M (1999) Dehydroepiandrosterone in the treatment of erectile dysfunction: a prospective, double-blind, randomized, placebo-controlled study. *Urology* 53:590–594; discussion:594–595

Roth MY, Page ST, Lin K, Anawalt BD, Matsumoto AM, Marck B, Bremner WJ, Amory JK (2011) The effect of gonadotropin withdrawal and stimulation with human chorionic gonadotropin on intratesticular androstenedione and DHEA in normal men. *J Clin Endocrinol Metab* 96:1175–1181

Schmidt PJ, Daly RC, Bloch M, Smith MJ, Danaceau MA, St Clair LS, Murphy JH, Haq N, Rubinow DR (2005) Dehydroepiandrosterone monotherapy in midlife-onset major and minor depression. *Arch Gen Psychiatry* 62:154–162

Sen A, Hammes SR (2010) Granulosa cell-specific androgen receptors are critical regulators of ovarian development and function. *Mol Endocrinol* 24:1393–1403

Shifren JL, Braunstein GD, Simon JA, Casson PR, Buster JE, Redmond GP, Burki RE, Ginsburg ES, Rosen RC, Leiblum SR, Caramelli KE, Mazer NA (2000) Transdermal testosterone treatment in women with impaired sexual function after oophorectomy. *N Engl J Med* 343:682–688

Shufelt C, Bretsky P, Almeida CM, Johnson BD, Shaw LJ, Azziz R, Braunstein GD, Pepine CJ, Bittner V, Vido DA, Stanczyk FZ, Bairey Merz CN (2010) DHEA-S levels and cardiovascular disease mortality in postmenopausal women: results from the National Institutes of Health – National Heart, Lung, and Blood Institute (NHLBI)-sponsored Women's Ischemia Syndrome Evaluation (WISE). *J Clin Endocrinol Metab* 95:4985–4992

Sklar CA, Kaplan SL, Grumbach MM (1980) Evidence for dissociation between adrenarche and gonadarche: studies in patients with idiopathic precocious puberty, gonadal dysgenesis, isolated gonadotropin deficiency, and constitutionally delayed growth and adolescence. *J Clin Endocrinol Metab* 51:548–556

Solerte SB, Fioravanti M, Vignati G, Giustina A, Cravello L, Ferrari E (1999) Dehydroepiandrosterone sulfate enhances natural killer cell cytotoxicity in humans via locally generated immunoreactive insulin-like growth factor 1. *J Clin Endocrinol Metab* 84:3260–3267

Spencer JB, Klein M, Kumar A, Azziz R (2007) The age-associated decline of androgens in reproductive age and menopausal Black and White women. *J Clin Endocrinol Metab* 92:4730–4733

Srinivasan M, Irving BA, Frye RL, O'Brien P, Hartman SJ, McConnell JP, Nair KS (2010) Effects on lipoprotein particles of long-term dehydroepiandrosterone in elderly men and women and testosterone in elderly men. *J Clin Endocrinol Metab* 95:1617–1625

Stanway SJ, Delavault P, Purohit A, Woo LW, Thurieau C, Potter BV, Reed MJ (2007) Steroid sulfatase: a new target for the endocrine therapy of breast cancer. *Oncologist* 12:370–374

Stickney DR, Ahlem CN, Morgan E, Reading CL, Onizuka N, Frincke JM (2011) Phase I and phase II clinical trials of androst-5-ene-3beta,7beta,17beta-triol. *Am J Transl Res* 3:275–283

Strous RD, Maayan R, Lapidus R, Stryjer R, Lustig M, Kotler M, Weizman A (2003) Dehydroepiandrosterone augmentation in the management of negative, depressive, and anxiety symptoms in schizophrenia. *Arch Gen Psychiatry* 60:133–141

Sugino M, Ohsawa N, Ito T, Ishida S, Yamasaki H, Kimura F, Shinoda K (1998) A pilot study of dehydroepiandrosterone sulfate in myotonic dystrophy. *Neurology* 51:586–589

Sunkara SK, Coomarasamy A (2011) Androgen pretreatment in poor responders undergoing controlled ovarian stimulation and in vitro fertilization treatment. *Fertil Steril* **95**:e73–e74; author reply:e75

Suzuki T, Suzuki N, Daynes RA, Engleman EG (1991) Dehydroepiandrosterone enhances IL2 production and cytotoxic effector function of human T cells. *Clin Immunol Immunopathol* **61**:202–211

Suzuki T, Suzuki N, Engleman EG, Mizushima Y, Sakane T (1995) Low serum levels of dehydroepiandrosterone may cause deficient IL-2 production by lymphocytes in patients with systemic lupus erythematosus (SLE). *Clin Exp Immunol* **99**:251–255

Svec F, Porter JR (1998) The actions of exogenous dehydroepiandrosterone in experimental animals and humans. *Proc Soc Exp Biol Med* **218**:174–191

Tomlinson JW, Holden N, Hills RK, Wheatley K, Clayton RN, Bates AS, Sheppard MC, Stewart PM (2001) Association between premature mortality and hypopituitarism. West Midlands Prospective Hypopituitary Study Group. *Lancet* **357**:425–431

Topor LS, Asai M, Dunn J, Majzoub JA (2011) Cortisol stimulates secretion of dehydroepiandrosterone in human adrenocortical cells through inhibition of 3betaHSD2. *J Clin Endocrinol Metab* **96**:E31–E39

Trivedi DP, Khaw KT (2001) Dehydroepiandrosterone sulfate and mortality in elderly men and women. *J Clin Endocrinol Metab* **86**:4171–4177

van Niekerk JK, Huppert FA, Herbert J (2001) Salivary cortisol and DHEA: association with measures of cognition and well-being in normal older men, and effects of three months of DHEA supplementation.

Psychoneuroendocrinology **26**:591–612

van Thiel SW, Romijn JA, Pereira AM, Biermasz NR, Roelfsema F, van Hemert A, Ballieux B, Smit JW (2005) Effects of dehydroepiandrostenedione, superimposed on GH substitution, on quality of life and insulin-like growth factor I in patients with secondary adrenal insufficiency: a randomized, placebo-controlled, cross-over trial. *J Clin Endocrinol Metab* **90**:3295–3303

van Vollenhoven RF, Engleman EG, McGuire JL (1994) An open study of dehydroepiandrosterone in systemic lupus erythematosus. *Arthritis Rheum* **37**:1305–1310

van Vollenhoven RF, Park JL, Genovese MC, West JP, McGuire JL (1999) A double-blind, placebo-controlled, clinical trial of dehydroepiandrosterone in severe systemic lupus erythematosus. *Lupus* **8**:181–187

Villareal DT, Holloszy JO (2004) Effect of DHEA on abdominal fat and insulin action in elderly women and men: a randomized controlled trial. *JAMA* **292**:2243–2248

Villareal DT, Holloszy JO (2006) DHEA enhances effects of weight training on muscle mass and strength in elderly women and men. *Am J Physiol Endocrinol Metab* **291**: E1003–E1008

Villareal DT, Holloszy JO, Kohrt WM (2000) Effects of DHEA replacement on bone mineral density and body composition in elderly women and men. *Clin Endocrinol (Oxf)* **53**:561–568

von Muhlen D, Laughlin GA, Kritz-Silverstein D, Bergstrom J, Bettencourt R (2008) Effect of dehydroepiandrosterone supplementation on bone mineral density, bone markers, and body composition in older adults: the DAWN trial. *Osteoporos Int* **19**:699–707

Waxenberg SE, Drellich MG, Sutherland AM (1959) The role of

hormones in human behavior. I. Changes in female sexuality after adrenalectomy. *J Clin Endocrinol Metab* **19**:193–202

Weiss EP, Shah K, Fontana L, Lambert CP, Holloszy JO, Villareal DT (2009) Dehydroepiandrosterone replacement therapy in older adults: 1- and 2-y effects on bone. *Am J Clin Nutr* **89**:1459–1467

Williams MR, Ling S, Dawood T, Hashimura K, Dai A, Li H, Liu JP, Funder JW, Sudhir K, Komesaroff PA (2002) Dehydroepiandrosterone inhibits human vascular smooth muscle cell proliferation independent of ARs and ERs. *J Clin Endocrinol Metab* **87**:176–181

Wiser A, Gonen O, Ghetler Y, Shavit T, Berkovitz A, Shulman A (2010) Addition of dehydroepiandrosterone (DHEA) for poor-responder patients before and during IVF treatment improves the pregnancy rate: a randomized prospective study. *Hum Reprod* **25**:2496–2500

Wit JM, Langenhorst VJ, Jansen M, Oostdijk WA, van Doorn J (2001) Dehydroepiandrosterone sulfate treatment for atrichia pubis. *Horm Res* **56**:134–139

Wolf OT, Neumann O, Hellhammer DH, Geiben AC, Strasburger CJ, Dressendorfer RA, Pirke KM, Kirschbaum C (1997) Effects of a two-week physiological dehydroepiandrosterone substitution on cognitive performance and well-being in healthy elderly women and men. *J Clin Endocrinol Metab* **82**:2363–2367

Wolf OT, Naumann E, Hellhammer DH, Kirschbaum C (1998) Effects of dehydroepiandrosterone replacement in elderly men on event-related potentials, memory, and well-being. *J Gerontol A Biol Sci Med Sci* **53**:M385–390

Wolkowitz OM, Reus VI, Keebler A, Nelson N, Friedland M, Brizendine L, Roberts E (1999) Double-blind treatment of major depression with dehydroepiandrosterone. *Am J Psychiatry* **156**:646–649

Wolkowitz OM, Kramer JH, Reus VI, Costa MM, Yaffe K, Walton P, Raskind M, Peskind E, Newhouse P, Sack D, De Souza E, Sadowsky C, Roberts E (2003) DHEA treatment of Alzheimer's disease: a randomized, double-blind, placebo-controlled study. *Neurology* **60**:1071–1076

Yakin K, Urman B (2011) DHEA as a miracle drug in the treatment of poor responders; hype or hope? *Hum Reprod* **26**:1941–1944

Yen SS, Morales AJ, Khorram O (1995) Replacement of DHEA in aging men and women. Potential remedial effects. *Ann N Y Acad Sci* **774**:128–142

Young J, Couzinet B, Nahoul K, Brailly S, Chanson P, Baulieu EE, Schaison G (1997) Panhypopituitarism as a model to study the metabolism of dehydroepiandrosterone (DHEA) in humans. *J Clin Endocrinol Metab* **82**:2578–2585

Zhai G, Teumer A, Stolk L, Perry JR, Vandenput L, Coviello AD, Koster A, Bell JT, Bhasin S, Eriksson J, Eriksson A, Ernst F, Ferrucci L, Frayling TM, Glass D, Grundberg E, Haring R, Hedman AK, Hofman A, Kiel DP, Kroemer HK, Liu Y, Lunetta KL, Maggio M, Lorentzon M, Mangino M, Melzer D, Miljkovic I, Nica A, Penninx BW, Vasan RS, Rivadeneira F, Small KS, Soranzo N, Uitterlinden AG, Volzke H, Wilson SG, Xi L, Zhuang WV, Harris TB, Murabito JM, Ohlsson C, Murray A, de Jong FH, Spector TD, Wallaschofski H (2011) Eight common genetic variants associated with serum DHEAS levels suggest a key role in ageing mechanisms. *PLoS Genet* **7**: e1002025

Zwain IH, Yen SS (1999) Neurosteroidogenesis in astrocytes, oligodendrocytes, and neurons of cerebral cortex of rat brain. *Endocrinology* **140**:3843–3852

The state-of-the-art in the development of selective androgen receptor modulators

Ravi Jasuja, Mikhail N. Zacharov, and Shalender Bhasin

21.1 Introduction

Selective androgen receptor modulators (SARMs) are a class of androgen receptor (AR) ligands that bind the androgen receptor and display tissue-specific activation of AR signaling (Bhasin *et al.* 2006; Narayanan *et al.* 2008; Bhasin and Jasuja 2009). The impetus for the development of SARMs was instigated by observations that testosterone administration has potential beneficial effects on the skeletal muscle, bone, erythropoiesis, mood and sexual function, and that the anabolic effects of testosterone are dose related. The therapeutic applications are limited by uncertainty about the potential adverse effects of testosterone on cardiovascular events and the prostate (Bhasin *et al.* 2006; Narayanan *et al.* 2008; Bhasin and Jasuja 2009). Therefore, pharmacophores that can activate androgen signaling and achieve beneficial therapeutic effects without the potential adverse effects would be attractive as therapeutic agents for a variety of clinical disorders. Although much of the SARM discovery effort is currently focused on their development as function-promoting anabolic therapies for limitations associated with sarcopenia (age-related loss of muscle mass and strength), frailty, acute illness and other chronic conditions, such as COPD, end-stage renal disease, AIDS wasting syndrome and many types of cancers, they may also be useful in the treatment of other medical conditions such as anemia, osteoporosis, autoimmune rheumatic disorders and androgen replacement in individuals at high risk of prostate cancer, and for male contraception and to promote cutaneous wound healing (Bhasin *et al.* 2006; Narayanan *et al.* 2008; Bhasin and Jasuja 2009).

Structurally, SARMs can be categorized into steroidal and non-steroidal SARMs. Many potent steroidal SARMs were developed during the 1940s and 1950s by modifying the chemical structure of the testosterone molecule. The pioneering efforts of scientists at Ligand Pharmaceuticals and the University of Tennessee ushered in the modern era of non-steroidal SARMs (Bhasin *et al.* 2006; Narayanan *et al.* 2008; Bhasin and Jasuja 2009). The Ligand team was the first to develop a series of cyclic quinolinones that had anabolic activity on the skeletal muscle, and tissue selectivity (Edwards *et al.* 1998; Hamann *et al.* 1999; van Oeveren *et al.* 2006; 2007; Miner *et al.* 2007; Higuchi *et al.* 2007). Dalton and Miller, at the University of Tennessee, discovered that aryl-propionamides with structural similarities to bicalutamide and hydroxyflutamide could activate AR-dependent transcriptional activity and had preferential anabolic effects on the muscle relative to the prostate (Dalton *et al.* 1998; He *et al.* 2002). Since then, most of the major pharmaceutical

Testosterone: Action, Deficiency, Substitution, ed. Eberhard Nieschlag and Hermann M. Behre, Assoc. ed. Susan Nieschlag. Published by Cambridge University Press. © Cambridge University Press 2012.

Structure-activity relationship	Compounds	Chemical structure
Removing 19-methyl increases anabolic activity	19-nortestosterone (nandrolone) series of compounds	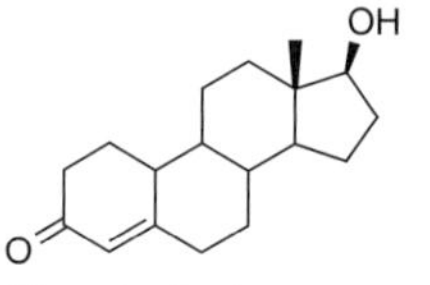 19-nortestosterone
17-α alkyl substitutions retard first-pass presystemic metabolism	Many orally active steroidal androgens have 17-α alkyl substitutions	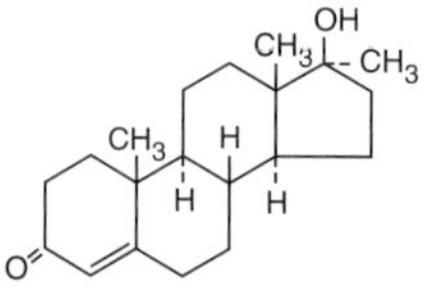 17α-methyltestosterone
17-α alkyl substitutions increase anabolic activity	7α-methyl, 9-nortestosterone	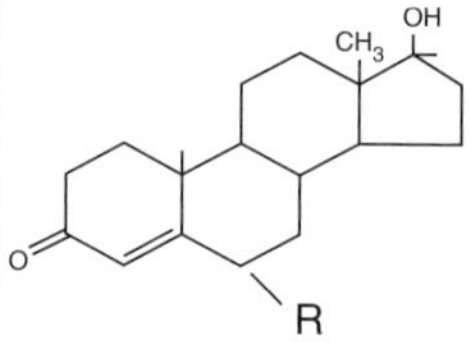 7α-alkyl,19-nortestosterone
Esterification of 17β-hydroxyl group increases hydrophobicity and extends duration of in vivo action	Testosterone enanthate, cypionate and undecanoate	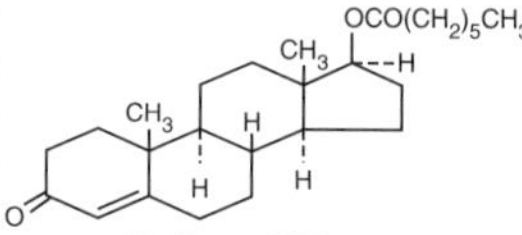 $C_{26}H_{40}O_3$ MW 400.6 Testosterone enanthate

Fig. 21.1 Structure-activity relationship of steroidal SARMs. Reproduced with permission from Bhasin and Jasuja (2009).

houses and many biotechnology companies have supported SARM discovery programs. The development of non-steroidal SARMs during the past 15 years has been guided by a discovery approach that has been based on high-throughput screening of pharmacophore libraries using assays that are steered by pharmacophore binding to AR and transactivation of AR-dependent reporter genes. This approach has differed substantially from that used in the discovery of the steroidal SARMs in the 1940s and 1950s, which was based on an understanding of the structure-activity relationships. As pharmaceutical and biotechnology companies have led the developmental effort related to the discovery of non-steroidal SARMs, much of this research remains unpublished and unavailable for critical peer appraisal.

21.2 Structural classes of SARMs

Structurally, SARMs can be classified into steroidal and non-steroidal. Functionally, these compounds can be categorized as pure agonists, pure antagonists and partial agonists. Most of the SARMs that have advanced to phase I and II human trials are partial agonists: they are potent agonists in the muscle and bone, but weak agonists in the prostate (Bhasin *et al.* 2006; Narayanan *et al.* 2008; Bhasin and Jasuja 2009).

21.3 Structure-activity relationships of steroidal SARMs

While the structure-activity relationships of the steroidal SARMs were elucidated seven decades ago (Bhasin *et al.* 2006; Bhasin and Jasuja 2009; Hoffman *et al.* 2009), only limited information about non-steroidal SARMs has been published (Fig. 21.1).

17α-alkyl substitution by retarding the presystemic metabolism of testosterone extends its half-life and makes it orally active (Dimick *et al.* 1961; Bhasin and Jasuja 2009; Hoffman *et al.* 2009). Thus, a number of oral androgens, such as 17α-methyltestosterone (Fig. 21.1), have 17α-alkyl substitution (Dimick *et al.* 1961). However, when administered orally, 17α-alkylated androgens are potentially hepatotoxic and markedly lower plasma HDL-C (Bhasin and Jasuja 2009; Hoffman *et al.* 2009).

The nandrolone series of molecules was synthesized based on the insight that the removal of the 19-methyl group increases the anabolic activity of testosterone (Murad and Haynes 1980; Fragkaki *et al.* 2009). Thus, a number of anabolic steroids are based on the 19-nor-testosterone backbone. Nandrolone is reduced by the steroid 5α-reductase enzyme in target tissues to a less potent androgen, dihydronandrolone. However, it serves only as a weak substrate for the CYP19 aromatase enzyme and is less susceptible to aromatization.

7α-alkyl substitutions make testosterone less susceptible to 5α-reduction and increase its tissue selectivity with respect to the prostate (Bhasin and Jasuja 2009). Thus, 7α-methyl, 19-nortestosterone has anabolic activity in the levator ani assay, but has a lower level of prostate effects (Kumar *et al.* 1992; Sundaram *et al.* 1994). A number of potent anabolic molecules in this series with varying alkyl groups have been investigated.

Testosterone is cleared rapidly from circulation and has a short half-life. The esterification of the 17β-hydroxyl group makes the molecule more hydrophobic and thereby retards its absorption from an oily depot injection. The longer the ester, the greater is its hydrophobicity, and the slower is the absorption of the ester from its oily depot into the circulation. When 17β-hydroxyl esters of testosterone are injected intramuscularly in an oily suspension, they are released slowly from the oil depot into the circulation (Snyder and Lawrence 1980; Sokol *et al.* 1982). The slow release of 17β-hydroxyl esters from the oil depot extends their duration of action. However, de-esterification of testosterone esters is not rate-limiting; the half-life of testosterone enanthate in plasma is similar to that of non-esterified testosterone. Similarly, esterification of nandrolone to form nandrolone decanoate increases its half-life.

Oxandrolone is an oral androgen derived from DHT that has a 17α-methyl substituent. The substitution of a second carbon with oxygen increases the stability of the 3-keto group and increases its anabolic activity. It does not undergo aromatization to an estrogen.

21.4 Non-steroidal SARMs

Many structural categories of SARM pharmacophores have been developed: aryl-propionamide (GTX, Inc.), bicyclic hydantoin (BMS), quinolinones (Ligand Pharmaceuticals), tetrahydroquinoline analogs (Kaken Pharmaceuticals, Inc.), benzimidazole, imidazolopyrazole, indole and pyrazoline derivatives (Johnson and Johnson), azasteroidal derivatives (Merck), and aniline, diaryl aniline and benzoxazepinones derivatives (GSK) (Fig.21.2; Bhasin *et al.* 2006; Narayanan *et al.* 2008; Bhasin and Jasuja 2009). This list is not exhaustive; additional structural categories surely exist but have not been published. We refer those who are interested in SARM structures to an excellent treatise on this topic by Narayanan *et al.* (2008).

Ligand compounds LGD-2226 and LGD-2941 are bicyclic 6-anilino quinolinone derivatives (van Oeveren *et al.* 2006; 2007; Miner *et al.* 2007). In the Hershberger assay using the castrated male rat (Hartsook and Hershberger 1961), these compounds stimulate the growth of levator ani muscle while exerting little effect on prostate size (Gao *et al.* 2004a; 2004b; 2005; Miner *et al.* 2007). These compounds also increase bone mass and strength, and bone architecture in ovariectomized female rats (Rosen and Negro-Vilar 2002; Kearbey *et al.* 2007; Miner *et al.* 2007). LGD-2226 maintains male reproductive behavior in the castrated rat model (Miner *et al.* 2007).

The team led by Dalton and Miller at the University of Tennessee developed novel SARMs, S1 and S4, by structural modifications of aryl-propionamide analogs bicalutamide and hydroxyflutamide. These compounds – S1 and S4 – bind AR with high affinity and demonstrate tissue selectivity in the Hershberger assay (Yin *et al.* 2003a; 2003b). When given at an appropriate dose, S4 fully restores the levator ani weight, muscle strength, BMD, bone strength and lean body mass, and suppresses LH and FSH (Gao *et al.* 2004a; 2004b; 2005; Kearbey *et al.* 2007), while only partially restoring prostate weight. S4 also prevents ovariectomy-induced bone loss in a female rat model of osteoporosis (Kearbey *et al.* 2007).

The hydantoin derivatives, developed by the BMS group (Hamann *et al.* 2007) have an A-ring structure that is similar to that of bicalutamide. The cyano or nitro group of these molecules interacts with Q711 and R752 (Manfredi *et al.* 2007; Ostrowski *et al.* 2007). The benzene ring or the naphthyl group, together with the hydantoin ring, overlaps the steroid plane, while the hydantoin ring nitrogen forms an H bond with N705. BMS-564929 binds AR with high affinity and high specificity (Manfredi *et al.* 2007; Ostrowski *et al.* 2007). BMS-564929 demonstrated

Chemotype	Structure	Examples
Aryl-propionamide analogs	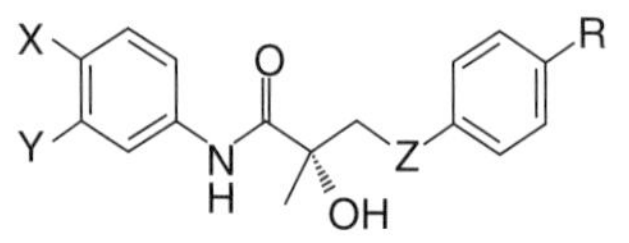	Ostarine, andarine
Bicyclic hydantoin analogs	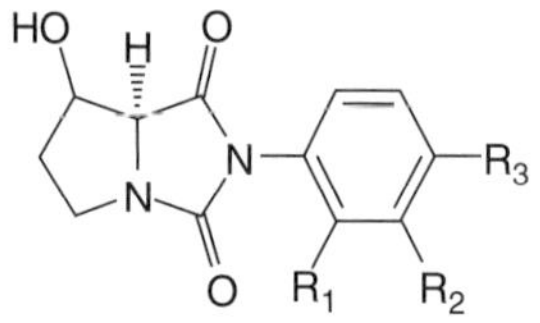	BMS-564929
Quinolinones	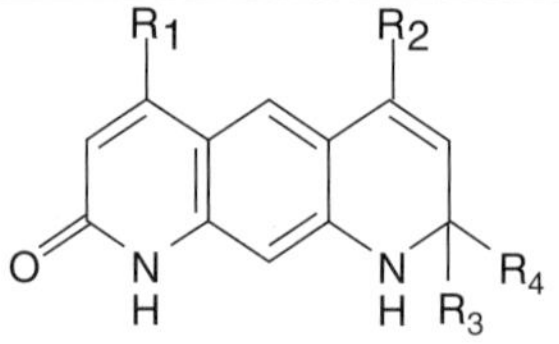	LGD-2226, LGD-2941
Tetrahydroquinoline analogs	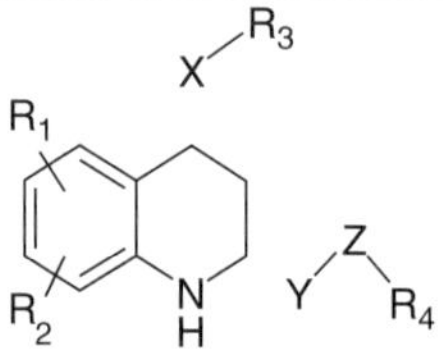	Kanen Pharmaceuticals, S-40503
Benzimidazoles	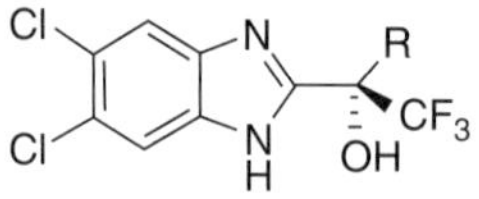	Johnson and Johnson's benzimadozole derivative
Butanamides	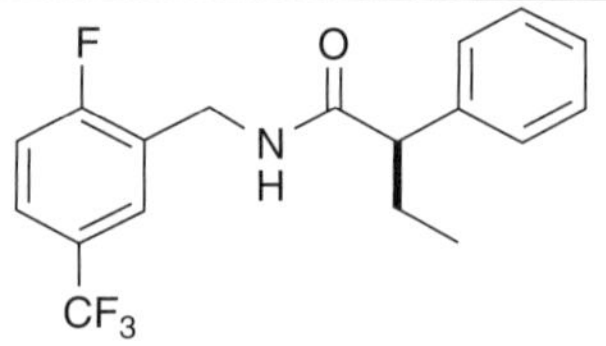	Merck SARM based on butanamide scaffold

Fig. 21.2 Various structural classes of non-steroidal SARMs. Reproduced with permission from Bhasin and Jasuja (2009).

anabolic activity in the levator ani muscle, and a high degree of tissue selectivity as indicated by a substantially higher ED50 for the prostate than for levator ani muscle (Hamann et al. 2007; Manfredi et al. 2007; Ostrowski et al. 2007). Hydantoin derivatives are potent suppressors of LH. BMS-564929 is orally available in humans, with a half-life of 8–14 hours (Manfredi et al. 2007; Ostrowski et al. 2007).

Hanada et al. (2003) at Kaken Pharmaceutical Co. reported a series of tetrahydroquinoline derivatives as AR agonists for bone. Although these compounds displayed high AR affinity and strong agonist activity in the prostate and levator ani, they demonstrated little selectivity between androgenic and anabolic tissues (Hanada et al. 2003). Significant in-vivo pharmacological activity was only observed at high subcutaneous doses (Hanada et al. 2003).

Merck scientists have developed a number of 4-azasteroidal derivatives and butanamides with anabolic activity in the muscle and bone and reduced activities in reproductive tissues and sebaceous glands (Schmidt et al. 2009). One such SARM, TFM-4AS-1, induces the expression of some androgen-dependent genes similar to DHT, and others to a lesser extent than DHT or not at all (Schmidt *et al.* 2009). TFM-4AS-1 does not promote the conformation required for interaction between the N-terminal and C-terminal domain, and displays tissue-selective agonistic activity on the muscle and bone while exhibiting reduced activity in the prostate and sebaceous glands (Schmidt *et al.* 2009). The scientists at Johnson and Johnson replaced the propionamide linker with cyclic elements such as pyrazoles, benzimidazoles, indoles and cyclic propionanilide mimetics (Ng *et al.* 2007). Additional compounds have been developed by other pharmaceutical companies (Narayanan *et al.* 2008).

21.5 Mechanisms of tissue-selective actions of SARMs

The expression profiles of androgen-dependent genes induced by tissue-selective SARMs differ from those induced by DHT (Narayanan *et al.* 2008; Schmidt *et al.* 2009). For instance, Narayanan *et al.* (2008) found that an aryl-propionamide SARM, S-22, and DHT differed significantly from each other in the recruitment of AR and its co-regulators to PSA enhancer. S-22 also differed from DHT in that it induced rapid phosphorylation of several kinases (Narayanan *et al.* 2008). Three general hypotheses have been proposed to explain the mechanisms that contribute to tissue-specific transcriptional activation and selectivity of the biological effects of SARMs (Bhasin *et al.* 2006; Narayanan *et al.* 2008; Bhasin and Jasuja 2009). These hypotheses are not mutually exclusive and it is possible that all three may be operative.

The coactivator hypothesis assumes that the repertoire of co-regulator proteins that associates with the SARM-bound AR differs from that associated with testosterone-bound AR, leading to transcriptional activation of a differentially regulated set of genes. According to the conformational hypothesis, ligand binding induces specific conformational changes in the ligand-binding domain (LBD), which modulates the surface topology and subsequent protein–protein interactions between AR and other co-regulators involved in genomic transcriptional activation or cytosolic proteins involved in non-genomic signaling (Bhasin *et al.* 2006; Narayanan *et al.* 2008; Bhasin and Jasuja 2009). Accordingly, the functional differences among the three ligand classes – agonists,

antagonists and SARMs – are reflected in conformationally distinct states with distinct thermodynamic partitioning. Differences in ligand-specific receptor conformation and protein–protein interactions could result in tissue-specific gene regulation, due to potential changes in interactions with androgen response elements (AREs), co-regulators or transcription factors. Ligand-induced protein–protein interactions contribute to interactions between the amino and carboxyl terminal ends of the AR (i.e. N/C interaction) and coactivator recruitment (Masiello *et al.* 2004). Both interactions are mediated by the interaction between the AF2 region of AR and the FxxLF or LxxLL binding motifs (Song *et al.* 2003). The hydrophobic groove present in the AF2 region of AR ligand-binding domain (AR-LBD) appears to be more favorable for phenylalanine binding, which suggests that the N/C interaction is preferred and may even be essential for agonist activity (Song *et al.* 2003; Narayanan *et al.* 2008).

Jasuja *et al.* (2009) used a variety of biophysical techniques, including steady-state second-derivative absorption and emission spectroscopy, pressure and temperature perturbations, and 4,4'-bis-anilino-naphthalene 8-sulfonate (bis-ANS) partitioning to determine the kinetics and thermodynamics of the conformational changes in AR-LBD after DHT binding. The results of these biophysical experiments are consistent with the conclusion that DHT binding leads to energetic stabilization of AR-LBD, and substantial rearrangement of residues distant from the ligand-binding pocket of AR (Jasuja *et al.* 2009). Dihydrotestosterone binding to AR-LBD involves biphasic receptor rearrangement including the population of a molten globule-like intermediate state (Fig.21.3; Jasuja *et al.* 2009). Although non-steroidal SARM-bound AR-LBD conformation has not been well characterized, Sathya *et al.* (2003) reported that some steroidal SARMs that have agonist activity in vitro induce an activating conformational change without facilitating N/C interactions. These data suggest that ligand-specific conformational change is achievable with synthetic ligands.

Bohl *et al.* (2007) reported that bicalutamide adopts a greatly bent conformation in the AR. Although the A-ring and amide bond of the bicalutamide molecule overlaps with the steroidal plane, the B-ring of bicalutamide folds away from the plane, pointing to the top of the ligand binding pocket (LBP), which forms a unique structural feature of this

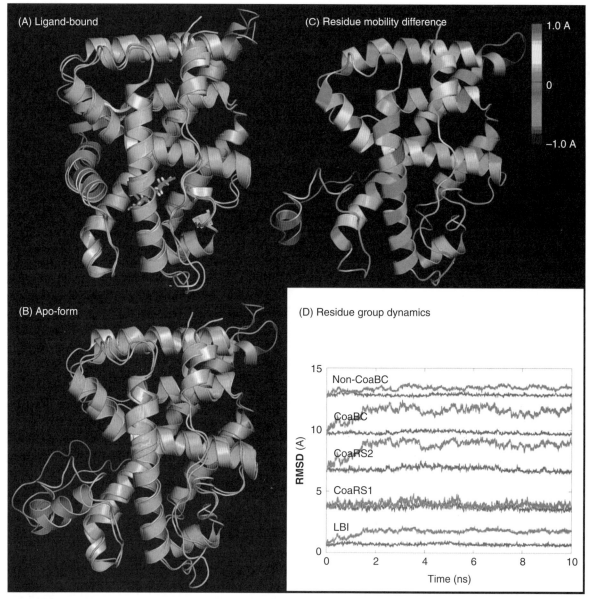

Fig. 21.3 See plate section for color version. Molecular modeling of AR-LBD upon ligand binding. The simulations were performed at 295.5 K and atmospheric pressure. (A, B) Superimposed representations of AR-LBD in the ligand-bound form and apo-form, respectively. Pink coloring shows the initial structures, and the pale green coloring shows the structures after 10 ns of simulations. (C) The AR-LBD apo-form colored by the difference between standard deviations of residue RMSDs (root mean square deviations) for LBD-R1881 complex and apo-form over 6–10 ns. Positive values correspond to greater mobility in the apo-form. (D) The predicted RMSDs for ligand-binding interface (LBI), coactivator recruitment surface 1 (CoaRS1), coactivator recruitment surface 2 (CoaRS2) and coactivator binding cleft (CoaBC). Red curves show RMSDs of helices in a ligand-bound structure, green curves in an apo-form structure. The groups of residues are defined as follows: LBI (V685, L701, N705, L707, Q711, L744, M745, M749, R752, Y763, F764, Q783, M787, F876, T877, L880, F891, M895), CoaRS1 (V713, V730, M734), CoaRS2 (E709, L712, V713, V715, V716, K717, K720, F725, R726, V730, Q733, M734, I737, Q738), CoaBC (helices 3, 3', 4, 5, 12), Non-CoaBC (helices 1, 6, 7, 8, 9, 10, 11). Reproduced with permission from Jasuja *et al.* (2009).

class of ligands (Bohl *et al.* 2007). The A-ring cyano group forms H bonds with Q711 and R752, similar to the 3-keto group in 5α-DHT (Bohl *et al.* 2007). The chiral hydroxyl group forms H bonds with L704 and

N705, mimicking ring C and the 17β-OH group in 5α-DHT (Bohl *et al.* 2007); these H bonding interactions are critical for high binding affinity. Favorable hydrogen bonding between ligand and the T877 side chain, structural features that mimic the 3-keto group of testosterone, and hydrophobic interactions are critical for the ligand to bind with high affinity and stimulate AR action (Bohl *et al.* 2007). The elucidation of the X-ray crystal structure of S1-bound AR has shown that W741 side chain is displaced by the B-ring to expand the binding pocket so that the compound orients towards the AF2 region (Bohl *et al.* 2007). The protein fold of the SARM-bound AR is the same for steroidal and non-steroidal SARMs (Bohl *et al.* 2007). It remains unclear how ligand–receptor interaction determines the agonist or antagonist activity of the ligand.

The unique conformation imparted by specific ligand-binding events allows the recruitment of a specific repertoire of AR co-regulator proteins which contribute to tissue-specificity of action. Tissue selectivity of SARMs might also be related to tissue-specific expression of co-regulator proteins (Heinlein and Chang 2002). We have investigated the molecular events that follow coactivator binding to AR, and the mechanisms that govern the sequence-specific effects of AR co-regulators are poorly understood (Zacharov *et al.* 2011). Using consensus coactivator sequence D11-FxxLF and biophysical techniques, we showed that coactivator association is followed by conformational rearrangement in AR-LBD that is enthalpically and entropically favorable, with activation energy of 29.8 ± 4.2 kJ/mol (Zacharov *et al.* 2011). Each coactivator induces a distinct conformational state in the dihydrotestosterone:AR-LBD:coactivator complex (Zacharov *et al.* 2011). Computational modeling revealed that the intramolecular rearrangements in AR-LBD backbone induced by the specific coactivators are different (Zacharov *et al.* 2011). These data suggest that coactivators may impart specificity in the transcriptional machinery by changing the steady-state conformation of AR-LBD. The data provide direct evidence that, even in the presence of the same ligand, AR-LBD can occupy distinct conformational states depending on its interactions with specific coactivators in the tissues; this coactivator-specific conformational gating may dictate subsequent binding partners and interaction with the DNA-response elements (Zacharov *et al.* 2011).

Testosterone actions in some androgenic tissues are amplified by its conversion to 5α-DHT (Russell and Wilson 1994); while its effects on some other tissues require its aromatization to estradiol. The non-steroidal SARMs do not serve as substrates for either the steroid 5α-reductases or the CYP19 aromatase. Some differences of the actions of SARMs from those of testosterone could be related to the inability of non-steroidal SARMs to undergo 5α-reduction or aromatization.

The tissue selectivity of SARMs could also be related to differences in their tissue distribution. Autoradiography studies with bicalutamide and hydantoin derivatives have not revealed the preferential accumulation of these SARMs in anabolic tissues (Hamann 2004). Differences in pharmacokinetics and metabolic clearance might also contribute to disparities in the in-vivo activities of SARMs with similar in-vitro binding affinity and transactivational potency.

21.6 Preclinical experience with first-generation non-steroidal SARMs

Preclinical proof-of-concept studies with a number of non-steroidal SARMs have revealed promising tissue selectivity (Gao *et al.* 2004a; 2004b; Bhasin *et al.* 2006; Kearbey *et al.* 2007; Miner *et al.* 2007; Narayanan *et al.* 2008; Bhasin and Jasuja 2009). Much of the preclinical data generated by pharmaceutical companies has remained unpublished; therefore, it is difficult to compare the relative potency and tissue selectivity of different SARMs, and the examples cited below from the published literature should not be viewed as evidence of exclusive or unique activity of a particular SARM.

However, it is apparent that many non-steroidal SARMs have achieved varying degrees of selectivity of anabolic action on the muscle relative to prostate and seminal vesicles (Gao *et al.* 2004a; 2004b; Bhasin *et al.* 2006; Kearbey *et al.* 2007; Miner *et al.* 2007; Ostrowski *et al.* 2007; Narayanan *et al.* 2008; Bhasin and Jasuja 2009; Schmidt *et al.* 2009). Although Hershberger assay based on the mass of levator ani muscle in castrated rodents has been used typically to determine the relative anabolic activity of SARMs (Hartsook and Hershberger 1961), some SARMs, such as the Ligand compounds, LGD-2226, LGD-2941 and LGD-4033, have been shown to stimulate the growth of other skeletal muscle groups, such as the plantaris, gastrocnemius and biceps brachii, as well (Miner *et al.* 2007). LGD-2226, LGD-2941 and LGD-4033 have also been shown to maintain measures of mating behavior in castrated male rats, including the number of mounts, intromissions and ejaculations, and copulatory efficiency (Miner *et al.* 2007). Several SARMs – Ligand Pharmaceuticals' LGD-2226,

LGD-2941 and LGD-4033 compounds, GTX's compound, ostarine, and Merck's compound, TFM-4AS-1 – have been reported to increase BMD, bone mass and strength, and restore bone architecture in ovariectomized female rodents (Miner *et al.* 2007; Kearbey *et al.* 2007; Schmidt *et al.* 2009). In intact rats, SARMs with agonist activity would be expected to inhibit LH and FSH and spermatogenesis, as has been reported for the S4 compound.

21.7 Early phase I and II SARM trials

A number of first-generation SARMs have advanced to phase I trials, and some are in phase II trials (Basaria *et al.* 2012). At the doses that have been tested, the first-generation SARMs have been reported to induce modest gains of 1.0 to 1.5 kg in fat-free mass and muscle strength, and small reductions in fat mass. At these doses, these compounds on which data have been reported in public forums have generally been well tolerated with minimal or no changes in liver enzymes and blood counts, and modest reductions in HDL cholesterol and triglycerides. However, it is possible that the next generation of SARM molecules will have greater potency and selectivity than the first-generation SARMs.

These compounds are being positioned for early efficacy trials for cancer cachexia, aging-associated functional limitations, sarcopenia, osteoporosis and frailty.

Also, SARMs that potently inhibit gonadotropins, but spare the prostate, would be attractive as candidates for male contraception. The use of SARMs for the treatment of androgen-deficiency syndromes in men has been proposed; the relative advantages of SARMs over testosterone for this indication are not readily apparent. Many biological functions of testosterone, especially its effects on libido and behavior, bone, and plasma lipids require its aromatization to estrogen; because the currently available SARMs are neither aromatized nor 5α-reduced, these compounds would face an uphill regulatory bar for approval as they would be required to show efficacy and safety in many more domains of androgen action than has been required of testosterone formulations.

21.8 Regulatory challenges to SARM development

In phase I and II trials, oral administration of the first-generation SARMs has been associated with reductions in HDL cholesterol. The suppression of HDL-C might reflect the combined effects of the oral route of administration and the lack of aromatization. It is possible that a systemic route of administration – transdermal or intramuscular – might attenuate the potential for HDL-C reductions.

Most of the first-generation non-steroidal SARMs are partial agonists (Gao *et al.* 2004a; 2004b): they compete with endogenous testosterone and, in intact animals, can antagonize the effects of testosterone on the prostate. Such SARMs with antagonistic or low intrinsic activity in prostate might be useful in the treatment of BPH or prostate cancer. The suppressive effects of this class of SARMs on gonadotropin secretion could have potential application for the development of male contraceptives (Gao *et al.* 2004a;2004b). Because the currently available SARMs are neither aromatized nor 5α-reduced, these compounds would face an uphill regulatory bar for approval as they would be required to show efficacy and safety in many more domains of androgen action than has been required of testosterone formulations.

The ability of SARMs to promote both muscle strength and bone mechanical strength constitutes a unique advantage over other therapies for osteoporosis that only increase bone density. By increasing muscle mass and strength, SARMs might also reduce fall propensity and thereby reduce fracture risk. Furthermore, the regulatory pathway for the approval of drugs for osteoporosis has been well delineated because of precedents set by previously approved drugs. In contrast, the pathway for approval of function-promoting anabolic therapies has not been clearly established.

Considerable effort is underway to generate a consensus around indications, efficacy outcomes in pivotal trials, and minimal clinically important differences in key efficacy outcomes; these efforts should facilitate efficacy trials of candidate molecules. In view of these uncertainties, the first-generation SARMs are being positioned for acute or subacute indications for grievous conditions, such as rehabilitation after a hip fracture or an acute illness, and cancer cachexia. Efficacy trials with short intervention durations for these acute and subacute indications would provide a substantially more favorable risk-to-benefit ratio than long-term trials for the prevention of more chronic conditions such as sarcopenia. The initial approval for short-term indications would also allow accumulation of safety data in clinical populations.

21.9 Key messages

- Non-steroidal SARMs are being developed as a new class of function-promoting anabolic therapies for functional limitations associated with frailty, acute and chronic illnesses, aging, cancer and cachexia, anemia and osteoporosis.
- The first-generation non-steroidal SARMs are partial agonists and have tissue-selective anabolic effects on the muscle and bone versus the reproductive tissues.
- The mechanisms of tissue-selective actions of SARMs are incompletely understood. Non-steroidal SARMs induce unique conformational changes in the AR ligand-binding domain, and recruit a unique

repertoire of co-regulator proteins to the liganded receptor, and thereby induce ligand-specific gene expression. The inability of non-steroidal SARMs to undergo 5α-reduction and aromatization, and differences in the tissue-specific expression of co-regulator proteins, may also contribute to their tissue selectivity.

- The efficacy trials of SARMs are just beginning, and initial trials have shown early evidence of safety and modest gains in lean body mass.
- Initial efficacy trials of SARMs are likely to be for short-term treatment indications for acute or subacute conditions associated with functional limitations.

21.10   References

Basaria S, Collins L, Dillon EL, Orwoll K, Storer TW, Miciek R, Ulloor J, Zhang A, Eder R, Zientek H, Gordon G, Kazmi S, Sheffield-Moore M, Bhasin S (2012) The safety, pharmacokinetics, and the effects of LGD-4033, a novel non-steroidal oral, selective androgen receptor modulator (SARM), in healthy young men. *J Gerontol A Biol Sci Med Sci*; in press

Bhasin S, Jasuja R (2009) Selective androgen receptor modulators as function promoting therapies. *Curr Opin Clin Nutr Metab Care* 12:232–240

Bhasin S, Calof OM, Storer TW, Lee ML, Mazer NA, Jasuja R, Montori VM, Gao W, Dalton JT (2006) Drug insight: testosterone and selective androgen receptor modulators as anabolic therapies for chronic illness and aging. *Nat Clin Pract Endocrinol Metab* 2:146–159

Bohl CE, Wu Z, Miller DD, Bell CE, Dalton JT (2007) Crystal structure of the T877A human androgen receptor ligand-binding domain complexed to cyproterone acetate provides insight for ligand-induced conformational changes and structure-based drug design. *J Biol Chem* 282:13648–13655

Dalton JT, Mukherjee A, Zhu Z, Kirkovsky L, Miller DD (1998)

Discovery of nonsteroidal androgens. *Biochem Biophys Res Commun* 244:1–4

Dimick DF, Heron M, Baulier EE, Jaylee MF (1961) A comparative study of the metabolic fate of testosterone, 17 alpha-methyl-testosterone. 19-nor-testosterone. 17 alpha-methyl-19-nor-testosterone and 17 alpha-methylestr-5(10)-ene-17 beta-ol-3-one in normal males. *Clin Chim Acta* 6:63–71

Edwards JP, West SJ, Pooley CL, Marschke KB, Farmer LJ, Jones TK (1998) New nonsteroidal androgen receptor modulators based on 4-(trifluoromethyl)-2(1H)-pyrrolidino[3,2-g] quinolinone. *Bioorg Medl Chem Lett* 8:745–750

Fragkaki AG, Angelis YS, Koupparis M, Tsantili-Kakoulidou A, Kokotos G, Georgakopoulos C (2009) Structural characteristics of anabolic androgenic steroids contributing to binding to the androgen receptor and to their anabolic and androgenic activities. Applied modifications in the steroidal structure. *Steroids* 74:172–197

Gao W, Reiser PJ, Kearbey JD, Phelps MA, Coss CC, Miller DD, Dalton JT (2004a) *Effects of Novel Selective Androgen Receptor Modulator (SARM) on Skeletal Muscle Mass and Strength in Castrated Male Rats.* The Endocrine Society, New Orleans

Gao W, Kearbey JD, Nair VA, Chung K, Parlow AF, Miller DD, Dalton JT (2004b) Comparison of the pharmacological effects of a novel selective androgen receptor modulator, the 5alpha-reductase inhibitor finasteride, and the antiandrogen hydroxyflutamide in intact rats: new approach for benign prostate hyperplasia. *Endocrinology* 145:5420–5428

Gao W, Reiser PJ, Coss CC, Phelps MA, Kearbey JD, Miller DD, Dalton JT (2005) Selective androgen receptor modulator treatment improves muscle strength and body composition and prevents bone loss in orchidectomized rats. *Endocrinology* 146:4887–4897

Hamann LG (2004) Discovery and preclinical profile of a highly potent and muscle selective androgen receptor modulator (SARM). 227th National Meeting of the American Chemical Society Medicinal Chemistry Division, March 28–April 1, Anaheim, CA

Hamann LG, Mani NS, Davis RL, Wang XN, Marschke KB, Jones TK (1999) Discovery of a potent, orally active, nonsteroidal androgen receptor agonist: 4-ethyl-1,2,3,4-tetrahydro-6-(trifluoromethyl)-8-pyridono[5,6-g]-quinoline (LG121071). *J Med Chem* 42:210–212

Hamann LG, Manfredi MC, Sun C, Krystek SR Jr, Huang Y, Bi Y, Augeri DJ, Wang T, Zou Y, Betebenner DA, Fura A, Seethala R, Golla R, Kuhns JE, Lupisella JA, Darienzo CJ, Custer LL, Price JL, Johnson JM, Biller SA, Zahler R, Ostrowski J (2007) Tandem optimization of target activity and elimination of mutagenic potential in a potent series of N-aryl bicyclic hydantoin-based selective androgen receptor modulators. *Bioorg Medl Chem Lett* **17**:1860–1864

Hanada K, Furuya K, Yamamoto N, Nejishima H, Ichikawa K, Nakamura T, Miyakawa M, Amano S, Sumita Y, Oguro N (2003) Bone anabolic effects of S-40503, a novel nonsteroidal selective androgen receptor modulator (SARM), in rat models of osteoporosis. *Biol Pharm Bull* **26**:1563–1569

Hartsook EW, Hershberger TV (1961) Effect of synthetic steroid or phenanthrene compounds upon weight gain and feed efficiency of rats. *ProcSocExp Biol Med* **106**:57–60

He Y, Yin D, Perera M, Kirkovsky L, Stourman N, Li W, Dalton JT, Miller DD (2002) Novel nonsteroidal ligands with high binding affinity and potent functional activity for the androgen receptor. *Eur J Med Chem* **37**:619–634

Heinlein CA, Chang C (2002) Androgen receptor (AR) coregulators: an overview. *Endocr Rev* **23**:175–200

Higuchi RI, Arienti KL, Lopez FJ, Mani NS, Mais DE, Caferro TR, Long YO, Jones TK, Edwards JP, Zhi L, Schrader WT, Negro-Vilar A, Marschke KB (2007) Novel series of potent, nonsteroidal, selective androgen receptor modulators based on 7H-[1,4]oxazino[3,2-g]quinolin-7-ones. *J Med Chem* **50**:2486–2496

Hoffman JR, Kraemer WJ, Bhasin S, Storer T, Ratamess NA, Haff GG, Willoughby DS, Rogol AD (2009) Position stand on androgen and human growth hormone use. *J Strength Cond Res* **23**(5 Suppl): S1–S59

Jasuja S, Ulloor J, Yengo CM, Choong K, Istomin AY, Livesay DR, Jacobs DJ, Swerdloff RS, Mikšovská J, Larsen RW, Bhasin S (2009) Kinetic and thermodynamic characterization of DHT-induced conformational perturbations in androgen receptor ligand binding domain. *Mol Endocrinol* **23**:1231–1241

Kearbey JD, Gao W, Narayanan R, Fisher SJ, Wu D, Miller DD, Dalton JT (2007) Selective androgen receptor modulator (SARM) treatment prevents bone loss and reduces body fat in ovariectomized rats. *Pharm Res* **24**:328–335

Kumar N, Didolkar AK, Monder C, Bardin CW, Sundaram K (1992) The biological activity of 7 alpha-methyl-19-nortestosteroneis not amplified in male reproductive tract as is that of testosterone. *Endocrinology* **130**:3677–3683

Manfredi MC, Bi Y, Nirschl AA, Sutton JC, Seethala R, Golla R, Beehler BC, Sleph PG, Grover GJ, Ostrowski J, Hamann LG (2007) Synthesis and SAR of tetrahydropyrrolo[1,2-b][1,2,5]thiadiazol-2(3H)-one 1,1-dioxide analogues as highly potent selective androgen receptor modulators. *Bioorg Medl Chem Lett* **17**:4487–4490

Masiello D, Chen SY, Xu Y, Verhoeven MC, Choi E, Hollenberg AN, Balk SP (2004) Recruitment of beta-catenin by wild-type or mutant androgen receptors correlates with ligand-stimulated growth of prostate cancer cells. *Mol Endocrinol* **18**:2388–2401

Miner JN, Chang W, Chapman MS, Finn PD, Hong MH, Lopez FJ, Marschke KB, Rosen J, Schrader W, Turner R, van Oeveren A, Viveros H, Zhi L, Negro-Vilar A (2007) An orally active selective androgen receptor modulator is efficacious on bone, muscle, and sex function with reduced impact on prostate. *Endocrinology* **148**:363–373

Murad F, Haynes RC (1980) Androgens and anabolic steroids. In: Goodman L, Gilman A (eds) *The Pharmacological Basis of Therapeutics*, 6th edn. McMilan Press, New York, pp 1448–1465

Narayanan R, Mohler ML, Bohl CE, Miller DD, Dalton JT (2008) Selective androgen receptor modulators in preclinical and clinical development. *Nucl Recept Signal* **6**:e010

Ng RA, Lanter JC, Alford VC, Allan GF, Sbriscia T, Lundeen SG, Sui Z (2007) Synthesis of potent and tissue-selective androgen receptor modulators (SARMs): 2-(2,2,2)-trifluoroethyl-benzimidazole scaffold. *Bioorg Medl Chem Lett* **17**:1784–1787

Ostrowski J, Kuhns JE, Lupisella JA, Manfredi MC, Beehler BC, Krystek SR Jr, Bi Y, Sun C, Seethala R, Golla R, Sleph PG, Fura A, An Y, Kish KF, Sack JS, Mookhtiar KA, Grover GJ, Hamann LG (2007) Pharmacological and X-ray structural characterization of a novel selective androgen receptor modulator: potent hyperanabolic stimulation of skeletal muscle with hypostimulation of prostate in rats. *Endocrinology* **148**:4–12

Rosen J, Negro-Vilar A (2002) Novel, non-steroidal, selective androgen receptor modulators (SARMs) with anabolic activity in bone and muscle and improved safety profile. *J Musculoskelet Neuronal Interact* **2**:222–224

Russell DW, Wilson JD (1994) Steroid 5 alpha-reductase: two genes/two enzymes. *Annu Rev Biochem* **63**:25–61

Sathya G, Chang CY, Kazmin D, Cook CE, McDonnell DP (2003) Pharmacological uncoupling of androgen receptor-mediated prostate cancer cell proliferation and prostate-specific antigen secretion. *Cancer Res* **63**:8029–8036

Schmidt A, Harada S-I, Kimmel DB, Bai C, Chen F, Rutledge SJ, Vogel RL, Sccafonas A, Gentile MA, Nantermet PV, McElwee-Witmer S, Pennypacker B, Massarachia P, Sahoo SP, Kim Y, Meissner RS, Hartman GD, Duggan ME, Rodan GA, Towler DA, Ray WJ (2009) Identification of anabolic selective androgen receptor modulators with reduced activities in the reproductive tissues and sebaceous glands. *J Biol Chem* **284**:36367–36376

Snyder PJ, Lawrence DA (1980) Treatment of male hypogonadism withtestosterone enanthate. *J Clin Endocrinol Metab* **51**:1335–1339

Sokol RZ, Palacios A, Campfield LA, Saul C, Swerdloff RS (1982) Comparison of the kinetics of injectable testosterone in eugonadal and hypogonadal men. *Fertil Steril* **37**:425–430

Song LN, Herrell R, Byers S, Shah S, Wilson EM, Gelmann EP (2003) Beta-catenin binds to the activation function 2 region of the androgen receptor and modulates the effects of the N-terminal domain and TIF2 on ligand-dependent transcription. *Mol Cell Biol* **23**:1674–1687

Sundaram K, Kumar N, Bardin CW (1994) 7 alpha-methyl-19-nortestosterone: an ideal androgen for replacement therapy. *Recent Prog Horm Res* **49**:373–376

van Oeveren A, Motamedi M, Mani NS, Marschke KB, Lopez FJ, Schrader WT, Negro-Vilar A, Zhi L (2006) Discovery of 6-N,N-bis (2,2,2-trifluoroethyl)amino-4-trifluoromethylquinolin-2(1H)-one as a novel selective androgen receptor modulator. *J Med Chem* **49**:6143–6146

van Oeveren A, Motamedi M, Martinborough E, Zhao S, Shen Y, West S, Chang W, Kallel A, Marschke KB, Lopez FJ, Negro-Vilar A, Zhi L (2007) Novel selective androgen receptor modulators: SAR studies on 6-bisalkylamino-2-quinolinones. *Bioorg Med Chem Lett* **17**:1527–1531

Yin D, Gao W, Kearbey JD, Xu H, Chung K, He Y, Marhefka CA, Veverka KA, Miller DD, Dalton JT (2003a) Pharmacodynamics of selective androgen receptor modulators. *J Pharmacol Exp Ther* **304**:1334–1340

Yin D, He Y, Perera MA, Hong SS, Marhefka C, Stourman N, Kirkovsky L, Miller DD, Dalton JT (2003b) Key structural features of nonsteroidal ligands for binding and activation of the androgen receptor. *Mol Pharmacol* **63**:211–223

Zacharov MN, Pillai BK, Bhasin S, Ulloor J, Istomin AY, Guo C, Godzik A, Kumar R, Jasuja R (2011)) Dynamics of coregulator-induced conformational perturbations in androgen receptor ligand binding domain. *Mol Cell Endocrinol* **341**:1–8

Chapter 22

The essential role of testosterone in hormonal male contraception

Eberhard Nieschlag and Hermann M. Behre

22.1 General prospects

22.1.1 Reasons for male contraception

Female contraception is very effective. Nevertheless, 40% of the 208 million pregnancies occurring worldwide in 2008 were unplanned, and half of the unintended pregnancies were terminated by abortion; an intervention that ended fatally for about 250 000 of these women (Singh *et al.* 2010). Although improved distribution and utilization of female contraceptive methods might ameliorate this situation, the contribution of a male contraceptive is well worth considering. Men enjoy the pleasures of sex, but can do little to contribute to the tasks of family planning – a pharmacological male contraceptive is perhaps long overdue. In addition, the risks of contraception would also be more fairly shared between women and men. Representative

Testosterone: Action, Deficiency, Substitution, ed. Eberhard Nieschlag and Hermann M. Behre, Assoc. ed. Susan Nieschlag. Published by Cambridge University Press. © Cambridge University Press 2012.

surveys have shown that a pharmacological male contraceptive would be acceptable to large segments of the population in industrialized nations, and would thus contribute to further stabilization of population dynamics. It might also help developing countries whose exponential population growth endangers economic, social and medical progress. Last but not least, male contraception can be considered an outstanding issue in the political field of gender equality.

22.1.2   Existing methods

Traditional male methods of contraception such as periodic abstinence or coitus interruptus are associated with a relatively high rate of unwanted pregnancy and also cause a disturbance in sexual activity. Condoms are the oldest barrier method available. However, when using condoms conception rates are relatively high, with 12 out of 100 couples conceiving during the first year of use (Pearl index = 12). Condom use has increased since the beginning of the AIDS epidemic, but more for protection from HIV infection and other sexually transmitted diseases than for contraceptive purposes.

Vasectomy is a safe and surgically relatively simple method for male contraception. The rate of unwanted pregnancy after vasectomy is less than 1%. The drawback to vasectomy is that it is not easily reversible. Achieving fatherhood after vasectomy requires either surgical reversal or sperm extraction from a testicular biopsy and intracytoplasmatic sperm injection into the ovum. Only about 50% of these men will become fathers in the end.

Given the disadvantages of these mechanical male methods, what then are the prerequisites for an ideal male contraceptive (Nieschlag *et al.* 2010)? It should be:

- as effective as comparable female methods
- acceptable to both partners
- rapidly effective
- independent of sexual act
- free of side-effects, especially without influence on masculinity, libido and potency
- without influence on progeny
- reversible in regard to fertility
- easily available and financially affordable.

22.1.3   New approaches to male contraception

Despite attempts to improve the existing methods, e.g. vas occlusion instead of surgical dissection, or the introduction of new materials (e.g. polyurethane) for condoms, the inherent disadvantages of these methods preventing sperm transport into the female tract persist, and must be replaced and/or supplemented by pharmacological methods. Post-testicular approaches to male contraception are still in the preclinical phase (Cooper and Yeung 2010). By investigating the molecular physiology of sperm maturation, epididymal function and fertilization, the aim is to identify processes that might be blocked by specific pharmacological agents with rapid onset of action. However, all substances investigated so far have shown toxic side-effects when interfering effectively with sperm function. At the moment then, only hormonal methods fulfill most of the requirements for a male contraceptive and are currently under clinical development.

All hormonal male contraceptives clinically tested to date are based on testosterone, either on testosterone alone or on a combination of testosterone with other hormones, in particular with either gestagens or GnRH analogs. Because of the essential role of testosterone, it is appropriate to include an overview on current hormonal approaches to male contraception in this volume on testosterone.

22.2   Principle of hormonal male contraception

The testes have an endocrine and an exocrine function: the production of androgens and of male gametes. Suppression of gamete production or interference with gamete function without affecting the endocrine function is the goal of endocrine approaches to male fertility regulation. However, since the two functions of the testes are interdependent, it has remained impossible so far to suppress spermatogenesis exclusively and reversibly without significantly affecting androgen synthesis.

Follicle-stimulating hormone and LH/testosterone are responsible for the maintenance of fully normal spermatogenesis (see Chapters 2 and 6; also Weinbauer and Nieschlag 1996). If only one of the two is eliminated, spermatogenesis will be reduced, but only in quantitative terms; i.e. fewer but normal sperm will be produced and azoospermia will not be achieved. This has been demonstrated in monkeys by the elimination of FSH by immunoneutralization, resulting in reduced sperm numbers but not in complete azoospermia (Srinath *et al.* 1983), which – at least until quite recently – was considered to be required for an effective male method. Therefore, even if new modalities for the selective suppression of FSH or FSH action should become available, it remains doubtful whether they would lead to a method for male contraception (Nieschlag 1986).

Until such results become available, the concept of azoospermia remains valid as a prerequisite for effective hormonal male contraception. However, as it is very difficult to achieve azoospermia uniformly in all volunteers participating in clinical trials for hormonal male contraception, and the pregnancy rates appear to be acceptably low if sperm counts drop below 1 million/ml, investigators active in the field reached a consensus that azoospermia or at least oligozoospermia i.e. <1 million/ml sperm should be the goal for an effective hormonal method (Nieschlag *et al.* 2007). To achieve this goal, not only FSH must be suppressed, but also intratesticular testosterone must be drastically reduced. Since testosterone alone can maintain spermatogenesis and much lower testosterone concentrations appear to be necessary for maintenance of spermatogenesis than previously considered, intratesticular testosterone must be depleted to such an extent that peripheral serum concentrations drop into the hypogonadal range. In order to maintain androgenicity, including libido, potency, male sex characteristics, psychotropic effects, protein anabolism, bone structure and hematopoiesis, testosterone levels in the general circulation have to be replaced, while the testes themselves are depleted of testosterone. However, even testes of volunteers achieving azoospermia show measurable testosterone concentrations, although reduced to 2% of normal, and volunteers developing azoospermia have low intratesticular levels similar to those suppressing only to oligozoospermia (see Chapter 6). Therefore, other factors must be of additional importance. Interestingly, the macaque monkey suppressed to azoospermia shows hardly any decrease in intratesticular testosterone, and elimination of FSH action appears to be more important than intratesticular testosterone (Weinbauer *et al.* 2001; Narula *et al.* 2002). For some time it was thought that the intratesticular conversion of testosterone to DHT is of importance in the maintenance of spermatogenesis and should be interfered with. However, the application of a 5α-reductase inhibitor did not additionally affect the suppression of spermatogenesis by testosterone alone (McLachlan *et al.* 2000). Recently, the number of CAG repeats in exon 1 of the androgen receptor has been found to determine the suppressibility of spermatogenesis, provided FSH and LH are well suppressed (von Eckardstein *et al.* 2002; Nieschlag *et al.* 2011).

This leads to the general principle of hormonal male contraception: namely the suppression of FSH and LH, resulting in depletion of intratesticular testosterone and cessation of spermatogenesis, while, at the same time, peripheral testosterone is substituted with an androgen preparation. This can be achieved by testosterone alone. However, since testosterone alone does not lead to azoospermia or severe oligozoospermia (<1 million/ml) in all individuals tested, testosterone needs to be combined with other substances suppressing pituitary gonadotropin secretion. As in female hormonal contraceptives, gestagens as pituitary-suppressing agents are being tested in men in combination with androgens. Gonadotropin-releasing hormone agonists, as well as antagonists, are also being explored as further possible combinations with androgens.

22.3 Testosterone alone

22.3.1 Testosterone enanthate

According to the principle outlined above, testosterone should be the first choice for hormonal male contraception since it not only suppresses pituitary LH and FSH secretion, but also replaces testosterone. Indeed, since the 1970s various investigations have been undertaken to suppress spermatogenesis with testosterone alone (Reddy and Rao 1972; Patanelli 1978). However, these were all surrogate studies, looking for sperm counts and not for pregnancies or rather for the prevention of pregnancies. Not until 1990 was an initial study testing this form of male contraception published by the WHO: the first study ever performed on the efficacy of hormonal male contraception (WHO 1990). Volunteers in 10 centers on four continents participated and received 200 mg testosterone enanthate intramuscularly per week. Those volunteers developing azoospermia within the first six months continued to receive injections for a further year. In this period (efficacy phase), couples refrained from using any further contraceptive methods. A total of 137 men reached the efficacy phase. During this period only one pregnancy occurred. This high rate of efficacy is well comparable to that of established female methods. This was a very encouraging result. However, only about two-thirds of all participants developed azoospermia. The other volunteers showed strong suppression of spermatogenesis, as evidenced by oligozoospermia (Waites 2003).

In order to answer the question of whether men developing oligozoospermia can be considered infertile, a second worldwide multicenter study followed (WHO 1996). In this study azoospermia again proved to be a most effective prerequisite for contraception. If sperm concentrations, however, failed to drop below 3×10^6/ml, resulting pregnancy rates were higher than when using condoms. When sperm concentrations decreased below 3×10^6/ml, which was the case in 98% of the participants, protection was not as effective as for azoospermic men, but was better than that offered by condoms.

Even if these WHO studies represented a breakthrough by confirming a principle of action (Waites 2003), they did not offer a practicable method. For a method requiring weekly intramuscular injections is not acceptable for broad use. Moreover, several months (on average four) were required before sperm production reached significant suppression. For this reason research concentrated on the development of long-acting testosterone preparations and on substances to improve overall effectiveness.

The WHO multicenter studies revealed an interesting phenomenon: the rate of azoospermia was greater in East Asian than in Caucasian men (WHO 1990; 1996). This finding was also confirmed by independent studies using testosterone enanthate injections in men in Indonesia (Arysad 1993), Thailand (Aribarg et al. 1996) and China (Cao et al. 1996).

22.3.2   Testosterone buciclate

Under the auspices of the WHO, a synthesis program identified testosterone buciclate as a testosterone ester with long-lasting effectiveness. First tested in monkeys and then in hypogonadal patients, it showed a long effective phase of three to four months after a single injection (see Chapter 15). A single injection of 1200 mg in a contraceptive study resulted in suppression of spermatogenesis comparable to that of weekly enanthate injections (Behre et al. 1995). Unfortunately, the WHO and the NIH, which jointly hold the patent on testosterone buciclate, were unable to find an industrial partner to further develop this promising ester for general use, so that its potential for male contraception has never been fully explored.

22.3.3   Testosterone undecanoate

22.3.3.1   Oral testosterone undecanoate

If testosterone is suited for contraception, the orally effective testosterone undecanoate should provide the male contraceptive "pill." This possibility was tested

in the early phase of development. However, even when high doses of 3×80 mg were taken daily for 12 weeks, only one of seven volunteers developed azoospermia (Nieschlag et al. 1978). Although this result was disappointing, the study demonstrated that stable levels of testosterone in serum are important to suppress pituitary gonadotropins.

22.3.3.2   Testosterone undecanoate in tea seed oil

While testosterone undecanoate was used as an oral preparation solely in the West, in China it has been marketed as an im preparation in tea seed oil for use in hypogonadism (see Chapter 5), and has more recently also been tested for male contraception. In a large multicenter efficacy study – the first completed since the WHO studies – involving 308 Chinese men given monthly injections of 500 mg testosterone undecanoate after a loading dose of 1000 mg, only 3% of the subjects did not suppress to azoospermia or severe oligozoospermia, and the remaining 97% induced no pregnancy (Gu et al. 2003).

The largest efficacy study to date was also performed in China, based on a loading dose of 1000 mg followed by monthly injections of 500 mg testosterone undecanoate. In this, 898 men entered the efficacy phase during which only 9 pregnancies were recorded. This represents a pregnancy rate of 1.1/100 person years (Gu et al. 2009). Thus, in China testosterone undecanoate provides better protection against pregnancy than condom use. Although injection intervals of four weeks appeared to be an achievement over the weekly injections of testosterone enanthate, the participants in a Chinese study considered the frequency of injections the most inconvenient part of this regimen (Zhang et al. 2006). Were testosterone undecanoate in castor oil also used in China this complaint could certainly be overcome.

22.3.3.3   Testosterone undecanoate in castor oil

In Caucasian men im testosterone undecanoate has not only been tested successfully for the treatment of male hypogonadism (see Chapters 14 and 15), but also in male contraception. Applying an improved galenic preparation of testosterone undecanoate (using castor oil instead of Chinese tea seed oil as vehicle), injection intervals could be spaced to six weeks, but, as with testosterone enanthate in weekly injections, only two-thirds of the volunteers achieved azoospermia (Kamischke et al. 2000a). Although this rate of azoospermia is not different from that achieved with testosterone enanthate alone, the longer injection interval represents a significant advantage. A later pharmacokinetic study concluded that eight-week intervals of 1000 mg injections would be sufficient for contraceptive purposes (Qoubaitary *et al.* 2006). Considering that 10- to 14-week intervals of 1000 mg testosterone undecanoate are required for substitution of hypogonadal men, about one-third more testosterone is required for contraception in normal volunteers.

Clinical studies to date have only included volunteers with so-called "normal" semen values by WHO standards. As a male contraceptive should be applicable to all interested men regardless of their semen parameters, how volunteers with subnormal semen parameters respond to hormonal male contraception has recently been investigated (Nieschlag *et al.* 2011). During a 34-week treatment phase the volunteers received injections of 1000 mg testosterone undecanoate in weeks 0, 6, 14 and 24. This was followed by a 24-week recovery and follow-up period. Twenty-three men with normal semen parameters and 18 with sperm counts below 20 million completed the trial. The normal volunteers showed the expected response, with 17 suppressing sperm counts below 1 million/ejaculate (13 showing azoospermia), and 6 not suppressing below 1 million sperm/ejaculate. By the end of the recovery period all sperm counts had returned to the range of starting values. The subnormal group showed a similar pattern with 13/18 (= 72%) men suppressing below 1 million/ejaculate (8/18 = 44% showing azoospermia) and the remaining 5/18 (= 28%) not suppressing sperm counts below 1 million/ejaculate. All sperm counts returned to the starting range. This demonstrated that, regarding suppressibility and reversibility, volunteers with normal and subnormal sperm counts display the same pattern. These results have a significant impact on the eligibility of men for hormonal contraception, as those with subnormal semen parameters would not need to be treated separately from those with normal parameters.

22.3.4 Testosterone pellets

Pellets consisting of pure testosterone are used for substitution in hypogonadism in some countries (see Chapter 15). In male contraceptive studies a one-time application showed efficacy comparable to weekly testosterone enanthate injections (Handelsman *et al.* 1992; McLachlan *et al.* 2000). The disadvantage of minor surgery required for insertion under the abdominal skin is compensated for by their low price and long duration of action. In further studies testosterone pellets have only been used in combination with other substances (see below).

22.3.5 19-Nortestosterone

When searching for preparations with longer-lasting effectiveness, 19-nortestosterone-hexoxyphenylpropionate was tested, the spectrum of effects of which is very similar to that of testosterone, and which has been used as an anabolic since the 1960s (molecular structure is shown in Fig.22.1). This 19-nortestosterone ester injected every three weeks enabled azoospermia to be reached by as many men as by testosterone enanthate. Thus the 19-nortestosterone ester is as effective as testosterone enanthate but allows a longer injection interval (Schürmeyer *et al.* 1984; Knuth *et al.* 1985; Behre *et al.* 2001). However, 19-nortestosterone is not fully equivalent to testosterone as it is converted to estrogens to a lesser degree than testosterone. Although no side-effects were detected in the trials using 19-nortestosterone, long-term untoward effects, e.g. on bones, cannot be excluded. In the light of newer, long-acting testosterone preparations, 19-nortestosterone appears less attractive for contraception.

22.3.6 7α-Methyl-19-nortestosterone

Another synthetic androgen with possible application in hypogonadism and in male contraception is 7α-methyl-19-nortestosterone (MENT). It has been tested in three doses of subdermal silastic implants in a multicenter study by the Population Council. In a dose-dependent fashion azoospermia can be achieved at the same rate as other testosterone preparations alone, i.e. in about two-thirds of the tested subjects; the advantage being that the effect of one set of implants may last for as long as one year (von Eckardstein *et al.* 2003). The potential of these implants alone or in combination with a gestagen is currently undergoing testing by the Population Council (New York).

22.4 Testosterone plus gonadotropin-releasing hormone analogs

22.4.1 Testosterone plus gonadotropin-releasing hormone agonists

In contrast to naturally occurring GnRH, GnRH agonists – after producing an initial stimulation

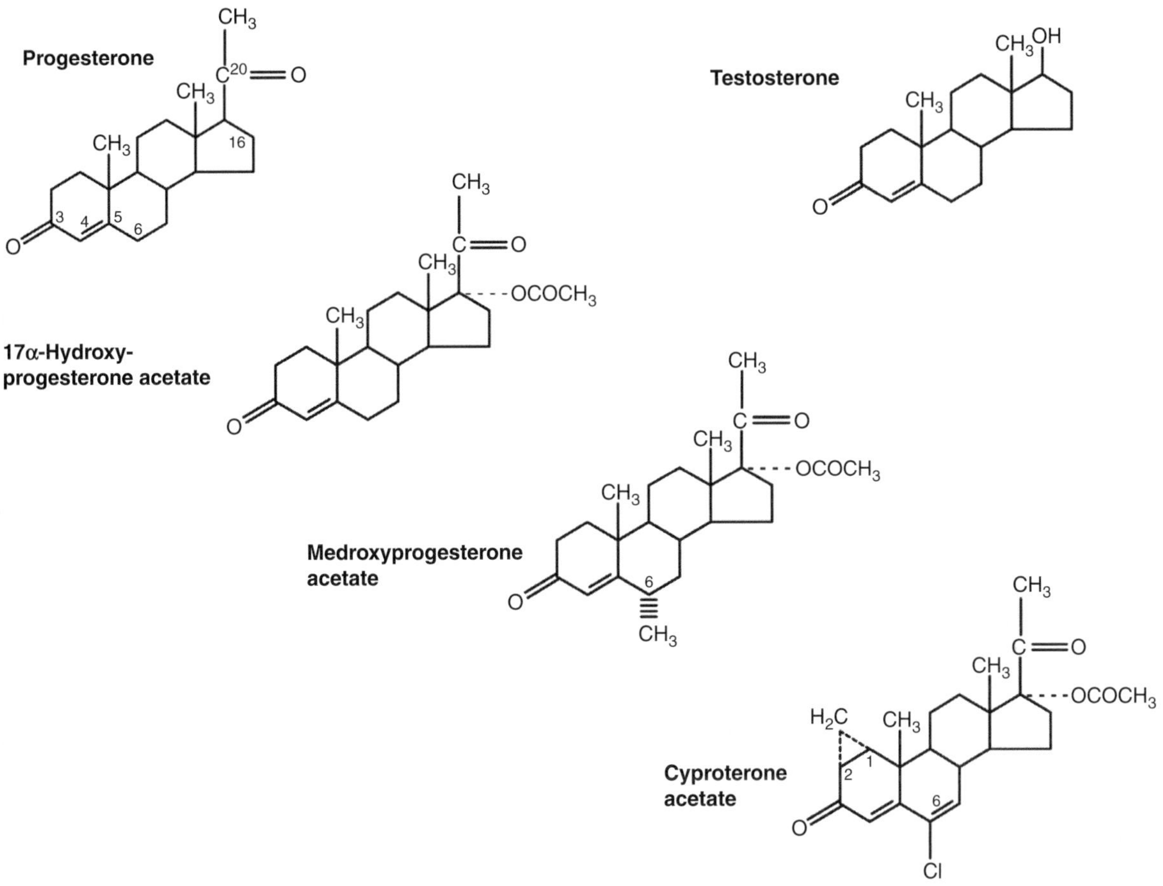

Fig. 22.1 Progestins derived from 17-hydroxyprogesterone tested in hormonal male contraception.

of gonadotropin release for approximately two weeks – lead to GnRH receptor downregulation and thereby to suppression of LH and FSH synthesis and secretion.

Between 1979 and 1992, 12 trials for hormonal male contraception using GnRH agonists, mostly in combination with testosterone, were published (for a review see Nieschlag *et al.* 1992). Altogether 106 volunteers participated in these trials. The GnRH agonists Decapeptyl (triptorelin acetate), buserelin and nafarelin were administered at daily doses of 5–500 μg/volunteer for periods of 10–30 weeks. In about 30% of men, sperm production could be suppressed below 5×10^6/ml, and azoospermia occurred in 21 men; while in the remaining volunteers, sperm numbers were only slightly reduced or remained unaffected. One explanation for the ineffectiveness of GnRH agonist plus androgen is the escape of FSH suppression after several weeks of GnRH agonist treatment (Behre *et al.* 1992; Bhasin *et al.* 1994).

Altogether, GnRH agonists in combination with testosterone did not prove useful in male contraception. At times it has been suggested that higher doses of the GnRH agonists should be used, but currently no further clinical studies appear to be under way.

22.4.2 Testosterone plus gonadotropin-releasing hormone antagonists

In contrast to GnRH agonists, GnRH antagonists produce a precipitous and prolonged fall of LH and FSH serum levels in men (e.g. Pavlou *et al.* 1989; Behre *et al.* 1994). It took much longer to develop GnRH antagonists that were suitable for clinical application than it did for GnRH agonists, and clinical trials using GnRH antagonists for male contraception started some 12 years later than those using agonists. To date, results have become available from five clinical trials using GnRH antagonists for male contraception (for review see Nieschlag and Behre 1996; Swerdloff *et al.* 1998; Behre *et al.* 2001).

Overall, 35 of the 40 volunteers (88%) who took part in these studies became azoospermic, most within three months. This is a much better rate of complete suppression than that produced by the administration of testosterone enanthate alone. Although studies in monkeys had suggested that delayed testosterone administration would increase the effectiveness of GnRH antagonists (Weinbauer *et al.* 1987; 1989), in men GnRH administration followed by delayed testosterone administration (azoospermia in 20/22 men) offered little advantage over concomitant GnRH and testosterone administration (azoospermia in 15/18 men). It should also be noted that, in the later studies with concomitant administration, all 14 volunteers became azoospermic (Pavlou *et al.* 1994; Behre *et al.* 2001). The major advantage of using GnRH antagonists is the short time required to achieve azoospermia; that is, within 6–8 weeks, which is considerably shorter than the mean of 17 weeks required in Caucasian men when testosterone alone was used (WHO 1995).

These results are promising. However, the antagonists and regimen tested so far require a daily injection, which makes them unacceptable for contraceptive purposes. Recently, modern GnRH antagonists for treatment of hormone-dependent prostate cancer became available that have to be injected only on a monthly basis (Boccon-Gibod *et al.* 2011). In addition, orally effective GnRH antagonists have been shown to suppress gonadotropins in normal men (Amory *et al.* 2009). The combination of these new GnRH antagonists with testosterone has the clear potential for effective hormonal contraception and should be tested in appropriate clinical trials in the near future.

It could be argued that the high price of GnRH antagonists may preclude their development as male contraceptives, which need to be affordable and in the same price range as comparable female methods. In order to shorten the period of use of GnRH antagonists, two studies have investigated the possibility of applying GnRH antagonists only in an initial suppression phase, and then continuing with the androgen alone (Swerdloff *et al.* 1998; Behre *et al.* 2001). Although successful in the monkey model (Weinbauer *et al.* 1994), studies in men produced contradictory results, so that this approach would require further experimentation.

22.5 Testosterone combined with progestins

The potency of gestagens to suppress gonadotropins is well known, and it was therefore obvious to combine testosterone with gestagens to achieve higher contraceptive efficacy. An overview of all studies using testosterone in combination with a progestin performed to date is given in Table 22.1, and the gestagen formulae are shown in Figs. 22.1 and 22.2.

Unfortunately, a systematic comparison of the different gestagens with regard to their contraceptive potency in males has never been performed. Even worse, a Cochrane Review analyzing 45 clinical trials came to the conclusion that the studies comprised too few volunteers, so that significant differences between the various steroid combinations could not be detected (Grimes *et al.* 2007). In the following, important studies are briefly summarized to highlight the cumbersome and often frustrating development of effective male contraception (Nieschlag 2009).

22.5.1 Testosterone or 19-nortestosterone plus depot medroxyprogesterone acetate

19-Norethisterone (norethindrone), medroxyprogesterone acetate (MPA), depot-MPA (DMPA), 17-hydroxyprogesterone capronate and megestrol acetate were used in early clinical trials initiated by the WHO (1972–1995) and the Population Council (Schearer *et al.* 1978) (molecular structures are in Figs.22.1 and 22.2). The most favorable combination was the monthly im injection of 200 mg DMPA plus 200 mg testosterone enanthate or testosterone cypionate; this combination gave the best results in suppressing spermatogenesis, and the incidence of untoward side-effects was low. Twelve volunteers were injected weekly with 200 mg 19-nortestosterone hexoxyphenylpropionate, followed by injections with the same dose every 3 weeks up to week 15. In addition, the volunteers were injected with 250 mg DMPA in weeks 0, 6 and 9. Azoospermia was achieved in 9 of 12 volunteers during the study course, while, in 3 of the remaining 4 volunteers, spermatogenesis was suppressed to single sperm, and, in one volunteer, to a sperm concentration of 1.3 million/ml.

The promising results prompted the WHO Task Force on Methods for the Regulation of Male Fertility

Table 22.1 Overview of studies on hormonal male contraception using either testosterone alone or in combination with progestins

Reference	Number of subjects	Ethnic origin	Androgen dose	Progestin dose	Azoospermia (n)	Severe oligozoospermia below 1 million/ml (n)	Oligozoospermia below 3 million/ml (n)
Testosterone alone							
WHO 1990	271	Mixed	TE 200 mg im/week	None	157	??	??
Behre et al. 1995	8	Caucasian	TB 1000 mg im once	None	3	—	—
Handelsman et al. 1992	9	Unknown	T pellets 1200 mg	None	5	4	0
Handelsman et al. 1996	10	Unknown	T pellets 400 mg	None	0	0	0
Handelsman et al. 1996	10	Unknown	T pellets 800 mg	None	4	0	0
Meriggiola et al. 1996	5	Caucasian	TE 100 mg im/week	None	5	0	0
Bebb et al. 1996	18	Caucasian	TE 100 mg im/week	None	6	4	1
WHO 1996	225	Mixed	TE 200 mg im/week	None	157	29	8
Zhang et al. 1999	12	Chinese	TU* 500 mg im/4 weeks	None	11	1	0
Zhang et al. 1999	12	Chinese	TU* 1000 mg im/4 weeks	None	12	0	0
Kamischke et al. 2000a	14	Caucasian	TU 1000 mg im/6 weeks	None	7	4	1
McLachlan et al. 2002	5	Not stated	TE 200 mg im/week	None	4 men ≤ 0.1 or azoospermia	4	0
von Eckardstein et al. 2003	35	Caucasian	MENT implants, 3 doses	None	10	—	3
Gu et al. 2003	305	Chinese	TU* 500 mg im/4 weeks	None	284	6	6

Gu et al. 2009	898	Chinese	TU* 500 mg im/4 weeks	None	855	—	43
Nieschlag et al. 2011	41	Caucasian	TU 1000 mg im/ 6, 14 and 24 weeks	None	25	9	—

Depot medroxyprogesterone acetate (DMPA)

Alvarez-Sanchez et al. 1977	8	Dominican republic	TE 250 mg im/week	DMPA 150 mg/4 weeks	4	3	1
Alvarez-Sanchez et al. 1977	10	Dominican republic	TE 250 mg im/week	DMPA 300 mg/4 weeks	7	2	0
Brenner et al. 1977	6	Caucasian	TE 200 mg im/week	DMPA 100 mg/4 weeks	1	2	1
Brenner et al. 1977	3	Caucasian	TE 200 mg im/week	DMPA 150 mg/4 weeks	1	0	0
Frick et al. 1977	12	Caucasian	TE 250 mg im/week	DMPA 100 mg im/4 weeks	6	4	0
Frick et al. 1977	6	Caucasian	T-propionate 4 rods	DMPA 100 mg im/4 weeks	2	0	0
Melo and Coutinho 1977	11	Brazilian	TE 200 mg im/week	DMPA 100–150 mg im/4 weeks	11 men ≤ 0.1 or azoospermia	0	??
Faundes et al. 1981	10	Dominican republic	TE 500 mg im/week	DMPA 150 mg/4 weeks	8	1	0
Frick et al. 1982	4	Caucasian	TE 500 mg/4 weeks	150 mg/4 weeks	4	0	0
Frick et al. 1982	5	Caucasian	TE 250 mg/2 weeks	75 mg/2 weeks	5	0	0
WHO 1993	45	Indonesian	19-Nortestosterone 200 mg im/3 weeks	DMPA 250 mg im/6 weeks	44	1	0
WHO 1993	45	Indonesian	TE 200 mg im/3 weeks	DMPA 250 mg im/6 weeks	43	2	0
Knuth et al. 1989	12	Caucasian	19-Nortestosterone 200 mg im/3 weeks	DMPA 250 mg im/6 weeks	6	4	2
Wu and Aitken 1989	10	Caucasian	TE 250 mg im/week	DMPA 200 mg/4 weeks	6	0	4
Pangkahila 1991	10	Indonesian	TE 100 mg im/week	DMPA 100 mg/4 weeks	10	0	0
Pangkahila 1991	10	Indonesian	TE 250 mg im/week	DMPA 200 mg/4 weeks	10	0	0
Handelsman et al. 1996	10	Not stated	T pellets 800 mg	DMPA once 300 mg im	9	0	1

Study	n	Ethnicity	Testosterone regimen	Gestagen/other regimen	5 men ≤ 0.1 or azoospermia		
McLachlan et al. 2002	5	Not stated	TE 200 mg im/week	DMPA once 300 mg im		5	0
Turner et al. 2003	53	Unknown	T pellets 800 mg/16 weeks	DMPA 300 mg im/12 weeks	49	2	0
Gu et al.2004	30	Chinese	TU* 1000 mg/8 weeks	DMPA 150 or 300 mg/8 weeks	28	1	1
Page et al. 2006	38	Not stated	T gel 100 mg/day	DMPA 300 mg/12 weeks ± GnRH antagonist	31	2	3
Levonorgestrel (LNG)							
Fogh et al. 1980	5	Caucasian	TE 200 mg/4 weeks	LNG 250 µg po/day	1	??	1
Fogh et al. 1980	5	Caucasian	TE 200 mg im/4 weeks	LNG 500 µg po/day	2	??	??
Bebb et al. 1996	18	Caucasian	TE 100 mg im/week	LNG 500 µg po/day	12	2	3
Anawalt et al. 1999	18	Caucasian	TE 100 mg im/week	LNG 125 µg po/day	11	5	1
Anawalt et al. 1999	18	Caucasian	TE 100 mg im/week	LNG 250 µg po/day	14	2	0
Ersheng et al. 1999	16	Chinese	TU 250 mg im/4 weeks	Sino-Implant 2 rods	6	0	1
Kamischke et al. 2000a	14	Caucasian	TU 1000 mg im/6 weeks	LNG 250 µg po/day	8	4	2
Gaw Gonzalo et al. 2002	20	Mixed	Testoderm TTS 2 patches/day	Norplant II 4 rods	7	5	2
Gaw Gonzalo et al. 2002	15	Mixed	Testoderm TTS 2 patches/day	LNG 125 µg po/day	5	1	1
Gaw Gonzalo et al. 2002	14	Mixed	TE 100 mg im/week	Norplant II 4 rods	13	1	0
Pöllänen et al. 2001	5	Caucasian	DHT gel 250 mg/day	LNG 30 µg po/day	0	0	1
Pöllänen et al. 2001	5	Caucasian	DHT gel 250 mg/day	Jardelle (LNG) 1 rod	0	0	0
Pöllänen et al. 2001	8	Caucasian	DHT gel 500 mg/day	Jardelle (LNG) 2 rods	0	0	0
Pöllänen et al. 2001	7	Caucasian	DHT gel 250 mg/day	Jardelle (LNG) 4 rods	0	0	0
Gui et al.2004	41	Chinese	TU* 500 or 1000 mg/8 weeks	LNG 4 implants	31	5	4
Anawalt et al.2005	41	Mixed	TE 100 mg/week	LNG 31 µg or 62 µg/day	25	13	2
Wang et al. 2006	19 / 21	Caucasian Chinese	T implants/15–18 weeks	LNG 4 implants	13 / 19	— / —	— / —
Wang et al. 2007	18	Chinese	TU* 500 mg/6 weeks	LNG 250 mg po/day	17	—	1

Norethisterone enanthate (NETE)

Study	N	Ethnicity	Testosterone	Progestin			
Kamischke et al. 2001	14	Caucasian	TU 1000 mg im/6 weeks	NETE 200 mg/6 weeks	13	0	0
Kamischke et al. 2002	14	Caucasian	TU 1000 mg im/6 weeks	NETE 200 mg/6 weeks	13	1	0
Kamischke et al. 2002	14	Caucasian	TU 1000 mg im/6 weeks	NETE 400 mg/6 weeks	13	1	0
Kamischke et al. 2002	14	Caucasian	TU 1000 mg im/6 weeks	NETA 10 mg po/day	12	2	0
Meriggiola et al. 2005	10	Caucasian	TU 1000 mg/8 weeks	NETE 200 mg/6 weeks	9	—	—
	8	Caucasian	TU 1000 mg/12 weeks	NETE 200 mg/12 weeks	3	—	—
Qoubaitary et al. 2006	10	Mixed	TU 750 mg/8 weeks	NETE 250 mg/8 weeks	5	2	1
	10	Mixed	TU 1000 mg/8 weeks	NETE 250 mg/8 weeks	10	—	—
CONRAD 2011		Mixed	TU 1000 mg/8 weeks	NETE 200 mg/8 weeks	—	—	—

Cyproterone acetate (CPA)

Study	N	Ethnicity	Testosterone	Progestin			
Meriggiola et al. 1996	5	Caucasian	TE 100 mg im/week	CPA 50 mg po/day	3	0	1
Meriggiola et al. 1996	5	Caucasian	TE 100 mg im/week	CPA 100 mg po/day	5	0	0
Meriggiola et al. 1998	5	Caucasian	TE 100 mg im/week	CPA 12.5 mg po/day	3	2	0
Meriggiola et al. 1998	5	Caucasian	TE 100 mg im/week	CPA 25 mg po/day	5	0	0
Meriggiola et al. 2002a	9	Caucasian	TE 100 mg im/week	CPA 5 mg po/day	6	3	0
Meriggiola et al. 2002a	7	Caucasian	TE 200 mg im/week	CPA 5 mg po/day	0	4	2
Meriggiola et al. 2003	24	Caucasian	TU 1000 mg/6 weeks	CPA 20 and 2 mg po/day	13	11	—

Desogestrel (DSG) or etonogestrel (ENG)

Study	N	Ethnicity	Testosterone	Progestin			
Wu et al. 1999	8	Caucasian	TE 50 mg im/week	DSG 300 µg po/day	8	0	0
Wu et al. 1999	7	Caucasian	TE 100 mg im/week	DSG 150 µg po/day	4	3	0
Wu et al. 1999	8	Caucasian	TE 100 mg im/week	DSG 300 µg po/day	6	0	1
Anawalt et al. 2000	7	Caucasian	TE 50 mg im/week	DSG 150 µg po/day	4	1	0
Anawalt et al. 2000	8	Caucasian	TE 100 mg im/week	DSG 150 µg po/day	8	0	0
Anawalt et al. 2000	8	Caucasian	TE 100 mg im/week	DSG 300 µg po/day	7	1	0
Kinniburgh et al. 2001	8	Caucasian	T pellets 400 mg/12 weeks	DSG 150 µg po/day	6	2	0
Kinniburgh et al. 2001	7	Caucasian	T pellets 400 mg/12 weeks	DSG 150 µg po/day	5	1	0

Study	n	Ethnicity	Androgen	Progestin			
Anderson et al. 2002a	9	Black	T pellets 400 mg/12 weeks	DSG 150 µg po/day	9	0	0
Anderson et al. 2002a	11	Mixed	T pellets 400 mg/12 weeks	DSG 150 µg po/day	9	0	1
Anderson et al. 2002a	8	Black	T pellets 400 mg/12 weeks	DSG 300 µg po/day	8	0	0
Anderson et al. 2002a	12	Mixed	T pellets 400 mg/12 weeks	DSG 300 µg po/day	8	0	0
Anderson et al. 2002b	14	Caucasian	T pellets 400 mg/12 weeks	Implanon (ENG) 1 rod	9	1	3
Anderson et al. 2002b	14	Caucasian	T pellets 400 mg/12 weeks	Implanon (ENG) 2 rods	9	4	0
Kinniburgh et al. 2002	15	Caucasian	T pellets 400 mg/12 weeks	DSG 300 µg po/day	15	0	0
Kinniburgh et al. 2002	18	Chinese	T pellets 400 mg/12 weeks	DSG 300 µg po/day	18	0	0
Kinniburgh et al. 2002	18	Chinese	T pellets 400 mg/12 weeks	DSG 150 µg po/day	11	2	2
Kinniburgh et al. 2002	13	Caucasian	T pellets 400 mg/12 weeks	DSG 150 µg po/day	11	2	0
Brady et al.2004	9	Not stated	T pellets 400 mg/12 weeks	Etonogestrel implants	9	2	—
Walton et al. 2007	16	Caucasian	T pellets 600 mg/12 weeks	Etonogestrel implants	11	2	—
	10	Caucasian	MENT implants	Etonogestrel implants	3	5	—
Mommers et al. 2008	134	Caucasian	TU 750 mg/12 weeks	Etonogestrel implants high dose	—	≈125	—
	112	Caucasian	TU 750 mg/10 weeks / TU 1000 mg/12 weeks	Etonogestrel implants low dose	—	≈100	—
Self-applicable							
Nieschlag et al. 1978	7	Caucasian	Andriol 240 mg po/day	None	1	0	0
Guerin and Rollet 1988	13	Caucasian	Andriol 160 mg po/day	NETA 10 mg po/day	7	2	3
Guerin and Rollet 1988	5	Caucasian	T gel 250 mg/day	NETA 5 mg po/day	4	1	0
Guerin and Rollet 1988	5	Caucasian	T gel 250 mg/day	NETA 10 mg po/day	5	0	0
Guerin and Rollet 1988	8	Caucasian	T gel 250 mg/day	MPA 20 mg po/day	5	0	1
Meriggiola et al. 1997	8	Caucasian	Andriol 80 mg po/day	CPA 12.5 mg po/day	1	3	2
Hair et al. 1999	4	Caucasian	Andropatch 2 patches/day	DSG 75 µg po/day	0	1	0
Hair et al. 1999	6	Caucasian	Andropatch 2 patches/day	DSG 150 µg po/day	3	0	0
Hair et al. 1999	7	Caucasian	Andropatch 2 patches/day	DSG 300 µg po/day	4	1	0

Büchter et al. 1999	12	Caucasian	Testoderm TTS 2 patches/day	LNG 250 µg po, later 500 µg	2	3	0
Gaw Gonzalo et al. 2002	19	Mixed	Testoderm TTS 2 patches/day	None	5	0	1
Pöllänen et al. 2001	2	Caucasian	DHT gel 250 mg/day	None	0	0	0
Soufir et al. 2011	35	Not stated	T gel 100–125 mg/day	MPA 2 × 10 mg daily	23	5	1

Source: updated from Kamischke and Nieschlag (2004).

Abbreviations: T, testosterone; TE, testosterone enanthate; TB, testosterone buciclate; TU*, testosterone undecanoate in tea seed oil; TU, testosterone undecanoate in castor oil; MENT, 7α-methyl-19-nortestosterone; NETA, norethisterone acetate; po, per os; ??, not known, can not be extracted from the paper.

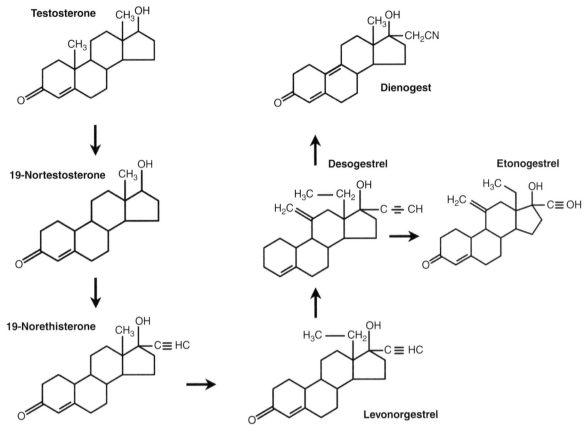

Fig. 22.2 Progestins derived from 19-nortestosterone tested in hormonal male contraception.

to launch a large-scale multicenter trial in five centers in Indonesia, comparing the effectiveness of testosterone enanthate, or 19-nortestosterone hexyoxyphenyl-propionate, in combination with DMPA (WHO 1993). Surprisingly, 43/45 and 44/45 subjects in the testosterone and the 19-nortestosterone groups respectively suppressed to azoospermia. Unfortunately, this study had failed to include groups treated with the androgens alone, so that it remained unclear whether the azoospermia rates of 97% and 98% were due to the combined treatment or could also be achieved by the androgens alone.

The latter possibility appears likely in the light of ethnic differences between Caucasian and East Asian men. Although ultimately effective, the disadvantage remains that it took almost 20 weeks to reach azoospermia or the lowest sperm counts in these volunteers. Thus, more rapid onset of sperm suppression is required.

A more recent study testing contraceptive efficacy and using either 200 mg testosterone enanthate given alone in weekly im injections or in combination with an injection of 300 mg DMPA showed that the suppression rate was not greater when DMPA was added (McLachlan et al. 2002). However, when subcutaneous testosterone implants of 200 mg were applied every four or six months in combination with 300 mg DMPA given every three months, 53/54 men achieved azoospermia or suppression below 1×10^{6} sperm/ml. During a 12-month efficacy phase with otherwise unprotected intercourse, no pregnancy occurred (35.5 person years) (Turner et al. 2003). The differences between the studies highlight the fact that obviously the kinetics of testosterone are very important, since the implants produce very stable serum levels and the testosterone enanthate injections cause high peaks and troughs. Although the combination of an implant with an injection every three months may not be ideal, this study was the first to demonstrate the contraceptive efficacy of a testosterone plus progestin combination.

In order to test whether one of the two steroid entities could be self-administered, the addition of a testosterone transdermal gel to the DMPA injections (300 mg/three months) was tested (Page *et al.* 2006). The results were comparable to those from trials where DMPA was combined with injectable testosterone.

In order to develop a self-applicable male hormonal contraceptive, Soufir *et al.* (2011) initiated an efficacy study combining transdermal testosterone (100–125 mg daily) with oral MPA (2 × 10 mg daily). Of the 35 eligible couples, 25 entered the efficacy phase, and all female partners together were exposed for 211 months to otherwise unprotected intercourse. The one pregnancy occurred in a couple that showed bad compliance. Numbers of participants and months of exposure are too low for statistical analysis, but the results show that a self-applicable male hormonal contraceptive is possible.

Recovery to baseline semen parameters appears to be rather slow in studies employing DMPA. This may be due to secondary depots of this progestin formed in the subcutaneous and abdominal fat, and requires special attention should studies be extended over several years.

22.5.2   Testosterone plus levonorgestrel

Levonorgestrel has been widely used for contraception in females, either orally or as an implant, and has proved safe and effective. Although early studies combining 0.5 mg levonorgestrel given orally with testosterone enanthate were not very encouraging (Fogh *et al.* 1980), later trials comparing testosterone enanthate (100 mg/week) alone with testosterone enanthate in combination with 0.5 mg levonorgestrel given orally showed that the combination resulted in more pronounced suppression of spermatogenesis than testosterone enanthate alone (Bebb *et al.* 1996).

Encouraged by the renewed interest in levonorgestrel, we conducted a self-administration trial combining oral levonorgestrel with a transdermal testosterone patch applied to the trunk (Büchter *et al.* 1999). Unfortunately the results were disappointing, as suppression of spermatogenesis was insufficient. We presume that the testosterone dose absorbed from the transdermal systems was too low and often impeded by inadequate adhesiveness to the skin of the systems (Büchter *et al.* 1999). The study

again emphasizes the need for steady serum testosterone levels to suppress gonadotropins, even when co-administered with a potent gestagen.

Similarly it was shown that the combination of 0.5 mg levonorgestrel given orally with transdermal DHT was quite ineffective; nor did the combination of transdermal DHT with levonorgestrel implants lead to sufficient suppression of spermatogenesis (Pöllänen *et al.* 2001).

When the long-acting testosterone preparation testosterone undecanoate (in castor oil) given at six-week intervals was combined with oral levonorgestrel, the progestin did not enhance the effect of testosterone undecanoate alone (Kamischke *et al.* 2000b). However, when levonorgestrel was administered in four capsules delivering about 160 µg levonorgestrel (Norplant II = Jadelle)/per day together with weekly injections of 100 mg testosterone enanthate, 93% of the subjects achieved azoospermia and all suppressed to oligozoospermia below 1×10^6/ml sperm (Gaw Gonzalo *et al.* 2002).

When MENT implants were combined with levonorgestrel implants in different doses, a clear dose-dependent effect could be observed, but it remains undetermined whether implants with sufficiently long duration can be manufactured. Non-biodegradable implants that have to be removed surgically from the implantation site when contraceptive protection is no longer required appear impractical for widespread use unless they can be left in situ for long periods (Wang *et al.* publication in preparation).

22.5.3   Testosterone plus cyproterone acetate

Animal studies and studies in sexual delinquents have shown that the antiandrogen cyproterone acetate, which can be considered a potent progestin, suppresses spermatogenesis, an effect exerted through suppression of pituitary gonadotropin secretion. In clinical trials using 5 to 20 mg cyproterone acetate per day for up to 16 weeks, sperm counts and motility were reduced markedly (Fogh *et al.* 1979; Moltz *et al.* 1980; Wang and Yeung 1980). Thus, cyproterone acetate appeared to be a possibility for male fertility control. However, decreases in serum testosterone levels to below normal were also observed. Some of the volunteers complained of fatigue, lassitude and decrease in libido and potency attributable to the diminished testosterone levels.

When, later, cyproterone acetate was combined with testosterone enanthate injections at even higher doses of 50 and 100 mg, it effectively suppressed spermatogenesis (Meriggiola *et al.* 1996), but even when lower doses of cyproterone acetate were administered, antiandrogenic effects prevailed and the volunteers showed decreased red blood, preventing this antiandrogenic gestagen from being an attractive combination for male contraception (Meriggiola *et al.* 1998). Although the attempt to create a male pill by co-administration of oral testosterone undecanoate with oral cyproterone acetate led to suppression of spermatogenesis, it had to be discontinued because of a decrease in hemoglobin and hematocrit caused by the antiandrogen (Meriggiola *et al.* 1997). However, when combining 1000 mg testosterone undecanoate every six weeks with 20 mg CPA daily initially, followed by only 2 mg CPA/day, the initial suppression of spermatogenesis could be maintained and antiandrogenic effects prevented (Meriggiola *et al.* 2003).

22.5.4   Testosterone plus dienogest

The latest progestin to be tested for male contraceptive purposes is the orally effective dienogest. This is another 19-norprogestin in which position 17 is not substituted by the common ethinyl group, but by a cyanomethyl group and a double bond is introduced in ring B. When given at 2, 5 or 10 mg doses over 21 days, 10 mg resulted in a suppression of gonadotropins comparable to 10 mg of cyproterone acetate. Semen parameters were not affected, as one would expect with this short application period (Meriggiola *et al.* 2002b). As dienogest displays only mild antiandrogenic activity, this substance may be a possible candidate for future trials. However, to date further testing has only been performed in rats (Misro *et al.* 2009).

22.5.5   Testosterone plus desogestrel or etonogestrel

Orally administered desogestrel, a levonorgestrel derivative, was evaluated in clinical trials using 300 µg/day combined with weekly injections of 50 or 100 mg testosterone enanthate for 24 weeks. A third group received 150 µg/day desogestrel and 100 mg testosterone enanthate per week intramuscularly.

While the group receiving 50 mg testosterone enanthate showed complete suppression of spermatogenesis, i.e. azoospermia, the other groups achieved only incomplete suppression. In the most effective group, total serum testosterone levels were found in the range of the lower limit of normal men, and this may explain why the volunteers complained of decreased sex drive, depression, fatigue and nocturnal sweating (Wu *et al.* 1999).

In a two-center study in Edinburgh and Shanghai, testosterone pellets (400 mg every three months) were combined with either 150 or 300 µg desogestrel/day orally (Kinniburgh *et al.* 2001). Azoospermia was achieved in all 28/28 men receiving the 300 µg desogestrel dose. Disregarding the fact that a combination of an implant with an oral pill might not offer a highly attractive option, these results are quite promising.

This group continued their investigations using etonogestrel, the active metabolite of orally active desogestrel, as an implant which was recently licensed for use as a female contraceptive (Implanon). Twenty-eight men received one or two etonogestrel implants which provide contraceptive protection in females for three years, but the implants were removed from the volunteers after six months. In addition, they received 400 mg testosterone pellets at the beginning of the study and after three months. Nine men in each group achieved azoospermia and, in the group with two implants, sperm counts fell to 0.1×10^6/ml in 13/14 men (Anderson *et al.* 2002b).

In the first (and so far last) industry-sponsored trial, Organon and Schering decided to test etonogestrel implants with testosterone undecanoate injections in various combinations (Mommers *et al.* 2008). This study involved 354 volunteers in seven treatment groups receiving either placebo or 750–1000 mg testosterone undecanoate every 10–12 weeks with two doses of etonogestrel, for 42–44 weeks. Ninety percent of treated men suppressed spermatogenesis to ≤1 million/ml ejaculate. Although the combination of an implant with injections may not appear too attractive for practical use, the study had a high success rate and could have formed the basis for a phase III efficacy study. Unfortunately, both companies discontinued their male contraception programs when they were taken over by other firms who were at that stage not interested in male contraception.

22.5.6   Testosterone plus 19-norethisterone

19-norethisterone, one of the earliest progestins derived from testosterone (Djerassi *et al.* 1954), is characterized by some undesirable androgenicity when given to women, which might be of advantage when administered to men. An early study with only a few volunteers using a combination of orally effective 19-norethisterone acetate with either a transdermal testosterone gel or oral testosterone undecanoate led to azoospermia in all volunteers (Guerin and Rollet 1988). Considering its properties and these promising results, it was surprising that it took another 10 years to investigate the use of 19-norethisterone more systematically.

In a pharmacokinetic study, single injections of 200 mg 19-norethisterone enanthate led to a marked suppression of the gonadotropins (FSH for 29 days), testosterone, SHBG and sperm (Kamischke *et al.* 2000b). When testosterone undecanoate became available in the form of im depot injections, it was combined with norethisterone enanthate, and volunteers achieved azoospermia or severe oligozoospermia in all but one. The additive effect to testosterone undecanoate alone was striking. An injected dose of 200 mg 19-norethisterone enanthate every six weeks was as effective as 400 mg, so that 200 mg appears to be a useful dose. Although 19-norethisterone acetate 10 mg given orally daily in combination with im testosterone undecanoate is as effective as injected norethisterone enanthate, the combination of the two steroids in one injection appears quite attractive (Kamischke *et al.* 2000a; 2001; 2002). In an ensuing dose-finding study, Meriggiola *et al.* (2005) showed that it might be possible to extend the injection intervals to eight weeks.

Based on these findings, the WHO, together with CONRAD, initiated a large-scale efficacy trial intended to include 440 couples in 11 centers worldwide. The men received 1000 mg testosterone undecanoate plus 200 mg norethisterone enanthate im every eight weeks. Although contraceptive efficacy appeared to be satisfactory, the study was prematurely suspended because of undesirable side-effects, especially depression and other mood changes, increase of sexual desire and pain at the injection site. These side-effects were not unexpected, but occurred more often that expected. Two "serious adverse events" (SAEs) were judged to be either possibly or probably related to the study regimen. By the time of the suspension of the study (April 5, 2011) 321 men had been enrolled into the study, 100 men had completed the 12-months efficacy phase and 103 men were still in the suppression or efficacy phase. All subjects continued to be followed until the end of the recovery phase (CONRAD 2011). Thus, this largest efficacy trial ever performed worldwide came to an unhappy end.

22.6   Side-effects of hormonal male contraception

Possible side-effects of hormonal male contraception might be caused by too high or too low testosterone levels or by additional substances. Decreased testicular volumes reflecting suppression of spermatogenesis are inherent to all hormonal methods, but not considered a serious effect by the volunteers as long as sexual function remains unaltered. In all major studies performed to date, sperm counts returned to normal levels (Liu *et al.* 2006). Weight gain is most likely an anabolic effect of testosterone. Due to the high peak serum testosterone levels caused by testosterone enanthate in the earlier studies, acne and mild gynecomastia could be observed in individual cases. Except for local skin reactions, side-effects of GnRH analogs are mainly attributable to decreased testosterone levels, not sufficiently compensated for by testosterone supplementation. Sweating and, in particular, nocturnal sweating is a feature of some added progestins.

Depending on the type and doses of progestin, significant decreases are observed in SHBG. This indicates the influence of progestins on liver function and may enhance the androgenicity of the testosterone preparation, since the unbound free fraction of testosterone in circulation may increase. Some of the effects seen when progestins are added may be due to this phenomenon. When adding levonorgestrel or 19-norethisterone acetate or enanthate an increase in prolactin is seen, which remains without biological significance. An increase in red blood was more pronounced when progestins were added to testosterone than when testosterone was given alone. Hemostasis is affected by testosterone alone (downregulation) and by progestin (in this case norethisterone) alone (upregulation), but given in combination, the effects appear to be neutralized (Zitzmann *et al.* 2002). In the suspended large WHO/CONRAD study, depression and other mood changes were the major complaints and it remains to be seen whether this was due to too little testosterone or whether this was a genuine effect of norethisterone.

22.7 Acceptability of hormonal male contraception

The acceptability of hormonal male contraception can definitely only be assessed when a final product becomes available. Nevertheless, it should be remembered that worldwide about 15% of all couples practicing contraception rely on male methods, albeit with varying preferences, and the proportion of men practicing contraception is increasing. Thus in the Netherlands the percentage of vasectomized men whose wives were of reproductive age rose from 2 to 10.5% from 1975 to 2008 and from 8 to 12.2% in the USA; the highest rates of vasectomized men are found in the United Kingdom and in New Zealand. Worldwide, however, only 2.7% of men are vasectomized. Similarly, the use of condoms for contraception varies from country to country with a worldwide average of 5.7%. It is to be expected that the percentage of men willing to practice contraception varies between cultures and with methods available. According to a survey in Hong Kong and Shanghai some years ago, half the men interviewed were willing to take a daily contraceptive pill; in Edinburgh and Cape Town two-thirds were willing to do so (Anderson and Baird 1997; Martin *et al.* 2000). Also acceptability in Australian men was found to be high (Weston *et al.* 2002). After more than 50 years of female oral contraception, the attitude of men towards new methods of male contraception has changed. Worldwide surveys showed men to be willing to use pharmacological contraceptive methods (Heinemann *et al.* 2005). In addition, "despite commonly expressed views to the contrary, most women would trust their male partners to use a hormonal method" (Glasier *et al.* 2000; Glasier 2010).

22.8 Outlook

While a large proportion of clinical research is driven by the pharmaceutical industry, in the case of male contraception industry fails. Without the long-range perspective and endurance of institutions and organizations such as the WHO, Population Council, the National Institute of Child Health and Human Development, some medical research councils and a few foundations, male contraception would long have been abandoned (Nieschlag 2009). The principle and effectiveness of hormonal male contraception has been demonstrated in many studies. The fact that the majority of clinical trials on hormonal male contraception have been published in high-ranking journals emphasizes the high priority the scientific community attributes to these endeavors. Investigators are so convinced of the validity of the concept of hormonal male contraception that they drafted recommendations for regulatory approval for male hormonal contraception at their annual summit meetings (since 1997) (Nieschlag and 10th Summit Meeting Group 2007). Little more would have been required to convince industry to bring this development to fruition. However, the recent suspension of the WHO/CONRAD study implies an unexpected setback in the entire development of hormonal male contraception. Unless clear mistakes in the design or the conduct of the study can be detected during the current analysis of the study, it will be very difficult to get the pharma industry back on track or to attract new funding.

On a more general note, comparing the situation with the development of the female pill, the lack of public advocacy for male contraception is striking. Male contraception lacks prominent advocates, as the development of female contraception benefited from personalities such as Margaret Sanger (1879–1966) and Katherine McCormick (1875–1967). Hormonal male contraception requires similar advocacy to finally result in a marketable product (Nieschlag 2009). However, it should not be forgotten that there is a fundamental sex difference in the perception of contraception. For women contraception means personally avoiding pregnancy with all of its medical, social and economic implications including the threat of death. In contrast, for men contraception is more of an intellectual issue regarding respect for the partner and avoiding financial, social and legal obligations of fatherhood. Without emotion, however, it remains difficult to attract protagonists campaigning for male contraception.

22.9 Key messages

- Testosterone-induced azoospermia leads to effective, safe and reversible male contraception. Suppression of spermatogenesis to below

1 million/ml sperm may still be compatible with protection from pregnancy.

- About two-thirds of Caucasian and almost all East Asian men reach azoospermia when given weekly testosterone enanthate injections or four- to six-weekly injections of testosterone undecanoate.
- In order to speed up suppression of spermatogenesis and increase the rate of azoospermia, testosterone is combined with either progestins or GnRH antagonists.
- All effective approaches tested so far require injections or implantations. Self-administered

modalities (oral or transdermal) require a high rate of compliance.

- Side-effects of hormonal contraception were rare and tolerable until the WHO/CONRAD study was prematurely suspended because of mood alterations, the reasons for which have to be clarified.
- Acceptability of a hormonal method as assessed by opinion polls is high.
- After academic research established the principle of hormonal male contraception, it remains to be seen whether the pharmaceutical industry will enter the field of male contraception again.

22.10   References

Alvarez-Sanchez F, Faundes A, Brache V, Leon P (1977) Attainment and maintenance of azoospermia with combined monthly injections of depot medroxyprogesterone acetate and testosterone enanthate. *Contraception* **15**:635–648

Amory JK, Leonard TW, Page ST, O'Toole E, McKenna MJ, Bremner WJ (2009) Oral administration of the GnRH antagonist acyline, in a GIPET-enhanced tablet form, acutely suppresses serum testosterone in normal men: single-dose pharmacokinetics and pharmacodynamics. *Cancer Chemother Pharmacol* **64**:641–645

Anawalt BD, Bebb RA, Bremner WJ, Matsumoto AM (1999) A lower dosage levonorgestrel and testosterone combination effectively suppresses spermatogenesis and circulating gonadotrophin levels with fewer metabolic effects than higher dosage combinations. *J Androl* **20**:407–414

Anawalt BD, Herbst KL, Matsumoto AM, Mulders TM, Coelingh-Bennink HJ, Bremner WJ (2000) Desogestrel plus testosterone effectively suppresses spermatogenesis but also causes modest weight gain and high-density lipoprotein suppression. *Fertil Steril* **74**:707–714

Anawalt BD, Amory JK, Herbst KL, Coviello AD, Page ST, Bremner WJ, Matsumoto AM (2005)

Intramuscular testosterone enanthate plus very low dosage oral levonorgestrel suppresses spermatogenesis without causing weight gain in normal young men: a randomized clinical trial. *J Androl* **26**:405–413

Anderson RA, Baird DT (1997) Progress towards a male pill. *IPPF Med Bull* **31**:1–5

Anderson RA, Van Der Spuy ZM, Dada OA, Tregoning SK, Zinn PM, Adeniji OA, Fakoya TA, Smith KB, Baird DT (2002a) Investigation of hormonal male contraception in African men: suppression of spermatogenesis by oral desogestrel with depot testosterone. *Hum Reprod* **17**:2869–2877

Anderson RA, Kinniburgh D, Baird DT (2002b) Suppression of spermatogenesis by etonogestrel implants with depot testosterone: potential for long-acting male contraception. *J Clin Endocr Metab* **87**:3640–3649

Aribarg A, Sukcharoen N, Chanprasit Y, Ngeamvijawat J, Kriangsinyos R (1996) Suppression of spermatogenesis by testosterone enanthate in Thai men. *J Med Assoc Thai* **79**:624–629

Arysad, KM (1993) Sperm function in Indonesian men treated with testosterone enanthate. *Int J Androl* **16**:355–361

Bebb RA, Anawalt BD, Christensen RB, Paulsen CA, Bremner WJ, Matsumoto AM (1996) Combined

administration of levonorgestrel and testosterone induces more rapid and effective suppression of spermatogenesis than testosterone alone: a promising male contraceptive approach. *J Clin Endocr Metab* **81**:757–762

Behre HM, Nashan D, Hubert W, Nieschlag E (1992) Depot gonadotropin-releasing hormone agonist blunts the androgen-induced suppression of spermatogenesis in a clinical trial of male contraception. *J Clin Endocr Metab* **74**:84–90

Behre HM, Böckers A, Schlingheider A, Nieschlag E (1994) Sustained suppression of serum LH, FSH and testosterone and increase of high-density lipoprotein cholesterol by daily injections of the GnRH antagonist Cetrorelix over 8 days in normal men. *Clin Endocr* **40**:241–248

Behre HM, Baus S, Kliesch S, Keck C, Simoni M, Nieschlag E (1995) Potential of testosterone buciclate for male contraception: endocrine differences between responders and nonresponders. *J Clin Endocr Metab* **80**:2394–2403

Behre HM, Kliesch S, Lemcke B, Nieschlag E (2001) Suppression of spermatogenesis to azoospermia by combined administration of GnRH antagonist and 19-nortestosterone cannot be maintained by 19-nortestosterone alone in normal men. *Hum Reprod* **16**:2570–2577

Bhasin S, Berman N, Swerdloff RS (1994) Follicle-stimulating hormone (FSH) escape during chronic gonadotropin-releasing hormone (GnRH) agonist and testosterone treatment. *J Androl* **15**:386–391

Boccon-Gibod L, van der Meulen E, Persson BE (2011) An update on the use of gonadotropin-releasing hormone antagonists in prostate cancer. *Ther Adv Urol* **3**:127–140

Brady BM, Walton M, Hollow N, Kicman AT, Baird DT, Anderson RA (2004) Depot testosterone with etonogestrel implants result in induction of azoospermia in all men for long-term contraception. *Hum Reprod* **19**:2658–2667

Brenner PF, Mishell DR Jr, Bernstein GS, Ortiz A (1977) Study of medroxyprogesterone acetate and testosterone enanthate as a male contraceptive. *Contraception* **15**:679–691

Büchter D, von Eckardstein S, von Eckardstein A, Kamischke A, Simoni M, Behre HM, Nieschlag E (1999) Clinical trial of transdermal testosterone and oral levonorgestrel for male contraception. *J Clin Endocr Metab* **84**:1244–1249

Cao J, Yuan J, Jin W (1996) Clinical trial of an anti-fertility method with testosterone enanthate in normal men. *Chung Hua I Hsueh Tsa Chih* **76**:335–337

CONRAD (2011) Male Hormonal Contraceptive Trial Ending Early: Innovative Study is a Collaboration of WHO and CONRAD, April 22, 2011. Available at: http://www. conrad.org/news-pressreleases-63. html (accessed Jan 20, 2012)

Cooper TG, Yeung CH (2010) Pharmacological approaches to male contraception. In: Nieschlag E, Behre HM, Nieschlag S (eds) *Andrology. Male Reproductive Health and Dysfunction*, 3rd edn. Springer-Verlag, Berlin, pp 589–599

Djerassi C, Miramontes L, Rosenkranz G, Sonheimer F (1954) Steroids LIV. Synthesis of 19-nor-17α-

ethinyltestosterone and 19-nor-17α-methyltestosterone. *J Am Chem Soc* **76**:4092–4094

Ersheng G, Cuihong L, Youlun G, Lamei L, Changhai H (1999) Inhibiting effects of sino-implant plus testosterone undecanoate on spermatogenesis in Chinese men. *Reprod Contracept* **10**:98–105

Faundes A, Brache V, Leon P, Schmidt F, Alvarez-Sanchez F (1981) Sperm suppression with monthly injections of medroxyprogesterone acetate combined with testosterone enanthate at a high dose (500 mg). *Int J Androl* **4**:235–245

Fogh M, Corker CS, Hunter WM, McLean H, Philip J, Schon G, Skakkebaek NE (1979) The effects of low doses of cyproterone acetate on some functions of the reproductive system in normal men. *Acta Endocrinol* **91**:545

Fogh M, Corker CS, McLean H (1980) Clinical trial with levonorgestrel and testosterone enanthate for male fertility control. *Acta Endocrinol* **95**:251–257

Frick J, Bartsch G, Weiske WH (1977) The effect of monthly depot medroxyprogesterone acetate and testosterone on human spermatogenesis. II. High initial dose. *Contraception* **15**:669–677

Frick J, Danner C, Kunit G, Joos H, Kohle R (1982) Spermatogenesis in men treated with injections of medroxyprogesterone acetate combined with testosterone enanthate. *Int J Androl* **5**:246–252

Gaw Gonzalo IT, Swerdloff RS, Nelson AL, Clevenger B, Garcia R, Berman N, Wang C (2002) Levonorgestrel implants (Norplant II) for male contraception clinical trials: combination with transdermal and injectable testosterone. *J Clin Endocr Metab* **87**:3562–3572

Glasier A (2010) Acceptability of contraception for men: a review. *Contraception* **82**:453–450

Glasier AF, Anakwe R, Everington D, Martin CW, van der Spuy Z, Cheng

L, Ho PC, Anderson RA (2000) Would women trust their partners to use a male pill? *Hum Reprod* **15**:646–649

Grimes DA, Lopez LM, Gallo MF, Halpern V, Nanda K, Schulz KF (2007) Steroid hormones for contraception in men. *Cochrane Database Syst Rev* **18**:CD004316

Gu Y, Liang X, Wu W, Liu M, Song S, Cheng L, Bo L, Xiong C, Wang X, Liu X, Peng L, Yao K (2009) Multicenter contraceptive efficacy trial of injectable testosterone undecanoate in Chinese men. *J Clin Endocrinol Metab* **94**:1910–1915

Gu YQ, Wang X-H, Xu D, Peng L, Cheng L-F, Huang M-K, Huang Z-J, Zhang G-Y (2003) A multicenter contraceptive efficacy study of injectable testosterone undecanoate in healthy Chinese men. *J Clin Endocr Metab* **88**:562–568

Gu YQ, Tong JS, Ma DZ, Wang XH, Yuan D, Tang WH, Bremner WJ (2004) Male hormonal contraception: effects of injections of testosterone undecanoate and depot medroxyprogesterone acetate at eight-week intervals in Chinese men. *J Clin Endocrinol Metab* **89**:2254–2262

Guerin JF, Rollet J (1988) Inhibition of spermatogenesis in men using various combinations of oral progestagens and percutaneous or oral androgens. *Int J Androl* **11**:187–199

Gui YL, He CH, Amory JK, Bremner WJ, Zheng EX, Yang J, Yang PJ, Gao ES (2004) Male hormonal contraception: suppression of spermatogenesis by injectable testosterone undecanoate alone or with levonorgestrel implants in Chinese men. *J Androl* **25**:720–727

Hair WM, Kitteridge K, Wu FCW (1999) A new male contraceptive pill/patch combination – oral desogestrel and transdermal testosterone: suppression of gonadotropins and spermatogenesis in men. In: The Endocrine Society's 81st Annual Meeting; 1999

June 12–15; San Diego, CA, USA; Poster P3–374

Handelsman DJ, Conway AJ, Boylan LM (1992) Suppression of human spermatogenesis by testosterone implants. *J Clin Endocr Metab* **75**:1326–1332

Handelsman DJ, Conway AJ, Howe CJ, Turner L, Mackey MA (1996) Establishing the minimum effective dose and additive effects of depot progestin in suppression of human spermatogenesis by a testosterone depot. *J Clin Endocrinol Metab* **81**:4113–4121

Heinemann K, Saad F, Wiesemes M, White S, Heinemann L (2005) Attitudes toward male fertility control: results of a multinational survey on four continents. *Hum Reprod* **20**:549–556

Kamischke A, Nieschlag E (2004) Progress towards hormonal male contraception. *Trends Pharmacol Sci* **25**:49–57

Kamischke A, Plöger D, Venherm S, von Eckardstein S, von Eckardstein A, Nieschlag E (2000a) Intramuscular testosterone undecanoate with or without oral levonorgestrel: a randomized placebo-controlled feasibility study for male contraception. *Clin Endocrinol* **53**:43–52

Kamischke A, Diebäcker J, Nieschlag E (2000b) Potential of norethisterone enanthate for male contraception: pharmacokinetics and suppression of pituitary and gonadal function. *Clin Endocrinol* **53**:351–358

Kamischke A, Venherm S, Plöger D, von Eckardstein S, Nieschlag E (2001) Intramuscular testosterone undecanoate and norethisterone enanthate in a clinical trial for male contraception. *J Clin Endocr Metab* **86**:303–309

Kamischke A, Heuermann T, Krüger K, von Eckardstein S, Schellschmidt I, Rübig A, Nieschlag E (2002) An effective hormonal male contraceptive using testosterone undecanoate with oral or injectable

norethisterone preparations. *J Clin Endocr Metab* **87**:530–539

Kinniburgh D, Anderson RA, Baird DT (2001) Suppression of spermatogenesis with desogestrel and testosterone pellets is not enhanced by addition of finasteride. *J Androl* **22**:88–95

Kinniburgh D, Zhu H, Cheng L, Kicman AT, Baird DT, Anderson RA (2002) Oral desogestrel with testosterone pellets induces consistent suppression of spermatogenesis to azoospermia in both Caucasian and Chinese men. *Hum Reprod* **17**:1490–1501

Knuth UA, Behre, HM, Belkien L, Bents H, Nieschlag E (1985) Clinical trial of 19-nortestosterone-hexoxyphenylpropionate (Anadur) for male fertility regulation. *Fertil Steril* **44**:814–821

Knuth UA, Yeung CH, Nieschlag E (1989) Combination of 19-nortestosterone-hexoxyphenylpropionate (Anadur) and depot-medroxyprogesterone-acetate (Clinovir) for male contraception. *Fertil Steril* **51**:1011–1018

Liu PY, Swerdloff RS, Christenson PD, Handelsman DJ, Wang C; Hormonal Male Contraception Summit Group (2006) Rate, extent and modifiers of spermatogenic recovery after hormonal male contraception: an integrated analysis. *Lancet* **367**:1412–1420

Martin CW, Anderson RA, Cheng L, Ho PC, van der Spuy Z, Smith KB, Glasier AF, Everington D, Baird DT (2000) Potential impact of hormonal male contraception: cross-cultural implications for development of novel preparations. *Hum Reprod* **15**:637–645

McLachlan RI, McDonald J, Rushford D, Robertson DM, Garrett C, Baker HW (2000) Efficacy and acceptability of testosterone implants, alone or in combination with a 5α-reductase inhibitor, for male hormonal contraception. *Contraception* **62**:73–78

McLachlan RI, O'Donnell L, Stanton PG, Balourdos G, Frydenberg M, DeKretser DM, Robertson DM (2002) Effects of testosterone enanthate plus medroxyprogesterone acetate on semen quality, reproductive hormones and germ cell populations in normal young men. *J Clin Endocrinol Metab* **87**:546–556

Melo JF, Coutinho EM (1977) Inhibition of spermatogenesis in men with monthly injections of medroxyprogesterone acetate and testosterone enanthate. *Contraception* **15**:627–634

Meriggiola MC, Bremner WJ, Paulsen CA, Valdiserri A, Incorvala L, Motta R, Pavani A, Capelli M, Flamigni C (1996) A combined regimen of cyproterone acetate and testosterone enanthate as a potentially highly effective male contraceptive. *J Clin Endocr Metab* **81**:3018–3023

Meriggiola MC, Bremner WJ, Costantino A, Pavani A, Capelli M, Flamigni C (1997) An oral regimen of cyproterone acetate and testosterone undecanoate for spermatogenic suppression in men. *Fertil Steril* **68**:844–850

Meriggiola MC, Bremner WJ, Costantino A, Di Cintio G, Flamigni C (1998) Low dose of cyproterone acetate and testosterone enanthate for contraception in men. *Hum Reprod* **13**:1225–1229

Meriggiola MC, Costantino A, Bremner WJ, Morselli-Labate AM (2002a) Higher testosterone dose impairs sperm suppression induced by a combined androgen-progestin regimen. *J Androl* **23**:684–690

Meriggiola MC, Bremner WJ, Costantino A, Bertaccini A, Morselli-Labate AM, Huebler D, Kaufmann G, Oettel M, Flamigni C (2002b) Twenty-one day administration of dienogest reversibly suppresses gonadotropins and testosterone in normal men. *J Clin Endocrinol Metab* **87**:2107–2113

Meriggiola MC, Costantino A, Cerpolini S, Bremner WJ, Huebler D, Morselli-Labate AM, Kirsch B, Bertaccini A, Pelusi C, Pelusi G (2003) Testosterone undecanoate maintains spermatogenic suppression induced by cyproterone acetate plus testosterone undecanoate in normal men. *J Clin Endocrinol Metab* **88**:5818–5826

Meriggiola MC, Costantino A, Saad F, D'Emidio L, Morselli Labate AM, Bertaccini A, Bremner WJ, Rudolph I, Ernst M, Kirsch B, Martorana G, Pelusi G (2005) Norethisterone enanthate plus testosterone undecanoate for male contraception: effects of various injection intervals on spermatogenesis, reproductive hormones, testis, and prostate. *J Clin Endocrinol Metab* **90**:2005–2014

Misro MM, Chaki SP, Kaushik MC, Nandan D (2009) Trials for development of once-a-month injectable, hormonal male contraceptive using dienogest plus testosterone undecanoate: dose standardization, efficacy and reversibility studies in rats. *Contraception* **79**:488–497

Moltz L, Römmler A, Post K, Schwartz U, Hammerstein J (1980) Medium dose cyproterone acetate (CPA): effects on hormone secretion and on spermatogenesis in man. *Contraception* **21**:393

Mommers E, Kersemaeker WM, Elliesen J, Kepers M, Apter D, Behre HM, Beynon J, Bouloux PM, Costantino A, Gerbershagen HP, Gronlund L, Heger-Mahn D, Huhtaniemi I, Koldewihn EL, Lange C, Lindenberg S, Meriggiola MC, Meuleman E, Mulder PFA, Nieschlag E, Perheentupa A, Solomon A, Väisälä L, Wu FC, Zitzmann M (2008) Male hormonal contraception: a double-blind, placebo-controlled study. *J Clin Endocrinol Metab* **93**:2572–2580

Narula A, Gu Y-Q, O'Donnell L, Stanton PG, Robertson DM, McLachlan RI, Bremner WJ (2002)

Variability in sperm suppression during testosterone administration to adult monkeys is related to follicle stimulating hormone suppression and not to intratesticular androgens. *J Clin Endocrinol Metab* **87**:3399–3406

Nieschlag E (1986) Reasons for abandoning immunization against FSH as an approach to male fertility regulation. In: Zatuchni GI, Goldsmith A, Spieler JM, Sciarra J (eds) *Male Contraception: Advances and Future Prospects.* Harper & Row, Philadelphia, pp 395–400

Nieschlag E (2009) Male hormonal contraception: love's labour's lost? (Editorial) *J Clin Endocrinol Metab* **94**:1890–1892

Nieschlag E, Behre HM (1996) Hormonal male contraception: suppression of spermatogenesis with GnRH antagonists and testosterone. In: Filicori M, Flamigni C (eds) *Treatment with GnRH Analogs: Controversies and Perspectives.* Parthenon, London, pp 243–248

Nieschlag E, Hoogen H, Bölk M, Schuster H, Wickings EJ (1978) Clinical trial with testosterone undecanoate for male fertility control. *Contraception* **18**:607–614

Nieschlag E, Behre HM, Weinbauer GF (1992) Hormonal male contraception: a real chance? In: Nieschlag E, Habenicht UF (eds) *Spermatogenesis – Fertilization – Contraception. Molecular, Cellular and Endocrine Events in Male Reproduction.* Springer, Heidelberg, pp 477–501

Nieschlag E; 10th Summit Meeting Group (2007) 10th Summit Meeting consensus: recommendations for regulatory approval for hormonal male contraception. October 22–23, 2006. *Contraception* **75**:166–167

Nieschlag E, Nieschag S, Behre HM (eds) (2010) *Andrology. Male Reproductive Health and Dysfunction*, 3rd edn. Springer-Verlag, Berlin

Nieschlag E, Vorona E, Wenk M, Hemker AK, Kamischke A, Zitzmann M (2011) Hormonal male contraception in men with normal and subnormal semen parameters. *Int J Androl* **34**:556–567

Page ST, Amory JK, Anawalt BD, Irwig MS, Brockenbrough AT, Matsumoto AM, Bremner WJ (2006) Testosterone gel combined with depomedroxyprogesterone acetate is an effective male hormonal contraceptive regimen and is not enhanced by the addition of a GnRH antagonist. *J Clin Endocrinol Metab* **91**:4374–4380

Pangkahila W (1991) Reversible azoospermia induced by an androgen-progestin combination regimen in Indonesian men. *Int J Androl* **14**:248–256

Patanelli DJ (ed) (1978) *Hormonal Control of Male Fertility (Workshop Proceedings)*, NIH Publication No. 78-1097. US Department of Health, Education, and Welfare (NIH), Bethesda, MD

Pavlou SN, Wakefield G, Schlechter NL, Lindner J, Souza KH, Kamilaris TC, Konidaris S, Rivier JE, Vale WW, Toglia M (1989) Mode of suppression of pituitary and gonadal function after acute or prolonged administration of a luteinizing hormone-releasing hormone antagonist in normal men. *J Clin Endocrinol Metab* **73**:1360–1369

Pavlou SN, Herodotou D, Curtain M, Minaretzis D (1994) Complete suppression of spermatogenesis by co-administration of a GnRH antagonist plus a physiologic dose of testosterone. In: *Proceedings of the 76th Meeting of the Endocrine Society, Anaheim, CA*, p 1324

Pöllänen P, Nikkanen V, Huhtaniemi I (2001) Combination of subcutaneous levonorgestrel implants and transdermal dihydrotestosterone gel for male hormonal contraception. *Int J Androl* **24**:369–380

Qoubaitary A, Meriggiola C, Ng CM, Lumbreras L, Cerpolini S, Pelusi G, Christensen PD, Hull L, Swerdloff RS, Wang C (2006) Pharmacokinetics of testosterone undecanoate injected alone or in combination with norethisterone enanthate in healthy men. *J Androl* 27:853–867

Reddy PR, Rao JM (1972) Reversible antifertility action of testosterone propionate in human males. *Contraception* 5:295–301

Schearer SB, Alvarez-Sanches F, Anselmo G, Brenner P, Coutinho E, Lathen-Faundes A, Frick J, Heinild B, Johansson EDB (1978) Hormonal contraception for men. *Int J Androl* **2** (Suppl 2):680–712

Schürmeyer T, Knuth UA, Belkien L, Nieschlag E (1984) Reversible azoospermia induced by the anabolic steroid 19-nortestosterone. *Lancet* **25**:417–420

Singh S, Sedh G, Hussain R (2010) Unintended pregnancy: worldwide levels, trends, and outcomes. *Stud Fam Plann* **41**:241–250

Soufir JC, Meduri G, Ziyyat A (2011) Spermatogenetic inhibition in men taking a combination of oral medroxyprogesterone acetate and percutaneous testosterone as a male contraceptive method. *Hum Reprod* 26:1708–1714

Srinath BR, Wickings EJ, Witting CH, Nieschlag E (1983) Active immunization with follicle stimulating hormone for fertility control: a 4 1/2-year study in male rhesus monkeys. *Fertil Steril* **40**:110–117

Swerdloff RS, Bagatell CJ, Wang C, Anawalt BD, Berman N, Steiner B, Bremner WJ (1998) Suppression of spermatogenesis in man induced by Nal-Glu gonadotropin releasing hormone antagonist and testosterone enanthate (TE) is maintained by TE alone. *J Clin Endocr Metab* 83:3527–3533

Turner L, Wishart S, Conway AJ, Liu PY, Forbes E, McLachlan RI, Handelsman DJ (2003)

Contraceptive efficacy of a depot progestin and androgen combination in men. *J Clin Endocr Metab* 88:4659–4667

von Eckardstein S, Schmidt A, Kamischke A, Simoni M, Gromoll J, Nieschlag E (2002) CAG repeat length in the androgen receptor gene and gonadotropin suppression influence the effectiveness of hormonal male contraception. *Clin Endocrinol* 57:647–655

von Eckardstein S, Noé G, Brache V, Nieschlag E, Croxatto H, Alvarez F, Moo-Young A, Sivin I, Kumar N, Small M, Sundaram K (2003) A clinical trial of 7α-methyl-19-nortestosterone implants for possible use as a long acting contraceptive for men. *J Clin Endocrinol Metab* **88**:5232–5239

Waites GMH (2003) Development of methods of male contraception: the impact of the World Health Organization Task Force. *Fertil Steril* 80:1–15

Walton MJ, Kumar N, Baird DT, Ludlow H, Anderson RA (2007) 7alpha-methyl-19-nortestosterone (MENT) vs testosterone in combination with etonogestrel implants for spermatogenic suppression in healthy men. *J Androl* **28**:679–688

Wang C, Yeung KK (1980) Use of low-dosage oral cyproterone acetate as a male contraceptive. *Contraception* 21:245

Wang C, Wang XH, Nelson AL (2006) Levonorgestrel implants enhanced the suppression of spermatogenesis by testosterone implants: comparison between Chinese and non-Chinese men. *J Clin Endocrinol Metab* **91**:460–470

Wang C, Cui YG, Wang XH, Jia Y, Sinha Hikim A, Lue YH, Tong JS, Qian LX, Sha JH, Zhou ZM, Hull L, Leung A, Swerdloff RS (2007) Transient scrotal hyperthermia and levonorgestrel enhance testosterone-induced spermatogenesis suppression in men through increased germ cell

apoptosis. *J Clin Endocrinol Metab* 92:3292–3304

Weinbauer GF, Nieschlag E (1996) The Leydig cell as a target for male contraception. In: Payne AH, Hardy MP, Russell LD (eds) *The Leydig Cell.* Cache River Press, Vienna, IL, pp 629–662

Weinbauer GF, Surmann FJ, Nieschlag E (1987) Suppression of spermatogenesis in a nonhuman primate (Macaca fascicularis) by concomitant gonadotropin-releasing hormone (GnRH) antagonist and testosterone treatment. *Acta Endocrinol* **114**:138–146

Weinbauer GF, Khurshid S, Fingscheidt U, Nieschlag E (1989) Sustained inhibition of sperm production and inhibin secretion induced by a gonadotropin-releasing hormone antagonist and delayed testosterone substitution in non-human primates (Macaca fascicularis). *J Endocrinol* **123**:303–310

Weinbauer GF, Limberger A, Behre HM, Nieschlag E (1994) Can testosterone alone maintain the gonadotropin-releasing hormone antagonist-induced suppression of spermatogenesis in the non-human primate? *J Endocrinol* **142**:485–495

Weinbauer GF, Schlatt S, Walter V, Nieschlag E (2001) Testosterone-induced inhibition of spermatogenesis is more closely related to suppression of FSH than to testicular androgen levels in the cynomolgus monkey model (Macaca fascicularis). *J Endocrinol* **168**:25–38

Weston GC, Schlipalius ML, Bhuinneain MN, Vollenhoven BJ (2002) Will Australian men use male hormonal contraception? A survey of a postpartum population. *Med J Aust* 176:204–205

WHO (1972–1995) *Special Programme of Research, Development and Research Training in Human Reproduction,* Annual and Biannual

Reports. World Health Organization, Geneva

WHO Task Force on Methods for the Regulation of Male Fertility (1990) Contraceptive efficacy of testosterone-induced azoospermia in normal men. *Lancet* **336**:955–959

WHO Task Force on Methods for the Regulation of Male Fertility (1993) Comparison of two androgens plus depot-medroxyprogesterone acetate for suppression to azoospermia in Indonesian men. *Fertil Steril* **60**:1062–1068

WHO Task Force on Methods for the Regulation of Male Fertility (1995) Rates of testosterone-induced suppression to severe oligozoospermia or azoospermia in two multinational clinical studies. *Int J Androl* **18**:157–165

WHO Task Force on Methods for the Regulation of Male Fertility (1996) Contraceptive efficacy of testosterone-induced azoospermia and oligozoospermia in normal men. *Fertil Steril* **65**:821–829

Wu FC, Aitken RJ (1989) Suppression of sperm function by depot medroxyprogesterone acetate and testosterone enanthate in steroid male contraception. *Fertil Steril* **51**:691–698

Wu FCW, Balasubramanian R, Mulders TMT, Coelingh-Bennink HJT (1999) Oral progestogen combined with testosterone as a potential male contraceptive: additive effects between desogestrel and testosterone enanthate in suppression of spermatogenesis, pituitary-testicular axis, and lipid

metabolism. *J Clin Endocr Metab* **84**:12–122

Zhang GY, Gu YQ, Wang XH, Cui YG, Bremner WJ (1999) A clinical trial of injectable testosterone undecanoate as a potential male contraceptive in normal Chinese men. *J Clin Endocrinol Metab* **84**:3642–3647

Zhang L, Shal IH, Liu Y, Vogelsong KM, Zhang L (2006) The acceptability of an injectable, once-a-month male contraceptive in China. *Contraception* **73**:548–553

Zitzmann M, Junker R, Kamischke A, Nieschlag E (2002) Contraceptive steroids influence the hemostatic activation state in healthy men. *J Androl* **23**:503–511

Chapter 23

Testosterone use in women

Susan R. Davis

23.1 Introduction

The role of testosterone in women and its potential as a therapeutic agent continues to attract controversy. Testosterone levels in women decline with age from the mid-reproductive years, and are low in women who have experienced surgical menopause, premature ovarian failure and hypopituitarism. The primary outcome of clinical trials on the effects of testosterone

Testosterone: Action, Deficiency, Substitution, ed. Eberhard Nieschlag and Hermann M. Behre, Assoc. ed. Susan Nieschlag. Published by Cambridge University Press. © Cambridge University Press 2012.

in women has been on treatment of female sexual dysfunction; notably that characterized by loss of sexual desire. There is substantial evidence that judicious testosterone therapy is effective for the treatment of loss of sexual desire in postmenopausal women and women approaching the late reproductive years, as well as women with ovarian or pituitary failure, with doses given that achieve circulating levels close to the physiological range for young reproductive women. The greatest body of clinical data is from studies of transdermal testosterone in postmenopausal women. The link between postmenopausal estrogen-progestin use and both breast cancer and cardiovascular disease has created a level of concern regarding any form of hormone use in women. Objective data show no adverse cardiovascular effects of transdermal testosterone therapy, and cumulative data from RCTs do not indicate increased cancer risk in women treated with testosterone. A recent Cochrane Review (Somboonporn et al. 2005) has thoroughly evaluated the evidence for the effects of testosterone added to estrogen therapy in postmenopausal women. This chapter reviews the physiology of testosterone in women, summarizes the findings from observational studies and clinical trials, and considers indications for use.

23.2 Physiology

23.2.1 Testosterone physiology in the female reproductive years

In healthy, young, reproductive-aged women testosterone circulates in nanomolar concentrations, in contrast to picomolar levels of estradiol. The production of testosterone in premenopausal women is of the order of 0.2 to 0.25 mg per day (Longcope 1986). Approximately half of the circulating testosterone is produced by the ovaries, with the remainder produced by peripheral conversion of pre-androgens to testosterone, with androstenedione being the main precursor. Whether there is direct secretion of testosterone by the adrenals continues to be debated. The pre-androgens, androstenedione and DHEA, are produced by both the ovaries and the adrenals, with the adrenals also being the main site of production of DHEAS. Circulating DHEAS is an important precursor for the ovarian intrafollicular production of testosterone and DHT (Haning et al. 1993). Whether the postmenopausal ovary continues to secrete testosterone remains contentious, as discussed below. Hence, there is ongoing debate

regarding elective bilateral oophorectomy in peri/postmenopausal women undergoing hysterectomy.

Testosterone can undergo 5α-reduction to form DHT. Dihydrotestosterone can then be converted to androstane-3α,17β-diol (3α-diol), which in turn can be glucuronidated at carbons 3 or 17 to form 3α-diol-3-glucuronide (3α-diol,3G) or 3α-diol-17-glucuronide (3α-diol,17G), of which 3α-diol,17G is the predominant form. Plasma 3α-diol,17G is a marker of peripheral androgen action and is significantly elevated in idiopathic hirsutism (Horton et al. 1982). Alternatively, testosterone can be aromatized to estradiol in extra-gonadal tissues including the brain, adipose tissue, vascular endothelium and bone (Simpson and Davis 2001). Therefore, maintenance of physiological circulating testosterone levels in women ensures adequate supply of substrate for estrogen biosynthesis in extra-gonadal sites, such as bone, in which high tissue estrogen concentrations may be physiologically important. That the primary source of estrogen in extra-gonadal sites is that produced locally from androgens also explains the apparent threshold dose of estrogen replacement after menopause below which bone loss continues, and the observation that, whereas standard estrogen replacement therapy has little effect on libido (Utian 1972; Campbell and Whitehead 1977), most parameters of sexuality improve when extremely high doses of estrogen are administered (Davis et al. 1995).

There is significant cyclicity in plasma levels of androstenedione and testosterone in regularly ovulating women, with increases in the mean circulating levels of both of these hormones in the middle third of the menstrual cycle (Mushayandebvu et al. 1996). This is followed by a second rise in androstenedione production by the corpus luteum during the late luteal phase. Ovarian androgens are produced by the thecal cells under the control of LH.

Under normal physiological conditions, only 1–2% of total circulating testosterone in women circulates unbound to plasma proteins. The rest is bound by sex hormone-binding globulin (SHBG) and albumin, with SHBG binding 66% of total circulating testosterone in healthy women (Dunn et al. 1981). The binding affinity for steroids bound by SHBG is DHT > testosterone > androstenediol > estradiol > estrone (Dunn et al. 1981). SHBG also weakly binds DHEA, but not DHEAS (Dunn et al. 1981). Therefore, variations in the plasma levels of SHBG will influence the amount of unbound testosterone. It is frequently stated that endogenous testosterone lowers, and estrogen increases, SHBG production. However, in-vitro studies show that extremely high levels of estradiol and testosterone are required to influence SHBG biosynthesis and release from the hepatocytes (Edmunds *et al.* 1990; Loukovaara *et al.* 1995). Taken together, in-vitro studies indicate no effect of estradiol and testosterone on hepatocyte SHBG production at physiological concentrations seen in women; high hepatic concentrations of estradiol, as seen with oral estrogen, might increase SHBG biosynthesis, but there are conflicting findings for effects of supraphysiological testosterone on hepatocyte SHBG production (Loukovaara *et al.* 1995). There is also a widely held belief that insulin suppresses SHBG production (Pugeat *et al.* 2000). However, insulin does not directly regulate SHBG gene expression in vitro, but rather fructose and glucose, as well as peroxisome-proliferator receptor gamma are key regulators of human SHBG biosynthesis (Selva *et al.* 2007; Selva and Hammond 2009). Fructose and glucose-induced lipogenesis reduces hepatocyte nuclear factor 4alpha levels, which in turn attenuate SHBG expression (Selva *et al.* 2007). This in part explains why SHBG is a sensitive biomarker of the metabolic disturbances associated with increased fructose consumption.

23.2.2 Physiological and non-physiological causes of lower testosterone levels in women

The main cause of lowered testosterone levels in women is the natural decline with age. The mean circulating levels of total and free testosterone decline continuously with increasing age from the early reproductive years, such that the levels of women in their forties are approximately half of those of women in their twenties, as shown in Fig. 23.1 (Zumoff *et al.* 1995; Davison *et al.* 2005a). Androstenedione and DHEAS levels also fall linearly with age (Davison *et al.* 2005a), and this may contribute to the decline in the level of their main metabolite, testosterone. In the late reproductive years there is failure of the mid-cycle rise in free testosterone that characterizes the menstrual cycle in young ovulating women (Mushayandebvu *et al.* 1996). This occurs despite preservation of normal free testosterone levels at other phases of the cycle. The mean plasma concentrations of testosterone in women transiting the menopause are also significantly lower than younger ovulating women sampled in the early follicular phase. Testosterone levels do not fall at menopause. Across the perimenopausal period total testosterone, androstenedione,

DHT and the ratio of total testosterone to SHBG do not change (Burger *et al.* 1995; Davison *et al.* 2005a).

Most studies indicate that the postmenopausal ovary in many women continues to produce testosterone. Acutely following oophorectomy there is a decline in testosterone, with both testosterone and androstenedione decreasing acutely by about 50% (Judd *et al.* 1994), and postmenopausal women who have undergone bilateral oophorectomy have been found to have lower total and free testosterone levels than women who have not (Laughlin *et al.* 2000; Davison *et al.* 2005a). Peripheral and ovarian vein sampling of women undergoing bilateral oophorectomy with and without GnRH therapy has demonstrated that the postmenopausal ovary is hormonally active and contributes significantly to the pool of testosterone in women (Judd *et al.* 1974; Sluijmer *et al.* 1995; Fogle *et al.* 2007). In contrast, other investigators believe that the postmenopausal ovary does not produce testosterone (Couzinet *et al.* 2001; Labrie *et al.* 2010). In a study comparing healthy postmenopausal women with and without oophorectomy and/or adrenalectomy, adrenalectomy was associated with total and bioavailable testosterone below the detection limit; whereas androstenedione was reduced but measurable, even in women who had undergone both oophorectomy and adrenalectomy (Couzinet *et al.* 2001). In this study the number of women providing data was small, and there was marked variability in testosterone levels. Another more recent study of oophorectomized and ovary-intact women has shown wide ranges of testosterone levels in these populations, and although an argument was mounted that the study demonstrated no direct contribution of testosterone from the postmenopausal ovary, this was not supported by the study data (Labrie *et al.* 2010).

Hysterectomy has also been associated with lower circulating testosterone in women (Laughlin *et al.* 2000; Davison *et al.* 2005a). Other iatrogenic causes of low testosterone include chemical oophorectomy; for example, the use of GnRH antagonists for the treatment of fibroids or endometriosis, postchemotherapy or radiotherapy, and the administration of oral estrogens or oral glucocorticosteroids. In general, circulating free testosterone is suppressed in women using either the combined oral contraceptive pill or oral estrogen as hormone replacement therapy (Mathur *et al.* 1985; Krug *et al.* 1994). This is a result of an increase in SHBG combined with suppression of LH production by the pituitary and, hence, decreased stimulus for the ovarian stromal production of

Total testosterone

DHEAS

Free testosterone

Androstenedione

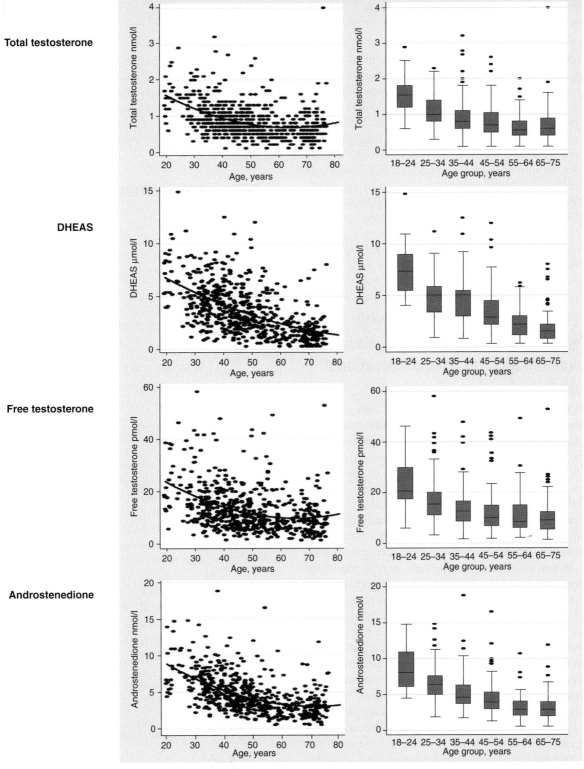

Fig. 23.1 Relationship between age and individual androgens in women (Davison *et al.* 2005a) with permission. To convert nmol/l to ng/dl or pmol/liter to pg/dl, divide by 0.0347; to convert µmol/liter to µg/dl divide by 0.027. Raw data are represented as scattergraphs with fitted regression curves. In the box and whisker plots, the box represents the interquartile range (IQR), the line in the box is the median. The whiskers extend to the upper and lower adjacent values. The upper adjacent value is defined as the largest data point ≤ the 75th percentile + 1.5 × IQR. The lower adjacent value is defined as the smallest data point ≥ the 25th percentile − 1.5 × IQR. Outliers are any values beyond the whiskers. DHEAS = dehydroepiandrosterone sulfate.

testosterone. These effects may be amplified in older women whose overall androgen production is declining. Treatment with oral glucocorticosteroids results in ACTH suppression and, hence, reduced adrenal androgen production (Abraham 1974). Total testosterone levels are significantly lower in premenopausal and postmenopausal women with hypopituitarism due to loss of both ovarian and adrenal androgen production (Miller *et al.* 2001; Zang and Davis 2008).

In the premenopausal years, other pathophysiological states such as hypothalamic amenorrhea and hyperprolactinemia are characterized by low circulating testosterone levels (Miller *et al.* 2007). Similarly, women with premature ovarian failure have lowered androgen levels (Kalantaridou *et al.* 2006).

23.3 Clinical associations with endogenous testosterone levels in women: findings from observational studies

Studies investigating relationships between endogenous testosterone levels and health outcomes are confounded by a number of factors. Androgens undergo substantial metabolism in extra-gonadal tissues (Labrie 1991), such that circulating blood levels in women may not accurately reflect tissue concentrations or tissue effects. Precise measurement of testosterone at very low concentrations has been an ongoing challenge for clinical research in this field (Taieb *et al.* 2003). Furthermore, as testosterone is an obligatory precursor for estrogen production, it is difficult to differentiate the independent effects of testosterone versus estrogen for pathophysiological outcomes. Also often disregarded is that studies evaluating testosterone action commonly report both total testosterone levels and the FAI. The FAI (total testosterone / SHBG × 100) is believed, by some, to reflect biologically active testosterone. Sometimes the term "bioavailable testosterone" is loosely used when unbound testosterone has been estimated by the FAI. SHBG levels vary substantially in women, with endogenous levels inversely linked to central adiposity and insulin levels (Nestler and Strauss 1991; Goodman-Gruen and Barrett-Connor 1997; Randolph *et al.* 2003). In the many studies in which total testosterone is not associated with the outcome of interest, but SHBG and the FAI or "bioavailable" testosterone are, the likelihood is that SHBG is driving the association.

Taking into consideration that endogenous hormone levels may be poor indicators of their clinical effects, various studies have attempted to delineate the relationships between testosterone and clinical characteristics including sexual function, well-being, cardiovascular disease (CVD) risk, insulin resistance and cognition.

23.3.1 Testosterone and sexual function

The relationships between androgens and sexual function were explored in a cross-sectional study of 1423 non-healthcare seeking women, aged 18 to 75 years, randomly recruited from the community via the electoral roll, of whom 1021 completed a validated sexual function questionnaire (Davis *et al.* 2005). Total and free testosterone levels were not related to sexual function scores. However, women aged 45 years or more with low sexual responsiveness had a greater likelihood of having a serum DHEAS value below the 10th centile for their age (odds ratio 3.9; 95% confidence interval 1.54–9.81; $p = 0.004$). For women aged 18 to 44 years, having low sexual desire, sexual arousal or sexual responsiveness was also associated with having a DHEAS value below the 10th centile for their age (Davis *et al.* 2005). As the normal range for serum DHEAS amongst young women is relatively large and a significant proportion of women with low DHEAS do not have low sexual function, a cutoff level below which women can be said to be more likely to have low sexual function could not be identified.

There is also evidence that testosterone is associated with vaginal health, with levels being inversely associated with vaginal atrophy in postmenopausal women (Leiblum *et al.* 1983). Testosterone has vasodilatory effects (Worboys *et al.* 2001), enhancing vaginal blood flow and lubrication with sexual arousal (Leiblum *et al.* 1983; Tuiten *et al.* 2000). These effects may be due to direct androgen actions or in part be due to estradiol biosynthesis from testosterone in the vascular bed (Harada *et al.* 1999). The clinical significance of this is that the complaint of vaginal dryness is usually attributed to estrogen deficiency, whereas failure to lubricate with sexual stimulation may require adequate androgen action.

23.3.2 Testosterone and well-being

Lowered well-being is a common complaint amongst women at midlife. However, evidence that low testosterone underpins diminished well-being is lacking. In a study in which 1224 premenopausal and postmenopausal women completed a validated psychological general well-being questionnaire, no relationship between overall well-being and total or free testosterone was identified (Bell *et al.* 2006).

23.3.3 Testosterone and cardiovascular disease

Observational studies consistently demonstrate that both endogenous testosterone and SHBG are inversely associated with increased CVD risk in women. In a cross-sectional, community-based study exploring the relationships between androgens and CVD risk markers, total testosterone was not associated with circulating lipid levels or CRP when age, smoking, alcohol, BMI and exercise were taken into account (Bell *et al.* 2007). For premenopausal women, free testosterone explained 1% of the variance in CRP. SHBG contributed significantly to variations in CRP, triglycerides and HDL-C in both pre- and post-menopausal women. Similarly other researchers have found a strong inverse relationship between SHBG and CRP when adjusting for other variables (Joffe *et al.* 2006).

The FAI, but not total testosterone, has been related to the metabolic syndrome and increased CVD risk (Golden *et al.* 2004; Sutton-Tyrrell *et al.* 2005). The FAI has been strongly associated with visceral fat in postmenopausal women, even after adjusting for insulin resistance (Janssen *et al.* 2010). The FAI and SHBG were interchangeable in their strength of association with visceral fat, whereas total testosterone was not related to visceral fat. Thus SHBG is the factor in the FAI associated with visceral fat, not testosterone. Similarly, in young to middle-aged women, SHBG levels, but not total or free testosterone, have been inversely associated with sub-clinical CVD (Calderon-Margalit *et al.* 2010) and coronary artery calcium (Ouyang *et al.* 2009). Thus SHBG, not testosterone, underpins the relationship between FAI and CVD risk factors in these studies.

Endogenous testosterone has been positively associated with brachial artery flow-mediated dilatation, a measure of endothelial function, in postmenopausal women (Montalcini *et al.* 2007). Free testosterone has been inversely associated with carotid intima-media thickness (Bernini *et al.* 1999), and total and free testosterone are inversely associated with internal carotid artery atherosclerosis (Debing *et al.* 2007). Most recently, prevalent CVD in older women has been associated with lower levels of androgen precursors and a higher estradiol-to-testosterone ratio (Naessen *et al.* 2010). Furthermore, women with a total testosterone level in the lowest quintile were observed to have the greatest risk for all-cause mortality and incident CVD, independent of traditional risk factors, over a 4.5-year follow-up period (Sievers *et al.* 2010). Polycystic ovarian syndrome (PCOS) is a common condition characterized by hyperinsulinemia and androgen excess. The largest observational study reporting the morbidity and mortality associated with this condition did not find an increase in coronary heart disease morbidity or mortality in women with PCOS, although these women had more CVD risk factors (Wild *et al.* 2000).

Taken together, observational studies indicate low, not high testosterone is associated with CVD risk in women.

23.3.4 Testosterone and osteoporosis

Testosterone appears to have skeletal effects, either via the AR or as a precursor for estradiol production in bone. Testosterone levels have been positively correlated with BMD in premenopausal and postmenopausal women (Slemenda *et al.* 1996; Rariy *et al.* 2011). For women aged 67 years or more, total testosterone is positively associated with BMD at the lumbar spine and hip, even after adjusting for estradiol, and free testosterone is positively associated with hip BMD, lean body mass, and body fat (Rariy *et al.* 2011).

To investigate the relationship between testosterone and hip fracture in postmenopausal women, 400 participants in the Women's Health Initiative Observational Study who experienced their first non-pathological hip fracture (median follow-up, seven years) were matched with 400 controls by age, ethnicity and baseline blood draw date (Lee *et al.* 2008). High endogenous testosterone was associated with a significantly decreased risk of hip fracture, independent of SHBG, serum estradiol concentration and other potential risk factors.

In women with anorexia nervosa, total and free testosterone levels, but not estradiol, are positively associated with bone volume fraction and trabecular thickness after controlling for BMI (Lawson *et al.* 2010). Androgen receptors have been demonstrated in human osteoblast-like cell lines, and androgens have been shown to directly stimulate bone cell proliferation and differentiation (Kasperk *et al.* 1989).

23.3.5 Testosterone and cognitive function

Testosterone has been reported to have neuroprotective properties (Rosario *et al.* 2009). Higher endogenous testosterone levels in premenopausal women have been linked with better performance in tasks of spatial and mathematical ability (Gouchie and Kimura 1991); whilst in elderly women higher testosterone levels have been associated with superior performance on verbal fluency and verbal memory tasks (Wolf and Kirschbaum 2002). Levels of testosterone in the human female brain during the reproductive years are several-fold greater than those of estradiol (Bixo *et al.* 1995). Within the brain testosterone exhibits neuroprotective effects including protection against oxidative stress, serum deprivation-induced apoptosis and soluble beta amyloid (Aβ) toxicity (Pike *et al.* 2009). Although some of these effects of testosterone are blocked by aromatase inhibition and thus appear to be estrogen-mediated, protection against Aβ toxicity appears to be AR-mediated (Pike *et al.* 2009). There is also evidence that endogenous androgens influence levels of Aβ, possibly by an AR-dependent mechanism involving upregulation of the Aβ-catabolizing enzyme neprilysin (Yao *et al.* 2008). In addition to having neuroprotective effects, testosterone has positive effects on endothelial function (Montalcini *et al.* 2007) and acts as a vasodilator (Worboys *et al.* 2001), such that testosterone-induced vascular effects may contribute to neuroprotective effects. As mild cognitive impairment precedes the development of dementia by several years, and a parallel is seen between the fall of testosterone levels in women and the rise in incidence of mild cognitive decline and dementia, further exploration of this association is warranted.

23.4 Effects of testosterone: findings from randomized, controlled trials

23.4.1 The use of testosterone for the treatment of female sexual dysfunction

There is no diagnostic lower limit for testosterone or free testosterone that can be used to classify a woman as androgen deficient (Davis *et al.* 2005). Thus the use of testosterone therapy for women is not based on an established link between symptoms and biochemistry, but rather clinical evidence that exogenous testosterone improves the most commonly reported sexual problems in women. These are sexual desire and arousal, pleasure and overall satisfaction (Laumann *et al.* 1999; Hayes *et al.* 2008). For most women, these problems are part of a continuum of the sexual experience, and are inextricably related. Recent studies evaluating the efficacy of testosterone for the treatment of female sexual dysfunction (FSD) have required participants to fulfill the diagnostic criteria of hypoactive sexual desire disorder (HSDD), which has been defined as "persistent or recurrent deficiency or absence of sexual thoughts and fantasies and/or desire for, or receptivity for, sexual activity, causing personal distress or interpersonal difficulties" (American Psychiatric Association 1994).

The controversies regarding the use of testosterone to treat HSDD are first whether this is a condition that merits pharmacological intervention and second whether testosterone, as a pharmacological intervention, is sufficiently effective and safe.

23.4.2 The need to treat hypoactive sexual desire disorder

Population-based data show that most women believe an active sex life is important for one's sense of well-being, and that higher levels of physical pleasure in sex are significantly associated with higher levels of emotional satisfaction. However, the prevalence of HSDD amongst postmenopausal women is of the order of 9 to 14%, with no differences between natural and surgically menopausal women (Shifren *et al.* 2008). The prevalence of this condition is consistent across developed and undeveloped countries (Tungphaisal *et al.* 1991; Dennerstein *et al.* 2006).

The impact of HSDD extends well beyond an individual's sexual life. Hypoactive sexual desire disorder is associated with diminished health-related QoL in both naturally and surgically menopausal women (Biddle *et al.* 2009). Women with HSDD are more likely to be depressed and dissatisfied with their home life, and with the emotional and physical relationships they have with their sexual partner. The overall effect of HSDD on quality of life in women with HSDD is similar in magnitude to that seen in adults with other common chronic conditions such as diabetes and back pain (Biddle *et al.* 2009). Women in the community who self-identify as being sexually dissatisfied have significantly lower well-being in comparison to women who self-identify as being satisfied with their sexual life (Davison *et al.* 2009). Aware of the importance of the sexual activity in the relationship, women commonly continue to engage in sexual activity despite experiencing little sexual desire or pleasure, or dyspareunia (Manderson 2005; Davison *et al.* 2008; Avis *et al.* 2009). Overall, loss of sexual desire for many women leads to lowered well-being and increased anxiety and personal distress, translating into relationship disharmony, often with an unavoidable negative ripple effect impacting other family members. Just as individuals seek treatment for other factors that impact negatively on their quality of life such as depression, women experiencing HSDD should be encouraged to discuss their problems with a healthcare provider.

23.4.3 Efficacy of testosterone for treatment of hypoactive sexual desire disorder: findings from randomized, controlled trials

The early studies demonstrating efficacy of testosterone in postmenopausal women with FSD were small and involved the use of testosterone implants (Burger *et al.* 1987) or injections (Sherwin and Gelfand 1987). They were not selective for women fulfilling the criteria of HSDD. A single-blind study that compared estradiol implants alone, versus estradiol plus testosterone implants, in postmenopausal women experiencing lowered libido, found sustained benefits of the addition of testosterone when women were assessed by a validated sexual function questionnaire every six months over two years (Davis *et al.* 1995). Similar benefits of oral methyltestosterone therapy were subsequently reported (Sarrel *et al.* 1998; Lobo *et al.* 2003; Warnock *et al.* 2005). However, concerns that oral methyltestosterone lowers HDL-C and may increase weight and visceral fat accumulation (Leao *et al.* 2006; Somboonporn *et al.* 2005) have resulted in diminished interest in its use and the development of non-oral testosterone therapies for women. The most extensively investigated therapy has been the transdermal testosterone patch (TTP) which delivers 300 μg of testosterone per day. Although the TTP as a treatment for HSDD was studied first in surgically menopausal women using oral estrogen, it has been shown to be efficacious in both naturally and surgically menopausal women taking oral and non-oral estrogen or not using concurrent estrogen.

A Cochrane Review concluded that the addition of testosterone to postmenopausal estrogen therapy improves sexual function in postmenopausal women (Somboonporn *et al.* 2005).

Research into the TTP followed the guidelines set out by the FDA. For evidence that testosterone therapy was an effective treatment for HSDD, the FDA required the primary outcome to be the frequency of satisfactory sexual events determined by the treated woman. Study participants were thus required to keep a daily diary documenting each sexual event and stating whether it was "satisfactory" or not. Women not in a monogamous ongoing relationship and women found to be depressed or experiencing poor relationship satisfaction were excluded from these recent large, randomized, placebo-controlled trials (RCTs).

As already stated, women who report being dissatisfied with their sexual life continue to engage in sexual activity, such that the total frequency of sexual engagement is a poor measure of a woman's sexual well-being (Manderson 2005). Further evidence for this is provided by a recent study which found that postmenopausal women who self-identified as being dissatisfied with their sexual well-being still recorded a median of five sexual events per month (Davison *et al.* 2008). Similarly, at baseline women recruited to a large, randomized, placebo-controlled trial of testosterone treatment for HSDD also reported on average five sexual events per month, with only 50% of these events being considered by the women as sexually satisfying (Davis *et al.* 2008a). Therefore, evaluation of treatment efficacy needs to include other aspects of sexual function important to the woman rather than just a count of total activities. Hence various questionnaires have been developed and validated to assess sexual desire, arousal, pleasure and other parameters of the female sexual response.

In two large studies of the TTP versus placebo in surgically menopausal women on oral estrogen therapy, the increase in the number of satisfying sexual events per month was from three times a month to five times per month with active therapy (Buster *et al.* 2005; Simon *et al.* 2005). There was an associated decline in personal distress, a key component of HSDD, which decreased by 65% and 68% in each of these two large studies with TTP 300 μg/day, compared with 40% and 48% with placebo (Fig. 23.2). All domains of sexual function (arousal, pleasure, orgasm, self-image, reduced concern,

(A)

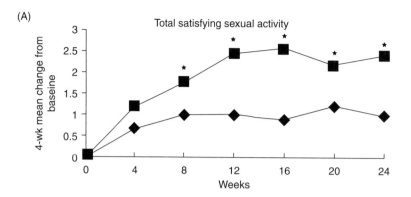

(B)

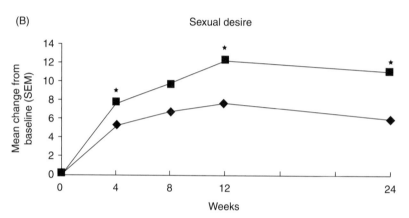

(C)

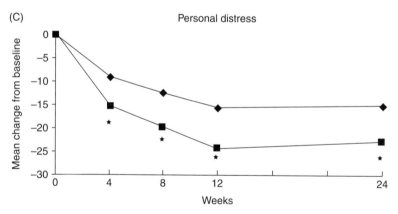

Fig. 23.2 Changes in four-week frequency of (A) total satisfying sexual activity, (B) sexual desire score and (C) personal distress score in postmenopausal women treated with a testosterone patch releasing 300 μg/day, 150 μg/day or placebo over 24 weeks. Symbols: ■, testosterone; ♦, placebo; *, $p \leq 0.05$ vs. placebo. (Simon *et al.* 2005, *with permission.*)

and responsiveness) also improved to a significantly greater extent with testosterone than with placebo. Naturally menopausal women with HSDD receiving a stable dose of oral estrogen had a mean increase from baseline in their four-week frequency of satisfying sexual events with TTP 300 μg/day of 1.92 (73%) compared with placebo (0.5, (19%)), accompanied by increases in the other domains of sexual function assessed (Fig. 23.3), and decreased distress (Shifren *et al.* 2006). Efficacy of TTP therapy has been shown

to be similar in postmenopausal women treated with transdermal estrogen and those not using any concurrent estrogen therapy in RCTs (Davis *et al.* 2006a; 2008a; Panay *et al.* 2010).

The general emphasis has been on the development of testosterone as a treatment for postmenopausal women. But testosterone levels do not decline with natural menopause. So, women who have lowered testosterone in their early postmenopausal years would have had lowered testosterone in

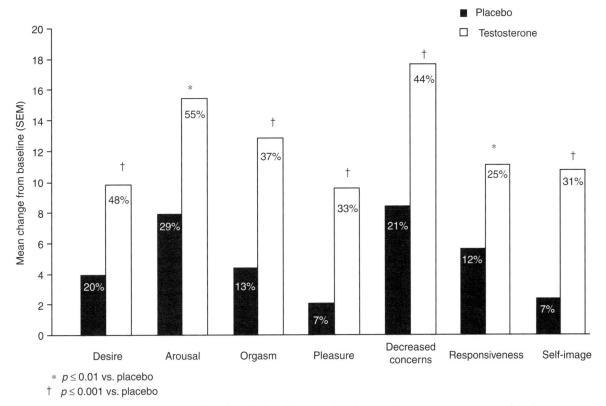

* $p \leq 0.01$ vs. placebo
† $p \leq 0.001$ vs. placebo

Fig. 23.3 Mean change from baseline in Profile of Female Sexual Function domain scores, by treatment group, at week 24 (intent-to-treat population). In naturally menopausal women on oral estrogen with and without transdermal testosterone therapy. (Shifren *et al.* 2006, *with permission.*)

their late reproductive years. Therefore, in patients with HSDD, the argument for treating women in their late reproductive years with testosterone is as strong as for treating naturally menopausal women with testosterone. Two randomized placebo-controlled trials have also shown that transdermal testosterone improves the frequency of satisfactory sexual events and other parameters of sexual well-being in older premenopausal women presenting with loss of libido (Goldstat *et al.* 2003; Davis *et al.* 2008b). Concern regarding the safety of testosterone in women who have the potential to conceive has limited its use in premenopausal women. However, restoration of testosterone levels to within the normal range for young healthy women would not virilize a female fetus. Indeed, the rise in SHBG in early pregnancy protects the fetus from maternal androgen exposure. Treatment with transdermal testosterone also has been shown to significantly improve sexual function in women with hypopituitarism (Miller *et al.* 2006).

Of note, when administered transdermally at doses that restore levels of free testosterone to those seen in healthy young women, the effects of testosterone on sexual function do not become manifest until about six to eight weeks of treatment. Transdermal testosterone appears to be less effective for women with an elevated SHBG level (> 160 pmol/l) (Shifren *et al.* 2006) or if used by women taking conjugated equine estrogens (Procter and Gamble Pharmaceuticals 2004).

With respect to the local vaginal effects of testosterone, there are some preliminary data that the vaginal application of testosterone, 300 μg/d, may alleviate dyspareunia in women with breast cancer, without raising circulating blood levels (Witherby *et al.* 2011). This merits further evaluation.

The mechanism of action of testosterone in terms of sexual function in women has not been extensively researched. In postmenopausal women treated with a stable dose of transdermal estradiol, the effects of testosterone therapy were unaltered by the concurrent administration of an aromatase inhibitor in an RCT, indicating that the therapeutic effect of testosterone on sexual desire and arousal is a consequence of direct androgen action, as opposed to the aromatization of testosterone to estradiol (Davis *et al.* 2006b).

Taken together, the available clinical evidence supports the efficacy of parenteral testosterone therapy as part of the management of lowered sexual desire and arousal in women who have undergone a comprehensive clinical evaluation to exclude other causes.

23.4.4 Effects of testosterone therapy on mood and well-being

Most large RCTs of testosterone versus placebo have included assessments of well-being in their design. A significant improvement in well-being, measured by a validated questionnaire, has only been observed in RCTs in which the study population had a baseline well-being score below that of the general population (Shifren *et al.* 2000; Goldstat *et al.* 2003; Davis *et al.* 2006a). Testosterone should not be considered a treatment option for mood disorders in women.

23.4.5 Effects of testosterone therapy on cardiovascular function and cardiovascular disease risk

Studies of testosterone administered by subcutaneous implant (Davis *et al.* 1995), transdermal patch (Simon *et al.* 2005; Davis *et al.* 2008a), spray (Davis *et al.* 2008b) or gel (Davis *et al.* 2006b) do not show any adverse effects in terms of altered lipid levels, CRP, glycosylated hemoglobin (HbA1c) or insulin sensitivity. However, HDL-C and apolipoprotein A1 levels decrease significantly when oral methyltestosterone is administered with oral estrogen (Barrett-Connor *et al.* 1999; Chiuve *et al.* 2004). Combined estrogen and methyltestosterone therapy is also associated with reduced plasma concentrations of apolipoprotein B, reduced LDL particle size, and increased total body LDL catabolism (Wagner *et al.* 1996). Similarly, oral testosterone undecanoate adversely affects lipoproteins and increases insulin resistance (Zang *et al.* 2006).

SHBG is a strong independent marker of insulin resistance and the risk of type 2 diabetes. Levels of SHBG do not change with transdermal testosterone therapy in studies over 26 to 52 weeks (Braunstein *et al.* 2005; Davis *et al.* 2008a). In women with documented congestive cardiac failure, treatment with the TTP releasing 300 µg of testosterone per day was associated with significant functional improvements assessed by peak oxygen consumption, distance walked over the six-minute walking test, muscle strength and insulin resistance, compared with placebo (Iellamo *et al.* 2010). None of the RCTs comparing the transdermal testosterone therapy with placebo have shown a difference in event rate for any CVD outcome, including venous thromboembolic events, versus placebo.

23.4.6 Effects on bone and lean mass

Small studies have shown that testosterone treatment will increase vertebral and hip BMD in postmenopausal women (Davis *et al.* 1995; Watts *et al.* 1995). In women of reproductive years with hypopituitarism, treatment with the TTP (300 µg daily) for 12 months resulted in significant increases in BMD at the hip and radius, and in lean body mass (Miller *et al.* 2006). Similarly, oral methyltestosterone has been shown to significantly increase BMD in women with Turner syndrome, versus placebo (Zuckerman-Levin *et al.* 2009). Whether testosterone therapy will prevent fractures has not been investigated.

Overall, studies evaluating the effects of testosterone on body composition in postmenopausal women report increased lean mass and reduced body fat. In postmenopausal women, testosterone implant therapy over two years increased lean body mass as assessed by DXA (Davis *et al.* 2000). Combined oral methyltestosterone with oral estrogen therapy results in increased lean mass, reduced percentage body fat and increased lower body strength compared to estrogen therapy alone (Dobs *et al.* 2002). In women with Turner syndrome, oral methyltestosterone increased total trunk lean body mass, whereas total fat mass decreased and the visceral fat and visceral-to-subcutaneous fat ratio, as evaluated by abdominal CT, did not change with testosterone compared with placebo (Zuckerman-Levin *et al.* 2009). In women with hypopituitarism, treatment with the TTP did not affect intra-abdominal or subcutaneous fat mass as measured by CT (Miller *et al.* 2006).

23.4.7 Effects of testosterone on cognition

High-quality RCT data for the effects of testosterone on cognitive performance in women are lacking.

Some studies have reported effects of a single dose (Aleman *et al.* 2004) or have been of short duration (Kocoska-Maras *et al.* 2011), such that the clinical significance of the findings is unclear. Other longer and larger studies mostly indicate a favorable effect of testosterone on cognitive performance, but the findings are not consistent and all have methodological limitations. A significant improvement in immediate and delayed verbal memory using the California Verbal Learning Test was observed in an open-label study of transdermal testosterone in postmenopausal women on estrogen therapy (Shah *et al.* 2006); whereas a negative effect on immediate but not delayed verbal memory was observed over 24 weeks with testosterone undecanoate as an oral therapy (Moller *et al.* 2010). In a study of oral estrogen alone or in combination with methyltestosterone, women receiving estrogen and methyltestosterone maintained a steady level of performance on the Building Memory task, whereas those receiving estrogen alone showed a decrease in performance (Wisniewski *et al.* 2002). An important consideration in terms of methodology is that all of the published studies of the effects of testosterone on cognitive performance have employed tests developed for cognitively impaired individuals, which are not sensitive to small changes in cognitive performance within the normal range for healthy women. Findings are also confounded by the well-documented practice effects observed when normally functioning individuals are exposed to the same test materials within a brief time interval. Studies using more sophisticated measures of cognitive performance developed for cognitively intact individuals, that are resistant to practice effects, are needed.

23.4.8   Use of testosterone for treatment of vulval lichen sclerosis

Vulval lichen sclerosis is a chronic skin condition characterized by pruritus, irritation, burning, dyspareunia and tearing. It most commonly occurs after the fifth decade. The typical appearance is porcelain-white papules and plaques, often with areas of ecchymosis or purpura affecting the vulval tissue. The mainstay of treatment for this condition is high-dose topical steroid cream, usually clobetasol propionate. Although testosterone cream has been recommended in the past, the findings have been inconsistent, and adverse androgenic effects have been reported (ACOG 2008).

23.5   Safety of testosterone therapy for women

23.5.1   Testosterone and adverse androgenic effects

The potential masculinizing effects of androgen therapy include development of acne, hirsutism, deepening of the voice and androgenic alopecia. These effects are dose related and are uncommon if supraphysiological hormone levels are avoided. Compared with placebo therapy, women treated with transdermal testosterone in various studies report a higher rate of androgenic adverse events, mainly attributable to increased hair growth (Fig. 23.4). However, withdrawal from research studies due to androgenic adverse events has not been seen to be greater in women treated with testosterone (Davis *et al.* 2008a). Hirsutism, androgenic alopecia and/or acne are relatively strong contradictions to androgen therapy.

23.5.2   Testosterone and breast cancer risk

The main concern of regulators and the community is whether testosterone therapy may influence breast cancer risk. Testosterone treatment results in growth-inhibitory and apoptotic effects in some, but not all, breast cancer cell lines, and, in rodent breast cancer models, despite the potential for testosterone to be aromatized to estradiol, testosterone action is generally antiproliferative and proapoptotic (Somboonporn and Davis 2004). It is of note that from the 1940s through until the 1970s, testosterone was used in the treatment of breast cancer (Adair and Herrmann 1946; Rieche and Wolff 1975).

For premenopausal women, data pertaining to testosterone and breast cancer risk is limited to findings from observational studies of endogenous hormone levels, as testosterone therapy is rare in premenopausal women, and the only RCTs undertaken have been too small to provide useful data. The significance of the available data is limited by failure to take into account timing of blood drawing in relation to the menstrual cycle or time of day, imprecision of assays used, and failure to take into account estradiol levels. Most studies do not demonstrate an association between testosterone and breast cancer risk in premenopausal women (Somboonporn and Davis 2004). One prospective, case control study

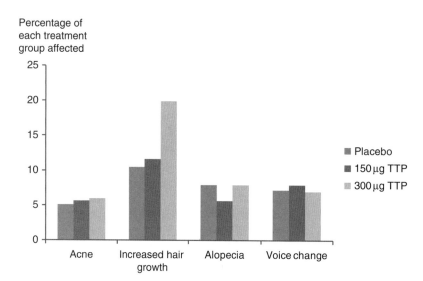

Percentage of
each treatment
group affected

Fig. 23.4 Effects of different doses of the transdermal testosterone patch on androgenic events over 12 months in postmenopausal women not using concurrent estrogen therapy. Adapted from Davis *et al.* (2008a). See plate section for color version.

has reported a relationship between testosterone and increased risk of subsequent breast cancer, although estradiol levels were not taken into account in the analysis (Dorgan *et al.* 2010). Despite PCOS being characterized by chronic estradiol and estrone exposure and androgen excess, women with PCOS do not have an increased risk of breast cancer (Coulam *et al.* 1983; Gammon and Thompson 1991; Anderson *et al.* 1997).

The older observational studies of endogenous testosterone and breast cancer risk in postmenopausal women are also limited by assay imprecision (Somboonporn and Davis 2004). More recent studies undertaken within the NSABP Cancer Prevention Trial (Beattie *et al.* 2006) and the Nurses' Health Study (Danforth *et al.* 2010) showed no significant association between breast cancer risk and any of the androgens measured.

Observational studies of women using methyltestosterone have produced mixed results. The Nurses' Health Study reported an increase in risk for current but not past users of methyltestosterone therapy up to 2002 (Tamimi *et al.* 2006). This was an older cohort (mean age 61.5 years). There were 29 cases of breast cancer in estrogen plus testosterone users and 3 cases in testosterone-only users in 5628 women-years of follow-up. Testosterone users were younger, leaner, more likely to have benign breast disease (55%) and consumed more alcohol than controls, and the indications for testosterone therapy were not known. In another study no significant effect on breast cancer risk of estrogen plus methyltestosterone use, versus

no use of hormone therapy, was reported (adjusted hazard ratio:1.42; 95% CI: 0.95–2.11) in the setting of 49% of users also being progestin users, compared with 11% of non-hormone users being past estrogen-progestin users (Ness *et al.* 2009). A third, large, case control study of women aged 50–64 years reported no effect of methyltestosterone use on breast cancer risk (Jick *et al.* 2009).

Cohort studies of women treated with either testosterone implants or transdermal testosterone do not show an increase in risk with testosterone therapy (Dimitrakakis *et al.* 2004; Davis *et al.* 2009a). There has been no evidence of an increased risk in association with duration of exposure and no evidence of altered risk in past users of testosterone therapy in the above-mentioned studies. Testosterone therapy does not alter mammographic density over 12 months (Davis *et al.* 2009b). No RCT has been of sufficient size or duration to provide definitive evaluable data for the impact of testosterone on breast cancer risk.

23.5.3 Testosterone and endometrial cancer risk

Endometrial cancer is more common amongst women with obesity (Lindemann *et al.* 2008), diabetes (Lindemann *et al.* 2008) and polycystic ovarian syndrome (PCOS) (Wild *et al.* 2000) and/or prolonged unopposed exposure to estrogen (Antunes *et al.* 1979) and agents which are estrogen-receptor agonists in the endometrium, such as tamoxifen (Thurlimann *et al.* 2005). There has been no association between free testosterone and endometrial cancer risk after adjustment for estrone and estradiol levels (Allen *et al.* 2008). Data pertaining to the effects of treatment with testosterone on the endometrium are limited. Tissue samples from female-to-male transsexuals treated with high-dose testosterone for, on average, three years prior to hysterectomy show inactive endometria, with expression of Ki-67 in the glands, stroma, and glands and stroma together being significantly lower than for controls (Perrone *et al.* 2009). Transdermal testosterone is associated with endometrial atrophy (Zang *et al.* 2007; Davis *et al.* 2008a), and no cases of endometrial hyperplasia or carcinoma have been diagnosed in clinical trials of testosterone therapy. Taken together, the available data do not indicate that treatment with testosterone significantly influences endometrial cancer risk.

23.5.4 Other safety concerns

None of the RCTs of testosterone implants or transdermal testosterone patch or gel have reported liver toxicity, polycythemia or other adverse metabolic effects. Sleep apnea has also not been reported in women receiving physiological doses of testosterone.

23.6 Appropriate candidates for testosterone therapy

23.6.1 Identifying women likely to benefit from testosterone therapy

Overall, women who present with HSDD from the late reproductive years and beyond are potential candidates for testosterone therapy. Physicians should specifically consider women who have experienced premature ovarian failure or surgical menopause, or who have adrenal insufficiency or hypopituitarism, as having a high likelihood of HSDD, as these are conditions characterized by low androgen production. Consideration should also be given to women who have experienced iatrogenic ovarian failure secondary to chemotherapy, radiotherapy or chemical ovarian suppression.

A recent study by Avis and others (Avis *et al.* 2009) provides a broad insight into sexual activity across the menopause. In this large cohort, 50% of postmenopausal women reported engaging in masturbation, with 17% of women reporting doing so once to twice a month and 10% at least once a week.

This form of sexual activity was most common amongst single, widowed and divorced women. The importance of this observation is that the desire to experience sexual well-being is not limited to women in relationships, and that sexual desire and capacity to be aroused is an important consideration for all women. Although most of the published studies of testosterone have required participants to be in established monogamous relationships, this should not be a requirement for consideration of testosterone therapy in clinical practice.

An array of physical, psychological, cultural and relationship factors influence sexual well-being and sexual function. Hence women presenting with the complaint of diminished sexual interest with or without impaired sexual responsiveness need a general psychological, physical and social health assessment. Commonly contributing factors include stress, fatigue, relationship issues, depression and medication side-effects. Although identification of such factors does not exclude a woman from consideration for treatment with testosterone, such factors need to be managed. For example, relationship issues are not uncommonly a consequence of a woman's diminished desire to engage in sexual activity, rather than the primary cause.

Loss of sexual desire is not uncommon amongst women using the combined oral contraceptive pill. Simply switching to another form of contraception will often improve sexual well-being in younger women. Concurrent use of the combined oral contraceptive pill did not appear to impede response to testosterone therapy (Davis *et al.* 2008b).

The use of antidepressants is commonly associated with impaired sexual function and may reflect either inadequate treatment of depression or a drug side-effect (Werneke *et al.* 2006). Unfortunately research into the adverse effects of antidepressants and many other drugs on sexual function in women is sorely lacking. Women who present primarily with arousal disorder and inability to achieve orgasm, but no significant loss of libido, in association with antidepressant therapy, may respond well to phosphodiesterase type 5 inhibitor therapy (Nurnberg *et al.* 2008). Whether testosterone therapy will benefit women with antidepressant-associated FSD is yet to be determined, as most studies of testosterone in women have excluded women with depression and users of antidepressants.

Table 23.1 Assessment of women presenting with sexual dysfunction

1. Medical history

- Current circumstances

- Relationship issues: consider referral for relationship counseling

- Employment and social engagement

- Sexual experiences and sexual health knowledge, including individual and partner's understanding of anatomy and sexuality and whether the women is experiencing sexual stimulation: consider referral for sexual counseling

- Health history, medications, drug use

2. Medical examination, including genital and pelvic examination, particularly for loss of sensitivity or pain disorders

3. Identify and manage health-related factors

  a. Mental health

    i. Body image and self-esteem

    ii. Experience of sexual abuse/trauma

    iii. Negative attitudes, inhibitions and anxieties, cultural and religious beliefs

  b. Physical health

  c. Medication side-effects, particularly antidepressants and antipsychotics

  d. Partner's mental and physical health

4. Consider testosterone therapy

Table 23.2 Contraindications to testosterone therapy in women

Pregnancy and lactation

Current use of antiandrogen therapy

Troublesome acne or hirsutism

Hormone-dependent malignancy current or past

SHBG level below the lower limit of normal

Free testosterone level in the mid-normal range for young women and above

23.6.2 Assessment of women presenting with low sexual desire

It is important that each woman be assessed in the context of her personal circumstances, partnership status, sexual experiences and cultural expectations (Table 23.1). It should not be assumed that a woman is experiencing adequate sexual stimulation, both physical and emotional, such that this does not need to be explored. Referral to either a psychologist or sexual counselor is often appropriate. Medical history needs to include general medical, psychosocial and urogynecological details and the use of all medications, both prescription and non-prescription. A medical examination should include a full genital and pelvic assessment, including assessment of sensitivity in women with loss of sensitivity or sexual pain.

Laboratory investigations should only be performed as indicated and might include exclusion of factors causing fatigue (iron deficiency, thyroid dysfunction and hyperglycemia). There is no point in measuring reproductive hormones in women taking the combined oral contraceptive pill, as it suppresses estradiol and testosterone production and increases SHBG.

As there is no level of testosterone, total or free, below which a woman can be diagnosed as being androgen deficient, the measurement of testosterone should not be used to indicate which women merit treatment. However, a testosterone level should be measured prior to therapy primarily to exclude women who may be at risk of side-effects if treated. Total testosterone is notoriously difficult to measure at lower levels, as seen in women, with sensitivity and precision (Davison *et al.* 2005b). Clinicians interested in this field of therapeutics should discuss with their pathology service the sensitivity and precision of the assays being employed. Ideally total testosterone (protein-bound and free testosterone) should be measured as well as SHBG, and from this free testosterone can be reliably estimated by the pathology service using the Sodergard equation (Sodergard *et al.* 1982). The measurement of free testosterone in women by direct "kit" assays is generally completely unreliable (Herold and Fitzgerald 2003). Abnormal levels can be found when androgen excess is not expected.

Contraindications to testosterone therapy are primarily related to increased risk of worsening existing acne, hirsutism or alopecia, pregnancy and lactation, and unknown effects on hormone-dependent cancer (Table 23.2). A low SHBG will enable more rapid clearance of administered testosterone, and hence increased risk of androgenic side-effects. Similarly women with a free testosterone level in the high-normal or above normal range for healthy young premenopausal women (Davison *et al.* 2005a) are at greater risk of overtreatment.

23.7 Treatment options

Available data indicate that the most physiological mode of delivery of testosterone is parenteral, and primarily as a transdermal formulation. To date the testosterone patch has only been approved for the treatment of surgically menopausal women using concurrent estrogen in European Union countries. A transdermal testosterone cream is available in Australia, with small studies showing efficacy in premenopausal and postmenopausal women (Goldstat *et al.* 2003; El-Hage *et al.* 2007). Increased hair growth over the application site is a problem for some women.

In some countries testosterone is available as testosterone pellets implanted subcutaneously under local anesthetics. Most commonly a dose of 50 mg is used (Davis *et al.* 1995). These implants usually remain effective for periods of four to six months, although there is considerable intraindividual and interindividual variation in their absorption and degradation. Therefore, repeat implantation should not be undertaken without confirmation that total testosterone corrected for SHBG, or free testosterone, has fallen back into the lower quartile of the normal female range. Otherwise, the risk of adverse androgenic effects is increased with the insertion of a new implant.

Other parenteral modes of delivery of testosterone under development include a transdermal metered-dose testosterone spray, a transdermal gel and an intranasal testosterone gel.

Neither oral testosterone undecanoate nor methyltestosterone can be recommended for women, as both may adversely affects lipids, and testosterone undecanoate may induce insulin resistance. Some clinicians undertake a clinical trial of im injections of testosterone esters 50–100 mg. This may or may not result in a clinical response over one to two weeks. A positive response supports the initiation of longer-term therapy. However, as peak levels are very supraphysiological, testosterone esters should not be considered a long-term treatment option.

There is extensive off-label prescribing of testosterone products, formulated for men, to treat women. As this approach may result in grossly elevated testosterone levels and androgenic effects, this practice cannot be condoned. Based on prescription and physician survey data, the number of physicians prescribing compounded testosterone formulations is increasing (Snabes and Simes 2009). Caution is urged, however, as there are no published pharmacokinetic or safety data or efficacy studies to validate this method of administration.

23.8 Conclusions

Testosterone has been widely used by women as an unapproved therapy for decades. In appropriate doses, it is effective for the treatment of low sexual desire in women approaching and following menopause. Large well-controlled trials have shown testosterone improves sexual desire, arousal, orgasm frequency, pleasure and overall satisfaction and decreases distress associated with FSD. It should also be considered in the management of women with premature ovarian failure and hypopituitarism. Possible beneficial effects of testosterone on fracture risk, cognitive function and cardiovascular function require further investigation.

Excessive therapy will clearly result in undesirable androgenic effects such as hirsutism and acne, although this is not common when treatment is aimed at achieving testosterone levels in the female range. The capacity for both the breast and endometrium to aromatize testosterone to estradiol underlies concern regarding the potential for testosterone therapy to increase the risk of breast and endometrial cancer. No RCT has been sufficiently large or of sufficient duration to clarify the effects of exogenous testosterone on cancer risk, although cumulative data from the RCTs conducted to date do not indicate an increase in risk.

Availability of approved testosterone therapies for women is limited to a few countries, and, in many of these, approved use is limited to specific populations. Thus many clinicians are forced to resort to adapting products approved for men or the prescription of compounded products. However, the extensive off-label prescribing of testosterone products for women raises serious safety concerns, and together with the evidence for the negative impact of FSD on quality of life, highlights the need for an approved testosterone formulation for women.

23.9 Key messages

- Levels of testosterone and DHT decline during the reproductive years, but do not change acutely across natural menopause.
- There is no cutoff level for testosterone or free testosterone below which women can be labeled as "androgen deficient."
- Transdermal testosterone therapy improves sexual desire, arousal and global sexual satisfaction in both premenopausal and postmenopausal women presenting with low sexual desire which causes them concern.
- Free testosterone levels are dependent on SHBG, which is highly responsive to the metabolic milieu, being suppressed in the setting of insulin resistance, hepatic steatosis and obesity.
- In circumstances in which total testosterone is not associated with health outcomes, such as cardiovascular disease, but free testosterone is, this is usually a consequence of low SHBG, not a direct androgen effect.
- Whether testosterone treatment increases the risk of breast cancer is still debated. There is no evidence that past users of testosterone have an increased risk of breast cancer and there are no signals that transdermal testosterone modifies breast cancer risk. Studies further evaluating this are underway.

23.10   References

Abraham GE (1974) Ovarian and adrenal contribution to peripheral androgens during the menstrual cycle. *J Clin Endocrinol Metab* **39**:340–346

ACOG (American College of Obstetrics and Gynecology) (2008) ACOG Practice Bulletin No. 93: diagnosis and management of vulvar skin disorders. *Obstet Gynecol* **111**:1243–1253

Adair FE, Herrmann JB (1946) The use of testosterone propionate in the treatment of advanced carcinoma of the breast. *Ann Surg* **123**:1023–1035

Aleman A, Bronk E, Kessels RP, Koppeschaar HP, van Honk J (2004) A single administration of testosterone improves visuospatial ability in young women. *Psychoneuroendocrinology* **29**:612–617

Allen NE, Key TJ, Dossus L, Rinaldi S, Cust A, Lukanova A, Peeters PH, Onland-Moret NC, Lahmann PH, Berrino F, Panico S, Larranaga N, Pera G, Tormo MJ, Sanchez MJ, Ramon Quiros J, Ardanaz E, Tjonneland A, Olsen A, Chang-Claude J, Linseisen J, Schulz M, Boeing H, Lundin E, Palli D, Overvad K, Clavel-Chapelon F, Boutron-Ruault MC, Bingham S, Khaw KT, Bueno-de-Mesquita HB, Trichopoulou A, Trichopoulos D, Naska A, Tumino R, Riboli E, Kaaks R (2008) Endogenous sex hormones and endometrial cancer risk in women in the European Prospective Investigation into Cancer and Nutrition (EPIC). *Endocr Relat Cancer* **15**:485–497

American Psychiatric Association (1994) *Diagnostic and Statistical Manual of Mental Disorders*. American Psychiatric Press, Washington, DC

Anderson KE, Sellers TA, Chen PL, Rich SS, Hong CP, Folsom AR (1997) Association of Stein-Leventhal syndrome with the incidence of postmenopausal breast carcinoma in a large prospective study of women in Iowa. *Cancer* **79**:494–499

Antunes C, Strolley P, Rosenshein N, Davies J, Tonascia J, Brown C, Burnett L, Rutledge A, Pokempner M, Garcia R (1979) Endometrial cancer and estrogen use. Report of a large case-control study. *N Eng J Med* **300**:9–13

Avis NE, Brockwell S, Randolph JF Jr, Shen S, Cain VS, Ory M, Greendale GA (2009) Longitudinal changes in sexual functioning as women transition through menopause: results from the Study of Women's Health Across the Nation. *Menopause* **16**:442–452

Barrett-Connor E, Young R, Notelovitz M, Sullivan J, Wiita B, Yang HM, Nolan J (1999) A two-year, double-blind comparison of estrogen-androgen and conjugated estrogens in surgically menopausal women. Effects on bone mineral density, symptoms and lipid profiles. *J Reprod Med* **44**:1012–1020

Beattie MS, Costantino JP, Cummings SR, Wickerham DL, Vogel VG, Dowsett M, Folkerd EJ, Willett WC, Wolmark N, Hankinson SE (2006) Endogenous sex hormones, breast cancer risk, and tamoxifen response: an ancillary study in the NSABP Breast Cancer Prevention Trial (P-1). *J Natl Cancer Inst* **98**:110–115

Bell R, Donath S, Davison S, Davis S (2006) Endogenous androgen levels and wellbeing: differences between pre- and postmenopausal women. *Menopause* **13**:65–71

Bell RJ, Davison SL, Papalia MA, McKenzie DP, Davis SR (2007) Endogenous androgen levels and cardiovascular risk profile in women across the adult life span. *Menopause* **14**:630–638

Bernini G, Sgro M, Moretti A, Argenio GF, Barlascini CO, Cristofani R, Salvetti A (1999) Endogenous androgens and carotid intimal-medial thickness in women. *J Clin Endocrinol Metab* **84**:2008–2012

Biddle AK, West SL, D'Aloisio AA, Wheeler SB, Borisov NN, Thorp J (2009) Hypoactive sexual desire disorder in postmenopausal women: quality of life and health burden. *Value Health* **12**:763–772

Bixo M, Backstrom T, Winblad B, Andersson A (1995) Estradiol and testosterone in specific regions of the human female brain in different endocrine states. *J Steroid Biochem Mol Biol* **55**:297–303

Braunstein GD, Sundwall DA, Katz M, Shifren JL, Buster JE, Simon JA, Bachman G, Aguirre OA, Lucas JD, Rodenberg C, Buch A, Watts NB (2005) Safety and efficacy of a testosterone patch for the treatment of hypoactive sexual desire disorder in surgically menopausal women: a randomized, placebo-controlled trial. *Arch Intern Med* **165**:1582–1589

Burger HG, Hailes J, Nelson J, Menelaus M (1987) Effect of combined implants of estradiol and testosterone on libido in postmenopausal women. *BMJ* **294**:936–937

Burger HG, Dudley EC, Hopper DL (1995) The endocrinology of the menopausal transition: a cross-sectional study of a population-based sample. *J Clin Endocrinol Metab* **80**:3537–3545

Buster JE, Kingsberg SA, Aguirre O, Brown C, Breaux JG, Buch A, Rodenberg C, Wekseman K, Casson P (2005) Testosterone patch for low sexual desire in surgically menopausal women: a randomized trial. *Obstet Gynecol* **105**:944–952

Calderon-Margalit R, Schwartz SM, Wellons MF, Lewis CE, Daviglus ML, Schreiner PJ, Williams OD, Sternfeld B, Carr JJ, O'Leary DH, Sidney S, Friedlander Y, Siscovick DS (2010) Prospective association of serum androgens and sex hormone-binding globulin with subclinical cardiovascular disease in young adult women: the "Coronary Artery Risk Development in Young Adults" women's study. *J Clin Endocrinol Metab* **95**:4424–4431

Campbell S, Whitehead M (1977) Oestrogen therapy and the menopausal syndrome. *Clin Obstet Gynaecol* **4**:31–47

Chiuve SE, Martin LA, Campos H, Sacks FM (2004) Effect of the combination of methyltestosterone and esterified estrogens compared with esterified estrogens alone on apolipoprotein CIII and other apolipoproteins in very low density, low density, and high density lipoproteins in surgically postmenopausal women. *J Clin Endocrinol Metab* **89**:2207–2213

Coulam CB, Annegers JF, Kranz JS (1983) Chronic anovulation syndrome and associated neoplasia. *Obstet Gynecol* **61**:403–407

Couzinet B, Meduri G, Lecce M, Young J, Brailly S, Loosfelt H, Milgrom E, Schaison G (2001) The post menopausal ovary is not a major androgen-producing gland. *J Clin Endocrinol Metab* **86**:5060–5065

Danforth KN, Eliassen AH, Tworoger SS, Missmer SA, Barbieri RL, Rosner BA, Colditz GA, Hankinson SE (2010) The association of plasma androgen levels with breast, ovarian and endometrial cancer risk factors among postmenopausal women. *Int J Cancer* **126**:199–207

Davis SR, McCloud PI, Strauss BJG, Burger HG (1995) Testosterone enhances estradiol's effects on postmenopausal bone density and sexuality. *Maturitas* **21**:227–236

Davis SR, Walker KZ, Strauss BJ (2000) Effects of estradiol with and without testosterone on body composition and relationships with lipids in post-menopausal women. *Menopause* **7**:395–401

Davis SR, Davison SL, Donath S, Bell RJ (2005) Circulating androgen levels and self-reported sexual function in women. *JAMA* **294**:91–96

Davis SR, van der Mooren MJ, van Lunsen RHW, Lopes P, Rees M, Moufarege A, Rodenberg C, Buch A, Purdie D (2006a) The efficacy and safety of a testosterone patch for the treatment of hypoactive sexual desire disorder in surgically menopausal women: a randomized, placebo-controlled trial. *Menopause* **13**:387–396

Davis SR, Goldstat R, Papalia MA, Shah SM, Kulkarni J, Donath S, Bell R (2006b) Effects of aromatase inhibition on sexual function and wellbeing in postmenopausal women treated with testosterone: a randomized placebo-controlled trial. *Menopause* **13**:37–45

Davis SR, Moreau M, Kroll R, Bouchard C, Panay N, Gass M, Braunstein GD, Linden-Hirschberg A, Rodenberg C, Pack S, Koch H, Moufarage A, Studd J (2008a) Testosterone for low libido in menopausal women not taking estrogen therapy. *N Eng J Med* **359**:2005–2017

Davis SR, Papalia MA, Norman RJ, O'Neill S, Redelman M, Williamson M, Stuckey BGA, Wlodarczyk J, Gard'ner K, Humberstone A (2008b) Safety and efficacy of a testosterone metered-dose transdermal spray for treatment of decreased sexual satisfaction in premenopausal women: a placebo-controlled randomized, dose-ranging study. *Annals Internal Med* **148**:569–577

Davis SR, Wolfe R, Farrugia H, Ferdinand A, Bell RJ (2009a) The Incidence of invasive breast cancer among women prescribed testosterone for low libido. *J Sex Med* **6**:1850–1856

Davis SR, Hirschberg AL, Wagner LK, Lodhi I, von Schoultz B (2009b) The effect of transdermal testosterone on mammographic density in postmenopausal women not receiving systemic estrogen therapy. *J Clin Endocrinol Metab* **94**:4907–4913

Davison SL, Bell R, Donath S, Montalto JG, Davis SR (2005a) Androgen levels in adult females: changes with age, menopause, and oophorectomy. *J Clin Endocrinol Metab* **90**:3847–3853

Davison SL, Bell R, Montalto JG, Sikaris K, Donath S, Stanczyk FZ, Davis SR (2005b) Measurement of total testosterone in women: comparison of a direct radioimmunoassay versus radioimmunoassay after organic solvent extraction and celite column partition chromatography. *Fertil Steril* **84**:1698–1704

Davison SL, Bell RJ, LaChina M, Holden SL, Davis SR (2008) Sexual function in well women: stratification by sexual satisfaction, hormone use, and menopause status. *J Sex Med* **5**:1214–1222

Davison SL, Bell RJ, La China M, Holden SL, Davis SR (2009) The relationship between self-reported sexual satisfaction and general wellbeing in women. *J Sex Med* **6**:2690–2697

Debing E, Peeters E, Duquet W, Poppe K, Velkeniers B, Van den Brande P (2007) Endogenous sex hormone levels in postmenopausal women undergoing carotid artery endarterectomy. *Eur J Endocrinol* **156**:687–693

Dennerstein L, Koochaki P, Barton I, Graziottin A (2006) Hypoactive sexual desire disorder in menopausal women: a survey of western European women. *J Sex Med* **3**:212–222

Dimitrakakis C, Jones R, Liu A, Bondy CA (2004) Breast cancer incidence in postmenopausal women using testosterone in addition to usual hormone therapy. *Menopause* **11**:531–535

Dobs AS, Nguyen T, Pace C, Roberts C (2002) Differential effects of oral estrogen versus estrogen-androgen replacement therapy on body composition in postmenopausal women. *J Clin Endocrinol Metab* **87**:1509–1516

Dorgan JF, Stanczyk FZ, Kahle LL, Brinton LA (2010) Prospective case-control study of premenopausal serum estradiol and testosterone levels and breast cancer risk. *Breast Cancer Res* **12**:R98

Dunn JF, Nisula BC, Rodbard D (1981) Transport of steroid hormones. Binding of 21

endogenous steroids to both testosterone-binding globulin and cortico-steroid-binding globulin in human plasma. *J Clin Endocrinol Metab* **53**:58–68

Edmunds SE, Stubbs AP, Santos AA, Wilkinson ML (1990) Estrogen and androgen regulation of sex hormone binding globulin secretion by a human liver cell line. *J Steroid Biochem Mol Biol* **37**:733–739

El-Hage G, Eden JA, Manga RZ (2007) A double-blind, randomized, placebo-controlled trial of the effect of testosterone cream on the sexual motivation of menopausal hysterectomized women with hypoactive sexual desire disorder. *Climacteric* **10**:335–343

Fogle RH, Stanczyk FZ, Zhang X, Paulson RJ (2007) Ovarian androgen production in postmenopausal women. *J Clin Endocrinol Metab* **92**:3040–3043

Gammon MD, Thompson WD (1991) Polycystic ovaries and the risk of breast cancer. *Am J Epidemiol* **134**:818–824

Golden SH, Ding J, Szklo M, Schmidt MI, Duncan BB, Dobs A (2004) Glucose and insulin components of the metabolic syndrome are associated with hyperandrogenism in postmenopausal women: the atherosclerosis risk in communities study. *Am J Epidemiol* **160**:540–548

Goldstat R, Briganti E, Tran J, Wolfe R, Davis S (2003) Transdermal testosterone improves mood, well being and sexual function in premenopausal women. *Menopause* **10**:390–398

Goodman-Gruen D, Barrett-Connor E (1997) Sex hormone-binding globulin and glucose tolerance in postmenopausal women. The Rancho Bernardo Study. *Diabetes Care* **20**:645–649

Gouchie C, Kimura D (1991) The relationship between testosterone levels and cognitive ability patterns. *Psychoneuroendocrinology* **16**:323–334

Haning JRV, Hackett R, Flood CA, Loughlin JS, Zhao QY, Longcope C (1993) Plasma dehydroepiandrosterone sulfate serves as a prehormone for 48% of follicular fluid testosterone during treatment with menotropins. *J Clin Endocrinol Metab* **76**:1301–1307

Harada N, Sasano H, Murakami H, Ohkuma T, Nagura H, Takagi Y (1999) Localized expression of aromatase in human vascular tissues. *Circ Res* **84**:1285–1291

Hayes RD, Dennerstein L, Bennett CM, Fairley CK (2008) What is the "true" prevalence of female sexual dysfunctions and does the way we assess these conditions have an impact? *J Sex Med* **5**:777–787

Herold DA, Fitzgerald RL (2003) Immunoassays for testosterone in women: better than a guess? *Clin Chem* **49**:1250–1251

Horton R, Hawks D, Lobo R (1982) 3 alpha, 17 beta-androstanediol glucuronide in plasma. A marker of androgen action in idiopathic hirsutism. *J Clin Invest* **69**: 1203–1206

Janssen I, Powell LH, Kazlauskaite R, Dugan SA (2010) Testosterone and visceral fat in midlife women: the Study of Women's Health Across the Nation (SWAN) fat patterning study. *Obesity (Silver Spring)* **18**:604–610

Jick SS, Hagberg KW, Kaye JA, Jick H (2009) Postmenopausal estrogen-containing hormone therapy and the risk of breast cancer. *Obstet Gynecol* **113**:74–80

Joffe HV, Ridker PM, Manson JE, Cook NR, Buring JE, Rexrode KM (2006) Sex hormone-binding globulin and serum testosterone are inversely associated with C-reactive protein levels in postmenopausal women at high risk for cardiovascular disease. *Ann Epidemiol* **16**:105–112

Judd HL, Judd GE, Lucas WE, Yen SSC (1974) Endocrine function of the postmenopausal ovary. Concentrations of androgens and estrogens in ovarian and peripheral venous blood. *J Clin Endocrinol* **39**: 1020–1024

Judd HL, Lucas WE, Yen SSC (1994) Effect of oopherectomy on circulating testosterone and androstenedione levels in patients with endometrial cancer **118**:793–798

Kalantaridou SN, Calis KA, Vanderhoof VH, Bakalov VK, Corrigan EC, Troendle JF, Nelson LM (2006) Testosterone deficiency in young women with 46, XX spontaneous premature ovarian failure. *Fertil Steril* **86**:1475–1482

Kasperk CH, Wergedal JE, Farley JR, Llinkhart TA, Turner RT, Baylink DG (1989) Androgens directly stimulate proliferation of bone cells in vitro. *Endocrinology* **124**:1576–1578

Kocoska-Maras L, Zethraeus N, Radestad AF, Ellingsen T, von Schoultz B, Johannesson M, Hirschberg AL (2011) A randomized trial of the effect of testosterone and estrogen on verbal fluency, verbal memory, and spatial ability in healthy postmenopausal women. *Fertil Steril* **95**:152–157

Krug R, Psych D, Pietrowsky R, Fehm HL, Born J (1994) Selective influence of menstrual cycle on perception of stimuli with reproductive significance. *Psychosom Med* **56**:410–417

Labrie F (1991) Intracrinology. *Mol Cell Endocrinol* **78**:C113–C118

Labrie F, Martel C, Balser J (2010) Wide distribution of the serum dehydroepiandrosterone and sex steroid levels in postmenopausal women: role of the ovary? *Menopause* **18**:30–43

Laughlin G, Barrett-Connor E, Kritz-Silverstein D, Von Muhlen D (2000) Hysterectomy, oophorectomy, and endogenous sex hormone levels in older women: the Rancho Bernado Study **85**:645

Laumann E, Paik A, Rosen RC (1999) Sexual dysfunction in the United States: prevalence and predictors. *Jama* **281**:531–544

Lawson EA, Miller KK, Bredella MA, Phan C, Misra M, Meenaghan E, Rosenblum L, Donoho D, Gupta R, Klibanski A (2010) Hormone predictors of abnormal bone microarchitecture in women with anorexia nervosa. *Bone* **46**:458–463

Leao LM, Duarte MP, Silva DM, Bahia PR, Coeli CM, de Farias ML (2006) Influence of methyltestosterone postmenopausal therapy on plasma lipids, inflammatory factors, glucose metabolism and visceral fat: a randomized study. *Eur J Endocrinol* **154**:131–139

Lee JS, LaCroix AZ, Wu L, Cauley JA, Jackson RD, Kooperberg C, Leboff MS, Robbins J, Lewis CE, Bauer DC, Cummings SR (2008) Associations of serum sex hormone-binding globulin and sex hormone concentrations with hip fracture risk in postmenopausal women. *J Clin Endocrinol Metab* **93**:1796–1803

Leiblum S, Bachmann GA, Kemmann E, Colburn D, Schwartzman L (1983) The importance of sexual activity and hormones. *Jama* **249**:2195

Lellamo F, Volterrani M, Caminiti G, Karam R, Massaro R, Fini M, Collins P, Rosano GM (2010) Testosterone therapy in women with chronic heart failure: a pilot double-blind, randomized, placebo-controlled study. *J Am Coll Cardiol* **56**:1310–1316

Lindemann K, Vatten LJ, Ellstrom-Engh M, Eskild A (2008) Body mass, diabetes and smoking, and endometrial cancer risk: a follow-up study. *Br J Cancer* **98**:1582–1585

Lobo R, Rosen RC, Yang H-M, Block B, Van der Hoop R (2003) Comparative effects of oral esterified estrogens with and without methyl testosterone on endocrine profiles and dimensions of sexual function in postmenopausal women with

hypoactive sexual desire. *Fertil Steril* **79**:1341–1352

Longcope C (1986) Adrenal and gonadal androgen secretion in normal females. *J Clin Endocrinol* **15**:213–228

Loukovaara M, Carson M, Adlercreutz H (1995) Regulation of production and secretion of sex hormone-binding globulin in HepG2 cell cultures by hormones and growth factors. *J Clin Endocrinol Metab* **80**:160–164

Manderson L (2005) The social and cultural context of sexual function among middle-aged women. *Menopause* **12**:361–362

Mathur RS, Landgreve SC, Moody LO, Semmens JP, Williamson HO (1985) The effect of estrogen treatment on plasma concentrations of steroid hormones, gonadotropins, prolactin and sex hormone-binding globulin in post-menopausal women. *Maturitas* **7**:129–133

Miller K, Sesmilo G, Schiller A, Schonfeld D, Burton S, Klibanski A (2001) Androgen deficiency in women with hypopituitarism. *J Clin Endocrinol Metab* **86**:561–567

Miller KK, Biller BM, Beauregard C, Lipman JG, Jones J, Schoenfeld D, Sherman JC, Swearingen B, Loeffler J, Klibanski A (2006) Effects of testosterone replacement in androgen-deficient women with hypopituitarism: a randomized, double-blind, placebo-controlled study. *J Clin Endocrinol Metab* **91**:1683–1690

Miller KK, Lawson EA, Mathur V, Wexler TL, Meenaghan E, Misra M, Herzog DB, Klibanski A (2007) Androgens in women with anorexia nervosa and normal-weight women with hypothalamic amenorrhea. *J Clin Endocrinol Metab* **92**: 1334–1339

Moller MC, Bartfai AB, Radestad AF (2010) Effects of testosterone and estrogen replacement on memory function. *Menopause* **17**:983–989

Montalcini T, Gorgone G, Gazzaruso C, Sesti G, Perticone F, Pujia A (2007) Endogenous testosterone and endothelial function in postmenopausal women. *Coron Artery Dis* **18**:9–13

Mushayandebvu T, Castracane DV, Gimpel T, Adel T, Santoro N (1996) Evidence for diminished midcycle ovarian androgen production in older reproductive aged women. *Fertil Steril* **65**:721–723

Naessen T, Sjogren U, Bergquist J, Larsson M, Lind L, Kushnir MM (2010) Endogenous steroids measured by high-specificity liquid chromatography-tandem mass spectrometry and prevalent cardiovascular disease in 70-year-old men and women. *J Clin Endocrinol Metab* **95**:1889–1897

Ness RB, Albano J, McTiernan A, Cauley J (2009) Influence of estrogen plus testosterone supplementation on breast cancer. *Arch Intern Med* **169**:41–46

Nestler JE, Strauss JF 3rd (1991) Insulin as an effector of human ovarian and adrenal steroid metabolism. *Endocrinol Metab Clin North Am* **20**:807–823

Nurnberg HG, Hensley PL, Heiman JR, Croft HA, Debattista C, Paine S (2008) Sildenafil treatment of women with antidepressant-associated sexual dysfunction: a randomized controlled trial. *Jama* **300**:395–404

Ouyang P, Vaidya D, Dobs A, Golden SH, Szklo M, Heckbert SR, Kopp P, Gapstur SM (2009) Sex hormone levels and subclinical atherosclerosis in postmenopausal women: the Multi-Ethnic Study of Atherosclerosis. *Atherosclerosis* **204**:255–261

Panay N, Al-Azzawi F, Bouchard C, Davis SR, Eden J, Lodhi I, Rees M, Rodenberg CA, Rymer J, Schwenkhagen A, Sturdee DW (2010) Testosterone treatment of HSDD in naturally menopausal women: the ADORE study. *Climacteric* **13**:121–131

Perrone AM, Cerpolini S, Maria Salfi NC, Ceccarelli C, De Giorgi LB, Formelli G, Casadio P, Ghi T, Pelusi G, Pelusi C, Meriggiola MC (2009) Effect of long-term testosterone administration on the endometrium of female-to-male (FtM) transsexuals. *J Sex Med* **6**:3193–3200

Pike CJ, Carroll JC, Rosario ER, Barron AM (2009) Protective actions of sex steroid hormones in Alzheimer's disease. *Front Neuroendocrinol* **30**:239–258

Procter and Gamble Pharmaceuticals (2004) Intrinsa® (testosterone transdermal system) NDA No. 21-769. Ed ACfRH Drugs. US Food and Drug Administration, Washington, DC

Pugeat M, Cousin P, Baret C, Lejeune H, Forest MG (2000) Sex hormone-binding globulin during puberty in normal and hyperandrogenic girls. *J Pediatr Endocrinol Metab* **13** (Suppl 5):1277–1279

Randolph JF Jr, Sowers M, Gold EB, Mohr BA, Luborsky J, Santoro N, McConnell DS, Finkelstein JS, Korenman SG, Matthews KA, Sternfeld B, Lasley BL (2003) Reproductive hormones in the early menopausal transition: relationship to ethnicity, body size, and menopausal status. *J Clin Endocrinol Metab* **88**:1516–1522

Rariy CM, Ratcliffe SJ, Weinstein R, Bhasin S, Blackman MR, Cauley JA, Robbins J, Zmuda JM, Harris TB, Cappola AR (2011) Higher serum free testosterone concentration in older women is associated with greater bone mineral density, lean body mass, and total fat mass: the cardiovascular health study. *J Clin Endocrinol Metab* **96**:989–996

Rieche K, Wolff G (1975) Comparison of testosterone decanoate, drostanolone and testololactone in disseminated breast cancer – a randomized clinical study. *Arch Geschwulstforsch* **45**:485–488

Rosario ER, Chang L, Head EH, Stanczyk FZ, Pike CJ (2009) Brain

levels of sex steroid hormones in men and women during normal aging and in Alzheimer's disease. *Neurobiol Aging* **32**:604–613

Sarrel P, Dobay B, Wiita B (1998) Estrogen and estrogen-androgen replacement in postmenopausal women dissatisfied with estrogen-only therapy. Sexual behavior and neuroendocrine responses. *J Reprod Med* **43**:847–856

Selva DM, Hammond GL (2009) Peroxisome-proliferator receptor gamma represses hepatic sex hormone-binding globulin expression. *Endocrinology* **150**:2183–2189

Selva DM, Hogeveen KN, Innis SM, Hammond GL (2007) Monosaccharide-induced lipogenesis regulates the human hepatic sex hormone-binding globulin gene. *J Clin Invest* **117**:3979–3987

Shah SM, Bell RJ, Savage G, Goldstat R, Papalia MA, Kulkarni J, Donath S, Davis SR (2006) Testosterone aromatization and cognition in women: a randomized, placebo-controlled trial. *Menopause* **13**:600–608

Sherwin BB, Gelfand MM (1987) The role of androgen in the maintenance of sexual functioning in oophorectomized women. *Psychosomatic Med* **49**:397–409

Shifren JL, Braunstein G, Simon J, Casson P, Buster JE, Red Burki RE, Ginsburg ES, Rosen RC, Leiblum SR, Caramelli KE (2000) Transdermal testosterone treatment in women with impaired sexual function after oophorectomy. *N Eng J Med* **343**:682–688

Shifren JL, Davis SR, Moreau M, Waldbaum A, Bouchard C, DeRogatis L, Derzko C, Bearnson C, Kakos N, O'Neill S, Levine S, Wekselman K, Buch A, Rodenberg C, Kroll R, Kroll M (2006) Testosterone patch for the treatment of hypoactive sexual desire disorder in naturally menopausal women: results from the INTIMATE NM1 study. *Menopause* 13:770–779

Shifren JL, Monz BU, Russo PA, Segreti A, Johannes CB (2008) Sexual problems and distress in United States women: prevalence and correlates. *Obstet Gynecol* 112:970–978

Sievers C, Klotsche J, Pieper L, Schneider HJ, Marz W, Wittchen HU, Stalla GK, Mantzoros C (2010) Low testosterone levels predict all-cause mortality and cardiovascular events in women: a prospective cohort study in German primary care patients. *Eur J Endocrinol* 163:699–708

Simon J, Braunstein G, Nachtigall L, Utian W, Katz M, Miller S, Waldbaum A, Bouchard C, Derzko C, Buch A, Rodenberg C, Lucas J, Davis S (2005) Testosterone patch increases sexual activity and desire in surgically menopausal women with hypoactive sexual desire disorder. *J Clin Endocrinol Metab* 90:5226–5233

Simpson ER, Davis SR (2001) Minireview: aromatase and the regulation of estrogen biosynthesis – some new perspectives. *Endocrinology* 142:4589–4594

Slemenda C, Longcope C, Peacock M, Hui S, Johnston CC (1996) Sex steroids, bone mass, and bone loss. A prospective study of pre-, peri- and postmenopausal women. *J Clin Invest* 97:14–21

Sluijmer AV, Heineman MJ, De Jong FH, Evers JL (1995) Endocrine activity of the postmenopausal ovary: the effects of pituitary down-regulation and oophorectomy. *J Clin Endocrinol Metab* 80:2163–2167

Snabes MC, Simes SM (2009) Approved hormonal treatments for HSDD: an unmet medical need. *J Sex Med* 6:1846–1849

Sodergard R, Backstrom T, Shanhag V, Carstensen H (1982) Calculation of free and bound fractions of testosterone and estradiol-17 beta to human plasma proteins at body temperature. *J Steroid Biochem* 16:801–810

Somboonporn W, Davis S (2004) Testosterone and the breast: therapeutic implications for women. *Endocrine Reviews* 25:374–388

Somboonporn W, Bell RJ, Davis SR (2005) Testosterone for peri and postmenopausal women. *Cochrane Database Syst Rev* 4: CD004509

Sutton-Tyrrell K, Wildman RP, Matthews KA, Chae C, Lasley BL, Brockwell S, Pasternak RC, Lloyd-Jones D, Sowers MF, Torrens JI (2005) Sex hormone-binding globulin and the free androgen index are related to cardiovascular risk factors in multiethnic premenopausal and perimenopausal women enrolled in the Study of Women Across the Nation (SWAN). *Circulation* 111:1242–1249

Taieb J, Mathian B, Millot F, Patricot MC, Mathieu E, Queyrel N, Lacroix I, Somma-Delpero C, Boudou P (2003) Testosterone measured by 10 immunoassays and by isotope-dilution gas chromatography-mass spectrometry in sera from 116 men, women, and children. *Clin Chem* 49:1381–1395

Tamimi RM, Hankinson SE, Chen WY, Rosner B, Colditz GA (2006) Combined estrogen and testosterone use and risk of breast cancer in postmenopausal women. *Arch Intern Med* 166:1483–1489

Thurlimann B, Keshaviah A, Coates AS, Mouridsen H, Mauriac L, Forbes JF, Paridaens R, Castiglione-Gertsch M, Gelber RD, Rabaglio M, Smith I, Wardly A, Price KN, Goldhirsch A (2005) A comparison of letrozole and tamoxifen in postmenopausal women with early breast cancer. *N Engl J Med* 353:2747–2757

Tuiten A, Von Honk J, Koppeschaar H, Bernaards C, Thijssen J, Verbaten R (2000) Time course of effects of testosterone administration on sexual arousal in women. *Arch Gen Psychiatry* 57:149

Tungphaisal S, Chandeying V, Sutthijumroon S, Krisanapan O, Udomratn P (1991) Postmenopausal sexuality in Thai women. *Asia Oceania J Obstet Gynaecol* 17: 143–146

Utian WH (1972) The true clinical features of postmenopausal oophorectomy and their response to estrogen replacement therapy. *S Afr Med J* 46:732–737

Wagner JD, Zhang L, Williams JK, Register TC, Ackerman DM, Wiita B, Clarkson TB, Adams MR (1996) Esterified estrogens with and without methyltesterone decrease arterial LDL metabolism in Cynomolgus monekys. *Arterioscler Thromb Vasc Biol* 16:1473–1480

Warnock JK, Swanson SG, Borel RW, Zipfel LM, Brennan JJ (2005) Combined esterified estrogens and methyltestosterone versus esterified estrogens alone in the treatment of loss of sexual interest in surgically menopausal women. *Menopause* 12:374–384

Watts NB, Notelovitz M, Timmons MC (1995) Comparison of oral estrogens and estrogens plus androgen on bone mineral density, menopausal symptoms and lipid-lipoprotein profiles in surgical menopause 85:529–537

Werneke U, Northey S, Bhugra D (2006) Antidepressants and sexual dysfunction. *Acta Psychiatr Scand* 114:384–397

Wild S, Pierpoint T, Jacobs H, McKeigue P (2000) Long-term consequences of polycystic ovary syndrome: results of a 31 year follow-up study. *Hum Fertil (Camb)* 3:101–105

Wisniewski A, Ngyuen T, Dobs AS (2002) Evaluation of high-dose estrogen and high-dose estrogen plus methyltestosterone treatment on cognitive task performance in postmenopausal women. *Horm Res* 58:150–155

Witherby S, Johnson J, Demers L, Mount S, Littenberg B, Maclean CD, Wood M, Muss H (2011) Topical testosterone for breast cancer patients with vaginal atrophy related to aromatase inhibitors: a phase I/II study. *Oncologist* 16:424–431

Wolf OT, Kirschbaum C (2002) Endogenous estradiol and testosterone levels are associated with cognitive performance in older women and men 41:259

Worboys S, Kotsopoulos D, Teede H, McGrath BP, Davis SR (2001) Evidence that parenteral testosterone therapy may improve endothelium-dependent and -independent vasodilation in postmenopausal women already receiving estrogen. *J Clin Endocrinol Metab* 86:158–161

Yao M, Nguyen TV, Rosario ER, Ramsden M, Pike CJ (2008) Androgens regulate neprilysin expression: role in reducing beta-amyloid levels. *J Neurochem* 105:2477–2488

Zang H, Davis SR (2008) Androgen replacement therapy in androgen-deficient women with hypopituitarism. *Drugs* 68:2085–2093

Zang H, Carlstrom K, Arner P, Hirschberg AL (2006) Effects of treatment with testosterone alone or in combination with estrogen on insulin sensitivity in postmenopausal women. *Fertil Steril* 86:136–144

Zang H, Sahlin L, Masironi B, Eriksson E, Linden Hirschberg A (2007) Effects of testosterone treatment on endometrial proliferation in postmenopausal women. *J Clin Endocrinol Metab* 92:2169–2175

Zuckerman-Levin N, Frolova-Bishara T, Militianu D, Levin M, Aharon Peretz J, Hochberg Z (2009) Androgen replacement therapy in Turner syndrome: a pilot study. *J Clin Endocrinol Metab* 94:4820–4827

Zumoff B, Strain GW, Miller LK, Rosner W (1995) Twenty-four hour mean plasma testosterone concentration declines with age in normal premenopausal women 80:1429–1430

Detection of illegal use of androgens and selective androgen receptor modulators

Wilhelm Schänzer and Mario Thevis

24.1 Introduction

Anabolic androgenic steroids (AAS) are known to be misused both in competitive and in non-competitive sports (Haupt and Rovere 1984; Wilson 1988; Yesalis *et al.* 1993). Moreover, it seems that AAS are becoming "social drugs," as even young people apply them as an expression of an improved "lifestyle."

The misuse of AAS in athletics has been observed for more than 50 years. The first rumors dated from 1954 and were attributed to weightlifters who seemed to have used testosterone (Wade 1972). By 1965 synthetic AAS had become widely popular among bodybuilders and weightlifters, but were also applied in other forms of sports.

By using these steroids, athletes hoped to increase muscle strength. Such improvements in muscle strength to increase physical performance in sport are naturally an essential effect of training. As AAS stimulate protein synthesis in muscle cells, athletes expect performance-enhancing effects beyond those brought about by training alone. At the end of the sixties, the first anti-doping rules were established by international sport federations (1967, International Cycling Union and 1968, International Olympic Committee – IOC), but only stimulants and narcotics were banned (Clasing 1992). At that time, the Medical Commission of the IOC was already aware of widespread misuse of AAS in sports. They were not banned because no reliable method was available to

Testosterone: Action, Deficiency, Substitution, ed. Eberhard Nieschlag and Hermann M. Behre, Assoc. ed. Susan Nieschlag.
Published by Cambridge University Press. © Cambridge University Press 2012.

detect them (Beckett and Cowan 1979). Under these circumstances the first methods for AAS detection were developed (Brooks *et al.* 1975; Ward *et al.* 1975), and in 1974 the Medical Commission of the IOC and the International Amateur Athletic Federation (IAAF) first banned the use of AAS. This prohibition encompassed only synthetic steroids, such as metandienone, stanozolol etc., and the use of endogenous steroids, e.g. testosterone, was not restricted. At that time athletes misused only synthetic AAS. The reason was that AAS were used in human medicine to treat catabolic conditions; scientific data obtained from animal studies led to the conclusion that synthetic AAS are more anabolic and less androgenic than testosterone itself (Kochakian 1976).

Whether athletes experience a positive performance-enhancing effect or not when using AAS has been discussed controversially for many years. Nowadays it is known that androgens have muscle growth-promoting effects in boys, in women and in hypogonadal men. It has never been proven that androgens, when administered in therapeutic doses, have positive effects on muscle growth in healthy adult men. The assumption that AAS have less effect on muscle growth in men is based on the fact that the androgen receptor in men is nearly completely saturated (Wilson 1996). However, high doses of androgens have been reported to exert muscle mass-enhancing effects (Bhasin *et al.* 1996). An unethical and secret program of hormonal doping of athletes in the former German Democratic Republic (GDR) was reported (Franke and Berendonk 1997), and performance-improving effects of AAS were elucidated.

The most frequently misused steroid in the GDR was Oral Turinabol (dehydrochloromethyl-testosterone, Fig. 24.1), which was used from 1968 onwards by nearly all male and female athletes. In later years the steroid mestanolone (the 17α-methylated dihydrotestosterone, 17β-hydroxy-17α-methyl-5α-androstan-3-one) was also regularly administered, which seemed to be more effective in promoting aggressiveness and allowed higher training cycles without much bodyweight increase (Franke and Berendonk 1997). Beside oral androgenic steroids, also injections of steroid esters (nor-testosterone and testosterone esters) were applied, mainly to female athletes. Interestingly, in the document of Franke and Berendonk (1997), further chlorinated steroids are listed which have been

developed but misused to a lesser extent, e.g. 11β-hydroxy-Oral Turinabol, also named as SXII. Concerning performance-enhancement effects, Franke and Berendonk (1997) quoted "a summary report to the Stasi on March 3, 1977 . . . (Stasi = Ministry of State Security) under the code name 'Technik,' (pp. 243–44))," which described the GDR results and concluded:

> The positive value of anabolic steroids for the development of a top performance is undoubted. Here are a few examples . . . Performances could be improved with the support of these drugs within four years as follows: Shot-put (men) 2.5–4 m; Shot-put (women) 4.5–5 m; Discus throw (men) 10–12 m; Discus throw (women) 11–20 m; Hammer throw 6–10 m; Javelin throw (women) 8–15 m; 400 m (women) 4–5 sec; 800 m (women) 5–10 sec; 1500 m (women) 7–10 sec . . . Remarkable rates of increase in performances were also noted in the swimming events of women . . . from our experiences made so far, it can be concluded that women have the greatest advantage from treatments with anabolic hormones with respect to their performance in sports . . . Especially high is the performance-supporting effect following the first administration of anabolic hormones, especially with junior athletes.

To control the (mis)use of synthetic AAS, urine samples of athletes collected after competition events were tested. As AAS are not used directly during competition but rather during training to increase muscle strength, athletes stopped administration of AAS before competition, switching to those AAS (e.g. stanozolol) they believed could not be detected, and to endogenous androgens, such as testosterone, which were not banned. Investigations of test samples from the Olympic Summer Games in 1980 in Moscow showed that 2.1% of male and 7.1% of female athletes had elevated testosterone levels (Zimmermann 1986) in urine, and the highest urinary testosterone levels were detected for women in swimming and track and field events. These results could only be explained by exogenous application of testosterone.

Donike developed a GC-MS method for detection of testosterone and epitestosterone excreted in urine, and proved that the ratio of testosterone to epitestosterone (T/E) is significantly increased after application of testosterone (Donike *et al.* 1983). Based on these results, sport federations also banned testosterone in 1984 and applied the T/E ratio measurements (cutoff level of six) to their rules. In 2006 the World

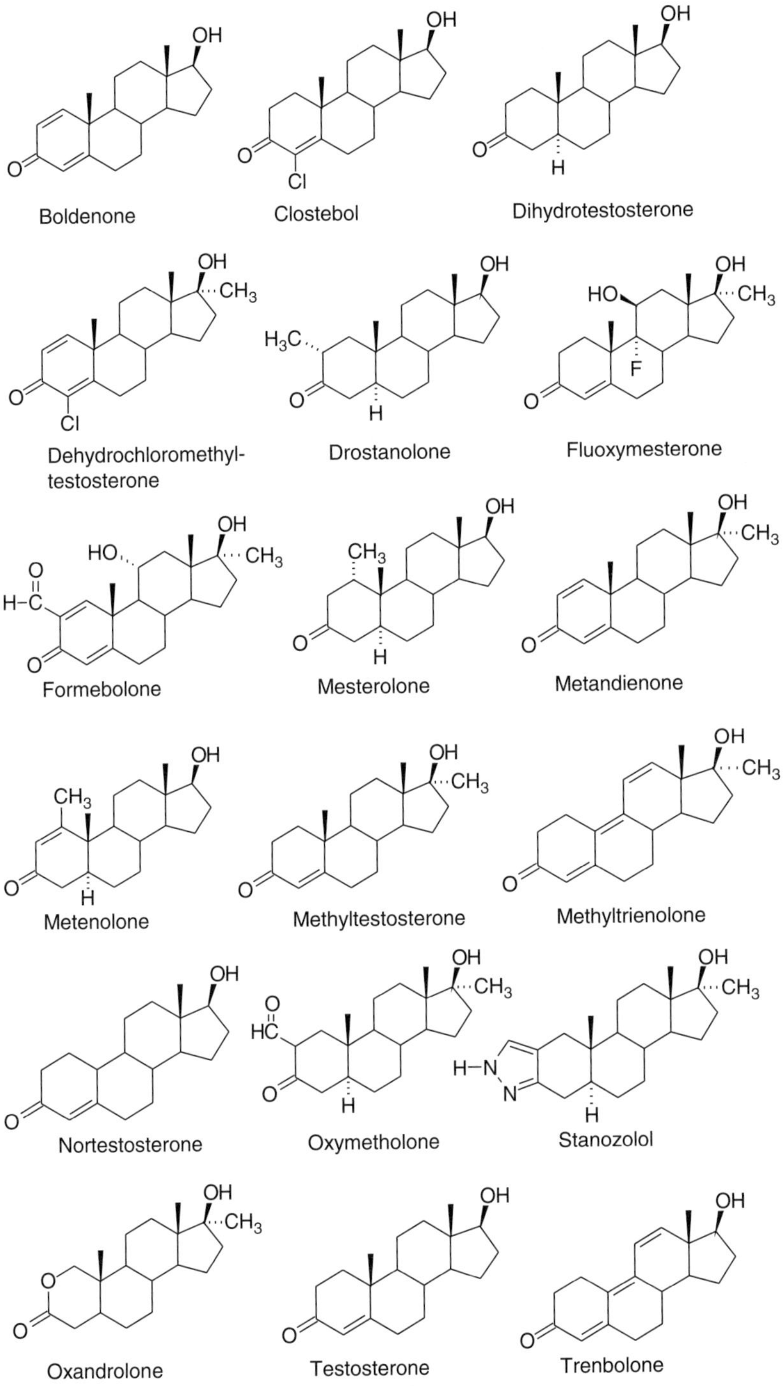

Fig. 24.1 Structural formulae of AAS which have been internationally detected in doping tests in sports.

Anti-Doping Agency (WADA) reduced the T/E ratio cutoff to four, and athletes with increased values will undergo follow-up investigations. In addition to the ban of testosterone, other endogenous androgens such as dihydrotestosterone, and prohormones of testosterone, dihydrotestosterone and nortestosterone, as well as new designer steroids, were added to the list of prohibited AAS during recent years.

24.2 Frequency of steroid hormone misuse

Considering this misuse of AAS, the question arises, to what extent are AAS really misused? Is it restricted to a few high-level performing athletes in sports or is it so extensive as to be regarded as a social drug problem? Available data derive:

1. from positive findings resulting from checking AAS doping in competition sports; and
2. from results of questionnaires concerning the use of AAS in non-competitive sports.

24.2.1 Androgen misuse in controlled competition sports

Androgen misuse in competition sports is investigated by laboratories which are accredited by the WADA. Each year the accredited laboratories (35 laboratories in 2011, worldwide) report the positive findings from the A-sample (see below) analyses. The annual testing frequency was about 207 500 samples for all laboratories from 2002 to 2010. In this time period a total number of 1 867 109 doping tests were analyzed by the WADA-accredited laboratories for Olympic and non-Olympic sports, and 9345 AAS were reported in different types of sport as positive findings. This represents 0.5% of all test samples. Compared to data from 1992–2001, the positive findings with AAS were 0.34% lower. Fig. 24.1 shows the chemical structure of misused steroids. The data indicate that the misuse of AAS is limited to a number of well-known AAS. Among the most frequent steroid hormones misused in controlled competitive sports are the synthetic steroids nortestosterone, stanozolol, metandienone and metenolone, and the endogenous steroid testosterone.

The detection of Oral Turinabol, the most widely used steroid in the former GDR, is based on identification of long-term excreted metabolites following hydroxylation at C-6, C-16, 17-epimerization and reduction of the 4,5 double bond to a 5β-configuration. The steroid is still of interest and in recent years it appeared on the black market, advertised as a new "reinvented" steroid. But the numbers of positive results in doping control are still low compared to the misuse of metandienone and stanozolol. In the time period from 2005 to 2009, approximately 29 doping violations were reported for Oral Turinabol worldwide in comparison to 1094 cases for stanozolol and 526 for metandienone.

24.2.2 Androgen misuse in non-competitive sports

In comparison to officially controlled competition sports, no analytical data from laboratories concerning the misuse of AAS are available for those areas of athletics and private life where no tests are performed. To overcome this lack of information, scientists have performed surveys; however, only a few publications are available. Yesalis et al. (1993) published results of investigations in the United States and calculated that one million Americans had used AAS some time in their lives, including about 250 000 in the past year. In 1993 a Canadian study (Canadian Centre for Drug-Free Sport 1993) confirmed that, in Canada, 80 000 young people between the ages of 13 and 18 had used AAS. A self-report questionnaire about the misuse of AAS among 13 355 Australian high-school students reported 3.2% of male and 1.2% of female users (Handelsman and Gupta 1997). Questionnaires from Switzerland were summarized by Kamber (1995), who concluded that AAS are a serious problem. A questionnaire from 16 000 recruits in Switzerland and 3700 women of the same age showed that 1.8% of the recruits and 0.3% of the women had administered AAS in 1993. Two surveys in Germany investigated the misuse of AAS in fitness studios mainly associated with bodybuilding. Boos et al. (1998) published a misuse rate of AAS of about 24% in males and 8% in females, and Striegel et al. (2006) reported a rate of 19.2% in male and 3.9% in female visitors in fitness centers.

Data concerning the most commonly misused AAS in non-controlled sports are only available via recommendations in magazines for bodybuilders, via "underground" handbooks (Taylor 1982; Duchaine 1989; Grundig and Bachmann 1995; Sinner 2009) and the internet and via confiscated, smuggled substances and those obtained from black-market sources. Frequently recommended AAS include boldenone undecylenate, drostanolone enanthate and propionate, fluoxymesterone, mesterolone, metandienone, metenolone acetate and enanthate, methandriol dipropionate, methyltestosterone, nortestosterone decanoate and other esters (hexylphenylpropionate, laurate, propionate and undecanoate), oxandrolone, oxymetholone, stanozolol, testosterone

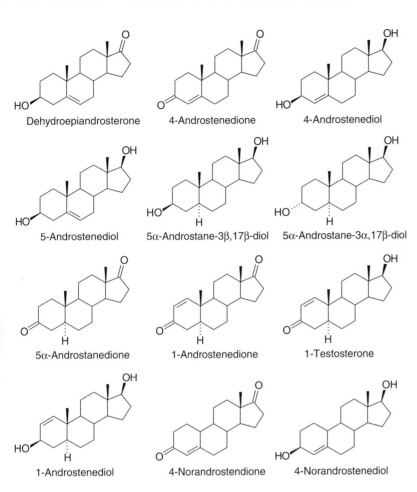

Fig. 24.2 Structural formulae of prohormones of testosterone, dihydrotestosterone and 1-ene steroids.

Dehydroepiandrosterone

4-Androstenedione

4-Androstenediol

5-Androstenediol

5α-Androstane-3β,17β-diol

5α-Androstane-3α,17β-diol

5α-Androstanedione

1-Androstenedione

1-Testosterone

1-Androstenediol

4-Norandrostendione

4-Norandrostenediol

in the form of different esters (cypionate, enanthate, heptylate, decanoate, hexanoate, isocaproate, isohexanoate, phenylpropionate, propionate and undecanoate) and trenbolone, trenbolone acetate.

These substances are largely identical with those products which were confiscated and distributed by the black market over the last 20 years.

24.3 Prohormones of androgens

Since 1999, prohormones of testosterone (e.g. dehydroepiandrosterone (DHEA, 3β-hydroxyandrost-5-en-17-one), 4-androstenedione (androst-4-ene-3,17-dione), 4-androstenediol (androst-4-ene-3β,17β-diol), 5-androstenediol (androst-5-ene-3β,17β-diol)) (Fig. 24.2), prohormones of dihydrotestosterone (5α-androstane-3β,17β-diol, 5α-androstane-3α,17β-diol, 5α-androstanedione (5α-androstane-3,17-dione)) (Fig. 24.2), steroids with 5α-androst-1-ene structure (1-androstenedione (5α-androst-1-ene-3,17-dione), 1-testosterone (17β-hydroxy-5α-androst-4-en-3-one), 1-androstenediol (5α-androst-1-ene-3β,17β-diol)) (Fig. 24.2), and prohormones of nortestosterone (4-norandrostenedione (estr-4-ene-3,17-dione), 4-norandrostenediol (estr-4-ene-3β,17β-diol)) (Fig. 24.2) have been marketed in the United States as nutritional supplements.

Steroids with 5α-androst-1-ene structure may be considered as prohormones of dihydrotestosterone, as the double bond at C1–2 is partly hydrogenated in human metabolism, but otherwise the compounds are not synthesized in the human body as intermediates of endogenously produced steroids and should be classified as designer steroids.

Prohormones are advertised as having effects similar to testosterone, dihydrotestosterone and nortestosterone because of a "high conversion rate" of prohormones to the physiologically effective steroids in the human body after oral, sublingual or buccal application. In contrast to such incorrect advertisements, only small amounts of the applied prohormone may be converted to the effective steroid. Indeed, for medical treatment prohormones are useless. Therefore companies providing prohormones recommend applying several times per day, especially before training or competition (high amounts (100 mg and more) of oral preparations of single prohormones, combinations of different prohormones and sublingual preparations). Published data (Leder et al. 2000) demonstrate that, in male persons, e.g. androstenedione 100 mg/day taken orally for seven days yielded no significant changes in serum testosterone levels compared to the control group, whereas 300 mg/day of androstenedione for seven days showed a significant increase in peak and AUC (area under curve) serum testosterone (AUC 34%), but with high interindividual variation. As prohormones are also used by females and adolescents, lower amounts of prohormones may yield physiological changes in serum testosterone levels; e.g. 100 mg androstenedione given orally to females yielded an increase in serum testosterone concentrations of up to 0.8 ng/ml (Kicman et al. 2003).

In a study with 19-norandrostenediol, a prohormone of 19-nortestosterone, by Schrader et al. (2006), an open-label, crossover trial with eight healthy male volunteers was conducted. After administration of capsules or sublingual tablets with 25 mg of 19-norandrostenediol, plasma concentrations of the pharmacologically active 19-nortestosterone were determined up to 5.7 ng/ml. The results demonstrate the importance of prohibiting prohormones such as 19-norandrostenediol, in particular, since plasma concentrations of nandrolone between 0.3 and 1.2 ng/ml have been reported to influence endocrinological parameters (Belkien et al. 1985).

The distribution of prohormones in the United States was not restricted until 2005 because these products have not been marketed as medications. But in 2005 prohormones were included in the list of controlled substances by the "Anabolic Steroid Control Act" to prohibit the illegal distribution of these substances. In Europe prohormones are considered unlicensed medications, and their distribution is banned. Nevertheless, control of the misuse of prohormones is difficult: products enter the European market via neighbor states, directly via airports and by internet or postal orders.

Additional new products have entered the market with a 1-ene structure, such as androsta-1,4-diene-3,17-dione, which is considered as a prohormone of the synthetic AAS boldenone (17β-hydroxyandrosta-1,4-dien-3-one), and steroids with a 5α-androst-1-ene structure (Fig. 24.2) which are marketed as prohormones.

24.4   Designer steroids

Designer steroids are anabolic steroids which are designed to be undetectable in drug testing but have anabolic effects similar to testosterone and other steroid-like performance-enhancing drugs. The most famous scandal with designer steroids was the Balco scandal in 2002 when the sports nutrition center, Bay Area Laboratory Co-operative (BALCO), in California (USA) provided a modified steroid to top-level athletes. This steroid was later identified as tetrahydrogestrinone (THG). The starting steroid was an already-banned anabolic androgenic steroid named gestrinone, which was chemically modified by the introduction of four hydrogen atoms at the C-17 ethinyl group (Fig. 24.3). The tetrahydrogestrinone so obtained remained undetectable until reference material was delivered to the IOC-accredited doping control laboratory in Los Angeles (Catlin et al. 2004). Further designer steroids such as norboletone (Catlin et al. 2002) and desoxymethyltestosterone (Madol, DMT) (Sekera et al. 2005) were distributed at the same time. Since that time, an increasing number of designer steroids, not explicitly synthesized for athletes, have also been illegally marketed and advertised as dietary supplements (Kazlauskas 2010; Parr and

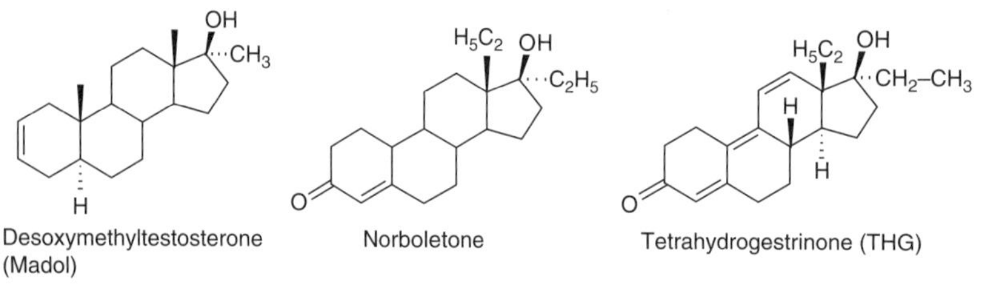

Fig. 24.3 Structural formulae of designer steroids Madol, norboletone and tetrahydrogestrinone.

Desoxymethyltestosterone (Madol)

Norboletone

Tetrahydrogestrinone (THG)

Schänzer 2010). None of these designer steroids is of interest for medical purposes. Depending on the country, they are illegally distributed. They are non-approved drugs and may cause severe side-effects.

24.5 Contamination of nutritional supplements with prohormones

Since 1999, the same time when prohormones were entering the market, nutritional supplements have become sporadically "contaminated" with prohormones. "Contamination" in this context signifies that a supplement contains substances which are not declared on the label. As the amount of "contamination" is low, less than 1 per mille of the product, it is assumed that the prohormones are not intentionally added to the supplements but may be contaminated due to poor quality control during the production of nutritional supplements and prohormones. Several athletes have been tested in the past with positive results for norandrosterone (main metabolite of nortestosterone and the main metabolite of the prohormones of nortestosterone such as norandrost-4-ene-3,17-dione and norandrost-4-ene-3β,17β-diol); the use of nutritional supplements which contained low traces of prohormones of nortestosterone led to positive results. In such a case the athlete has not intentionally applied a doping substance, but the sports federations consider the presence of norandrosterone in the urine sample as a doping offence for which the athlete is fully responsible.

To what extent nutritional supplements may be contaminated has been shown in different studies and by an international study supported by the IOC (Geyer *et al.* 2004). The latter study investigated 630 different nutritional supplements from 13 countries including the United States, Italy, France, Germany and Great Britain. Out of the 634 samples analyzed, 94 (14.8%) contained prohormones not declared on the label ("positive supplements"). Of these 94 positive supplements, 23 samples (24.5%) contained prohormones of nortestosterone and testosterone; 64 samples (68.1%) only contained prohormones of testosterone; 7 samples (7.5%) only contained prohormones of nortestosterone.

In relation to the total number of products purchased per country, most of the positive supplements (84%) originate from companies located in the United States. (The investigation was focused on nutritional supplements offered in western countries and which have been identified as a source for positive findings. The problem was clearly in connection with prohormones of testosterone and nortestosterone produced in the United States and was not aimed at products originating from Asian countries.)

The positive supplements showed anabolic androgenic steroid concentrations of 0.01 μg/g up to 190 μg/g. Excretion studies with application of supplements containing nortestosterone prohormones corresponding to a total uptake of more than 1 μg resulted in urinary concentrations of the nortestosterone metabolite norandrosterone above the cutoff limit (2 ng/ml urine) for several hours (positive doping result).

Positive doping tests caused by "contaminated" supplements with prohormones of only testosterone or dihydrotestosterone have not been proved, which is explainable by the low amounts of contamination and the applied tests, which have to differentiate between endogenous and exogenous origin of testosterone and which will not be influenced by ingestion of low amounts of prohormones or testosterone itself.

This problem of contaminated nutritional supplements with prohormones seems to have beeen reduced in recent years, as in 2005 the "Anabolic Steroid Control Act" in the United States banned the marketing and distribution of prohormones.

24.6 Detection of misuse of anabolic androgenic steroid hormones

24.6.1 Organization of doping tests

Doping control is organized by national and international sports federations and by the WADA for the different types of sports. Increasingly, national anti-doping programs are managing doping control via one overall organization. This strategy seems to be the most effective testing action, as any possible intention by individual sports federations to hide positive cases and to protect their athletes can be excluded. The IOC only performed doping tests during the Olympic winter and summer games, and it has no "out of competition testing program." This deficit has now been compensated for by WADA.

For a doping test, athletes are selected according to the rules of the responsible sports federation. The doping test is carried out in two steps. The first step includes the sample-taking procedure and transportation of the urine specimens to a WADA-accredited laboratory. In the following step the laboratory analyzes the sample for banned drugs. The sample-taking procedure is an important step. To avoid any manipulation, athletes have to deliver a urine sample under visual inspection by an accredited supervisor. The urine is divided into an A- and a B-sample; both samples are sealed and then transported to the laboratory. All steps during this procedure are documented and the athlete has to sign a protocol of the sample-taking procedure and sealing of samples. All handling of a urine specimen (sample-taking, transportation containers and laboratory tests) must be documented and is designated as "chain of custody." The laboratory is not in possession of the athlete's name corresponding to the urine sample, and all samples have code numbers. The reason for dividing the urine specimen into A- and B-samples is to guarantee the best chain of custody: if the A-sample is tested positive (the laboratory reports an adverse analytical finding), the B-sample can be analyzed on request of the athlete. For transparency the B-sample analysis will be performed in the presence of the athlete and his advisers. If the B-analysis confirms the A-result, the sample is considered as positive and the federation can impose sanctions on the athlete.

Doping test samples are analyzed by WADA-accredited laboratories. Laboratories seeking accreditation have to comply with the requirements for doping drug testing set by the WADA World-Anti-Doping Code. Additionally, the laboratory has to be accredited by a national accreditation body following the standard of ISO 17025. The laboratory must show that it has the capability to analyze all banned substances below the specified concentration limits within a controlled quality system.

The prerequisite for this accreditation system is a standardization of analytical techniques and detection limits of banned substances among the different laboratories. Information concerning new doping drugs and doping techniques is rapidly distributed in order to deal with new problems in a coordinated manner. Especially for the detection of synthetic AAS, which are misused mainly during training periods, the laboratory has to use highly sensitive methods.

At the present time, 35 WADA laboratories all over the world (20 in Europe, 4 in North America, 2 in South America, 6 in Asia, 1 in Australia and 2 in Africa) are accredited.

24.6.2 Detection and identification of misused anabolic androgenic steroids

Synthetic AAS were first banned in 1974. As no comprehensive analytical method for the detection of AAS in human urine was available at the beginning of the seventies, new methods had to be developed. The first methods were based on radioimmunoassay (RIA) techniques; for instance Brooks et al. (1975) developed an antiserum for metandienone with some cross-reactivity to other 17α-methyl steroids. The RIA techniques were discouraging for several reasons: the method did not consider the high degree of metabolism of AAS (therefore screening for the parent steroid was less successful), the antisera had only limited sensitivity for other steroids and the possibility of false positives, which was not acceptable for routine analysis. As early as 1975 Ward et al. presented a GC-MS method for the detection of the AAS metandienone, nortestosterone, norethandrolone and stanozolol. Nevertheless, the RIA technique was used as a screening method during the 1976 Olympic Games in Montreal and in Moscow in 1980, but confirmation of suspicious samples was performed by GC-MS. After 1981 all IOC-accredited laboratories used GC-MS as the main analytical tool for AAS identification (Donike et al. 1984; Massé et al. 1989; Schänzer and Donike 1993).

Analysis of AAS can be divided and described in two steps: first a sample preparation is performed with the aim to separate the banned substances from the biological matrix (urine) and to reduce biological interference (biological background). Sample preparation for AAS also includes a chemical modification (derivatization) of the isolated substances to improve their analytical detectability when gas chromatographic separation techniques are applied. The second step covers the analytical measurement, which is based on a physical principle, mainly on gas chromatography in combination with mass spectrometry (GC-MS) or tandem mass spectrometry (GC-MS/MS). Additionally, liquid chromatography and tandem mass spectrometry (LC-MS/MS) is used for AAS with poor gas chromatographic properties or which are sensitive to temperature.

The main advantage of chromatographic techniques such as GC-MS, GC-MS/MS and LC-MS/MS is the possibility of analyzing a high number of substances within one run. This minimizes costs and allows a high throughput of samples. In fact it is possible to run a maximum of 50 samples per day and per GC-MS instrument.

24.6.2.1 Metabolism

To a large extent, anabolic androgenic steroids are metabolized by phase I and phase II reactions, and only a few AAS are excreted unchanged in urine for a short period of time after administration. To detect the misuse of AAS which are not excreted in urine or only to a small extent, the analytical method cannot rely on monitoring only the parent steroid but must identify its metabolites. Detection of an AAS metabolite in urine is proof for the misuse of a banned anabolic androgenic doping substance. This presumes that the metabolite cannot be generated from endogenous steroids in the body compartment.

Metabolites of the most frequently misused anabolic steroids have been investigated by different working groups in recent years, and reviews have been published (Schänzer and Donike 1993; Schänzer 1996; Thevis and Schänzer 2010). Basically, the metabolism of AAS follows the metabolic pathways of the principal androgen testosterone. This includes reduction of the double bond at C4-C5 to form 5α- and 5β-isomers, the reduction of the 3-keto group to a 3α-hydroxy function and, in the case of 17β-hydroxy steroids with a secondary hydroxy group, the oxidation yielding a 17-keto function. Additionally, many AAS are metabolized by cytochrome P450 hydroxylation reactions, and steroids with hydroxy groups mainly at C-6β, C-16α and C-16β are produced. In the metabolism of stanozolol, a synthetic steroid with a condensed pyrazol ring on the steroid A-ring (Fig. 24.1), further hydroxylation occurs at C-4β and C-3$'$ of the heterocyclic ring. In general, in the course of phase I metabolism steroids are enzymatically transformed to more polar but pharmacologically inactive compounds. Phase I reactions are often followed by phase II processes, also known as phase II conjugation. In the case of AAS and their metabolites the reaction creates steroid conjugates with sulfate or glucuronic acid (Thevis et al. 2001). These highly polar compounds are then rapidly eliminated in the urine.

In the last 20 years excretion studies performed with 17α-methyl steroids have demonstrated that the metabolism of AAS is highly complex, and the detection of more than 20 metabolites after administration of one single AAS is not unusual. Similar results regarding the high number of metabolites are known for the metabolism of testosterone (Kochakian 1990).

24.6.2.2 Pharmacokinetics

A further important factor which has to be considered for detection of AAS is the pharmacokinetics of the parent compound and its excreted metabolites. As AAS are misused during training and the number of doping tests is limited, it is desirable to detect AAS as long as possible after their last administration. Analysis of the parent steroids and/or their metabolites, which are excreted very rapidly, is less effective for screening analysis than the detection of metabolites excreted long-term: these are steroids detectable for the longest possible period of time after administration (Schänzer et al. 1996; Schänzer et al. 2006). The main differences between the pharmacokinetics of AAS are caused by their pharmaceutical preparation and the kind of application. Depot preparations, e.g. 19-nortestosterone injected intramuscularly as its undecanoate ester (Deca-Duraboline®), are detectable in urine for several weeks; whereas most oral preparations are completely eliminated within a few days after intake. Once they became aware of these scientific data, athletes switched their doping activities to AAS with short elimination times and to steroids which were believed to be undetectable.

24.6.2.3 Sample preparation

For sample preparation of anabolic steroids it has to be considered that most of the AAS and their metabolites are excreted in conjugated form. Following sample preparation, unconjugated steroids can be separated by extracting an aliquot of urine (e.g. 2 ml) with a polar, organic, non-water-miscible solvent. Based on their polar and acidic character, conjugated steroids are not extractable and remain in the aqueous layer. These conjugates (mainly glucuronides) can be liberated by enzymatic hydrolysis of the urine specimen. The enzyme used can be added directly to the urine or to an isolate obtained via an absorber resin. Enzymatic hydrolysis is achieved completely using enzyme preparations with β-glucuronidase from *Escherichia coli* or β-glucuronidase/arylsulfatase from *Helix pomatia*. The "free" steroids are then extracted from the aqueous phase via a simple liquid extraction with tert-butyl methyl ether, or in the case of less polar steroids, with an alkane (e.g. n-pentane).

The first analysis is a screening procedure by which all banned AAS are detected in one single analytical run. Suspicious samples are confirmed by a second aliquot of the same urine specimen, which is isolated using a substance-specific isolation technique.

24.6.2.4 Derivatization

For GC-MS analysis based on the polar groups of AAS (hydroxy and keto groups), high interactions with polar functions of the gas chromatography column phase reduce the detectability of AAS at low concentrations. Derivatization of polar functions of AAS can lead to a distinct improvement in peak intensity and detection limit of the analytical method. The most frequently used derivatization methods are acylation (e.g. trifluoroacetylation) and silylation (e.g. trimethylsilylation). For doping analysis of AAS, silylation is the method of choice, and the introduction of a trimethylsilyl group to an AAS is the most common derivatization reaction, converting polar groups such as hydroxy and keto functions to less polar trimethylsilyl ethers with excellent gas chromatography behavior. For this kind of derivatization a respectable reagent MSTFA (N-methyl-N-trimethylsilyltrifluoroacetamide) was developed (Donike 1969). Additionally, the mass spectrum is generally changed to higher and more abundant molecular and fragment ions, which also improves the signal-to-noise ratio of the substance to be identified compared to the analytical and biological background. Therefore, derivatization for GC-MS and GC-MS/MS detection of substances isolated from biological fluids unequivocally yields a more accurate analytical result, which is an absolute requirement in view of the complex matrix and large number of possible interferences.

24.6.3 Detection of synthetic anabolic androgenic steroids

In some instances AAS are differentiated into endogenous and exogenous AAS according to their route of administration. The term "synthetic" should exemplify the fact that these AAS are not produced in the body: they are chemically synthesized and can only enter the circulating blood system by exogenous application. Anabolic androgenic steroids which are naturally synthesized in the glands of mammalian cells are called endogenous steroids, even though their application can be exogenous. As synthetic AAS and/or their metabolites are not present in the human organism, their identification in a urine sample of

an athlete constitutes the misuse of a banned steroid. The criteria for identification of a substance are based on the analytical method applied.

In GC-MS, GC-MS/MS and LC-MS/MS identification of synthetic AAS obtained from a urine specimen, it is mandatory to register a full mass spectrum, or a selected ion monitoring (SIM) profile of the main abundant fragment ions, or daughter ions generated by tandem MS experiments of a diagnostic precursor ion (SRM, selected reaction monitoring). The mass spectrometric data (MS spectrum, SIM profile or daughter ions) of the isolated substance should be in accordance with an authentic synthesized reference substance or, in the event that a synthesized reference metabolite is not available, with a well-characterized metabolite from an excretion study with the corresponding AAS. In addition to the MS data, the gas chromatography or liquid chromatography retention time of the isolated steroid has to be in accordance with the gas chromatography or liquid chromatography retention time of the reference substance. For this purpose, reference metabolites of AAS frequently *misused* but not commercially available were synthesized (Schänzer and Donike 1993).

As an example, Fig. 24.4 shows the criteria for a positive sample for a long-term excreted metabolite of metandienone:

- registration of a full mass spectrum which can be compared with the reference spectrum; or
- in case of low concentrations, a selected ion monitoring (SIM) profile with the main intense fragment ions of the metandienone metabolite 17,17-dimethyl-18-nor-5β-androst-1,13-dien-3α-ol.

To increase the efficiency of AAS misuse testing and to detect AAS for a longer period of time after administration, more selective and sensitive MS techniques have been used during the last decade. The main improvements were, first, installation of more sensitive and selective mass spectrometers, and second, by substance-specific sample preparation (Schänzer *et al.* 1996). The use of high-resolution mass spectrometry (HRMS) was announced to the public at the 1996 Olympic Games in Atlanta. This technique was established after 1992 in a few IOC-accredited laboratories. The advantage of HRMS became apparent before Atlanta when, during doping testing by the International Weightlifting Federation, more than 40 athletes were confirmed positive only by HRMS and not

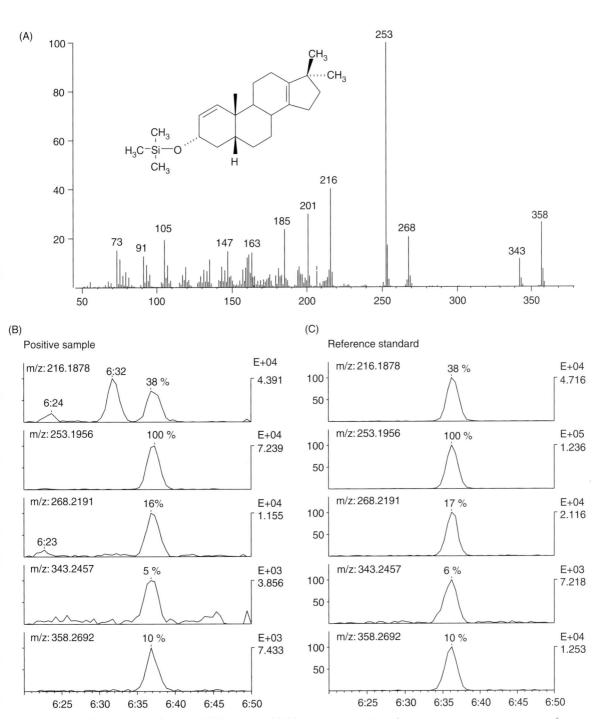

Fig. 24.4 Criteria for a positive confirmation: (1) The registered EI (electron impact ionization) mass spectrum, e.g. mass spectrum of an isolated metabolite of metandienone: 17,17-dimethyl-18-nor-5β-androsta-1,13-dien-3α-ol TMS, (A) has to be in accordance with the mass spectrum of an authentic reference substance, or (2) The main abundant fragment ions of the isolated substance show similar intensities (B) when selected ion monitoring (SIM) registration is applied in comparison to the intensities of the same fragments of the reference compound (C).

by the conventional MS technique. Following these results the IOC decided that it was necessary that accredited laboratories use more sophisticated equipment, such as HRMS or tandem mass spectrometry (MS-MS).

24.6.4 Detection of endogenous anabolic androgenic steroids

24.6.4.1 Indirect detection methods

The misuse of testosterone by athletes is also tested by GC-MS analysis of urinary extracts. The MS data alone does not distinguish exogenous (doping) from endogenous origin of testosterone. In 1983 Donike et al. developed a method to calculate urinary excreted testosterone by a ratio to 17-epitestosterone. Both isomeric steroid hormones are excreted mainly as glucuronides which are enzymatically hydrolyzed before GC-MS analysis. The urinary testosterone/epitestosterone ratio (T/E ratio) represents a relatively constant factor within an individual, and alterations under physical exercise have not been noted. Exogenous application of testosterone results in an increase in the urinary concentration of testosterone glucuronide, whereas epitestosterone glucuronide is not influenced. Based on measurements of large reference groups, Donike proposed a T/E ratio of 6 : 1 as a marker to handle a urine specimen suspicious for testosterone misuse. In 2006 the WADA reduced the ratio to 4 : 1. An increased T/E value (T/E > 4) is not immediately considered as a positive sample. Following the WADA rule, the athlete has to be further investigated and it has to be determined that the increased value is not caused by physical or pathological conditions. In practice this requires several test samples of the athlete and evaluation of previous tests in order to establish the athlete's individual T/E reference values (subject-based reference values). Additionally, analysis of the sample by IRMS (isotope ratio mass spectrometry) of carbon is applied to prove whether the $^{13}C/^{12}C$ ratio of the urinary excreted testosterone and its main metabolites is consistent with the endogenous production of testosterone (see Section 24.6.4.2).

Doping with DHT became public knowledge after the Asian Games in 1994, when seven athletes were tested positive for DHT misuse. The criteria for DHT doping are also based on statistical methods, and population-based reference values with limits for the

ratios of DHT/epitestosterone, DHT/etiocholanolone, 5α-androstane-3α,17β-diol/5β-androstane-3α,17β-diol, and androsterone/etiocholanolone were established (Kicman et al. 1995; Donike et al. 1995). Nowadays suspicious samples are also forwarded to IRMS analysis to prove the exogenous origin of DHT and/or its main metabolites.

24.6.4.2 Direct detection method: gas chromatography–combustion–isotope ratio mass spectrometry (GC-C-IRMS)

The T/E ratio results can be supported by gas chromatography–combustion–isotope ratio mass spectrometry (GC-C-IRMS). This method was first introduced by Becchi et al. in 1994 and has been adopted by other research groups (Aguilera et al. 1996; Horning et al. 1997; Shackleton et al. 1997; Flenker et al. 2008) with distinct modifications. A review of GC-C-IRMS in dope analysis has been presented by Cawley and Flenker (2008).

The principle of IRMS is the precise measurement of the $^{13}C/^{12}C$ isotope ratio of organic compounds. This method became practical for trace analysis in doping control when instruments combining gas chromatography and isotope ratio mass spectrometry were developed. Isotopes are elements with the same number of protons but different numbers of neutrons. Carbon occurs in three kinds of isotopes: ^{12}C (6 protons and 6 neutrons) with a frequency of approximately 98.9%, ^{13}C (6 protons and 7 neutrons) at a rate of 1.1% and ^{14}C (6 protons and 8 neutrons), a radioactive isotope with a half-life of 5760 years (used in determination of age), in traces. In the course of synthesizing organic compounds, ^{12}C atoms react slightly faster than ^{13}C atoms. This effect results in a reduction of the ^{13}C amount compared to ^{12}C. The $^{13}C/^{12}C$ ratio is calculated in per mille (delta ^{13}C (‰)) relative to a reference gas with a standardized $^{13}C/^{12}C$ ratio. The delta-value becomes more negative when the ^{13}C portion is reduced, which occurs during synthetic pathways. For isotope measurement, urinary excreted steroids have to be isolated to high purity. For gas chromatographic separation, derivatization is applied using acetylation of steroids with the aim of improving gas chromatography peak shape, or analysis refers to the underivatized steroids.

Steroids are separated by gas chromatography followed by complete oxidation to carbon dioxide in a combustion chamber. The carbon dioxide is then introduced to the mass spectrometer where the exact masses m/z 44 for $^{12}CO_2$ and m/z 45 for $^{13}CO_2$ are independently registered. For this kind of isotope ratio measurement, a minimum of 5–10 ng of a steroid has to be used to obtain precise data. The $^{13}C/^{12}C$ ratio can be estimated with an accuracy of $\pm 0.0002\%$ (± 0.2 per mille to the $^{13}C/^{12}C$ ratio of the reference gas).

A direct proof of exogenous testosterone application is possible as the delta-values are decreased to -28 ppm after administration, in comparison to -18 to -24 ppm (depending on the nutrition of the athlete) before intake. This method is also effective when ethnic differences influence testosterone metabolism, e.g. in Asians who have low T/E ratios, and when a testosterone application will not necessarily exceed the T/E ratio cutoff (de la Torre *et al.* 1997). Exogenous testosterone also influences the $^{13}C/^{12}C$ ratio of the metabolites of testosterone. Based on these data it was proved that precursors within the synthetic pathway of testosterone, such as pregnane-diol, pregnanetriol (metabolites of progesterone and 17α-hydroxyprogesterone) and cholesterol are not influenced by exogenous testosterone, whereas testosterone and its metabolites have decreased delta-values indicating exogenous application.

The IRMS method can additionally be applied to detect and identify doping with other endogenous AAS such as dihydrotestosterone and DHEA.

24.7 Selective androgen receptor modulators (SARMs)

24.7.1 General aspects

Selective androgen receptor modulators (SARMs) have received considerable attention from the doping control community since determined medicinal research outlined their potential beneficial properties for the treatment of various diseases (Gao and Dalton 2007; Kilbourne *et al.* 2007; Mohler *et al.* 2008; 2009; Bhasin and Jasuja 2009). Due to the major goal of developing ligands that induce anabolism specifically in muscle and bone tissue, a misuse of SARMs (comparable to the illicit use of steroidal and other non-steroidal agents) in elite and amateur sport cannot be excluded. A great variety of drug candidates based on considerably different pharmacophores has been prepared and investigated in preclinical or clinical trials, and new drug entities are continuously published, demonstrating the unconfined interest in novel anabolic agents allowing for a separation of anabolic and androgenic effects. Arylpropionamide-derived SARMs represent one of the most advanced classes of compounds, which are complemented by bicyclic hydantoin-, quinolinone-, tetrahydroquinolinone-(Nagata *et al.* 2011), carbazole-(Miller *et al.* 2010), as well as 4-aza-steroid-derived compounds (Schmidt *et al.* 2010) (Fig. 24.5), as recently reviewed by Mohler *et al.* (2009). Selective androgen receptor modulator – based drugs might offer new alternative therapeutic strategies towards the treatment of disease-associated muscle wasting, osteoporosis, anemia and different classifications of muscular dystrophies; however, concerns about an illicit use infiltrating the world of sports arose and were supported by recent findings of non-approved drug candidates on the black market (Thevis *et al.* 2009; 2011). Consequently, since January 2008, the entire class of androgen receptor modulators has been prohibited in sports according to the anti-doping regulations of the WADA (2010), although no SARM product has yet been officially launched. Nevertheless, such therapeutics may be particularly attractive to athletes as they presumably offer the desired anabolic effects without typical undesirable effects commonly associated with anabolic androgenic steroid (mis)use.

24.7.2 Analytical approaches

For sports drug testing purposes, numerous detection methods have been established during recent years, and several approaches targeting the intact compounds as well as in-vitro, in-vivo or chemically derived metabolites were reported (Thevis *et al.* 2006; 2007a; 2008a; 2008b; 2008c; 2010; Thevis and Schänzer 2008). Most of these methods are based on liquid chromatography–(tandem) mass spectrometry (LC-MS(/MS)), as the structural diversity of SARMs represents a key factor in sample preparation and analysis of this class of emerging drugs. As depicted in Fig. 24.5, all representatives of SARMs comprise polar functions that lead to positive (2-quinolinones) or negative (arylpropionamides, bicyclic hydantoins) charges during the analytical process. Moreover, the metabolic fate of most compounds is yet to be fully elucidated. Solid-phase extraction (SPE) and liquid-liquid extraction (LLE) were chosen for first studies

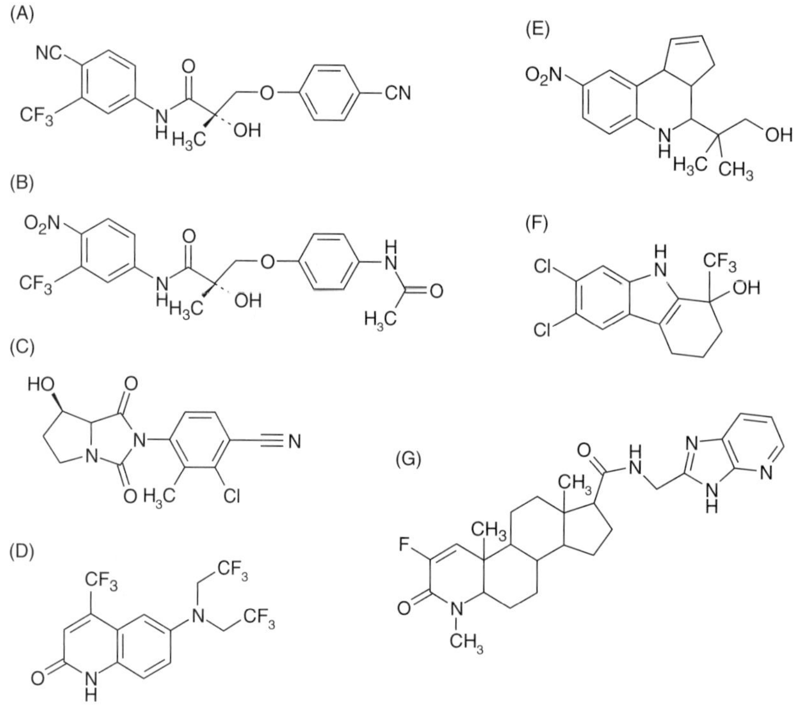

Fig. 24.5 Chemical structures of selected representatives of SARMs with arylpropionamide (S-22, A, and Andarine, B), bicyclic hydantoin (BMS-564929, C), quinoline (LGD-2226, D), tetrahydroquinoline (E), carbazole (RAD35101, F), and 4-aza-steroid (MK-0773, G) -derived nuclei.

on the detection of SARMs in doping control analysis, followed by LC-ESI-MS/MS (liquid chromatography with electrospray ionization–tandem mass spectrometry) analysis, which enabled the detection of 1 ng/ml of arylpropionamide-derived SARMs from urine specimens. The simultaneous measurement of precursor ion scans on most common product ions derived from the conserved nucleus, or high resolution/high accuracy MS targeting these core fragment ions following "all ion fragmentation" (e.g. by in-source collision-induced dissociation), complemented the assay to allow for a comprehensive screening for related drugs as well as their metabolites (Thevis *et al.* 2006; Thomas *et al.* 2010). The bicyclic hydantoin BMS-564929 (Fig. 24.5C) was also extracted from spiked urine samples using SPE, but due to a poorly acidic nature and limited proton affinity, methanol adduct formation under negative ESI conditions was employed to allow detection limits of 5–20 ng/ml (Thevis *et al.* 2007b). In contrast, 2-quinolinone-derived SARMs (Fig. 24.5D) were isolated from urine specimens by means of common LLE, and LC-MS/MS using positive ESI enabled the detection of 0.2 ng/ml (Thevis *et al.* 2007a).

24.8 Outlook

Improvement in the fight against doping was achieved by: national and international founding of national anti-doping agencies and the World Anti-Doping Agency independent of sport organizations; the development and improvement of more efficient detection methods supported by national and international research grants; the legalization of anti-doping actions by national laws to allow police investigations.

For analysis of AAS, the general strategy is to improve sensitivity to detect exogenous AAS, by GC-MS(MS) or LC-MS(MS), possibly several weeks after the last application. Currently this appears to be the best approach, as the efficiency of testing programs for athletes in out-of-competition periods in countries with less democratic structures is questionable.

For the misuse of endogenous AAS, a program is planned by WADA referred to as "The Athlete's Biological Passport." This program is a follow-up of continuous testing of athletes to establish their individual steroid profile data, in general, for testosterone and its main metabolites. This program is not entirely new as the T/E ratio testing has been well established for over 20 years. The program will cover all athletes, not only athletes with elevated T/E ratio, i.e. greater than four.

The implementation of new technologies especially in MS has yielded improvements in selectivity and sensitivity for the detection of banned substances. Beside the use of urine as biological matrix, current tests are including more and more blood samples. Methods for hair analysis of AAS have been developed and may be used in the future, too. Other matrices such as saliva or even breath may be of interest as well. Preventive doping research may focus on these matrices, keeping in mind the strong improvements in MS.

The fight against doping, which has been in the hands of sport organizations for more than 40 years, was improved when several countries implemented independent anti-doping agencies and set in force anti-doping laws which allow police investigations in the case of an anti-doping rule violation in sport, or in case of strong suspicions of practicing with doping substances or doping methods. In general such regulations prohibit the distribution of doping substances and methods to athletes. The aim is not to punish the athletes but those persons responsible for providing the banned substances, e.g. trainers, physicians, other individuals of the healthcare system and dealers.

However, the key elements in the international anti-doping fight remain the doping control of athletes, including chemical analysis of samples. Support by national anti-doping rules is appreciated, and police investigations can help to provide additional data to support actions against doping structures independent of anti-doping sport regulations. These should be considered as synergistic measures to improve the anti-doping fight in sport.

24.9 Key messages

- Misuse of androgens in competitive sports has been banned since 1974 and is tested by WADA-accredited laboratories.
- Androgens are used by athletes during training to improve muscle strength.
- Non-therapeutic hormones such as prohormones of testosterone and nortestosterone and designer steroids have been marketed as nutritional supplements since 1999.
- Positive doping cases have been proved to originate from the use of nutritional supplements "contaminated" with prohormones of nortestosterone.
- Testosterone, nortestosterone, stanozolol and metandienone represent the most frequently misused AAS in controlled sports.
- Synthetic androgens are extensively metabolized, and doping tests are focused on urinary excreted metabolites.
- Doping with endogenous steroids is controlled by indirect methods; e.g. testosterone misuse is tested by a ratio of testosterone to epitestosterone (4 : 1). Samples with elevated ratios are followed up by additional studies to exclude physiological and pathological influences.
- Direct methods, such as gas chromatography–combustion–carbon isotope ratio mass spectrometry have become available to identify doping with endogenous steroids unambiguously.
- Selective androgen receptor modulators are designed to tissue-selectively stimulate or inhibit the androgen receptor.
- Due to their non-steroidal structure, SARMs are not subject to metabolic degradation by typical steroid-metabolizing enzymes such as 5α-reductase.

24.10 References

Aguilera R, Becchi M, Casabianca H, Hatton CK, Catlin DH, Starcevic B, Pope HG Jr (1996) Improved method of detection of testosterone abuse by gas chromatography/combustion/isotope ratio mass spectrometry analysis of urinary steroids. *J Mass Spectrom* 31: 169–176

Becchi M, Aguilera R, Farizon Y, Flament MM, Casabianca H, James P (1994) Gas chromatography/combustion/isotope-ratio mass spectrometry analysis of urinary steroids to detect misuse of testosterone in sport. *Rapid Commun Mass Spectrom* 8: 304–308

Beckett AH, Cowan DA (1979) Misuse of drugs in Sport. *Brit J Sports Med* 2: 185–194

Belkien L, Schurmeyer T, Hano R, Gunnarsson PO, Nieschlag E (1985) Pharmacokinetics of 19-nortestosterone esters in normal men. *J Steroid Biochem* 22: 623–629

Bhasin S, Jasuja R (2009) Selective androgen receptor modulators as function promoting therapies. *Curr Opin Clin Nutr Metab Care* 12: 232–240

Bhasin S, Storer TW, Berman N, Callegari C, Clevenger B, Phillips J, Bunell TJ, Tricker R, Shirazi A, Casaburi R (1996) The effects of supraphysiologic doses of testosterone on muscle size and strength in normal men. *J Med* **335**: 1–7

Boos C, Wulff P, Kujath P, Bruch HP (1998) Medikamentenmissbrauch im Freizeitsport. *Deutsches Ärzteblatt* **95**(16): A953–A957

Brooks RV, Firth R, Summer NA (1975) Detection of anabolic steroids by radio immunoassay. *Br J Sports Med* **9**: 89–92

Canadian Centre for Drug-Free Sport (1993) News Release – Over 80,000 young Canadians using anabolic steroids. CCDFS, Montreal

Catlin DH, Ahrens BD, Kucherova Y (2002) Detection of norbolethone, an anabolic steroid never marketed, in athletes' urine. *Rapid Commun Mass Spectrom* **16**: 1273–1275

Catlin DH, Sekera MH, Ahrens BD, Stracevic B, Chang YC, Hatton CK (2004) Tetrahydrogestrinone: discovery, synthesis, and detection in urine. *Rapid Commun Mass Spectrom* **18**: 1245–1249

Cawley AT, Flenker U (2008) The application of carbon isotope ratio mass spectrometry to doping control. *J Mass Spectrom* **43**: 854–864

Clasing D (1992) *Doping – verbotene Arzneistoffe im Sport*. Gustav Fischer Verlag, Stuttgart

de la Torre X, Segura J, Yang Z, Li Y, Wu M (1997) Testosterone detection in different ethnic groups. In: Schänzer W, Geyer H, Gotzmann A, Mareck-Engelke U (eds) *Proceedings of the 14th Cologne Workshop on Dope Analysis 1996*. Sport und Buch Strauß, Cologne, pp 71–89

Donike M (1969) N-Methyl-N-trimethylsilyl-trifluoracetamid, ein neues Silylierungsmittel aus der Reihe der silylierten Amide. *J Chromatogr* **42**: 103–104

Donike M, Bärwald KR, Klostermann K, Schänzer W, Zimmermann J (1983) Nachweis von exogenem Testosteron. In: Heck H, Hollmann W, Liesen W, Rost R (eds) *Sport:*

Leistung und Gesundheit. Deutscher Ärzte Verlag, Cologne, pp 293–298

Donike M, Zimmermann J, Bärwald KR, Schänzer W, Christ V, Klostermann K, Opfermann G (1984) Routine Bestimmung von Anabolika im Harn. *Deutsch Z Sportmed* **1**: 14–23

Donike M, Ueki M, Kuroda Y, Geyer H, Nolteernsting E, Rauth S, Schänzer W, Schindler U, Völker E, Fujisaki M (1995) Detection of dihydrotestosterone (DHT) doping: alteration in the steroid profile and reference ranges for DHT and its 5α-metabolites. *J Sports Med Phys Fitness* **35**: 235–250

Duchaine D (1989) *Underground Steroid Handbook II*. Technical Books, Venice, FL

Flenker U, Güntner U, Schänzer W (2008) Delta[13]C-values of endogenous urinary steroids. *Steroids* **73**: 408–416

Franke WW, Berendonk B (1997) Hormonal doping and androgenization of athletes: a secret program of the German Democratic Republic government. *Clin Chem* **43**: 1262–1279

Gao W, Dalton JT (2007) Expanding the therapeutic use of androgens via selective androgen receptor modulators (SARMs). *Drug Discov Today* **12**: 241–248

Geyer H, Parr MK, Mareck U, Reinhart U, Schrader Y, Schänzer W (2004) Analysis of non-hormonal nutritional supplements for anabolic-androgenic steroids – results of an international study. *Int J Sports Med* **25**: 124–129

Grundig P, Bachmann M (1995) *World Anabolic Review 1996*. Sport Verlag Ingenohl, Heilbronn

Handelsman DJ, Gupta L (1997) Prevalence and risk factors for anabolic-androgenic steroid abuse in Australian high school students. *Int J Androl* **20**: 159–164

Haupt HA, Rovere GD (1984) Anabolic steroids: a review of the literature. *Am J Sports Med* **12**: 469–484

Horning S, Geyer H, Machnik M, Schänzer W, Hilkert A, Oeßelmann J (1997) Detection of exogenous testosterone by 13C/12C analysis. In: Schänzer W, Geyer H, Gotzmann A, Mareck-Engelke U (eds) *Proceedings of the 14th Cologne Workshop on Dope Analysis 1996*. Sport und Buch Strauß, Cologne, pp 275–283

Kamber M (1995) Mitteilung in Doping – Information und Prävention. *Maggelingen* **7**: 4–7

Kazlauskas R (2010) Designer steroids. In: Thieme D, Hemmersbach P (eds) *Doping in Sports*. Handbook of Experimental Pharmacology, Vol. 195, Springer, Heidelberg, pp 155–185

Kicman AT, Coutts SB, Walker CJ, Cowan DA (1995) Proposed confirmatory procedure for detecting 5α-dihydrotestosterone doping in male athletes. *Clin Chem* **41**: 1617–1627

Kicman AT, Bassindale T, Cowan DA, Dale S, Hutt AJ, Leeds AR (2003) Effect of androstenedione ingestion on plasma testosterone in young women; a dietary supplement with potential health risks. *Clin Chem* **49**: 167–169

Kilbourne EJ, Moore WJ, Freedman LP, Nagpal S (2007) Selective androgen receptor modulators for frailty and osteoporosis. *Curr Opin Investig Drugs* **8**: 821–829

Kochakian CD (1976) *Anabolic-Androgenic Steroids*. Springer-Verlag, Berlin

Kochakian CD (1990) A steroid review: metabolite of testosterone; significance in the vital economy. *Steroids* **55**: 92–97

Leder BZ, Longcope C, Catlin DC, Ahrens B, Schoenfeld DA, Finkelstein JS (2000) Oral androstenedione administration and serum testosterone concentrations in young men. *JAMA* **283**: 779–782

Massé R, Ayotte C, Dugal R (1989) Integrated methodological approach to the gas chromatographic mass spectrometric analysis of anabolic steroid metabolites in urine. *J Chromatogr* **489**: 23–50

Miller CP, Bhaket P, Muthukaman N, Lyttle CR, Shomali M, Gallacher K, Slocum C, Hattersley G (2010) Synthesis of potent, substituted carbazoles as selective androgen receptor modulators (SARMs). *Bioorg Med Chem Lett* **20**: 7516–7520

Mohler ML, Bohl CE, Narayanan R, He Y, Hwang DJ, Dalton JT, Miller DD (2008) Nonsteroidal tissue-selective androgen receptor modulators. In: Ottow E, Weinmann H (eds) *Nuclear Receptors as Drug Targets.* Wiley-VCH, Weinheim, pp 249–304

Mohler ML, Bohl CE, Jones A, Coss CC, Narayanan R, He Y, Hwang DJ, Dalton JT, Miller DD (2009) Nonsteroidal selective androgen receptor modulators (SARMs): dissociating the anabolic and androgenic activities of the androgen receptor for therapeutic benefit. *J Med Chem* **52**: 3597–3617

Nagata N, Miyakawa M, Amano S, Furuya K, Yamamoto N, Inoguchi K (2011) Design and synthesis of tricyclic tetrahydroquinolines as a new series of nonsteroidal selective androgen receptor modulators (SARMs). *Bioorg Med Chem Lett* **21**: 1744–1747

Parr MK, Schänzer W (2010) Detection of the misuse of steroids in doping control. *J Steroid Biochem Mol Biol* **121**: 528–537

Schänzer W (1996) Review – metabolism of anabolic androgenic steroids. *Clin Chem* **42**: 1001–1020

Schänzer W, Donike M (1993) Metabolism of anabolic steroids in man: synthesis and use of reference substances for identification of anabolic steroid metabolites. *Anal Chim Acta* **275**: 23–48

Schänzer W, Delahaut P, Geyer H, Machnik M, Horning S (1996) Longterm detection and identification of metandienone and

stanozolol abuse in athletes by gas chromatography/high resolution mass spectrometry (GC/HRMS). *J Chormatogr B* **687**: 93–108

Schänzer W, Geyer H, Fußhöller G, Halatcheva N, Kohler M, Parr MK, Guddat S, Thomas A, Thevis M (2006) Mass spectrometric identification and characterization of a new long-term metabolite of metandienone. *Rapid Commun Mass Spectrom* **10**: 2252–2258

Schmidt A, Kimmel DB, Bai C, Scafonas A, Rutledge S, Vogel RL, McElwee-Witmer S, Chen F, Nantermet PV, Kasparcova V, Leu CT, Zhang HZ, Duggan ME, Gentile MA, Hodor P, Pennypacker B, Masarachia P, Opas EE, Adamski SA, Cusick TE, Wang J, Mitchell HJ, Kim Y, Prueksaritanont T, Perkins JJ, Meissner RS, Hartman GD, Freedman LP, Harada S, Ray WJ (2010) Discovery of the selective androgen receptor modulator MK-0773 using a rational development strategy based on differential transcriptional requirements for androgenic anabolism versus reproductive physiology. *J Biol Chem* **285**: 17054–17064

Schrader Y, Thevis M, Schänzer W (2006) Quantitative determination of metabolic products of 19-norandrostenediol in human plasma using gas chromatography/ mass spectrometry. *Drug Metab Dispos* **34**: 1328–1335

Sekera MH, Ahrens BD, Chang YC, Starcevic B, Georgakopoulos C, Catlin DH (2005) Another designer steroid: discovery, synthesis, and detection of 'madol' in urine. *Rapid Commun Mass Spectrom* **19**: 781–784

Shackleton CH, Phillips A, Chang T, Li Y (1997) Confirming testosterone administration by isotope ratio mass spectrometric analysis of urinary androstanediols. *Steroids* **62**: 379–387

Sinner D (2009) *Anabole Steroide – Das Schwarze Buch 2010.* BMS Verlag, Gronau, Germany

Striegel H, Simon P, Frisch S, Roecker K, Dietz K, Dickhuth HH, Ulrich R (2006) Anabolic ergogenic substance users in fitness-sports: a distinct group supported by the health care system. *Drug Alcohol Depend* **81**: 11–19

Taylor WN (1982) *Steroids and the Athlete.* McFarland & Company, London

Thevis M, Schänzer W (2008) Mass spectrometry of selective androgen receptor modulators. *J Mass Spectrom* **43**: 865–876

Thevis M, Schänzer W (2010) Synthetic anabolic agents: steroids and nonsteroidal selective androgen receptor modulators. In: Thieme D, Hemmersbach P (eds) *Doping in Sports.* Handbook of Experimental Pharmacology, Vol. 195. Springer, Heidelberg, pp 99–126

Thevis M, Opfermann G, Schmickler H, Schänzer W (2001) Mass spectrometry of steroid glucuronide conjugates. I. Electron impact fragmentations of 5α-/5β-androstan-3α-ol-17-one glucuronides, 5α-estran-3α-ol-17-one glucuronide and deuterium-labelled analogues. *J Mass Spectrom* **36**: 159–168

Thevis M, Kamber M, Schänzer W (2006) Screening for metabolically stable aryl-propionamide-derived selective androgen receptor modulators for doping control purposes. *Rapid Commun Mass Spectrom* **20**: 870–876

Thevis M, Kohler M, Maurer J, Schlörer N, Kamber M, Schänzer W (2007a) Screening for 2-quinolinone-derived selective androgen receptor agonists in doping control analysis. *Rapid Commun Mass Spectrom* **21**: 3477–3486

Thevis M, Kohler M, Schänzer W (2007b) Mass spectrometry of new growth promoting drugs: hydantoin-derived selective androgen receptor modulators and growth hormone secretagogues. In: Schänzer W, Geyer H, Gotzmann A,

Mareck U (eds) *Recent Advances in Doping Analysis*. Sport und Buch Strauß, Cologne, pp 263–272

Thevis M, Kohler M, Schlörer N, Fusshöller G, Schänzer W (2008a) Screening for two selective androgen receptor modulators using gas chromatography-mass spectrometry in doping control analysis. *Eur J Mass Spectrom (Chichester, Eng)* **14**: 153–161

Thevis M, Kohler M, Thomas A, Schlörer N, Schänzer W (2008b) Doping control analysis of tricyclic tetrahydroquinoline-derived selective androgen receptor modulators using liquid chromatography/electrospray ionization tandem mass spectrometry. *Rapid Commun Mass Spectrom* **22**: 2471–2478

Thevis M, Lohmann W, Schrader Y, Kohler M, Bornatsch W, Karst U, Schänzer W (2008c) Use of an electrochemically synthesised metabolite of a selective androgen receptor modulator for mass spectrometry-based sports drug testing. *Eur J Mass Spectrom (Chichester, Eng)* **14**: 163–170

Thevis M, Geyer H, Kamber M, Schänzer W (2009) Detection of the arylpropionamide-derived selective androgen receptor modulator (SARM) S-4 (Andarine) in a black-market product. *Drug Test Anal* **1**: 387–392

Thevis M, Thomas A, Fusshöller G, Beuck S, Geyer H, Schänzer W (2010) Mass spectrometric characterization of urinary metabolites of the selective androgen receptor modulator andarine (S-4) for routine doping control purposes. *Rapid Commun Mass Spectrom* **24**: 2245–2254

Thevis M, Geyer H, Thomas A, Schänzer W (2011) Trafficking of drug candidates relevant for sports drug testing: detection of non-approved therapeutics categorized as anabolic and gene doping agents in products distributed via the Internet. *Drug Test Anal* **3**: 331–336

Thomas A, Guddat S, Kohler M, Krug O, Schänzer W, Petrou M, Thevis M (2010) Comprehensive plasma-screening for known and unknown substances in doping controls. *Rapid Commun Mass Spectrom* **24**: 1124–1132

WADA (2010) *The 2010 Prohibited List*. World Anti-Doping Agency, Montreal. Available at: www.wada-ama.org/Documents/World_Anti-Doping_Program/WADP-Prohibited-list/WADA_Prohibited_List_2010_EN.pdf (accessed Jan 14, 2010)

Wade N (1972) Anabolic steroids: doctors denounce them, but athletes aren't listening. *Science* **176**: 1399–1403

Ward RJ, Lawson AM, Shackleton CHL (1975) Screening by gas chromatography–mass spectrometry for metabolites of five commonly used anabolic steroid drugs. *Br J Sports Med* **9**: 93–97

Wilson JD (1988) Androgen abuse by athletes. *Endocr Rev* **9**: 191–199

Wilson JD (1996) Androgens. In: Hardmann JG, Limbird IE, Molinoff PB, Ruddon RW, Goodman Gilman A (eds) *Goodman and Gilman's The Pharmacological Basis of Therapeutics*, 9th edn. McGraw Hill, New York, pp 1441–1457

Yesalis CE, Kennedy NJ, Kopstein AN, Bahrke MS (1993) Anabolic-androgenic steroid use in the United States. *JAMA* **270**: 1217–1221

Zimmermann J (1986) *Untersuchungen zum Nachweis von exogenen Gaben von Testosterone*. Thesis, German Sports University, Cologne. Hartung-Gorre Verlag, Konstanz

Sequelae of doping with anabolic steroids

Elena Vorona and Eberhard Nieschlag

25.1 Introduction: the dimension of the problem

Since ancient times substances have been consumed and methods applied to enhance physical performance in athletic activities. Since the 1950s anabolic androgenic steroids (ASS) have played a dominant role in "doping," the modern designation for such generally unsanctioned manipulations. Although many other hormones and drugs are also used for doping, e.g. GH, hCG, thyroid hormones, erythropoietin, SARMs, amphetamines, β-receptor agonists, diuretics, cocaine etc., and gene doping is on the horizon, AAS still dominate the field (see Chapter 24). AAS are not only used in high-performance competitive athletics, but also in amateur and popular sports, fitness training and bodybuilding, so that the number of users is astonishingly high, indicating that AAS indeed produce the desired effects, perceived or real, in the consumer (Hartgens and Kuipers 2004).

As there are no effects of medications without side-effects, it is not surprising that a number of unwanted sequelae are attributed to the use of AAS.

In sharp contrast to the great number of AAS users stands the fact that the possible side-effects of AAS have not been evaluated in randomized controlled trials (RCTs), which are the gold standard in modern evidence-based medicine. There are various reasons for this. None of the AAS (nor any other substance) has been approved by regulatory agencies for the purpose of doping and therefore subjected to the usual regulatory scrutinization which requires proper toxicology and RCTs. Anabolic androgenic steroid doses used for doping are 5 to 20 times greater than clinically applied doses – i.e. doses which would only be used during drug development in toxicological animal studies but not in clinical trials. As the use of AAS is illicit, it would be extremely difficult to enroll current users in RCTs as they would not admit AAS use and would reject revealing their identity. In addition, most AAS users also simultaneously administer other drugs, often of unknown purity and at undefined doses. This makes it very difficult to establish any causal relationship between a specific substance and side-effects. This is illustrated by a

Testosterone: Action, Deficiency, Substitution, ed. Eberhard Nieschlag and Hermann M. Behre, Assoc. ed. Susan Nieschlag.
Published by Cambridge University Press. © Cambridge University Press 2012.

27-year old Olympic athlete who died in 1987 from toxic multiple organ failure: 102 drugs were identified in her body; among others, stanozolol, aspirin, diclofenac, metamizol, codeine and heparin (Fischer-Solms 2009). Retrospective systematic analyses are also lacking, as, again, former consumers do not come forward, especially if they were champions and medal winners, except in a few rare cases. Often they also just forget what they were taking and at what doses; or they never knew.

In the former German Democratic Republic (GDR), a systematic nationwide doping program existed for high-performance athletics. The major anabolic androgenic steroid used in that program was chlordehydromethyltestosterone (Oral Turinabol). This had primarily an anabolic effect, which leads to a distinct gain of muscle mass during intensive training. Its only slight androgenic effect explained its widespread use by female athletes. The active ingredient is metabolized in the body quite rapidly and was not detectable in blood in doping tests five to seven days after withdrawal of AAS. Production of endogenous testosterone in males during its use was not significantly influenced, and was again fully intact a short time after discontinuation of the drug. The normal dose in male athletes was 20–40 mg/day; females took 5–20 mg/day. Some athletes took considerably higher amounts of the agents (up to 100 mg daily; Sinner and Bachmann 2004).

The full dimension of this program became evident only after the collapse of the regime in 1989 (Berendonk 1991; Franke and Berendonk 1997; Steinigen 2003). It has been estimated that altogether about 10 000 athletes were involved in this program. In 2002 the German Federal Parliament passed a law (Dopingopferhilfegesetz; DOHG) to financially compensate former GDR athletes for any demonstrable physical damage caused by doping. This situation in Germany is unique insofar as a state-supported program organized the doping. Affected athletes now demand compensation from the Federal Republic of Germany as the legal successor of the GDR. This places the athlete in an awkward position, as he/she needs to demonstrate causal relationships between doping and possible disease; particularly because of the absence of any systematic studies concerning the long-term effects of doping, in particular AAS.

Furthermore the effects and side-effects of AAS are dependent on the genetic makeup of the user as well as on body weight, duration of administration

and the dose applied. For example, it has been shown that changes in testosterone levels in men were associated with dose-dependent and region-specific changes in adipose tissue and lean body mass in the extremities and trunk (Woodhouse et al. 2004). Similarly, side-effects of clinical doses of testosterone are modulated by the polymorphism of the AR (Zitzmann and Nieschlag 2007). Supraphysiological serum testosterone concentrations not only reduced subcutaneous fat, but led to a significant loss of adipose tissue from the smaller, deeper intermuscular fat stores (Bhasin et al. 1996).

Another critical question is whether the influences of AAS are the same in male and female athletes. Except for the typical sex-dependent effects (e.g. dysmenorrhea, clitoral hypertrophy and breast atrophy in women, and testicular atrophy, azoospermia and gynecomastia in men), it is generally assumed that AAS act similarly in men and women, but this remains unclear.

The following summary of side-effects is based on extrapolation from effects observed in patients treated with AAS and on descriptions of individual cases or groups of cases, mainly retrospective and hardly ever controlled.

25.2 Side-effects of anabolic androgenic steroids in both sexes

25.2.1 Skin

Anabolic androgenic steroids act through the AR, presenting in epidermal and follicular keratinocytes, sebocytes, sweat gland cells, dermal papilla cells, dermal fibroblasts, endothelial cells and genital melanocytes. The use of AAS can very rapidly lead to cutaneous changes in previously unaffected athletes through affection of e.g. sebaceous gland growth and differentiation, hair growth, epidermal barrier homeostasis and wound healing (Zouboulis et al. 2007). The AR polymorphism appears to play a role in the severity of the symptoms (Zouboulis et al. 2007).

The most frequent skin manifestations are acne vulgaris, oily skin, seborrhea, striae, hirsutism and male pattern alopecia (Walker and Adams 2009). Over 50% of athletes taking part in a questionnaire aiming to identify unsupervised AAS regimens and side-effects of AAS reported acne (Evans 1997). After elimination of the causal agent these changes are mostly reversible. To speed up recovery antiandrogen therapy with cyproterone acetate or spironolactone might be tried (Zouboulis *et al.* 2007). However, severe forms of anabolic androgenic steroid-induced acne conglobata will leave extensive scarring on the affected skin areas (Gerber *et al.* 2008).

After acne, striae distensae as a result of rapid muscular hypertrophy, supported by AAS intake, is the most prevalent skin side-effect in athletes, especially in bodybuilders. Over 40% of athletes complained about stretch marks of the skin (Parkinson and Evans 2006), with typical localization in the musculus pectoralis or upper arm region. After discontinuation of drug misuse striae can persist as white streaks (Wollina *et al.* 2007).

25.2.2 Blood

Administration of testosterone and anabolic steroids to healthy men causes temporary activation of the coagulation system as well as of fibrinolysis. Both changes were reversed after discontinuation of the drug (Kahn *et al.* 2006). For example, testosterone can increase the activity of thromboxanA2 receptors and thrombocyte aggregation, and thereby also the risk of thrombosis. Simultaneously the activity of the fibrinolytic system rises, in particular of antithrombin III and of protein S (Ferenchick *et al.* 1995; Shapiro *et al.* 1999). Levels of plasmin–α2-antiplasmin complex (PAP, terminal marker of fibrinolysis), of factor XIIc and of antithrombin sank significantly in males who received testosterone undecanoate as depot injections (Zitzmann *et al.* 2002). Hormone replacement therapy containing androgens decreased the plasminogen-activator-inhibitor-1 (PAI-1) in premenopausal women, leading to improved fibrinolytic activity (Winkler 1996).

Changes of the hemostatic system during testosterone therapy have also been investigated in female transsexuals (female-to-male) who received 250 mg testosterone enanthate injections every two weeks over an extended period of time (Toorians *et al.* 2003). This therapy had a slight antithrombotic effect.

Anabolic androgenic steroids cause a significant increase of erythrocytes and hemoglobin concentration (Alén 1985; Clasing and Müller 2008; Sjöqvist *et al.* 2008; Nieschlag *et al.* 2010), which constitutes part of the intended effects as it increases oxygen transport. However, increases in the hematocrit above 52% may lead to thrombosis and apoplexy, especially in older subjects. To what extent the AR

polymorphism that modifies the erythropoiesis-stimulating effect of testosterone in substituted patients is of influence in athletes is not known (Zitzmann and Nieschlag 2007).

25.2.3 Heart and vessels

It has been demonstrated that long-term AAS users had an altered electrophysiological capacity of the myocardium, with a significantly higher incidence of abnormal electrocardiograms post-exercise (e.g. extension of QRS complex >114 ms, arrhythmias, including atrial fibrillation, ventricular fibrillation, ventricular tachycardia, supraventricular and ventricular ectopic beats) compared with controls (Achar *et al.* 2010; Sculthorpe *et al.* 2010).

Anabolic androgenic steroids can often cause concentric left ventricular myocardial hypertrophy, the extent of which seems to be dose related (Dickerman *et al.* 1998; Karila *et al.* 2003). It has been shown that AAS exert a long-standing hypertrophic effect on the myocardium. Here there are no significant differences between current and previous AAS users (De Piccoli *et al.* 1991; Di Bello *et al.* 1999; Vogt *et al.* 2002). Anabolic androgenic steroids seem not to influence systolic heart function. However, as anabolics affect the diastolic function of the left ventricle, this serves as a criterion for differentiation between physiologic, training-induced hypertrophy and a pathological myocardium (Caso *et al.* 2006; Kindermann 2006).

The athlete's heart is characterized by moderate proportional myocardial hypertrophy without functional limitations. Training without AAS does not lead to thickened heart chamber walls. The pathological left ventricular myocardial hypertrophy, developing under AAS intake, is often associated with restricted diastolic function of the affected heart chamber, probably caused by increasing myocardial fibrosis. The second diagnostic criterion is the thickness of the left ventricular myocardium seen on echocardiography. A heart chamber wall thickness of more than 13 mm is suspicious of pathological myocardial hypertrophy or AAS misuse (Dickerman *et al.* 1998; Kindermann 2006). A left ventricular hypertrophy can be detected on echocardiography several years after AAS withdrawal (Achar *et al.* 2010). Although myocardial hypertrophy seems to be reversible, impaired diastolic function of the left ventricle and the decreased inotropic capacity of the myocardium are irreversible (Turillazzi *et al.* 2011).

It has been reported that uncontrolled AAS misuse can cause a significantly higher incidence of cardiac death in apparent healthy young athletes. This concerns mainly powerlifters and bodybuilders taking very high AAS doses, often as a mixture with other drugs. In his dissertation, Kistler (2006) described effects of AAS misuse on the human organism, based on autopsy data of 10 young bodybuilders (mean age 33.7 years) who took unsupervised mixtures of drugs to enhance performance. In four cases the cause of death was acute cardiac dysfunction. In all 10 cases the mean heart weight of 517 g was significantly higher than the mean physiological heart weight. Furthermore, in all cases chronic ischemic changes of the myocardium were found histologically. It is also notable that in almost all cases arteriosclerosis of the coronary vessels and atheromatosis of the arteria carotis and aorta were found, despite the relatively young age of the athletes.

Some cases of dilatative cardiomyopathy have been described in healthy young bodybuilders during intake of AAS. In all cases it was uncontrolled high-dose AAS misuse, particularly in combination with other drugs (Schollert and Bendixen 1993; Clark and Schofield 2005). In individuals with a genetic disposition for dilatative cardiomyopathy using AAS it becomes specifically difficult to disentangle causal relationships. It is suggested that approximately 30% of dilatative cardiomyopathy cases show a familial accumulation. In most cases the inheritance is autosomal dominant, rarely X-chromosomal or autosomal-recessive. Because the probability of manifestation and gene expression have a high variability, some other predictive and environmental factors (e.g. viral infections or stress) can be responsible for the development of the cardiomyopathy (Maisch et al. 2005).

It has not been definitely clarified whether AAS cause arterial hypertension. In some cases AAS abuse led to a long-term (up to one year) elevation of blood pressure (Achar et al. 2010). Arterial hypertension induced by AAS abuse can persist up to one year after discontinuation of drug intake.

High doses of AAS, especially in cases of simultaneous consumption of several preparations, can cause reduction of the HDL fraction of cholesterol and increase of LDL cholesterol (Hartgens et al. 2004; Kindermann 2006; Bonetti et al. 2008). These effects on lipoprotein levels can be noted approximately two months after the beginning of ASS use. Only several months after discontinuation of the administration does the lipid status return to normal. After long-standing use atherosclerosis and consequential coronary heart disease, cerebral vessel disease or peripheral arterial obstructive disease could hypothetically develop, but this has not been proven.

It should be remembered here that during the last decade a number of studies have appeared which reverse the role of testosterone from a risk factor for cardiovascular diseases to a cardioprotective agent (see Chapter 10). However, this applies to testosterone doses in the physiological range and can certainly be different if excessive AAS doses are applied.

25.2.4 Liver

Changes of the liver structure have been described, mainly in cases of chronic misuse of the 17α-alkylated AAS, e.g. methyltestosterone, metandienone, oxandrolone, stanozolol (Turillazzi et al. 2011). Because of their liver toxicity, 17α-alkylated androgenic steroids are considered obsolete for clinical use (at least in Europe) (Nieschlag 1981), but continue to be available illegally for doping purposes. As a direct toxic effect on hepatocytes with ultrastructural cell damage, oxidative stress leading to increased ROS (reactive oxygen species) production could play a role in the hepatotoxicity of AAS.

Changes often observed are intrahepatic cholestasis, peliosis hepatis (lacunar blood-filled cavities, which come from central veins or from focal necrosis of hepatocytes) and proliferative changes of the liver structure such as focal-nodular hyperplasia and liver adenomas (Nieschlag 1981; Rolf and Nieschlag 1998; Nakao et al. 2000).

A causal connection between AAS misuse and hepatocellular carcinoma has been described mostly in patients with other severe liver diseases (Giannitrapani et al. 2006; Clasing and Müller 2008). It has been hypothesized that AAS could play a key role in the development of steatosis hepatis, inhibiting the normal process of steroid biosynthesis and leading to cholesterol storage (Turillazzi et al. 2011).

A slight increase of transaminases is mostly reversible, and several weeks after discontinuation of AAS normal ranges are achieved (Basaria 2010).

25.2.5 Bones and muscles

Anabolic androgenic steroids given in childhood or adolescence cause an acceleration of bone maturation in young athletes. At the end of puberty, activation of the endochondrial bone formation leads to premature closure of the growth zones with growth retardation (Rolf and Nieschlag 1998; Przkora *et al.* 2005; Sjöqvist *et al.* 2008). Anabolic androgenic steroids including testosterone support radial bone growth and distinct periost formation. This also explains the larger cross-section size of male compared to female bones (Vanderschueren *et al.* 2004; Lindberg *et al.* 2005; see Chapter 7).

Under acute intake of AAS rhabdomyolysis has been observed, with acute renal failure as a possible complication.

Athletes often strain their musculoskeletal system acutely and to an extreme extent over long periods, resulting in a high incidence of complaints, injuries and disorders in joints, tendons, bones and muscles. These may become chronic so that the former athlete suffers long after discontinuing high-performance sports – and AAS abuse. There are, however, no appropriate investigations documenting a negative impact of AAS on the musculoskeletal system, and it is even suspected that AAS could possibly prevent more severe damage.

25.2.6 Kidneys

Renal disorders have been described mostly after long-term AAS use, and range from a slight increase of serum creatinine to acute renal failure as a complication of rhabdomyolysis. It has been hypothesized that the interindividual differences concerning the grade of side-effects depend on the genetically programmed function of the uridine diphosphate glucuronosyltransferase (UGT) enzymes, which provide glucuronidation of steroids, the first phase of the deactivation and elimination pathway of AAS (Deshmukh *et al.* 2010). Histologically, a focal segmental glomerulosclerosis with tubular atrophy and interstitial fibrosis can be found with long-term abuse (Turillazzi *et al.* 2011). Mild forms of renal dysfunction with elevation of serum creatinine, blood urine nitrogen and uric acid without sclerotic/fibrotic morphological changes often return to normal ranges after discontinuation of AAS (Turillazzi *et al.* 2011).

Conversely, testosterone and other AAS have been used for over 25 years for anemia treatment in patients with chronic kidney insufficiency before erythropoietin became available for clinical use. However, the doses used were in the normal clinical range and far below those in AAS abuse. The general condition and the serum parameters of the malnourished patients with chronic renal failure improved due to reduction of catabolism (Johnson 2000; see Chapter 17).

25.2.7 Tumors

There is no indication that testosterone in replacement doses has any effect on tumor development or growth, except in the prostate where it stimulates growth of an existing carcinoma (see Chapter 13). However, there are no reports about a relationship between current or former AAS abuse and prostate carcinoma.

The most feared malignant disease after long-term AAS intake is hepatocellular carcinoma. The possible cause of tumor development in the case of abuse of 17α-alkylated AAS is direct hepatotoxicity; in the case of AAS underlying aromatization (endogenous testosterone), a toxic effect of estrogens on hepatic tissue is discussed. It has been observed that human hepatocellular carcinoma tissue has elevated aromatase activity. Attempts to treat unresectable hepatocellular carcinoma with tamoxifen did not lead to positive results (Giannitrapani *et al.* 2006).

25.2.8 Behavior

Headaches, sleeplessness, increased irritability and depressive mood status were described following AAS abuse (Turillazzi *et al.* 2011). A study in women described complaints of depressive mood after discontinuation of AAS, persisting several weeks thereafter (Gruber and Pope 2000). Anabolic androgenic steroids abusers have an affinity for developing alcohol or opioid dependence (Basaria 2010). It has been suggested that there are at least three etiological mechanisms of developing AAS dependence: body image disorders such as "muscle dysmorphia"; an experience of dysphoria or depression after attempting to discontinue misuse, based on hypogonadotropic hypogonadism; and possible hedonic effects of AAS (Kanayama *et al.* 2010).

25.2.9 Causes of sudden death under anabolic androgenic steroids

In most cases of sudden cardiac death of young athletes, the cause was previously undiagnosed congenital heart failure (Sullivan *et al.* 1998). As further possible causes the following are discussed: coronary spasms due to inhibition of NO release; premature coronary arteriosclerosis due to increased atherogenesis; thrombotic coronary arterial occlusion due to increased blood platelet aggregation and/or an increase of hematocrit and blood viscosity; as well as direct cardiotoxic effects with impairment of mitochondria and myofibrils and associated destruction of the myocytes and their replacement by fibrous tissue (Dickerman *et al.* 1995; Sullivan *et al.* 1998; Fineschi *et al.* 2001; Kistler 2006).

The above mentioned study describing autopsy results and chemical-toxicological findings of 10 young bodybuilders showed that 5 athletes died because of acute cardiac dysfunction due to myocardial infarction (see Section 25.2.3). Further old infarctions ($n = 4$) and chronic ischemic myocardial changes ($n = 10$) were found. Noteworthy was the fact that AAS abusers had an affinity to consume other substances. In 8 of 10 cases concomitant medication was detected in blood and/or urine samples or in the hair. In three cases acute intoxication with opioids, benzodiazepines, alcohol and Rohypnol (flunitrazepam) was the cause of death (Kistler 2006).

25.3 Specific side-effects in men

Due to negative feedback in the regulation of the hypothalamic-pituitary-gonadal axis, AAS can cause a reversible suppression of spermatogenesis up to azoospermia (Knuth *et al.* 1989; Rolf and Nieschlag 1998). As the spermatogenic tissue constitutes about 95% of the testes, its atrophy is followed by shrinkage of the testes. After cessation of AAS intake spermatogenesis and testicular volumes recover within months. During intake, the users may be infertile to various degrees, often being unaware of the causal relationship. Proper diagnosis may be impeded by the fact that these men may not wish to admit abuse, neither to their physician nor to their partner, and an insistent exploration is required. Low LH, FSH and testosterone (in cases where testosterone is not used as the AAS) point to the suppressed pituitary-testicular axis (Fronczak *et al.* 2011). Should spermatogenesis not recover after cessation of use, a pre-existing fertility disorder is more likely than damage caused by the AAS. In order to hasten recovery, sometimes hCG is prescribed without any proof of effectiveness. It should be mentioned here that the suppression of the pituitary and spermatogenesis by testosterone is exploited in approaches to male hormonal contraception (see Chapter 22).

Considering the great number of teenage boys using AAS, the question arises as to whether AAS application in boys around puberty may be harmful to spermatogenesis. Although systematic investigations in pubertal AAS users are lacking, treatment of over-tall boys with high doses of testosterone for reduction of final height provides an analogy. Initially it was suspected that this treatment would be harmful to the testes and leave permanent damage. However, when the proper control groups were co-investigated, the incidence of subnormal semen parameters was the same in both groups (Lemcke *et al.* 1996; Hendriks *et al.* 2010), indicating that at this age the testes are not different from adult men in their capacity to recover from suppression.

In cases of high-dose intake of aromatizable AAS, bilateral gynecomastia in men can develop with a prevalence of 20–30% (O'Sullivan *et al.* 2000). Concurrent use of ER or aromatase inhibitors has been applied to counteract this development. In cases of a persistent, therapy refractory gynecomastia, a liposuction with mastectomy may be required (Babigian and Silverman 2001; Hartgens and Kuipers 2004).

After abrupt discontinuation of AAS abuse athletes can show temporary signs of hypogonadotropic hypogonadism, such as decreased libido, ED and depression (Basaria 2010).

The single case of a former GDR weightlifter has been reported who used Oral Turinabol at high doses (up to 20 tablets per day) from 18 to 23 years of age. He developed gynecomastia under the treatment and was, at the age of 32, operated on for a unilateral intratesticular leiomyosarcoma (Froehner *et al.* 1999). As these tumors are extremely rare and have been described in hamsters after treatment with testosterone propionate and diethylstilbestrol (Kirkham and Algard 1965), the authors suspected a causal relationship between AAS abuse and the sarcoma. As this remains the only reported case, the pathogenesis of the tumor is unclear.

25.4 Effects of anabolic androgenic steroids in women

In females, dysmenorrhea, secondary amenorrhea with anovulation and, as their consequence, infertility are the changes most often caused by AAS abuse. A large study with the aim of evaluating the side-effects of testosterone administration in therapeutic doses in women showed that there were no significant differences concerning the frequency of cerebro-vascular diseases, coronary heart disease, mamma carcinoma, deep venous thrombosis/lung embolism, diabetes mellitus or acute hepatitis between women receiving testosterone therapy and the control group (Van Staa and Sprafka 2009; see also Chapter 23).

Changes of the reproductive system due to suppression of the hypothalamic-pituitary-gonadal axis, such as dysmenorrhea, secondary amenorrhea with anovulation and reduction of breast size are reversible. It can take weeks or months up to complete recovery of the axis. In some cases it has been reported that after cessation of AAS administration in women it can take up to two years until testosterone concentrations in serum dropped to normal levels (Urman et al. 1991). Concerning possibly irreversible side-effects of AAS use in women, such as clitoris hypertrophy, there is no documented experience.

25.4.1   Hirsutism

Hirsutism is the most frequent and reversible side-effect of AAS use in women (Braunstein 2007). The degree of increased facial or body hair growth depends on the dose and duration of AAS excess and can be described according to the hirsutism score by Ferriman–Gallwey, established in 1961. Based on the intensity of hair growth in nine face/body areas, hirsutism can be diagnosed as mild, moderate and severe (Ferriman and Gallwey 1961). In some cases it has been reported that after AAS administration in women it could take up to two years until testosterone concentrations in serum dropped to normal levels and hirsutism disappeared (Urman et al. 1991).

25.4.2   Deepening of the voice

Deepening of the voice is part of the virilization that AAS can cause in women. In contrast to acne, hirsutism, alopecia, mammary atrophy and clitoral hypertrophy, deepening of the voice tends to be irreversible (Kindermann 2006). These effects of androgens in women have been described repeatedly (Bauer 1973; Wirth 1979; Strauss et al. 1985; Baker 1999). Lowering of the voice is caused by growth of the larynx in girls and by thickening of the vocal chords in women after puberty. The voice change can be so pronounced that on the telephone women may be mistaken for men. It is accompanied by hoarseness which may intensify upon longer use of the voice.

This dysarthria may become a problem for teachers, actors and singers who are professionally dependent on their voices. Such voice alterations are also observed with endogenous elevation of testosterone levels, e.g. CAH (Nygren et al. 2009) or in women sensitive to the androgenic action of some oral contraceptives. As changes of the voice are mostly irreversible, application of AAS or other steroids has to be suspended at the earliest sign of symptoms.

25.4.3   The question of breast cancer

The question about the effect of exogenous androgens on the development of breast cancer has been discussed controversially in the scientific literature. The lack of controlled studies contributes to the uncertainties so that indirect evidence from other clinical situations has to be referred to.

Experience with long-term hormonal therapy in transsexuals (female to male) aiming at virilization (standard therapy: testosterone enanthate 250 mg im every second week or testosterone undecanoate 1000 mg every 10–12 weeks for two to three years before surgical therapy, e.g. mastectomy, ovariectomy and hysterectomy, and for years after that) shows no increased risk for breast cancer (Gooren et al. 2008; Mueller and Gooren 2008). Since the 1970s, when the first hormonal therapy of transsexuals was documented, only one clinical case has been reported; in this case a mamma carcinoma of the residual breast tissue developed 10 years after bilateral mastectomy and continuous testosterone therapy (Burcombe et al. 2003).

The polycystic ovary syndrome (PCOS) is characterized by a significant increase of the testosterone concentration in blood, and often serves as a model for long-term testosterone exposure in women. Studies showed that the risk for breast cancer in these women does not increase (Somboonporn and Davis 2004).

Exogenous androgens are partially metabolized in the breast tissue to estrogens. However, not all synthetic androgens are subject to aromatization; e.g. tibolone and its metabolites cannot be aromatized (de Gooyer et al. 2008). This also applies to the metabolism of Oral Turinabol (chlordehydromethyltestosterone) unless taken in extremely high doses (see Section 25.3): the molecule is not aromatized, so that estrogenic side-effects become clinically not relevant (Kley 2004).

A large randomized study showed that postmenopausal women who received estrogens exclusively did not have an increased risk of mamma carcinoma, in contrast to women who received an estrogen/gestagen combination (Anderson *et al.* 2004). The age of the patient and the duration of estrogen therapy are considered as risk factors for the development of breast cancer in women. Comparable results have also been shown in other studies (Magnusson *et al.* 1999; Million Women Study Collaborators, 2003). However, women who at the time point of the evaluation received hormone replacement therapy (estrogen or estrogen/gestagen preparations), in comparison to women who had never taken hormonal drugs, had a higher risk for the development of breast cancer. Women who in the past received hormonal therapy did not have a higher risk for mamma carcinoma.

It has also been shown that the additional administration of testosterone during hormonal replacement therapy in postmenopausal women (estrogen/gestagen preparations) inhibited the proliferation of breast cells and thereby decreased the risk of mamma carcinoma (Hofling *et al.* 2007).

In vitro, in animals and also in postmenopausal patients, androgens (e.g. testosterone, DHT) blocked proliferation of breast cells caused by estrogens and expression of ER genes (Lapointe *et al.* 1999; Zhou *et al.* 2000; Andò *et al.* 2002; Ortmann *et al.* 2002; Dimitrakakis *et al.* 2004). The antiproliferative and proapoptotic action of androgens is probably mediated through the AR, despite the potential of testosterone to metabolize to estrogens (Somboonporn and Davis 2004). Before these interrelations were known, advanced stages of mamma carcinoma had even been treated with testosterone from the 1940s until the 1970s (Van Winkle 1949; Labhart 1978). The underlying clinical experience was that testosterone inhibits rather than supports a mamma carcinoma.

Mutations in *BRCA1* and *BRCA2* genes (breast cancer genes) can exhibit a higher risk for the development of a mamma carcinoma.

In conclusion, there are no appropriate epidemiological studies which clearly document or negate a causal connection between the administration of AAS in young female athletes and the development of mamma carcinoma later in life. There is also no accumulation of case reports which would argue for such a connection. Indirectly one can assume that use of AAS (e.g. Oral Turinabol) at young ages cannot be causal for breast cancer.

25.5   Conclusion

As shown in this chapter, AAS abuse can result in minor and major sequelae, most reversible; some irreversible and severe. Unfortunately, the negative and deserved image of AAS is often applied to testosterone when used for a clinical indication. Proper studies are lacking, and medical knowledge of the field is predominantly based on case reports, so that causal relationships are often difficult to establish. Nevertheless, athletes, bodybuilders and fitness studio customers appear to have only vague knowledge of the side-effects of AAS, which they often belittle in the light of the relatively few severe long-term problems in relation to the vast number of AAS abusers and the fact that AAS contribute significantly to performance and success. More education about the possible sequelae of AAS abuse is mandatory to prevent negative long-term effects. At the same time the medical profession should pay more attention to the endocrinology of physical activity and sports, and should research the question of why athletes have the desire to use AAS, and whether they may need some sort of androgen substitution to reach the goals they set for themselves. Thereby medicine could contribute to the problem beyond doping control and bring androgen abuse from the illicit darkness to the light of knowledge, resulting in healthy cooperation between athletics and medical research.

25.6   Key messages

- Anabolic androgenic steroid effects and side-effects depend on dose, sex and weight of the athlete, duration of intake and combination with other drugs.
- Due to the illicit nature of AAS abuse, controlled clinical trials on the short- and long-term undesired side-effects of AAS are lacking, so that a causal relationship between AAS abuse and assumed sequelae is often difficult to establish.
- Anabolic androgenic steroids cause a temporary activation of the coagulation system as well as fibrinolysis.
- The most frequent AAS effect on the cardiovascular system is left ventricular myocardial hypertrophy with impairment of diastolic function.

- Effects on the liver (cholestasis, peliosis) are associated with a chronic misuse of the 17α-alkylated AAS.
- Anabolic androgenic steroids do not increase the incidence of malignant tumors, with a possible exception of 17α-alkylated AAS induced hepatocellular carcinoma.

- Anabolic androgenic steroid abuse does not contribute to the development of mammary carcinoma.
- Most AAS effects are reversible.
- In unclear clinical situations the possibility of AAS abuse should be taken into consideration.

25.7 References

Achar S, Rostamian A, Narayan SM (2010) Cardiac and metabolic effects of anabolic-androgenic steroid abuse on lipids, blood pressure, left ventricular dimensions, and rhythm. *Am J Cardiol* **106**:893–901

Anderson GL, Limacher M, Assaf AR, Anderson GL, Limacher M, Assaf AR, Bassford T, Beresford SA, Black H, Bonds D, Brunner R, Brzyski R, Caan B, Chlebowski R, Curb D, Gass M, Hays J, Heiss G, Hendrix S, Howard BV, Hsia J, Hubbell A, Jackson R, Johnson KC, Judd H, Kotchen JM, Kuller L, LaCroix AZ, Lane D, Langer RD, Lasser N, Lewis CE, Manson J, Margolis K, Ockene J, O'Sullivan MJ, Phillips L, Prentice RL, Ritenbaugh C, Robbins J, Rossouw JE, Sarto G, Stefanick ML, Van Horn L, Wactawski-Wende J, Wallace R, Wassertheil-Smoller S (2004) Effects of conjugated equine estrogen in postmenopausal women with hysterectomy: the Women's Health Initiative randomized controlled trial. *JAMA* **291**:1701–1712

Alén M (1985) Androgenic steroid effects on liver and red cells. *Br J Sports Med* **19**:15–20

Andò S, De Amicis F, Rago V, Carpino A, Maggiolini M, Panno ML, Lanzino M (2002) Breast cancer: from estrogen to androgen receptor. *Mol Cell Endocrinol* **193**:121–128

Babigian A, Silverman RT (2001) Management of gynecomastia due to use of anabolic steroids in bodybuilders. *Plast Reconstr Chir* **1**:240–242

Baker J (1999) A report on alterations to the speaking and singing voices of four women following hormonal therapy with virilizing agents. *J Voice* **13**:496–507

Bauer G (1973) Klinik der Stimmstörungen. In: Biesalski P (ed) *Phoniatrie*. Thieme-Verlag, Stuttgart, pp 165–172

Basaria S (2010) Androgen abuse in athletes: detection and consequences. *J Clin Endocrinol Metab* **95**:1533–1543

Berendonk M (1991) *Doping-Dokumente. Von der Forschung zum Betrug*. Springer-Verlag, Berlin

Bhasin S, Storer TW, Berman N, Callegari C, Clevenger B, Phillips J, Bunnell TJ, Tricker R, Shirazi A, Casaburi R (1996) The effects of supraphysiologic doses of testosterone on muscle size and strength in normal men. *N Engl J Med* **335**:1–7

Bonetti A, Tirelli F, Catapano A, Dazzi D, Dei Cas A, Solito F, Ceda G, Reverberi C, Monica C, Pipitone S, Elia G, Spattini M, Magnati G (2008) Side effects of anabolic androgenic steroids abuse. *Int J Sports Med* **29**:679–687

Braunstein GD (2007) Safety of testosterone treatment in postmenopausal women. *Fertil Steril* **88**:1–16

Burcombe RJ, Makris A, Pittam M, Finer N (2003) Breast cancer after bilateral subcutaneous mastectomy in a female-to-male transsexual. *Breast* **12**:290–293

Caso P, D'Andrea A, Caso I, Severino S, Calabrò P, Allocca F, Mininni N, Calabrò R (2006) The athlete's heart and hypertrophic cardiomyopathy: two conditions which may be misdiagnosed and coexistent. Which parameters should be analysed to distinguish one disease from the other? *J Cardiovasc Med (Hagerstown)* **7**:257–266

Clark BM, Schofield RS (2005) Dilated cardiomyopathy and acute liver injury associated with combined use of ephedra, gamma-hydroxybutyrate and anabolic steroids. *Pharmacotherapy* **25**:756–761

Clasing D, Müller RK (2008) *Dopingkontrolle*, 5th edn. Sportverlag Strauß, Cologne

de Gooyer ME, Oppers-Tiemissen HM, Leysen D, Verheul HA, Kloosterboer HJ (2008) Tibolone is not converted by human aromatase to 7alpha-ethynylestradiol (7alpha-MEE): analyses with sensitive bioassays for estrogens and androgens and with LC-MSMS. *Steroids* **68**:235–243

De Piccoli B, Giada F, Benettin A, Sartori F, Piccolo E (1991) Anabolic steroid use in body builders: an echocardiographic study of the left ventricle morphology and function. *Int J Sports Med* **12**:408–412

Deshmukh N, Petroczi A, Barker J, Szekely AD, Hussain I, Naughton DP (2010) Potentially harmful advantage to athletes: a putative connection between UGT2B17 gene deletion polymorphism and renal disorders with prolonged use of anabolic androgenic steroids. *Subst Abuse Treat Prev Pol* **5**:1–7

Di Bello V, Giorgi D, Bianchi M, Bertini A, Caputo MT, Valenti G, Furioso O, Alessandri L, Paterni M, Giusti C (1999) Effects of anabolic-androgenic steroids on weight-lifters' myocardium: an ultrasonic videodensitometric study. *Med Sci Sports Exerc* **31**:514–521

Dickerman RD, Schaller F, Prather I, McConathy WJ (1995) Sudden cardiac death in a 20-year-old bodybuilder using anabolic steroids. *Cardiology* **86**:172–173

Dickerman RD, Schaller F, McConathy WJ (1998) Left ventricular wall thickening does occur in elite power athletes with or without anabolic steroid use. *Cardiology* **90**:145–148

Dimitrakakis C, Jones RA, Liu A, Bondy CA (2004) Breast cancer incidence in postmenopausal women using testosterone in addition to usual hormone therapy. *Menopause* **11**:531–535

Evans NA (1997) Gym and tonic: a profile of 100 male steroid users. *Br J Sports Med* **31**:54–58

Ferenchick GS, Hirokawa S, Mammen EF, Schwartz KA (1995) Anabolic-androgenic steroid abuse in weight lifters: evidence for activation of the hemostatic system. *Am J Hematol* **49**:282–288

Ferriman DM, Gallwey JD (1961) Clinical assessment of body hair growth in women. *J Clin Endocrinol* **21**:1440–1447

Fineschi V, Baroldi G, Monciotti F, Paglicci Reattelli L, Turillazi E (2001) Anabolic steroid abuse and cardiac sudden death: a pathologic study. *Arch Pathol Lab Med* **125**:253–255

Fischer-Solms H (2009) Spitzensport: Doping in Ost und West. In: Stiftung Haus der Geschichte der Bundesrepublik Deutschland, *Wir gegen uns: Sport im geteilten Deutschland*. Primus-Verlag, Darmstadt, pp 111–121

Franke WW, Berendonk B (1997) Hormonal doping and androgenization of athletes: a secret program of the German Democratic Republic government. *Clin Chem* **43**:1262–1279

Froehner M, Fischer R, Leike S, Hakenberg OW, Noack B, Wirth MP (1999) Intratesticular leiomyosarcoma in a young man after high dose doping with Oral-Turinabol. *Cancer* **86**:1571–1575

Fronczak CM, Kim ED, Barqawi AB (2011) The insults of illicit drug use on male fertility. *J Androl* Jul 28 [Epub ahead of print]

Gerber PA, Kukova G, Meller S, Neumann NJ, Homey B (2008) The dire consequences of doping. *Lancet* **372**:656

Giannitrapani L, Soresi M, La Spada E, Cervello M, D'Alessandro N, Montalto G (2006) Sex hormones and risk of liver tumor. *Ann N Y Acad Sci* **1089**:228–236

Gooren LJ, Giltay EJ, Bunk MC (2008) Long-term treatment of transsexuals with cross-sex hormones: extensive personal experience. *J Clin Endocrinol Metab* **93**:19–25

Gruber A, Pope HG Jr (2000) Psychiatric and medical effects of anabolic-androgenic steroid use in women. *Psychother Psychosom* **69**:19–26

Hartgens F, Kuipers H (2004) Effects of androgenic-anabolic steroids in athletes. *Sport Med* **34**:513–554

Hartgens F, Rietjens G, Keizer HA, Kuipers H, Wolffenbuttel BH (2004) Effects of androgenic-anabolic steroids on apolipoproteins and lipoprotein (a). *Br J Sports Med* **38**:253–259

Hendriks AE, Boellaard WP, van Casteren NJ, Romijn JC, de Jong FH, Boot AM, Drop SL (2010) Fatherhood in tall men treated with high-dose sex steroids during adolescence. *J Clin Endocrinol Metab* **95**:5233–5240

Hofling M, Hirschberg AL, Skoog L, Tani E, Hägerström T, von Schoultz B (2007) Testosterone inhibits estrogen/progestogen-induced breast cell proliferation in postmenopausal women. *Menopause* **14**:183–190

Johnson CA (2000) Use of androgens in patients with renal failure. *Semin Dial* **13**:36–39

Kahn NN, Sinha AK, Spungen AM, Bauman WA (2006) Effects of oxandrolone, an anabolic steroid, on hemostasis. *Am J Hematol* **81**:95–100

Kanayama G, Brower KJ, Wood RI, Hudson JI, Pope HG Jr (2010) Treatment of anabolic-androgenic steroid dependence: emerging evidence and its implications. *Drug Alcohol Depend* **109**:6–13

Karila TA, Karjalainen JE, Mäntysaari MJ, Viitasalo MT, Seppälä TA (2003) Anabolic androgenic steroids produce dose-dependant increase in left ventricular mass in power athletes, and this effect is potentiated by concomitant use of growth hormone. *Int J Sports Med* **24**:337–343

Kindermann W (2006) Kardiovaskuläre Nebenwirkungen von anabol-androgenen Steroiden. *Herz* **31**:566–573

Kirkham H, Algard FT (1965) Characteristic of an androgen/estrogen dependent leiomyosarcoma of the ductus deferens of the Syrian hamster. I. In vivo. *Cancer Res* **25**:141–146

Kistler L (2006) *Todesfälle bei Anabolikamissbrauch. Todesursache, Befunde und rechtsmedizinische Aspekte*. Dissertation for Doctor of medicine at the Medical Faculty of the Ludwig-Maximilian University in Munich

Kley HK (2004) Anabole Steroide – pharmakologische Wirkung der Dopingmittel. In: Clasing D (ed) *Doping und seine Wirkstoffe. Verbotene Arzneimittel im Sport*. Spitta Verlag, Balingen, pp 64–84

Knuth UA, Maniera H, Nieschlag E (1989) Anabolic steroids and semen parameters in bodybuilders. *Fertil Steril* **52**:1041–1047

Labhart A (1978) *Klinik der inneren Sekretion*, 3rd edn. Springer-Verlag, Heidelberg, pp 1039–1040

Lapointe J, Fournier A, Richard V, Labrie C (1999) Androgens down-regulate bcl-2 prooncogene expression in ZR-75-1 human breast cancer cells. *Endocrinology* 140:416–421

Lemcke B, Zentgraf J, Behre HM, Kliesch S, Bramswig JH, Nieschlag E (1996) Long-term effects on testicular function of high-dose testosterone treatment for excessively tall stature. *J Clin Endocrinol Metab* 81: 296–301

Lindberg MK, Vandenput L, Movèrare Skrtic S, Vanderschueren D, Boonen S, Bouillon R, Ohlsson C (2005) Androgens and the skeleton. *Minerva Endocrinol* 30:15–25

Magnusson C, Baron JA, Correia N, Bergström R, Adami H-O, Persson I (1999) Breast cancer risk following long-term oestrogen and oestsrogen-progestin-replacement therapy. *Int J Cancer* 81:339–344

Maisch B, Richter A, Sandmöller A, Porting I, Pankuweit S (2005) Inflammatory dilated cardiomyopathy (DCMI). *Herz* 30:535–544

Million Women Study Collaborators (2003) Breast cancer and hormone-replacement therapy in the Million Women Study. *The Lancet* 362:419–427

Mueller A, Gooren L (2008) Hormone-related tumors in transsexuals receiving treatment with cross-sex hormones. *Europ J Endocrinol* 159:197–202

Nakao A, Sakagami K, Nakata Y, Komazawa K, Amimoto T, Nakashima K, Isozaki H, Takakura N, Tanaka N (2000) Multiple hepatic adenomas caused by long-term administration of androgenic steroids for aplastic anemia in association with familial adenomatous polyposis. *J Gastoenterol* 35:557–562

Nieschlag E (1981) Ist die Anwendung von Methyltestosteron obsolet? *Dtsch Med Wochenschr* 106:1123–1125

Nieschlag E, Behre HM, Nieschlag S (eds) (2010) *Andrology. Male*

Reproductive Health and Dysfunction, 3rd edn. Springer-Verlag, Berlin, pp 437–455

Nygren U, Södersten M, Falhammar H, Thorén M, Hagenfeldt K, Nordenskjöld A (2009) Voice characteristics in women with congenital adrenal hyperplasia due to 21-hydroxylase deficiency. *Clin Endocrinol* 70:18–25

Ortmann J, Prifti S, Bohlmann MK, Rehberger-Schneider S, Strowitzki T, Rabe T (2002) Testosterone and 5 alpha-dihydrotestosterone inhibit in vitro growth of human breast cancer cell lines. *Gynecol Endocrinol* 16:113–120

O'Sullivan AJ, Kennedy MC, Casey JH, Day RO, Corrigan B, Wodak AD (2000) Anabolic-androgenic steroids: medical assessment of present, past and potential users. *Med J Aust* 173:323–327

Parkinson AB, Evans NA (2006) Anabolic androgenic steroids: a survey of 500 users. *Med Sci Sports Exerc* 38:644–651

Przkora R, Jeschke MG, Barrow RE, Suman OE, Meyer WJ, Finnerty CC, Sanford AP, Lee J, Chinkes DL, Mlcak RP, Herndon DN (2005) Metabolic and hormonal changes of severely burned children receiving long-term oxandrolone treatment. *Ann Surg* 242:384–389

Rolf C, Nieschlag E (1998) Potential adverse effects of long-term testosterone therapy. *Baillieres Clin Endocrinol Metab* 12:521–534

Schollert PV, Bendixen PM (1993) Dilated cardiomyopathy in a user of anabolic steroids. *Ugeskr Laeger* 155:1217–1218

Sculthorpe N, Grace F, Jones P, Davies B (2010) Evidence of altered cardiac electrophysiology following prolonged androgenic anabolic steroid use. *Cardiovasc Toxicol* 10:239–243

Shapiro J, Christiana J, Frishman W (1999) Testosterone and other anabolic steroids as cardiovascular drugs. *Am J Ther* 6:167–174

Sinner D, Bachmann M (2004) *Anabole Steroide. Das schwarze Buch.* BMS Verlag, Gronau, pp 47–49, 561–563

Sjöqvist F, Garle M, Rane A (2008) Use of doping agents, particularly anabolic steroids, in sports and society. *Lancet* 371:1872–1882

Somboonporn W, Davis SR (2004) Testosterone effects on the breast: implications for testosterone therapy for women. *Endocr Rev* 25:374–388

Steinigen J (2003) *Zivilrechtliche Aspekte des Dopings aus der Sicht des Spitzensportlers.* Weißensee Verlag, Berlin

Strauss RH, Liggett MT, Lanese RR (1985) Anabolic steroid use and perceived effects in ten weight-trained women athletes. *JAMA* 253:2871–2873

Sullivan ML, Martinez CM, Gennis P, Gallagher EJ (1998) The cardiac toxicity of anabolic steroids. *Prog Cardiovasc Dis* 41:1–15

Toorians A, Thomassen M, Zweegman S, Magdeleyns E, Tans G, Gooren L, Rosing J (2003) Venous thrombosis and changes of hemostatic variables during cross-sex hormone treatment in transsexual people. *J Clin Endocrinol Metab* 88:5723–5729

Turillazzi E, Perilli G, Di Paolo M, Neri M, Riezzo I, Fineschi V (2011) Side effects of AAS abuse: an overview. *Mini Rev Med Chem* 11:374–389

Urman B, Pride SM, Yuen BH (1991) Elevated serum testosterone, hirsutism, and virilism associated with combined androgen-estrogen hormone replacement therapy. *Obstet Gynecol* 77:595–598

Vanderschueren D, Vandenput L, Boonen S, Lindenberg M, Bouillon R, Ohlsson C (2004) Androgens and bone. *Endocr Rev* 25:389–425

Van Staa TP, Sprafka JM (2009) Study of adverse outcomes in women using testosterone therapy. *Maturitas* 62:76–80

Van Winkle W Jr (1949) The action of steroid hormones in mammary cancer. *Radiology* **53**:530–539

Vogt AM, Geyer H, Jahn L, Schänzer W, Kübler W (2002) Cardiomyopathy associated with uncontrolled self medication of anabolic steroids. *Z Kardiol* **91**:357–362

Walker J, Adams B (2009) Cutaneous manifestations of anabolic–androgenic steroid use in athletes. *Int J Dermatol* **48**:1044–1048

Wollina U, Pabst F, Schönlebe J, Abdel-Naser MB, Konrad H, Gruner M, Haroske G, Klemm E, Schreiber G (2007) Side-effects of topical androgenic and anabolic substances

and steroids. A short review. *Acta Dermatoven APA* **16**:117–122

Winkler U (1996) Effects of androgens on haemostasis. *Maturitas* **24**:147–155

Wirth G (1979) *Stimmstörungen*. Dtsch Ärzteverlag, Cologne

Woodhouse LJ, Gupta N, Bhasin M, Singh AB, Ross R, Phillips J, Bhasin S (2004) Dose-dependent effects of testosterone on regional adipose tissue distribution in healthy young men. *J Clin Endocrinol Metab* **89**:718–726

Zhou J, Ng S, Adesanya-Famuiya O, Anderson K, Bondy CA (2000) Testosterone inhibits estrogen-induced mammary epithelial proliferation and suppresses

estrogen receptor expression. *FASEB J* **14**:1725–1730

Zitzmann M, Nieschlag E (2007) Androgen receptor gene CAG repeat length and body mass index modulate the safety of long-term intramuscular testosterone undecanoate therapy in hypogonadal men. *J Clin Endocrinol Metab* **92**:3844–3853

Zitzmann M, Junker R, Kamischke A, Nieschlag E (2002) Contraceptive steroids influence the hemostatic activation state in healthy men. *J Androl* **23**:503–511

Zouboulis CC, Chen WC, Thornton MJ, Qin K, Rosenfield R (2007) Sexual hormones in human skin. *Horm Metab Res* **39**:85–95

Index